Seventh Edition

Pharmacy Practice for Technicians

Skye A. McKennon
Robert J. Anderson

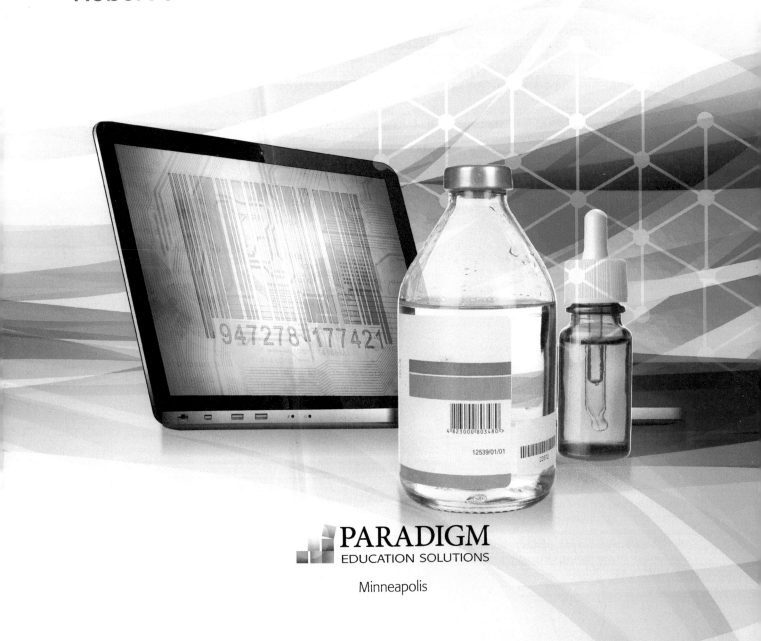

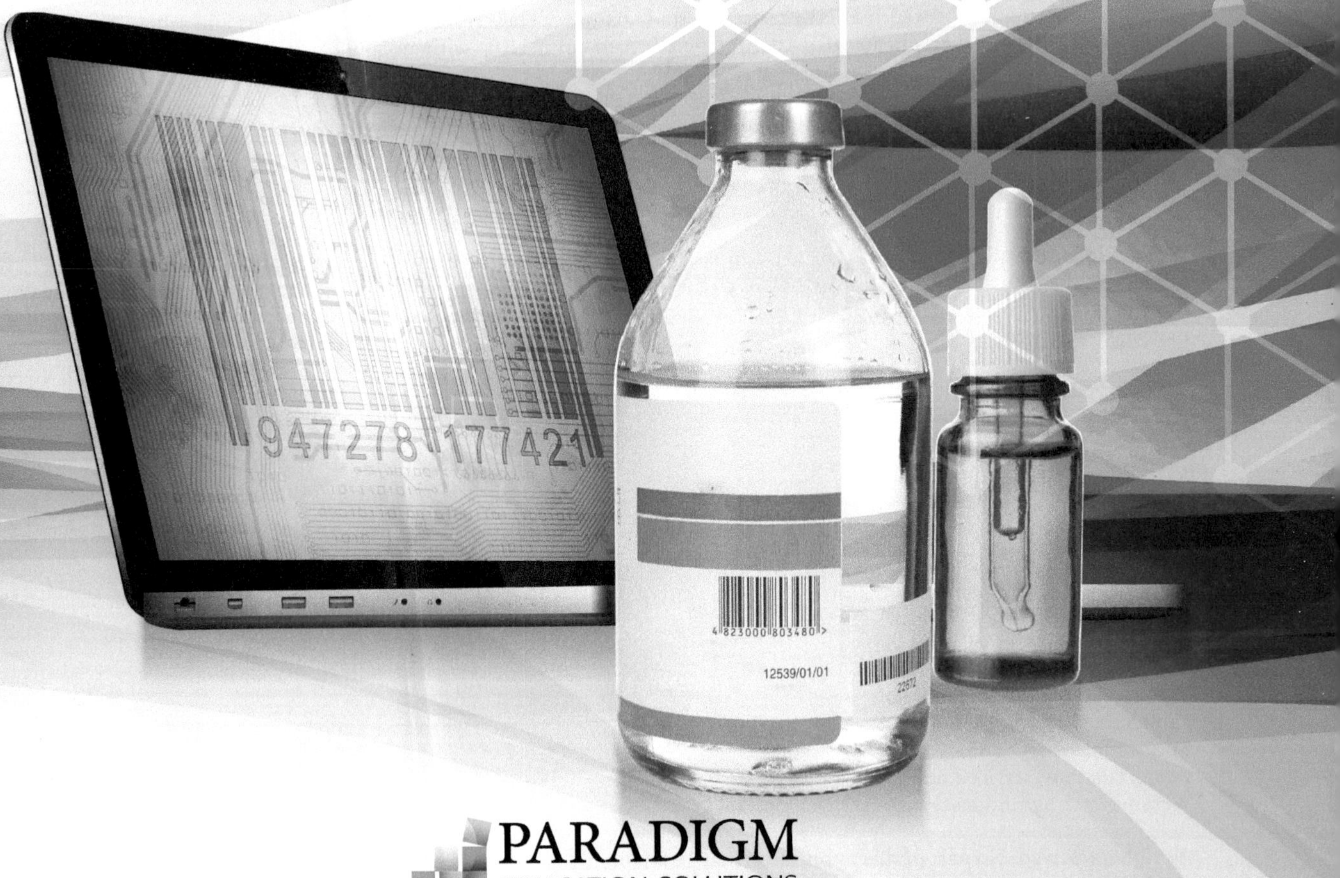

PARADIGM
EDUCATION SOLUTIONS
Minneapolis

VP of Content Management: Christine Hurney
Director of Content Development: Carley Fruzzetti
Developmental Editor: Brian Farrey-Latz
Director of Production: Timothy W. Larson
Production Editors: Melora Pappas, Emily Tope
Senior Design and Production Specialist: Julie Johnston
Copy Editor: Anne Ketchen
Proofreader: Margaret P. Roeske
Indexer: Terry Casey
Digital Projects Manager: Tom Modl
Digital Products and Onboarding Supervisor: Ryan Isdahl
VP Marketing: Lara Weber McLellan
Associate Product Manager: Shealan Pream

Cover Photo Credit: © fad1986/iStock (laptop); © archibald1221/iStock (blue barcode) © urfinguss/iStock (clear bottle); © Vasilyev Alexander/iStock (brown dropper bottle)
Cover Illustration Credit: © traffic_analyzer/iStock
Interior Photo Credits: Following the index.

ISBN 978-0-76389-301-9 (print)
ISBN 978-0-76389-482-5 (digital)

7900 Xerxes Avenue S, STE 310
Minneapolis, MN 55431-1118
Email: customerservice@ppij.com
Website: ParadigmEducation.com

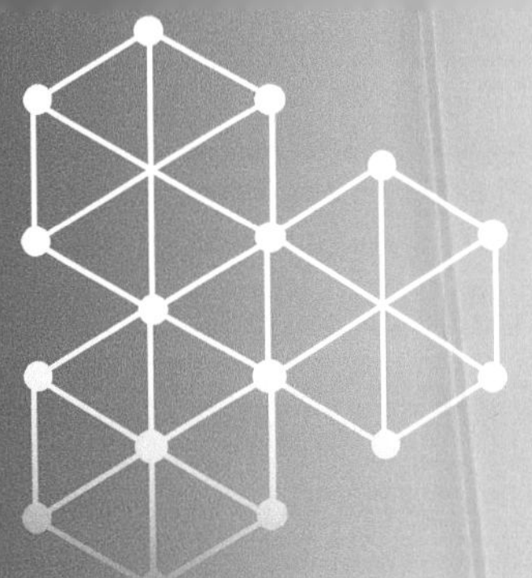

BRIEF CONTENTS

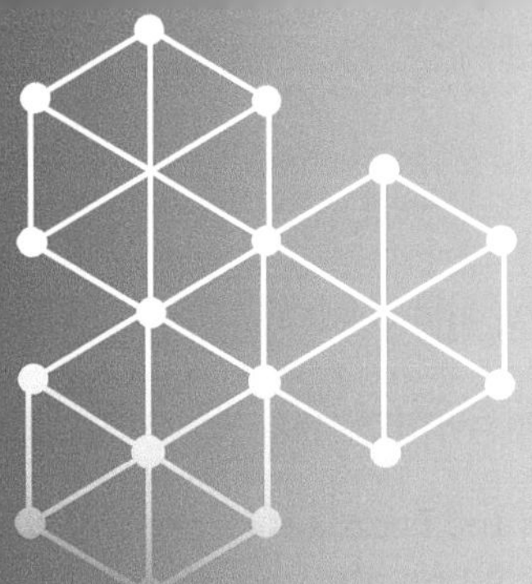

CONTENTS

Chapter 12
Infection Control, Aseptic Technique, and Cleanroom Facilities............489

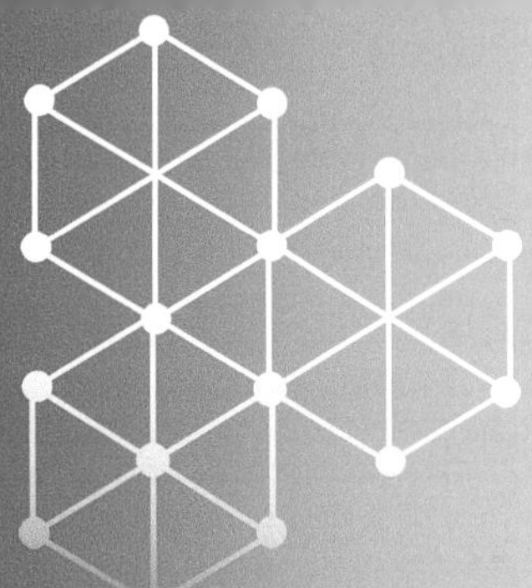

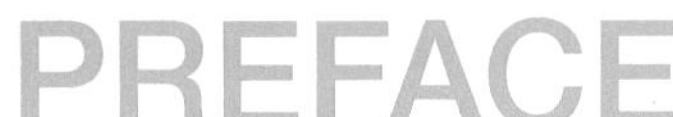

PREFACE

Pharmacy Practice for Technicians: What Makes This New Edition Exciting?

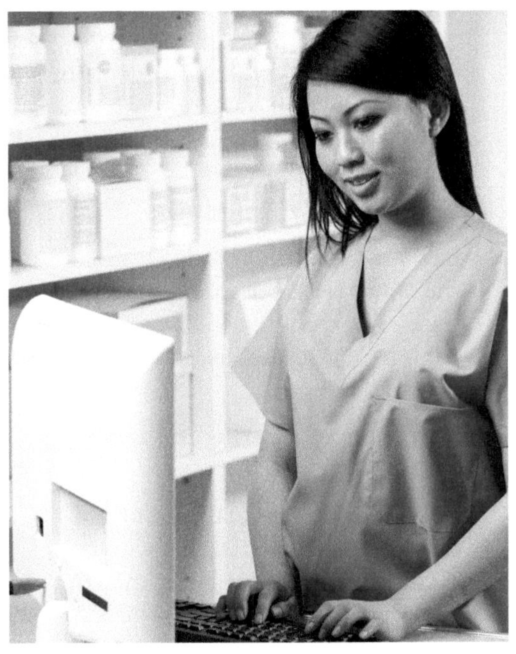

Since the field of pharmacy is changing so swiftly, your course content has to be cutting-edge and geared toward your success! You want to build knowledge to conquer a certification exam and establish a skills base for exceptional, safe service to patients. As a well-trained pharmacy technician, you will be best able to continually advance in your career once you are in the field. *Pharmacy Practice for Technicians*, Seventh Edition, has been dramatically updated to help you accomplish these goals. The Seventh Edition features include:

- Alignment with the latest ASHP curriculum standards, covering accreditation topics in a logical order with easy-to-understand language
- The web-based Cirrus learning platform to assemble all student and instructor resources in one easy-access location
- Leading topics in pharmacy, such as Medication Therapy Management (MTM), the ASHP Practice Advancement Initiative (PAI), interoperability, informatics, and more
- Updates on new standards for sterile, nonsterile, and hazardous compounding–as detailed in recent revisions for *USP* Chapters <795> and <797> (rev. 2019)
- Expanded sections on pharmacy law and ethical decision making
- Focus on career planning and stepping stones for advanced practice specialties
- Increased coverage of professionalism and soft skills, communication, and cultural awareness
- Luminous design and more images for enhanced readability and retention
- Extensive instructor input included for every phase of the new edition development
- New in-class review material and digital resources

Pharmacy Practice for Technicians, Seventh Edition, is designed to work in concert with Paradigm's *Pharmacy Labs for Technicians*, Fourth Edition, for hands-on practice or to stand alone as a comprehensive introductory course for pharmacy technician programs.

Study Assets: A Visual Walk-Through

Print and eContent

The courseware is available in print and online. The online resources include Watch and Learn Lessons containing video and text to help students understand the material in whichever manner works best. The course content includes a variety of features created to assist students in learning the concepts and skills needed by pharmacy technicians.

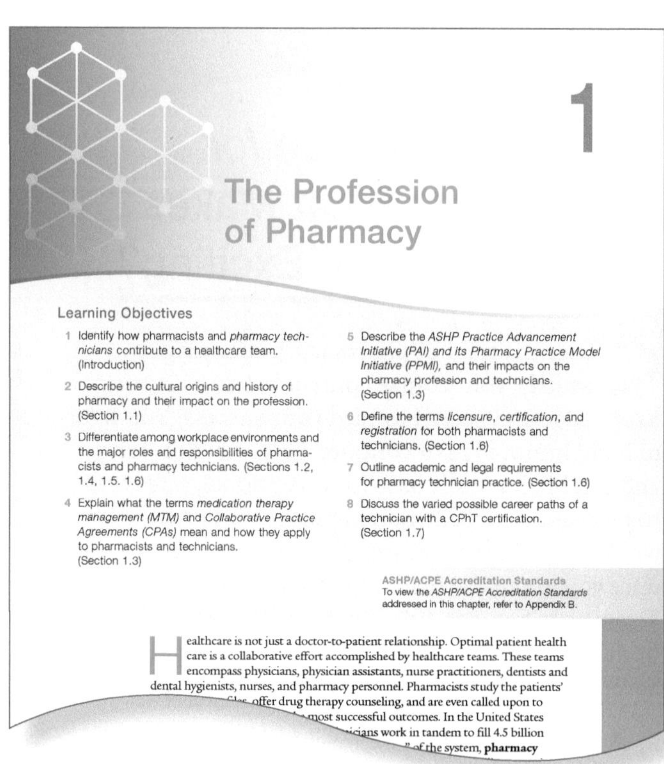

1

The Profession of Pharmacy

Learning Objectives

1 Identify how pharmacists and *pharmacy technicians* contribute to a healthcare team. (Introduction)

2 Describe the cultural origins and history of pharmacy and their impact on the profession. (Section 1.1)

3 Differentiate among workplace environments and the major roles and responsibilities of pharmacists and pharmacy technicians. (Sections 1.2, 1.4, 1.5. 1.6)

4 Explain what the terms *medication therapy management (MTM)* and *Collaborative Practice Agreements (CPAs)* mean and how they apply to pharmacists and technicians. (Section 1.3)

5 Describe the *ASHP Practice Advancement Initiative (PAI) and its Pharmacy Practice Model Initiative (PPMI)*, and their impacts on the pharmacy profession and technicians. (Section 1.3)

6 Define the terms *licensure*, *certification*, and *registration* for both pharmacists and technicians. (Section 1.6)

7 Outline academic and legal requirements for pharmacy technician practice. (Section 1.6)

8 Discuss the varied possible career paths of a technician with a CPhT certification. (Section 1.7)

ASHP/ACPE Accreditation Standards
To view the *ASHP/ACPE Accreditation Standards* addressed in this chapter, refer to Appendix B.

Healthcare is not just a doctor-to-patient relationship. Optimal patient health care is a collaborative effort accomplished by healthcare teams. These teams encompass physicians, physician assistants, nurse practitioners, dentists and dental hygienists, nurses, and pharmacy personnel. Pharmacists study the patients' … offer drug therapy counseling, and are even called upon to … most successful outcomes. In the United States … work in tandem to fill 4.5 billion … of the system, **pharmacy**

Learning Objectives

Each chapter begins with a list of the major concepts students should learn after reading the chapter and completing the exercises.

ASHP/ACPE Accreditation Standards

An author-created mapping of chapter-specific topics to industry standards for pharmacy technician training is provided in Appendix B.

In the Real World

Feature boxes highlight how the skills and concepts learned in the course will be important when working as a pharmacy technician.

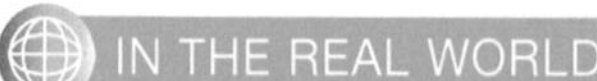

With expanding pharmacy patient care services and the increasing volume and complexity of pharmaceuticals, a certified technician graduating from an accredited program is an essential member of the healthcare team and an invaluable assistant in helping pharmacists provide medication services to patients and providers in all practice settings. The US Bureau of Labor Statistics forecasts a positive demand for pharmacy technician positions with 12% growth through 2026.

- act as a cashier, stock shelves, and handle inventory (sometimes handling procurement)
- assemble patient medication profiles and histories; check them for accuracy
- prepare online insurance claim forms, reconcile billing with copays and other insurance requirements
- run automated equipment for high-volume drug processing and packaging
- prepare nonsterile, sterile, and hazardous medications
- in the hospital, work with the nursing staff, fill and deliver medication orders, repackage medications, and restock automated medication dispensing machines in the hospital floor units
- …ication supplies in special packaging

Visually Engaging Study Tools

Figures, diagrams, tables, and photographs enhance visual learning and aid retention of course content.

TABLE 7.3 Parts of a Prescription

Part	Description
Prescriber information	Name, address, telephone number, and other information identifying the prescriber; NPI and DEA numbers; and, sometimes, the state license number
Date	Date on which the prescription was written; this date may differ from the date on which the prescription was received
Patient information	Full name, address, telephone number, and date of birth of the patient
℞	Symbol ℞, from the Latin word *recipere* meaning "to take"
Inscription	Medication prescribed, including generic or brand name, strength, and amount
Subscription	Instructions to the pharmacist on dispensing the medication
Signa	Directions for the patient to follow (commonly called the sig)
Addi[illegible]	[illegible]ditional instructions that the prescriber deems necessary

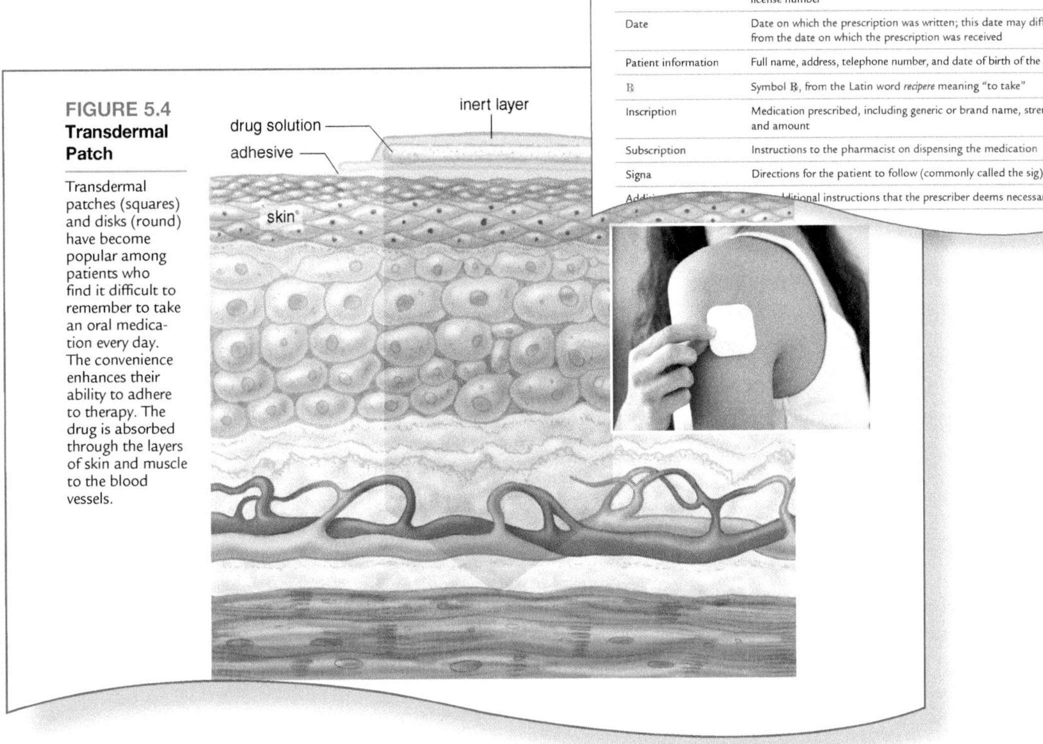

FIGURE 5.4 Transdermal Patch

Transdermal patches (squares) and disks (round) have become popular among patients who find it difficult to remember to take an oral medication every day. The convenience enhances their ability to adhere to therapy. The drug is absorbed through the layers of skin and muscle to the blood vessels.

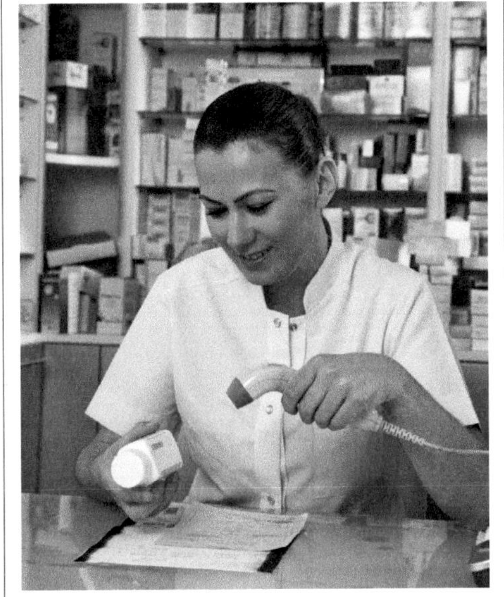

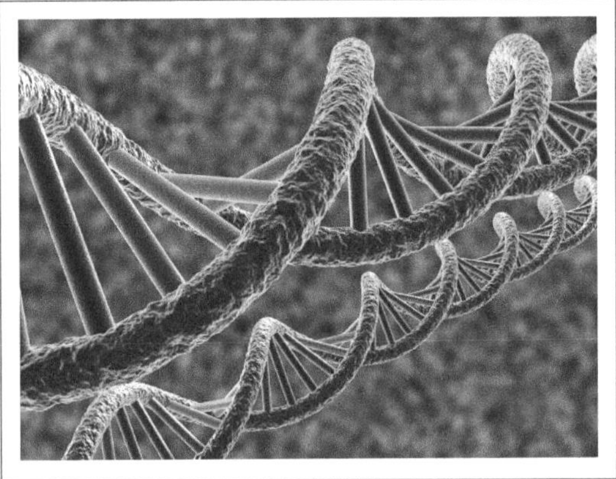

Margin Reminders

Short tips and hints spotlight important information related to chapter content.

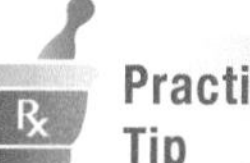

Provides reminders about key elements.

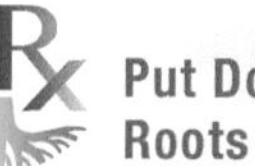

Offers word origins to make terms memorable.

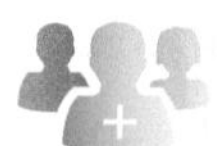

Gives advice on professional and soft skills.

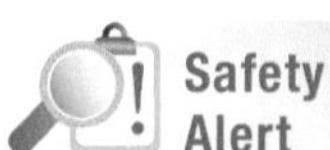

Calls out warnings to avoid problems.

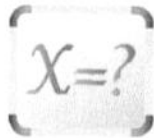

Supplies calculating hints.

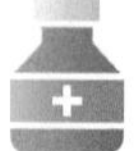

Highlights interesting tidbits.

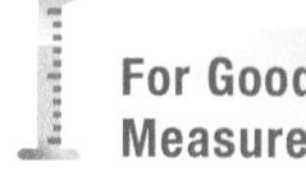

Assists in accuracy with measuring counsel.

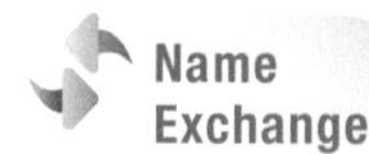

Reminds about items with two names, such as brand and generic drugs.

Review and Assessment

Each chapter ends with a set of resources that includes a summary of key concepts, a quick quiz to check understanding of course content, and critical thinking and research challenges.

Review and Assessment

CHAPTER SUMMARY

- Pharmacy technicians are part of the health-care team, assisting the pharmacist in management of medication therapies.
- The profession of pharmacy has ancient roots, dating to the use of herbal medicines
- The primary mission of the pharmacy profession today is to assist patients in achieving overall wellness and favorable outcomes with their medication therapies and to safeguard the public health—technicians share in this mission.

Appendices

Additional resources support student learning with succinct, at-a-glance reference materials. These include:

- Appendix A: Common Pharmacy Abbreviations and Acronyms
- Appendix B: ASHP/ACPE Accreditation Standards*

Glossary

Chapter key terms are presented in bold and are contextually defined when introduced in each chapter. The terms and their formal definitions are compiled in a course-level glossary.

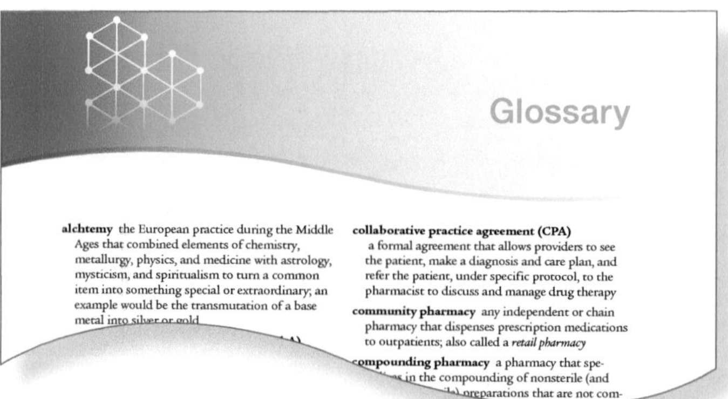

*Appendix B identifies the *ASHP/ACPE Accreditation Standards* associated with the chapter content. This list is meant for guidance purposes only and was created by the author of this text. Neither ASHP nor ACPE has participated in or had any role in creating the list of standards or any other content that is included in this book.

cirrus™ The Cirrus Solution

Elevating student success and instructor efficiency

Powered by Paradigm, Cirrus is the next-generation learning solution for teaching pharmacy technician students the concepts and skills needed to become successful employees valued by patients, colleagues, and supervisors. Cirrus seamlessly delivers complete course content in a cloud-based learning environment that puts students on the fast track to success. Students can access their content from any device, anywhere, through a live internet connection. Because Cirrus is platform-independent, students receive the same learning experience whether they are using PCs, Macs, or Chromebook computers. Cirrus also provides access to all the *Pharmacy Technician Series* content. This content is delivered in a series of scheduled assignments that report to a grade book, thus tracking student progress and achievement.Compatible with Canvas, D2L, and Blackboard, Cirrus is exportable through LTI for flexible learning using a school's LMS.

Cirrus Student eResources

Concepts and Training

The Concepts and Training section provides students with access to the complete contents of the printed book in both Watch and Learn Lessons and the eBook. Watch and Learn Lessons present each section of the courseware with a corresponding video covering the key concepts and topics. Read the content, watch the video, and then assess understanding using the corresponding quiz.

Review and Assessment

The Review and Assessment section reinforces and assesses student learning, allowing students to self-monitor their progress and engage more deeply with the material. This section includes the following features:

- Chapter Summary provides a list of key points from the chapter.
- Check Your Understanding provides a gradable, multiple-choice quiz on chapter content.
- Make Connections offers critical-thinking scenarios and research opportunities.
- Flash cards help students study key terms related to common generic and brand-name drugs, key historical figures and legislation, important federal and state agencies and pharmacy organizations that oversee pharmacy practice, and additional core content.
- Chapter practice quiz provides students with an opportunity to assess their understanding of chapter content by answering multiple-choice questions.

Cirrus Instructor eResources

Designed to support *Pharmacy Practice for Technicians*, Seventh Edition, the Instructor eResources include materials to help instructors plan their course, teach the content, and assess student progress and mastery. Accessed through Cirrus and visible only to instructors, these resources are categorized into two areas: Planning resources and Delivery and Assessment resources.

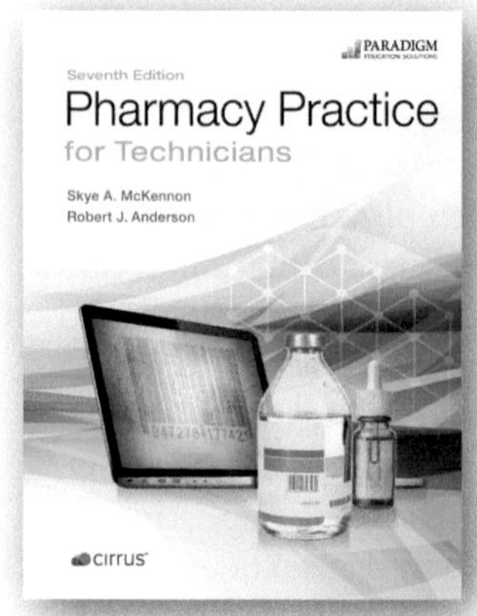

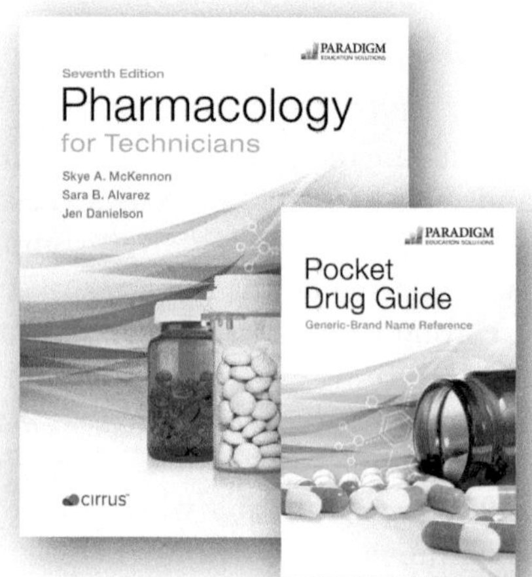

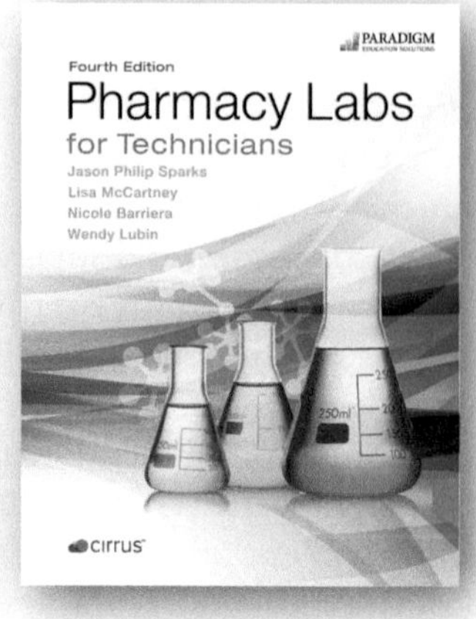

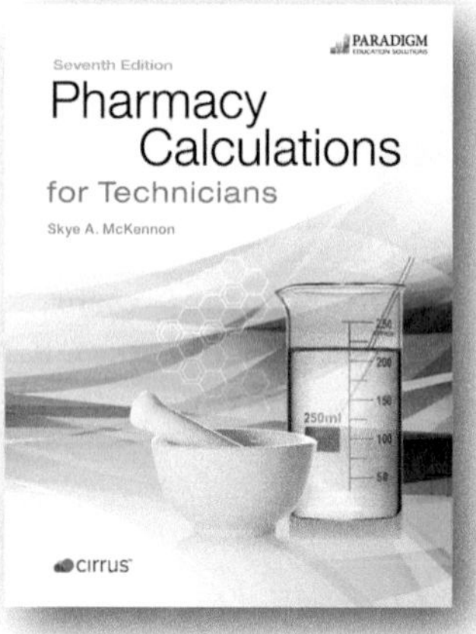

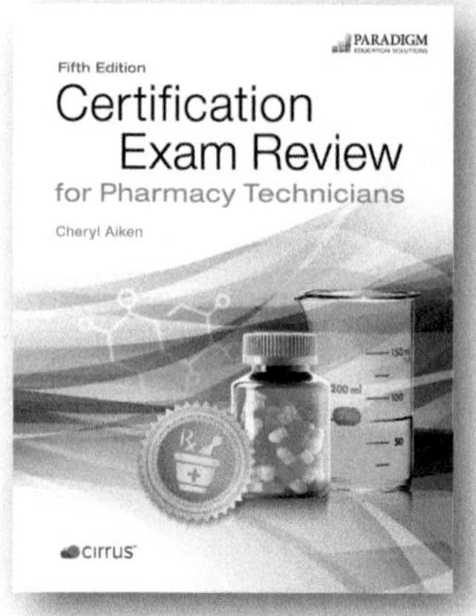

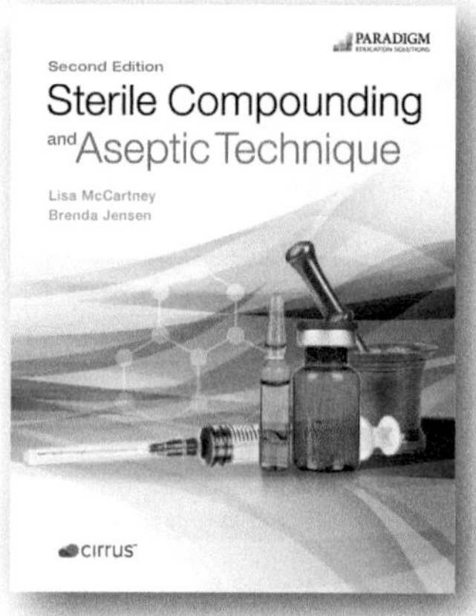

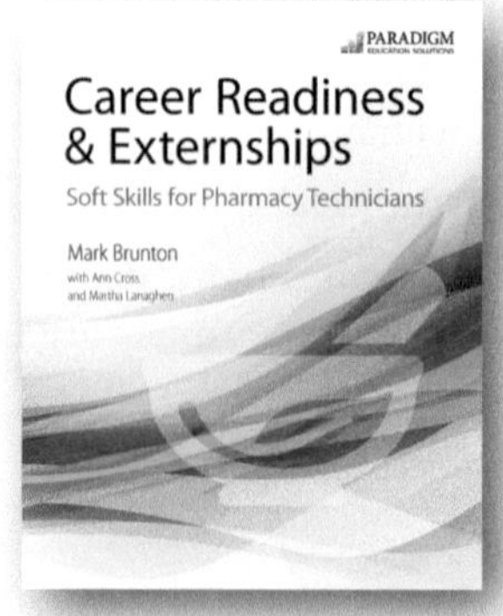

Paradigm's Comprehensive Pharmacy Technician Series

In addition to *Pharmacy Practice for Technicians*, Seventh Edition, Paradigm offers other courseware designed specifically for the pharmacy technician curriculum and integrated in the Cirrus learning environment:

- *Pharmacology for Technicians*, Seventh Edition
- *Pocket Drug Guide: Generic Brand Name Reference*
- *Pharmacy Labs for Technicians*, Fourth Edition
- *Pharmacy Calculations for Technicians*, Seventh Edition
- *Certification Exam Review for Pharmacy Technicians*, Fifth Edition
- *Sterile Compounding and Aseptic Technique*, Second Edition
- *Career Readiness & Externships: Soft Skills for Pharmacy Technicians*

Related Health Career Solutions

Additional offerings in Paradigm's Health Career line of courses are particularly useful for pharmacy technicians:

- *What Language Does Your Patient Hurt In? A Practical Guide to Culturally Competent Care*, Third Edition
- *Medical Terminology: Connecting through Language*
- *Medical Terminology Pocket Guide*
- *Pharmacology Essentials for Allied Health*
- *Exploring Electronic Health Records*, Second Edition
- *Emergency & Disaster Preparedness for Health Professionals,* Second Edition, with pharmacy specific eChapter
- *Introduction to Health Information Management*

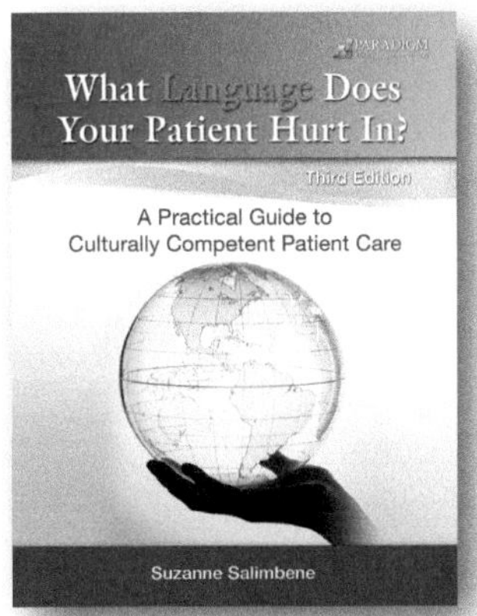

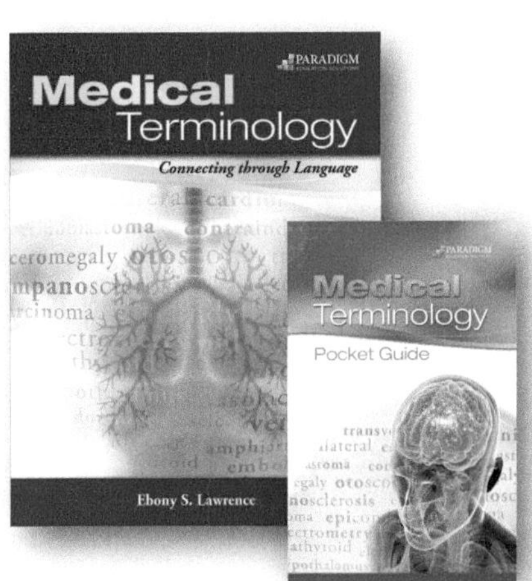

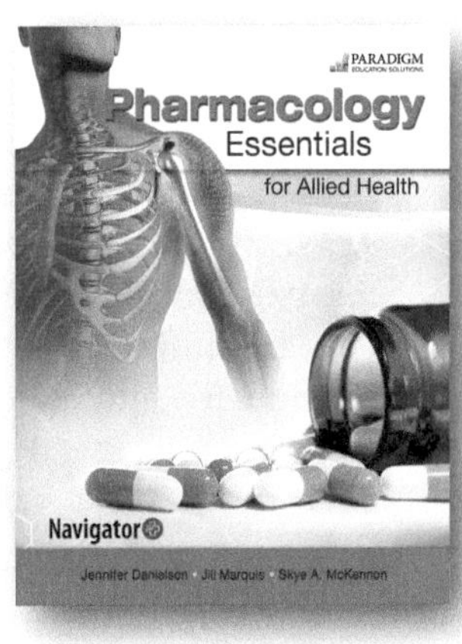

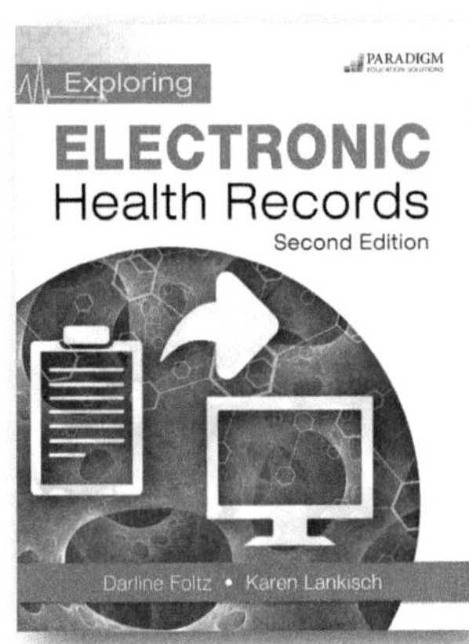

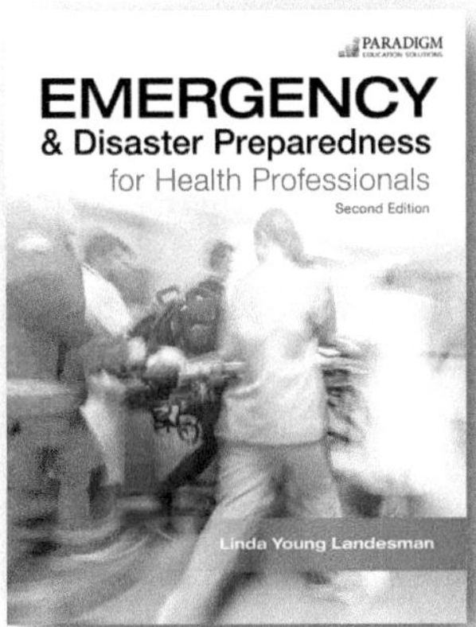

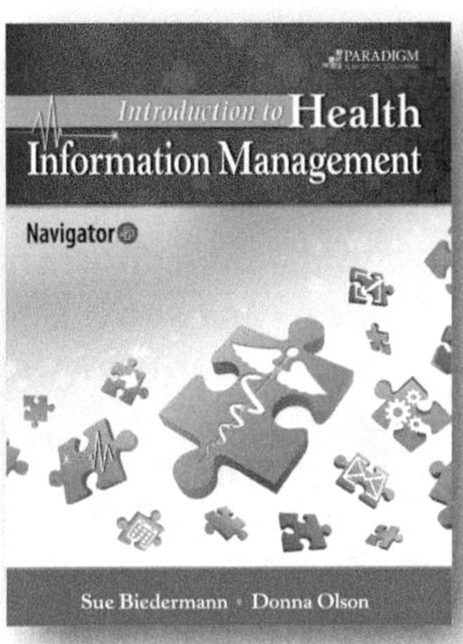

About the Authors

Skye A. McKennon

Skye A. McKennon is a licensed pharmacist, board-certified pharmacotherapy specialist (BCPS), group exercise instructor, certified lifestyle coach, and preventionist. Dr. McKennon completed her bachelor's degree and doctor of pharmacy (PharmD) degree from Washington State University. She also completed postdoctoral residency training at Swedish Medical Center in Seattle, Washington.

Dr. McKennon has practice experience in the institutional and ambulatory pharmacy settings. Notably, she was instrumental in the development of a lipid management clinic at Evergreen Health. Her passion for teaching and education led her to faculty positions at the University of Washington School of Pharmacy and at the Washington State University College of Pharmacy. Courses designed and directed by Dr. McKennon include applied pharmacotherapeutics, institutional pharmacy practice, and diabetes prevention. She has been both an instructor and a guest lecturer of various courses for pharmacy and other health science students, including therapeutics, pharmacotherapy for older adults, global health brigades, and law and ethics.

Dr. McKennon has presented her work at international and national symposiums such as the Seventh International Conference on Interprofessional Practice and Education as well as the American Association of Colleges of Pharmacy annual meeting and the Academy of Integrative Health and Medicine annual meeting. She has authored four pharmacy textbooks and written chapters in textbooks for a variety of health science audiences. Dr. McKennon is also a contributor to her regional pharmacy community and regularly provides live and online continuing education.

Robert J. Anderson

Robert J. Anderson, PharmD, has more than 40 years of experience in academia and pharmacy practice, having worked in both independent and chain community pharmacies. Dr. Anderson is a past member of the United States Pharmacopeia (USP) Expert Committee. Professor Emeritus at the Southern School of Pharmacy at Mercer University in Atlanta, Georgia, he is currently a part-time community pharmacist and author. Dr. Anderson has served as an associate director for the Department of Pharmaceutical Services at the University of Nebraska Medical Center in Omaha, Nebraska, and as a clinical pharmacy specialist at Kaiser Permanente, Southeast Region, in Atlanta. He is coauthor on the third, fourth, fifth and sixth editions of *Pharmacy Practice for Technicians*, as well as on the second and third editions, and upcoming fourth edition (2017) of *Certification Exam Review for Pharmacy Technicians*. He has been a guest lecturer in clinical pharmacology at several state nurse practitioner programs and has written chapters in *Clinical Pharmacology and Therapeutics* and *Handbook of Nonprescription Drugs* and also served on the editorial boards of *Family Practice Recertification* and *American Journal of Managed Care Pharmacy*. He is president of RJA Consultants, LLC for legal consulting.

About the Experts

Several exceptional instructors and content specialists reviewed and contributed to this program's textbook and digital resources to help ensure accuracy and appropriate instructional approaches. Special thanks are due to these individuals who shared their vast expertise and passion for the profession:

Content Area Expert Reviewers

Amanda Daniels, BS, CPhT (all chapters)
Pharmacy Technology Clinical Coordinator/Instructor, Atlanta Technical College

Irene Villatoro, Ph.T.R, CPh.T, B.S. (all chapters)
Program Director, San Jacinto College North

Kurstin M. Peplinski BS, CPhT, CSPT (Chapters 12, 13)
Fairview Pharmacy Services

Assessment Reviewer

Sarah Lawrence, PharmD, MA, BCGP
Independent Pharmacy Educational Consultant

Acknowledgments

The quality of this body of work is a testament to the feedback we have received from many instructors, additional contributors, and series survey respondents.

Irene Villatoro, Ph.T.R, CPh.T, B.S.
(all chapters)
Program Director
San Jacinto College North

Nicole Barriera, CPhT
Pikes Peak Community College

Mark Brunton, CPhT, MSHE
Northwest Career College

Kevin Hope, RPh
Clinical Pharmacy Education Specialist
freeCE

Anne LaVance, CPhT
Delgado Community College

Wendy Almeda Lubin BS, CPhT
Front Range Community College

Nader Rassaei,MD,MA,BS, CPhT
El Paso Community College

Andrea Redman, Pharm D, BCPS
Emory Healthcare

Hannah Brooke Stokely, BS, CPhT
Southeastern Institute, Pfeiffer Institute

Veronica Velasquez BA, PhTR, CPhT
Austin Community College

Special Acknowledgment

Pharmacy Practice for Technicians was originally authored by Don. A. Ballington, MS, whose high-quality training materials for pharmacy technicians serves as the foundation for Paradigm's *Pharmacy Technician Series.*

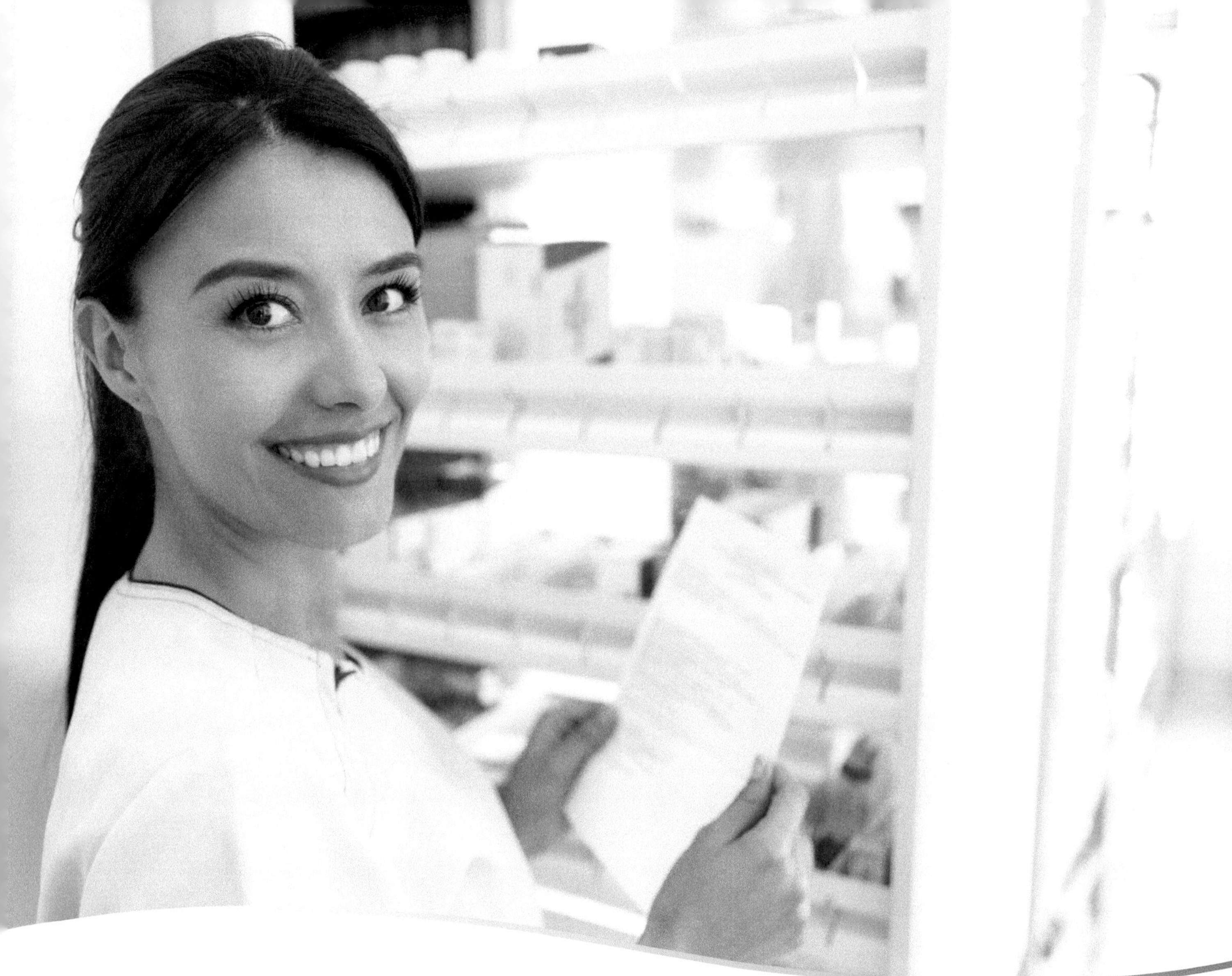

UNIT 1 Principles of Pharmacy Practice

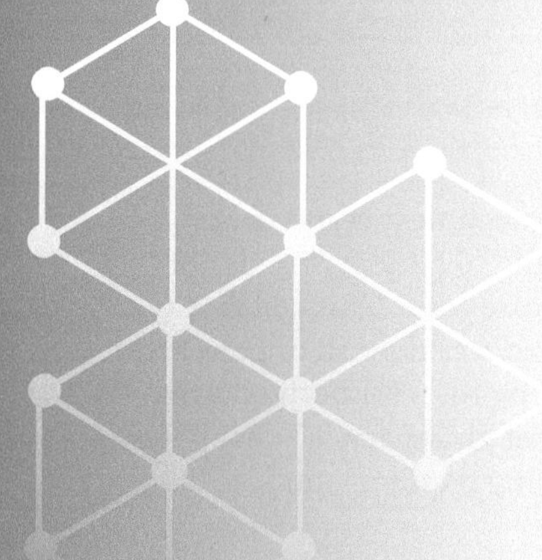

1

The Profession of Pharmacy

Learning Objectives

1. Identify how pharmacists and *pharmacy technicians* contribute to a healthcare team. (Introduction)
2. Describe the cultural origins and history of pharmacy and their impact on the profession. (Section 1.1)
3. Differentiate among workplace environments and the major roles and responsibilities of pharmacists and pharmacy technicians. (Sections 1.2, 1.4, 1.5. 1.6)
4. Explain what the terms *medication therapy management (MTM)* and *Collaborative Practice Agreements (CPAs)* mean and how they apply to pharmacists and technicians. (Section 1.3)
5. Describe the *ASHP Practice Advancement Initiative (PAI) and its Pharmacy Practice Model Initiative (PPMI),* and their impacts on the pharmacy profession and technicians. (Section 1.3)
6. Define the terms *licensure*, *certification*, and *registration* for both pharmacists and technicians. (Section 1.6)
7. Outline academic and legal requirements for pharmacy technician practice. (Section 1.6)
8. Discuss the varied possible career paths of a technician with a CPhT certification. (Section 1.7)

ASHP/ACPE Accreditation Standards
To view the *ASHP/ACPE Accreditation Standards* addressed in this chapter, refer to Appendix B.

Healthcare is not just a doctor-to-patient relationship. Optimal patient health care is a collaborative effort accomplished by healthcare teams. These teams encompass physicians, physician assistants, nurse practitioners, dentists and dental hygienists, nurses, and pharmacy personnel. Pharmacists study the patients' medication profiles, offer drug therapy counseling, and are even called upon to monitor these therapies for the most successful outcomes. In the United States today, pharmacists and pharmacy technicians work in tandem to fill 4.5 billion prescriptions each year. Often called the "backbone" of the system, **pharmacy technicians** do the hands-on work of gathering information and filling prescriptions and medication orders, while **pharmacists** oversee, check, and approve work, and educate providers and patients about drugs and supplements, including best uses, side effects, and interactions.

Pharmacists could not offer reliable drug-therapy counseling and monitoring without the assistance of educated, well-trained, and certified pharmacy technicians. Pharmacy technicians are responsible for many functions in a pharmacy beyond just helping to fill the prescriptions.

Like other technicians in healthcare—such as radiology technicians and dental technicians—pharmacy technicians play a key role in attending to patients' needs and tamping down, or at least slowing, pharmacy-related healthcare costs. This collaborative work environment improves efficiency and potentially reduces the risk of preventable and costly medication errors. To understand the emerging roles for both pharmacists and technicians, it is helpful to understand the history of pharmacy, contemporary workplaces, and current education and licensing requirements.

1.1 The Origins of the Profession

In early civilizations, sickness or disease was often thought to be a form of punishment or a curse by demons or evil spirits. To rid the victims of ill health, relatives would call upon a priest, shaman, or medicinal healer to identify the spiritual cause and then determine the appropriate remedy. At the same time, these civilizations carried with them deep knowledge of medicinal plants and herbal remedies. Early recipes for drug preparations were freely mixed with prayers, chants, incantations, and rituals. Many indigenous healers on every inhabited continent continue these practices, holding great knowledge about medicinal plants in their cultural heritages. Contemporary drug companies are seeking this knowledge for new medications.

Over time, the pharmacy profession evolved into a scientific pursuit involving the compounding and dispensing of medications and drug information. In the wake of this shift from an art to a science, pharmacy has moved from the back rooms of village **apothecary** shops to a variety of medical practice settings that cater to specific patient populations with medication needs.

Pharmacy practitioners have evolved from ancient medicinal healers and alchemists to educated and trained pharmacists and technicians who rely on quality assurance, safety standards, and technology to ensure the well-being of their patients and customers.

Early Medications and Formularies

The use of drugs in the healing arts by all cultures is as old as human history. Archaeologists exploring the remains of the ancient city-states of Mesopotamia (near present-day Iraq and Iran) unearthed clay tablets listing hundreds of medicinal preparations from various sources, including plants, animals, and minerals. Early inhabitants used the trial-and-error method to compile medicine lists known as **pharmacopeias**, or *dispensatories*. Medicine lists are still an important part of pharmacy practice. Current-day drug lists used by insurance carriers and healthcare systems are called **drug formularies**.

The most famous early formulary was the 110-page Ebers Papyrus (1500 BCE) containing more than 700 prescriptions for ailments that affected early Egyptian cultures.

Eastern Medicine Roots

The use of botanicals as tools of healing became the basis of **traditional Eastern medicine**, which continues especially in China, Japan, and India. Many of these herbal treatments are widely used in Western cultures today; for example, ginseng is used to enhance energy. A well-known figure who laid the foundation for traditional Eastern medicine is Sushruta.

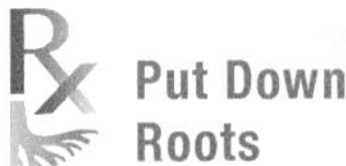
Put Down Roots

The word *pharmacy* comes from the ancient Greek word *pharmakon*, meaning "drug or remedy."

Sushruta was a Hindu surgeon from the sixth century BCE who wrote a medicinal work called the *Sushruta Samhita.* This work discussed hundreds of surgical procedures, over 1,000 medical conditions, and the medicinal use of over 500 plants. Sushruta's collection of medicinal recipes is one of the three foundational texts of Indian traditional medicine called Ayurveda. Ayurveda is a holistic approach to medicine that includes a patient's spiritual well-being. In **Ayurvedic medicine**, physicians prescribe treatments such as herbs, exercise, and diet and lifestyle changes to maintain a balance of natural forces in the body.

Western medicine moved away from its religious roots into a dependence upon observation, theories and hypotheses, and scientific experimentation.

Greek Roots

Much of contemporary Western medicine and pharmacy practice finds itself indebted to some key early Greek physicians.

Hippocrates Ancient Greeks were the first culture to shift to a more classical scientific approach. The famous Greek physician **Hippocrates** (ca. 460–370 BCE) believed that illness had a physical explanation and was not the result of possession by evil spirits or disfavor with the gods. He thought that the body's four "humors," or liquid systems, (blood, phlegm, yellow bile, and black bile) must be in the correct balance to maintain optimal health. His hypothesis formed the origins of the theory of bodily systems and scientific observation practiced today.

During his lifetime, Hippocrates published more than 70 medical texts that scientifically categorized diseases, their signs and symptoms, and their treatments. He is also credited with establishing a lexicon for medical terminology that healthcare professionals still use. Because of his many contributions to the practice of Western medicine, Hippocrates is known as the "Father of Modern Medicine." He is also known for the Hippocratic Oath—the "do no harm" vow taken by medical practitioners to uphold the highest standards of medical ethics.

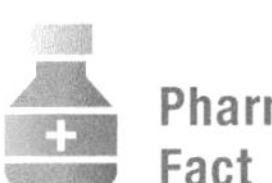
Pharm Fact

Dioscorides cataloged more than 1,000 substances—mainly botanicals—that had medicinal value.

Dioscorides Another early Greek physician, **Pedanius Dioscorides** (40–90 CE), is credited with writing one of the world's greatest pharmaceutical texts: *De Materia Medica* (*On Medical Matters*). Written in the first century CE, Dioscorides's text includes descriptions of herbal remedies and their usage, side effects, quantities, dosages, and storage guidelines. Dioscorides gathered his knowledge of medicinal herbs and minerals as a soldier serving in the Roman army.

As he traveled across the European continent, he collected samples of herbs that he later studied and tested for potential medicinal properties. For 15 centuries, *De Materia Medica* served as the standard reference for drugs; it is considered the forerunner of current pharmacological references, such as the *US Pharmacopeia–National Formulary (USP-NF)* and the *Prescribers' Digital Reference.*

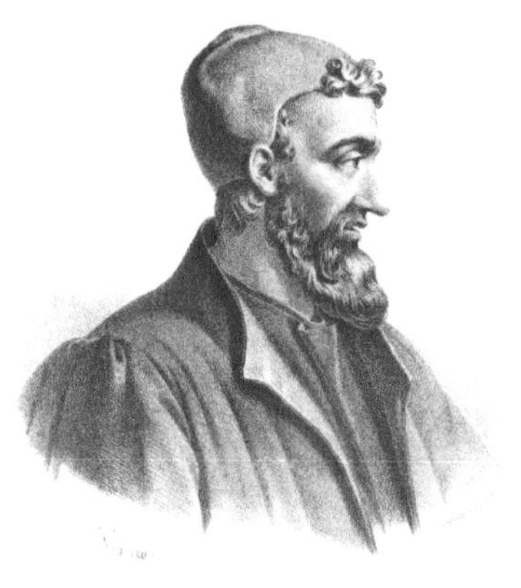
Galen is considered the "Father of Pharmacy" for extracting, identifying, and classifying active ingredients from natural sources.

Galen Like Dioscorides, **Claudius Galen** (130–216 CE) was a notable Greek physician. He pioneered the practice of dissecting animals to study organs and anatomy, and he extracted active healing ingredients from plants, analyzing and organizing their medicinal effects on the body. His work led to the coining of the term **galenical pharmacy**—the extraction of active ingredients into compounding substances, such as juices, saps, and oils.

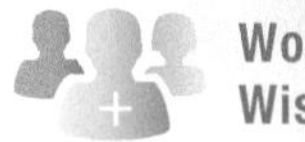

Work Wise

Prayers and medicine remain linked for many individuals, religions, and cultures; respect and sensitivity are always needed. Some scientific studies associate prayer with health benefits.

From these, Galen created recipes for medicines like ointments and drops. For his extensive body of work and writings in the pharmaceutical sciences, including *De Methodo Medendi (On the Healing Method)*, Galen is considered to be the "Father of Pharmacy."

Arabic Medicine Roots

Arab civilizations drew upon their own cultural knowledge and that of the Greeks. The Arabic Muslim communities were among the first cultures to develop a list of drugs with dosage formulations for tablets, syrups, and extracts, and to regulate the state-run pharmacies for care of patients.

The twin brothers **Cosmas and Damian** (approximately 270–303 CE) are symbolic links between the Arab and Greek worlds of medicine and pharmacy. The brothers were Arab Christians living in Syria under Roman rule. They practiced healing and medicine (both surgery and pharmacy) for no charge because they wanted to heal and serve even the poorest patients. They were beheaded by the Romans for being Christians and came to be revered as patron saints of medicine and pharmacy throughout the Middle East and Europe.

The Middle Ages: Ethics and Institutions

During the Middle Ages (approximately 500 to 1400 CE), the profession of pharmacy in both the European and Persian empires was evolving with deep ethical roots of healing service. From the late 700s CE on, the Islamic governments in Egypt and Jerusalem established hospitals to care for the sick. The great Al-Mansur Hospital in Cairo in the 1200s served the rich and poor and had separate wings for different kinds of surgery and care. It also trained both men and women to care for the sick. Caring for the poor is an ongoing concern today for pharmacists and pharmacy technicians, who help those on limited means find ways to afford their medications.

In Europe, since there were no healthcare systems or printing presses, Christian monasteries became storehouses of knowledge as the monks studied and copied manuscripts. Monasteries of monks and abbeys of nuns used the accumulated knowledge of healing to serve the community in many ways. They grew gardens of herbs for food and medicine. These hospitable monastic facilities provided free medicines and healthcare, thus serving as additional precursors to today's charity hospitals, community healthcare clinics, and public health departments.

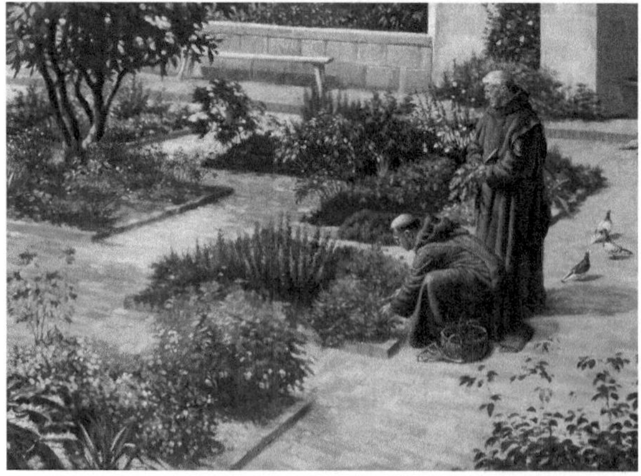

As the poor had no access to physicians or even apothecaries, religious orders of monks and nuns invited the poor into their monasteries or guesthouses for healing and care. The assisting novices were early hospital technicians.

A number of Jewish-Arab physicians had a significant impact on the progress of pharmacy practice and ethics in Northern Africa. **Moses ben Maimon** (Maimonides, 1135–1204 CE), who served the sultan in Cairo, gathered vast amounts of accumulated knowledge into books. He wrote about common illnesses and focused on moderation, healthy living, and illness prevention. Maimon emphasized a sense of humble servitude toward the poor and rich. His prayer to accomplish this was passed on to pharmacy professionals for centuries, even being used in their graduation ceremonies in the United States in the early 20th century. His prayer, other spiritual practices, and the Hippocratic medical oath underpin the contemporary emphasis on professional ethics in pharmacy and medicine.

Put Down Roots

Drug is related to the 14th-century Dutch words *droge waere*, which translates as "dry goods" and came to mean "dried herbs and spices."

Apothecary is derived from the Latin word *apotheca*, a storage place associated with dry goods, herbs, and wine.

The Pharmacy Shop

In Western Europe by the 11th and 12th centuries, physicians were often their own pharmacists or chemists and they owned the dispensary that distributed drugs to patients. Pharmacies were commonly under the authority of the College of Physicians or a similar professional group of doctors who followed the traditions of Greek, Roman, and Arab medical practices. However, in 1241, Sicily enforced the Edict of Salerno that forbade physicians from running pharmacists' shops and required medications to be produced by a qualified chemist in a registered shop. This pioneering concept took a long time to become standard practice.

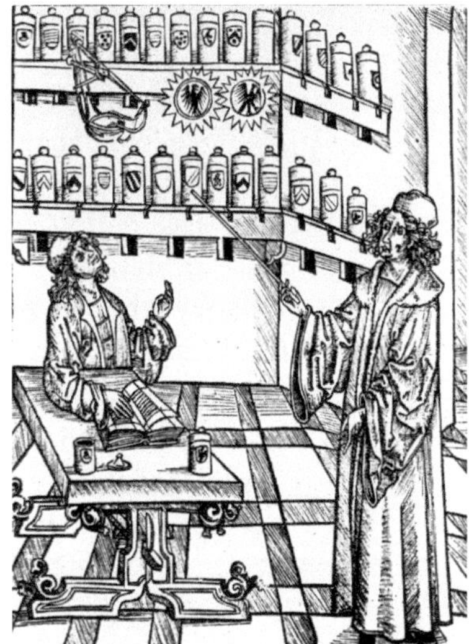

This woodcut of an early pharmacy technician, who was an apprentice for a master chemist, is from *A Pharmaceutical Lesson* by Hieronymus Brunschwig.

Since only the upper class could afford to consult with a physician, most "common folk" turned to midwives who gathered medicinal plants from the fields, or to wine and spice shopkeepers who also sold herbal medicines from plants and substances from more distant places. An **apothecary** store concept was developing. The cheapest remedies it stored and sold came from the herbs or plants growing in the surrounding countryside, such as foxglove (*Digitalis purpurea*) for heart problems.

Most apothecaries had a back room that resembled a small chemistry laboratory where the store chemists could experiment with and compound various formulations. Leeches were also collected and used in bloodletting in an effort to draw out the illness in the blood and balance the bodily fluids. Leeches are still used to keep blood flowing to a wound to help with the healing process. Toxic minerals and noxious tasting plants were used in purging compounds.

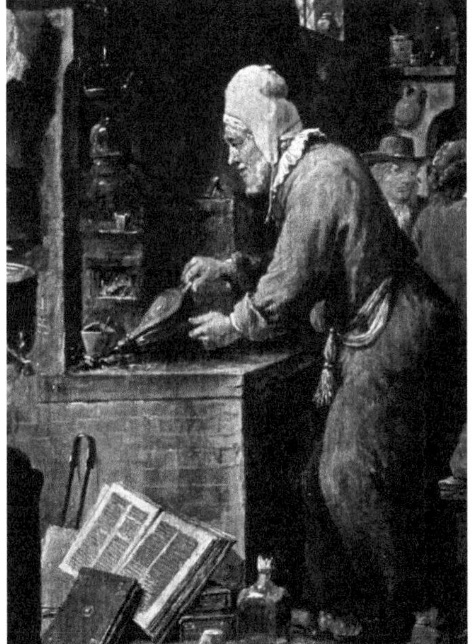

This painting, called *The Alchemist*, is by David Teniers the Younger (1582–1649) and is displayed at the Prado Museum in Madrid. Alchemists often depended upon assistants.

The First Guilds

Trade guilds (a cross between a trade union and a professional organization) developed in Europe with a system of apprentices in training to join each profession. The chemist and apothecary apprentices were the early pharmacy technicians. For centuries, English apothecaries belonged to the Grocers Guild. Interestingly, many pharmacies today are located in large grocery and mega-stores.

The Renaissance Alchemy and Apothecary Guilds

Greek, Roman, and Arab scientific influences were less emphasized in Europe during the Renaissance (about 1350–1650 CE). This period saw the rise of pharmacists moving into **alchemy**, which combined chemistry, metallurgy, physics, and medicine with elements of astrology and mysticism. The alchemists' goals were to find the most valuable essences to turn something ordinary into something with supernatural or supervaluable properties. For instance, alchemists would attempt to change base metals—such as iron, nickel, or lead—into silver or gold and seek medicinal elixirs or minerals as keys to undying youth.

By 1617 in Britain, the apothecaries had split from the Grocers Guild and joined with the doctors working as medicinal compounders to start their own more specialized guild. This new apothecary guild set standards, determined membership in the profession, and oversaw the training and length of apprenticeships. (The first London apothecary guild was called the Worshipful Society of Apothecaries.) Formalized universities and educational programs in chemistry and medical sciences grew out of these early guild efforts. The state boards of pharmacy and professional pharmacy associations of today (discussed later in the chapter) are considered the offspring of these medieval pharmacy guilds.

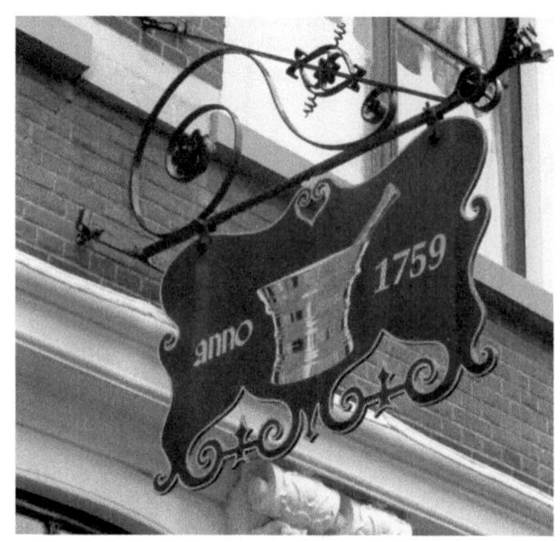

The Scientific Revolution and Exploration

In the 17th century, scientific methods were once again emphasized. University students in Western Europe studied the Greek and Latin classics. Scholars pursued and published scientific research, advancing medicine, and pharmacy. It is not surprising that these scholars and researchers borrowed words or word parts from the ancient languages for their new discoveries. Their lexicon—based on Greek and Latin root words, prefixes, and suffixes—remains at the heart of many medical terms today.

As European explorers brought back exotic plants and spices, the list of medicinal agents used in Europe grew. Medicinal practitioners and chemists needed to be skilled not only in biology and chemistry, but also in botany as they created new medicinal agents from these newly introduced natural substances. Rudimentary research to determine the efficacy of these new botanical drugs was initiated.

In North America during the early period of colonization (early 1600s to late 1700s), **herbal medicine** was widely practiced by Native Americans, and the newcomers learned medicinal uses of the local plants from them. Herbs such as purple coneflower (used to prevent infection), wild ginger (used to treat a stomachache), and saw palmetto (used to treat prostate problems) were common natural remedies. These herbs, along with herbal remedies from the world at large, continue to be sought-after cures, especially as more individuals embrace the practice of holistic and natural medicine.

Among the early colonists in what is now the United States and Canada, there were very few pharmacists. Predictably, the medical profession in settler colonies followed the European model, albeit at a much slower pace. Gradually the profession of medicine separated from that of pharmacy, and the apothecary shop became an independent entity owned and operated by the pharmacist.

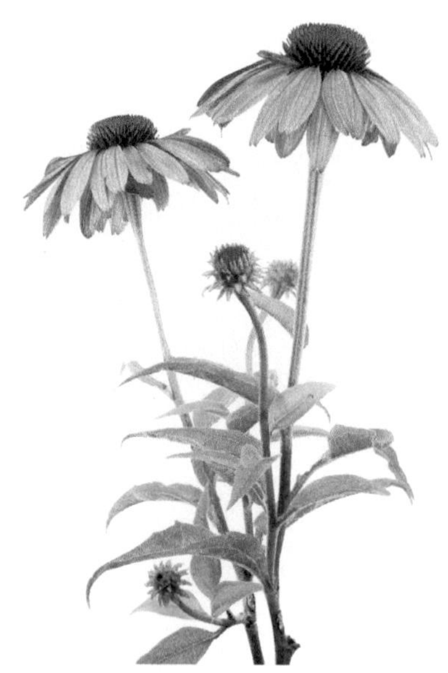

Extracts from the *Echinacea* plant (purple coneflower) are still used today to build immunity and prevent infection.

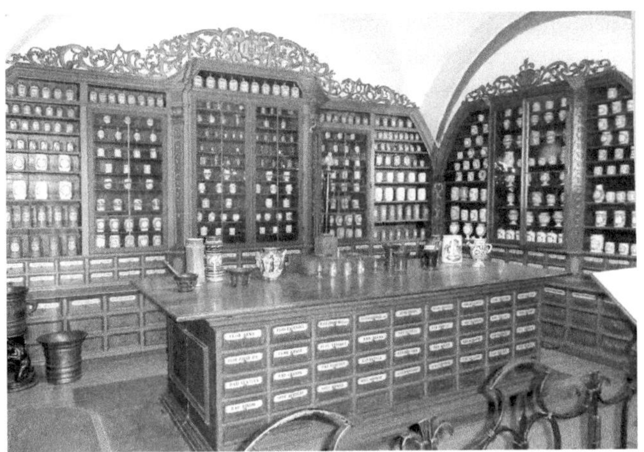

This image is of a German apothecary preserved at the German Pharmacy Museum in Heidelberg Castle.

Early Pharmaceutical Manufacturing and the Need for Standards

By the 1800s, the pharmacist, or chemist, was becoming increasingly recognized as a specialized provider of healthcare in Europe and North America. Physicians had begun to refer patients to the chemists to get their prescribed drug recipes compounded. Chemists relied on their own knowledge and experiences to formulate liquids and powders and to make their own capsules and tablets. Subsequently, they would package and label the drugs in containers and then dispense these medications to patients. For common illnesses, patients went to the chemist for common cures, just as we go to the drug store for over-the-counter (OTC) drugs.

Every physician or pharmacist had favorite formulas or recipes for compounding their medicinal products, though many recipes were similar. Concerned by these varying recipes, a group of eleven physicians convened in 1820 in Washington, DC, to list the standard compounding recipes for the common drugs used in the United States. They called the list the *US Pharmacopeia (USP).*

Updates of this early drug formulary are now released annually *(US Pharmacopeia-National Formulary [USP-NF]),* written by the organization that grew out of this meeting. It is now an independent, nonprofit organization called the **US Pharmacopeial Convention (USP)** that sets quality standards for prescription medications, over-the-counter (OTC) drugs, homeopathic drugs, and dietary supplements. The USP also sets the quality standards for the compounding of both nonsterile, sterile, and hazardous medications; these standards are now widely recognized by the US government and accreditation organizations.

The First American Pharmacy Schools and Associations

Though Europe had schools for pharmacy, the United States had none. In 1822, two years after the formation of the USP, the Philadelphia College of Pharmacy became the first school in the young nation to offer courses in the pharmaceutical sciences and to grant pharmacy-specific diplomas. Up until this time, no formal schooling was required; one simply became a pharmacist after completing an apprenticeship in an apothecary. (Apprenticeships were the common method for learning a trade at this time.)

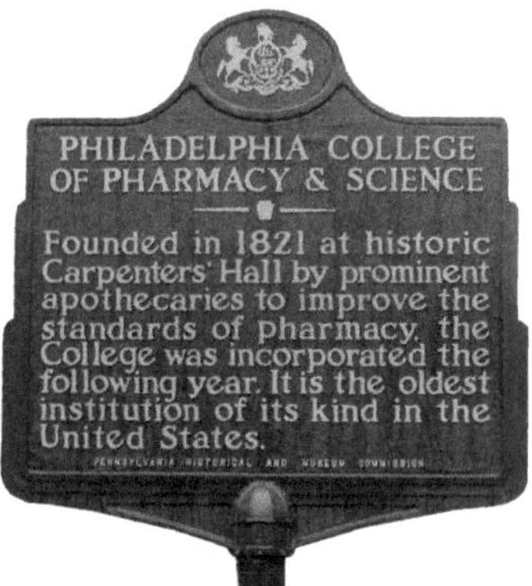
PHILADELPHIA COLLEGE
OF PHARMACY & SCIENCE
Founded in 1821 at historic Carpenters' Hall by prominent apothecaries to improve the standards of pharmacy, the College was incorporated the following year. It is the oldest institution of its kind in the United States.

In 1852, the American Pharmaceutical Association, now known as the **American Pharmacists Association (APhA)**, was organized to help establish professional practice standards and address the problem of varying qualities and recipes of imported drugs. The APhA called for standards for drug ingredients, compounding, and dosages, and encouraged state governments to regulate the pharmacy profession by requiring pharmacy apprentices to pass formal certification examinations to obtain licensure to practice as pharmacists.

Additional universities worldwide began to offer formal education and degree programs in pharmacy, most focusing on the study of **pharmacognosy** (the study of the medicinal functions of natural products and chemicals of animal, plant, and mineral origins). Pharmacists in training still spent time as apprentices in apothecaries.

By the late 1800s, large-scale pharmaceutical manufacturing had begun, especially in Europe where universities often worked with manufacturers to have their new laboratory compounds developed and produced. Although many pharmacists continued to rely on herbal extracts as ingredients in their compounded preparations, they began slowly to sell mass-manufactured, artificial chemical preparations as well. For example, in 1899, the German pharmaceutical manufacturer Bayer synthesized aspirin from acetylsalicylic acid and mass-produced it instead of extracting and compounding the salicylic acid from willow-tree bark. Aspirin is still popular today, not only as a remedy for headache, pain, and inflammation, but also as a medication to reduce blood clots in high-risk heart patients.

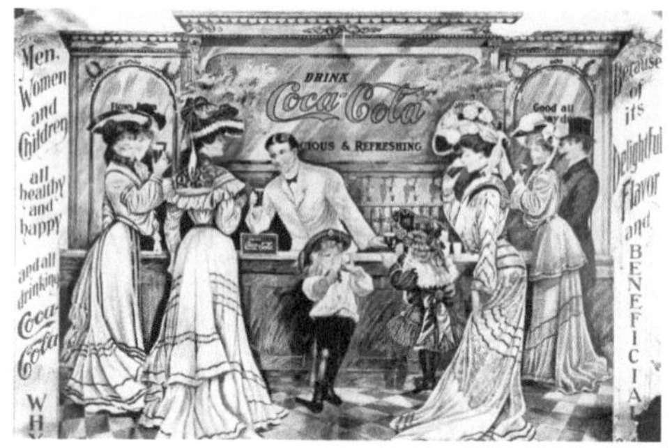

While men socialized in bars, women and children went to drug stores and ice cream parlors for refreshments. During Prohibition, almost every drug store had a soda fountain selling drinks, such as Coca-Cola and Pepsi-Cola, which technicians often served.

Compounding Commercial Success Stories

For much of the 19th and 20th centuries in the United States, it was common to find pharmacy soda fountains. Pharmacists added fruit-flavored syrups to carbonated water, and some even concocted recipes or formulations for refreshing new beverages to attract customers. For example, in 1886, John Pemberton, a pharmacist in Atlanta, Georgia, began to sell a compounded tonic called Coca-Cola, which obviously became wildly popular. Its name was derived from one of its ingredients: cocaine. For more than two decades, the Coca-Cola formula contained this plant alkaloid until growing concerns over the harmful and addictive effects of cocaine forced its manufacturer to replace it with caffeine.

In 1893, another pharmacist, Caleb Bradham in North Carolina, created a similar carbonated drink later called Pepsi-Cola. Technicians would assist in making the drinks as the soda "jerks," or servers. The carbonated drinks mass-produced today had their origins at the corner drug store soda fountains. Though the soda fountains faded away in the 1960s with the rise of bottled and canned drinks, these pharmacist-created fountain drinks remain mainstays globally.

1.2 The 20th-Century Evolution of Pharmacy Education and Practice

As the number of formalized pharmacy programs increased, the need for a pharmacy curriculum and practice standards did too. Within the last century, formalized practice and programs have evolved through four stages of development.

The Traditional Era of Compounding Pharmacists

During the first half of the 1900s, more than 80% of all prescriptions were compounded by pharmacists. For instance, Walgreens started out as a corner drug store in 1901, run by Charles R. Walgreen on the South Side of Chicago, selling medications and other valued retail items. With no formal pharmacy education, he had trained under prominent pharmacists to learn the science and art of compounding. Though one *could* study in a university pharmacy program, there were no educational requirements to take the pharmacist examination until 1920. As long as applicants completed a three- or four-year apprenticeship in a pharmacy, they were eligible for the exam. This is similar to the current situation for pharmacy technicians in some states.

Many pharmacy assistants worked alongside the pharmacists in apothecaries or small corner drug stores and hospitals, and they, too, received only on-the-job training. In the corner drug stores, pharmacy assistants also worked as cashiers and stocking clerks. During and after World War II, the need for hospital care for wounded soldiers increased the need for hospital drugs, pharmacists, and trained pharmacy assistants.

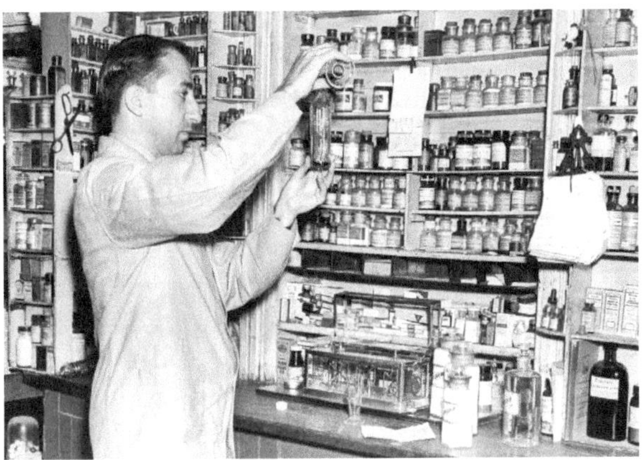

Prior to World War II, many pharmacists compounded their own preparations from oils, tinctures, and other essences from natural sources.

The American Society of Hospital Pharmacists (ASHP) formed during World War II to meet needs for standards and professional support particularly suited to hospitals, which included the need for trained assistants. Recognizing the volume of help required at the war front and in veterans hospitals, the US Department of Defense started formal training programs for medics and pharmacy technicians. After fulfilling the terms of their service, many military pharmacy medics became trained pharmacy technicians in nonmilitary hospital settings back home.

The Scientific Era of Drug Development

Following WWII and in the early 1950s, pharmaceutical manufacturers, such as Eli Lilly, Merck, and Pfizer, expanded laboratory research, leading to many new mass-marketed drugs (such as new antibiotics, hormones, vaccines, and cancer-fighting chemicals) in various dosage formulations. Companies began mass-marketing these laboratory drugs and making them available to corner drug stores.

Pharmacy Education

As drug production moved from the pharmacist's shop to the assembly line, the pharmacist increasingly became more of a retail merchant selling premanufactured products. Consequently, pharmacists had to keep abreast and become much more

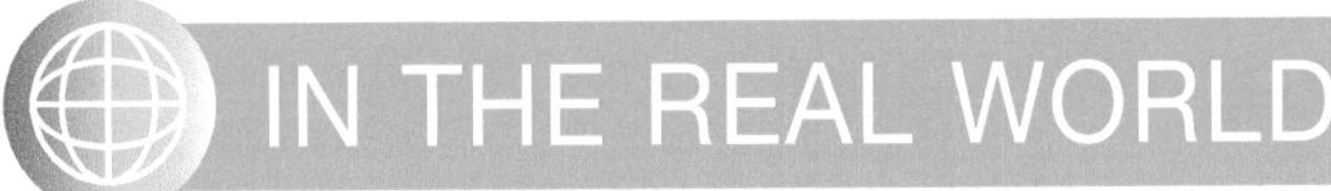

Pharmacy compounding is nearly a lost art. Of all prescriptions written, fewer than 1% are accomplished by hand compounding. The pharmacy personnel who work on compounding generally require specialized training in nonsterile, sterile, and hazardous compounding (see Chapters 10, 12, and 13).

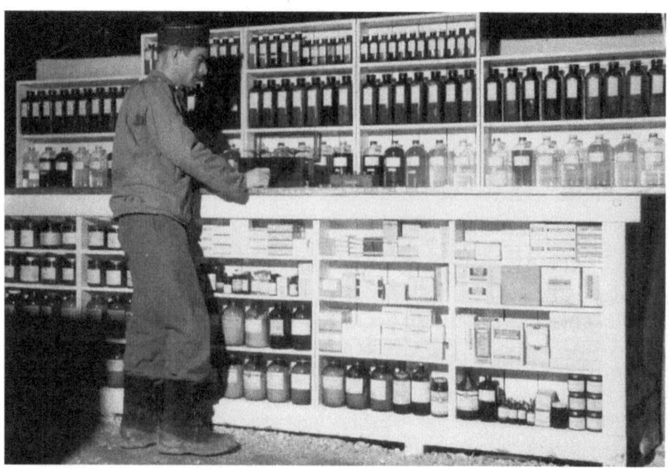

In March 1944, this Pharmacy Officer in Teano, Italy, at the 8th Evacuation Hospital, is filling a soldier's prescription. The US Department of Defense was the first institution to offer formal training for pharmacy technicians.

knowledgeable about new drugs, their uses, side effects, and interactions—the emerging field of **pharmacology**. The necessity of a more formalized higher-education program for pharmacists became clear.

Universities and colleges expanded their curricula and offered four-year degree programs that included prerequisite science courses. In addition to biology, physics, medicinal chemistry, anatomy, and physiology, pharmacists were required to complete courses in both pharmacognosy and pharmacology. Most courses were accompanied by work experience in an on-campus laboratory that often included a simulated pharmacy. Students also gained practical experience by working as interns in community and hospital pharmacies during summers and holidays. Both academic coursework and intern hours were required to take the state licensure examination.

By 1960, a five-year Bachelor of Science Pharmacy degree (which included two years of pre-pharmacy course work and three years of professional studies) was the minimum standard for pharmacist programs in the United States. Additional science courses were developed and added to the pharmacy curriculum, including **pharmaceutics**—the study of how drug dosage formulations are manufactured and released in the body.

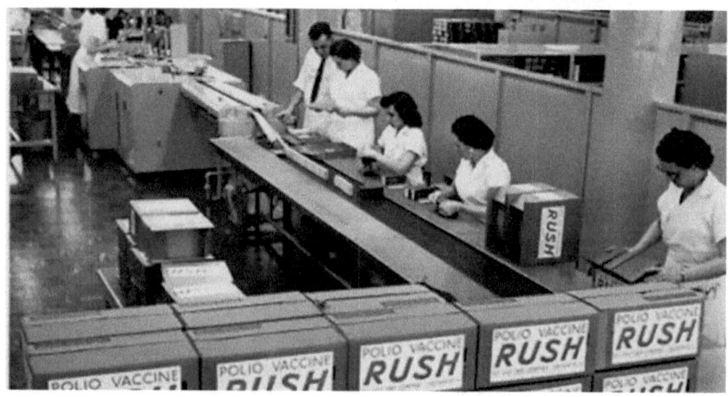

This 1955 image shows workers at the Eli Lilly and Company manufacturing unit carefully packaging and applying labels to the Salk polio vaccine vials, which were rushed to the childhood immunization program in order to stop the polio epidemic (discussed in Chapter 3).

Pharmacy Technician Training

In a complementary way, the ASHP and the US Department of Health and Welfare were pushing for hospitals and junior colleges to begin training pharmacy technicians to continue the supply of educated pharmacy aides. In 1968, the first formal hospital training programs began. ASHP assisted in developing national program guidelines. The military and large university hospital pharmacies were early adopters of the pharmacy technician's role, and these institutions still depend heavily on them today.

The Education-Retail Gap

By the late 1960s, many US pharmacy students had begun to feel that there was a gap between their highly scientific schooling and the everyday realities of a community pharmacist. Until 1969, it was not considered ethical for a pharmacist to label the medication vials with the drug name or discuss the potential side effects of the medication with the patient. The pharmacist had to devote the bulk of their energies to completing routine tasks, running the business, and filling and dispensing drugs, rather than sharing information on drugs and interacting with patients and other healthcare professionals. To meet this educational gap, structured on-the-job

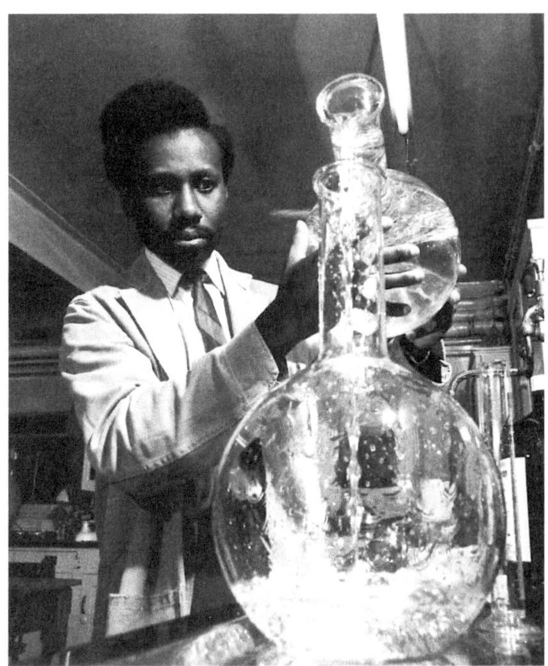

This pharmacy technician is working in the hospital pharmacy in London Hospital, Whitechapel, in 1968. Pharmacy technician training programs were just beginning in US hospitals.

internships gradually became more of a required component of pharmacy programs so that students also learned the job's retail aspects.

As for pharmacy assistants in community settings, they were mostly aides attending to cashiering and stocking; few assistants had educational training and credentials. Trained technicians were generally employed in hospitals.

The Clinical Era of Patient and Technician Education

In 1973, the American Association of Colleges of Pharmacy established a study to consider the contemporary pharmacy mission. The 1975 Millis Commission report, *Pharmacists for the Future*, emphasized the role of pharmacists in sharing knowledge with patients and providers about drug use. The Millis Commission report (named after Dr. John Millis, the study director) led to a new focus on clinical or *patient-oriented pharmacy*. In this new clinical role, the pharmacist advises patients and healthcare providers about the appropriateness and effects of specific drugs.

This new role particularly suited the **managed care** model of healthcare, or **health maintenance organizations (HMOs)**, that were gaining popularity in the 1970s and 1980s. In an HMO insurance plan, all the providers and facilities are under the oversight and salaried employment of the insurance company. The purpose of an HMO is to facilitate preventive care and overall health rather than have patients come in for emergencies; emergency care and hospitalizations are very costly in the short- and long-term, and often represent the worst-case scenario for a patient. HMOs found they could cut costs by developing their own best practice protocols and drug formularies, and utilizing group purchasing of drugs and medical devices.

HMO patient members primarily use the HMO's staff providers, facilities, pharmacies, and drug lists, making it easier for healthcare professionals to share patients and information. In an HMO setting, physicians can work closely with clinically trained pharmacists to consult with patients on wellness counseling, drug therapy for pain and chronic diseases, and other prescribed drug therapies. Along with teaching hospitals, HMOs became the earliest implementers of the clinical care model for pharmacists. Early on, HMO specialty pharmacists were trained to provide services that often included education, ordering of laboratory tests, and adjusting patient dosages.

Cashiering may not be directly involved with healing, but ill patients and distressed family members particularly appreciate kind, understanding customer service as they are in states of worry, illness, or confusion over medications.

Hospital Pharmacy Technician Training

To free up time for hospital pharmacists to serve in this expanded role, formalized in-service training programs for pharmacy technicians were developed that focused on the preparation of medications. Technicians, following ASHP training guidelines, learned to assist in the preparation of sterile **intravenous (IV) solutions**—which are delivered directly as liquid medication in a patient's vein—and fill medication orders without compromising patient safety. This allowed time for the specialty trained pharmacists to make daily hospital rounds with physicians, consult with patients, and monitor prescribed therapies.

Community Pharmacy Technician Training

Along with a push for training pharmacists for an expanded clinical role, there was a push for greater training of community pharmacy technicians. In 1979, the American Association of Pharmacy Technicians formed, and the Massachusetts College of Pharmacy began offering a pharmacy technician training program. In 1981, Michigan became the first state to use an examination to test the qualifications of a pharmacy technician.

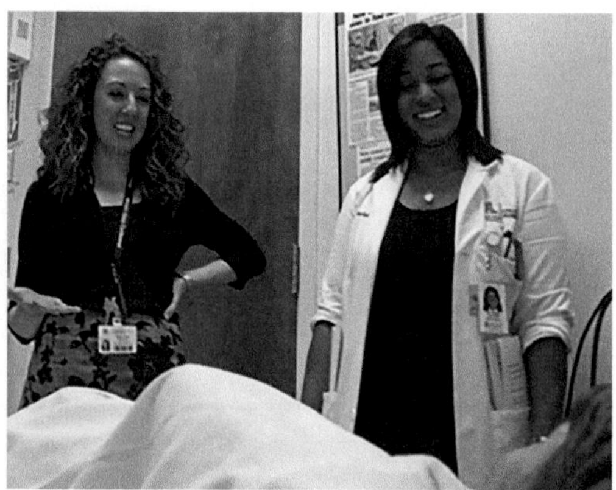

This pharmacist brings a student from the College of Pharmacy at Arizona State University on patient rounds to learn patient care.

The Computer and Pharmaceutical Counseling Era

In the 1980s, computers were moving into pharmacy practice, replacing the typewriters of yesteryear. There was a slow learning curve as both pharmacists and technicians had to be trained on new hardware and software.

Over the last three decades, the software has greatly improved, with new innovations improving safety and productivity. Alongside pharmacy automation came the expansion of generic drugs and drug insurance programs. Prior to this, most drugs were brand name only and paid for in cash. With computerized entry of prescription orders and insurance billing information, the need for computer-educated and pharmacy-trained technicians grew even greater.

In 1990, Drs. Charles Hepler and Linda Strand built upon the Millis Commission report with a new framework for clinical pharmaceutical care; the report further expanded the professional mission to also include responsibility for counseling one-on-one with patients in choosing and using pharmaceuticals to ensure positive outcomes for drug therapy. The mission statements of many pharmacy organizations started to integrate this philosophy.

More colleges of pharmacy adopted the six-year PharmD degree program (two years undergraduate science program and four years professional along with internships). New courses were developed, such as **pharmacokinetics** (individualizing doses of drugs based on absorption, distribution, metabolism, and excretion from the body), **biochemistry** (applying chemistry to biological processes), **therapeutics**, and **pathophysiology**. Therapeutics is the study of applying pharmacology to the treatment of illness and disease states, whereas pathophysiology is the study of diseases and illnesses affecting the normal functions of the body.

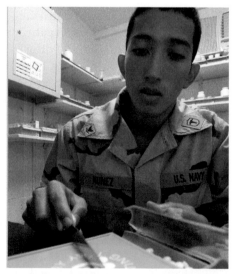

Navy Hospital Corpsman 3rd Class Esteban Nunez Ide, a pharmacy technician, counts out tablets for a naval patient's prescription dosage.

More schools of pharmacy, community colleges, and vocational schools began adding pharmacy technician programs. Illinois joined Massachusetts and Michigan in requiring an examination to become a pharmacy technician, and ASHP organized a national conference on the emerging role of the pharmacy technician in light of the changing role of the pharmacist. In 1989, the first conference for pharmacy technician educators was organized, followed by the formation of the **Pharmacy Technician Educators Council (PTEC)**. PTEC not only offered instructor networking support but increasingly became a forum to develop and share a pharmacy technician curriculum, educational resources, and instructional materials. It continues this networking and support, advocating to increase the credentialing, recognition, and responsibilities of pharmacy technicians and leading the way in best technician practices.

As the pharmacy profession was expanding and evolving into many new areas, such as geriatric and mental health drug therapies, the American Society of Hospital Pharmacists (ASHP) was also broadening its organizational scope. In 1995 it changed its name to the **American Society of Health-System Pharmacists** (still abbreviated ASHP). Since then it has represented the interests of pharmacists and pharmacy technicians for best practice in hospitals, health maintenance organizations, long-term care facilities, home care, and other components of healthcare.

1.3 Medication Therapy Management in the 21st Century

The trends of an aging population and increased dependence on drugs and supplements for healthcare have continued into the new century. The potential for dangerous side effects, overuse, and harmful medication interactions has risen exponentially. Providers and pharmacists recognized they had only partial information about the supplements and drugs (including OTC drugs and alcohol) that patients were using and the drug reactions the patients had in the past.

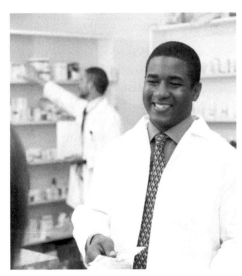

The pharmacist, with the support of the pharmacy technician, works to ensure positive outcomes for drug therapy through careful medication counseling and monitoring when appropriate.

Insufficient patient information was leading to great safety issues as well as overall inefficiencies, waste, and other problems. From this arose the push for electronic health records for shared health information among care providers and more education about drugs and their interactions from the pharmacist. The pharmacist was the ideal professional to act as a counselor and case manager to help patients choose, use, and monitor their drugs in a more holistic manner for the best health outcomes. This is called **medication therapy management (MTM)**.

The growing costs of drugs and adoption of generic drugs and drug formularies by insurance companies (following the lead of HMOs) raised new questions about drug equivalencies and compatibilities. Patients and prescribers didn't know which drugs were covered by insurance and which were not. Pharmacy personnel needed to be a source of this information, which added to the advantage of pharmacists overseeing patient medication therapy management.

MTM includes a review of all medications, supplements, and OTC products used by a patient; this review helps identify and address any potential problems. Other MTM practices include recommending a less costly drug to a physician; identifying potential serious drug-drug interactions, side effects, or adverse reactions; and counseling patients on the importance of wellness activities and adhering to a prescribed drug therapy to better control their diseases. MTM patient-pharmacist interactions and the amount of pharmacist time they require are gradually being recognized and reimbursed by insurance companies because they have been proven to result in better health outcomes and less waste from ineffective or problematic medication use. Pharmacy technicians are assisting in MTM with some technicians even specializing in medical assistant advocacy.

Collaborative Practice Agreements

As the patient care role of the pharmacist advanced, formal relationships between pharmacists and prescribers were created. One such relationship is called a Collaborative Practice Agreement (CPA). **Collaborative Practice Agreements**, or CPAs, are formal agreements where licensed providers (such as physicians) make a diagnosis, supervise patient care, and refer patients to a pharmacist for protocol-based care.

Under CPAs, pharmacists can independently provide specific patient care functions after a diagnosis and referral is made by a prescriber. CPA services may include patient assessment as well as selecting, initiating, administering, monitoring, and adjusting medication regimens. Almost all states now allow some form of CPA. The Centers for Disease Control and Prevention (CDC) encourages the use of CPAs as studies show pharmacist involvement in the healthcare team improves patient care. These expanded services would be difficult for a pharmacist to perform without the support of pharmacy technicians. Technicians address the ongoing needs of the pharmacy, including scheduling of patient appointments, obtaining medication histories, reconciling medications, and prior authorization assistance.

Note that CPAs are not required for pharmacists to provide many patient care services, such as performing medication reviews, counseling patients, providing disease screening, and referring to other providers.

Pharmacy Practice Model Initiative

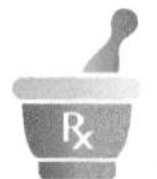

Practice Tip

Alert, focused, and willing technicians help pharmacists stay focused on patient care with fewer distractions, providing them the time they need to answer patients' questions sufficiently and offer them counsel.

In order for pharmacists to provide expanded patient care services, they require support and assistance to fulfill other pharmacy-related responsibilities. Pharmacists need the help of trained pharmacy technicians. Hence a related movement to improve patient outcomes was developed by the ASHP called the **Pharmacy Practice Model Initiative (PPMI)**. The PPMI required the education and certification of pharmacy technicians and encouraged implementation of pharmacy practices that will not only improve the quality of healthcare, but also lower its costs through enhanced roles, education, and responsibilities for both pharmacists and pharmacy technicians. The overall mission was to further empower the pharmacy team with better tools "to take responsibility for patient outcomes." The ASHP has expanded the scope of its offerings for reform and assessment, calling it the **Practice Advancement Initiative (PAI)**.

Advanced Technician Practice

An essential part of the PAI is the utilization of emerging advanced technician positions, including technician supervisor, Tech Check Tech, informatics or business administration specialist, and insurance or medical assistance advocacy specialist.

A more complete listing of advanced positions can be found at https://PharmPractice7e.ParadigmEducation.com/AdvRoles. Pharmacy technicians may also find expanded roles in documenting clinical monitoring statistics, inventory control and management, or quality and safety monitoring.

Pharmacy technicians may also get specialized training and/or certificates in IV infusions, nonsterile and sterile compounding and aseptic technique, chemotherapy and hazardous compounding, pediatric medication preparation, and prenatal or parenteral nutrition. These advanced technician roles are being implemented in various institutional (especially hospital) and community settings across the country, varying from state to state. For a glimpse at this future, see the Advanced Technician case studies at https://PharmPractice7e.ParadigmEducation.com/PAI. More information on career options is provided in the final chapter.

1.4 Contemporary Pharmacy Settings

As already described, there are both community pharmacies and institutional pharmacies. An overview of some of the common settings within these categories can provide you with a sense of the career scope for where technicians work.

Community Pharmacies

Community pharmacies, which are also called *retail pharmacies,* are the "drug stores" that include not only pharmaceuticals but supplements, durable medical equipment (such as crutches, splints, slings, syringes), cosmetics, stationery, gifts, and other miscellaneous purchases.

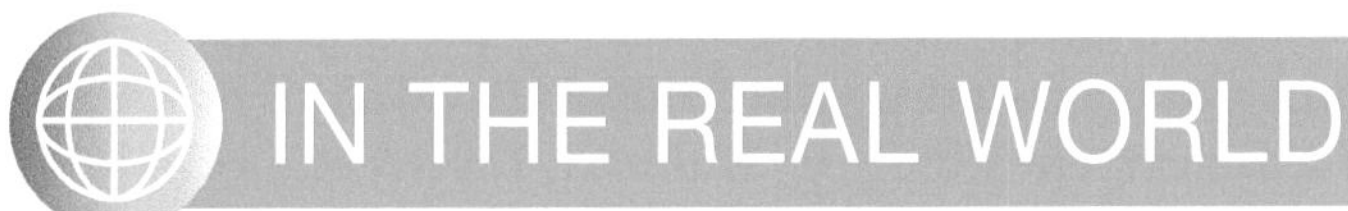

In the 1980s, the Goodrich Pharmacies in Central Minnesota established an agreement with local physicians to offer drug substitution counseling. Since then, the practice of Goodrich pharmacists counseling patients has grown dramatically. Through collaborative practice agreements (CPAs), Goodrich offers expanded patient care services to area patients and employees of the University of Minnesota, among others. To provide expanded patient care services, Goodrich depends on educated pharmacy technicians. Goodrich hosts internships and externships for pharmacist and technician students from the local university and technical and community colleges.

Goodrich Pharmacy stores also offer simple health services to general customers, such as vaccines; chronic disease management and cessation of smoking classes; low-cost screenings for high cholesterol, high blood pressure, asthma, and diabetes; and health education classes. Their customer MTM services include an information-gathering consultation, creation of a personalized care plan with treatment and goals, and continuous follow-up on patient progress. They remind patients, "The most expensive medication is the one you take incorrectly."

In community pharmacy settings, pharmacy technicians tend to have more direct patient contact than in other settings. Community pharmacies can also offer off-site pharmaceutical delivery services to assisted living and nursing homes, which provide institutional services predominantly to older adults or disabled residents who can no longer provide care for themselves at home. These facilities may also be tailored for those with debilitating diseases or conditions, such as Alzheimer's disease, stroke, or amyotrophic lateral sclerosis. Community pharmacies generally come in five main kinds: independent, chain, institutional, HMOs, and mail-order.

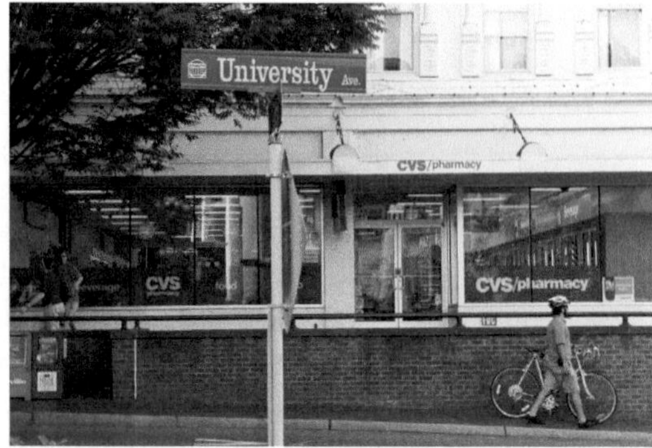

Many metropolitan areas have one or more community pharmacies that provide pharmacy services 24 hours a day, seven days a week.

Independent Pharmacies

These drug stores are usually owned and operated by a pharmacist or group of pharmacists. The pharmacist-owner makes the decisions about the practice, the range of retail products offered, standards, and technician responsibilities. They also decide to what degree they want to offer expanded patient care services. Some independent pharmacies may decide to become "compounding only" pharmacies of products individualized or not readily available commercially.

Chain Pharmacies

These retail operations consist of four or more stores run by a regional or national corporation that makes the decisions about customer initiatives and employee standards. They have the stand-alone corner drug store model (e.g., Walgreens, CVS, Rite Aid) or are a division of a department store (e.g., Walmart, Target) or grocery store (e.g., Kroger, Publix). These stores are usually in metropolitan areas and have a great deal of automation. Some have established walk-in clinics staffed by prescribers (such as nurse practitioners) for basic health assessments, specialty clinics for HIV/AIDS, or educational services on chronic illnesses or the cessation of smoking.

Institutional Community Pharmacies

More and more healthcare organizations, such as hospitals, clinics, and universities, are opening their own community pharmacies since patients like to have a one-stop experience. Operation and employment decisions do not come from the specific pharmacists that work there, but from the healthcare organization that runs them.

Health Maintenance Organizations (HMO)

In pharmacies run by an HMO, there are no insurance claims to fill out. Patient-related costs are paid as part of the network with its established fees. Prescribers, nurses, and pharmacists all have direct access to electronic medical records for each patient. Communications on best care plans are shared with the healthcare team. There is a formulary of approved drugs to help control costs and inventory.

Mail-Order or Warehouse Production Pharmacies

These are highly automated and are often run by large retail chain pharmacies, HMOs (for refills), insurance companies, and the Veterans Administration (VA). Technicians have contact with patients over the phone and through online interactions. They check prescriptions for accuracy and completeness, and process them for pharmacy approval and mailing. The technicians utilize sophisticated automation in an assembly-line environment. This growing pharmacy production and warehousing approach often has better pay and benefits for some technician positions because of the high volume. The technicians may also process insurance claims (if the pharmacy is not run by an HMO) and handle stocking and inventory duties. Mail-order pharmacies often dispense medications in 90-day increments.

Institutional Pharmacies

Institutional pharmacies are pharmacies organized under a corporate structure that follow specific rules and regulations for accreditation. They service healthcare facilities, such as the following: hospitals, long-term care facilities, home healthcare pharmacies, and specialty compounding pharmacies.

Hospital Pharmacies

Approximately one-fourth of all technicians work in a **hospital pharmacy** to supply patients with their hospital-prescribed medications. Together, the pharmacists and technicians prepare 24- to 72-hour drug dosage supplies and oversee an extensive floor stock inventory. Many work in a completely sterile cleanroom setting to prepare IV solutions. HMOs may have their own hospitals and have institutional pharmacies within them. University hospitals may also have pharmacy research laboratories.

Long-Term Care Facilities

Pharm Fact

Some early medicines had alcohol or "spirits" in them. Now some states have pharmacies that also sell alcohol.

In assisted living facilities (ALF) and skilled nursing facilities (SNF), both medical and residential care are provided, offering round-the-clock care, often entailing sterile IV solutions. Facilities that treat mental health patients suffering from acute or chronic psychiatric disorders or patients with traumatic brain or spinal injuries requiring in-patient rehabilitation also sometimes have on-site pharmacies.

Home Healthcare Pharmacy

The institutional delivery of medical, nursing, and pharmacy services and supplies to patients in their homes is **home healthcare**. Also part of this institutional pharmacy service are deliveries to home **hospice care** and **palliative care**—which are focused on supplying pain relief and quality of life for those who have terminal conditions (hospice) or serious, ongoing painful debilitating illnesses (palliative). Treating patients in their own homes is less costly than in a hospital, generally more pleasant, and less uprooting for the patient.

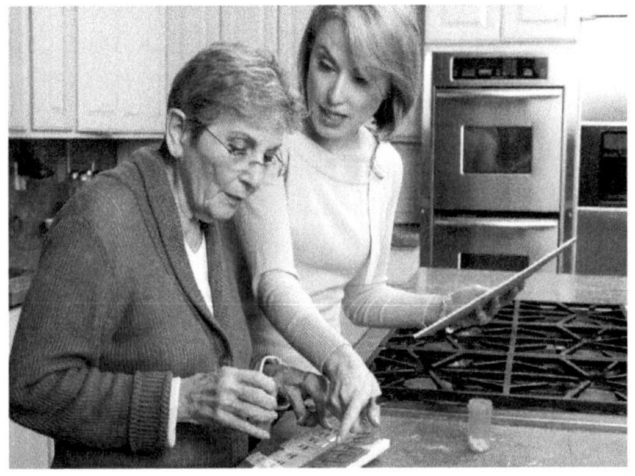

Pharmacists and pharmacy technicians work with nurses to provide medications for nursing homes, hospice settings, and homebound patients.

The pharmacist and pharmacy technicians work to provide IV infusions and oral medications, and they often need to be available for emergencies at odd hours. The medications are prepared and then picked up by or delivered to the attending nurse, who then dispenses the medications, educates the patient or patient's caregiver on use, and monitors the patient's progress. If the home healthcare system does not have its own pharmacy, it often contracts with specialty compounding or community pharmacies for services.

Specialty Compounding Pharmacies

Sterile compounding pharmacies specialize in sterile compounds such as IV solutions, parenteral nutrition, and injections. **Hazardous compounding pharmacies** utilize toxic substances that are chemical, biological, or radioactive (**nuclear pharmacies**). There are more than 100 diagnostic and therapeutic uses for such compounds, including cancer treatments. These pharmacies are typically located off-site and managed by one of several specialty pharmaceutical manufacturers. Because of the unique equipment and inherent hazards, these pharmacies are staffed by pharmacists and technicians with advanced training.

FIGURE 1.1 Practice Settings for Today's Pharmacist

Technicians work where pharmacists work. Trends suggest a gradual increase in chain and mail-order pharmacies at the expense of independent community pharmacies. Long-term care and home healthcare pharmacies are expected to increase along with the aging US population.

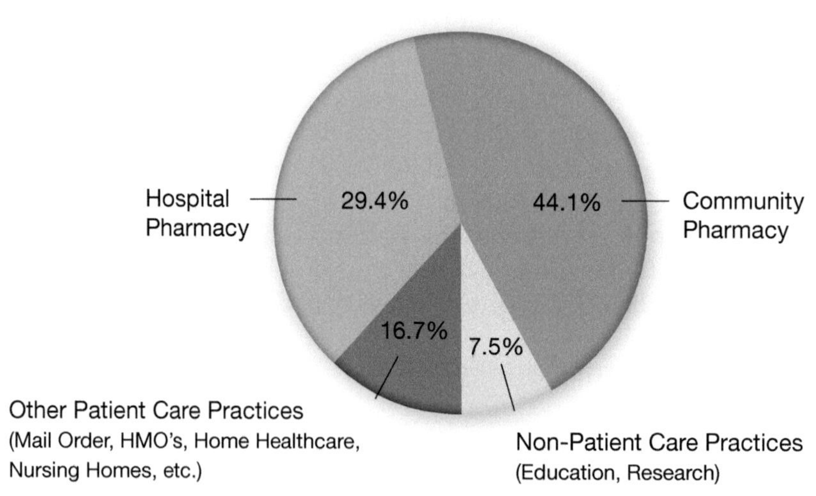

Source: 2014 National Pharmacist Workforce Study by the American Association of Colleges of Pharmacy

1.5 The Roles and Responsibilities of a Pharmacist

The role of pharmacists and technicians has always been to safeguard and enhance the health of the patients whom they serve. What has changed is the complexity of this task. Pharmacists assume more patient care responsibilities and subsequently more liability. Today, with the vast number of medications on the market, pharmacists need to be vigilant in detecting an error in the prescribing and dosing of a medication, a problematic combination of drugs, a dangerous use of a drug (such as the use of a cancer-causing drug or a drug that can cause birth defects if used by a pregnant patient), and any interactions of a medication with food, drink, or other medications. A pharmacist must also be watchful for any adverse reaction that is reported by patients.

Technicians aid pharmacists in this vigilance and must feel empowered to ask questions when they see something out of the ordinary or amiss.

Although pharmacists still supervise the dispensing and compounding of medications, they are increasingly spending more time doing the following tasks:

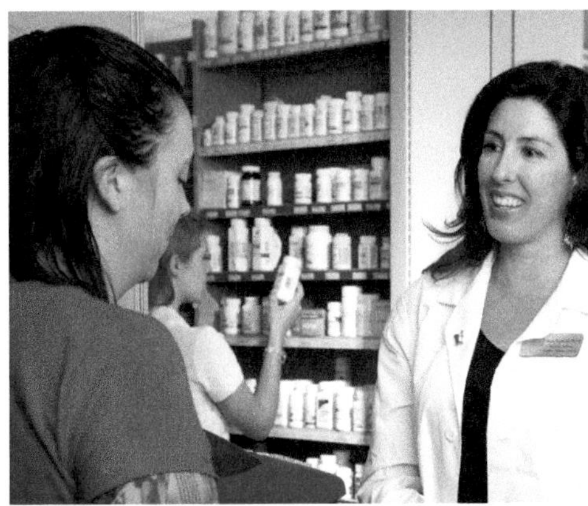
When dispensing a prescription medication, the pharmacist plays an important role in educating a patient about side effects, potential interactions with other medications, and dosing schedules.

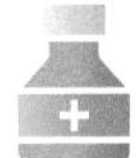
Pharm Fact

Since 2000, there has been an increase of over 60% in new pharmacy schools in the United States, which have opened to address expected pharmacist shortages.

- assessing information on a patient's medical, medication, and allergy history
- checking age-appropriate dosing for medication and potential duplications of therapy
- counseling patients on possible side effects and adverse reactions
- screening patients for chronic diseases such as hypertension and diabetes
- ensuring positive outcomes to therapy for hypertension, diabetes, asthma, and high cholesterol
- counseling patients on computer alerts for interactions with prescription and OTC drugs and dietary supplements
- screening and treating patients with illnesses that can be safely self-medicated
- assisting and supporting motivated patients to quit smoking
- providing consumers with recommendations on OTC drugs, vitamins, minerals, herbs, and dietary supplements
- providing up-to-date and accurate information to all prescribers as a drug therapy expert
- dispensing information on proper use of medical supplies and equipment, especially for diabetics
- educating on and monitoring the safe use of controlled substances
- vaccinating high-risk patients for preventable diseases such as influenza, pneumonia, and shingles

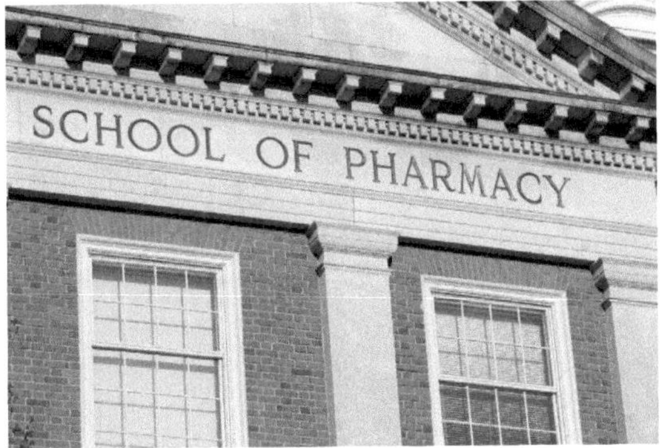

All US schools of pharmacy now offer the equivalent of at least four years of professional education and experiential training, in addition to at least two years of undergraduate science courses.

Educational Requirements of a Pharmacist

Pharmacy personnel shortages are projected due to both an aging population that requires more prescriptions and the pharmacist's expanded counseling role. Some pharmacy technicians go on to pursue pharmacy degrees, having gained valuable experience that helped shape and validate their career goals.

For a pharmacy degree, all US pharmacy colleges/schools offer a doctorate of pharmacy or PharmD. In Canada, pharmacy students graduate with a Bachelor of Science degree in Pharmacy or a Doctorate of Pharmacy, depending on their program.

IN THE REAL WORLD

The Centers for Medicare & Medicaid Services conservatively estimates that the cost of healthcare in the United States is $3.5 trillion per year, or approximately 18% of the GDP. Healthcare costs associated with an aging population and technological innovations are projected to increase, becoming 20% of the GDP within the next decade.

According to IMS Health (a healthcare information service), the segment of funds invested in prescriptions in the United States in 2017 was $450 billion; the cost and number of prescriptions continue to rise. It is estimated that 4.78 billion prescriptions will be dispensed in the United States in the year 2021. In Canada, with a far smaller population, currently 500 million prescriptions are being filled annually, with their number also increasing.

Many pharmacy schools in the United States prefer that students enter with a bachelor's degree, but it is not a requirement. Pre-pharmacy undergraduate coursework typically consists of anatomy, biology, calculus, chemistry, microbiology, physics, and statistics. A pharmacy applicant typically completes an online application and takes the Pharmacy College Admission Test (PCAT).

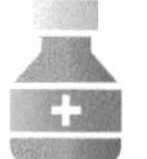

Pharm Fact

The typical successful pharmacy school applicant in the United States has a prior degree (typically in biology or chemistry), a grade point average (GPA) of 3.5–4.0, good scores on the PCAT (>400), experience in pharmacy and community service projects, excellent communication skills, and self-motivation.

Several colleges allow incoming students to apply to zero- to six-year pharmacy programs. Zero-to-six-year pharmacy programs admit students without prerequisites or PCAT results. A student enrolls in the pharmacy program and completes both their prerequisite courses and pharmacy school courses within 6 years. Acceptance into a pharmacy school has become intensely competitive. Many schools require an on-site personal interview with both faculty members and current pharmacy students.

Once accepted at a university, pharmacy students generally find the coursework extremely challenging. Basic and clinical science courses are combined with practice or internship time in community and hospital pharmacies interspersed at different times throughout the curriculum. The last year is spent working at various practice sites as a healthcare team member learning patient care skills. At graduation, it is traditional for all graduates to recite the Oath of a Pharmacist, affirming "I promise to devote myself to a lifetime of service to others through the profession of pharmacy" and vowing to relieve suffering and improve the welfare of others, among other honorable promises.

The pharmacist is ultimately responsible and liable for the pharmacy technician's work. All prescriptions and medication orders must be checked by the pharmacist.

Licensing of a Pharmacist

A licensed pharmacist must complete a designated number of intern hours (within and/or outside the academic program) and then pass a national standardized examination, including a state-specific law examination (laws differ between states). Though licensure is state-specific, a process for reciprocation (recognizing other state licenses) exists through the National Association of Boards of Pharmacy (NABP), permitting practice in different states. Pharmacists who work in a government facility, such as a VA hospital, are required to have a valid license in only one state.

A pharmacy license must be renewed annually or biannually, depending on the state. Most states require the completion of a designated number of continuing education credits (commonly 30 units every two years) for relicensure.

1.6 The Roles and Responsibilities of a Pharmacy Technician

A pharmacy technician is an individual who has been trained to work under the oversight of a pharmacist to fullfill pharmacy activities that do not require the direct judgment of a pharmacist—for example, the physical assembling or compounding of a prescription. A central defining feature of the pharmacy technician's job is accountability to the pharmacist. Technicians are not legally allowed to counsel a patient on medications or fill a prescription alone. Medication and dispensing errors—such as entering incorrect data from the prescription or selecting the wrong drug, dose, or dosage form—can cause serious reactions, and even death, if not detected. The pharmacist, then, takes final responsibility (and liability) for the pharmacy technician's actions. However, a certified technician assists the pharmacist in checking and rechecking prescriptions to ensure accuracy and safety.

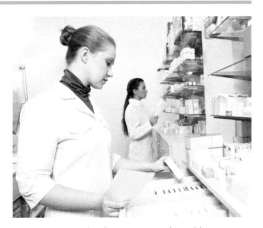

In recent years, both *US News and World Report* and *Forbes* have named pharmacy technicians in the "best jobs" categories for people trying to break into healthcare positions. They considered growing market demand, initial entry and upward mobility, median annual earnings, and opportunities to pursue part-time work in order to continue pursuing higher education.

The responsibilities of technicians vary according to the needs of the pharmacy workplace. The duties a technician may perform depend on education, state laws, and the workplace but may include the following:

- input prescriptions in the computer system; check accuracy
- prepare prescribed prescriptions—retrieve, weigh, pour, count, measure, and at times mix, count tablets, and label bottles
- deliver medications to patients in some settings
- engage with customers in answering phones, handling patient questions (not prescription-related), and referring patients to the pharmacist for medication counseling
- contact physicians' offices with refill requests and assist in safety/quality checks
- act as a cashier, stock shelves, and handle inventory (sometimes handling procurement)
- assemble patient medication profiles and histories; check them for accuracy

IN THE REAL WORLD

With expanding pharmacy patient care services and the increasing volume and complexity of pharmaceuticals, a certified technician graduating from an accredited program is an essential member of the healthcare team and an invaluable assistant in helping pharmacists provide medication services to patients and providers in all practice settings. The US Bureau of Labor Statistics forecasts a positive demand for pharmacy technician positions with 12% growth through 2026.

- prepare online insurance claim forms, reconcile billing with copays and other insurance requirements
- run automated equipment for high-volume drug processing and packaging
- prepare nonsterile, sterile, and hazardous medications
- in the hospital, work with the nursing staff, fill and deliver medication orders, repackage medications, and restock automated medication dispensing machines in the hospital floor units
- prepare medication supplies in special packaging

A Pharmacy Technician's Education

Since 1983, ASHP has been responsible for the accreditation of pharmacy technician training programs. All the Department of Defense (DOD) military training programs for pharmacy technicians (or specialists) in all branches of the service are now ASHP-accredited. Pharmacy technician roles in the DOD are standardized and not subject to state pharmacy laws and regulations. There are currently over 250 accredited pharmacy technician programs in the United States, based mostly in vocational, technical, and community colleges. Approximately 12,000 students of accredited programs graduate each year, similar to the number of annual pharmacist graduates. As there is for pharmacists, there is also an oath of service for technicians. More information on an oath of service ethics and the professionalism of pharmacy technicians is in Chapter 15.

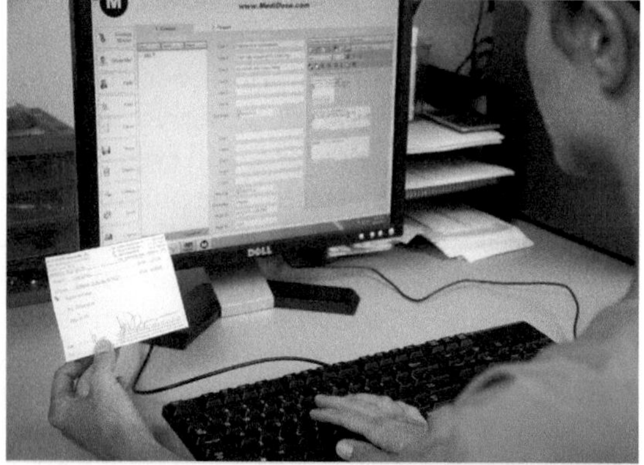
An important function of the pharmacy technician is to accurately input prescribed medications into the computer.

The ASHP-accredited coursework covers various topics:

- introduction to practice
- medical terminology
- pharmacology
- inpatient and outpatient dispensing procedures and record keeping

- pharmacy calculations
- sterile and nonsterile compounding techniques and aseptic techniques
- pharmacy laws and regulations
- communications, professionalism, and customer service

To learn more about the ASHP Model Curriculum, visit: https://PharmPractice7e.ParadigmEducation.com/ASHPModelCurriculum.

FIGURE 1.2
State Requirements for Pharmacy Technicians

As states make regulations for certification and licensing, most are requiring Pharmacy Technician Certification Board (PTCB) certification. A growing number, though, are allowing that of "another approved certifying agency," which generally means the Exam for the Certification of Pharmacy Technicians (ExCPT). In a few states, such as Michigan, passing the modules and exams from a chain pharmacy store-approved program (such as from Walgreens, CVS, Meijer, Rite Aid, Kroger, Omnicare, and a few others), will suffice for a license. These certifications, however, may not be sufficient for hospital practice.

CPhT Map and Technician Regulatory Snapshot

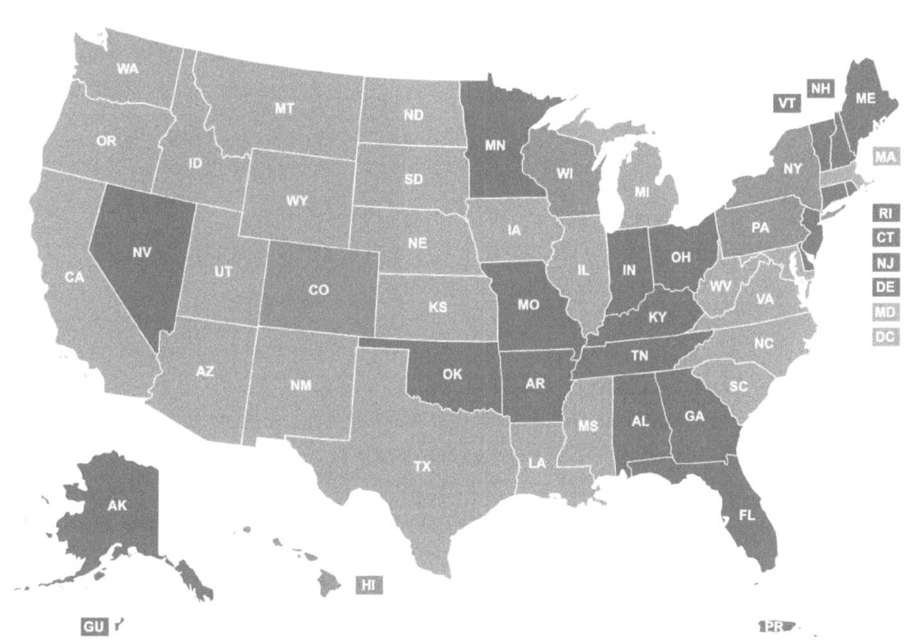

Legend

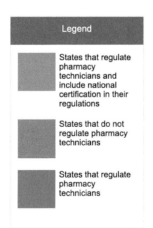

- States that regulate pharmacy technicians and include national certification in their regulations
- States that do not regulate pharmacy technicians
- States that regulate pharmacy technicians

PTCB's National Certification Program

Figures are current as of December 31, 2017.

Since 1995, the Pharmacy Technician Certification Board has granted 648,710 certifications.

This map represents the 282,155* PTCB Certified Pharmacy Technicians (CPhTs) who were active at the end of December 2017. All 50 states and DC accept PTCB Certification. Forty-five states and DC regulate pharmacy technicians; 24 states and DC include national certification in their regulations.

*Total also includes active CPhTs in Canada and the Virgin Islands.

Credentialing of Pharmacy Technicians

According to a survey from the National Association of Boards of Pharmacy (NABP), the term *pharmacy technician* is now used in laws and regulations in 47 states and is also recognized in the provinces of Canada. Being a pharmacy technician today does not simply mean having a job in a pharmacy; rather, it is a chosen career path in which the technician is a recognized paraprofessional. Key to attaining that recognition is gaining the state-required credentials. (See Figure 1.2.)

A **credential** is simply a documented piece of evidence of one's qualifications. Credentials for a pharmacy technician may include **licensure, registration**, and/or **certification**. However, the specific credential requirements to practice vary widely from state to state. The requirements for practice are set up by each state board of pharmacy.

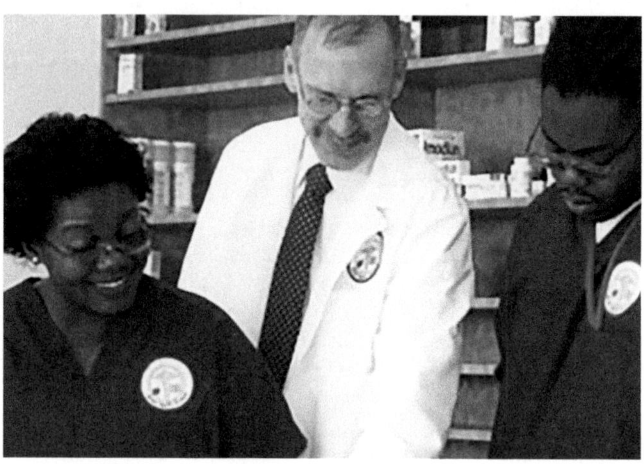

The combination of classroom instruction, online learning, hands-on training, and independent study should help you pass the certification examination to earn your CPhT credential.

Since 2014, the **Pharmacy Technician Accreditation Commission (PTAC)**—a collaboration between the ASHP and the American Council on Pharmaceutical Education (ACPE)—was formed to review and accredit all future pharmacy technician education and training programs. This accrediting body utilizes the ASHP accreditation standards that went into effect in 2014 and follow the ASHP Model Curriculum. The content of this book has been designed to fit those standards and cover the essential topics in the field.

There are also numerous nonaccredited pharmacy technician training programs that vary in content, duration, and rigor. Nonaccredited pharmacy technician programs are often suited to fit the state's requirements and local workplace and economic realities. Credentials for program graduates may include a certificate of completion or an associate degree. Professional pharmacy organizations, such as the ASHP, have long advocated for the development of uniform educational standards that follow a model curriculum to establish consistency among graduates. Consistency can build trust and encourage employers to offer greater responsibility and pay.

Canada has more consistency in technician training programs than the United States. The Pharmacy Examining Board of Canada sets the standards for all registered pharmacy technicians. The student must enroll in a program accredited by the Canadian Council for Accreditation of Pharmacy Programs (CCAPP). The student must also complete a structured field training program prior to being allowed to take an examination.

State Registration

In the majority of states, pharmacy technicians are required to be "registered," or listed on the state's official list of pharmacy technicians. Registration generally means that an individual must sign up with a state agency, such as the state board of

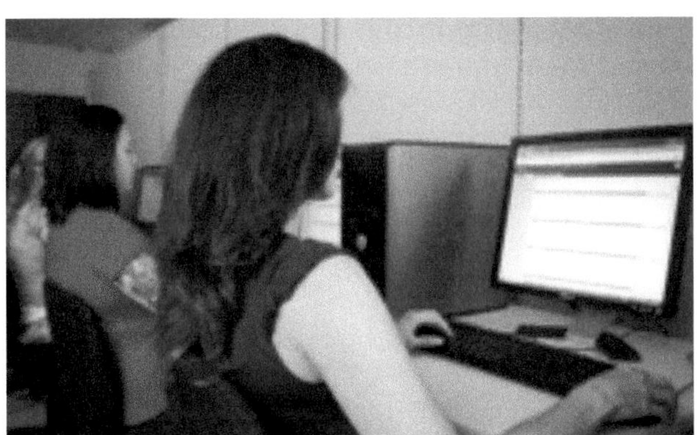

Certification examinations are taken online and are immediately scored. More and more states are requiring that technicians pass the examination to practice.

pharmacy, before starting to practice in any licensed pharmacy. Pharmacy technicians who are not registered, or have allowed their registration to lapse, cannot legally work in a pharmacy in these states.

A majority of states also have training requirements, but are not yet standardized across the states. One of the main reasons for registration is to report and keep track of any serious disciplinary action (stealing drugs or money, etc.) before the disciplined technician applies for another pharmacy technician job or is hired at another pharmacy within or outside the state. If a technician changes employment within the state, they must notify the board of pharmacy. Registration cannot be reciprocated or transferred to another state. States have varying continuing education requirements for annual reregistration.

National Certification and Certification Exams

Some states require certification. Certification is the process by which a nongovernmental association grants recognition to an individual who has met certain predetermined qualifications specified by that profession. For pharmacy technicians, this requires passing an examination—either the **Pharmacy Technician Certification Board (PTCB)** Exam or the **Exam for the Certification of Pharmacy Technicians (ExCPT)**—and being awarded the title of **Certified Pharmacy Technician (CPhT)**. Certification is like an academic degree and is generally valid and transferable to all states. If a CPhT moves to another state to practice, the CPhT credential would be valid, but the CPhT would be responsible for state registration and knowing and following the laws and continuing education requirements of the new state.

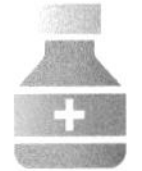

Pharm Fact

There are approximately 300,000 active CPhTs in practice in the United States, Canada, and the Virgin Islands.

Pharmacy Technician Certification Exam (PTCE)

The most popular and recognized national certification is the **Pharmacy Technician Certification Exam (PTCE)**, sponsored by the PTCB. The examination grew out of an effort by two states (Michigan and Illinois), the ASHP, and the American Pharmacy Association to develop technician standards. The board developed the PTCE based on task analyses of the actual work of pharmacy technicians in both the retail and hospital pharmacy settings. In 2001, the National Association of Boards of Pharmacy joined this effort to offer a certification program for pharmacy technicians.

The PTCE for pharmacy technician certification is recognized in all 50 states and the District of Columbia. Since 1995, the PTCB has granted nearly 650,000 certifications. PTCB **recertification** requires proof of completion of continuing education (20 hours over two years), especially in the areas of patient safety and pharmacy laws.

The Exam for Certification of Pharmacy Technicians (ExCPT)

An alternative test evolved out of the efforts of the National Community Pharmacists Association, National Association of Chain Drug Stores, and the **National Healthcareer Association (NHA)**. The ExCPT is offered through the NHA. Although the examination is similar in content to the PTCE, it has more focus on community pharmacies and is not yet recognized in all states.

Clearly, there is a need for all states to have more consistency in technician training and examination requirements. The National Association of Boards of Pharmacy is working toward this goal in its Model State Pharmacy Act and Model Rules initiative for all states. To become PTCB-certified after 2020, technicians will have to graduate from an ASHP/ACPE-accredited program and successfully pass the PTCE. This is not too dissimilar from the requirements for pharmacist licensure, just at a different level.

State License

If a license (or in most cases, registration) is required for a pharmacy technician to practice in a state, the state board may require a national examination and certification *plus* passing an examination on state-specific pharmacy laws, graduating from an accredited program, and/or having experience. The state may also accept workplace training and registration in an official state registry. The state board of pharmacy should be consulted for specific state requirements.

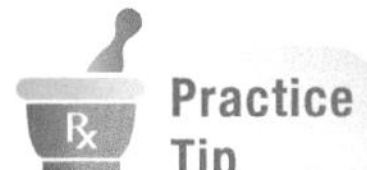

Practice Tip

Check your state's pharmacy technician requirements at the state website, or if your program has access to the latest edition, check the *Survey of Pharmacy Law.*

The state board also makes the laws on the workload distribution and outlines the allowable ratio of pharmacists to technicians and the responsibilities of the technicians. For example, in South Carolina, a certified pharmacy technician is allowed to take down notes about a new prescription or refill a prescription over the phone and confirm it with the pharmacist; in most other states that must be done by the pharmacist. Many states stipulate a maximum ratio of technicians (including pharmacy interns) to pharmacists, which varies from 2:1 to 6:1. The ratio may be dependent on the number of certified pharmacy technicians employed at a site. Some states may use a higher technician-to-pharmacist ratio if at least one technician is certified.

Workplace Credential Requirements

Community pharmacies increasingly expect their technicians to be certified by taking one of the technician certification examinations. Certification may be a requirement for initial employment (especially in large hospitals) or strongly encouraged within the first year of employment. The cost of taking the certification examination is commonly reimbursed by employers. There are often strong financial reasons for becoming certified. Hospital pharmacies require certification and will often expect prior experience or advanced training, especially if the technician will be working with sterile IV products and chemotherapy.

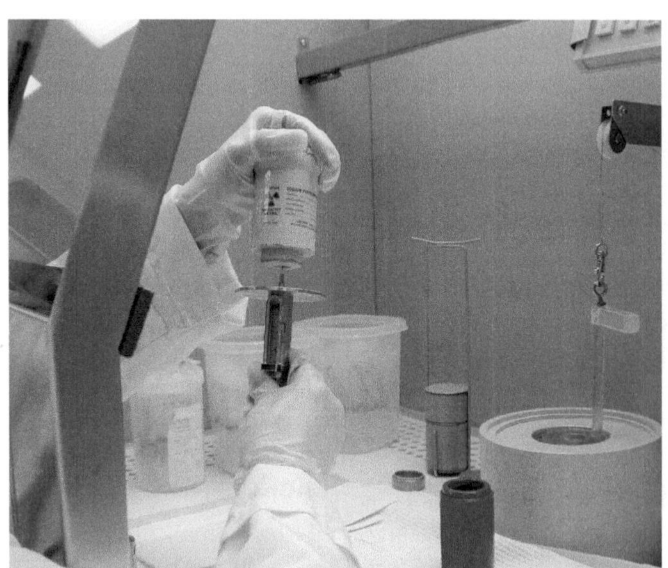

A pharmacy technician with a specialized certification in nuclear pharmacy prepares a sterile, radioactive medication using special equipment and protective shields.

To stay updated or certified, continuing education credits are required; topics may include managed healthcare, therapeutic issues, inventory control, patient interactions, pharmacy law, interpersonal skills, and drug distribution. Visit https://PharmPractice7e.ParadigmEducation.com/ASHP.

In specialized areas of practice—such as nonsterile compounding, sterile compounding, chemotherapy, or nuclear pharmacy—the pharmacy technician generally must have additional training. There will be more discussion on this throughout various chapters.

1.7 Professional Outlook for Pharmacy Technicians

Job roles, advancement opportunities, and pay scales vary considerably, depending on whether the position is in a chain pharmacy versus an independent pharmacy, a small hospital versus a larger university hospital or other institutional practice setting, such as a mail-order warehouse, HMO pharmacy, or home healthcare setting.

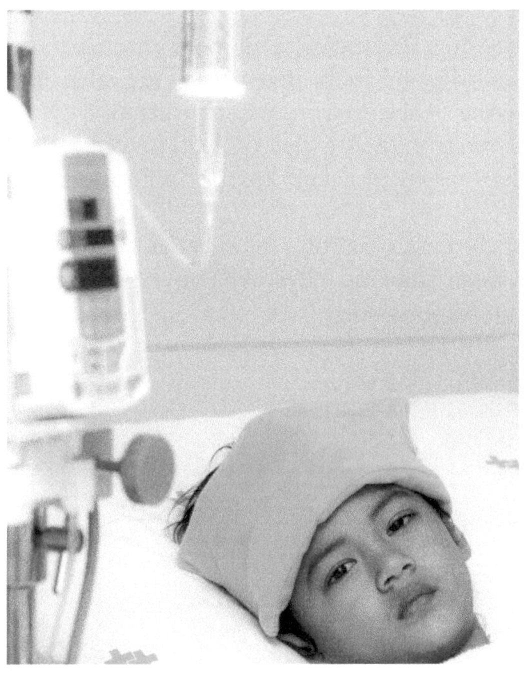

This child is recovering in a pediatric intensive care unit, assisted by IV fluid therapy prepared by a technician and approved by a pharmacist. Specialty training and certificates can be attained in IV infusion and in pediatric and prenatal medication preparations.

Job Realities for a Pharmacy Technician

As states vary in their credentialing requirements, they also vary in their pay scales; pharmacy technicians should check pay scales in their areas. For example, California has traditionally had one of the higher pay scales among US states.

For a full-time pharmacy technician, the annual salary range is approximately $20,000 to $53,000 per year, depending on education, experience, and the state's average cost of living. Working for the federal government in VA hospitals and other facilities is one of the higher paying options, as are hospitals. Many pharmacists and technicians feel that the salary and benefits for technicians in many work settings are currently too low. It is hoped that, in the future, graduates from an accredited pharmacy training program (coupled with a nationally recognized and integrated certification) can expect an improved salary and benefit package with a lower turnover in the profession. As noted, some technicians are moving into advanced technician roles; in some areas, technicians can earn specialty certifications that can increase their pay and responsibilities. Technician roles will be discussed in more detail in Chapter 16.

Your Professional Path

As you have seen, the role of a pharmacy technician is a varied one, with increasing options in the workplace setting and different specialties. After practicing for a number of years in one area, you may choose to branch off into another area within the field. Hospital or institutional settings often offer the greatest range of opportunities. Many educators and students are seeking to "stack" their certifications in healthcare expertise, gaining certifications in, for example, healthcare coding, phlebotomy, and Basic Life Support (BLS, formerly CPR) to make themselves more marketable and able to expand their responsibilities and pay range. Some pharmacies already require BLS certification.

You may also consider pursuing a related area or higher level of professional education. You can use your experience as a pharmacy technician as a first step to becoming a licensed or registered nurse, medical assistant or phlebotomist, retail or office manager, dental hygienist or dentist, pharmacist, or even a physician. Through this course, you may want to ask yourself:

1. What are my short-term goals for being a pharmacy technician?
2. What are my long-term goals?
3. What aspects do I like about the field?
4. What strengths can I offer?

Working through your school, you will want to seek out externships, which are short workplace or job shadowing experiences, or student internships. ASHP requires technicians to have experiences in both community and institutional settings, so that you can have better knowledge of the field.

Whatever the path, you are a key player on a healthcare team in all pharmacy settings. Your work, upon which pharmacists depend, helps determine the health and welfare of your patients. The executive director of the Pharmacy Certification Technician Board, USAF Retired Colonel Everett B. McAllister, MPA, RPh, told *Pharmacy Times* in 2015, "In many ways, pharmacy technicians are the backbone of the pharmacy operation."

He commented on the importance of the emerging roles for experienced technicians to support a successful pharmacy team and advised, "Everyone on the team is here to take care of patients: that's our main responsibility."

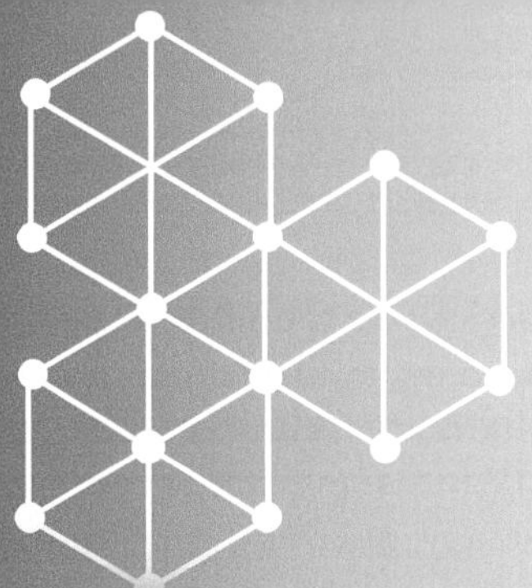

Review and Assessment

CHAPTER SUMMARY

- Pharmacy technicians are part of the healthcare team, assisting the pharmacist in management of medication therapies.
- The profession of pharmacy has ancient roots, dating to the use of herbal medicines with prayers and rituals for healing.
- Pharmacy practice has evolved from the art of compounding natural herbal drugs to the science of dispensing manufactured synthetic medications and herbal supplements, and counseling about their proper use.
- Pharmacists at one time were not required to be formally educated or pass an examination to practice. As their role grew in responsibility, states required more standard education and licensing for pharmacists, as is happening for pharmacy technicians today.
- Assistants have long been part of the profession of healing with medications. The first technicians learned on the job from chemists and pharmacists. Some were apprentices training to become pharmacists/chemists.
- The first formally trained US pharmacy technicians were trained by the Army as medics in WWII.
- Hospitals were the first nonmilitary institutions to formally train pharmacy technicians and require certification.
- The primary mission of the pharmacy profession today is to assist patients in achieving overall wellness and favorable outcomes with their medication therapies and to safeguard the public health—technicians share in this mission.
- Pharmacy technicians work in a variety of community, institutional, and warehouse settings. Their full responsibilities vary according to the setting, their education, state regulations, and the individual workplace. Technicians carry out a wide range of duties under pharmacist oversight and approval.
- In addition to dispensing medication, the pharmacy profession has a clinical function of patient counseling and care. In medication therapy management (MTM), the pharmacist educates providers and patients about appropriate drugs and their usage, side effects and medication interactions, insurance formularies, and other issues, and then monitors the therapies. The pharmacy technician assists the pharmacist in these duties to effectively carry out these professional responsibilities.

- Collaborative Practice Agreements (CPAs) detail formal relationships between pharmacists and prescribers that allow for expanded pharmacist-provided patient care services. CPAs allow pharmacists to provide services such as selecting, administering, monitoring, and adjusting medication regimens. Technicians support the pharmacist in many aspects of providing expanded patient care services.
- Standardized formal educational training programs and opportunities to become a certified pharmacy technician are becoming essential in most states and may be a requirement in all states in the future.
- Advanced practice and specialized training and certification are available and needed for specific pharmacy technician jobs, such as preparing IV infusions, sterile compounding, chemotherapy, nuclear compounding, and other areas.
- Becoming a pharmacy technician can be a stepping-stone to other careers within pharmacy and allied health careers.

CHECK YOUR UNDERSTANDING

Take a moment to review what you have learned in this chapter and answer the following questions.

1. What is a formulary, and where did the concept originate?
   a. compilation of drug compounding tools from Ancient Greece
   b. book of herbal medicines from Italy
   c. scrolls of medicinal practices in China
   d. drug list on papyrus in Mesopotamia
2. What country was the forerunner in developing a logical, scientific-based approach to medical practice?
   a. India
   b. Italy
   c. Greece
   d. Germany
3. Which pharmacy organization required pharmacist apprentices to pass a formal certification exam in order to obtain a license to practice pharmacy?
   a. US Pharmacopeial Convention (USP)
   b. American Pharmacy Association (APhA)
   c. American Society of Health-System Pharmacists (ASHP)
   d. National Association of Boards of Pharmacy (NABP)
4. Formalized pharmacy technician training programs were first initiated by the
   a. Department of Defense.
   b. Philadelphia College of Pharmacy.
   c. University of Michigan College of Pharmacy.
   d. Illinois Pharmacists Association.

5. The emergence of the pharmaceutical industry threatened to reduce the role of the pharmacist to that of a
   a. compounder of medications.
   b. retail drug merchant.
   c. pharmaceutical scientist.
   d. toxicologist.

6. Which state/federal region became the first to use an examination to test the qualifications of a technician?
   a. Minnesota
   b. Washington, District of Columbia
   c. Ohio
   d. Michigan

MAKE CONNECTIONS

Take a moment to consider what you have learned in this chapter and respond thoughtfully to the following prompts. Note that some of these activities will require internet access.

1. Compare and contrast the roles of a pharmacist to the roles of a pharmacy technician. Where do you see redundancies? Why do you think this is?
2. Research the state board of pharmacy qualifications for your home state plus four other states and review where they overlap and where they diverge. What stands out most to you about where the qualifications are similar?

The online course includes additional review and assessment resources.

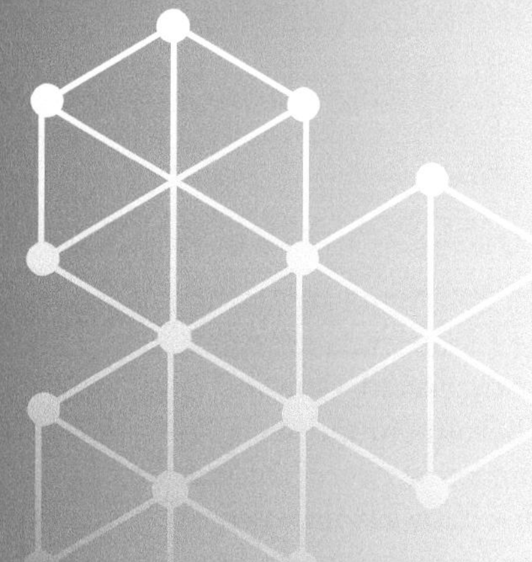

2 Pharmacy Law, Regulations, and Standards

Learning Objectives

1. Outline an overview of governmental pharmacy oversight in the US. (Section 2.1)
2. Define the terms *laws, regulations, standards*, and *professional ethics*. (Section 2.2)
3. Summarize how drug injuries and deaths lead to protective legislation. Describe significant federal drug laws in the 20th century and their effects on pharmacy practice in the United States. (Section 2.3)
4. Outline the different roles of government regulatory agencies and professional organizations—such as the Food and Drug Administration, Drug Enforcement Administration, and US Pharmacopeial Convention—in creating standards and enforcing laws and regulations. (Section 2.4)
5. Explain the role of state boards of pharmacy and the differences between state and federal laws as they apply to pharmacy. Paraphrase how the strictest rule is applied. (Section 2.4)
6. Define the specific legal term *standard of care* and its application to the pharmacist and pharmacy technician. (Section 2.6)
7. Explain the differences between criminal and civil law, how these laws affect the pharmacy profession, and the varying levels of liability of pharmacists and pharmacy technicians. (Section 2.7)
8. Explain and provide examples of the potential for legal actions against a pharmacy technician related to negligence, malpractice, or the law of agency and contracts. (Section 2.7)

ASHP/ACPE Accreditation Standards

To view the *ASHP/ACPE Accreditation Standards* addressed in this chapter, refer to Appendix B.

To be an effective pharmacy technician, you will need to understand the legal context in which you will practice. A variety of mechanisms control the practice of pharmacy, including a wide range of laws and ensuing regulations passed by federal, state, and local governmental entities. These legal mechanisms ensure that pharmaceutical manufacturers bring safe products to market, and that pharmacy personnel provide safe and effective care to consumers while staying safe themselves. In addition, various professional organizations have established standards that guide the manufacture of pharmacy products and the conduct of pharmacists and pharmacy technicians.

Any violations of pharmacy laws and standards may lead to adverse patient consequences—such as medication complications, injury, and even death—as well as personal consequences—such as legal action, loss of employment, and, in rare extreme cases, fines or jail. This chapter provides an overview of the complex system of interrelated pharmacy laws, regulations, and standards.

2.1 Pharmacy Oversight

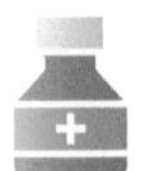

Pharm Fact

The most popular antibiotic dispensed in Mexico without a prescription is penicillin.

During the 19th century, the manufacture of drugs in the United States was unregulated. Medicines did not have to be proven safe or effective to be marketed. Opium and many of its extracts—such as morphine, codeine, and even heroin—found their way into medicines and were widely touted as cure-alls. These medicines were hawked by boisterous charlatans who would take their traveling medicine shows from town to town to proclaim the latest "miracle cure." There were no labeling regulations and no research to support the claims. In addition to opium extracts, these potions generally contained a high content of alcohol to make the customer "feel better." Not only were these medications addictive, but they occasionally caused injury or death.

By the advent of the 20th century, there were major concerns about these rogue medicines and about the purity of drugs imported from other countries. As a result, laws, oversight agencies, and professional organizations evolved to protect the public.

Laws and regulations related to drug approvals and pharmacy practice are generally stricter in the United States than in other countries. For example, in Mexico, you may be able to get many drugs without a prescription that would require a prescription in the United States, including some antibiotics. Such lax drug control seems astonishing to American pharmacy professionals in light of the distinct possibility of inappropriate use, poor quality, adverse reactions, and problematic drug interactions. Issues related to stringent US drug laws continue to be debated publicly because of the ongoing illegal importation of drugs from Canada and Mexico.

Governmental agencies and professional organizations that exercise controls on the contemporary practice of pharmacy include the following:

- federal, state, and local legislative bodies, such as the US Congress, state legislatures, and municipal governing councils, and the federal and state courts that uphold their laws
- federal and state regulatory agencies, including the following:
  - Food and Drug Administration (FDA)
  - Drug Enforcement Administration (DEA)
  - Occupational Safety and Health Administration (OSHA)
  - Federal Trade Commission (FTC), which has authority over business practices, such as direct-to-consumer drug advertising
  - Health Care Financing Administration (HCFA) of the Department of Health and Human Services (HHS) and the Center for Medicare & Medicaid Services (CMS). The CMS has authority over reimbursement under the Medicare and Medicaid government drug insurance programs

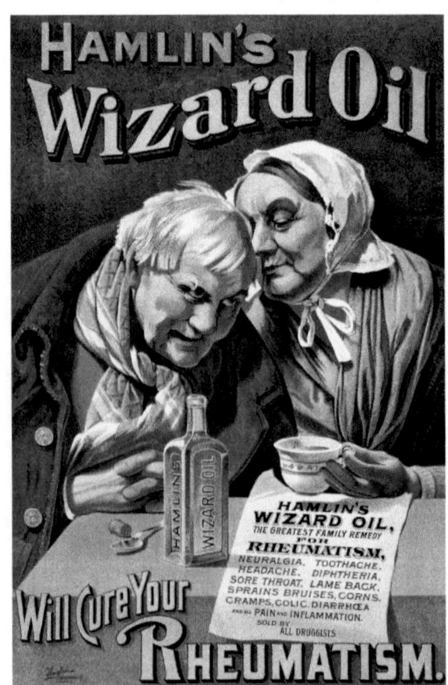

In the late 1880s, there was no control over the sale of pharmaceutical products. Thus, consumers were unprotected.

- ~ State boards of health and welfare agencies that budget for the provision of drugs needed by low-income or disabled individuals
- ~ Centers for Disease Control and Prevention (CDC)

- US Pharmacopeial Convention (USP)
- professional organizations including the following:
  - ~ Joint Commission (a professional hospital and healthcare system organization)
  - ~ National Association of Boards of Pharmacy (NABP)
  - ~ Individual state boards of pharmacy
  - ~ American Pharmacists Association (APhA)
  - ~ American Society of Health-System Pharmacists (ASHP)
  - ~ International Pharmaceutical Federation, National Pharmacy Technician Association, and American Association of Pharmacy Technicians
- individual businesses, companies, corporations, and institutions, such as community pharmacies, hospitals, nursing home facilities, and home healthcare organizations

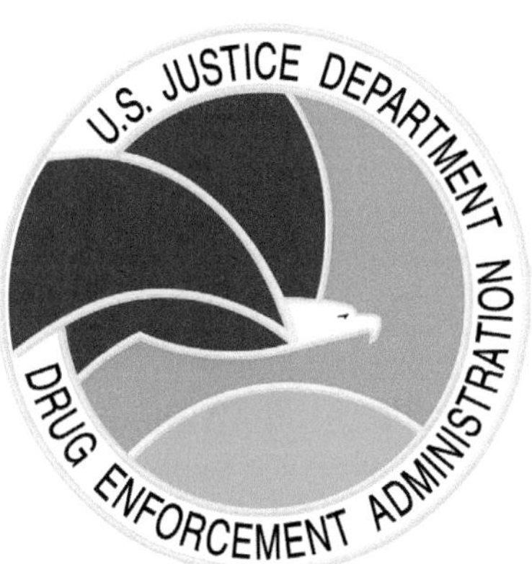

This seal represents the Drug Enforcement Administration, the federal regulatory agency that enforces the Controlled Substances Act.

2.2 Types of Oversight

To understand how these various oversight bodies function, one needs to recognize the different levels of legal and nonlegal influences, and how they work together.

Laws

A **law**, also known as a statutory law, is an overall rule that is passed by the legislative branches of federal, state, and local governments to guide conduct. Combined, the multilevel system of laws establishes the *minimum* acceptable standards to protect the public.

Regulations

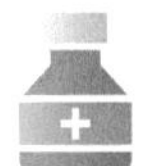

Pharm Fact

The state boards of pharmacy write the rules and advocate that the state legislatures pass them. Legislators are not required to follow a board's recommendations.

Regulations are a set of written rules and procedures that exist to carry out a law. For example, the FDA, a federal governmental agency, has published regulations on the drug approval process, generic drug substitution, patient counseling, and adverse reaction reporting systems. A violation of any FDA regulation is a breaking of federal law. Another national government agency, the Drug Enforcement Administration (DEA), has rules regulating the distribution, storage, documentation, and filling of prescriptions for controlled substances or legally restricted drugs. The federal programs of Medicare and Medicaid have regulations as well that are put in place for pharmacists and pharmacy technicians who dispense and bill prescriptions for older adults and low-income and disabled patients.

Within each state, the board of pharmacy oversees additional pharmacy rules that must be followed within its borders. As discussed in Chapter 1, licensure, registration, and certification requirements for pharmacy technicians vary from state to state. When there is a conflict between a state and a federal law or regulation, the more stringent law or regulation *always* applies.

Practice Tip

Many ethical dilemmas arise for pharmacists and technicians in the course of everyday practice. If they do not live up to professional ethics and standards, they risk causing patient harm, even death, and also losing their jobs. (Ethical dilemmas will be addressed in Chapter 15.)

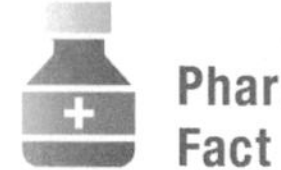

Pharm Fact

Due to growing public concern, during the developmental stages of the Pure Food and Drug Act, the manufacturer of Coca-Cola changed the key ingredient of its product from cocaine to caffeine.

Standards

A **standard** is a a guideline, benchmark, or desired level of quality to serve as the expected norm for a product or professional performance. Standards exist for drug products, individual professional conduct, and both community and institutional pharmacies—including hospitals, HMOs, nursing homes, and mail-order warehouses. For example, the US Pharmacopeial Convention (USP)—a nongovernmental professional organization—works with scientists to set ingredient and manufacturing standards that must be met by pharmaceutical companies before their new drug products can be submitted to the FDA. The USP also sets national standards for pharmacies preparing sterile and nonsterile preparations.

Ethics

Whereas laws and the resulting regulations represent the minimum level of legal oversight to protect the public, and professional standards represent quality in practice, professional **ethics** encompasses the higher realm of ideals, values, and missions that are held by professions and individual practitioners. Pharmacists and technicians are encouraged to abide by the oaths and the code of ethics set out by their professional organizations to achieve the *highest* standards of practice and care for patients as opposed to the minimum. This united professional goal to seek the best outcomes for patients helps hold healthcare professionals accountable for their decisions and actions in the workplace. It helps patients trust in the pharmacy profession as a whole as well as trust in individual pharmacists and pharmacy technicians. If a legal challenge is made related to an individual's professional actions or choices, they are compared with the accepted practices of other professionals in the field.

Hospitals and other healthcare companies generally establish mission statements and ethical codes of conduct for the facilities and their employees too. Following these established codes of ethics in one's personal and workday actions is an essential part of professionalism, which will be covered in greater detail in Chapter 15.

2.3 History of US Statutory Pharmacy Law and Oversight

To fully understand the maze of laws, agencies, and organizations that oversee drugs and the field of pharmacy on federal, state, and local levels, one needs to know the history of how they evolved. The following sections highlight, in chronological order, the major statutory laws affecting the profession of pharmacy.

Pure Food and Drug Act of 1906

Beginning in 1820, the US Congress began depending upon the new pharmacy professional organization, the USP, for standardization of ingredients in drug formulations. However, problems persisted with the use of dangerous ingredients, false marketing claims, and inaccurate labeling. The purpose of the Pure Food and Drug Act of 1906 was to address these problems and prohibit the sale or interstate transportation of adulterated or misbranded food and drugs. Labels could no longer legally contain false information about the strength or purity of the drugs. The act proved difficult to enforce, though, because the government had to prove that a drug was unsafe or contaminated, rather than the manufacturer having to prove that it was safe and pure.

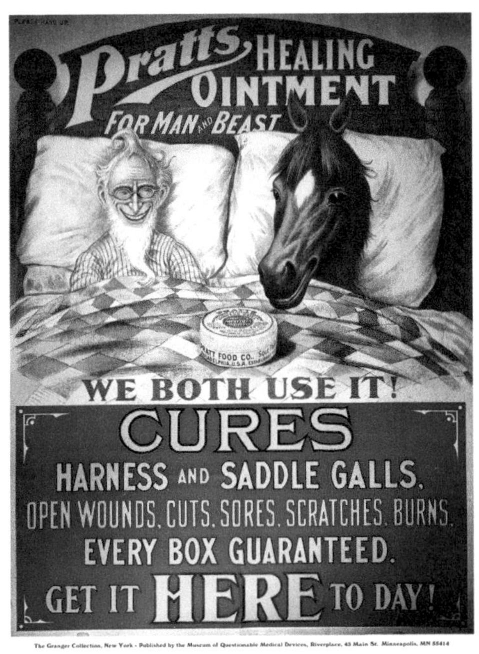

Marketers prior to the 1906 Pure Food and Drug Act could make any claims they wanted to help sell their medications.

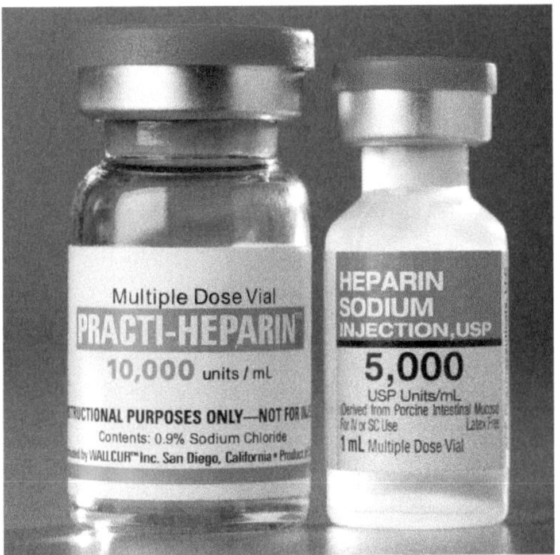

Vials of imported blood thinner (heparin) from China were found to be counterfeits. Unlike the sterile vials shown here, these adulterated products were contaminated by chondroitin sulfate and resulted in 149 deaths from adverse drug reactions.

Food, Drug, and Cosmetic Act of 1938

In 1937 more than 100 individuals died as the result of poisoning from a sulfa drug product that contained diethylene glycol, a toxic chemical used in antifreeze. The drug manufacturer, the S. E. Massengill Company, was unaware of diethylene glycol's poisonous nature, and the drug was marketed without being tested in animals or humans. Because of this tragedy, the Federal Food, Drug, and Cosmetic (FD&C) Act of 1938 was passed, becoming one of the most important pieces of legislation in pharmaceutical history. This legislation created the **Food and Drug Administration (FDA)**, a new government agency to ensure that pharmaceutical manufacturers obtain approval before releasing any new drug. From this point on, manufacturers were required to file a **new drug application (NDA)** with each new drug and provide study data to show that the product was safe for use by humans.

Unfortunately, this act did not require proof that a drug was effective or useful for the purpose for which it was sold. But the FDA did have the power to conduct inspections of manufacturing plants to ensure their compliance with safety and purity standards.

The act clarified the definitions of adulterated and misbranded drugs. An **adulterated product** became broadly defined as a product that differs from quality standards in drug strength, quality, or purity. For example, an adulterated product may be a prescription drug, over-the-counter (OTC) drug, or dietary supplement that is contaminated with other drugs or chemicals. The contaminating elements may or may not be harmful. For instance, certain dietary supplements have recently been found to be contaminated with other drugs, requiring their withdrawal from the market. Mail-order drugs from a Canadian website have been found to be manufactured in countries other than indicated, and adulterated with dangerous ingredients not labeled.

A **misbranded product**, on the other hand, is defined as a product whose label includes false statements about the identity or ingredients of the container's contents. Pharmaceutical manufacturers have been found guilty and paid hefty fines for promoting "off-label" medical uses of approved prescription drugs. For example, a drug may be

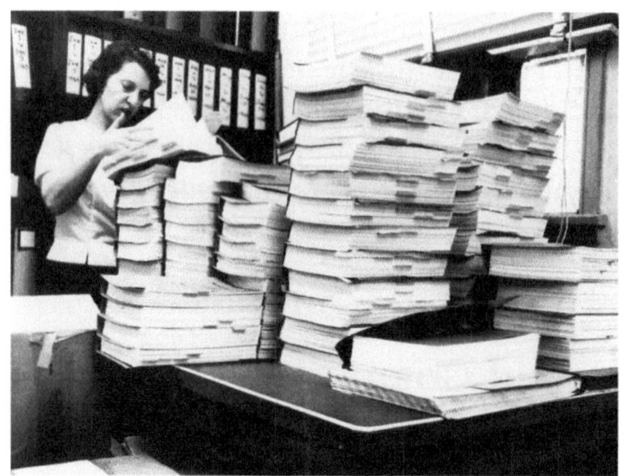

In the early 1960s, FDA chemist Lee Geismar helped review the studies for thalidomide's new drug application. Here she is chest deep in assessing the research for another new drug.

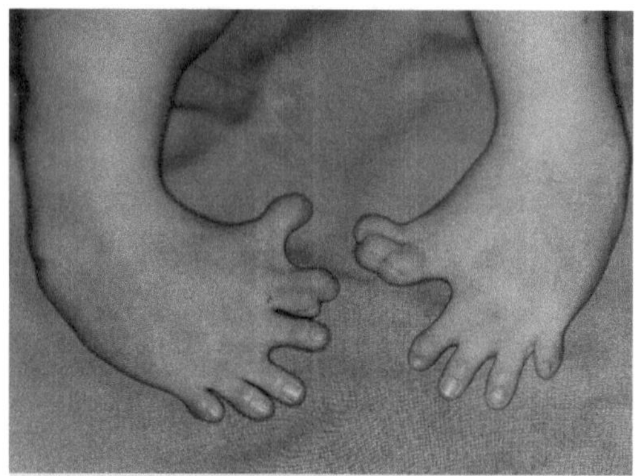

The effects of thalidomide on a child in the womb due to the mother's intake during pregnancy caused extremely stunted growth in the child's limbs before birth and afterwards.

FDA approved for high blood pressure, but a manufacturer's sales representatives may decide to promote its use to doctors for treatment of Alzheimer's disease even though there is little or no scientific evidence to support that indication and no FDA approval for it. The FDA is as busy today as in 1938 in addressing the many challenges of drug adulteration and misbranding.

Durham-Humphrey Amendment of 1951

The FD&C Act of 1938 was amended in 1951. The Durham-Humphrey Amendment established the distinction between so-called **legend drugs** (or prescription drugs that are labeled "Rx only" on the medication stock bottle), which require prescribers' directions, and **patent drugs** (OTC, nonprescription drugs), which require only adequate manufacturers' label directions. The prescription drug containers do not have to include "adequate directions for use" on their labels if instead they display the warning "Caution: Federal Law Prohibits Dispensing without a Prescription" and are accompanied by the required consumer information sheets from the prescriber and the manufacturer.

The amendment also authorized pharmacists to be able to take refill prescriptions for some substances over the telephone verbally rather than in writing. It set out guidelines as to which prescriptions can or cannot be refilled this way. Drugs with abuse potential were omitted to prevent false prescriber calls.

IN THE REAL WORLD

Today, more than 80% of drug ingredients are manufactured overseas in a complex supply chain often beyond FDA jurisdiction. Contaminated, subpotent (less effective), or counterfeit medications can enter the supply chain at several levels, from the production of raw ingredients to the point of retail sale. In the recent past, a counterfeit version of Avastin (bevacizumab), a cancer drug, was imported and then pulled by the FDA from the market.

Adulterated cough medicines containing a toxin (interestingly, diethylene glycol again) were distributed in Panama, which resulted in many deaths. Subpotent counterfeit medications misbranded as real ones have occasionally been discovered in the United States as well, adversely affecting patient health. In response, the FDA has established agreements with over 60 countries to work together for drug purity and safety.

Kefauver-Harris Amendments of 1962

The Kefauver-Harris Amendments of 1962 were passed in response to the birth of thousands of infants—mostly in Europe—with severe abnormalities resulting from mothers who had taken a new tranquilizer called **thalidomide** while they were pregnant. The amendments required drug manufacturers to file an investigational new drug application with the FDA and provide in-depth drug-animal studies before initiating clinical trials in humans. The clinical trials had to prove that the drugs were not only safe for humans, but also *effective*. Once all the extensive trials were completed (typically taking 7–10 years) and the results proved that the product was both safe and effective, the manufacturer could then be granted FDA approval to market the product. To compensate for innovation and research costs, the government issued patent protection for brand-name products for a designated length of time.

Put Down Roots

A patent is a legal protection to the ownership and use in the marketplace of a specific drug formulation, invention, idea, brand name, or logo. Patent protection for drug formulations from copycat drugs and generics lasts 20 years, with some extensions for special cases.

Comprehensive Drug Abuse Prevention and Control Act of 1970

The Comprehensive Drug Abuse Prevention and Control Act of 1970, commonly referred to as the **Controlled Substances Act (CSA)**, was created to combat and control drug abuse and to supersede previous federal laws regarding drug abuse. The act classified drugs with potential for abuse as **controlled substances**, or drugs that are restricted because of a risk for abuse and dependence. The controlled substances were then ranked into five levels of restriction, or **schedules** (see Table 2.1).

This controlled substance schedule, from most restrictive to least, continues to be used as follows:

- Schedule I drugs are not commercially available or legally dispensed in the United States due to their high potential for abuse and addiction.
- Schedule II drugs may be prescribed, but they are the most highly regulated drug category and no refills are allowed.
- Schedule III, IV, and V drugs generally have progressively less abuse and addiction potential than Schedule II drugs, but they *have quantity and time limits on refills*.

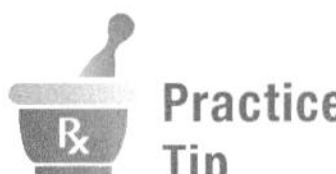

Practice Tip

Most controlled substance prescriptions are handwritten and signed by the prescriber. E-prescribing of controlled substances is also allowed, provided that both the prescriber and the pharmacy use DEA-approved software. In an emergency situation, a prescriber may phone in a C-II prescription, but a physical prescription must be provided within 7 days.

Filling prescriptions for controlled substances requires great attention to the regulations for ordering, filling, documenting, storing, and disposal. The specific requirements and steps for dispensing controlled substances will be covered in Chapter 14, as well as mentioned in the chapters on community and hospital dispensing (Chapters 7 and 11, respectively). Technicians need to study and carefully practice these requirements.

The CSA paved the way for more concerted government efforts against addictive drugs. On July 1, 1973, President Richard Nixon used an executive order to establish the DEA. This order consolidated the multiple agencies that had previously been working against illegal drug use into a new agency in the Department of Justice. The DEA would serve to work within the nation and with other nations for what President Nixon termed "an all-out global war on the drug menace."

The DEA classifies new drugs into the appropriate schedule (using data and input from the FDA and drug manufacturers). It also, at times, reevaluates drugs that have been on the market for some time to determine whether they should be changed to a scheduled drug. For example, there was concern about the overuse and abuse of the generic narcotic hydrocodone in combination products such as Lortab, Vicodin, and Norco. Consequently, the DEA reclassified these drug products from Schedule III to Schedule II in October 2014.

TABLE 2.1 Drug Schedules Under the Controlled Substances Act of 1970

Schedule	Manufacturer's Label	Abuse Potential	Accepted Medical Use	Examples
I	C-I	Highest potential for abuse	For research only; must have license to obtain; no accepted medical use in the United States	heroin (diacetylmorphine), lysergic acid diethylamide (LSD), tetrahydrocannabinols (THC)
II	C-II	High possibility of abuse, with use potentially leading to severe psychological or physical dependence	Dispensing severely restricted; cannot be prescribed by telephone except in an emergency; e-prescribing allowed with DEA aproved authorized digital signature; no refills on prescriptions	morphine; oxycodone; meperidine; hydromorphone; hydrocodone combination products (hydrocodone combined with acetaminophen, aspirin, or ibuprofen); fentanyl; methylphenidate; dextroamphetamine
III	C-III	Moderate to low potential for physical and psychological dependence	Prescriptions can be called in and refilled up to five times within six months if authorized by physician	codeine combination products (codeine combined with acetaminophen, aspirin, or ibuprofen); ketamines; anabolic steroids
IV	C-IV	Low potential for abuse and low risk of dependence	Same as for Schedule III	benzodiazepines, phenobarbital, carisoprodol, tramadol
V	C-V	Lower potential for abuse than Schedule IV and consist of preparations containing limited quantities of certain narcotics	Some sold without a prescription, depending on state law; if so, purchaser must be over age 18 and is required to sign a log and present a photo ID	liquid codeine combination cough preparations, diphenoxylate/atropine, pregabalin

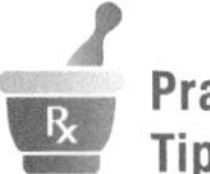

Practice Tip

While medical cannabis (or marijuana) is legal in many states, it is still illegal under federal law. At the time of publication, most cannabis products were considered Schedule I by the DEA. This is an example where federal and state laws differ.

Individual states may have additional guidelines for the prescribing and dispensing of controlled substances. State boards of pharmacy may advocate to their legislatures to reclassify prescription drugs as scheduled drugs or move a scheduled drug to a more restrictive schedule level to curb drug abuse in their region. Oral nasal decongestants, such as those containing pseudoephedrine (Sudafed) and ephedrine, and cough medicines containing codeine are available in most states as restricted OTC drugs. In other states, they may be registered as Schedule III drugs. As noted, the strictest rule always applies because that is the best way to protect the public health in a region and in the nation as a whole. All laws are written to set out only the minimum standard for safety, not the highest and most restrictive. If there is cause to have a more restrictive law in a specific state or the nation, then that rule overrides all.

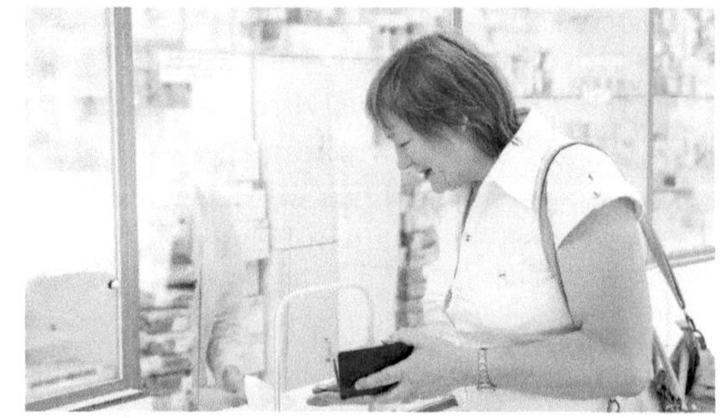

In pharmacies, prescription drugs and select OTC drugs must be stored in a locked and secured area, with a pharmacist always on duty during facility open hours.

The Controlled Substances Act was also significant as it determined who may have the authority to prescribe controlled substances. Prescribers must now be authorized and monitored by the DEA jurisdiction in which they are licensed. Practitioners who may be licensed include physicians, physician assistants, nurse practitioners (advanced practice nurses), dentists, veterinarians, podiatrists, and psychiatrists. Physician assistants and nurse practitioners working under the direct supervision of a collaborating physician can also prescribe some controlled substances under the supervising provider's DEA number.

In all cases, prescriptions must be written for a legitimate medical purpose based on the practitioner's professional practice. For example, a dentist may write a narcotic prescription for dental pain but not for back- or cancer-related pain. A prescription for some controlled substances from a foreign physician (for example, a practicing physician in Canada or Mexico) cannot be filled in the United States because the prescriber must have a DEA license, which is available only to licensed prescribers in the United States. In addition, some pharmacies may not be licensed to fill a Schedule II prescription written by an out-of-state physician without verification, even if the prescriber has a valid DEA license.

Poison and Prevention Packaging Act of 1970

To prevent accidental childhood drug poisonings, the Poison Prevention Packaging Act was passed in 1970. This act, enforced by the Consumer Product Safety Commission, required that most OTC and prescription drugs be packaged in **child-resistant containers** that cannot be opened by 80% of children under age 5, but can be opened by 90% of adults. Upon request from a patient, a drug may be dispensed in a normal container. In fact, the patient—not the prescriber—can make a blanket request that all drugs be dispensed to them without child-resistant containers. This blanket request is often made by older patients and those with severe rheumatoid arthritis. Medications commonly dispensed in non-child-resistant containers include the antibiotic azithromycin (or Zithromax Z-pak), Medrol Dosepak, birth control pills, sublingual nitroglycerin tablets, and metered-dose inhalers.

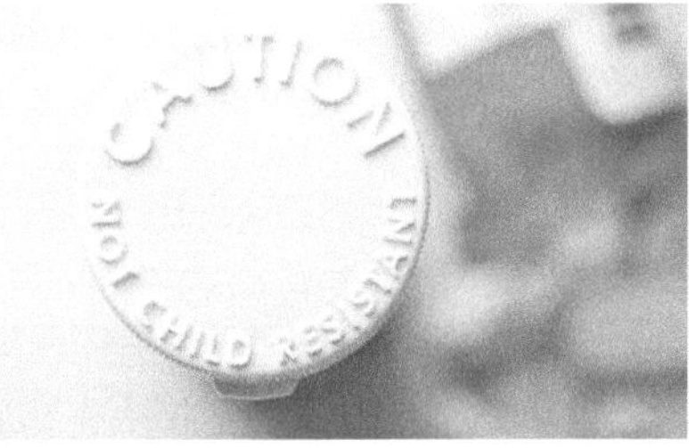

Unless specifically requested by the customer, medications are dispensed in child-resistant containers to prevent accidental poisonings.

For non–child-resistant containers, technicians should remind patients to place these medications out of reach if young children live in or visit their homes.

Drug Listing Act of 1972

The Drug Listing Act of 1972 gave the FDA the authority to compile a list of currently marketed drugs and assign them each a numbered code. Every new drug is also assigned a unique and permanent product signifier known as a **National Drug Code (NDC) number**. It consists of 10 or 11 characters that identify the manufacturer or distributor, the drug formulation, and the size and type of its packaging, in that order.

The FDA requests—*but does not require*—that the NDC number appear on all drug labels, including the labels on prescription containers (see Figure 2.1). Using this code, the FDA is able to maintain a database of drugs by use, manufacturer, and active ingredients. It can track newly marketed, discontinued, and remarketed drugs. This barcoded information is widely used today to double-check the accuracy of prescriptions filled by automation. Insurance companies also use the NDC number in processing pharmacy reimbursements.

FIGURE 2.1 Manufacturer Drug Label

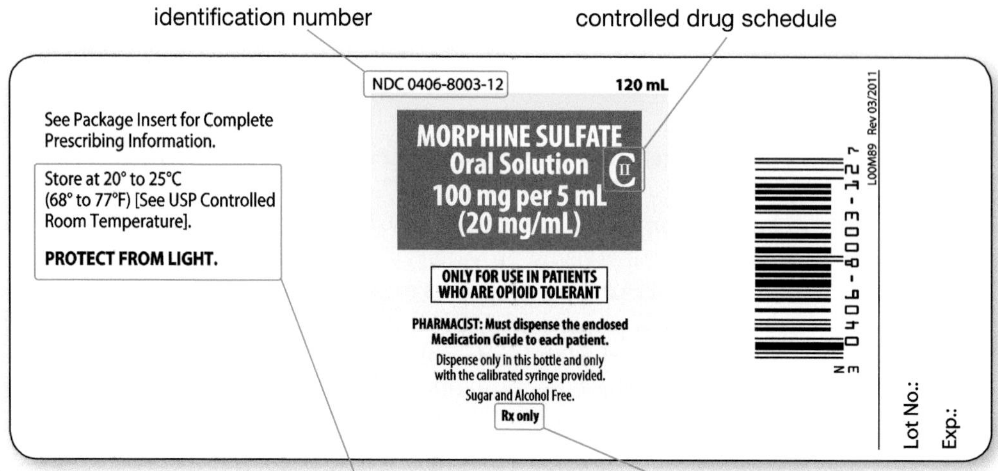

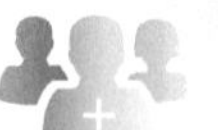

Work Wise

Patients often become frustrated by the confusion over generic and brand-name drugs. Listening to their concerns and explaining the differences and similarities can help them better understand their medications.

Orphan Drug Act of 1983

An **orphan drug** is a drug that is intended for patients suffering from a rare disorder (a condition that affects fewer than 200,000 people). Because developing and marketing these kinds of drugs can be prohibitively expensive, the Orphan Drug Act of 1983 provides the manufacturers tax incentives and grants them a longer time period to have the exclusive licenses to market these drugs. The FDA also moves these drugs faster through the approval process to get them swiftly to patients in need.

Since 1983, more than 500 orphan drugs have been FDA approved for treatment of rare diseases, most of which involve a genetic defect. For example, cystic fibrosis (CF) is a genetic disease that affects the lungs and other organs and often leads to premature death. With the act's support of orphan drugs, CF patients now have treatments available for an improved quality of life and a longer life span. Another group of orphan drugs— statins—were initially developed in 1985 in response to a rare genetic defect known as homozygous familial hypercholesterolemia. Today, statins are commonly prescribed medications for millions of patients with high cholesterol levels.

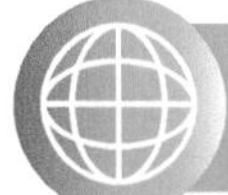

IN THE REAL WORLD

Cystic fibrosis (CF) affects approximately 1 in 10,000 people. In people with CF, a special protein (called the cystic fibrosis transmembrane conductance regulator) does not work correctly. The dysfunctional protein is unable to help move chloride—a component of salt—to the cell surface. This allows mucus in various organs—especially the lungs—to become thick and sticky. Drug treatments with special aerosolized antibiotics, biotechnology agents, and pancreatic enzymes to assist in digestion have markedly improved the life expectancy of patients with CF. There are over 50 orphan CF drugs, including Pulmozyme (dornase alpha) and aerosolized tobramycin. The financial incentives, patent and legal protections, and accelerated FDA approvals resulting from the adoption of the Orphan Drug Act allowed for the development of these drugs. Visit https://PharmPractice7e .ParadigmEducation.com/Orphan for more examples.

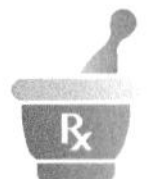

Practice Tip

More than 80% of prescriptions dispensed in community pharmacies are generic drugs. Generic drugs can be substituted for the related brand name drug in every state—unless the prescriber writes "brand only" or "do not substitute."

Drug Price Competition and Patent Term Restoration Act of 1984 (Hatch-Waxman Act)

Prior to the 1980s, drugs with **brand names** were the ones most prescribed, dispensed, and recognized by prescribers and patients. The proliferation of brand name drugs was the result of many state anti-substitution laws passed to combat similar but counterfeit drugs. However, by 1984, mounting pressure by lawmakers, pharmacists, and consumers to reduce healthcare costs led to the passing of the Drug Price Competition and Patent Term Restoration Act. This legislation, also known as the Hatch-Waxman Act, streamlined the process to approve equally effective drugs with nonproprietary names, or generic names.

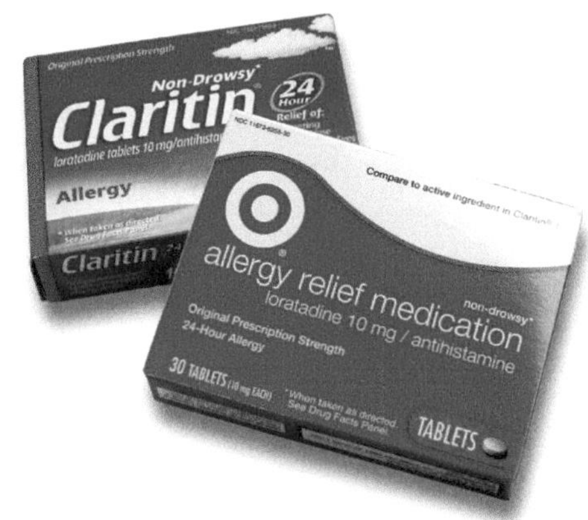

The rise in availability of cheaper, generic drugs was due in part to the Drug Price Competition and Patent Term Restoration Act of 1984.

Generic drugs are required to be comparable to their brand-name counterparts in intended use, quality, performance, safety, strength, route of administration, and dosage form. Since the original drug manufacturers handled the research studies, and the brand name drugs established a public track record of safety, the generic drugs are not required to go through the same rigorous scientific review for safety and effectiveness. However, they must demonstrate **bioequivalence** (similar strength and outcomes) to the brand-name product. (The concept of bioequivalence will be discussed in detail in Chapter 3.) The growth and expansion of generic manufacturers can be traced to the Hatch-Waxman Act.

The Hatch-Waxman Act also extended the length of the proprietary patent licenses for the brand-name drugs. The extended patent protection time allows the manufacturers to recoup the research and development costs, providing an incentive to research new drugs.

Once the patent expires, any manufacturer is allowed to copy and market a competing generic drug, which is clearly much less costly than developing the original. Since medications are labeled by both their generic names and their brand names (and, at times, by their chemical names), pharmacy personnel, including technicians, must be familiar with the various names for the related medications. (See Table 2.2 for examples of the different names for bioequivalent medications.)

TABLE 2.2 Different Names for One Drug

Type of Name	Drug Name
Chemical name	p-isobutylhydratropic acid
Generic name	ibuprofen
Brand name	Advil, Motrin, Motrin IB

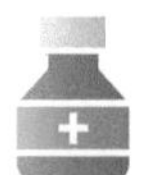

Pharm Fact

In 2014, Congress passed the Designer Anabolic Steroid Act, which added numerous new substances to the anabolic controlled substances list originally created in the 1990 act. The new bill also added serious penalties for mislabeling steroids to avoid detection.

Prescription Drug Marketing Act of 1987

Manufacturers distribute drugs through large distributors, which then work through smaller regional and state distributors and warehouses. Independent distributors and warehouses can purchase their own drug supplies to store for times of local shortages in the regular distribution system or to sell independently. Problems arose in this system. For example, foreign counterfeit drugs were being sold as brand name drugs by independent companies, and some distribution companies were taking their foreign sales returns and selling them in the United States. Unethical sales representatives were taking drug samples meant for providers and distributing them as prescription products. Warehouses were selling products at wholesale prices, undercutting the safe processes of pharmacy dispensers.

Due to concerns over the safety and competition issues raised by these secondary distribution markets, the Prescription Drug Marketing Act of 1987 required that all drug wholesalers be licensed by the states. The act also prohibited the sale, trading, or distribution of drug samples to persons other than those licensed to prescribe them. The reimportation of a drug into the United States by anyone except the manufacturer was prohibited as well.

Drug reimportation continues to be a political and economic issue. For example, many citizens travel across the Canadian border to fill their prescriptions or receive their prescriptions through the mail from Canadian drug wholesalers. US pharmaceutical manufacturers have threatened to reduce the supply of drugs to Canada if the practice of illegal reimportation to the states continues. Many Canadians also are concerned, fearing medication shortages and the abuse of prescription drugs within their own country from lax mail-order companies. The Medicare Modernization Act of 2003 (discussed later in the chapter) has helped to mitigate but not eliminate the drug reimportation problem—it adopted and has encouraged participation in Medicare Part D drug insurance plans, thus lowering costs to seniors, who are a major market for Canadian drugs.

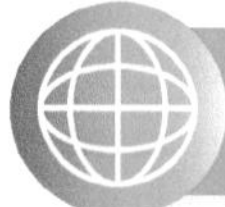

IN THE REAL WORLD

The dispensing of generic drugs has been a major factor in containing the high cost of pharmaceuticals, with savings ranging from 30% to 80% of brand-name counterparts. In 2012, US patients together saved $193 billion dollars by using generics, though generic prices are now rising exponentially. Although generic drugs are considered similar and effectively equal to brand drugs, it is important to realize that they are not exactly the same. FDA criteria require that the medically active ingredients found in the bloodstream after use must not be much less or more than 5% of the amount found after the brand-name drug. However, the added ingredients in generic drugs can be different and often are, and these ingredients can affect the drug's responsiveness in different patients. How quickly or slowly the drug acts can also vary.

Consequently, providers, pharmacists, and pharmacy technicians must understand that generics are not precise replicas of the brand name drugs. Patients should be careful to watch for specific outcomes and side effects to make sure that they have the right drug for their needs.

Anabolic Steroids Control Act of 1990

Anabolic steroids, or synthetic drugs that mimic the human hormone testosterone, have become widely known due to their misuse by popular professional athletes. These steroids are used to build muscle mass, enhancing the strength—and, ultimately, the performance—of the users. Anabolic steroids have a long list of serious adverse effects and can cause permanent damage. Prior to 1990, these drugs were illegally manufactured, imported, and sold on the black market. However, there were no stiff criminal penalties. Some anabolic drugs were included as ingredients in loosely regulated dietary supplements. Congress passed the Anabolic Steroids Control Act of 1990, which designated anabolic steroids as a Schedule III class of drugs on par with codeine. This provided regulated prescriptive access to patients who needed the steroids for pain or other uses while allowing the FDA to enforce steroid drug standards, confiscating and prosecuting those responsible for illegal use, product distribution, and imports.

To help enforce the Anabolic Steroids Control Act, many professional sports organizations employ random drug testing. Since anabolic steroids are Schedule III drugs, prescriptions for these steroids—such as testosterone gels, patches, and injections—can be refilled a maximum of only five times or for up to six months from the date written, whichever comes first. This is similar to regulations for many nerve and sleep medications.

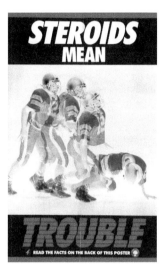

This FDA educational poster warns about the dangers of steroids.

Omnibus Budget Reconciliation Act of 1990

To help address the rising costs of pharmaceutical expenditures for Medicaid, the Omnibus Budget Reconciliation Act of 1990 (OBRA-90) required that, in order to receive Medicaid funding, each state had to establish a Drug Utilization Review (DUR) Board. The board's job has been to establish a state Medicaid preferred drug list and set standards for pharmacist-to-patient education and counseling. The act also required that pharmacy personnel engage in "a review of drug therapy before each prescription is filled or delivered to an individual . . . typically at the point of sale. . . . The review shall include screening for potential drug therapy problems due to therapeutic duplication, drug-disease contraindications, drug-drug interactions (including serious interactions with nonprescription OTC drugs), incorrect drug dosage or duration of treatment, drug-allergy interactions, and clinical abuse/misuse." OBRA-90 made the DUR and medication management therapy (MTM) a necessity for Medicaid patients, setting a standard for other patients as well.

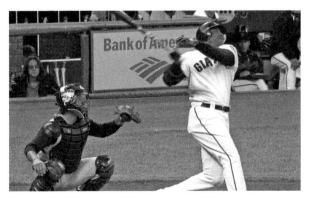

Barry Bonds, apparently under the influence of anabolic steroids, hit more career home runs than any other player in baseball history. However, he did not receive the Baseball Hall of Fame award his first year of eligibility because he was convicted in 2011 (upheld in 2013) of obstructing justice by denying knowledge of his steroid use.

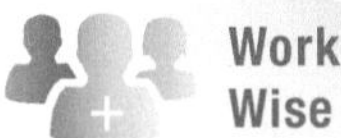

Work Wise

Many patients take drugs for granted without understanding their real effects. They do not understand the value of medications. Informed technicians can help explain some of these benefits while directing them to pharmacists for medication counseling.

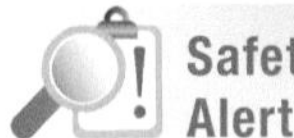

Safety Alert

The FDA does not regulate dietary supplements for purity or safety unless problems have arisen.

For these services, pharmacists need accurate records and information. OBRA-90 required pharmacy personnel to make reasonable efforts to collect, update, and record all pertinent patient information and medication history. A pharmacist must review the patient profile before filling each prescription and then offer to provide drug therapy screening and medication counseling. This offer must be documented, noting whether the counseling was accepted or refused. Technicians often handle or assist in this documentation process.

Dietary Supplement Health and Education Act of 1994

The Dietary Supplement Health and Education Act was passed in 1994. It provides definitions and guidelines on dietary supplements, including vitamins, minerals, herbs, and nutritional supplements. This legislation states that supplement manufacturers—unlike those of prescription and OTC drugs—are *not required* to provide proof of efficacy or standardization to the FDA. The manufacturers simply have to prove consumer safety and make truthful claims. The labels and marketing may not make claims of curing or treating ailments; they may state only that the products are supplements to support health.

While dietary supplements are sold alongside nonprescription drug products, many consumers think that they go through the same approval processes and rigor in their regulatory oversight. Pharmacy technicians should be prepared to explain the significant distinctions. The FDA may only review false claims of supplements and monitor safety issues that have arisen in public use and statements. If claims of medical treatments or miracle cures are made, the FDA can require manufacturers to provide scientific research and proof, similar to requirements for prescription and nonprescription drugs. Still, some manufacturers manage to tweak the verbiage of their labels to skirt this regulation—for example, using the tagline "for a healthy heart" rather than "to lower cholesterol."

If the FDA does want to remove a dietary supplement from the market for safety reasons, it may do so. However, it must first hold public hearings, and the burden of proof is upon the FDA to demonstrate that the dietary supplement is unsafe. The drug ephedra, or its herbal counterpart ma huang, was an ingredient in many weight-loss products. In 2004, the drug was removed from the market by the FDA as a result of multiple reports of serious adverse reactions and some deaths. The following year, the lower courts overruled the FDA's action, but in 2006 the Court of Appeals upheld the FDA action, thus removing all ephedra products from the US market.

IN THE REAL WORLD

In 2015, the FDA withdrew the Pyrola Advanced Joint Formula dietary supplement as it was found to be contaminated with diclofenac (a prescription pain and anti-inflammatory drug) and chlorpheniramine (an antihistamine). The FDA publishes a comprehensive list of dietary supplement withdrawals on its website: www.fda.gov.

More recently, the FDA has warned consumers of fraudulent claims made for "all natural" weight-loss supplements. Claims such as "magic pill," "melt your fat away," and "diet and exercise not required" should raise red flags. Several of these products have been found to be tainted with weight-loss prescription drugs. Thus, they are potentially dangerous and considered misbranded by the FDA. Within the past 20 years, more than 40 weight-loss products have been withdrawn from the market.

Health Insurance Portability and Accountability Act of 1996

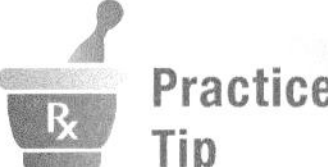

Every new patient should receive and sign a copy of the pharmacy's Privacy Agreement to be in compliance with the HIPAA statute. All patients need to re-sign it annually. Technicians often provide this form.

The **Health Insurance Portability and Accountability Act (HIPAA)** of 1996 included many provisions that directly affect all healthcare facilities and personnel, including pharmacy technicians. One provision is to ensure the portability of moving health insurance from one employer to another, as indicated by the act's name. So an emphasis was put on being able to communicate medical records electronically, using national codes for prescribers and pharmacy providers.

Perhaps the greatest effect of HIPAA on pharmacy technicians regards the handling of medical records, including personal prescription profiles. HIPAA placed safeguards to protect the confidentiality of patient health records. All healthcare facilities must provide a document to each patient that states the data privacy policy. It must also collect and save evidence of the patient's acknowledgment that the HIPAA privacy document was received.

Pharmacy personnel, including technicians, also must follow certain protocols for assembling and organizing patient profiles, andv, under penalty of law, take care not to reveal any information about any patient outside the pharmacy workplace. They may not discuss or transmit prescription data to anyone other than the patient, parents of children under 18, and appropriate healthcare providers. Every pharmacy must train its employees on patient data privacy, and this training must be renewed on an annual basis. Failure to comply with HIPAA regulation is grounds for immediate termination. (For more information, see Chapter 15.)

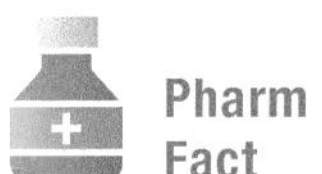

The 2005 **Patient Safety and Quality Improvement (PSQI) Act** promoted mechanisms for patient safety and continuous quality improvement in healthcare facilities. It encouraged the creation of **Patient Safety Organizations (PSOs)** that can collect confidential information on medical errors to develop systematic changes for safety.

Food and Drug Administration Modernization Act of 1997

The 1997 **Food and Drug Modernization Act** was enacted to update drug approval processes, streamlining them to accelerate the time until the release of newly patented and manufactured drugs. It also necessitated that the FDA regulate medical devices and required that biological drug products go through similar new drug approval processes.

Before this act, no specific federal or state laws governed the practice of small-batch pharmacy compounding. One provision of this legislation allows pharmacists to compound nonsterile (and/or sterile) medications for individuals if these medications meet established USP standards. This allows the compounders to skip the intensive FDA requirements for newly manufactured drugs so that they can offer more personally tailored prescription products for people with special concerns (such as pediatric and geriatric patients) and health conditions (such as severe allergies). The act outlines major situations where pharmacists or small-scale facilities do not have to adhere to the large-scale Current Good Manufacturing Practices, product labeling directions for use, or drug approval applications. These exceptions do not undermine the safety and efficacy of compounded products (p.52), but simply allow pharmacies to create personalized drugs for individuals and small groups of patients with specific needs.

The Food and Drug Administration Modernization Act also updated prescription drug labeling. Products labeled with "Caution: Federal Law Prohibits Dispensing without a Prescription" were changed to read "Rx only." The law also authorized fees, paid by the applicant drug manufacturer, to be added to a new drug application to provide additional resources to the FDA to process and accelerate the review and approval of new drugs.

Medicare Prescription Drug, Improvement, and Modernization Act of 2003

The Medicare Prescription Drug, Improvement, and Modernization Act, also called the **Medicare Modernization Act (MMA)**, updated the Medicare system and initiated the option of a prescription drug insurance program, called Medicare Part D, especially suited to patients with economic hardships or patients needing high-cost medications. The MMA also launched the Medicare Part C program, or the Medicare Advantage program, as a comprehensive healthcare insurance program option. Pharmacy technicians must be knowledgeable about Medicare programs since technicians are often involved in educating patients on their options.

The MMA and Medicare Part D encourage pharmacists to provide—and get reimbursed for—annual in-depth reviews of the medication profiles and ongoing therapies of Medicare patients taking high-cost medications or experiencing certain chronic health conditions. The purpose of this review is to add a safety feature to prevent adverse reactions and drug interactions (and costly hospitalizations) and to have the pharmacist look for ways to reduce medication costs. A lesser-known MMA provision allows for the development of health savings accounts for patients under age 65. This will be discussed in more detail in Chapter 8 on insurance.

Combat Methamphetamine Epidemic Act of 2005

Because common OTC ingredients are used to illegally manufacture **methamphetamine** (known as *meth*)—a highly addictive stimulant—Congress passed the Combat Methamphetamine Epidemic Act. The act reclassified all products containing the chemical pseudoephedrine (PSE) and ephedrine, found in products such as oral and nasal decongestants and combination sinus and allergy medications. It restricted the amount that can be purchased at one time or in any 30-day period.

All PSE products are now required to be stored behind the counter, and the purchaser has to present legal identification for purchase. The legislation also dictated that a log must be kept of all sales of PSE products and that all pharmacy employees, including technicians, had to complete a training program for the handling of PSE products. The DEA works with state agencies to enforce this act. (For additional information and procedures for the pharmacy technician to legally sell these OTC products, see Chapter 9.)

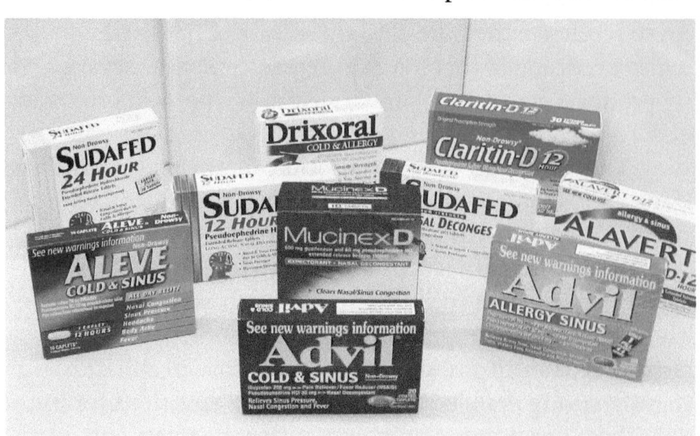

These are just a sampling of the over-the-counter drugs containing pseudoephedrine and/or ephedrine that are restricted by the 2005 Combat Methamphetamine Epidemic Act.

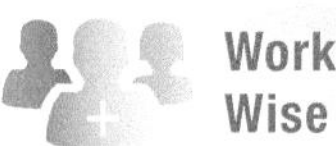

Work Wise

Patients and customers often share strong thoughts about politics and healthcare when talking to pharmacy personnel. To be professional, listen carefully but refrain from voicing a personal opinion. Choose your words carefully and respectfully, sticking to the facts of pharmacy practice.

Patient Protection and Affordable Care Act of 2010

The Patient Protection and Affordable Care Act of 2010, commonly known as the **Affordable Care Act (ACA)**, mandated healthcare coverage under threat of personal penalties for all US citizens (see Figure 2.2). The ACA increased access to healthcare for more than 32 million uninsured citizens and individuals with preexisting medical conditions who were previously declared uninsurable. It required states to provide health insurance options to those who were not covered, with federal funding assistance to those who needed it, and to offer catastrophic insurance coverage for individuals with high-cost illnesses.

Each state plan funded by the ACA must provide patients with a preferred drug list. This list helps ensure that patients are aware of which drugs are covered by their insurance and which are not. This is an area where medication therapy counseling from a pharmacist is particularly useful and often crucial.

The ACA also allowed healthcare systems and physician groups to form pilot healthcare teams, or **Accountable Care Organizations (ACOs)**, to serve Medicare Part D patients and to study team effectiveness in patient health outcomes and cost reductions. ACOs are groups of prescribers, pharmacists, and other providers, hospitals, and healthcare facilities that work together in a coordinated manner to seek out measurable improvements in patient outcomes. ACOs must include pharmacists, and each provider in the ACO must have full access to patient records so that they can communicate with each other for integrated patient care. ACOs are models of cooperative practice agreements. Technicians, especially advanced or specialist pharmacy technicians, often assist by helping assemble medication histories and by doing medication reconciliation, insurance formulary reconciliation, and medication assistance advocacy.

Studies are ongoing on the cost-benefit ratios to of the ACA different sectors. In 2015, the Supreme Court upheld the legality of the ACA. However, legal battles continue surrounding the ACA. Additional healthcare reform measures are being considered by government agencies, healthcare specialists, and all political parties.

Drug Quality and Security Act of 2013

The **Drug Quality and Security Act (DQSA)**, also known as the Compounding Quality Act, passed as a result of a contaminated medication that was compounded in 2012 by a small Massachusetts facility and then widely distributed to out-of-state physicians' offices, resulting in numerous patient deaths and injuries in a total of 20 states. Prior to this act, the regulatory oversight of small-batch medication compounding was handled solely by the states in which the substances were compounded and their pharmacy boards.

The overall goal of the DQSA is to better protect patients from drugs contaminated in the compounding process and sold in a different state, as well as to provide protection from counterfeit or stolen drugs. It established an electronic tracking system to trace drugs from ingredient sources through compounding and distribution processes. This tracking improves the ability to detect and swiftly remove harmful drugs from the public. The DQSA states that all small-scale pharmaceutical production should be compounded by a licensed pharmacist in a registered outsourcing facility. The facility must follow all state pharmacy requirements, and it is encouraged to register annually with the FDA as well, designating the pharmacist-in-charge and paying a fee.

FIGURE 2.2
Key Features of the Affordable Care Act

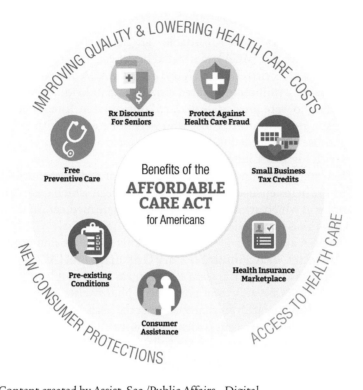

Content created by Assist. Sec./Public Affairs - Digital Communications Division

Benefits for Women

Providing insurance options, covering preventive services, and lowering costs.

Young Adult Coverage

Coverage available to children up to age 26.

Strengthening Medicare

Yearly wellness visit and many free preventive services for some seniors with Medicare.

Holding Insurance Companies Accountable

Insurers must justify any premium increase of 10% or more before the rate takes effect.

The compounding facility, however, must still comply with the Current Good Manufacturing Processes outlined by the USP and be subject to inspections by the FDA or its agents. When sterile processes are required, cleanroom standards must be followed in terms of facilities and procedures. Every six months, the pharmacy must report all the drugs and ingredients that were compounded to the Department of Health and Human Services and immediately report any adverse reactions from the pharmacy's compounded medications to the FDA. However, registration with the FDA is voluntary and costly to compounding facilities due to the terms of the legislation.

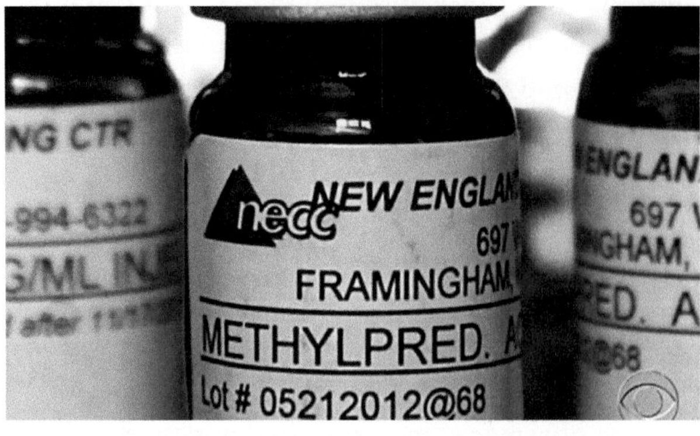

The New England Compounding Center sold a fungus-tainted, injectable steroid to healthcare facilities throughout the United States, resulting in deaths and injuries. It took the FDA 684 days to collect the information to warn providers to pull the medication, prompting the enactment of the DQSA.

Many problems have still not been eliminated. In 2013, a New Jersey compounding pharmacy, Med Prep Consulting, was temporarily shut down for mold found in injectable pharmaceutical solutions. To enhance consistency in patient safety, all states need to mandate that all compounding activities be in compliance with USP standards on sterile and nonsterile compounding. Also, all pharmacy personnel must be educated, certified, and licensed, plus have specialty training and certification in sterile compounding and aseptic technique. Texas led the way in 2015 by requiring that all pharmacy technicians, who already must be certified to practice, have additional certification in sterile processing and aseptic technique.

IN THE REAL WORLD

In 2012, 64 patients died in nine states as a result of a solution of methylprednisolone acetate (a steroid used for controlling pain) contaminated with fungus that was injected directly into the patients' spinal cords. The contaminated injections led to complications, including fungal meningitis. The drug was manufactured by the New England Compounding Center (NECC) in Massachusetts. Another 753 patients in 20 states were seriously injured. The unclean pharmacy facilities at NECC were running without FDA approval. Mold was discovered in the "cleanroom." A 2013 CBS *60 Minutes* investigation, "Lethal Medicine Linked to Meningitis Outbreak," uncovered the excruciating damage the surviving victims were still undergoing. It can be seen at https://PharmPractice7e.ParadigmEducation.com/LethalMedicine.

These incidents show the essential importance of sterile compounding and following precise aseptic technique and facility standards. They also show the value of the pharmacist and technician not rushing and cutting corners on sterile procedures. In December 2014, a federal jury indicted 14 NECC employees on 131 charges, including murder for two of the individuals, and also racketeering, fraud, conspiracy, and other crimes. A federal judge in 2015 approved a $200 million civil settlement for damages to victims and their families.

2.4 National Oversight Agencies and Organizations

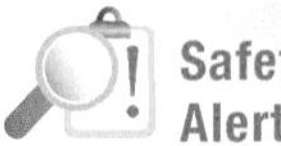

The FDA regulates OTC labeling, so that it is understandable to a layperson.

The laws, acts, and amendments previously discussed in this chapter provide the minimum level of acceptable standards for a broad scope of issues, offering a basic structure for the safe use of drug products and for the practice of pharmacy. Federal and state government agencies, along with nongovernmental organizations, work to ensure that the regulations required to fulfill these laws are established, reviewed, updated as needed, and enforced.

Food and Drug Administration

The FDA's Office of Medical Products and Tobacco oversees drugs. Within this office are several agencies pertinent to the practice of pharmacy: the Center for Drug Evaluation and Research (CDER), the Office of Pediatric Therapeutics, the Center for Devices and Radiological Health, the Center for Biologics Evaluation and Research (vaccinations), and the Office of Orphan Products Development. The profession of pharmacy is most affected by the CDER, which is primarily involved in the following tasks:

- new drug development and review
- generic drug review
- OTC drug review
- post-drug approval activities

As a public safety watchdog, the FDA enforces its regulations, including those for truth in advertising for food and drug packaging, labeling, advertising, and marketing. The FDA has been known to ask a manufacturer to cancel advertising

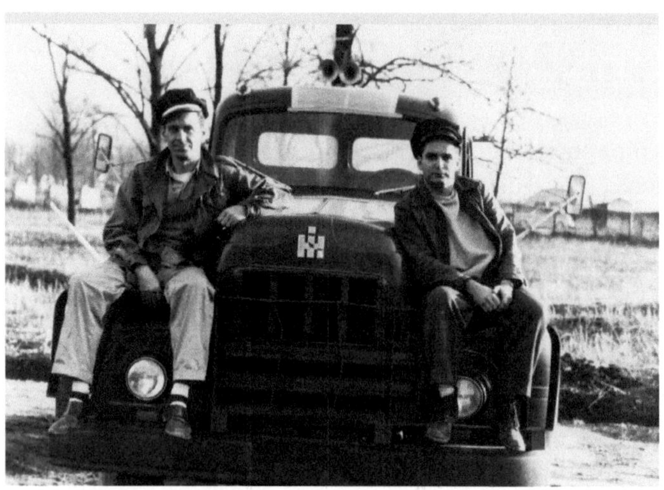

Throughout its history, the FDA has striven to keep the public safe—through legislation, laboratory oversight, public education presentations, and undercover drug inspections. Here are two undercover FDA agents in the mid 1950s, William Hill and Charles Eisenberg, ready to intercept illegally trucked and sold amphetamines and barbiturates.

campaigns and even to instruct the manufacturer to present a new advertising campaign to clear up any misconceptions. The ads and labels of OTC medications undergo the same level of FDA scrutiny to make all of the information readable and understandable to laypersons.

The FDA is also responsible for the annual publishing of *Approved Drug Products with Therapeutic Equivalence Evaluations*, better known as the Orange Book (available online). It identifies all drugs that are approved for both their safety and efficacy. This reference is used by drug wholesalers and in pharmacies primarily to make sure that generic products can be safely substituted for brand-name products.

The FDA offers two online publications, the Purple Book and the Green Book. The Purple Book (*Lists of Licensed Biological Products with Reference Product Exclusivity and Biosimilarity or Interchangability Evaluations*) is a guide to approved bioengineered drugs. The Green Book *(FDA Approved Animal Drug Products)* is a guide to drugs for use in veterinary medicine. There will be more discussion on these references in Chapter 4.

US Pharmacopeial Convention

The FDA works with the US Pharmacopeial Convention (USP)—an independent, nonprofit, scientific organization—and uses its quality standards for prescription drugs, OTC drugs, and dietary supplements. Their annual book of standards, or compendium, is called the ***US Pharmacopeia–National Formulary (USP–NF)***. All new drugs approved by the FDA must meet applicable *USP–NF* standards. The USP also has important works on dietary supplements, homeopathic products, and sterile and hazardous compounding standards.

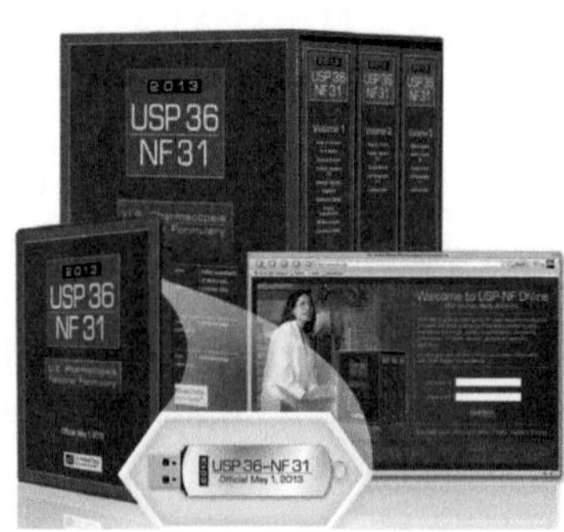

The *US Pharmacopeia-National Formulary* is an important reference for pharmacists and pharmacy technicians.

Drug Enforcement Administration

The **Drug Enforcement Administration (DEA)** is the primary agency responsible for enforcing the laws regarding potentially addictive controlled substances, both illegal and legal. Every pharmacy, healthcare institution, warehouse, or business involved in any way with controlled substances must be registered with the DEA so that it can track the ingredients and control the drugs. One of the DEA's functions is to inspect all medical facilities, including pharmacies, where suspicious activity is detected. The DEA works with state drug and narcotic agencies responsible for routine unannounced physical inspections; in addition, the local agency investigates issues of unsafe prescribing, dispensing, or forging of controlled drug prescriptions. The DEA can track the flow of narcotics from manufacturer to warehouse to pharmacy to patient.

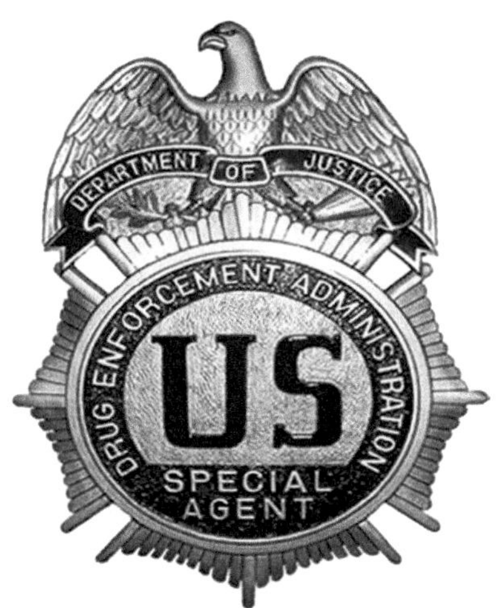

The Drug Enforcement Administration investigates suspect increases in drug usage.

The DEA—with the help of each state board of pharmacy and its agents—also keeps a close watch on prescribing and dispensing trends. For instance, any sudden increase in scheduled drug usage by a particular pharmacy (or in prescriptions by a particular physician) may trigger an investigation. Therefore, pharmacy personnel, including technicians, must be diligent in their handling and record keeping of controlled substances, as the misuse of these drugs has become a growing problem. Patient profiles must be carefully reviewed to monitor any overzealous use of controlled substances.

Through audits, the DEA can determine if a pharmacy warehouse, for instance, is dispensing controlled substances outside the scope of its licensed registration. In a much publicized case in 2012, the DEA suspended the license of a Florida wholesaler for two years, claiming that the company neglected its primary responsibility to prevent the diversion of controlled substance medications from legal prescriptions to illegal distribution at two chain drug stores. These two pharmacies dispensed over forty times the usual amount of an extended-release form of oxycodone (OxyContin), a strongly addictive Schedule II opioid drug. Drug wholesalers generally set monthly limits on the quantities of scheduled drugs they will send to individual pharmacies. It is not uncommon for a wholesaler to refuse to sell and send high volumes of medications, such as alprazolam (Xanax) or tramadol (Ultram), to a community pharmacy at the end of the calendar month if they are near their limit. In such cases, if the drug is needed, the pharmacist or technician must identify an alternate source.

National Council for Prescription Drug Programs

The **National Council for Prescription Drug Programs (NCPDP)** is a not-for-profit organization of members in the pharmacy service industry that issues six-digit NCPDP Processor ID Numbers (BINs), which pharmacies and pharmaceutical providers use for online electronic records transmissions. Similarly, prescribers and pharmacies each have a **National Provider Identifier (NPI)**, a unique 10-digit number, issued by the Centers for Medicare & Medicaid Services for government reimbursement. Pharmacies use these numbers in their FDA and DEA interactions and in ordering, purchasing, and tracking their medications, and in processing third-party prescription claims to insurance. The NCPDP has issued unique identifying numbers to more than 70,000 pharmacies. In addition to these numbers, it has established industry standards to facilitate online e-prescribing and exchanges of health information between pharmacies and medical offices. Also, pharmacists are eligible to request an NCPDP number, which may be needed for future pharmacy clinical service reimbursements.

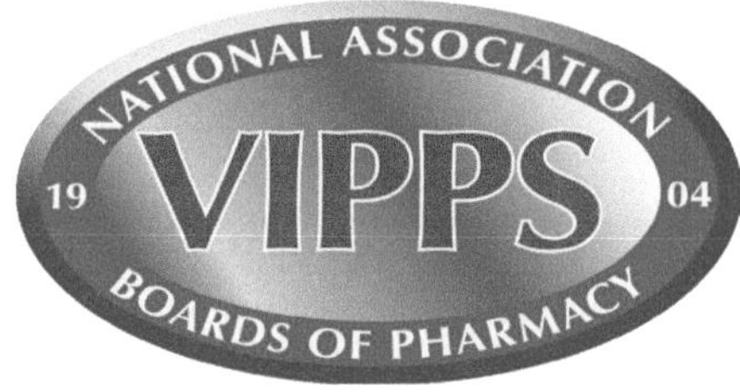

This seal of approval appears on accredited online pharmacy websites indicating that they meet nationally approved standards of pharmacy practice and are complying with the state standards for their location.

National Association of Boards of Pharmacy

The **National Association of Boards of Pharmacy (NABP)** is the only professional organization that represents all 50 state boards of pharmacy. NABP has developed a model for state practice acts and regulations to help individual state boards of pharmacy build their own regulations. Their *Model State Pharmacy*

Act and Model Rules of the National Association of Boards of Pharmacy streamlines the best of the differing pharmacy laws enacted in individual states to provide model language to the state boards of pharmacy. NABP has no legal regulatory authority but offers resources to assist state pharmacy boards as they put into place their laws, requirements, oversight, and enforcement.

NABP also operates the **Verified Internet Pharmacy Practice Sites (VIPPS)**, an accreditation program for internet pharmacies recognized by 17 states. With thousands of rogue internet drug outlets—known as fake online pharmacies—distributing counterfeit and unapproved drugs, VIPPS was developed in 1999 to help patients in the United States find legitimate internet pharmacies. The VIPPS program addresses such issues as protection of the patient's privacy, authentication and security of prescription orders, adherence to a recognized assurance policy, and provision of meaningful consultation between patients and pharmacists. NABP also performs an on-site survey of each VIPPS applicant's pharmacy facility. NABP then posts a list of VIPPS online pharmacies, which can be found at https://PharmPractice 7e.ParadigmEducation.com/NABP.

Only legitimate internet pharmacies and pharmacy-related websites qualify for ".pharmacy" domains. When patients find a site ending in ".pharmacy," they will know that it is a safe and legal online pharmacy that has been vetted through NABP's ".pharmacy" standards. ".Pharmacy" sites operating in a non-US country will also be vetted against that country's laws, regulations, and pharmacy practice standards. More information and a list of approved entities with registered ".pharmacy" domain names, is available at https://PharmPractice7e.ParadigmEducation.com/SafePharmacy.

Practice Tip

Remember that laws and regulations vary from state to state. When a conflict occurs between a state and a federal law or regulation, the more stringent law or regulation always applies. Get to know your state laws.

State Boards of Pharmacy

Governor-appointed leaders from the pharmacy community and consumer representatives make up the membership of each **state board of pharmacy**. The selected pharmacists generally represent community, hospital, and other areas of pharmacy practice. These boards work with the state departments of health and advise state legislators on pharmacy laws and regulations. Each state board is also responsible for overseeing the inspection of all new pharmacies and maintains a database of all active pharmacist licenses (and those of pharmacy technicians if required). Most states include the annual registration of pharmacy technicians in their database. They set the legal pharmacist-to-pharmacy technician ratio as well as oversee the licenses and certifications.

Some state boards specifically authorize the scope of technician practice, whereas other states define what the technician may do by detailing what the pharmacist must do. In these states, *by default, duties not legally mandated to the pharmacist may be*

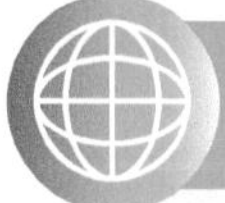

IN THE REAL WORLD

Pharmacy corporations or community pharmacies may elect to enforce more stringent control policies than those mandated by the state. For example, some pharmacies in locations experiencing high rates of drug abuse or OTC drug recreational use may implement a store policy requiring a written prescription from a licensed provider for the selling and dispensing of any OTC Schedule V drug.

carried out by the technician. For instance, many states allow any pharmacy technician to compound intravenous (IV) solutions under a pharmacist's supervision, whereas other states require pharmacy technicians to be specially certified. Still other states restrict IV solution preparation only to pharmacists.

Each state has its own drug enforcement agency that works with the regional DEA and may have different priorities. As noted, the state boards of pharmacy often implement their own regulations that are more rigorous than the federal standards, especially in terms of controlled substances. For example, most states allow some mechanism for filling emergency narcotic pain-relieving medication for terminally ill hospice patients, but some do not.

For noncontrolled drugs, there are variances in state regulations as well. Typically a foreign physician (e.g., from Canada or Mexico) may not prescribe drugs to be filled in US pharmacies. However, some boards of pharmacy in states adjacent to the Canadian or Mexican border may allow dispensing if certain conditions are met. Even the dispensing of insulin syringes may be limited by state boards—some states require a prescription for the syringes in an effort to discourage illicit drug use.

Occupational Safety and Health Administration

The **Occupational Safety and Health Administration (OSHA)** is an agency of the Department of Labor. Its primary mission is to ensure the safety and health of US workers. It establishes and enforces workplace regulations and standards; provides training, outreach, and education; and encourages continual improvement in workplace safety and health.

Pharmacy facilities must follow OSHA legal standards and regulations for their facility and processes, with all employees complying. OSHA even offers a video of a hospital pharmacy practice area and various elements to consider for safety at https://PharmPractice7e.ParadigmEducation.com/OSHAvideo.

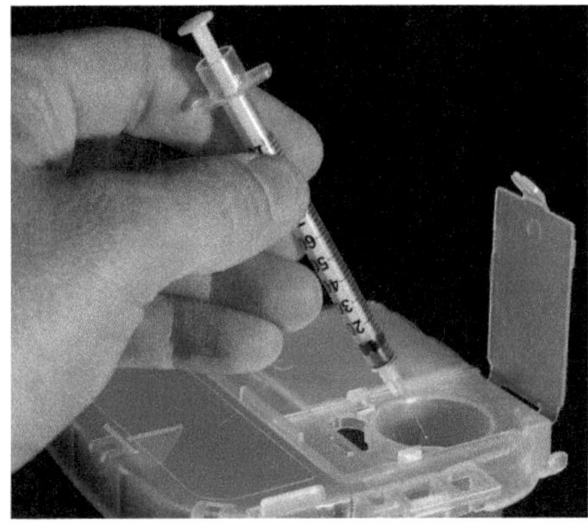

Technicians must follow OSHA rules to safely dispose of syringes to prevent the transmission of communicable diseases such as hepatitis and HIV. OSHA has many rules for hazardous compounding to protect staff from toxic exposure.

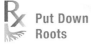

Put Down Roots

Epidemic grew from the Greek word *epi*, "among," and *demos*, "people." *Pan*, in Greek, means "all," giving us the word *pandemic*, a disease that affects all people, or an international epidemic.

Centers for Disease Control and Prevention

This federal agency, under the Department of Health and Human Services, provides guidelines to protect the public from large-scale health issues and illnesses. The Centers for Disease Control and Prevention (CDC) grew out of an army effort to fight malaria a century ago, which is still part of its work. The CDC works to fight infectious diseases to stop **epidemics** (regional widespread contagious diseases) and **pandemics** (globally widespread epidemics), sexually transmitted diseases, food-borne diseases, and other contagious illnesses. In addition, it focuses on educational awareness about health, disease, and addiction prevention, as well as environmental health, occupational safety and health, and injury prevention.

Many vaccinations and prescriptions have been developed for these preventive health goals. Pharmacy technicians encounter CDC guidance in such things as hand hygiene practices and temperatures for vaccine refrigeration. Hospitals, because so many sick patients gather there, have to be particularly concerned about contagious diseases. This will be covered in the hospital practice unit in Chapter 12. The CDC makes recommendations, not regulations.

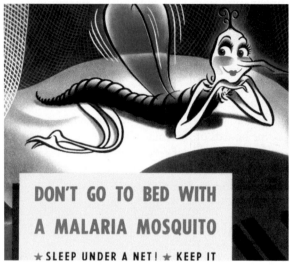

Theodor Geisel, before he became the beloved Dr. Seuss, used his talents to make posters and films for army troops. This poster was made for the Malaria Control in War Areas program, which evolved into the CDC.

State Departments and Boards of Health

Each state also has its own department or board of health to oversee the public health of state citizens. These entities can establish their own regulations for infectious diseases and other health issues that can indirectly affect pharmacy practice. For instance, they can choose to quarantine certain individuals or set up vaccine clinics under emergency situations. They may enlist the help of pharmacies in working against state epidemics or public health threats. For instance, in 2014, Governor Andrew Cuomo convened a gathering of state agencies and major hospitals to have an emergency response plan for the Ebola health alert. In this, pharmacists and technicians would have the job of preparing increased medications within the hospitals but not direct patient contact.

2.5 Drug and Professional Standards

As discussed, many healthcare and pharmacy professional organizations are involved in setting **professional standards**. Some work hand in hand with legal and enforcement agencies, offering guidelines for practice to offer the best care and fulfill the laws.

US Pharmacopeia Pharmacy Practice Standards

In addition to setting quality standards for drugs, the USP has also developed standards for practice by pharmacists and pharmacy technicians. Many standards relate to and affect compounding practices. For example, the *USP–NF* has General Chapters <795> (nonsterile) and <797> (sterile), which set standards involving the storage, packaging, and preparation of nonsterile and sterile compounded preparations. *USP–NF* has an additional electronic publication: *USP Compounding Compendium.*

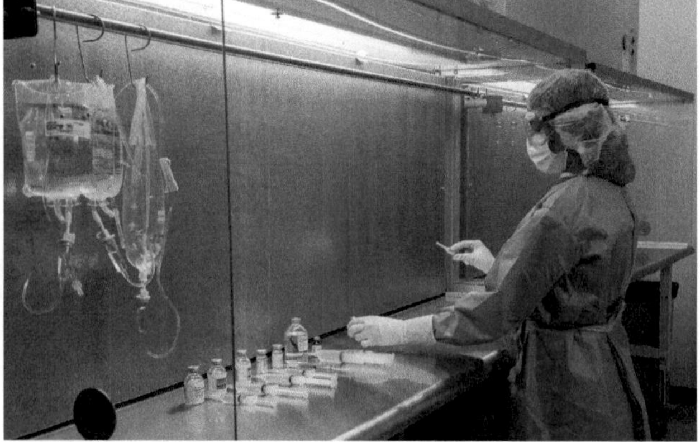

The pharmacist and technician must follow USP standards in the compounding of nonsterile (as shown here) and sterile medications.

The most current USP standards need to be incorporated and

continually updated into the policies and procedures of compounding pharmacies and the practices of technicians and pharmacists working in these areas and cleanrooms. The USP standards are being adopted by many divisions of the government and organizations that provide **accreditation**, the status achieved by meeting the quality standards and requirements designated by the accrediting organization, including state boards of pharmacy and the Joint Commission. *USP* Chapters <795> and <797> are discussed in more detail in Chapters 10, 12, and 13.

In addition, *USP* General Chapter <800> addresses the handling of hazardous substances in compounding, storage, shipping, and other handling methods. Hazardous substances include chemotherapy drugs but extend beyond them. The USP practices must be applied not only for the protection of the patients, but also for the technicians and other staff. These practice standards were updated in 2019. An introduction to hazardous compounding is found in Chapter 13.

The Joint Commission

The **Joint Commission** is a nongovernmental, nonprofit professional healthcare association that sets high standards of care for hospitals and other healthcare institutions. It provides rigorous inspections of their facilities in its approval processes for official accreditation. Although accreditation is voluntary under the law, many insurance carriers and governmental agencies require it for hospitals to receive reimbursement.

2.6 Legal Responsibilities of Pharmacy Personnel

Though all these laws and standards can seem overwhelming, procedures to adhere to them are built into the everyday practices of pharmacy, so the laws need not be difficult to remember and follow. Each facility manager is responsible for ensuring that the correct processes are established and personnel are trained. The pharmacists—who have to make judgments in the filling and dispensing of drugs, counseling patients, and overseeing the work of technicians—have the majority of the burden of liability. Yet all personnel work as a team in a pharmacy and are responsible for the parts they play. As pharmacy technicians shift into greater roles of responsibility, elements of liability shift with them. They must feel confident asking questions when situations or processes seem amiss or neglected to prevent problems.

No specific federal definition of the pharmacy technician's role yet exists, and no uniform definition has been adopted by all states. Rather, the technician's responsibilities are under constant review and change as states recognize the extending roles of pharmacists and automation and the need to adjust the technician's role to keep up with the needs and demands of the field, patients, and laws. Technicians can make the difference between life and death for patients in many situations by their conduct, and they always need to keep this idea foremost in their minds as they work.

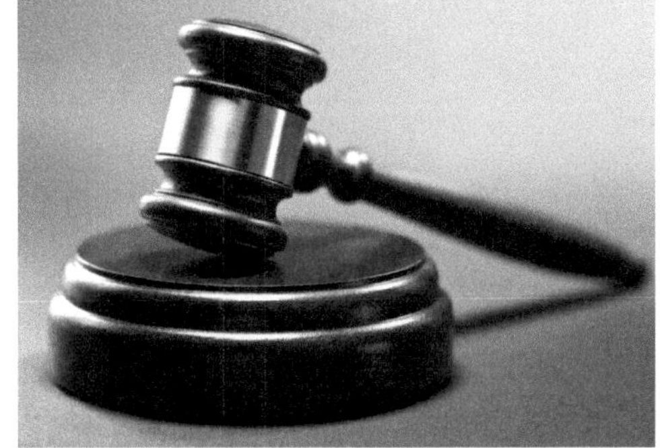

Serious violations of laws, regulations, or ethics by pharmacy technicians may result in loss of job, suspension or revocation of professional ability to practice, or criminal or civil penalties.

As a technician-in-training, you should visit the website of your state pharmacy board and talk to your instructors to get to know state-specific statutes and regulations. Some states will test you on them in order for you to be allowed to practice. Other references that are useful in comparing duties from state to state include the following:

- *Pharmacy Law Digest*
- Annual NABP *Survey of Pharmacy Law*
- Pharmacy Technician Certification Board website

2.7 The Courts and Pharmacy Professionals

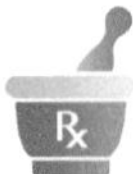

Practice Tip

You can find access to many different state pharmacy boards by clicking on the map at https://PharmPractice7e.Paradigm Education.com/PPMI assessment. You can also visit the websites of each state pharmacy board.

When a legal problem arises involving a pharmacy practice, the courts often become involved. The courts are separated between those established to resolve issues between the government and offending parties—**criminal law** cases—and those between citizens—**civil law** cases. In both criminal and civil courts, the party (person or group) filing the case is called the **plaintiff**, and the entity (person or group) being sued, or whom the case is against, is called the **defendant**.

The plaintiff is responsible for providing sufficient evidence to prove their case, which is referred to as **burden of proof**. The standard, or level, of proof must eliminate **reasonable doubt**, which is a doubt about the guilt of a defendant that arises or remains after thorough consideration of the evidence or lack thereof. This means that the prosecutor or plaintiff must provide enough evidence that the party committed the offending act to convince a jury "beyond any reasonable doubt". In civil cases, the burden of proof is not as high; it is that a "preponderance of evidence" points to a decision, or an accumulation of facts favors one side enough to decide upon the case.

The type of punishment in both kinds of court cases is dependent upon many factors, including the severity of the violation, the effects, and the type of case it is: criminal or civil. In the criminal case, the defendant might face monetary fines, probation, loss of professional license or ability to practice, or prison. The civil case might result in monetary awards to the plaintiff.

Criminal Violation of Pharmacy Laws and Regulations

When pharmacy violations occur under any level of law—federal, state, or local—a government prosecutor or public representative often brings a case against the suspected party. Such a case is filed using phrases like *State v. Jessica Smith, PharmD.* Examples of violations include providing controlled substances to people without prescriptions or for nonprescription purposes or substituting the wrong drug. It is the prosecutor's duty to see that society is protected from practitioners who violate the law. For instance, in 2002, when a Missouri pharmacist was convicted of tampering, adulterating, and misbranding cancer chemotherapy drugs, he was convicted of 20 felony counts and sentenced to 17–30 years in jail without parole. In addition, 307 civil lawsuits were filed against him, including 100 wrongful death suits.

Before court, the state board of pharmacy reviews pharmacy cases, and lesser cases are generally settled out of court. The board applies varying levels of consequences based on the offenses (see Table 2.3 for examples). It determines whether the defendant's license should be revoked, suspended (with voluntary surrender of license for the time period), not reissued, or the person be put on probation.

If evidence of alcohol or drug abuse is proven, the state board may require successful completion of a drug rehabilitation program or some other actions before the license can be reinstated, with random drug screening afterwards (see Table 2.3 for examples). As demonstrated in the Missouri case, if the severity of the offense and/or victim outcome merits it, the state board can ask for a criminal investigation, which can lead to indictment (formal criminal charge) and a trial, with criminal penalties of fines, probation, and/or jail time. Incarceration is rarely the punishment unless the acts in question were particularly deliberate and egregious, had an extreme outcome, or were clearly negligent (even an accident).

TABLE 2.3 Samples of California State Disciplinary Actions

Offense	Action
Personal misuse of drugs or alcohol; improper possession of controlled substances for sale; criminal offense with controlled substances; fraudulent acts, etc.	Revocation of license, along with such options as a requirement for drug rehabilitation or mental health counseling prior to reinstatement Minimum 90 days suspension with 3 to 5 years probation and public reprimand; board fees paid by violator
Emergency refill without prescriber authority; improper substitution of generic drug; or dispensing in incorrectly labeled container	One year probation with optional terms that can be added
Unlawful possession or disposal of needle or syringe; unprofessional conduct, etc.	Three-year probation

Civil Laws and Pharmacy Personnel

In cases where a criminal offense resulted in personal injury or damages, the victim or the victim's family may also sue the party in civil court for monetary damages. The plaintiff is responsible for the burden of proof. If this situation occurs, the violator may be tried in two different courts, criminal and civil, as in the case of the Missouri pharmacist presented earlier. If there is not sufficient evidence to prove the criminal case beyond reasonable doubt, those who have been harmed may file a civil case. There are two main types of civil court actions pertinent to pharmacy: torts (which include negligence and malpractice) and contracts.

Torts and Personal Injuries

In civil law, a tort refers to personal injuries. **Torts** address wrongs that one citizen commits against another, with the injured party suing the party that caused the injury (e.g., *Edgar Gonzales v. Dave's Drug Store and Dave Jones, RPh*). The most common tort in the medical/pharmacy arena is **negligence**, or carelessness, not acting as a reasonably prudent person would in the same situation. **Malpractice**, defined as improper, illegal, or neglectful professional activity, is a form of negligence. Other examples of torts include slander (using spoken words to speak falsely of another), libel (using written words to falsely represent another), assault (threatening another with bodily harm), and battery (causing bodily harm to another). For example, if a pharmacist or pharmacy technician speaks to a customer disparagingly about the professional competence of another healthcare professional, that pharmacist or technician may be found guilty of slander.

IN THE REAL WORLD

In February 2006 in Cleveland, Ohio, Emily Jerry, a bright-eyed two-year old, had just finished chemotherapy. Her tumor seemed gone, but her physician wanted one more round of chemotherapy to make sure. There was a backlog of hospital pharmacy orders, the computers were not working properly, and staffing was inadequate. A pharmacy technician, feeling rushed, made a chemotherapy compounding error (24 times the prescribed chemotherapy solution concentration). The technician told the pharmacist that she might have made an error. Pressured for time, the pharmacist did not check it carefully, and Emily Jerry died in great pain.

The state board revoked the pharmacist's license, and he was indicted on charges of reckless homicide and involuntary manslaughter (unintentional death). He received six months in jail, six months under house arrest, 400 hours of community service, and thousands of dollars in court costs. The technician, who had no academic study or certification, was not prosecuted.

The bereaved family founded the Emily Jerry Foundation, dedicated to saving lives by reducing preventable medical errors. The foundation has pushed for greater education and certification for pharmacy technicians. In Ohio, they passed Emily's Act in 2009, which requires that pharmacy technicians be at least 18 years of age, be certified and registered, and face disciplinary actions for errors. The foundation and the National Pharmacy Technician Association have been pushing for Emily's Act to be integrated into every state and to become federal law.

Emily's father, Christopher Jerry, told ***Pharmacy Times***, "I believe in hindsight that my little Emily's short life here on Earth was truly meant to save tens of thousands of lives going forward. I want to get technicians around the nation to continue to rally, and to let them know that I want to be their voice. If we all unite together on a national level, we will have a much more powerful voice to elevate the profession." Visit the Emily Jerry Foundation website to learn more: https://PharmPractice7e.ParadigmEducation.com/EmilyJerry.

A patient may sue the healthcare provider for malpractice when a professional fails to offer the minimum standard of care that results in injury. The legal **standard of care** is the level of care or established practices commonly expected of a particular kind of healthcare provider in the local community. Standard of care is based on:

- comparisons with the actions of other similarly educated healthcare professionals in the same situation and geographic area
- compliance with existing written guidelines, protocols, or policies and procedures
- expert testimony of healthcare professionals provided by the plaintiff or the defense

Only those healthcare providers who work in the same geographic area and have the same level of training would be compared for this specific standard of care. For example, a Denver pharmacist or technician would not be compared with those in Boston because local practices and protocols may differ. They would, however, be compared with other pharmacists or technicians working in the Denver area. Likewise, the job performance of a certified technician with advanced education and training practicing in Atlanta would be compared with other certified technicians in Atlanta. Because of the educational training, the technician would be held to a higher standard in a court of law than a noncertified technician.

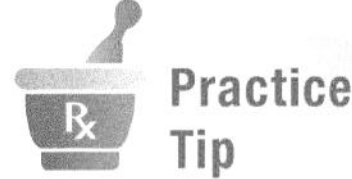

Practice Tip

Generally technicians are not brought to court because of actions done within their job description since they are under a pharmacist's approval. However, as technicians grow more educated, trained, are certified, and are given greater responsibilities, they are also growing more susceptible to litigation.

Negligence and Burden of Proof When a case of negligence or malpractice is brought, the burden is on the plaintiff to prove the **four Ds of negligence**: duty, dereliction, damages, and direct cause. The plaintiff must first prove that the defendant *had a duty* to provide care, or that there was a written or implied contract for care between the two parties. The plaintiff must then prove that the defendant *was derelict* or lacking in this duty, that this *caused actual damages* to the plaintiff, and that the damages were *directly caused* by the defendant's derelict conduct. There must be a "preponderance of the evidence" that it is more likely that the defendant is guilty of the accused act than not.

If the defendant is found guilty, then they will be ordered to pay a monetary award to the plaintiff. It is not possible, however, for the defendant to be sent to prison through a civil court. Hospitals, residential facilities, pharmacies, most practicing pharmacists, and some pharmacy technicians carry professional liability insurance to protect their business and personal assets from civil lawsuits involving negligence or malpractice.

Legal Outcomes Several levels of negligence or malpractice may be determined during an investigation and subsequent trial. If two or more causes or circumstances add to the assessment of negligence and resulting personal injury to the patient, then a case of contributory negligence may be determined. For example, if the physician and pharmacist were both responsible for the patient's injury, then each may be found guilty. The plaintiff's award may be broken down proportionally according to the judge's or jury's assessment of comparative negligence.

In this instance, if the physician was found to be more responsible than the pharmacist, then the award may be broken down wherein the physician must pay 70% and the pharmacist 30% of the damages awarded. Cases even exist in which the patient is found to have contributed to his or her own injury (for example, not taking medication as directed) and is thus found to be comparatively negligent. In this type of case, the plaintiff's total award may be reduced by a certain percentage depending on the judge's or jury's determination.

Law of Agency and Contracts

The **law of agency and contracts** is based on the Latin term *respondeat superior*, which translates to "let the master answer," referring to the employee-employer relationship. An employee is, in effect, an "agent" for an employer and may enter into contracts on the employer's behalf. This is an important agreement in the healthcare setting. For example, in a medical office, a nurse generally acts as a physician's agent with patients; in the pharmacy, technicians act as agents for the pharmacist or pharmacy. This principle means not only that an implied contract exists in the healthcare setting, but also that the contract is just as valid as any verbal agreement or written contract drawn up by a physician or a pharmacist.

In a pharmacy, the exchange of a prescription between a patient and a pharmacy technician who agrees to fill the prescription is considered an implied contract. By accepting the prescription for filling, the pharmacy and its personnel are now obligated to provide the patient with a service. If a mistake is made, then the pharmacy and/or pharmacist may be held liable, even though the pharmacist was not specifically the one

IN THE REAL WORLD

The following are real-life examples of preventable medication errors in the pharmacy. Training and experience are necessary to protect the public from these types of errors.

- In 1997, a technician failed to dilute a dose of injectable enalapril that a doctor had prescribed to control the blood pressure of a premature infant. The child received a 750-mcg dose instead of a 6-mcg dose and suffered neurological damage at Boston Children's Hospital. In the 2002 civil suit, the pharmacist, pharmacy supervisor, and technician were sued. They were covered under the hospital's malpractice insurance.
- In Florida, a teenage pharmacy technician, who was not formally trained or certified, typed in a dosage that was ten times the prescribed dose (by including an additional zero). This resulted in the death of a mother of three children. The state appeals court upheld a $26 million settlement against the chain pharmacy. The error could have been discovered by a routine check of the prescription by the pharmacist, but the prescription was not carefully checked; the pharmacy may also have been negligent in utilizing a young untrained technician.
- In Maryland, a pharmacy technician inadvertently gave someone else's medication to the wrong patient; the patient took the medication and died, and the pharmacy settled out of court. A similar case in Texas with the wrong drug being dispensed resulted in a costly hospitalization and a lawsuit against the pharmacy.

who accepted the prescription and entered into the contract to provide the service.

Therefore, the pharmacist (or pharmacy, in the case of a chain) must answer for all of the acts of their employees. However, a pharmacy technician can still be held liable if it can be proven that the technician overstepped the limitations of their position, such as by dispensing a prescription drug without a check by the supervising pharmacist.

Invasion of privacy is another pharmacy violation that may result in a civil lawsuit. Medical and prescription records, including those generated in the pharmacy, are considered the physical property of the facility that produced them. However, the information contained in them is the patient's property. It may not be divulged without the patient's consent to any nonmedical person, another provider, or an organization, unless by **subpoena**, a legal order.

If a member of the pharmacy staff violates patient privacy, the pharmacy is held responsible. Breaking HIPAA privacy laws is a federal criminal offense. HIPAA violations may carry heavy fines to the pharmacy and immediate termination of employment for the violator, including technicians. Confidentiality of medical information is further discussed in Chapter 15.

2.8 Ramifications for Technicians

As you have learned, the field of pharmacy is guided and protected by a fabric of interwoven laws, regulations, and standards. Knowing why the laws were enacted can help you remember them and take them seriously. Fortunately, these professional and legal expectations are integrated into everyday staff procedures.

Carefully following the established practice procedures in any pharmacy setting is extremely important because people's lives depend on your knowledge and skills as well as the knowledge and skills of the pharmacist. That's why your education as a pharmacy technician is so important. What you do or don't do makes a difference—not only to the patients and those you work with, but also to yourself both professionally and legally.

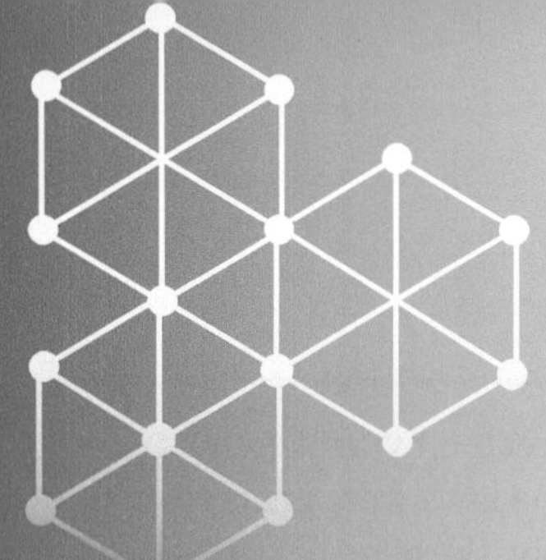

Review and Assessment

CHAPTER SUMMARY

- Numerous governmental agencies and professional organizations protect the public by overseeing the manufacture, dispensing, and use of drugs to ensure quality and prevent harm to others.
- Interrelated laws, regulations, standards, and ethics guide the practice of pharmacy technicians and pharmacists.
- Laws affecting pharmacy practice grew out of problems that harmed the public. These laws are important to know because they still have effects on pharmacy practices and procedures today.
- The Pure Food and Drug Act of 1906 and the Food, Drug, and Cosmetic Act of 1938 addressed problems of adulterated and misbranded drug products. The FD&C established the Food and Drug Administration, and future acts have outlined and expanded its role in drug and dietary supplement oversight.
- The FDA depends upon the standards for drug ingredients and procedures for drug preparation and pharmacy compounding procedures set by the US Pharmacopeial Convention (USP) in the *US Pharmacopeia–National Formulary (USP–NF)* and other USP resources.
- The Drug Price Competition and Patent Term Restoration Act of 1984, also known as the Hatch-Waxman Act, streamlined the process to approve equally effective drugs with nonproprietary names, or generic names.
- The Comprehensive Drug Abuse Prevention and Control Act of 1970 established schedules for controlled substances, with regulatory oversight provided by the DEA.
- The Health Insurance Portability and Accountability Act (HIPAA) of 1996 established standards of privacy that determine many pharmacy practices involving medication dispensing and patient medication information that technicians must know and follow.
- The Medicare Modernization Act of 2003 provided a voluntary drug insurance program to patients eligible for Medicare benefits called Medicare Part D.
- The Affordable Care Act of 2010 mandated that all US citizens must eventually have healthcare coverage.
- The deaths of patients in many states from a nonsterile facility and compounding practices led to the passage of the Drug Quality and Security Act. It also alerted states to the need for requiring facilities, pharmacists, and technicians to adhere to the most current USP sterile compounding and aseptic technique standards.

- OSHA protects the employee from unprotected handling of syringes and hazardous substances and other unsafe practices.
- State boards of pharmacy create their own drug regulations that must be known and followed; where state and federal laws differ, the strictest rule applies, which is often the state regulation. Pharmacy technicians must know and rigidly adhere to state regulations.
- State boards of pharmacy license and register pharmacies and pharmacists. They also determine the level of education, experience, certification, and registration that pharmacy technicians need in order to practice.
- The legal status of pharmacy technicians and their allowable duties vary from state to state, but technicians must always act under the direct supervision of licensed pharmacists.
- Criminal law and courts cover violations that harm the public or break laws; such violations can result in imprisonment, fines, restitution, and other penalties.
- Civil law and courts address harm or damage to other citizens and result in monetary settlements and other reparations.
- State pharmacy boards have the power to take administrative actions against those who violate state pharmacy laws, regulations, and standards.
- Technicians who do not follow best practices can kill or injure people with their momentary negligence, so continual focus and safety vigilance must be in mind. They can also lose their jobs, be fined, suspended, or face other sanctions.
- Violations of patient confidentiality by pharmacy technicians and other personnel can result in both legal repercussions and immediate termination of employment.

CHECK YOUR UNDERSTANDING

Take a moment to review what you have learned in this chapter and answer the following questions.

1. A benchmark or desired normal level of quality for a product or professional performance is called a(n)
   a. statutory law.
   b. ethical dilemma.
   c. standard.
   d. regulation.
2. Legislated rules and procedures that exist to maintain minimum public safety standards is the definition of
   a. regulations.
   b. ethics.
   c. criminal laws.
   d. professional policies.
3. Following a code of high professional standards is an example of
   a. ethics.
   b. criminal laws.
   c. civil laws.
   d. regulations.
4. The Drug Enforcement Administration (DEA) classifies controlled prescription drugs for greater or lesser access. The DEA reclassified which of the following controlled substances from a Schedule III to a Schedule II drug for greater control?
   a. tramadol
   b. anabolic steroids
   c. hydrocodone combination products
   d. liquid codeine cough preparations

5. Which of the following drugs is exempt from "child-resistant" containers?
   a. hydrocodone tablets
   b. nitroglycerin sublingual tablets
   c. ibuprofen tablets
   d. amoxicillin tablets

6. To be approved as a generic drug, the pharmaceutical manufacturer must prove
   a. safety.
   b. bioequivalence.
   c. efficacy.
   d. affordability.

MAKE CONNECTIONS

Take a moment to consider what you have learned in this chapter and respond thoughtfully to the following prompts. Note that some of these activities will require internet access.

1. CBD oil has seen increased popularity as a potential pain reliever. Using what you know of Federal government regulations and state laws involving cannabis, argue which agency (if any) should provide oversight into the oil's production and why.
2. Review the four Ds of negligence and research the Emily Jerry case. Argue how all four Ds apply to the Jerry case against the pharmacist.

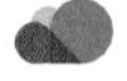 The online course includes additional review and assessment resources.

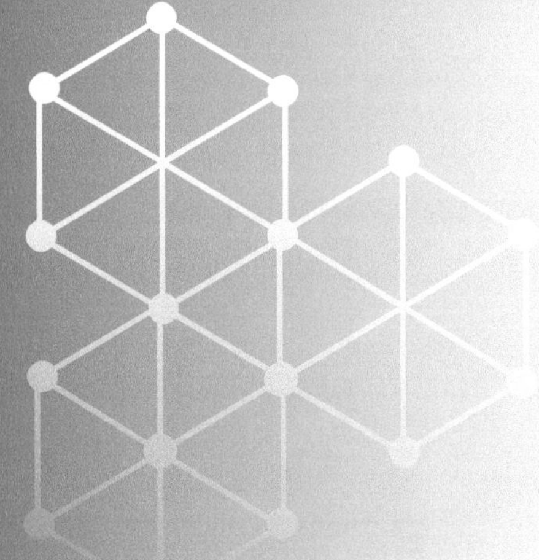

3

Drug and Supplement Development

Learning Objectives

1. Define the term *drug* and distinguish between prescription drugs, over-the-counter (OTC) drugs, homeopathic drugs, and dietary supplements. (Section 3.1)
2. Discuss the different classifications of drug uses: therapeutic, prophylactic, destructive, pharmacodynamic, and diagnostic. (Section 3.2)
3. Describe germ theory and how it has affected the development of sterile compounding and key drug types, such as vaccines, antibiotics, and antivirals. (Section 3.3)
4. Explain the roles of probiotics, vitamins, and nutrition in wellness. (Section 3.3)
5. Describe the discoveries that led to today's hormone and mental health drugs and the dangerous side effects when abused. (Section 3.3)
6. Describe how poisons from World War I and World War II became used in cancer drug therapies and why it is key that technicians follow US Pharmacopeial Convention (USP) practices for hazardous drug compounding. (Section 3.3)
7. Understand the significance of genetics on new drugs for diagnosis and treatment of diseases. (Section 3.3)
8. Explain ingredient sources, the differences between active and inert drug ingredients, and why careful checking of medication histories must be done to avoid problematic allergy and medication interactions. (Section 3.4)
9. Discuss the differing processes and roles of the Food and Drug Administration (FDA) and the USP in the approval of new and investigational pharmaceutical products, generic drugs, over-the-counter drugs, homeopathic drugs, and dietary supplements. (Sections 3.5, 3.6, 3.7, 3.8)

ASHP/ACPE Accreditation Standards
To view the *ASHP/ACPE Accreditation Standards* addressed in this chapter, refer to Appendix B.

Past centuries saw pharmacy and medicine evolve from strictly herbal medicines to a broad range of medications and dietary supplements. We often forget how medical and pharmaceutical advances over the last one hundred years have completely transformed people's average life span and quality of life. Most of us take for granted having drugs that help control contagious diseases, hormonal imbalances, cancer, pain, and chronic diseases, such as hypertension, asthma, and diabetes. We can also forget the dangers of medications that have not been carefully evaluated and approved, or that interact with other drugs.

Because new drug developments are built upon the scientific framework provided by earlier groundbreaking discoveries, it is important to know a little about the history of key discoveries to understand their effects on pharmacy practice today. This chapter considers these developments, the definition of drugs and other medications, and their classified uses and types of ingredients. It also explains the differences in the approval processes for prescription drugs, OTC drugs, homeopathic medications, and dietary supplements.

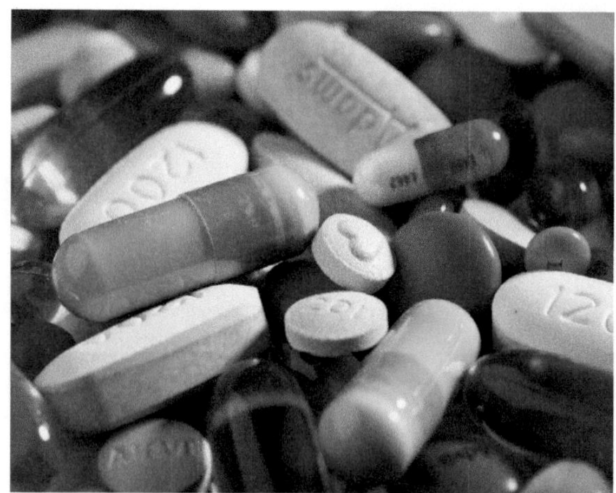

Medication has the ability to transform lives by helping to control or cure illness, pain, organ failure, cancer, and contagious and chronic diseases.

3.1 What Is a Drug?

FIGURE 3.1
Sample Prescription

A handwritten prescription should contain all the necessary information for the technician and pharmacist to fill it, and it should be signed by the provider. Most prescriptions are now e-prescriptions, but they still require the same elements.

Rx
Simona Brushfield, MD
2222 IH-35 South
Austin, TX 78703
(512) 555-1212 fax: (512) 555-1313

DOB Sept 12, 1953 DEA# ______
Pt. name Miguel Espinoza Date 01/15/2026
Address 7583 E 11th St
Austin, TX 78705

Humalog
100 units/mL Vial
1 vial
12 units subQ qAM;
18 units subQ qPM pc

Refill PRN times (no refill unless indicated)
Simona Brushfield, MD MD
______ License #

Laypeople generally think of drugs as only those substances manufactured by a pharmaceutical drug company for their medicinal effects, or narcotics that can be easily abused.

However, all drugs fall into one of three broad categories as designated by the FDA: prescription, over-the-counter (OTC), and homeopathic.

A **prescription drug**, formerly known as a *legend drug*, is a drug that can be legally dispensed to a patient only upon the receipt of a state-licensed healthcare provider's directive via an **e-prescription** (online electronic prescription) or a handwritten, faxed, or authorized verbal prescription. Consequently, all prescription drugs are labeled with the legend "Rx" (see Figure 3.1).

The prescription must have the provider's name, address, phone number, date written, and signature to be considered legal. The 10-digit National Provider Identifier (NPI) is often included for insurance purposes, and, for all controlled prescriptions, especially Schedule II drugs, the prescriber's Drug Enforcement Administration (DEA) number is required. This information, along with the patient's name, address, and date of birth, and the drug's name, dosage, duration, and prescribing date are all key parts of a prescription (see Figure 3.1). These elements will be covered in greater detail in the section on community pharmacy dispensing in Chapter 7.

An **over-the-counter (OTC)** drug is a medication that may be sold without a prescription. A **homeopathic** product uses minute dilutions of natural substances purportedly to stimulate the body's immune system.

Vitamins, minerals, herbs, and protein, energy, and nutritional drinks (which are also pharmacy health offerings) are not considered drugs by the FDA but rather **dietary supplements**.

3.2 Classifications for Drugs

Today's drugs are used not only to treat and cure illnesses, but also to aid in their diagnosis and even prevent or delay their onset. Because medications serve a variety of purposes in a patient's healthcare regimen, pharmacy technicians must be knowledgeable about the intended functions of commonly used medications; this knowledge can help them to recognize when something seems amiss in a prescription order. Medications are used for therapeutic, prophylactic, destructive, pharmacodynamic, and diagnostic purposes.

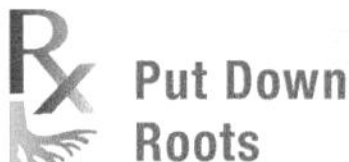

Put Down Roots

Therapeutic comes from the Greek word *therapeutikos*, to minister to or treat medically.

Therapeutic Agents

A **therapeutic agent** is a medication that targets a specific need in the body. Therapeutic agents are categorized according to the following functions:

Maintain Health

These prescription and OTC drugs as well as supplements of vitamins and minerals provide mild beneficial effects, support regular organ and cell functions, and help to regulate metabolism, or otherwise contribute to the maintenance of normal growth and functioning of the body. Specific examples include the use of the herbal supplement melatonin to help facilitate sleep or the use of baby aspirin to control clotting in patients at risk for a heart attack.

Relieve Symptoms

Examples of these medications include anti-inflammatory drugs, such as naproxen, used to treat fever, pain, or inflammation; narcotics to treat and prevent severe pain in terminally ill patients with cancer; and diuretics or water tablets to control excess fluid or control high blood pressure.

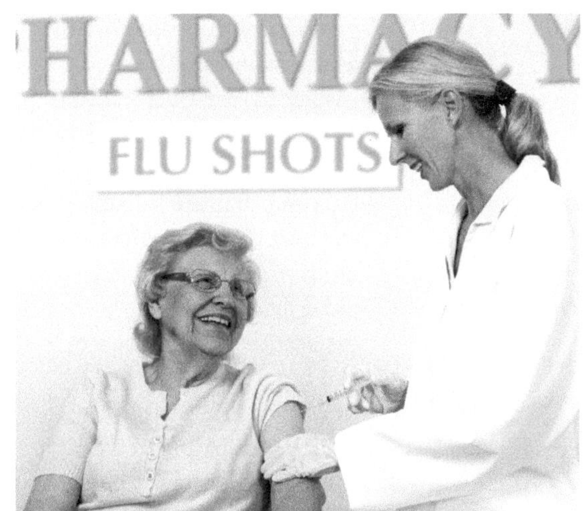

Many pharmacists administer flu, pneumonia, and shingles vaccines to prevent diseases.

Combat Illness

These medications include, for example, antibiotics to treat pneumonia, strep throat, or infections of the bladder or ear. Although antiviral medications do not cure HIV/AIDS, they may allow the immune system to remain sufficiently intact so as to delay disease progression. Drugs for Alzheimer's disease will not cure the patient, but they may delay both disease progression and loss of independence of the patient.

Reverse Disease Processes

These medications work to halt the decline of health and then improve bodily and mental processes; they include drugs that address depression, blood pressure, or cholesterol levels.

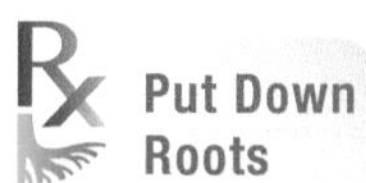

Put Down Roots

Prophylactic comes from the Greek *pro,* which means "before" or "in front of," and *phulsasin,* which means "to guard."

Prophylactic Agents

A **prophylactic agent** prevents illness or disease from occurring. Examples of prophylactic agents include the antiseptic and germicidal (germ-fighting) liquid chemicals used for preoperative hand washing procedures. Vaccines are used to prevent the onset of diseases, such as influenza (flu), pneumonia, shingles, tetanus, measles, mumps, rubella, chicken pox, poliomyelitis, meningitis, and hepatitis. Pharmacists are becoming increasingly involved in the administration of the influenza, pneumonia, shingles, and other vaccines to older adults and other high-risk individuals.

In certain situations, antibiotics (drugs to fight the growth of microorganisms) are prophylactic agents as well. For example, a patient who has a history of rheumatic fever may be given a large single dose of an antibiotic one hour prior to a dental procedure, or hunters going into areas infested with deer ticks may be prescribed antibiotics. This preventive action decreases the patient's risk for acquiring a serious bacterial infection.

Destructive Agents

A **destructive agent** works to kill specific living elements, such as bacteria, fungi, viruses, or abnormal cancer cells. Many antibiotics, especially those given in high doses and/or as intravenous (IV) infusions, are **bactericidal agents**, meaning that they kill rather than inhibit bacteria that are sensitive to these drugs. Penicillin is an example of a bactericidal drug (though resistance by some bacterial organisms has developed over the years). Another example of a destructive agent is radioactive iodine, which is used to destroy thyroid cells to reduce excess hormone secreted by the thyroid gland.

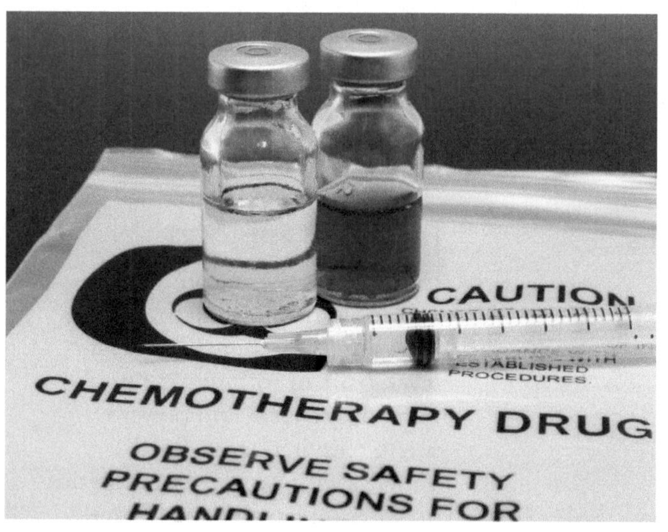

Traditional cancer drugs are destructive agents that kill both cancer and normal cells. Newer therapies are more selective.

Different antineoplastic drugs are used in combination to slow the growth of cancer cells at different phases of their cell growth cycles. Unfortunately, most of these drugs cannot effectively distinguish cancer cells from normal cells, so side effects often include hair loss, depression of the immune system, and ulcerations of the mouth or gastrointestinal (GI) tract. As cancer treatments have become more finely targeted, side effects have become somewhat less intense and long-lasting.

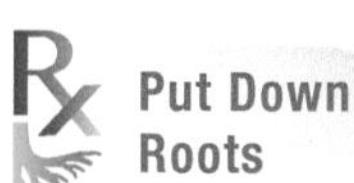

Put Down Roots

Pharmacodynamic comes from the Greek words *pharmakon,* drug, and *dynamic,* force or power.

Pharmacodynamic Agents

A **pharmacodynamic agent** is a medication that alters body functioning in a desired way. Pharmacodynamic agents can be used, for example, to stimulate or relax muscles, to dilate or constrict pupils, or to increase or decrease blood glucose levels. The caffeine found in coffee, tea, or a soft drink is considered a pharmacodynamic agent because it stimulates the nervous system, allowing the consumer to remain alert.

Other examples of these medications include decongestants for nasal stuffiness, oral contraceptives that depress hormones to prevent pregnancy, expectorants to thin fluid or loosen mucus in the respiratory tract, anesthetics to cause numbness or loss of consciousness, glucagon to increase blood glucose levels in patients with diabetes, and digoxin to increase heart muscle contraction or slow heart conduction in patients with heart disease.

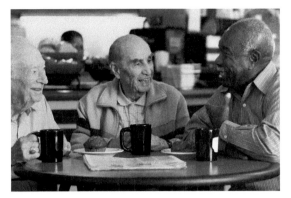

Caffeine is an example of a pharmacodynamic agent that can increase alertness.

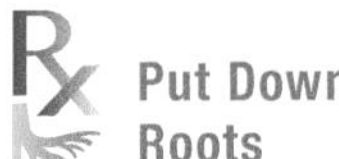

Put Down Roots

Diagnostic comes from the Greek word *diagnostikos,* meaning "to distinguish."

Diagnostic Agents

A **diagnostic agent** is a substance that helps healthcare providers diagnose a medical condition. These can be dyes or chemicals containing radioactive elements that are used to help healthcare professionals visualize or track the state or actions of cells, organs, and systems. Unstable radioactive elements give off energy in the form of radiation. These agents act as tracers, helping healthcare practitioners pinpoint, diagnose, and treat certain disorders. They are commonly used for imaging and functional studies of the brain, thyroid, lungs, liver, gallbladder, kidneys, and blood. The radiation exposure from the single use of an irradiated tracer is minimal.

3.3 Major Scientific Discoveries in Medicine and Drug Therapies

The varied uses of medications arose out of scientific discoveries in the related fields of medicine and pharmacy. This section highlights landmark discoveries that have had an outstanding impact and lasting effects on drug use, development, and the practice of pharmacists and technicians.

Drugs from the Science of Germ Theory

Contagious disease outbreaks and deaths from certain types of contaminated medications are the result of microorganisms, and contemporary prevention practices are based on the science of germ theory. In the late 1700s, scientists were just beginning to understand the existence of **microorganisms (microbes)**–microscopic or one-celled organisms–and their role in causing illness. These microbes include bacteria, viruses, fungi (including mold species), and protozoa, which will be discussed in greater detail in Chapter 12. An understanding of the role of microbes in causing illness developed into the **germ theory of disease**. Groundbreaking discoveries in germ theory led the way to vaccines, antibiotics, and the aseptic (germ-free) techniques used today.

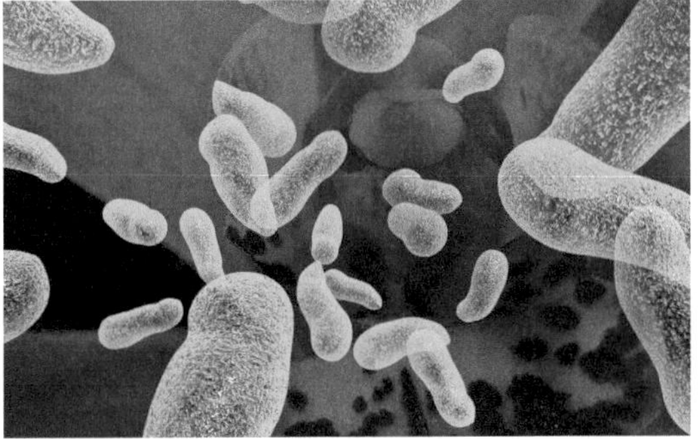

This computerized image shows microscopic bacteria.

Put Down Roots

The words *anti-body, antibiotics,* and *antigen* all come from the Greek prefix *antí*, meaning "against."

Smallpox—The First Vaccination

A major cause of premature deaths globally in the 1700s, much as heart disease and cancer are today, was a disease called smallpox. It was caused by various strains of the smallpox virus. Those lucky enough to survive were left scarred with pox marks over their faces and limbs, and were often made blind. No one knew how to prevent or cure smallpox. When explorers and armies from Europe brought it with them to the Americas, the disease decimated the Native American nations who lived here.

Dr. Edward Jenner observed that dairy workers previously exposed to cows with cowpox didn't get smallpox. Jenner theorized that cowpox exposure triggered people's bodies to provide special protection, or **immunity**, to the smallpox virus. So in 1796, Jenner tried introducing a tiny portion of matter from a cowpox lesion under the skin of a healthy individual and discovered that person did not contract smallpox later—despite being exposed. Jenner called the inoculation procedure a *vaccination*, from the Latin word *vaccinus*, meaning "from cows," leading to the term **vaccine**.

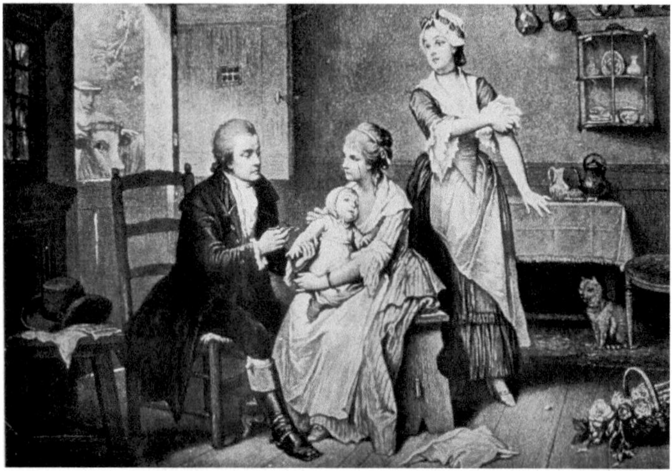

This etching, *Vaccinating the Baby*, by Ed Hamman, shows a traveling doctor giving a smallpox vaccination to an infant.

Vaccines work by introducing specific disease-causing dead or weakened live microorganisms or their toxins into the body. These **antigens**, or foreign substances, naturally cause the body to fight back, creating **antibodies** that can then neutralize the disease and foreign toxins. Jenner's smallpox vaccine was refined and proved so successful that it was developed into one of the world's first public health vaccines. The reason we don't see the devastation of smallpox today is that it was the first infectious disease in history to be completely eradicated worldwide in 1979.

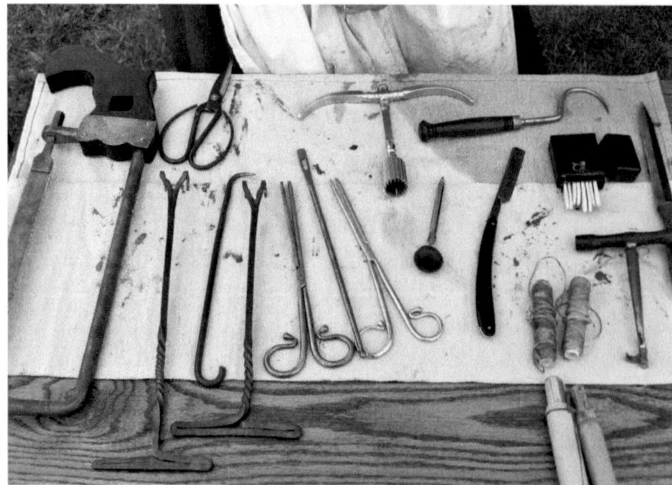

Surgical tools during the Civil War were reused over and over on different patients. Surgeons were even known to wipe off their knives and saws on their boots.

The Necessity of Cleanliness and Sterility

During the American Civil War (1861–1865), more soldiers died than in any other US war (and more died than in many wars combined). About one-fourth of the soldiers on each side died, and many more were injured and had amputations. Microorganisms killed far more soldiers than weapons—for every three soldiers killed in battle, five died of disease. With 620,000 soldiers killed from both sides (360,000 Union soldiers and 260,000 Confederate), it is estimated that more than one-fourth who died did it right in camp, from starvation, overcrowding, spoiled food, exposure, contaminated water, and insect bites. Consider that in the Union army alone, it is estimated that

IN THE REAL WORLD

Life expectancy for both men and women in the United States in 1900 was in the low 40s. It was even shorter in earlier years, in part due to infectious diseases. Contemporary childhood vaccines now protect against many of these once deadly infectious diseases, such as measles, mumps, rubella, chicken pox, pneumonia, hepatitis, diphtheria, tetanus, and pertussis. Life expectancies are presently nearly double: The United States averages 79 years; Canada, 82 years; and China, 76 years.

As more prophylactic vaccines are developed, however, questions arise about the administration of multiple vaccines at one time, the best timing and ages for administration (especially with infants), interactions with other drug therapies or individual body chemistries, and testing processes. Studies are ongoing to determine best practices and any potential side effects. The Centers for Disease Control and Prevention (CDC) collects data on vaccine reactions through the Vaccine Adverse Event Reporting System (VAERS), which will be further described in Chapter 14.

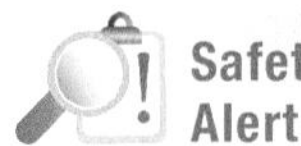

It is important for pharmacy technicians to be up-to-date on their own vaccinations and to reassure patients that the benefits of vaccine protection outweigh the small risk of adverse reactions (such as injection site redness and soreness).

nearly 45,000 Union soldiers lost their lives due to diarrhea, chicken pox, mumps, tuberculosis, yellow fever, measles, and malaria, which alone claimed over 10,000 Union soldiers.

In addition, army field surgeons did not know that they should wash their hands before surgery, and they commonly did multiple limb amputations with the same cutting instruments. They also thought that pus was good medicine, and transferred it from one patient to the next. Complications from tetanus, gangrene, blood poisoning (or sepsis), and many other forms of bacterial infection often killed those who had survived battle.

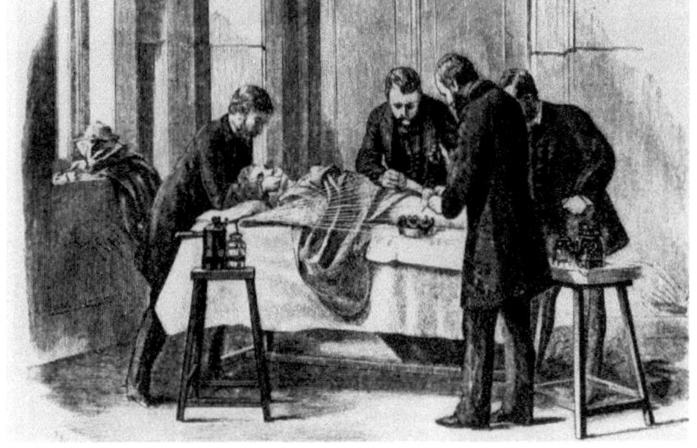

Lister used a mist of carbolic acid, the predecessor of our antibiotic spray-cleaning fluids, to disinfect the operating area before surgery, affording a huge improvement to patient recovery.

During the Civil War years, a French scientist named Louis Pasteur proved that diseases can be caused by germs, or microorganisms. He experimented with heating milk to the point where the germs were killed and then keeping it cold so that no additional germs could multiply. This process of "pasteurization" and then chilling transformed food safety, and it proved that germs do exist, though not in time to help most Civil War soldiers. However, by 1864, some surgeons were learning to control gangrene infections by pouring carbolic acid (very painful but effective) or iodine on the wounds, and female nurses—a rare but growing group at the time—brought cleanliness and clean bandages to the hospitals.

Joseph Lister, an English surgeon, applied Pasteur's work to surgery and medicine. Lister knew that carbolic acid (or phenol) killed bacteria, so in 1867, he began spraying the surgical room and soaking surgical dressings in a mild carbolic

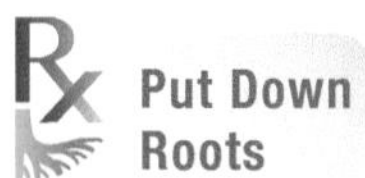

Put Down Roots

Septic, which means "infection," comes from the Greek word *septikos*, which means "rotten or characterized by putrefaction." The Greek *anti-* means "against" while *a-* means "without" or "free of." So, we get *antiseptic*, which fights against germs and *infection*, to achieve a condition that is aseptic, without germs.

acid solution to prevent infection. He also developed other **antiseptic**, or germ-fighting, protocols for surgery, including handwashing and gowning procedures. Lister's sterile practices formed the basis of **aseptic technique**—processes to protect patients from harmful germs—which have been improved upon and are still in use in pharmacies, hospitals, operating rooms, and army field hospitals. (In addition to his surgical technique, Lister developed the antiseptic mouthwash Listerine.)

Diseases Carried by Insects and Other Animals

Besides vaccines, sanitation, and aseptic techniques, other methods for disease prevention were needed. In 1897, Ronald Ross demonstrated that infectious diseases such as malaria were caused by microorganisms passed on by mosquitoes in tropical climates. Using mosquito netting, quinine (which inhibited the malaria microorganism), and vaccines for malaria and yellow fever became essential public health tactics for workers building the Panama Canal. These disease prevention techniques are still essential for anyone living, working, or visiting tropical areas today. Bubonic plague is carried by rodents, and Lyme disease is carried by deer ticks. Both of these diseases are treated with antibiotic drugs.

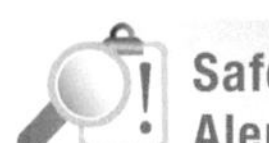

Safety Alert

Many people are allergic to penicillin. Always check a patient's drug allergy history when receiving a prescription for penicillin or one of its derivatives. Make sure to effectively clean counting trays after contact with penicillin or its derivatives.

Antibiotic Drug Development

Antibiotic drugs are medications that kill or inhibit the growth of bacteria. German physician Robert Koch and his team were able to isolate and identify the individual bacterial microbes causing anthrax, tuberculosis, and cholera in the 1880s and 1890s. Their work led the way to the study of other microorganisms—including viruses, fungi, and protozoans—and eventually to the development of drugs that target them.

Penicillin—The First True Antibiotic

The first antibiotic drug, penicillin, was discovered by accident in 1928. After returning to his research lab at the end of a long vacation, Dr. Alexander Fleming noticed that many of his bacterial culture petri dishes were contaminated by fungus. In these dishes, bacteria had not grown around the mold. Fleming isolated an extract from the bacteria-killing *Penicillium* fungus genus, so he named the new mold-based drug *penicillin*. Penicillin saved many soldiers' lives during World War II, and, in 1945, this antibiotic drug was mass-produced and marketed.

Penicillin and its derivatives are now the most widely used antibiotics in the world, and there are hundreds of other oral and injectable synthetic antibiotics.

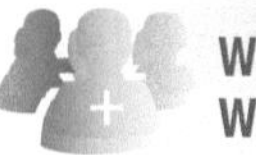

Work Wise

Fear and public shame have been historically attached to the disease of HIV/AIDS. Because it is a harsh diagnosis to receive, it is particularly important to be professional and courteous to patients with HIV/AIDS.

Combating Viruses: HIV/AIDS Challenges

Viruses are smaller than bacteria and have no cell structure of their own. They attach themselves to the cells of humans and other mammals to survive and multiply. You can be vaccinated against a virus, but antibiotics will not work against them, which has caused difficulties in dealing with outbreaks of viral diseases.

In the early 1980s, the emergence of a formidable virus—the human immunodeficiency virus (HIV)—was recognized when epidemiologists noted an outbreak of rare pneumonias and cancers in New York City. In 1983, HIV was independently isolated and verified by the Pasteur Institute in France and the National Cancer Institute in the United States. This virus progressively attacked the immune system and caused the development of acquired immunodeficiency syndrome, or AIDS. Transmitted through the exchange of bodily fluids during sexual contact, contaminated injection supplies used for intravenous drug use, or tainted blood transfusions, HIV quickly

IN THE REAL WORLD

One of the most destructive twentieth-century diseases was polio from poliovirus. Even President Franklin Delano Roosevelt was affected by the disease, which was characterized by muscle weakness and paralysis. Children often caught the virus swimming, and, if they survived, they might require braces, crutches, wheelchairs, or iron lungs (to help breathing) the remainder of their lives. In 1952, more than 21,000 cases of the most serious form of polio—paralytic polio—were reported in the United States alone, and there was no cure.

Then in 1953, the US physician Dr. Jonas Salk created an injectable vaccine from animal poliovirus cultures. Mass immunization programs for US children began in 1955. By 1957, there were only 2,500 US cases, and, by 1965, only 61. Polio was declared eradicated in all of the Americas in 1994, in the Western Pacific in 2000, in Europe in 2002, and in Southeast Asia in 2014. The countries of Afghanistan, Nigeria, and Pakistan continue to struggle. Worldwide, cases have dropped from hundreds of thousands to under 500 today, providing hope for total eradication. Today the inactivated polio vaccine is administered in four doses to children at 2 months, 4 months, and 6 to 18 months, with a booster dose at 4 to 6 years.

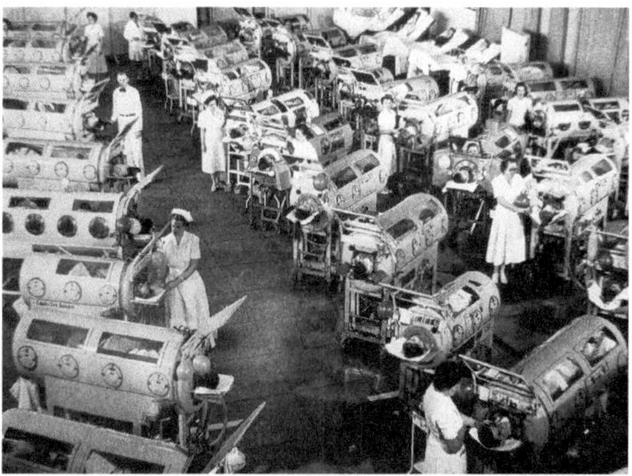

Patients who lost use of their lungs from the poliovirus had to use a ventilator, commonly called an iron lung.

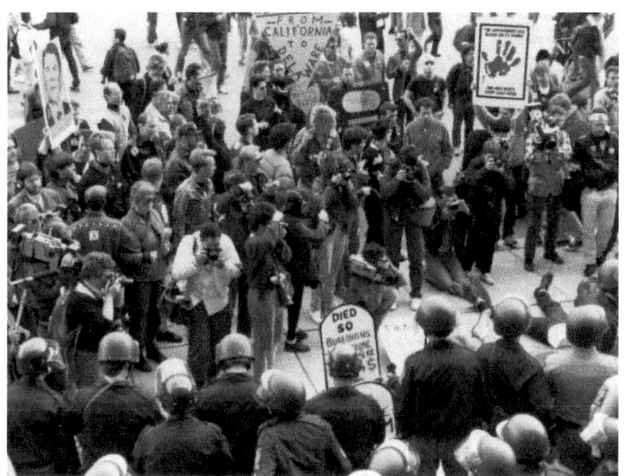

The AIDS Coalition to Unleash Power (ACT UP) rallied at FDA headquarters in 1988, demanding that the FDA release investigational drugs to try to treat dying AIDS patients.

grew to be a worldwide issue. Intense virus-fighting medications had to be developed. Zidovudine, the first **antiviral drug** to treat HIV, was approved by the FDA in 1987. Further studies demonstrated that one drug alone was insufficient to fight HIV due to the rapid development of viral resistance. Since 1987, many additional oral and injectable HIV drugs that attack the virus at different stages of its replication process have been developed.

Currently, combination therapy involving three or four drugs is common. Medications given to pregnant HIV-infected patients have been shown to be effective in reducing the transmission of the virus to the newborn at delivery from 100% to 5%. HIV medications can reduce the risk of transmission after exposure.

IN THE REAL WORLD

In the early days of the disease, a diagnosis of HIV or AIDS was virtually considered a death sentence. Today approximately 40,000 new cases of HIV/AIDS are reported each year, with more than 1.1 million people living with the disease in the United States alone. For these patients, regimented medication therapy allows many of them to lead near-normal lives.

Practice Tip

It is extremely important for the pharmacist and the technician to monitor the refill frequency on HIV drugs to delay the development of viral resistance. If an irregularity in refill timing is noted, the technician should alert the pharmacist to the need for counseling.

Probiotics and Encouraging Positive Microorganisms

Not all microorganisms are bad for one's health. In fact, contemporary science has found that many types of bacteria may be essential for good health. It has been long understood that live bacteria in yogurt, aged cheeses, and fermented foods can assist in digestive health. In 1907, Nobel Prize winner Élie Metchnikoff suggested that good digestion is dependent upon the interreactions of the bacteria in the digestive system. He believed that encouraging these positive microbes may help fight the infections of negative ones. This **probiotic** germ theory is one in which live microbes are used or encouraged to produce positive health benefits.

Many health supplements have been created to encourage the right conditions for positive microbes. Physicians and pharmacists often recommend yogurt or probiotics during a course of antibiotic therapy. Community pharmacies can be particularly helpful in promoting overall health and wellness by understanding probiotics, staying up to date on the latest research, and offering reputable probiotic products for patients.

The Power of Healthy Nutrition and Vitamins

Encouraging the right conditions for organs to function well has also been found to be important. Diseases and organ malfunction can be caused by vitamin deficiencies. In the 1900s, scientists found that a lack of vitamin C caused the disease of scurvy. Scurvy causes spongy gums, loose teeth, joint pain, muscle weakness, blood loss, and eventually death. A lack of vitamin D causes rickets (bone softening and warping); and a lack of vitamin B1 causes beriberi (neuron damage, weakness, pain, and, eventually, death).

Scientists are finding new nutritional connections all the time, and physicians regularly tell patients to eat a healthy diet rich in various vitamins to maintain health and address or prevent various diseases. Mineral salts rich in iron are used for the treatment of iron deficiency, and potassium is used for electrolyte replacement therapy. These supplemental therapies are additional ways to help the body function naturally. Informed pharmacy staff can help consumers understand the role of vitamins.

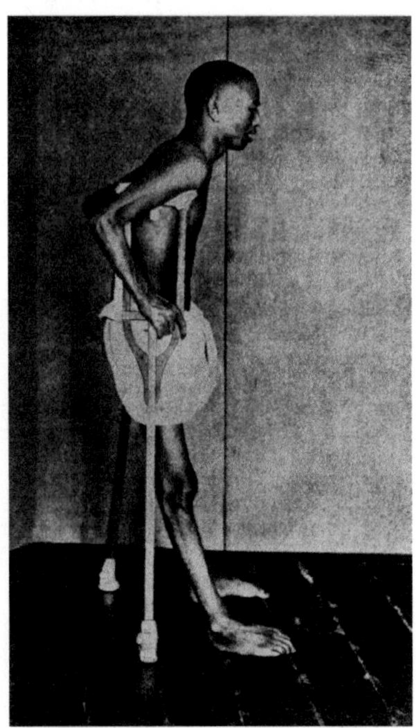

Beriberi was a common disease caused by lack of vitamin B1, or thiamine, which may be found in many types of beans, peas, lentils, barley, brown rice, and sunflower seeds, among other foods.

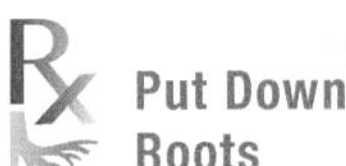

Put Down Roots

Hormone comes from the Greek word *hormon*, meaning "to set in motion" or "impel."

Discoveries of Key Hormones and Hormonal Drug Therapies

Scientists in the early 1900s started to explore the effects of organ secretions on bodily functions. **Hormones** are the body's secretions released by glands into the circulatory system that have specific regulatory effects on organs and other tissues. The last century brought new drug development in synthesized hormones, such as insulin, thyroid, and sex hormones, such as estrogen, progestin, and testosterone.

What if insulin and birth control medications were not available today? It is hard to comprehend the impact these discoveries have had not only on our health , but on our society. In the United States, it is estimated that more than 6 million patients with diabetes are staying alive and living normal lives while taking one or more types of insulin, much of it grown from cells in manufacturing laboratories. Today, over 100 million women worldwide use a form of oral contraception, colloquially referred to as "the pill").

Insulin—A Lifesaver

Once, contracting diabetes, known as the "sugar disease," was a terminal diagnosis. In the 1920s, research had shown a connection between problems with the pancreas and the disease of diabetes. The Canadian scientist, doctor, and Nobel Prize winner Sir Frederick Banting worked with his assistant Charles Best to try to isolate the pancreatic secretion that helps the body regulate sugar levels. They worked with diabetic dogs that were kept alive with an extract from the pancreas, which Banting and Best called *isletin* (named after the islets of Langerhans—pancreatic regions that secrete the hormone), simplified to **insulin**. In 1922, after insulin was isolated and purified, Banting and Best came to a hospital wing where comatose diabetic children were moving toward death. Their parents sat by their bedsides in tears or quiet sadness. As the two doctors moved through the room, injecting the patients, one by one the children started to awaken, and their families came alive, too, with joy. The effects of the insulin seemed miraculous, to say the least.

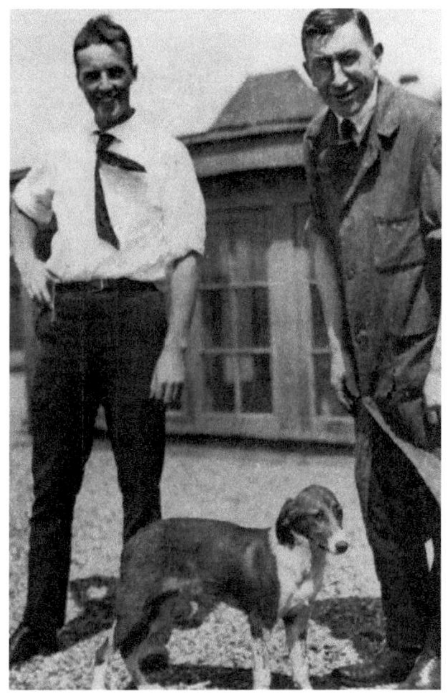

Charles H. Best (left) and Dr. Frederick Banting (right) in 1921 stand with a beagle that had been successfully treated with what would be called *insulin*.

Practice Tip

The educational materials on proper usage and potential side effects from the pharmaceutical manufacturer must always accompany the dispensing of birth control.

The Birth Control Pill

Another famous hormone drug is the oral contraceptive. Up until the mid-twentieth century, birth control was a taboo subject, and some state laws even prohibited teaching about contraceptive methods in medical schools. In the 1930s, the female sex hormones estrogen and progesterone and their functions were identified. Though funding was scarce and the hormones were difficult and expensive to develop, research continued in the hands of a few passionate scientists and activists. In 1960, the first birth control medication was approved by the FDA—Enovid—which had high doses of estrogen and progesterone. It worked but had dangerous and painful side effects.

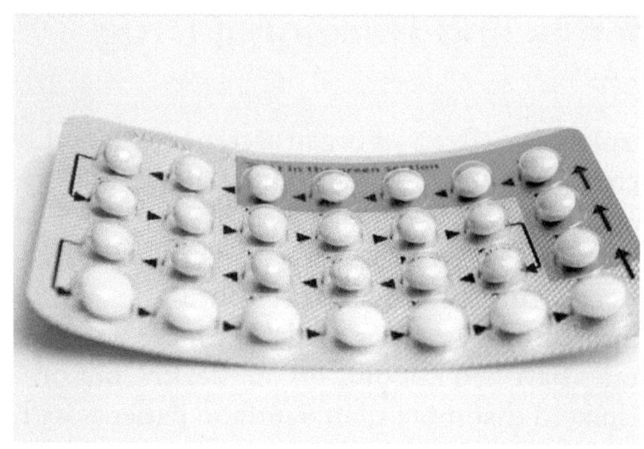

Oral contraceptives had a major effect on women's reproductive choices and helped fuel women's liberation in the 1960s.

Levels were lowered, and combinations refined to safe levels. There are now many brands and generics available on the market, including emergency contraception (sometimes referred to as the "morning after" pill) that is available without a prescription. In the future, other birth control options may become available over the counter. However, they must be used with care, remembering that they do have side effects and may not fit an individual's body chemistry. Side effects include but are not limited to nausea, thromboembolism (otherwise known as blood clots), cardiovascular disease, depression, and weight gain. Different types of hormonal contraception have different side-effect profiles.

Other Important Drug Discoveries

The last half of the twentieth century gave us many more significant medical and drug discoveries, especially in the areas of mental health, cancer chemotherapy, and gene therapy.

Work Wise

Patients with mental health conditions sometimes feel stigmatized. They must be made to feel particularly welcomed and respected, so that they are willing to continue to take their medications.

Development of Drugs for Mental and Cognitive Health

Prior to the 1950s, mental distress and illnesses were treated in misguided and often painful or cruel ways, including punishment; imprisonment; ice-cold baths; induced vomiting, bleeding, comas, or seizures; physical or emotional isolation or restraint; brain surgeries to remove sections or make openings; and electric shock treatment. Chlorpromazine (Thorazine) was the first official US **psychopharmaceutical drug** used to treat mental health diseases, which was approved by the FDA for schizophrenia in 1954. Though it was effective, it wasn't the magic bullet people had hoped for, as there were many dangerous side effects. It is seldom prescribed today, yet it opened the way for greater research into the effects of other drugs on the brain's cognitive, emotional, and social functioning.

Depression has long been a debilitating mental health disorder that can ruin lives and lead to suicide. In 1987, the FDA approved fluoxetine (Prozac) for treatment of depression. It provided major improvements over other medications as it could be taken once daily with fewer side effects. Because it could lift the spirits of people struggling painfully with depression, it became known as the "happy pill." However, as with any drug, fluoxetine has its side effects and concerns. It is only one of many antidepressants, sleep aids, mood

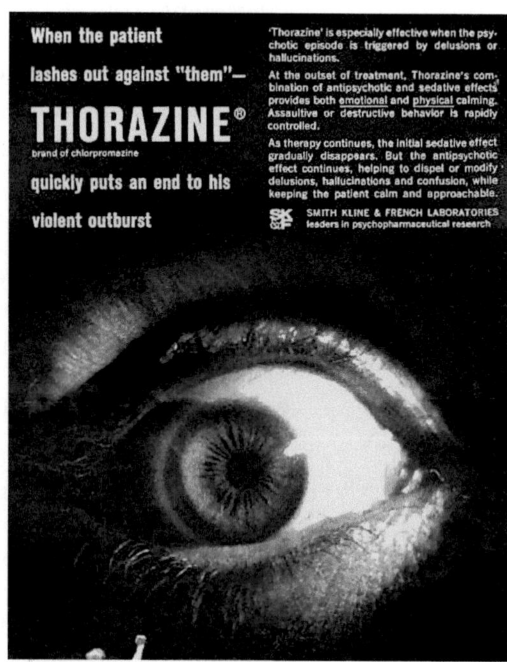

When the patient
lashes out against "them"—
THORAZINE®
brand of chlorpromazine
quickly puts an end to his
violent outburst
'Thorazine' is especially effective when the psychotic episode is triggered by delusions or hallucinations.
At the outset of treatment, Thorazine's combination of antipsychotic and sedative effects provides both emotional and physical calming. Assaultive or destructive behavior is rapidly controlled.
As therapy continues, the initial sedative effect gradually disappears. But the antipsychotic effect continues, helping to dispel or modify delusions, hallucinations and confusion, while keeping the patient calm and approachable.
SMITH KLINE & FRENCH LABORATORIES
leaders in psychopharmaceutical research

This is a 1962 ad for Thorazine (chlorpromazine), the first official US mental health drug.

Practice Tip

Beware: Adderall and Ritalin are commonly being over- or under-used, abused, or shared with those who do not have a legal prescription, especially by young people. It is important that patients do not take the effect of these drugs lightly and that they are directed to pharmacists for monitoring and counseling.

balancers, cognitive enhancers, and other mind-modulating drugs that are improving the lives of more than 54 million people worldwide struggling with mental illness.

A common problem diagnosed in contemporary children is attention deficit hyperactivity disorder (ADHD). Drug therapies using amphetamine/dextroamphetamine (Adderall) and methylphenidate (Ritalin), which are mind-focusing stimulants, have helped these children increase their ability to pay attention, stay focused on activities, and control behavioral issues.

However, it must be remembered that most drugs used to treat ADHD are legal amphetamines. Amphetamine-like drugs are a group of Schedule II controlled substances that serve as stimulants to the central nervous system. Illegal amphetamines or amphetamine derivatives, such as methamphetamine, go by the street names speed, uppers, or crank. All amphetamines, whether prescribed or not, are habit forming and can cause dependence and addiction. Drugs used to treat ADHD can cause side effects, dependence, and addiction and must be used with caution.

Turning Poisons into Cancer-Fighting Treatments

In the 1900s, a cancer diagnosis meant a premature and painful death with almost no relief. Families could do little but support their loved ones and brace for the inevitable. However, hope came from an unexpected place: weapons of war.

In World War I, mustard gas burned the faces and skin of soldiers, and, in World War II, nuclear radiation bombs killed or caused radiation sickness and cancers in the Japanese citizens of Hiroshima and Nagasaki. During and after World War II, scientists and physicians began to experiment with these devastating substances in **antineoplastic drugs**, which use toxins to poison the cancer cells. Dysfunctional cancer cells grow much faster than normal cells, taking over a bodily organ or system. To do so, they absorb nutrients more quickly than other cells. But they also absorb toxins faster, which has the desired effect of killing the cancer cells. Unfortunately, the toxins also kill some of the normal cells and make someone sick, which is why there are intense side effects of hair loss, nausea, vomiting, and immune cell suppression.

Early chemotherapy treatments were a painful race for time. Which would happen first: would the treatment kill the cancer cells? Or would the side effects kill the patient, or would the cancer prevail and kill the patient? Remissions were common, but the cancer often won. However, as cancer drugs and radiation became more targeted and used along with antibiotics and other drugs that boosted the body's immune system, survival rates became much higher. Now many children with leukemia often progress through childhood and go on to live healthy lives, and cancer survivors celebrate their freedom from the disease.

Because these anticancer substances are so poisonous, technicians must be particularly careful in their dispensing, compounding, storage, and disposal. More will be discussed in Chapter 13 on hazardous compounding.

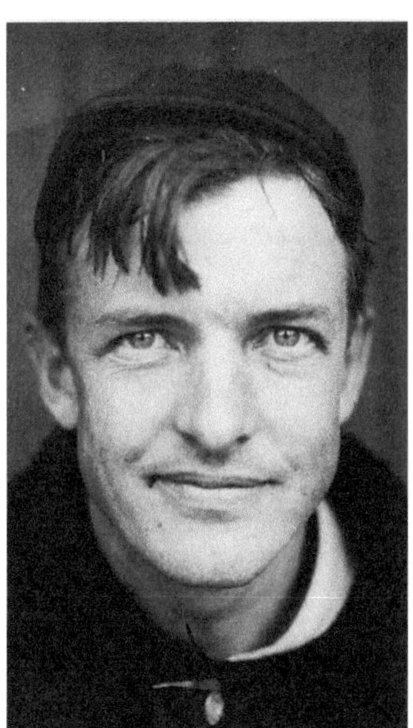

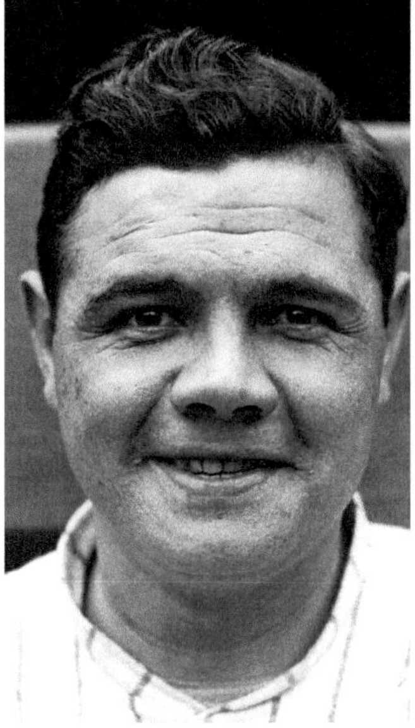

Famous Baseball Hall of Fame pitcher Christy Mathewson (left) died from exposure to mustard gas in World War I, and Babe Ruth (right) received cancer treatments that were made from nitrogen mustard, a similar compound, in the late 1940s.

Unraveling Human Genetics

Much of our recent success in drug development is due to a better understanding of human genetics, or the biological codes in cells that determine an organism's distinct inherited features. In 1953, the British physicist Francis Crick and American biologist James Watson were awarded a Nobel Prize for providing a model of the double-helix structure of the genetic strands of **deoxyribonucleic acid (DNA)**. DNA is carried in the center of each cell and is made up of atomic matter that carries codes to direct the growth of the cell.

A **gene** is a distinct segment of DNA that determines a specific individual characteristic, such as blue eyes or brown hair. A defect in one's DNA may increase the risk for developing certain diseases. Unraveling the DNA code and identifying the particular genes that affect specific diseases may make it easier to prevent or treat those diseases more effectively. Identifying a defective gene for a specific disease can assist in genetically designing a drug remedy for that disease, such as new forms of insulin for diabetes; clotting factors for hemophilia; potent anti-inflammatory drugs for rheumatoid arthritis; and drugs for combating viral and bacterial infections, anemia, and some cancers.

The development of **genetically engineered** drugs, drugs designed by manipulating genes in living substances to affect the genes in certain patient cells, has led to a new field of study that blends two scientific areas: pharmacology and genomics (or genetic molecular biology). Known as **pharmacogenomics**, it aims to design and produce drugs that cater to each individual's genetic makeup.

For example, blood thinners are metabolized by patients at different rates, thus altering the pharmacological and toxic effects of the drugs. Genetic engineering could design a blood thinning drug personalized to the patient's genes to produce the intended effects without the adverse reactions.

Biotechnology is the field of study that combines the sciences of biology, chemistry, and immunology to produce unique synthetic drugs with specific therapeutic effects. For cancer, new target-specific biotechnology drug treatments are making the difference between life and death, extending the quality of life without the debilitating side effects of earlier treatments. Research continues on personalized medications that tailor a drug, dose, and schedule to a specific disease in a specific patient. Because pharmacy technicians and pharmacists compound the correct ingredients and percentage for each patient, they are key links in the process of hope for cancer patients.

Generic biotechnology drugs that function in similar ways as brand-name biologically engineered drugs are called **biosimilars** and **interchangeables** (biosimilars that can legally be substituted for the brand). Biogenetically engineered and biosimilar drugs can be manufactured from many original living sources, such as the cells of humans, animals, microorganisms, or yeasts.

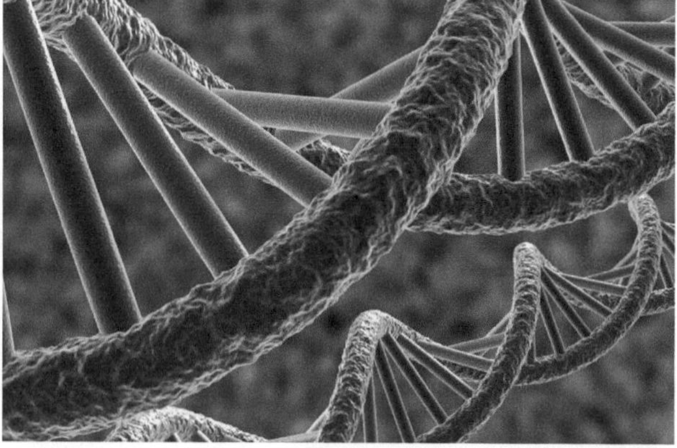

This computerized image of DNA shows the twisting ladder-like structure of genetic material. Scientists study the DNA's chemical composition. Some new drugs swap deficient gene sections and proteins with effective ones.

3.4 Drug Ingredients and Sources

Within a wide range of complex drugs and supplements, there is also a wide range of ingredients. Some are key therapeutic ingredients, and others support the actions, stability, or administration of the key ingredients. The **active ingredients** are the biochemically active components that exert the desired effects—for example, eradicating bacteria or viruses, lowering blood pressure or cholesterol, or controlling heart rates.

Most medications contain one or more active ingredients as well as several inactive or inert supporting ingredients. An **inert ingredient** has little or no physiological effect. Common inert ingredients include those that are needed to stabilize the tablet, capsule, or liquid formulation; those that provide the raw material for many topical creams and ointments; those that ensure sterility of injectable products; or those masking the unpleasant taste of some unpleasant oral medications for pediatric patients. These inert ingredients, such as coloring agents or preservatives, can sometimes cause an allergic reaction in a sensitive individual, which is why they must be listed. They are also sometimes called inactive ingredients.

Drug ingredients are derived from various sources and can be classified as natural, synthetic (created artificially), synthesized (created artificially but in imitation of naturally occurring substances), semisynthetic (containing both natural and synthetic components), and biologically engineered (containing genetic materials). Drugs made from natural agents that people are allergic to must be identified so that patients with allergies are not given these drugs.

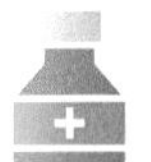

Pharm Fact

Over 600,000 crabs are captured each spring to donate 30% of their blue blood. It is used to reveal and isolate certain bacteria and help clot hemophiliac blood. Sadly, the crab populations are declining, with 10%–30% lost from blood harvesting.

Natural Sources

Many drugs are derived from naturally occurring biological products, such as single-celled organisms, plants, animals and humans, or minerals. In addition to penicillin and insulin, many other modern-day drugs are derived from natural sources. Even substances from viper venom have been used in medications to fight high blood pressure. Many drugs are from rainforest plant extracts, and PharmaMar, a Spanish drug company, has found almost 100 antitumor compounds from ocean life. Cultures of natural organisms can be grown in laboratories. Some of the natural sources of drugs and their benefits to treatment of diseases are included below:

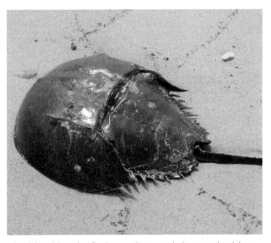

The blue blood of a horseshoe crab is so valuable to medicine that crabs are captured so that a small bit of their blood can be donated before they are sent back to the sea.

- Taxol interferes with growth capabilities of cancer cells (particularly breast cancer) and comes from the bark of the Pacific yew tree.
- Streptomycin, an antibiotic used to treat tuberculosis, is from the bacterium *Streptomyces griseus*.

- Vincristine, a drug that inhibits growth of leukemia and other cancer cells, comes from the periwinkle plant in the rainforests of Madagascar.
- Limulus amebocyte lysate is a compound from the horseshoe crab's blue blood that causes clots in the presence of bacterial toxins. It is used to test drugs, vaccines, and surgical implants to ensure that they are germ-free. It also helps the blood of hemophiliacs, whose blood does not clot.
- Armour Thyroid, a medication for poorly functioning thyroids, is an extract from desiccated (dried) pig thyroids.
- Somatotropin is a human growth hormone from cell lines of the human brain, now often synthesized to imitate the hormone.

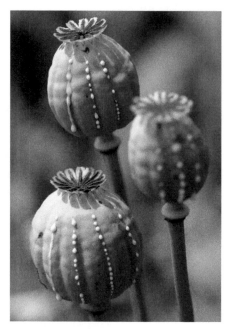

Morphine, codeine, paregoric, and heroin trace their source to the opium poppy.

Laboratory Sources

In pharmaceutical manufacturing, many naturally occurring substances have been created or combined with chemical or other ingredients in a laboratory setting. Drugs are classified as synthetic (chemical ingredients), synthesized (chemical ingredients made to imitate a naturally occurring agent), semisynthetic (chemical and natural ingredients together), and biogenetically engineered.

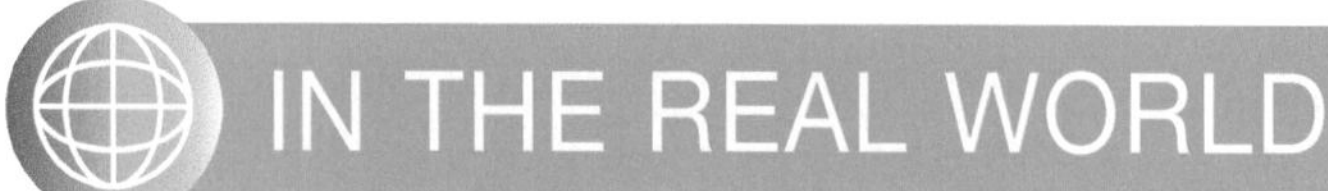

IN THE REAL WORLD

Synthetic and synthesized drugs have found their way into the illegal drug market. "Designer drugs" are produced in home chemistry laboratories by modifying the chemical structure of existing drugs.

For example, a semisynthetic version of marijuana exerts a similar an effect similar to the natural product but produces more intense hallucinations. Methamphetamine, also known as "meth" or "speed," is another example of an illegally synthesized drug. Because meth is produced from common decongestants made from pseudoephedrine and ephedrine, community pharmacies are required by law to place restrictions on the sale of products containing this key ingredient. (This is discussed in more detail in Chapter 9.)

Innocent-sounding street names of some dangerous designer drugs are spice, K2, bath salts, plant food, incense, fake weed, and Yucatan fire.

Synthetic Drugs

A **synthetic drug** is a drug that has been created in the laboratory from a series of chemical reactions to produce a specific pharmacological effect. Phenobarbital—a drug prescribed for seizure, nerve, or headache disorders—is an example of a synthetic chemical compound.

Synthesized Drugs

Ephedrine and aspirin are considered **synthesized drugs**, or laboratory drugs developed to mimic the pharmacological action of the naturally occurring sources—the Chinese herb ma huang and the white willow (weeping willow) tree, respectively.

Semisynthetic Drugs

Semisynthetic drugs are natural substances combined with laboratory substances designed to (1) improve the efficacy of the natural product; (2) reduce its side effects; (3) overcome medicinal obstacles; or (4) broaden the scope of its uses. Many current antibiotics, such as amoxicillin, are modifications of existing natural drugs, such as penicillin. These antibiotics are more effective against different strains of bacteria or bacteria that have developed resistance to the natural product.

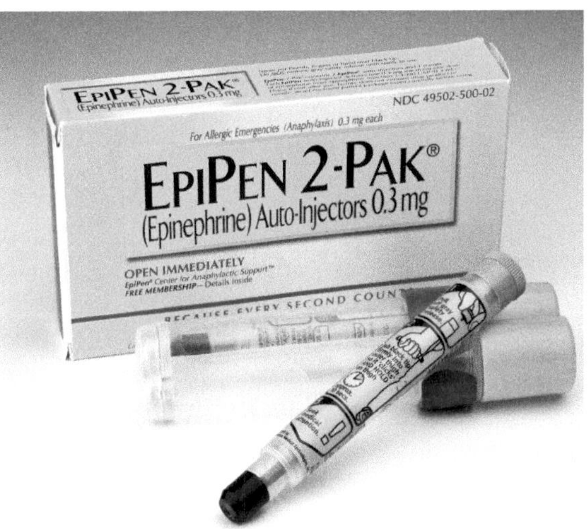

EpiPens contain epinephrine hydrochloride, a lifesaving, injectable synthesized drug used to mimic the actions of the hormone adrenaline for responding to severe allergic reactions, such as from bee stings. EpiPens are often dispensed in packages of two.

Biogenetically Engineered Drugs

Biogenetically engineered drugs are derived from the use of biotechnology to produce unique drugs with specific therapeutic effects, such as the slowing of Alzheimer's disease. Humulin is

IN THE REAL WORLD

Thalidomide was used in 46 countries to alleviate morning sickness in pregnant women, and was later linked to causing birth defects. It was not approved in the United States because FDA drug inspector Frances Oldham Kelsey and her team were not convinced that it had been adequately tested for this new therapeutic use. They refused to approve the medication. Oldham Kelsey's courage in standing up for safety and caution against the prevailing thought can inspire technicians to speak up and ask questions of the pharmacists, even asking them to query prescribers if something about a drug or dosage seems out of the ordinary or unsafe.

an artificial, slow-acting hormone—structurally identical to human insulin—which was developed with DNA technology applied to non-disease-producing laboratory strains of bacteria. Similarly, Novolin is a synthesized insulin using a special strain of baker's yeast. Both of these insulins are fast-acting and major improvements on an earlier generation of insulins from animal sources that caused more allergic skin reactions.

3.5 The Prescription Drug Approval Process

The question then is, how do all the different medicinal drugs get developed, manufactured, and approved as safe and effective for patients to use?

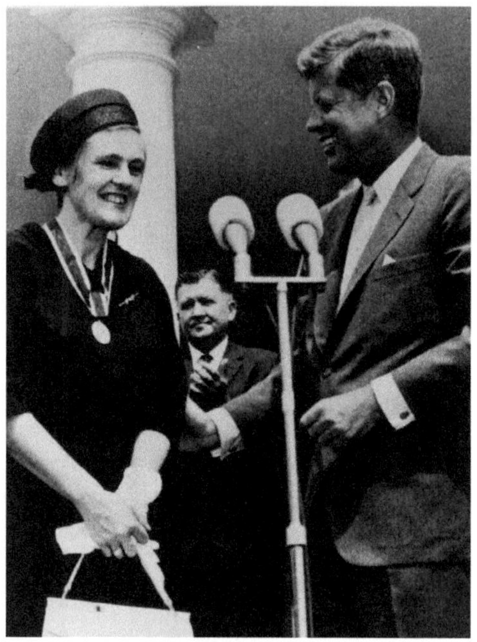

President John F. Kennedy awarded Frances Kathleen Oldham Kelsey the President's Award for Distinguished Federal Civilian Service in 1962 for her scientific and ethical stance on thalidomide that saved thousands of children from disfigurement and handicaps. She was later inducted into the National Women's Hall of Fame.

Investigational New Drug Application

As noted in Chapter 2, a pharmaceutical company must do extensive preclinical laboratory research on animals before an **investigational new drug (IND) application** can be officially initiated with the FDA. In its application, the developer must offer a compelling case for the human need for the drug, the results of the animal studies, an explanation of how the drug would be manufactured, and a detailed description of the proposed clinical studies on humans.

The research study must then be submitted and approved by the **Institutional Review Board (IRB)** of the university or hospital where the research will be conducted before the human clinical studies are allowed to begin. The IRB, also known as the Human Use Committee, is comprised of scientists and practitioners from various disciplines, plus consumers. The committee must review, approve, and monitor all medical research involving humans. The proposed studies must meet both scientific and ethical standards to be approved. In most cases each study participant must sign an **informed consent form**—a document that states the purpose and risks of the research in easily understandable terms.

After the IND is approved by the FDA, non-FDA scientists conduct three phases of human clinical studies as part of the drug approval process.

- Phase 1 is the initial study or trial of the new drug, usually completed on a small number of healthy volunteers (typically 20 to 80) over the span of months. The main purpose is to gather sufficient data concerning potential side effects and how the drug is metabolized and excreted. The data are used to design future clinical trials.

- The Phase 2 study aims to evaluate the effectiveness as well as the safety of a drug for a specific indication or disease state. Phase 2 studies also involve a small number of patients (typically in the hundreds) and are well controlled and closely monitored by the FDA. Phase 2 usually lasts from several months up to several years.
- If the results of Phase 1 and Phase 2 studies are promising, Phase 3 studies are conducted in larger clinical trials (larger groups) to better assess the overall benefits and risks of the investigational drug on patients (see Figure 3.2). Phase 3 studies typically involve thousands of study participants and last one to four years.

FIGURE 3.2 The FDA Drug Approval Process

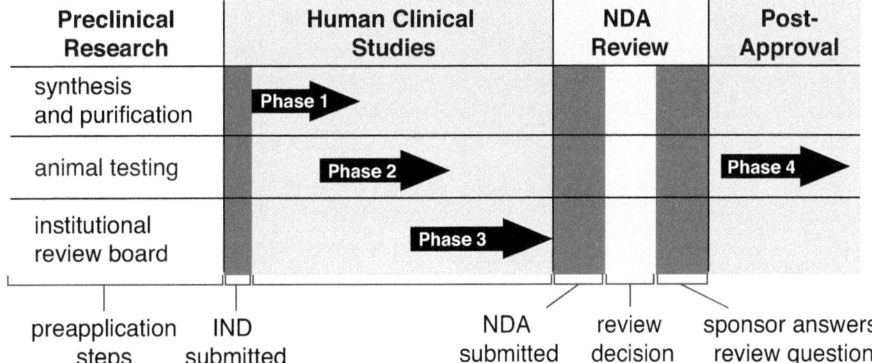

New Prescription Drug Application for Brand Name Drugs

If the investigational drug shows promise after Phase 3 studies are completed, the pharmaceutical manufacturer can submit a **new drug application (NDA)** to the FDA. In the NDA, the applicant must prove the case for both the safety and the effectiveness of the drug before they are permitted to market it. The results of the scientific studies are evaluated by an independent advisory panel of experts, and recommendations are forwarded to the FDA. If the benefit of the drug outweighs the risk, the drug is generally approved. The FDA may request that additional studies be completed. The drug approval process takes a year or longer in most cases. Occasionally, when a medication appears to be very promising early on in testing, the FDA may opt to fast-track the drug and grant early approval. Recent examples of this accelerated process can be seen with the quick approval of drugs to treat patients with HIV or cancer.

Drug development is risky as well as costly. Out of 5,000 to 10,000 screened compounds, only 250 enter preclinical research testing, 5 enter human clinical trials, and 1 new compound is approved by the FDA. The cost of developing a new drug is more than $1 billion, and it can sometimes take as long as 15 to 20 years of research and development to bring a new medication from the laboratory to the pharmacy shelf.

While Phases 1, 2, and 3 of a clinical trial are designed to predict safety of a new drug, serious and unexpected adverse effects can occur after a drug is on the market. For these reasons, a postmarketing safety system is in place, often referred to as Phase 4. Phase 4 requires a drug manufacturer to periodically submit safety data to the FDA. If patients are concerned about safety of drugs, you may want to help them understand the safety checks built into the FDA drug approval process.

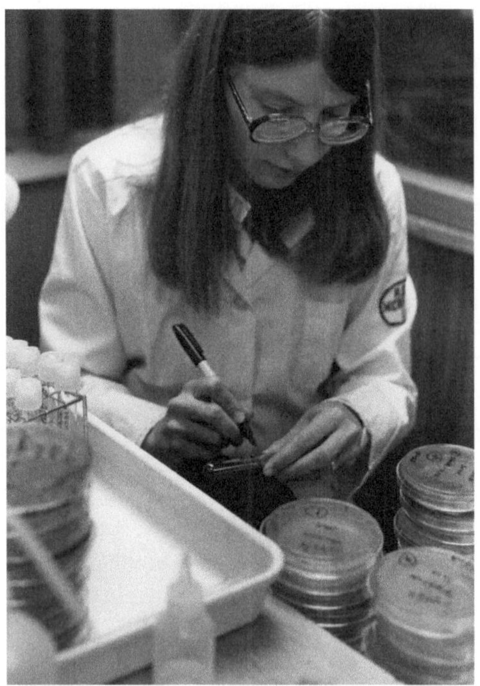

Concerned over resistance to antibiotics because of overuse, FDA researchers tested the effectiveness of various antibiotics on bacteria in 1978. This same concern continues today among many researchers.

Abbreviated Approvals for Generic Drugs

As discussed in Chapter 2, a generic drug contains the same active ingredients as the brand name product and delivers the same amount of medication in the same way and amount of time. Once the patent is due to expire on a brand name drug, a generic pharmaceutical company may submit an **abbreviated new drug application** to the FDA for approval.

Generic drug applications are termed "abbreviated" because they are not required to include the preclinical (animal) and clinical (human) data to establish safety and effectiveness. Instead, the generic applicants must scientifically demonstrate that their product is bioequivalent, or performs in the same manner as an already approved brand name drug. The drug patent for esomeprazole (sold under the brand name Nexium) expired in 2014.

Currently, esomeprazole is commercially available from several manufacturers who have formulated bioequivalent products. With fewer required studies, generic drugs are far less expensive and require much less time to get to the market.

One way scientists demonstrate bioequivalence between brand name and generic drugs is to measure the generic drug's **bioavailability**—that is, the rate and extent to which a drug reaches the bloodstream in healthy users and exerts the targeted pharmacological effect. Bioavailability involves how a drug is absorbed, metabolized, distributed, or eliminated from the objective data necessary to compare the generic product with that of the innovator (brand name) drug.

IN THE REAL WORLD

In October 2015, a new drug designed to boost sexual desire in women was released called Addyi (generic ingredient flibanserin). It exemplifies some of the issues of any new drug. The drug was turned down twice for release by the FDA (as the effects did not seem impressive) and had some specialists petitioning against it. It is now only being released with boxed warnings (warnings that highlight dangerous effects of a drug) and will not be dispensed without patients completing an online questionnaire to show that they understand the potential side effects. This drug is a tablet that must be taken daily for weeks or even months before the positive effects start to manifest. It works on the brain chemicals associated with appetite and moods. However, taking the pill and drinking alcohol can cause extremely low blood pressure and fainting. It has the additional side effects of nausea and dizziness. Also, since it may be prescribed for premenopausal women, the drug effects on pregnancy should be identified and provided to the consumer.

The FDA has developed special regulations for the approval of generic versions of expensive brand-name biotechnology drugs. Unlike for other generic drugs, biosimilars (biologically and therapeutically similar drugs) must demonstrate no clinically meaningful differences in safety and effectiveness when compared to the reference product. The first biosimilar drug was approved by the FDA in 2015, and there were no interchangeable drugs for legal substitution at that point.

3.6 Nonprescription Drug Approval Process

Since nonprescription medications and supplements are not considered as potent, potentially dangerous, or addictive as prescription drugs, the FDA does not require as intensive an approval process for them.

Over-the-Counter Drug Approvals

Most OTC drugs are meant for self-limited conditions (conditions that could resolve themselves on their own) that are usually dependent upon self-diagnosis for short-term therapy. Other OTC drugs, such as baby aspirin or allergy medicines, may be used on a long-term basis with physician permission.

To get approval to bring an OTC drug to market, the manufacturer has to submit a new drug application with a specific dose and indication. The FDA must check to see that the drug is safe and effective for use when the labeled directions on the container are followed with regard to dose, frequency, precautions and contraindications, and duration of therapy. After some brand-names prescription medications were proven to have a safe track record and the manufacturer's patent had nearly expired, the FDA approved an abbreviated new drug application for OTC sales. Examples of such drugs include ibuprofen (Advil), naproxen (Aleve), loratadine (Claritin), cetirizine (Zyrtec), and esomeprazole (Nexium). (See Table 3.1 for common drugs soon to have their patents expire.) When directions are followed, these drugs have been proven relatively safe and effective. When used inappropriately, these drugs can cause harmful side effects, adverse reactions, and interactions with prescription drugs.

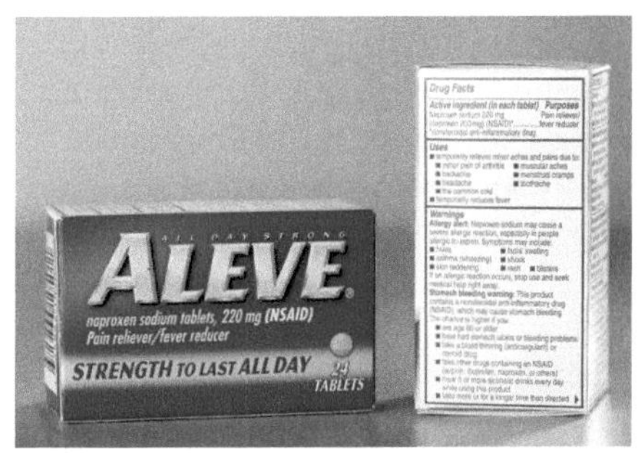

All OTC drugs must include "Drug Facts" labeling for the consumer to safely self-medicate with the product.

TABLE 3.1 Common Drugs with Patent Expiration Years

Brand Name Drug	Generic Drug	Therapeutic Use	Expected Patent Expiration Year
Janumet	sitagliptin/metformin	Type 2 diabetes	2022
Revlimid	lenalidomide	multiple myeloma	2022
Januvia	sitagliptin	Type 2 diabetes	2022
Perforomist	formoterol	Asthma and COPD	2021
Pradaxa	dabigatran	Prevention of blood clots	2021
Chantix	varenicline	Smoking cessation	2020

It is important for OTC drugs to have adequate product labeling, written in easily understood terms, as patients may have no contact with a pharmacist or typed physician instructions. The FDA-required labels contain a prominent "Drug Facts box that lists the active ingredients, purposes, and uses of the product, along with any warnings and directions, including age-appropriate dosing. This "Drug Facts" box allows the consumer to compare active ingredients and assess the benefits and risks of various OTC products. The labels of all OTC drugs must also include a toll-free number to report adverse effects. Also, due to patient allergies and hypersensitivities, the FDA requires manufacturers to list all inert ingredients (as well as the active ingredients) on product package inserts and on bottles of OTC products.

This image is of a homeopathic medication label.

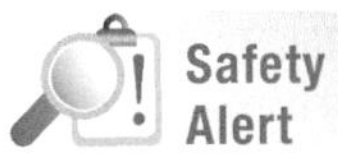

Most homeopathic medications are available without a prescription, so label directions must be read carefully.

Homeopathic Approvals

The FDA regulates homeopathic therapies like OTC drugs for accurate labeling, but the FDA does not evaluate them for safety or effectiveness. If the manufacturers meet certain conditions and standards set by the USP and the **Homeopathic Pharmacopoeia of the United States/Revision Service (HPRS)**, a compendium of standards and research created by the American Institute of Homeopathy, the FDA allows them to be marketed without agency preapproval.

Homeopathic therapy packaging must contain:

- an NDC (National Drug Code) number
- a list of the active and inactive ingredients (all of which must be on the approved list of the HPRS)
- the targeted condition
- the number of times an active ingredient has been diluted
- directions for use

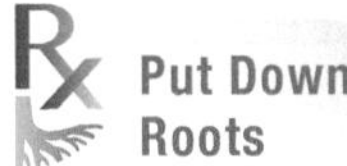

Homeopathic comes from the Greek word *homeo*, meaning "like," and *patheia* or *pathos*, meaning "disease" or "feeling."

Dietary Supplements

A dietary supplement is considered a food rather than a drug, so it has different legal oversight. Dietary supplements, including vitamins, minerals, and herbs, can be very helpful for many people to maintain a healthy lifestyle, especially when they are not eating a balanced diet rich in fruits and vegetables. However, consumers should be aware that the quality of many products has been suspect when tested by independent consumer laboratories. Unlike for prescription and OTC drugs, manufacturers of these products are not required to follow USP standards—though voluntary participation is strongly encouraged by the FDA. This means that the manufacturer must label all active and inactive ingredients and cannot make deceptive claims to prevent or cure disease.

Whereas other organizations may provide supplement testing and quality seals, or claim that they do, the USP is the only standard-setting organization for supplements recognized in US federal law. The organization's standards were acknowledged as the legal standards in the 1994 Dietary Supplement Health and Education Act. Though the FDA does not require manufacturers of supplements to have their products USP certified, it will prosecute them for misbranding if their products display the USP-verified mark or claim to be certified when they are not.

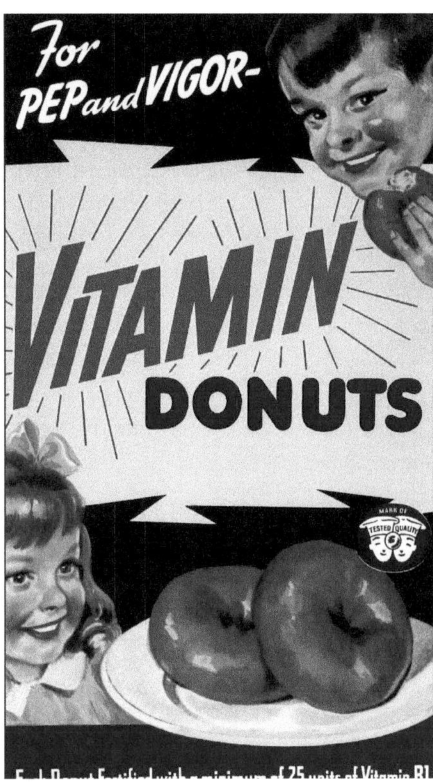

Though many advertisements tried to work vitamins into foods, the FDA did *not* approve of sales claims for vitamin-enriched donuts.

The USP-verified mark on a dietary supplement label tells consumers that the product quality has been verified under the rigorous **USP Dietary Supplement Verification Program**. This means that the dietary supplement:

- contains the ingredients listed on its label in the declared potency and amounts
- does not contain harmful levels of contaminants
- will break down and release ingredients into the body within a specified period
- has been made according to current US FDA good manufacturing practices

Though dietary supplements are not considered drugs by the FDA, the agency indirectly regulates them. The FDA is allowed to intervene only when proven safety concerns exist. Manufacturers are required to submit data to the FDA on all serious adverse events. The FDA publishes safety alerts and advisories, recalls, outbreaks, and emergency listings online for pharmacists and technicians to review.

Dietary supplements are also regulated by the **Federal Trade Commission (FTC)**. Created in 1914, this agency protects the US consumer from deceptive advertising practices in the marketplace. Though the FDA has primary responsibility for prescription and OTC drug labeling, the FTC regulates the labeling and advertising claims of dietary supplements. A company must be able to substantiate any product claims made in its labeling or advertising. For example, the following are some issues that have been investigated by the FTC:

- an herbal supplement that implied it prevented colds
- a dietary supplement that claimed to be effective in the treatment of arthritis symptoms
- a mineral that said that it improved athletic performance
- "miracle" weight-loss product that promised a loss of 15 pounds in 8 weeks
- a weight-loss product that did not reveal that it could cause serious increases in blood pressure

3.7 National Drug Code Number

Under the Drug Listing Act of 1972, discussed in Chapter 2, once a brand name or generic drug receives FDA approval, it is assigned a unique **National Drug Code (NDC) number** that appears on all drug stock labels as well as on the prescription labels. An NDC number is also assigned to any OTC, homeopathic, or dietary supplement on the market. As shown in Figure 3.3, the 10- to 11-character NDC number is made up of the following parts:

- a four- or five-digit labeler code, identifying the manufacturer or distributor of the drug
- a three- or four-digit product code, identifying the drug (active ingredient and its dosage form)
- a one- or two-digit package code, identifying the packaging size and type

Pharmacists and technicians use the NDC number to check that the correct drug is entered into the computer and dispensed. The pharmacy technician then focuses on the product and package code for filling the prescription, insurance reimbursement, and inventory control.

FIGURE 3.3 **NDC Number and Bar Code**

For both of these packages of Vistaril the first four digits of the NDC number (0069) indicate the manufacturer (Pfizer Labs) and the second four the product: 5420 indicates the drug is hydroxyzine pamoate, 50 mg oral capsules; 5410 indicates the same drug, 25 mg oral capsules. The last two numbers identify the packaging size (66), 100 capsules each.

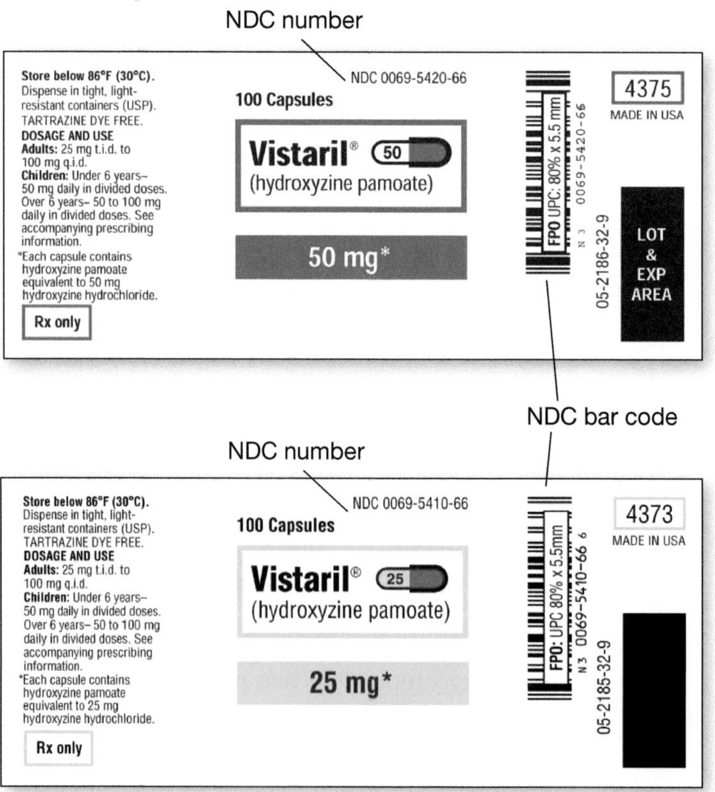

3.8 FDA Medication Safety Surveillance

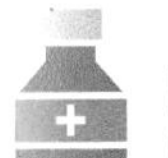
Pharm Fact

Students may also hear the phrase 'black box warning,' which is another way to say boxed warning.

Although every medication goes through a rigorous approval process, consumers should keep in mind that all drugs—prescription, OTC, and homeopathic, and all dietary supplements—have a risk of toxicity. In recognition of this fact, the FDA continues to gather information about any serious adverse reactions from approved medications. An **adverse drug reaction (ADR)** is defined as a negative consequence to a patient from taking a particular drug. Indeed, despite many years of research and clinical studies, some medications that enter the marketplace will still place individual patients at risk for a serious adverse reaction—an event that may not always be preventable or predictable. Even after millions of prescriptions are written (or vaccine doses administered) for patients of all ages, rare adverse effects may suddenly appear in the general population.

To protect the public's safety, the FDA requires that drug manufacturers develop an information resource for pharmacy personnel, called the package insert (PI), including boxed warnings about any possibilities of an extreme ADR. **Boxed warnings** (which show up in patient, provider, and pharmacy personnel reference materials from the manufacturer, FDA, and drug reference collections) highlight dangerous side effects, interactions, and use of drugs. These boxed warnings must also be included in the patients' information printout accompanying the medication. The FDA also established a nationwide surveillance system to serve as a conduit for reporting serious effects of certain medications. This **Adverse Event Reporting System (AERS)** is a centralized database that gathers and stores information from two separate programs: MedWatch for drugs and Vaccine Adverse Event Reporting System (VAERS) for vaccines. These will be covered in greater depth in Chapter 14 on safety. The FDA uses the collected information (with privacy protected) to track problems or issues that were not apparent when the medications and vaccinations were in clinical trials.

The recognition of a potential problem does not always mean that the product will be removed from the market. Many times, other initiatives are implemented to reduce or eliminate a safety risk—such as improving prescribing information, increasing awareness by educating healthcare professionals or the public, or perhaps simply changing the name of the drug or labeling. However, if significant incidents of ADRs come forth for any drug or vaccine, the FDA has the power to issue a **drug recall** (pull it off the market) with a marked level of urgency. Technicians and pharmacists must watch for these FDA recalls and immediately pull the products from their inventory, alerting patients when appropriate.

To avoid problems like those that occurred with thalidomide and other drugs, the FDA recognizes the need to do more prevention work with the high-risk drugs it has approved. It requires the manufacturers to develop Medication Guides, which provide patients with written consumer information on the high risks and proper uses of the drugs they have received. Medication Guides go beyond the usual patient instruction sheets.

However, some drugs require more detailed verbal and written communications *and* more focused patient monitoring. These drugs usually carry a high risk for serious adverse reactions if used inappropriately or by specific vulnerable populations. In these identified cases, the FDA requires that a **risk evaluation and mitigation strategy (REMS)** be developed by the drug manufacturers to ensure that the benefits of their drug outweigh the risks. For example, isotretinoin, a drug for severe acne, can cause serious birth defects if used inappropriately. Doctors and pharmacists must take special precautions to prevent pregnant or potentially pregnant women from using the drug.

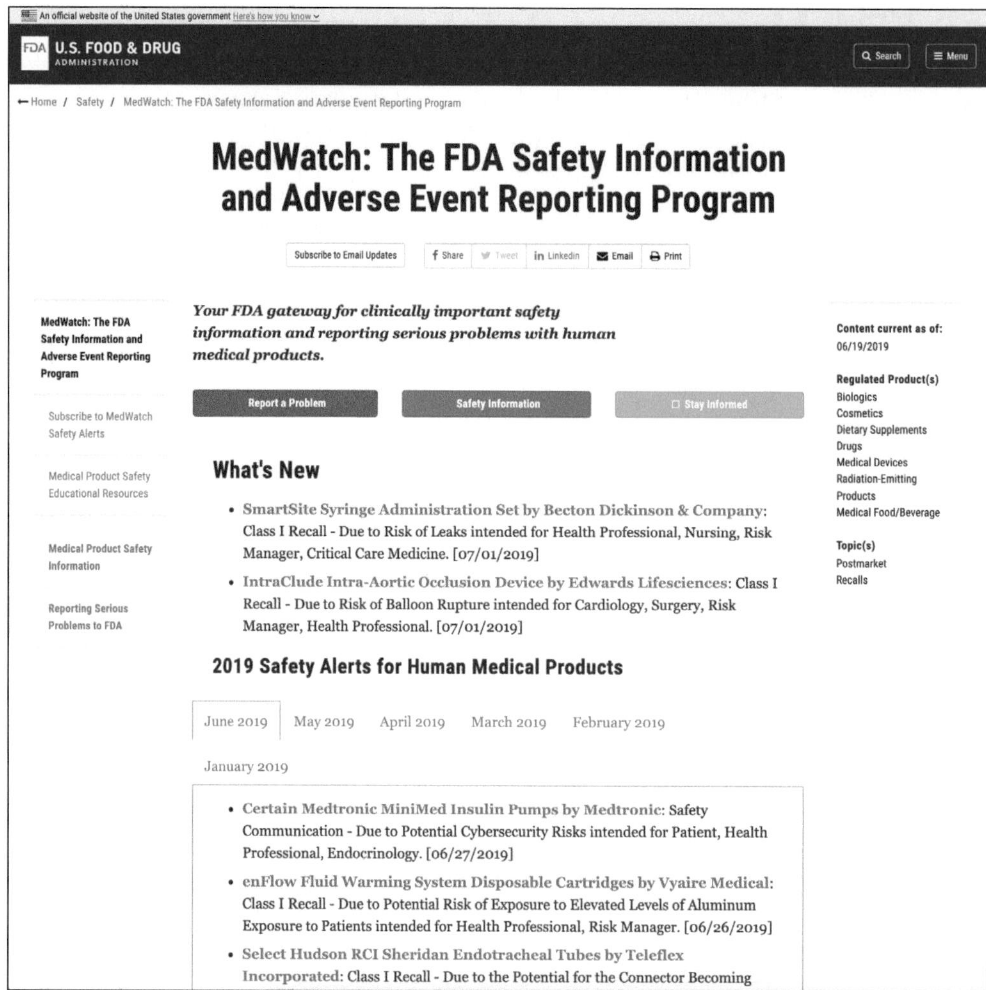

The FDA MedWatch website has the latest safety information on prescription drugs.

Drug manufacturers maintain a centralized database to monitor each patient more closely on these high-risk drugs and must make periodic assessment reports to the FDA on the status of the REMS for each drug. (Particular REMS will be discussed in Chapter 14.) Each prescriber and pharmacy must register with the pharmaceutical manufacturer and agree to the REMS policies and procedures before dispensing any of these drugs.

3.9 Applying an Understanding of Drugs

Though pharmacy technicians are not legally allowed to counsel patients, they do handle the daily filling and stocking of prescriptions as well as answer customers' retail questions. You, as a technician, need to be aware of the generic and brand names of drugs, their different medical purposes, why labels and warnings are important, and how the FDA oversees different pharmacy products. Knowing that certain drug products meet strict FDA requirements or USP standards can reassure patients of their safety and effectiveness when used appropriately. You can also help explain to customers why brand name products cost more than generics.

In a broader sense, by knowing some of the highlights of key drug developments, you can have a better understanding of how drugs work and how they have helped transform people's lives over the last century and a half. Taken appropriately, drugs have dramatically improved health, extended life expectancy, and alleviated suffering from disabling diseases, and they continue to do so. Taken inappropriately, drugs can cause serious side effects, adverse reactions (even disablement and death), interactions with other drugs, and inadequate treatment of the targeted medical condition. As a member of the pharmacy team, you will be an essential part of the educational process that makes the appropriate, safe use of drugs a priority.

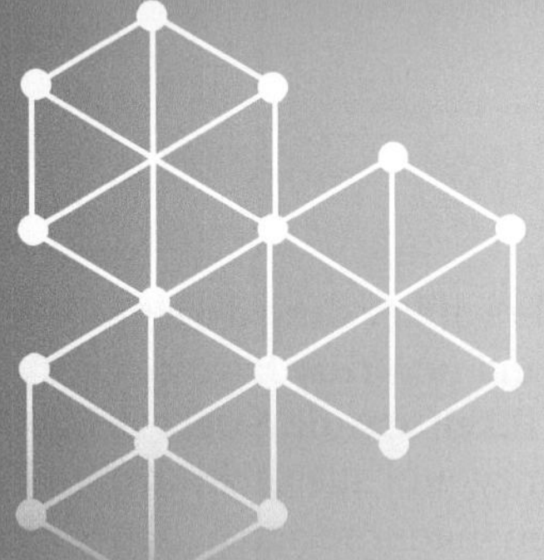

Review and Assessment

CHAPTER SUMMARY

- Drugs are classified by the FDA and regulated differently as prescription, OTC, or homeopathic drugs. Dietary supplements are considered foods, not drugs.
- Drugs are designed to have specific purposes: therapeutic, prophylactic, pharmacodynamic, destructive, and diagnostic.
- The identification of microorganisms as a cause of infectious illnesses is the basis for the germ theory of disease, which resulted in an emphasis on cleanliness and sterility in medicine and in the creation and administration of medications.
- Understanding germ theory led to the development of lifesaving vaccines, aseptic technique (used especially in the operating suites and hospital pharmacy), and the development of antibiotics and antivirals.
- Major drug developments in the past century include insulin, oral contraceptives, and mental health drugs.
- Many cancer drugs are destructive agents (with the first ones arising from agents used in war weapons), which is why following special safety procedures for chemotherapy and other hazardous compounding is so important.
- A relatively recent development–the unraveling of the human genetic code–has led to development of new biotechnology drugs and more targeted drug therapies.
- Drugs are classified as synthetic (chemical ingredients), synthesized (chemical ingredients made to imitate the naturally occurring agent), semisynthetic (chemical and natural ingredients together), and biogenetically engineered.
- The new prescription drug approval process consists of different phases of preclinical animal and clinical human studies, leading to submission of a new drug application to the FDA.
- For approximately every 10,000 new drugs studied, only one product will be approved by the FDA at a research cost of more than $1 billion.
- Generic drug approval processes are abbreviated because the brand name drug manufacturers did the extensive animal and human studies, and the drugs have track records. Generic drugs must show bioequivalence to the brand name products.
- The FDA regulates OTC and homeopathic drugs too, but with different approval processes. All drugs must follow USP standards and have extensive and easily understood labeling for consumers' use.
- The NDC number is assigned by the FDA and is specific for each manufacturer, drug product, dose, and package size. It is important in preventing medication errors and in executing drug recalls.

- The FDA monitors adverse effects of drugs and vaccines through its MedWatch and VAERS postmarketing surveillance programs. All healthcare personnel are encouraged to report any adverse effects from drugs or vaccines that they know about.
- Drug manufacturers, with the encouragement of the FDA, develop Medication Guides and REMS for select high-risk drugs to minimize serious adverse side effects. Pharmacy personnel must provide the information and/or follow the REMS guidelines to protect the public.
- The FDA can order drug recalls. Pharmacy personnel must watch for recalls, and respond by removing the drugs from the inventory and, if appropriate, contacting patients.Take a moment to review what you have learned in this chapter and answer the following questions.

CHECK YOUR UNDERSTANDING

1. Which of the following classifications of drugs undergoes the most extensive FDA approval process?
   a. homeopathic medications.
   b. prescription drugs
   c. dietary supplements
   d. OTC drugs
2. To bill insurance for a prescription of penicillin, a pharmacy technician will need the prescriber's
   a. DEA number
   b. NPI number
   c. NDC number
   d. state medical license number
3. Which drug classification is comprised of antineoplastic drugs?
   a. therapeutic agents
   b. diagnostic agents
   c. prophylactic agents
   d. destructive agents
4. With the help of pharmacy technicians, many pharmacists are now administering vaccines in community pharmacies. A vaccine is an example of a
   a. therapeutic agent.
   b. prophylactic agent.
   c. diagnostic agent.
   d. destructive agent.
5. A radiopharmaceutical used for imaging is an example of a
   a. therapeutic agent.
   b. diagnostic agent.
   c. pharmacodynamic agent.
   d. prophylactic agent.
6. Who discovered the first antiseptic used in sterilizing surgical rooms?
   a. Dr. Edward Jenner
   b. Dr. Francis Crick and Dr. James Watson
   c. Sir Alexander Fleming
   d. Dr. Joseph Lister

MAKE CONNECTIONS

Take a moment to consider what you have learned in this chapter and respond thoughtfully to the following prompts. Note that some of these activities will require internet access.

1. Consider the different purposes for drugs (therapeutic, prophylactic, destructive, pharmacodynamic, and diagnostic agents). Go through the over-the-counter aisles at your local pharmacy and find examples of as many types of agents as you can. Which types aren't available OTC?
2. Practice explaining the different phases of clinical drug trials and FDA safety checks to assure a nervous patient with concerns they have about the dangers of a new drug they are trying.

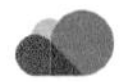
The online course includes additional review and assessment resources.

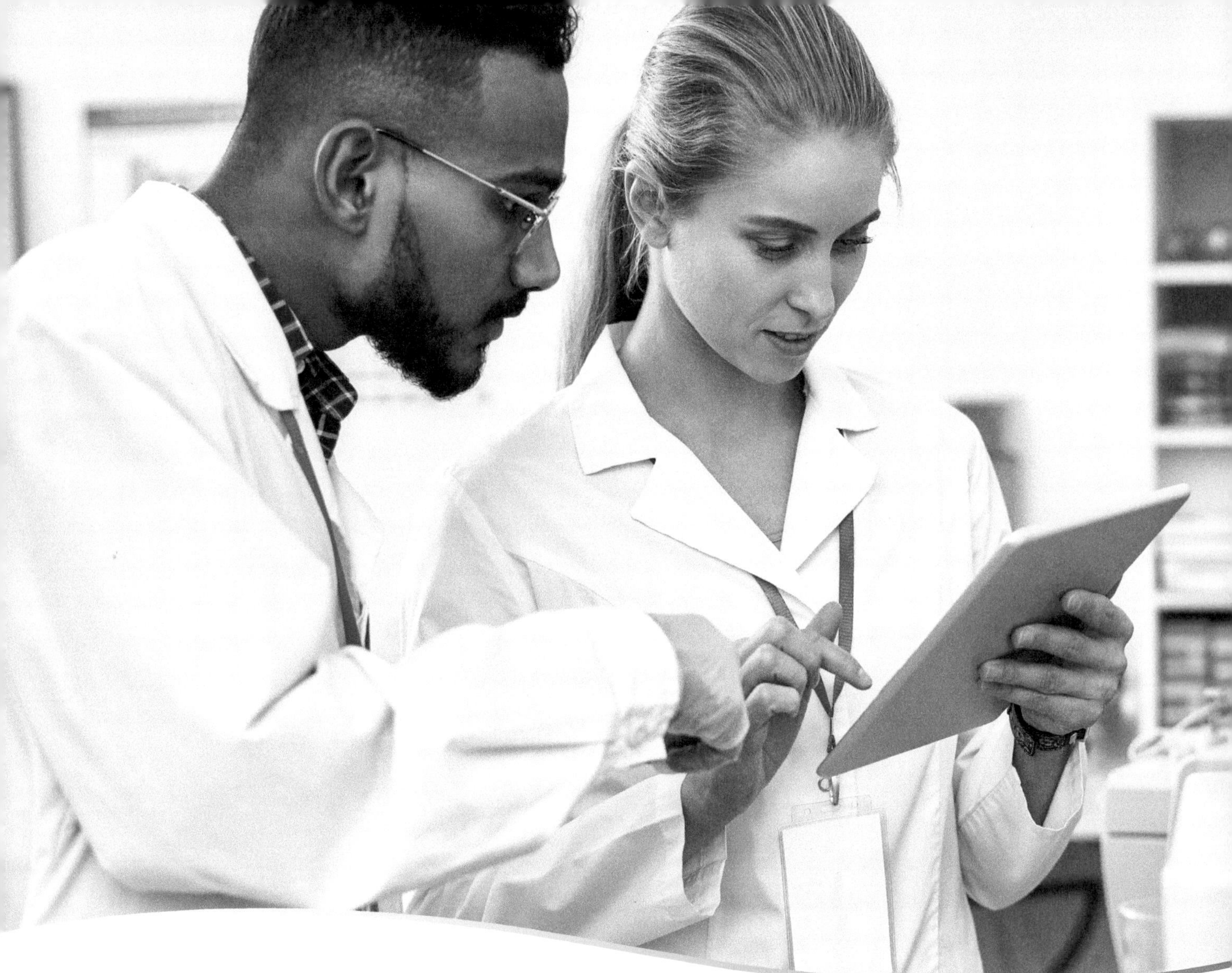

UNIT 2 Introduction to Pharmacy Skills

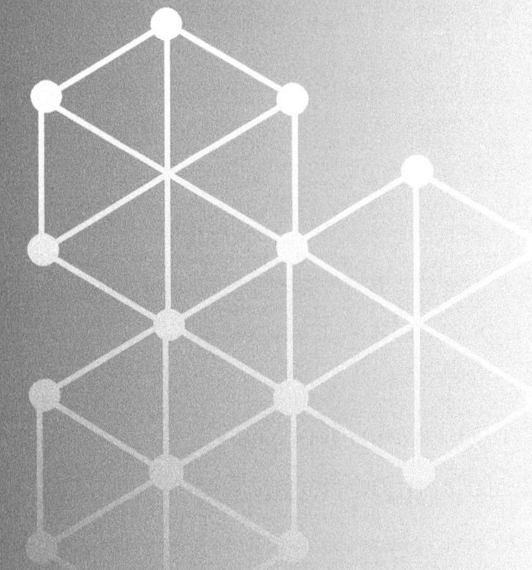

4

Introducing Pharmacology

Learning Objectives

1 Define the scope of the field of pharmacology and its areas of scientific study. (Section 4.1)

2 Explain the concepts of pharmaceutical indications and contraindications. (Section 4.2)

3 Discuss the concepts of pharmaceutical and therapeutic equivalency and how they relate to the dispensing of generic and alternative drugs. (Section 4.3)

4 Discuss the concepts of biosimilars and interchangeable biological drugs. (Section 4.3)

5 Explain how drugs are organized by anatomical systems in pharmacology. (Section 4.4)

6 Recognize the common anatomical categories of drugs and the most requested classes, brand names, and generics within these categories. (Sections 4.5–4.14)

7 List key drug reference guides. (Section 4.15)

ASHP/ACPE Accreditation Standards
To view the *ASHP/ACPE Accreditation Standards* addressed in this chapter, refer to Appendix B.

Though a healthy lifestyle remains the cornerstone of good health, drugs can serve to heal, maintain healthy processes, and supply missing bodily substances. **Pharmacology** is the science of drugs and their interactions with the organ systems of living animals.

There are over 2,000 drugs on the market, many in multiple formulations, and that is not even counting experimental research drugs! It is nearly impossible to memorize every single drug, which is why there are computer aids and pharmacists to depend upon. However, you will need a solid knowledge base. This chapter introduces you to drug categorization by anatomical systems along with the most commonly used pharmacy drugs in these categories with their generic drug equivalents. Alternative drug products, biosimilars, and interchangeable biologic drugs will also be explained.

Many of you may find the challenges of this chapter overwhelming at first. Do not be dismayed as this is only an overview, and you will recognize many brand name drugs from personal experiences and media advertising. You can study these and other drugs in more depth as you move through your studies and career. Knowledge of common drugs will become second nature as you gain on-site experience in the community and/or hospital pharmacy.

4.1 What Is the Scope of Pharmacology?

Put Down Roots

Pharmacology comes from the Greek word *pharmakon,* or "drug," and the Latin suffix *logia,* or "study of." *Toxicology,* then, is the study of *toxikon*—"arrow poison" in Greek—or poisons.

In its broadest sense, pharmacology includes the study of drugs and how they work. It encompasses specialized scientific disciplines, including the following:

- **therapeutics**–appropriate use of drugs for targeted medicinal purposes
- **pharmacodynamics**–biochemical, physiologic, and molecular effects of drugs on the body
- **toxicology**–symptoms, detection and treatment of poisonous effects and side effects
- **pharmaceutics**–various dosage forms and routes of administration and their drug-releasing capabilities
- **pharmacokinetics**–movement of drugs within the body: absorption, distribution, metabolism, and elimination (ADME) of drugs from the body, and harmful drug interactions
- **pharmacognosy**–natural sources of drugs and herbs

This chapter will present some aspects of the therapeutics, pharmacodynamics, and toxicology of common drugs and their classes. The pharmacokinetics of drugs are less applicable to a technician's work and will not be addressed in this book. There will, however, be mention of some of the ways these drugs are administered and their dosage forms (pharmaceutics). Greater explanation of pharmaceutics will be offered in the next chapter (Chapter 5). You will also find an introduction to common herbal medicines, supplements, and vitamins (pharmacognosy) in Chapter 9.

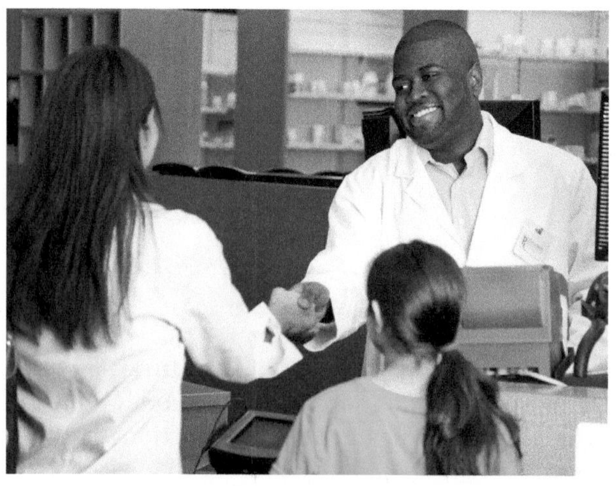

Customers trust their pharmacists for up-to-date information about drugs, and the pharmacists depend upon their technicians to know how to help fill patient prescriptions.

It takes pharmacists numerous years of studying the basic and applied elements of pharmacology for thousands of drugs before they can even begin to practice. That is why patient questions about drugs must always be directed to the pharmacist. However, the more you know, the more confidence you will have in performing the expanding role of a pharmacy technician.

4.2 Essential Knowledge for Technicians

When a pharmacy technician enters a prescription into the computer or pulls a drug from stock, it helps to be familiar with both the brand and generic names and their common dosage forms. Many names, dosages, and formulations are very similar and confusing if one doesn't have a basic understanding of pharmacology.

Without any familiarity, dangerous medication errors can occur. In many cases, prescribers write a prescription for a brand name drug–which is often easier to remember and spell–though a generic drug will be dispensed. So the pharmacy technician must be aware of the correct substitutions and situations when generic drugs can be legally substituted for brand name drugs and when they cannot.

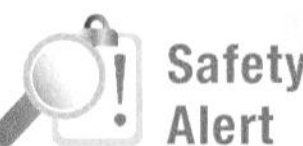

Safety Alert

Some drugs at higher doses can have a paradoxical effect. This may be a pain medication causing pain or an antidepressant causing suicidal panic. Prescribers, pharmacists, and technicians must ask about and be on the alert for any mention from patients about these kinds of dangerous side effects.

Besides recognizing common drugs and their generic substitutions, technicians should know the primary **indications** for the drugs, or the common intended uses, to treat specific diseases. For instance, a patient may call in to request a refill on their blood pressure medication, but they cannot remember, spell, or even pronounce the drug name correctly and do not have the prescription number readily available. How will the pharmacy technician know which medication in the patient's profile to refill without a basic knowledge of the indications of various drugs?

Technicians and pharmacists must also be aware of the **contraindications** of each drug— the specific situations *in which a drug should not be used* because it will be harmful to a patient. Say that same patient comes in for a refill, and the patient's medication history says that a new prescription for Nitrobid (nitroglycerin) has been added to the patient's record since the last refill. The contraindication for the antihypertensive drug refill says that it should not be given to patients who are taking nitroglycerin. The technician, seeing this, must then query the pharmacist and perhaps even the provider or provider's nursing assistant to see what should be done.

Additionally, one has to remember that, for every intended drug action, there are related unintended reactions, or **side effects**, that must *always* be considered. They can be mild or severe, such as varying intensities of nausea, constipation, diarrhea, itchiness and other skin reactions, drowsiness, pain, muscle aches, headaches, shakiness, and numbness. Though less common, technicians should also be aware of **paradoxical drug reactions** or effects. A paradoxical drug reaction occurs when use of a medication has the opposite effect from what is normally expected.

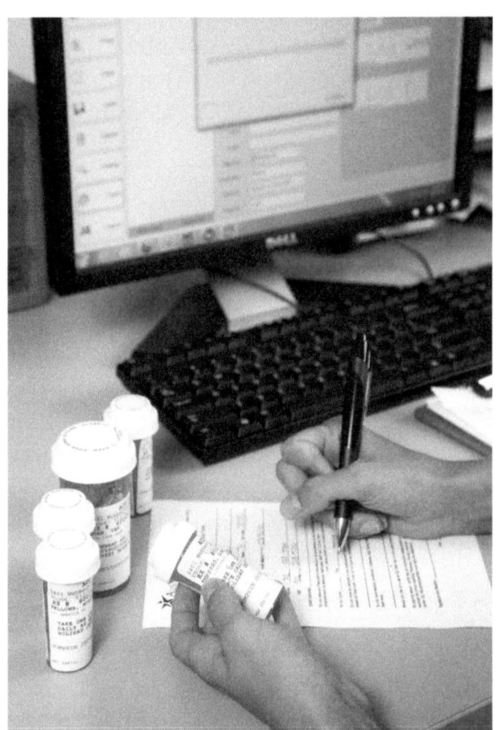

Technicians need to read prescriptions and medication profiles very carefully for each small detail—spelling dosages, indications, contraindications, potential interactions, and side effects. If something is amiss, they must question the pharmacist and, at times, the provider or assisting nurse.

Drug interactions occur when a drug affects the intended indication of another medication or reacts poorly with it. Interactions can happen between a drug and another prescribed (or nonprescribed) drug, food, or multiple drugs. Drugs in combination can cause many difficulties as they react together, and their side effects build up. In some cases patients are on multiple medications for chronic conditions and suffer from the side effects of drug. When one or more of the interacting drugs are discontinued, these patients find that their symptoms and overall health improve, in some cases dramatically. A drug can also interact badly with over-the-counter (OTC) and homeopathic drugs. Even vitamin, nutrient, or herbal supplements can interfere with or enhance the potency of a drug, or cause intense reactions; so the vitamins and supplements a patient is taking must be added to the patient profile and also considered. Finally, a drug to address one disease might worsen another disease or condition the patient is experiencing.

Adverse drug events (ADEs) are injuries or harmful responses due to the use of a drug. ADEs can arise from side effects, contraindications, allergic reactions, wrong use, or the results of combining a drug with one or more other medications, vitamins, or herbal supplements. ADEs account for approximately 125,000 hospital admissions each year, according to statistics from the US Department of Health and Human Services in 2014. These events can range in severity from an extremely unpleasant experience of shaking, vomiting, hives, and other occurrences, to paralysis, blindness, and death.

That is why technicians must look so carefully at the patient profile of medications, allergies, history of use, and software alerts. The pharmacist watches most specifically for these things and makes the final decisions, but the technician serves as the first line of inquiry and defense against prescription errors. This is why knowing more about common drugs and their indications and contraindications is important for pharmacy technicians.

4.3 Prescription Drug Substitutions

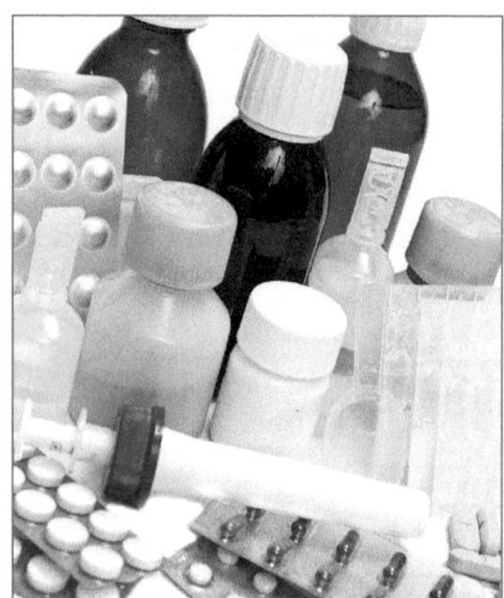

Medications come in different forms. To be a substitution, the drugs must have the same dosage forms.

As noted in earlier chapters, pharmacists or pharmacy technicians in all states are permitted (or in some cases required) to substitute a lower-cost generic drug in place of a higher-cost brand name drug for a specific indication as long as the generic drug is considered bioequivalent. Unless otherwise noted in this chapter, you will find the brand name drug listed as a proper name with the first letter capitalized and the generic drug/ingredient not capitalized. Sometimes, however, a generic drug will be mentioned with the brand name in parentheses. There are also generic drug brands.

Pharmaceutically and Therapeutically Equivalent Drug Products

For a specific generic drug to be considered as a bioequivalent for a brand drug by the Food and Drug Administration (FDA), it must be both pharmaceutically and therapeutically equal, though not necessarily identical in appearance.

Pharmaceutically Equivalent

To meet the US Pharmacopeia–National Formulary (USP–NF) standards for strength, quality, purity, and identity, each generic drug is formulated to contain the same amount of active ingredient in the same dosage form as the original, FDA-approved, brand name drug. This makes the two drug products **pharmaceutically equivalent**. However, these generic drug products *may differ* in characteristics such as shape, scoring configuration, packaging, inert ingredients (including colorings, flavors, and preservatives), expiration time, and—within certain limits—labeling. A vast majority of all FDA-approved drugs have a pharmaceutically equivalent generic product. A common example is the generic drug lisinopril 20 mg for treating high blood pressure. The dosage unit may look different (i.e., have different markings) than the brands Zestril or Prinivil, but the drug is absorbed in a similar manner.

Therapeutically Equivalent

Each generic drug *also* needs to be **therapeutically equivalent**, or provide the same medicinal benefit at the same dosage rates with the same degree of safety under the conditions specified in the labeling as the name brand version. This means that clinical trials show that the generic offers equal results in terms of safety and efficacy, compared to the brand name. The generic depends upon the long track record and earlier clinical studies of the brand name for FDA approval. In the example above, the pharmaceutically equivalent generic of lisinopril should lower blood pressure similarly to the brand product. If a generic drug is both pharmaceutically *and* therapeutically equivalent, it is considered generally "substitutable" for the brand name product by the technician and pharmacist without prior approval of the physician.

Pharmaceutical Alternative Drug Products

Generic drugs are not available for all brand name drugs (as some patents have not yet expired). Instead, **pharmaceutical alternative** drug products contain the same active therapeutic ingredients but different salts (for example, metoprolol succinate rather than metoprolol tartrate) or that come in different dosage forms (a tablet rather than a capsule or an immediate-release tablet rather than an extended-release tablet). These pharmaceutical alternatives may be recommended but *cannot be substituted* without physician approval. Thus, for a prescription of 100 mg of metoprolol succinate (an extended-release formulation), a pharmacy technician cannot substitute 100 mg of metoprolol tartrate (an immediate-release formulation). Although the active ingredients and dose are identical, the salts (succinate versus tartrate) and the release characteristics of the drugs differ. For this reason, this type of substitution is not permitted unless specifically prescribed.

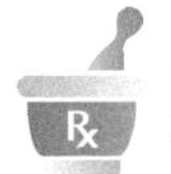

Practice Tip

On each prescription, watch for provider notes. "Brand medically necessary," "brand necessary," and "dispense as written" (DAW) all mean the same thing—no substitutions without authorization!

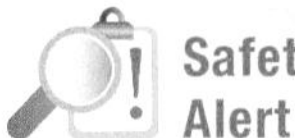

Safety Alert

Always remember that generics and brand names, though substitutable, *are not exactly alike*. The different formulations may affect patients differently, so when dispensing refills, listen for any patient concerns about substitutions to pass on to the pharmacist.

Brand Names Versus Generics

Some physicians do not like to substitute generics even if the medications are considered pharmaceutically and therapeutically equivalent. Just as with brand name drugs, not all patients will respond similarly to a specific generic drug. That is because each patient has a slightly different biological chemistry, and the formulations of inert ingredients affect patients differently. This often occurs with thyroid prescriptions written by an endocrinologist. The prescriber is permitted by law to write "brand medically necessary" on the prescription. Especially on new prescriptions, pharmacy technicians should look for and dispense only the drug specifically written in the prescription. This is a similar directive to a prescriber's "dispense as written" (DAW).

Because brand names are more recognizable, they are often more trusted. The patient may request a brand name drug even if the prescriber did not write "brand medically necessary" or "DAW" on the prescription. The patient's request would be indicated by writing "DAW2" on the prescription for insurance processing. This generally results in a higher copay, so the technician must make sure that the patient is aware of this. Then the patient should be referred to the pharmacist if they still want the brand name drug.

Conversely, a patient may request a lower-cost generic even though the physician wrote "brand necessary." A call to the physician's office will be necessary to approve the generic over the brand name drug.

When refilling a prescription, it is important that the pharmacy technician review the patient profile to see if a brand name or generic product was previously dispensed. For certain medications (such as thyroid hormone replacers or blood thinners), it is not good practice for the patient to keep switching between brand name and generic products even when they are bioequivalent and therapeutically equivalent. Laboratory results often slightly differ though the brand name and generic product are prescribed at the same dose. This is something the technician can explain to the patients, referring them to the pharmacist if necessary.

IN THE REAL WORLD

The dispensing of generic drugs is a major factor in containing the high cost of pharmaceuticals, with a cost savings of 30% to 80% over brand name counterparts. However, as brands are being developed, costs are rising there too. For instance, in seven months (from October 2013 to April 2014), the cost of the generic asthma medication albuterol sulfate rose from $11 for two tablets to $434 and the antibiotic doxycycline hyclate from an average of $20 per bottle to $1,849! Even so, generic drugs have considerably slowed the rate of cost increases on pharmaceuticals–but it is difficult to tell now by how much. In the same way, biosimilars are projected to save over $5 billion in healthcare costs over the next decade as more expensive biotechnology drugs come off patent.

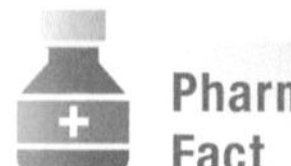

Pharm Fact

The FDA *Orange Book* first appeared in October 1980. Since it was near Halloween, the staff chose orange for the cover color, and the nickname stuck. For the biological drug guide, one staff member simply suggested purple, giving rise to the *Purple Book*.

The FDA Orange Book

A technician or pharmacist is not expected to remember *all* the pharmaceutical and therapeutic equivalencies or which are legal substitutions in what situations. The pharmacy software will help make these considerations clear and offer alerts. The online **FDA Orange Book** (officially known as the *Approved Drug Products with Therapeutic Equivalence Evaluations*)–is the official legal source for drug equivalency information in the United States. The web publication found at: https://PharmPractice7e.ParadigmEducation.com/OrangeBook provides information on generic substitution of drugs that may have many different brand name or generic manufacturer sources. It lists all the drug products the FDA considers to be (or not to be) therapeutically equivalent to other pharmaceutically equivalent products. It covers not only generic substitutions and alternatives, but also brand name alternatives at different dosages.

The Orange Book lists the doses that may be safely substituted. For example, two brand-name antihypertensive drugs for extended (24 hours) blood pressure control are Adalat CC and Procardia XL. They *cannot be substituted* for each other due to different drug-release characteristics. There are, however, generic manufactured drugs using the active ingredient nifedipine that are compatible with either or both that can be substituted (see Table 4.1). However, each manufacturer's formulation of salts or other ingredients offers different drug characteristics. Not every generic of the same active ingredient is the same. Some are appropriate as a substitution of one brand formulation and some for another. It depends on the drug formulation and its release characteristics, such as delayed or extended release.

TABLE 4.1 Generic Drugs Therapeutically Equivalent to Adalat CC and Procardia XL

Generic Drug (Trade)	Dosage	Manufacturer
nifedipine (Adalat CC)	30 mg, 60 mg	Par
nifedipine (Adalat CC or Procardia XL)	30 mg, 60 mg	Valeant
nifedipine (Adalat CC or Procardia XL)	30 mg, 60 mg, 90 mg	Mylan, Novast, Osmotica, Sun Pharma, TWI, Zydus

For example, the Par generic formulations of nifedipine in doses of 30 mg and 60 mg can be substituted for Adalat CC. The Mylan, Novast, Osmotica, Sun Pharma, TWI, and Zydus versions can be used for either Adalat CC or Procardia XL. In most cases, the software your pharmacy or drug wholesaler utilizes will cross-reference the FDA-approved generic equivalents of a given brand name drug.

As you learn drug names, it will be easier to remember them if you can remember them in families. The generic names of certain classes of drugs for specific indications often share the same suffix at the end. A great resource list of generic drug name prefixes, roots, and suffixes can be found at https://PharmPractice7e.ParadigmEducation.com/TakerX. Table 4.2 provides a sample.

TABLE 4.2 Sample of Common Generic Name Suffixes with Drug Class/Category

Suffix	Generic Examples	Class/Category
-artan	losartan, olmesartan, valsartan	Angiotensin receptor blocker
- afil	sildenafil, tadalafil, verdenafil	Phosphodiesterase inhibitor
-cillin	amoxicillin, ampicillin, nafcillin	Penicillin derivatives
-dipine	amlodipine, nicardipine, nifedipine	Calcium channel blockers
-erol	albuterol, formoterol, salmeterol	Bronchodilators
-floxacin	ciprofloxacin, levofloxacin, moxifloxacin	Fluoroquinolones
-lol	atenolol, metoprolol	Beta-blockers
-one	dexamethasone, methylprednisolone, prednisone	Corticosteroid
-prazole	esomeprazole, lansoprasole, pantoprazole	Proton pump inhibitors
-pril	benazepril, enalapril, lisinopril	Angiotensin converting enzyme inhibitors
-statin	atorvastatin, rosuvastatin, simvastatin	Statins (HMG-CoA reductase inhibitors)
-tidine	famotidine, ranitidine	Histamine-2 antagonists
-tropium	ipratropium, tiotropium	Anticholinergics
-zepam	diazepam, lorazepam, temazepam	Benzodiazepines

Biologically Comparable Drug Products

Biological drugs (including genetically engineered drugs) come from a variety of live or once-live sources, including animals, humans, and microorganisms such as yeast, bacteria, and fungi. These drugs are usually expensive injectable drugs used to treat genetic disorders, blood disorders related to cancer or chemotherapy, and inflammatory diseases, such as rheumatoid arthritis. These biological drug products tend to have larger and more complex molecules than most chemical compounds. When a brand-name biological drug is patented and FDA approved, it becomes the **biological reference product** for all similar biological drug products to come because it is the original drug that went through the extensive clinical trials for safety and effectiveness. A biological drug patent lasts 12 years.

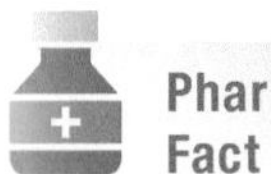

Pharm Fact

As of early 2019, the FDA had approved 19 biosimilar drugs. Different states have different rules. To see a summation of the fall 2018 state rules, go to https://PharmPractice7e.ParadigmEducation.com/NCSL.

Because biological drugs come from living matter or organisms, they *cannot be chemically reproduced with exactitude*. Therefore a generic version could not be specifically designated as pharmaceutically or therapeutically equivalent. That is why biological drug substitutions are handled differently. Instead of bioequivalent drugs, the FDA has evaluated and approved biosimilar drugs, which are similar though not identical to the parent innovator drugs. Some of these can be tested to be designated as **interchangeable biological drugs**, which are both biosimilar and have been proven to offer similar therapeutic results. These interchangeables can therefore be legally substituted for the biological reference products in prescriptions.

Biosimilar Drugs

Biosimilar drugs are deemed by the FDA as biologically comparable or sufficiently like the reference products in therapeutic methods. They have been proven to address the same indications with the same **pharmaceutical mechanism of action**, or precise ways that the active ingredients exert their influence on the body. They must also have the same administration routes, dosage forms, conditions of use, and levels of quality and strength as the original. (See Figure 4.1.)

FIGURE 4.1 **Sample Production Process of a Biological Reference Product**

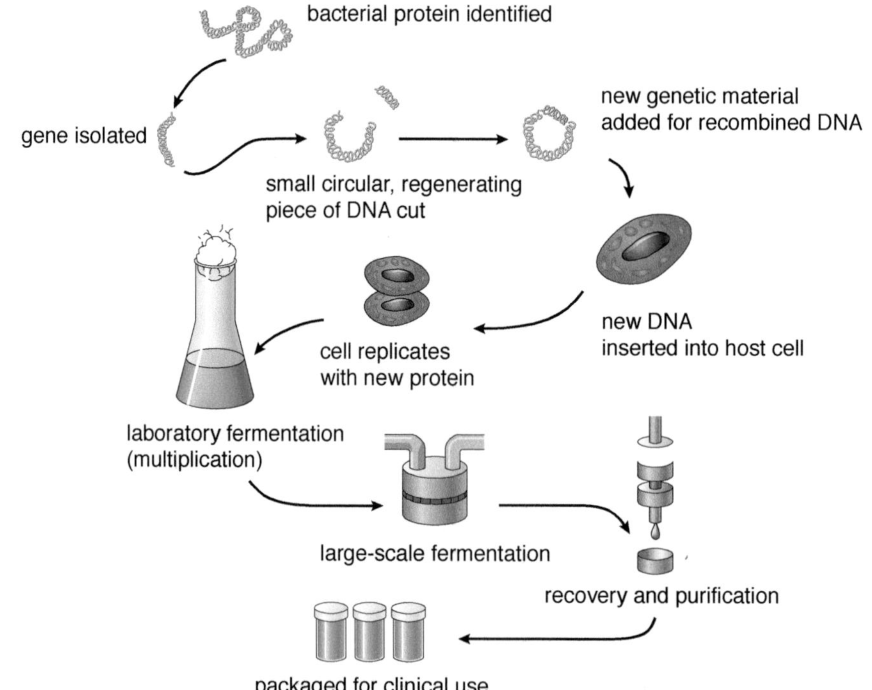

A biosimilar drug must demonstrate no substantial differences in terms of safety, purity, and potency from the original drug, but it may not yet have proven to provide the same clinical effectiveness as the original. Biosimilars that have been FDA-approved can be considered by physicians as alternative drug products for the related biological drug brands. However, the laws governing pharmacy substitution of a biosimilar for a biological brand vary from state to state. Some states allow substitution by the pharmacy as long as the prescriber and patient are notified.

IN THE REAL WORLD

While pharmacists are allowed to substitute generic drugs for another therapeutically equivalent generic drug in most cases, the same is not always true for biosimilar drugs. While the FDA carries out the scientific review of biosimilar products, it does not determine whether a biosimilar can be substituted for the innovator product. The FDA has deemed this decision up to individual state boards of pharmacy. Some states may permit a pharmacist to substitute a biosimilar product without prescriber authorization. Other states do not allow this change. Check with your state board of pharmacy for biosimilar substitution laws.

Interchangeable Biological Drug Products

To be designated an interchangeable biological drug, a biological drug must be biosimilar to the reference drug *and must exert the same therapeutic effect.*

The pharmaceutical manufacturer must present scientific data from clinical trials to the FDA indicating that the innovative interchangeable drug product can deliver similar results with the same effectiveness and safety as the reference drug. In addition, there can be no greater risk posed in switching from the reference drug to the interchangeable product.

If all these criteria are met for the FDA to approve the biosimilar as an interchangeable biological drug, pharmacists and technicians may be able to legally substitute it for the prescribed biological brand without contacting the physician for approval, as in a generic drug substitution. However, it is up to the discretion of each state whether or not to allow this substitution.

Practice Tip

Remember that biological drugs are from live or once-live organisms. Biologically interchangeable and biosimilar drugs are never bioequivalent to the patented formulation, unlike most generic drugs, which are bioequivalent.

The FDA Purple Book

Just as the *Orange Book* is a reference for therapeutically equivalent drugs, there is also a reference for interchangeable biological drug products. The online reference is published by the FDA and is titled Purple Book: *Lists of Licensed Biological Products with Reference Product Exclusivity and Biosimilarity or Interchangeability Evaluations.* Since that is quite a mouthful, it is just called the Purple Book. It currently has two FDA lists:

- Over 100 licensed biological drug products that specifically include natural substances (that may be alive), such as allergenic extracts, blood and blood components, gene therapy products, human tissues, and cellular products used in transplantation, vaccines, and more
- Over 275 licensed biologically engineered (bioengineered) or biotechnical (biotech) drug products, such as enzymes, protein growth enhancers, and antibodies developed as targeted cancer therapies

As biosimilars and interchangeables start to move through the approval processes, they will be included in the Purple Book. The FDA also publishes the Green Book: *FDA Approved Animal Drug Products* for veterinary-oriented substances. Because some of these animal drugs can be purchased at pharmacies, this is a valuable reference for pharmacists and technicians. Other common pharmaceutical references will be listed at the end of this chapter.

4.4 Anatomical Classification of Drugs

To study and remember some of the generic and brand name drugs you will encounter, it is often easiest to consider them according to their classification by anatomical system or organ and/or by their pharmaceutical action. For example, metoprolol ER (Toprol XL) and lisinopril (Prinivil, Zestril) are in the cardiovascular (heart-blood system) category, and both are used to treat high blood pressure, but each lowers the blood pressure in a different way. That is, the mechanism of action, or method, of pharmacological action is different. Many patients may require two or more drugs—with different mechanisms of action—to provide adequate blood pressure control.

Drug Facts and Comparisons® (F&C) is a primary reference for considering drugs by their anatomical classifications and finding the generic substitutions. It provides factual, up-to-date information on drug product availability, indications, administration and dose, pharmacological actions, contraindications, warnings, precautions, adverse reactions, overdoses, and patient instructions. It is available as a hardbound copy and as an online subscription.

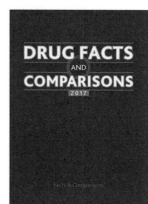

Drug Facts and Comparisons is a commonly used drug information resource. Pictured above is a hardbound copy, but the publication is also available online.

The rest of this chapter discusses the classifications in the same order that they are presented in the *F&C*:

- Central Nervous System (CNS) Agents
- Cardiovascular Agents
- Systematic Anti-Infective Agents
- Endocrine and Metabolic Agents
- Respiratory Agents
- Gastrointestinal Agents
- Renal and Genitourinary Agents
- Hematologic Agents
- Biotechnology Drugs
- Miscellaneous Drugs

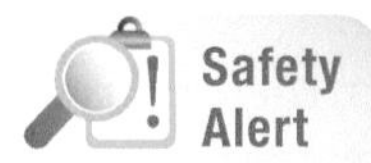

Make sure to read all boxed warnings as you get to know the drugs you will be working with.

Explaining how each drug mentioned in this chapter exactly works is beyond the scope of this overview. However, gaining a recognition of how drugs are pharmaceutically categorized for dispensing and becoming familiar with generic and brand drug names and their common indications is an essential component of the technician learning process and successfully passing the Pharmacy Technician Certification Exam. You will learn more about these in the community dispensing section of Chapter 7. Boxed warnings (which show up in patient, provider, and pharmacy personnel reference materials from the manufacturer, FDA, and drug reference collections) highlight dangerous side effects, interactions, and use.

4.5 Central Nervous System Agents

A key category in the *F&C* is the central nervous system (CNS), which consists of specialized nerve cells called **neurons** located in the brain and spinal cord. Neurons communicate with each other primarily through chemicals known as **neurotransmitters**. Prescribed drugs often alter the neurotransmitter activity at the neuron level to produce medicinal effects, which also can produce side effects that must be considered.

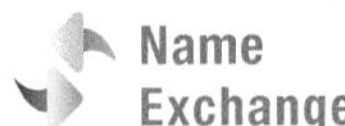

Put Down Roots

Analgesia comes from the Greek *algein*, "to feel pain," with the prefix *an*, meaning "not." It means to not feel pain or to result in painlessness.

Name Exchange

APAP is an abbreviation for nonnarcotic acetaminophen. The abbreviation comes from the active ingredient acetyl-paraami-nophenol. When combined with a narcotic, APAP often offers better relief for pain than either drug alone and at lower doses.

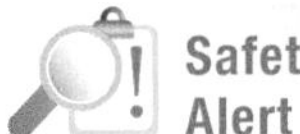

Safety Alert

Oxycodone is a potent Schedule II drug that is available as both an immediate-release generic drug and a long-acting brand name drug (OxyContin). It is important for the pharmacy technician to distinguish between the short- and long-acting formulations when entering the drugs into the computer to avoid medication errors.

Analgesic and Anti-Inflammatory Agents

Analgesic medications are used to relieve or reduce pain, whereas **anti-inflammatory drugs** work to reduce swelling. Multiple common medications in the subcategory of analgesic and anti-inflammatory agents act upon the CNS and nerves (see Table 4.3).

Narcotic Analgesics

Narcotics are pain relieving drugs that may substantially affect mood and behavior. Narcotics are highly addictive with particular contraindications and restrictions of use since they can cause a great deal of harm if misused. Narcotics have the following effects:

- **analgesia**, relieves or reduces pain
- **sedation**, allays anxiety and causes drowsiness
- **euphoria**, produces feelings of extreme high mood and energy
- **dysphoria**, develops feelings of anxiety, disordered thoughts, hyperfear, restlessness, malaise, or hallucinations

All narcotics are listed by the DEA as controlled substances because they are potentially addictive, meaning they may cause greater tolerance (need for higher doses for the same effects), physical and psychological dependence, and addiction. (There will be more on this in Chapter 14.)

Common narcotic analgesics are the **opiates**, which are drugs from the opium poppy plant, including heroin (illegal), morphine, and codeine. **Opioids** are synthetically made narcotics that offer opium-like effects of reduced perception and reaction to pain, and increased pain tolerance. Opioids often include opium elements but are chemically designed to have varied or extended opium-like effects. Medications that fall into this category include hydrocodone, oxycodone, and other related drugs (note the suffix - *codone*). **Adjuvant medications** are helper medications. They are not strictly used for pain, but they help in pain management and may be prescribed along with a pain reliever. Some common adjuvants are antidepressant and antiseizure medications, muscle relaxants, sedatives, or sleep-enhancing drugs.

Hydrocodone is the generic name for a powerful opioid narcotic pain reliever. Hydrocodone combination drugs (Lortab, Norco, and Vicodin) are by far the most popular prescribed pain medications. Hydrocodone drug combinations are Schedule II drugs with no refills permitted.

Oxycodone (OxyContin, Roxicodone) offers strong, narcotic pain relief. Many hydrocodone, oxycodone, and codeine preparations also contain acetaminophen, which increases their analgesic effects.

In the hospital setting, injections of fentanyl, morphine, and hydromorphone (Dilaudid) are commonly used for temporary relief of severe pain. For terminally ill hospice or cancer patients, around-the-clock narcotics—administered via infusion pumps, as liquids, or in controlled-release solid dosage forms or patches—are commonly and appropriately used to provide comfort and pain relief.

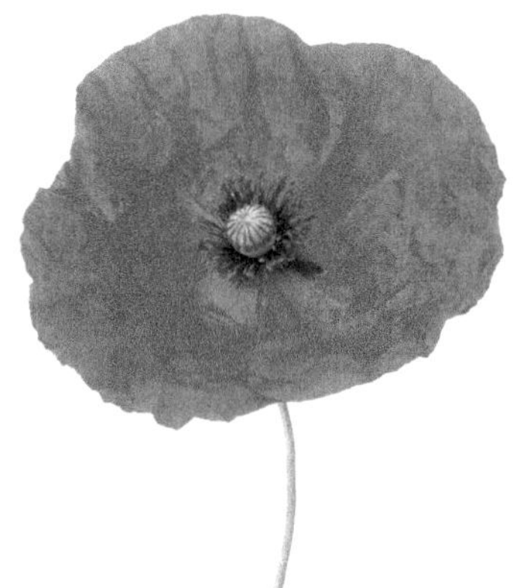

Opiates come from the Middle Eastern opium poppy plant (*Papaver somniferum*). The familiar red corn poppy (*Papaver rhoeas*) from Flanders Fields is related but does not contain hallucinogens.

Narcotic analgesics can cause stomach upset and constipation. Therefore it is recommended that these medications be taken with food, and if constipation occurs, a stool softener or short-term laxative may be recommended. Narcotic analgesics are generally considered CNS depressants, and they can cause drowsiness. **Depressants** are drugs meant to reduce activity and nervous action; they include sedatives, tranquilizers, and sleep inducers. It is best to avoid using them with other CNS depressants, such as psychiatric medications, OTC sleeping medications, or alcohol. As described, narcotic analgesics relieve pain, but they also have the potential for misuse (called opioid use disorder). Medication-assisted treatment of opioid use disorder typically includes opioid agonists. Opioid agonists include methadone (Dolophine) and buprenorphine (Subutex). Paradoxically, methadone can also be prescribed for pain management. When methadone is prescribed for the treatment of opioid abuse, it is administered in a controlled setting with direct observation of ingestion. This means methadone for the treatment of opioid use disorder is not dispensed in a typical community pharmacy. However, methadone used as an analgesic may be dispensed in a community or hospital pharmacy. Buprenorphine is usually administered in combination with naloxone (Suboxone, Bunavail, Zubsolv, Cassipa). Buprenorphone/naloxone side effects include sedation, headache, nausea, constipation, and insomnia.

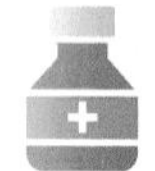

Pharm Fact

Though nasal corticosteroids, such as fluticasone propionate (Flonase), are found to be effective for some upper bronchial tract infections, they are not found to reduce symptoms of the common cold. They can even extend sore throat symptoms.

Non-Narcotic Analgesics

Acetaminophen (Tylenol) is a non-narcotic analgesic found in many prescription and OTC products. It is used for children and adults as a fever reducer and pain reliever (for headache and arthritis) that will not upset the stomach. It is considered generally safe to use during pregnancy. However, large total daily doses of acetaminophen (such as more than three grams per day or 5–6 extra-strength tablets per 24 hours) for the average person can damage the liver, especially if combined with alcohol.

Additional nonnarcotic pain relief medications include lidocaine (Lidoderm) and tramadol (Ultram). Lidocaine is a localized pain reliever that numbs sensation in a specific area. It is available as a patch that is worn for 12 hours and then removed for 12 hours. Tramadol is a narcotic-like substance that is frequently prescribed as around-the-clock pain medication. It was reclassified as a Schedule IV drug in 2014 by the DEA. It should not be taken with alcohol, narcotics, or sedatives, or if these have been used in the last few hours. These nonnarcotic pain relief medications may reduce the dose or frequency of the more potent and addicting narcotic medications.

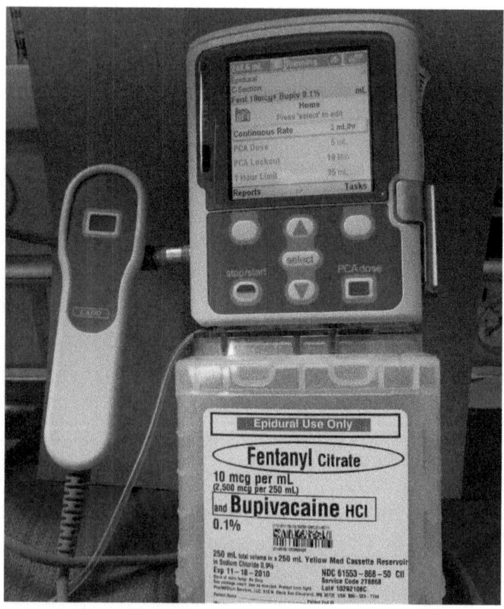

A hand-controlled analgesia pump allows patients to regulate the amount of pain medication they receive. This results in better pain control.

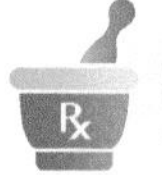

Practice Tip

Careful spelling counts! Many drugs are made of similar base compounds and often share some similar lettering patterns. Not being exact in computer keyboarding or failing to check prescriptions can lead to dangerous medication errors.

Anti-Inflammatory Medications

These drugs fight swelling. A number of anti-inflammatory drugs are **steroids**, or complex synthetic substances that can resemble human hormones. **Corticosteroids**, such as cortisone and prednisone, resemble the hormone cortisol, and can be targeted to reduce the body's natural mechanisms of swelling and white blood cell production. Short-term uses of steroids can be effective, but they can be detrimental if used long-term. That is why they are dangerous. These anti-inflammatory agents are described more fully in the discussion of endocrine agents later in this chapter.

The common anti-inflammatory drugs listed in Table 4.3 are often called **nonsteroidal anti-inflammatory drugs (NSAIDs)** and include ibuprofen and naproxen. NSAIDs come in a variety of common prescription and OTC forms. NSAIDs are not only used to deal with short-term pain and headaches but also chronic conditions, such as rheumatoid arthritis, migraines, and backaches. In conditions where swelling and pain are linked, many of the medications, such as ibuprofen (Motrin), handle both. If a patient is allergic to aspirin, an NSAID cannot be used.

TABLE 4.3 **Common Analgesic and Anti-Inflammatory CNS Agents**

Generic Name	Trade Name	Classification
Pain Relief		
acetaminophen	Tylenol, Panadol, Anacin	Nonnarcotic analgesic
buprenorphine/naloxone	Suboxone, Subutex (no naloxone)	Narcotic analgesic/antagonist
codeine	various trade names	Narcotic analgesic
fentanyl	Duragesic, Actiq	Narcotic analgesic
hydrocodone/APAP	Lortab, Norco, Vicodin	Narcotic analgesic
hydromorphone	Dilaudid	Narcotic analgesic
lidocaine	Lidoderm	Anesthetic analgesic
morphine	Kadian, MS Contin	Narcotic analgesic
oxycodone	OxyContin, Roxicodone	Narcotic analgesic
oxycodone/APAP	Percocet, Endocet	Narcotic analgesic
tramadol/APAP	Ultracet, Ultram (no APAP)	Central analgesic
Anti-Inflammatory		
celecoxib	Celebrex	COX-2 inhibitor
ibuprofen	Advil, Motrin	NSAID
meloxicam	Mobic	NSAID
naproxen	Aleve, Naprosyn	NSAID

NSAID = nonsteroidal anti-inflammatory drug

Anti-inflammatory agents are nonnarcotics but can cause serious gastrointestinal (GI) bleeding if taken in large doses for an extended period of time, especially in older individuals. It is recommended that NSAIDs always be taken with food, milk, or a snack. These drugs may negate the beneficial blood-thinning effects of aspirin when taken at the same time. Celecoxib (Celebrex) is less likely to cause GI side effects and bleeding, but it is much more costly. If a patient is allergic to sulfa drugs (drugs containing sulfur derivatives), celecoxib is contraindicated, or not recommended.

Adjuvant Medications

Adjuvant medications are helper medications. They are not strictly used for pain, but they help in pain management and may be prescribed along with a pain reliever. Some common adjuvants are antidepressant and antiseizure medications, muscle relaxants, sedatives, or sleep-enhancing drugs. The individual adjuvant medications will be discussed with their appropriate body system in this chapter.

Antianxiety and Hypnotic CNS Agents

Antianxiety and hypnotic drugs are **psychoactive drugs**, medications targeted to modify the brain functions to influence mood, perception, and consciousness. **Hypnotic** drugs are those that induce sleep. The commonly dispensed antianxiety and sleep medications listed in Table 4.4 are also CNS depressants; they have the same limitations as the narcotic analgesics, such as not mixing them with psychiatric medications, OTC sleeping medications, or alcohol.

The psychoactive drugs in the **benzodiazepine (BZD)** family (the "benzos") are used to treat anxiety, panic attacks, seizures, and insomnia. They include diazepam (Valium), and lorazepam (Ativan). Benzodiazepines generate some degree of physical or psychological dependence if used long-term.

The non-benzodiazepine sedatives zolpidem (Ambien) and eszopiclone (Lunesta) may also bring about physical or psychological dependence. Due to their dependence profile, benzos and the aforementioned non-benzodiazepines sedatives have been classified at the Schedule IV level. Refills of Schedule IV drugs must occur within six months of the original prescription date, and are limited to five refills. Prescriptions must also be monitored for early refills and abuse. Most medications with strong dependence profiles are recommended for short-term or "as-needed" use. In practice, though, many are used on a long-term, routine basis for anxiety or insomnia. The non-benzodiazepine sedatives have warnings for abnormal thoughts, CNS depression, and an increase in hazardous sleep-related activities (such as sleep-driving).

TABLE 4.4 Common Antianxiety and Hypnotic Agents

Generic Name	Trade Name	Classification
Antianxiety		
alprazolam	Xanax	Benzodiazepine
clonazepam	Klonopin	Benzodiazepine
diazepam	Valium	Benzodiazepine
lorazepam	Ativan	Benzodiazepine
Anti-insomnia		
eszopiclone	Lunesta	Non-benzodiazepine
temazepam	Restoril	Benzodiazepine
zolpidem	Ambien	Non-benzodiazepine

Antipsychotic and Antidepressant Agents

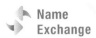

Name Exchange

The British term *adrenaline*, or the "stress" hormone (triggering the fight-or-flight response), is known in American and international healthcare communities as epinephrine. So adrenaline is epinephrine, and noradrenaline is norepinephrine.

Antipsychotic and **antidepressant** drugs (see Table 4.5) often act on neurotransmitters, such as **serotonin**, **norepinephrine**, and **dopamine**, to achieve a therapeutic effect. Serotonin is a hormonal neurotransmitter that affects memory, mood, appetite, sexual desire and function. It is thought that too little serotonin can lead to **depression**—a common but serious disorder that can affect mood, thinking, or ability to engage in daily activities, such as working, eating, or sleeping. Too much serotonin can lead to agitation, high heart rates, and confusion.

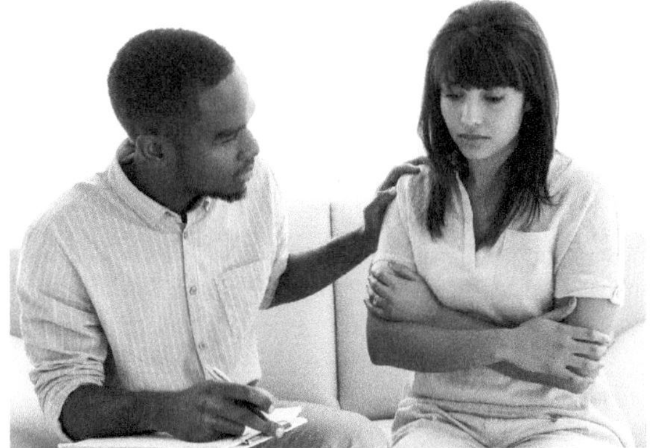

Treatment for depression may involve a combination of medication and psychotherapy.

Norepinephrine is considered the "stress hormone" that helps us address challenges with increased breathing, blood pressure, and sugar levels, but too much can lead to overstressing the system and psyche.

Dopamine is associated with movement, sexual desire, motivation, pleasure, and enjoyment. Modulating one or more of these elements to assist patients in living their everyday lives well is the purpose of antidepressant and antipsychotic drugs.

It is possible for antipsychotic and antidepressant drugs to work for a period of time and then lose their effectiveness as the body develops a tolerance. Also, some drugs can **bioaccumulate**, or collect in the fat cells of the body, resulting in the development of side effects after taking a drug for some time. Patient education and adherence are important while taking antipyschotics and antidepressants; a patient may experience **withdrawal symptoms**—or adverse reactions such as anxiety, sweating, nausea, shaking—if the drug is stopped abruptly. These drugs should always be tapered off.

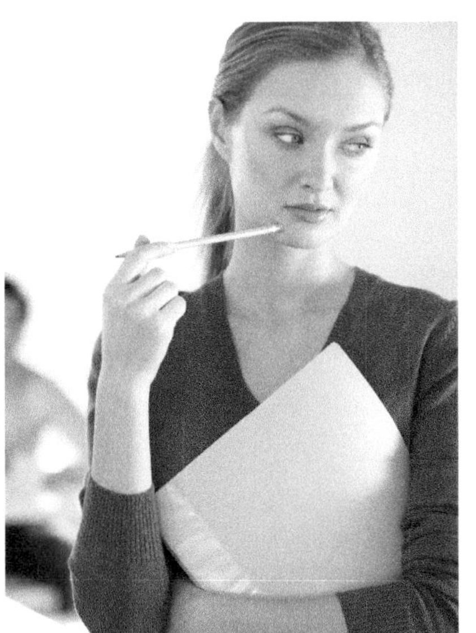

Anxiety, depression, and other mental health conditions can separate people from their friends and loved ones. Medications can sometimes relieve the symptoms so that patients may reconnect and lead more satisfying, normal lives.

Antipsychotics

Antipsychotic drugs are used to manage disordered thought and personality behaviors, such as delusions, hallucinations, mania, and severe agitation, which manifest themselves in diseases like schizophrenia and bipolar disorder. These drugs can also be used to treat severe anxiety and depression. Major depressive disorder or depression (intense, prolonged sadness) is dangerous, sometimes leading to suicide, and can accompany other mental health conditions.

The first antipsychotic drugs developed, including chlorpromazine (Thorazine) and thioridazine (Mellaril), were used to treat schizophrenia. The drugs are rarely prescribed today because of the higher incidence of side effects, such as blurred vision, dry mouth and related dental problems, and dementia-like symptoms. Other drugs and formulations have encountered success with fewer difficult side effects due to the blockage of certain brain functions.

Safety Alert

The antidepressant Celexa is often confused with the arthritis treatment Celebrex (brand name for the generic drug celecoxib). That is why it is so important to watch for correct spelling.

Aripiprazole (Abilify), olanzapine (Zyprexa), quetiapine (Seroquel), and risperidone (Risperdal) are considered **atypical antipsychotic drugs** because they target specific neurotransmitters. By balancing the levels of these hormone transmitters, the brain seems to function more effectively, and depression often remits. The atypical antipsychotic drugs are often used to enhance the antidepressant effect of traditional antidepressants. In addition to modulating **bipolar disorder** (excessively low mood, energy, and activity) and **mania** (excessively high mood, energy, and activity), these drugs are used in adults to treat **schizophrenia** (mental and emotional fragmentation and faulty reality perception) and severe agitation. However, these drugs may cause or aggravate diabetes and high cholesterol. They should be used cautiously in older adults due to potential cardiovascular adverse reactions. If the patient experiences any rigidity, tremor, or involuntary muscle twitching, the physician should be notified immediately. Alcohol should not be used while taking these drugs.

Antidepressants

Twelve of the most common CNS agents being used in the United States today are used primarily for the treatment of depression. As shown in Table 4.5, these drugs have various classifications and mechanisms of action. Although all the common medications listed are used to treat depression, the specific type and dose must be individually tailored to each patient to achieve the correct therapeutic response. Antidepressants carry boxed warnings because of the increased risk of suicidal thoughts and behavior in children, adolescents, and young adults. The generic

TABLE 4.5 Common Antipsychotic and Antidepressant CNS Agents

Generic Name	Trade Name	Classification
Antidepressants		
aripiprazole	Abilify	Atypical antipsychotic
citalopram	Celexa	SSRI
escitalopram	Lexapro	SSRI
fluoxetine	Prozac	SSRI
olanzapine	Zyprexa	Atypical antipsychotic
paroxetine	Paxil, Paxil CR	SSRI
quetiapine	Seroquel	Atypical antipsychotic
risperidone	Risperdal	Atypical antipsychotic
sertraline	Zoloft	SSRI
trazodone	Desyrel	Serotonin reuptake inhibitor/ antagonist
venlafaxine	Effexor, Effexor ER	SNRI
Antidepression, Pain Relief		
amitriptyline	Elavil	Tricyclic antidepressant
duloxetine	Cymbalta	SNRI, DA reuptake inhibitor

SSRI = selective serotonin reuptake inhibitor; SNRI = serotonin-norepinephrine reuptake inhibitors; DA = dopamine amitriptyline (Elavil) is an older antidepressant drug that offers a mild tranquilizing, soothing result. It is still used for depression, to enhance the effect of pain medications, and to prevent migraine headaches. This drug commonly causes drowsiness and is sometimes prescribed to treat insomnia. Amitriptyline can cause a dry "cotton" mouth and blurry vision.

Trazodone has a different mechanism of action from some of the other drugs but is also used as an antidepressant. It can also cause drowsiness and is sometimes prescribed for enhancing sleep. It has similar side effects of dry mouth, vision changes, and some hangover-like effects the next morning. Patients taking trazodone should avoid sun exposure, and males should be warned about the risk of priapism, or aprolonged painful erection. In some patients, trazodone can cause cramps in ankles and feet and some loss of small motor function after prolonged use.

Selective serotonin reuptake inhibitors (SSRIs) are antidepressants that block the reabsorption of serotonin so that more of the secreted serotonin circulates for positive effects. Several antidepressants, including the famous Prozac, generically known as fluoxetine, work in this way. Drugs like fluoxetine, venlafaxine (Effexor), and duloxetine (Cymbalta) may cause insomnia if given at bedtime. Venlafaxine and duloxetine should be used cautiously in patients with hypertension as they can elevate blood pressure.

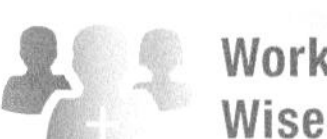

Since many patients on ADHD medications are children, their parents naturally are worried and have numerous questions and concerns. You cannot counsel them, but you can refer them to the pharmacist and answer billing and insurance questions.

Several prescription (and some OTC) drugs, such as tramadol (Ultram) and cyclobenzaprine (Flexeril), can cause unsafe levels of serotonin when used with certain antidepressants such as fluoxetine (Prozac), sertraline (Zoloft), and paroxetine (Paxil), causing confusion and agitation. Alcohol should not be used with these drugs either.

Miscellaneous CNS Agents

The diagnosis of **attention deficit hyperactivity disorder (ADHD)** is on the rise in pediatric patients. It manifests itself in difficulty focusing or concentration, overactivity, and difficulty in impulse control. Ironically, the usually prescribed drugs, such as methylphenidate and amphetamines, stimulate rather than depress the CNS, and this actually helps support the brain in focusing attention and behavior. Common side effects are insomnia and loss of appetite. Medications for ADHD should be taken in the morning or early afternoon.

Safety Alert

ADHD medications can be abused. Many of these medications are Schedule II drugs and need to be dispensed carefully. As a pharmacy technician, it is important for you to exercise caution and to dispense ADHD medications in accordance with laws and regulations for the safety of yourself and your patients.

Methylphenidate is available as both an immediate-acting drug (Ritalin) and as a longer-acting drug (Concerta). Amphetamines, or "uppers" as they have been called, are very dangerous because of their addictive qualities. The popular Adderall and Adderall XR (short- and long-acting formulations) are combinations of amphetamine salts. Lisdexamfetamine (Vyvanse) is also prescribed for ADHD. Due to the amphetamine content of these drugs, the DEA places them in the Schedule II category—no refills are authorized without a new prescription.

Unfortunately, drugs to treat ADHD may be abused. Patients might share their ADHD medications with friends who want to "focus" on a test or desire extra energy. Abuse of ADHD drugs is an evolving problem.

To slow the progression of moderate to severe Alzheimer's disease, other CNS agents, such as memantine (Namenda) and donepezil (Aricept), are used. These potent medications alter brain chemistry in an effort to generate the desired therapeutic response. Memantine is sometimes used in combination with donepezil, but drowsiness is a common side effect. Donepezil is metabolized in the liver so it is susceptible to drug interactions. The main side effects of donepezil are gastrointestinal, such as diarrhea, nausea, and vomiting. Additional drugs that help regulate or stimulate the CNS are listed in Table 4.6.

TABLE 4.6 Miscellaneous Central Nervous System Agents

Generic Name	Trade Name	Classification	Indication
amphetamine salts	Adderall	CNS stimulant	ADHD
carisoprodol	Soma	Skeletal muscle relaxant	Muscle spasms
cyclobenzaprine	Flexeril	Skeletal muscle relaxant	Muscle spasms
gabapentin	Neurontin	Anticonvulsant, analgesic	Pain, seizures
lisdexamfetamine	Vyvanse	CNS stimulant	ADHD
memantine	Namenda	Brain receptor antagonist	Alzheimer's disease
methylphenidate	Concerta, Ritalin	CNS stimulant	ADHD
metoclopramide	Reglan	Prokinetic agent	GERD, gastroparesis
ondansetron	Zofran	Serotonin receptor antagonist	Nausea, vomiting
pregabalin	Lyrica	Anticonvulsant, analgesic	Pain, seizures
promethazine	Phenergan	Antidopaminergic, antihistamine	Nausea
ropinirole	Requip	Dopamine agonist	Restless legs, Parkinson's
sumatriptan	Imitrex	Serotonin agonist	Migraine headache
tizanidine	Zanaflex	Alpha2-adrenergic agonist	Muscle spasms
topiramate	Topamax	Unknown	Migraine headache, weight loss, epilepsy

ADHD = attention-deficit/hyperactivity disorder; CNS = central nervous system; GERD = gastroesophageal reflux disease

Epilepsy is a disease where a patient suffers from **seizures**, which are spasms caused by overfiring of the neurons of the brain and nervous system. Seizures come in varying levels of severity. Patients are given **anticonvulsant** (antiseizure) medications to calm the nervous system by inhibiting the overly rapid and excessive firing of neurons. The most common drugs used to treat active seizures are benzodiazepines, such as lorazepam (Ativan) and clonazepam (Klonopin), which are also antianxiety drugs.

Gabapentin (Neurontin) and pregabalin (Lyrica) were initially used to control seizures. Today, though, these drugs are primarily used to reduce nerve pain associated with diabetes, chronic pain, shingles, and spinal cord injuries. Pregabalin is sometimes prescribed for fibromyalgia, or severe chronic muscle fatigue. The most common side effects of these drugs are drowsiness, dizziness, and swelling of the ankles. OTC antacids, such as Mylanta or Maalox, interfere with the absorption of gabapentin. It is recommended that pregabalin be administered at least one hour before or two hours after the patient takes antacids.

Muscle relaxants, which reduce muscle strain and pain, include carisoprodol (Soma) and cyclobenzaprine (Flexeril). These are commonly prescribed with narcotic analgesics and antianxiety drugs. They are indicated for short-term treatment of muscle spasms; however, they are often used long-term.

Promethazine (Phenergan) is commonly used in tablet, liquid, injection, or suppository forms for the treatment of nausea and vomiting from a viral illness or migraine headache.

Sumatriptan (Imitrex) is available in various dosage formulations to treat an occasional severe migraine headache. It must be used with caution in patients with heart disease and women of childbearing potential.

Metoclopramide (Reglan) is used to treat heartburn and slow stomach emptying in patients with diabetes as well as severe nausea and vomiting resulting from chemotherapy. It is commonly given 30 minutes prior to each meal and at bedtime; it can cause some severe abnormal muscle movement with long-term use. Ondansetron (Zofran), also used for stomach distress from chemotherapy, is available as an oral disintegrating tablet (ODT), as a syrup, and as an injection for pediatric patients or those too sick to swallow tablets. Ropinirole (Requip) is commonly prescribed at bedtime to treat "restless legs syndrome" (involuntary twitching of the legs). Common side effects with all these drugs are drowsiness and dizziness; as with most CNS drugs, alcohol must be avoided.

4.6 Cardiovascular Agents

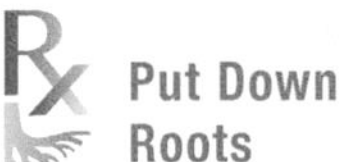

The term *cardiovascular* comes from the Greek *kardia*, meaning "heart," and the Latin vasculum, meaning "pertaining to the conveyance of circulating fluids."

Heart disease is a major health threat in the United States and includes conditions such as hypertension. The complications of untreated or undertreated hypertension include kidney failure, stroke, and heart attack. The risk of heart disease may be partly genetic, but hypertension is often the result of lifestyle choices as well, such as smoking, unhealthy food choices, being overweight, and lack of exercise. Elevated cholesterol is an important risk factor for cardiac disease and general heart disease.

Antihypertensive Agents

Antihypertensive agents work to lower blood pressure by dilating blood vessels, slowing heart rate, and increasing the elimination of fluids from the body (see Table 4.7). Often, more than one drug is needed to reach the desired blood pressure range, usually below 140 mm Hg for the systolic reading. Drugs known as **calcium channel blockers (CCBs)** stop calcium from entering the cells of the heart and blood vessels, making them more flexible and able to relax and widen, lessening blood pressure. The most commonly prescribed CCB is amlodipine (Norvasc), and it can cause headache, fast heart rate, and sometimes ankle swelling.

Beta-adrenergic blockers (beta blockers) are antihypertensive drugs for heart conditions that help regulate the blood pressure–raising effects of the hormone epinephrine (also known as adrenaline), which makes the heart beat faster. Beta-blockers can make the heart beat slower and with less force; they include atenolol, metoprolol, and the newest agent, nebivolol. Some are also used for glaucoma and migraine prevention.

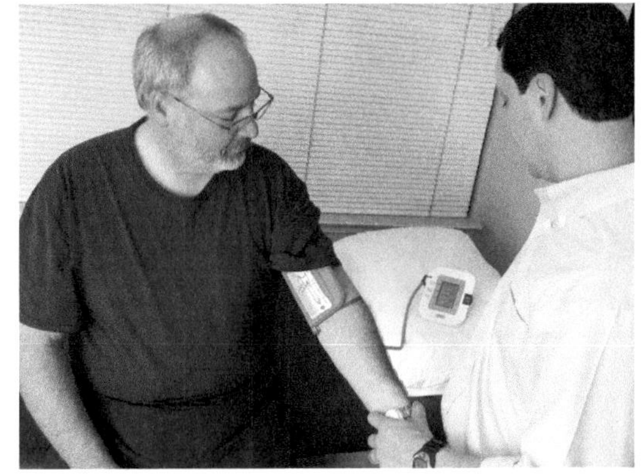

Monitoring blood pressure is an important component of hypertension therapy to assess how effective or necessary a prescription is.

TABLE 4.7 Common Antihypertensive Cardiovascular Agents

Generic Name	Trade Name	Classification
Hypertension		
amlodipine	Norvasc	Calcium channel blocker
atenolol	Tenormin	Beta-adrenergic blocker
metoprolol	Lopressor, Toprol	Beta-adrenergic blocker
nebivolol	Bystolic	Beta-adrenergic blocker
Hypertension, Heart Failure		
benazepril	Lotensin	ACE inhibitor
enalapril	Vasotec	ACE inhibitor
lisinopril	Prinivil, Zestril	ACE inhibitor
losartan	Cozaar	ARB
olmesartan	Benicar	ARB
ramipril	Altace	ACE inhibitor
valsartan	Diovan	ARB

ACE = angiotensin converting enzyme; ARB = angiotensin receptor blocker

Metoprolol succinate is available in an extended-release dosage form; metoprolol tartrate is available in an immediate-release dosage form. As discussed earlier, these different salts cannot be interchanged. They are generally well tolerated, but a patient must not run out of these medications–if the drug is withdrawn for 48 to 72 hours, blood pressure can rebound to unsafe levels, leading to severe chest pain or even a heart attack. Patients with diabetes who are prone to low blood sugar (hypoglycemia) must use these drugs with caution because the drugs can mask symptoms of low blood sugar.

Diuretics, which reduce water retention, are also prescribed for high blood pressure. They are addressed in the **renal** (kidney) section later in this chapter.

Angiotensin-converting enzyme (ACE) inhibitors reduce blood pressure and prevent heart failure by blocking or reducing the liver production of an enzyme that constricts the blood vessels. Their first cousins, **angiotensin receptor blockers (ARBs)**, block the absorption of the enzyme. Both ACEs and ARBs help keep the vessels more open, resulting in better blood flow and lower blood pressure. Both drugs also protect the kidneys from the damage caused by diabetes and hypertension. However, ACE inhibitors and ARBs can cause the body to retain potassium and must be used with caution in patients also taking potassium supplements, potassium-sparing diuretics (see Table 4.16 later in this chapter), or patients with declining kidney function.

The most common side effect of ACE inhibitors is a drug-induced dry cough caused by buildup of bradykinin, an irritating chemical, in the lungs. If the cough continues, an ARB is usually prescribed instead of an ACE. The most serious adverse effect of ACE inhibitors is **angioedema**, a swelling under the skin that can be a life-threatening allergic reaction, manifested by swelling of the tongue, lips, or eyes. If

Put Down Roots

Lipo comes from the Greek lipos, meaning "fat." Words like lipids (fats, like cholesterol in the blood), lipoproteins (groups of proteins carrying fats in the blood), lipidemia (excess fat in the blood), and hyperlipidemic (too much fat in the blood system) all come from this root.

these symptoms present themselves, the drug must be discontinued immediately, and the patient should be referred to emergency care.

Antihyperlipidemic (Cholesterol-Lowering) Agents

Antihyperlipidemic drugs are drugs that treat hyperlipidemia, a condition marked by elevated cholesterol, phospholipids, and/or triglycerides (discussed later) in the blood. Cholesterol itself is made in the body and absorbed through the ingestion of foods and beverage. Hyperlipidemia is problematic because it can cause cardiovascular disease and coronary artery blockage.

In the bloodstream, cholesterol is packaged in various molecules. **Low-density lipoproteins (LDLs)** are thought of as the "bad" cholesterol and contribute to artery blockages. In contrast, **high-density lipoproteins (HDLs)**—the "good" cholesterol—work to break up blockages in the blood vessels. **Triglycerides** are another type of fat found in the bloodstream consisting of three lipids combined. Triglycerides contribute to artery blockage. Patients' medical histories and risk factors are used to determine medical targets for cholesterol levels.

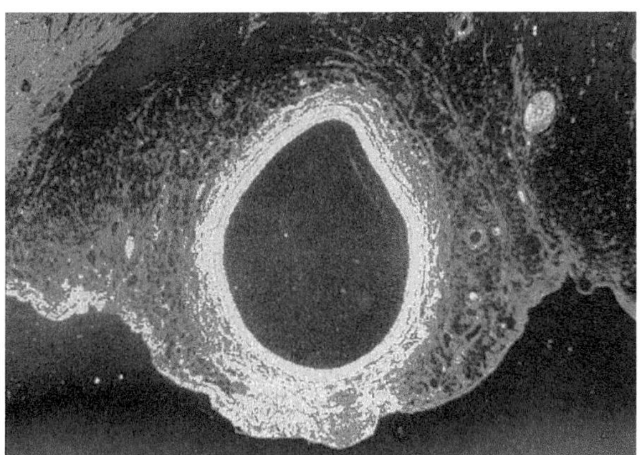
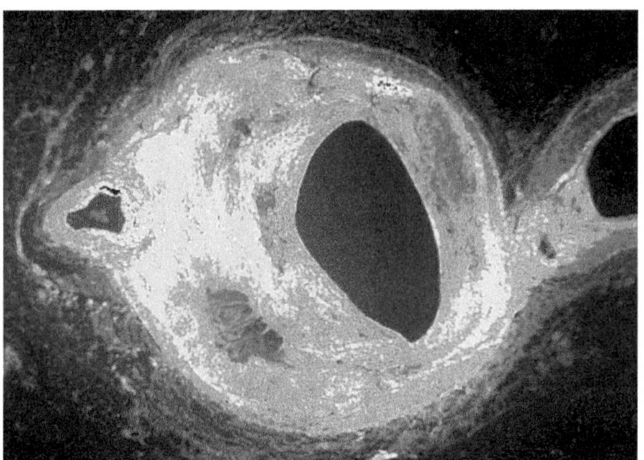

The cross-section of the artery on the right is healthy, while the one on the left is constricted from the cholesterol, calcium, and plaque that have collected on the artery's lining, narrowing the passageway for blood flow.

Put Down Roots

Hyperlipidemia comes from the Greek *hyper* (high amounts or excess), lipos (fat), and haima (blood), meaning "a condition with an excess of fatty acids or lipids."

Commonly used antihyperlipidemic agents (see Table 4.8) are referred to as **statins** because of their common suffix. Statins prevent the production of LDL by blocking a key enzyme in the liver that makes it. The official name of statins is HMG-CoA reductase inhibitors. (You can see why "statins" is so much easier to remember!) Statin drugs vary in name, dose, and potency but can lower LDL cholesterol up to 50% or more. Some statins should not be taken with grapefruit juice as this may decrease metabolism of the drug and increase the risk of side effects. Muscle fatigue is a common side effect, especially when these drugs are combined with other agents.

Niacin has lost popularity due to several trials questioning its benefit. Ezetimibe is now prescribed more frequently. Ezetimibe (Zetia) is an antihyperlipidemic categorized as a cholesterol absorption inhibitor, which works to prevent cholesterol absorption from the GI tract. Ezetimibe works to lower LDLs and triglycerides. Side effects with ezetimibe are usually mild and include abdominal cramps and diarrhea. Ezetimibe is sold by itself and in combination with other antihyperlipidemic drugs.

TABLE 4.8 Common Antihyperlipidemic Cardiovascular Agents

Generic Name	Trade Name	Classification
Cholesterol- and Triglyceride-Reducing		
atorvastatin	Lipitor	Statin
ezetimibe	Zetia	Cholesterol absorption inhibitor
fenofibrate	TriCor, Trilipix	Decreases triglycerides
lovastatin	Mevacor	Statin
niacin	Niaspan	Decreases triglycerides
omega-3 fatty acid	Epanova, Lovaza, Vascepa	Decreases triglycerides
pravastatin	Pravachol	Statin
rosuvastatin	Crestor	Statin
simvastatin	Zocor	Statin
simvastatin/ezetimibe	Vytorin	Statin/cholesterol absorption inhibitor

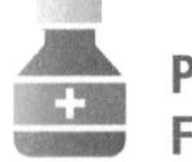

Pharm Fact

Salmon is very high in omega-3 fatty acids and can help naturally increase the body's HDLs and lower the body's triglycerides.

Fenofibrate (TriCor, Trilipix) lowers triglycerides directly and is usually well tolerated. However, it must be used with caution with statins, warfarin, and other blood thinners.

Omega-3 fatty acids, often found in fish oil supplements, are effective in lowering triglycerides. Omega-3 fatty acids can be found in OTC fish or algae oil supplements. Prescription forms are also available, such as Epanova, Lovaza, and Vascepa.

Miscellaneous Cardiovascular Agents

In addition to drugs that control high blood pressure and cholesterol, other agents (see Table 4.9) are used to treat abnormal heartbeats, heart failure, and angina pectoris (severe chest pain).

TABLE 4.9 Common Miscellaneous Cardiovascular Agents

Generic Name	Trade Name	Classification	Indication
carvedilol	Coreg	Alpha/beta blocker	Heart failure
digoxin	Lanoxin	Inotropic agent	Heart failure
isosorbide	Imdur, Ismo, Isordil	Vasodilator	Angina pectoris, heart failure

The agents for heart failure all work differently and are sometimes used in combination with each other or with the ACE inhibitors or ARBs discussed previously. Carvedilol (Coreg) is commonly used as a primary drug in the treatment of heart failure. It has a dual pharmacological blocking action to lower demands on a compromised heart. It is also available as a controlled-release dosage formulation (Coreg CR). All beta- blockers must be used with caution in patients with asthma and chronic obstructive pulmonary disease (COPD), characterized by increasing breathlessness or in combination with drugs that lower heart rate.

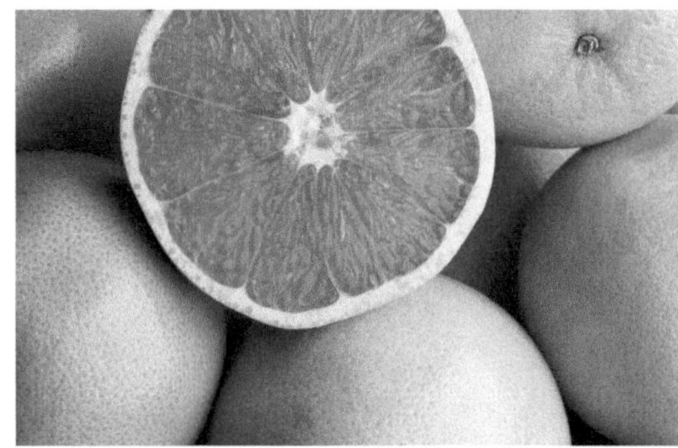
Patients on certain statins should be advised to avoid grapefruit and grapefruit products because they decrease metabolism of the statin and increase side effects.

Digoxin (Lanoxin) is an older drug that helps a weak heart beat stronger. While the drug is in use, the patient's serum blood levels should be monitored to prevent toxic levels and side effects, including abnormal heart rhythms (arrhythmias). The drug can slow down the heart rate and cause nausea and vomiting when toxic levels are reached, especially if blood potassium levels are low.

Isosorbide (Imdur, Ismo, Isordil) belongs to the nitrate family. Nitrates dilate the blood vessels, particularly those of the heart, increase oxygen and blood flow, to relieve chest pain, and/or reduce the workload on the heart. Nitrates can cause headaches and a dangerous drop in blood pressure when combined with erectile dysfunction drugs, including the well-known brands of Viagra, Levitra, and Cialis. Nitroglycerin is the most commonly known drug of this group. Nitroglycerin is often taken at the first sign of chest pain, with repeated doses every five minutes for three doses. If chest pain continues, the patient is advised to take a crushed aspirin tablet and go to the emergency room as quickly as possible. Nitroglycerin sublingual (under the tongue) tablets are sensitive to air and light and should be replaced every 3 to 6 months. Due to its emergency use, nitroglycerin should never be dispensed in a child-resistant container.

4.7 Systemic Anti-Infective Agents

Anti-infective agents include antibiotics, sulfa drugs, antifungals, and antivirals (see Table 4.10). Because microorganisms are living beings, they adapt to whatever drug agents we use against them and can become **resistant**, or immune to them. It is essential, then, that patients are advised to take the full dosage for the full time and not quit when the symptoms stop. The end of symptoms does not mean the microorganisms are all dead. They merely are weakened to the point that they cannot cause symptoms. The more technicians understand this, the more they can help patients understand the importance of following their prescription.

Practice Tip

For patients on antibiotics, pharmacy personnel should stress the importance of completing the entire course of therapy to reduce the incidence of antibiotic resistance and recurring infections.

Antibiotics

Antibiotics kill or weaken bacteria and commonly cause gastrointestinal side effects, such as diarrhea, as well as yeast infections. Doctors and pharmacists often advise patients to eat yogurt with live cultures (probiotics) to offset these side effects. If yeast infections develop and persist, patients may require treatment with OTC or prescription drugs. Also, with many antibiotics and sulfa drugs, the patient should take precautions in the sun because these agents cause sun sensitivity.

TABLE 4.10 Common Anti-Infective Agents

Generic Name	Trade Name	Classification
Infection		
amoxicillin	Amoxil	Aminopenicillin
amoxicillin-clavulanate	Augmentin	Aminopenicillin
ampicillin-sulbactam	Unasyn	Aminopenicillin
azithromycin	Z-Pak	Macrolide
cefazolin	Ancef	Cephalosporin
ceftazidime	Fortaz, Tazicef	Cephalosporin
ceftriaxone	Rocephin	Cephalosporin
cephalexin	Keflex	Cephalosporin
ciprofloxacin	Cipro	Fluoroquinolone
ertapenem	Invanz	Carbapenem
gentamicin	generic only	Aminoglycoside
levofloxacin	Levaquin	Fluoroquinolone
meropenem	Merrem	Carbapenem
moxifloxacin	Avalox	Fluoroquinolone
nafcillin	generic only	Penicillinase-resistant penicillin
penicillin	Veetids, Pen VK	Natural penicillin
sulfamethoxazole-trimethoprim	Bactrim, Septra	Sulfonamide
vancomycin	Vancocin	Glycopeptide
Acne-related Infection		
clindamycin	Cleocin	Lincosamide
doxycycline	Doryx, Vibramycin	Tetracycline
metronidazole	Flagyl	Antiprotozoan
Fungal Infection		
fluconazole	Diflucan	Antifungal
Viral Infection		
acyclovir	Zovirax	Antiviral
oseltamivir	Tamiflu	Antiviral
valacyclovir	Valtrex	Antiviral

IN THE REAL WORLD

A nearly completed course of antibiotics might kill nearly all bacteria that cause a particular disease, but the surviving bacteria then reproduce, creating more resistant bacteria by natural selection, decreasing the effectiveness of the antibiotic. Consequently, stronger doses of the antibiotic or additional drugs need to be prescribed, which, in turn, creates a higher risk of side effects. An example of this chain-reaction effect can be seen with the antibiotic amoxicillin. Due to drug resistance, the required dose of amoxicillin to treat ear infections in children has doubled in the past 30 years. A more serious example in the hospital environment is the development of methicillin-resistant Staphylococcus aureus (MRSA), which can be so unresponsive to antibiotics that it can cause death.

Some kinds of antibiotics may lower the effectiveness of oral contraceptives, so patients of child-bearing potential must be made aware of this.

Penicillins and Cephalosporins

Among the most common anti-infective drugs is the first antibiotic—penicillin (Veetids, Pen VK) and its derivatives, such as amoxicillin (Amoxil) and amoxicillin-clavulanate (Augmentin). Penicillins are commonly used to treat upper respiratory, sinus, and ear infections in children and adults. Ampicillin/sulbactam (Unasyn) and nafcillin (only generic is available) are used to treat infections resistant to traditional penicillins. It is important to ask about penicillin allergies.

The **cephalosporin antibiotics** are antibiotics synthesized to be like penicillin. They are generally well tolerated. Fewer than 5% of those allergic to penicillin develop a rash with cephalosporins, but the patient (or parent) should be advised of the possibility. However, if the patient has an anaphylactic reaction (severe allergy) to penicillins, cephalosporins should be avoided too. Each of the different cephalosporins—such as cefazolin (Ancef), ceftazidime (Fortaz, Tazicef), ceftriaxone (Rocephin), and cephalexin (Keflex)—is effective against different microorganisms. With the exception of cephalexin, most cephalosporins are administered by the intramuscular or intravenous route. These drugs are frequently used in both the community and hospital settings.

Macrolides, Lincosamides

Safety Alert

It is important for the technician to double check the allergy history in the patient profile prior to dispensing any antibiotic prescription.

For individuals with penicillin-related allergies, other antibiotics are also commonly used, such as azithromycin (Z-Pak, or Zithromax). Azithromycin works by stopping bacteria from making their own proteins. It is commonly prescribed in tablet (Z-Pak) or suspension form for the treatment of upper respiratory infections in children and adults. Azithromycin has the advantage of a one-, three-, or five-day course of therapy (instead of a two-week or

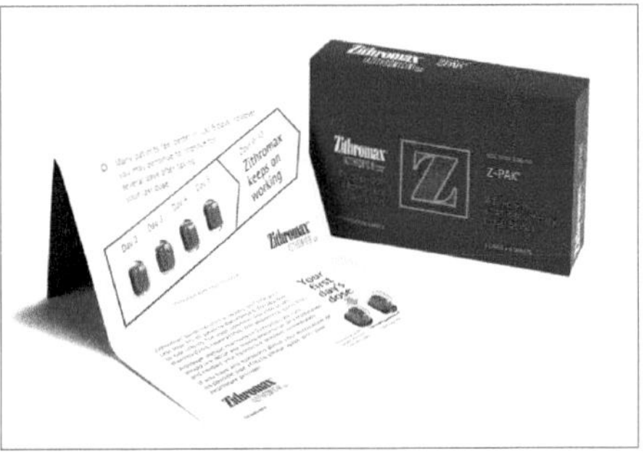

Azithromycin (Z-Pak, or Zithromax) is often used as an antibiotic for people with penicillin-related allergies.

longer regime), which may improve patient adherence. The drug should be taken with a meal or snack to lessen GI side effects. Unlike some antibiotic suspensions, which should be refrigerated, this one can be kept at room temperature. Azithromycin commonly interacts with other drugs, so the medication profile and use must be particularly assessed by the pharmacist.

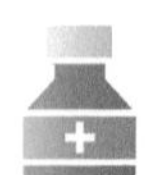

Pharm Fact

Since common colds are usually caused by viruses, antibiotics are not effective against them.

Clindamycin, belonging to the lincosamide family, is particularly effective to fight post-surgery infections caused by anaerobic bacteria (those that do not require oxygen for growth). It is administered intravenously in hospitals and in other dosage forms in the community pharmacy after dental surgery. Clindamycin is typically tolerated by patients who are allergic to penicillin, but it can cause ongoing diarrhea. If patients develop bloody diarrhea, they should contact their physician immediately. Clindamycin is also available topically for the treatment of acne.

Metronidazole is also used intravenously in the hospital after surgery as an agent against protozoa and anaerobic microorganisms. It is frequently prescribed as an oral tablet for five to seven days to treat vaginal infections as well. The use of alcohol with this drug could cause severe nausea, elevated heart rate, vomiting, and warmth/redness under the skin, and even death. Metronidazole is available in topical formulations for the treatment of acne.

Fluoroquinolones

The fluoroquinolones are a class of potent antibiotics that include ciprofloxacin (Cipro), levofloxacin (Levaquin), and moxifloxacin (Avalox). They *should not be taken with milk, dairy products, or antacids.* In rare but serious cases, they can cause ruptured tendons or severe tendinitis with strenuous exercise. The Medication Guide describes this reaction to consumers. As with many drugs, they are available as an injection in hospitals for serious infections as well as eye and ear drops. Ciprofloxacin and levofloxacin may interact with diabetes medications for lowering blood sugar, which can drop blood sugar to dangerous levels.

Tetracyclines

Doxycycline (Doryx, Vibramycin) is an all-purpose antibiotic commonly used to treat various bacterial infections, including pneumonia and acne. It is in the family of **tetracycline antibiotics**. These *must not* be taken by pregnant or nursing patients, those on oral contraceptives, or children younger than 8 years of age because they cause irreversible damage to teeth and bones. In addition, they must not be taken at the same time as dairy products, antacids, iron, or calcium supplements. Patients should particularly avoid sun exposure as they may burn more quickly.

Sulfa Drugs

In addition to antibiotics, sulfa drugs (sulphur-based medications) also fight bacterial infections as well as some fungal infections. The most commonly prescribed sulfa drug is a combination of sulfamethoxazole and trimethoprim (Bactrim, Septra), which when combined have mutually beneficial effects on fighting bacteria. This drug is commonly used to treat urinary tract infections (UTIs) and ear infections. Sulfa drugs should be taken with large quantities of water and must be used cautiously with blood thinners and other drugs. Sunscreen precautions should be recommended.

Other Antibiotics

Vancomycin (Vancocin) is the common drug of choice to treat **methicillin-resistant *Staphylococcus aureus* (MRSA)**—the bacterium responsible for many hard-to-treat infections in the hospital. If the MRSA infection is vancomycin-resistant, meropenem (Merrem) and other antibiotics serve as alternatives. Gentamicin (only generic is available) is an intravenous antibiotic that is frequently used in combination with other antibiotics to treat serious infections. Kidney function and drug blood levels must be carefully monitored with both vancomycin and gentamicin to adjust dosing. At toxic levels, these drugs can cause some degree of hearing loss; care must be taken to ensure accurate dosing levels.

Metronidazole is also used intravenously in the hospital after surgery as an agent against protozoa and anaerobic microorganisms. It is frequently prescribed as an oral tablet for five to seven days to treat vaginal infections as well. The use of alcohol with this drug could cause severe nausea, elevated heart rate, vomiting, and warmth/redness under skin, and even death. So as with other IV anti-infective agents, alcohol of any kind must be avoided for up to 72 hours after last use. Metronidazole is available in topical formulations for acne.

Antifungals and Antivirals

The antifungal drug fluconazole (Diflucan) is commonly prescribed as a one-time or short-term oral treatment for fungal yeast infections. For viral herpes infections, acyclovir (Zovirax) and valacyclovir (Valtrex) are used topically (Zovirax Ointment), orally, and intravenously. Oseltamivir (Tamiflu) is an antiviral drug used for flu outbreaks in both children and adults.

4.8 Endocrine and Metabolic Agents

The **endocrine** system is the network of glands that secrete hormones into the circulatory system to regulate bodily functions, including metabolism, or the processes of producing energy from nutrition. Various endocrine and metabolic agents are frequently prescribed in the community pharmacy. These drugs vary from hormones and birth control medications to drugs that treat bone loss, diabetes, thyroid conditions, inflammatory diseases, and gout (see Table 4.11).

TABLE 4.11 **Common Hormonal Agents**

Generic Name	Trade Name	Classification
Hormone Replacement Therapy		
conjugated estrogens	Premarin	Sex hormone
Contraceptive		
ethinyl estradiol-drospirenone	Gianvi	Hormonal contraceptive
ethinyl estradiol-etonogestrel	NuvaRing	Hormonal contraceptive
ethinyl estradiol-norgestimate	TriNessa, Tri-Sprintec	Hormonal contraceptive
ethinyl estradiol-norelgestromin	Ortho Evra, Xulane	Hormonal contraceptive
ethinyl estradiol-norethindrone	Loestrin 24 Fe	Hormonal contraceptive

Practice Tip

Patients need to be reminded that antibiotics may interfere with oral contraceptives.

Estrogens and Contraceptives

In menopausal and postmenopausal patients or those who have had a hysterectomy, reproductive hormone production drops dramatically, and can cause hot flashes, insomnia, and emotional imbalance. Hormone replacement therapy with estrogen is often used to reduce the symptoms. Short-term use in low doses has been shown to be safe and effective. The major side effect of estrogens is nausea, and there is a concern about the increase in the risk of stroke and cancer with long-term (over five years) use.

Many prescription contraceptive medications are available on the market. Most contain reproductive hormone combinations of **estrogen** and a progestin (a synthesized **progesterone**) to simulate pregnancy and work by preventing ovulation, preventing implantation of fertilized eggs, and/or altering cervical mucus. Some oral contraceptive packets contain tablets with different hormone amounts for each week of the month. Most oral contraceptive therapies include three weeks of active medication and one week of placebo or iron tablets. Contraceptive medications are quite effective if taken properly and are generally well accepted and tolerated. Many oral contraceptives fool the body into thinking it is already pregnant through hormone messengers. Users may experience some of the weight gain and mood swings of pregnancy.

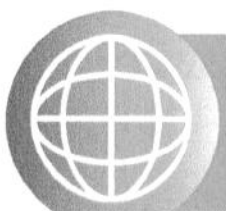

Safety Alert

If patients mention severe side effects from oral or hormonal contraceptive, such as intense depression or breakthrough bleeding, recommend that they immediately consult the pharmacist and their provider.

In patients over age 35 who smoke, birth control medications may increase the risk of a stroke. The FDA mandates that manufacturers provide and pharmacists dispense a Medication Guide with each oral or hormonal contraceptive prescription. NuvaRing is a once-a-month birth control device (in place for three weeks, out for one week) where hormones are slowly released intravaginally through a self-inserted ring dispenser; this drug should be refrigerated when stored. Ortho Evra and Xulane are contraceptive patches that also slowly release hormones through the skin. They are about the size of a Band-Aid and are worn on the buttock, abdomen, upper torso, or upper outer arm and is changed once a week.

IN THE REAL WORLD

Oral contraceptives have been widely available over the past 50 years. Today, with an estimated 100 million womenworldwide on oral contraceptives, there are many different combinations of brand and generic options. Some have different amounts of estrogen and progesterone during each week of the menstrual cycle. When taken appropriately, the drug is 91%+ effective in preventing pregnancy, and it is also useful in treating patients with irregular or painful menstrual cycles.

Hormonal contraceptives can sometimes cause headache, nausea, breakthrough bleeding, decreased sex drive, and mood swings; in most cases, the side effects may just occur initially. In some cases, another combination with different hormone components may need to be tried. If mood swings and depression are severe, patients should consider going off the medication while trying a non-hormonal treatment for contraception or adjusting the type and formulation of the hormone therapy.

Antidiabetic Agents

Diabetes is one of the fastest growing chronic diseases in the world, especially in the United States. Diabetes is caused by insufficient secretion of the hormone insulin by the pancreas for processing sugar. Type 1 diabetes was previously known as juvenile diabetes because it is often diagnosed in children and young adults. In type 1 diabetes, the body has stopped producing insulin, so patients always require insulin injections. Approximately 5% of patients with diabetes have this form.

In type 2 diabetes, formerly called adult onset diabetes, the body either becomes resistant to insulin or does not produce enough insulin to maintain normal blood sugar levels. Most patients with diabetes have this form, and it comes in a spectrum of severity. There is a link between the incidence of type 2 diabetes and the rise in consumption of processed foods with high levels of sugar. There is also a link to unhealthy lifestyles that put stress on the pancreas. Typically patients need nutrition and lifestyle changes as well as medications to adequately treat type 2 diabetes (see Table 4.12).

TABLE 4.12 **Common Diabetes-Controlling Agents**

Generic Name	Trade Name	Classification
glipizide	Glucotrol	Sulfonylurea
glyburide	DiaBeta, Micronase	Sulfonylurea
insulin aspart	Novolog	insulin
insulin detemir	Levemir	insulin
insulin glargine	glargine Lantus, Toujeo	insulin
insulin lispro	Humalog	insulin
linagliptin	Tradjenta	DPP-4 inhibitor
metformin	Glucophage	Biguanide
pioglitazone	Actos	Thiazolidinedione
sitagliptin	Januvia	DPP-4 inhibitor

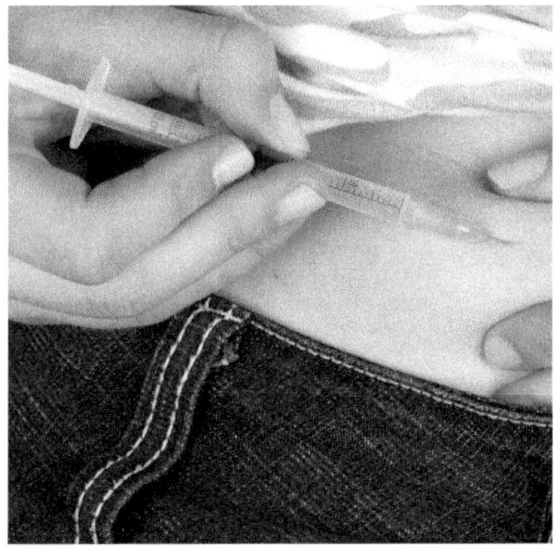

This patient is using a syringe to inject herself with insulin. Insulin pens can also be used for convenient injection. (See Chapter 5.)

Agents for Type 1 Diabetes

Drug therapy for type 1 diabetes relies on insulin. Many types of insulin are available. Rapid-release insulins—insulin aspart (Novolog), lispro (Humalog), and glulisine (Apidra)—are recommended to be taken 15 minutes prior to meals. The effects of short-acting insulins (with an "R" in their names) typically reach peak effect within an hour or two. Intermediate-acting insulins usually have an "N" in their names, as in Humulin N or Novolin N. Some rapid-release insulins can be sold without a prescription. Long-acting insulins—insulin glargine (Lantus, Toujeo), detemir (Levemir), and degludec (Tresiba)—are commonly used. These insulins do not peak; they provide a constant amount of glucose lowering over a 24-hour period. Insulins can be used separately or as mixtures of faster and slower release products. Insulin can be dispensed in a vial or in prefilled pen devices.

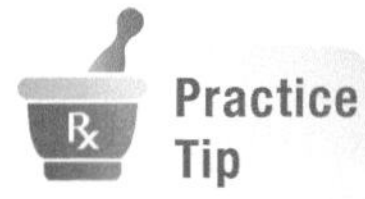

Practice Tip

Insulins lose their potency if stored unrefrigerated for more than 28 days. The patient should be advised to date insulin and replace it every 4 weeks if stored at room temperature.

Agents for Type 2 Diabetes

Medication therapy for type 2 diabetes may include insulin as well as a variety of other agents. All drugs for type 2 diabetes work to modulate or lower blood sugars but by different mechanisms of action. Often more than one drug is needed to attain blood sugar target levels.

One of the most common **antidiabetic drugs** is the **sulfonylureas**, a class of drugs that stimulates the cells of the pancreas to produce more insulin—think of squeezing a sponge to imagine the action. Sulfonylurea drugs include glimepiride (Amaryl), glipizide (Glucotrol), and glyburide (DiaBeta, Micronase). Patient blood sugars have to be monitored carefully (often self-monitored) to avoid hypoglycemia (low blood sugar) when using sulfonylureas. Sulfonylurea drugs can cause sensitivity to the sun and may interact poorly with other drugs, such as the antibiotic ciprofloxacin.

Other diabetes drugs have varying chemical bases for different types of actions. Metformin (Glucophage) is the most frequently prescribed type 2 diabetes drug. It is available in both an immediate-release and extended-release form. Metformin should be taken with food, and the patient may need to take a vitamin B12 supplement while taking long-term metformin. Sitagliptin (Januvia) became a treatment for type 2 diabetes in 2006. It is most effective at controlling blood sugars after a meal. It is sometimes prescribed as Janumet, a combination of sitagliptin and metformin. Linagliptin (Tradjenta) is similar to sitagliptin that is also available in combination with other antidiabetic drugs. Pioglitazone (Actos) must be used with caution in patients with heart failure.

Miscellaneous Endocrine Agents

The body has numerous other hormonal glands and metabolic mechanisms that can malfunction and may require medication (see Table 4.13).

Osteoporosis

For the treatment of bone loss, or osteoporosis, **bisphosphonates**, such as alendronate (Fosamax), are used. Bone loss often occurs in postmenopausal women or men

TABLE 4.13 Common Miscellaneous Endocrine and Metabolic Agents

Generic Name	Trade Name	Classification
Osteoporosis, Hypercalcemia		
alendronate	Fosamax	Bisphosphonate
Hypothyroidism		
levothyroxine	Levoxyl, Synthroid	Thyroid hormone
Hyperthyroidism		
methimazole	Tapazole	Thyroid reduction
Anti-Inflammatory		
allopurinol	Zyloprim	Xanthine oxidase inhibitor
methylprednisolone	Medrol Dosepak	Corticosteroid
prednisone	Deltasone	Corticosteroid

over age 75 who do not receive enough calcium. Bisphosphonates slow down the cells that break down bone, and they are most commonly taken once weekly or monthly. To increase absorption and minimize esophageal erosions in care-facility patients, these drugs must be taken first thing in the morning. It's also important to take these with water only and while standing, which present a problem for bedridden patients.

Thyroid Disorders

Thyroid problems can arise, especially as people age. The thyroid hormones are released by the thyroid gland. These hormones influence energy levels and metabolism, growth, body temperature, muscle strength, appetite, and the health of many organs.

Hypothyroidism occurs when the thyroid is not active enough and does not produce adequate amounts of thyroid hormone. People with this condition have very low energy or a great deal of fatigue. Hypothyroidism is very common with age, especially in women. Hypothyroidism is a treatable disease. Prescribers and some patients may request a brand name drug, such as Synthroid (generic levothyroxine), due to better tolerance or a more reliable therapeutic effect. If Synthroid is prescribed as "brand necessary," it is considered a Dispense as Written (or DAW) prescription when billing an insurance provider. Thyroid replacement medications should be taken in the morning or on an empty stomach to increase absorption. They must not be taken at the same time as dairy, antacids, iron, or calcium, or within two hours of ingestion of these substances.

Hyperthyroidism is the opposite condition, where the thyroid is overstimulated and active. It is less common than hypothyroidism but can be more dangerous. It can lead to racing heartbeats and anxiety, bulging eyes, and even blindness. A common medication used to treat it is methimazole (Tapazole).

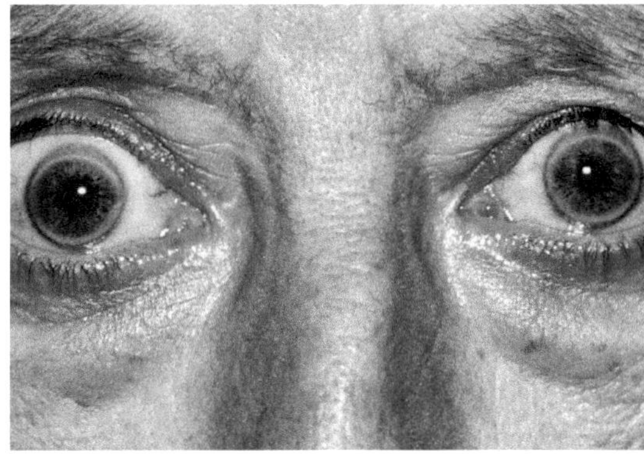

Protrusion of the eyeballs, known as exophthalmos, is a symptom of hyperthyroidism, or overactive thyroid.

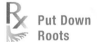

Put Down Roots

Hyper- comes from the ancient Greek *hupér,* meaning "over," while *hypo-* comes from the ancient Greek *hupo,* meaning "under."

Inflammatory Conditions

Patients can be plagued with various inflammatory diseases and illnesses, such as rheumatoid arthritis, asthma, allergic reactions, poison ivy/oak, ulcerative colitis, Crohn's disease, and gout (a painful swelling of the joints due to an accumulation of uric acid). **Cortisol** is a hormone that the adrenal glands naturally produce that helps the body reduce inflammation, among other things. The corticosteroids are synthetic versions of cortisol and include prednisone (Deltasone) and methylprednisolone (Medrol Dosepak).

Corticosteroids are usually prescribed for short-term use because prolonged use can increase the risk of high blood pressure and blood sugar, increase in appetite and weight gain, muscle weakness and bruising, glaucoma or cataracts, stomach ulcers, and hallucinations. It is important to note that corticosteroids are not the same types of steroids as the anabolic steroids used by athletes that can be more dangerous and damaging. Some patients with chronic inflammatory conditions may be on lifelong therapy or may use high doses for a short time for acute flare-ups. Corticosteroids should be taken with food and may interfere with blood sugar or blood-thinning medications.

4.9 Respiratory Agents

Practice Tip

Patients need to be reminded to keep inhalers and nebulizers clean and to rinse their mouths after using corticosteroids to prevent a fungal infection in the mouth called thrush.

Shortness of breath, wheezing, and decreased oxygen in the blood can be caused by asthma, chronic obstructive pulmonary disease (COPD), allergies, and coughing that constricts the airways and causes inflammation. To aid breathing, the airways need to relax. Table 4.14 lists examples of common respiratory drugs used for relaxing and opening the airways.

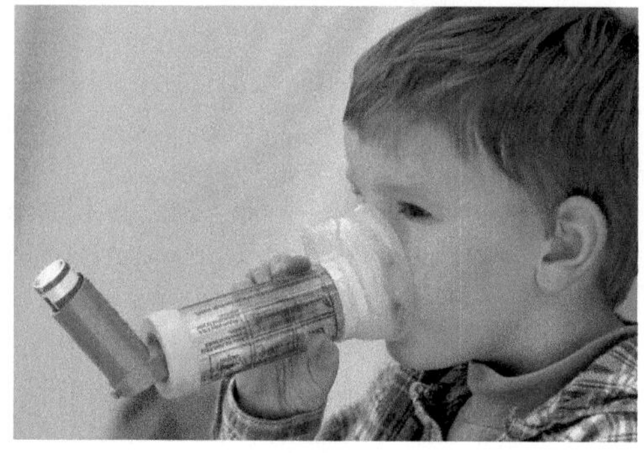

This child is using a metered-dose inhaler (MDI) with a spacer (the clear tube) for increased penetration into the tissue of the lungs.

TABLE 4.14 Common Respiratory Agents

Generic Name	Trade Name	Classification
Asthma, COPD		
albuterol	ProAir, Ventolin, Proventil	Bronchodilator
budesonide/formoterol	Symbicort	Inhaled steroid/bronchodilator
fluticasone/salmeterol	Advair	Inhaled steroid/bronchodilator
formoterol	Foradil	Bronchodilator
levalbuterol	Xopenex	Bronchodilator
salmeterol	Serevent	Bronchodilator
COPD		
ipratropium	Atrovent	Anticholinergic
ipratropium/albuterol	Combivent, DuoNeb	Anticholinergic/bronchodilator
tiotropium	Spiriva	Anticholinergic
Asthma, Allergy		
budesonide	Pulmicort	Inhaled corticosteroid
formoterol	Foradil	Bronchodilator
fluticasone	Flonase, Flovent	Inhaled corticosteroid
mometasone	Asmanex	Inhaled corticosteroid
montelukast	Singulair	Leukotriene receptor antagonist
salmeterol	Serevent	Bronchodilator

Agents for Asthma and COPD

Albuterol (ProAir, Ventolin, and Proventil) and its chemical cousins–levalbuterol (Xopenex), formoterol (Foradil), and salmeterol (Serevent)–all work in different ways to open the breathing passageways (bronchodilators) and lungs of patients with asthma or COPD. Albuterol is the fastest-acting bronchodilator and should be used for acute attacks. Albuterol may be prescribed as a tablet, syrup, metered-dose inhaler (MDI), propellant spray for inhaling, or sterile solution for a nebulizer. (The differences between an inhaler and a nebulizer will be explained in Chapter 5.)

The side effects of albuterol and its derivatives include increased heart rate and blood pressure. Overuse may cause patients to develop a tolerance so that other medications need to be considered.

Put Down Roots

The term *bronchodilator* comes from the Greek *bronchos* meaning "windpipe" and the Latin *dilatare* meaning "to widen."

The mixed formulations of budesonide/formoterol (Symbicort) and fluticasone/salmeterol (Advair) combine a passage-opening substance with a corticosteroid that reduces the swelling that causes difficulty breathing in asthma and COPD. Decreasing inflammation should reduce the number of acute attacks and the need for the use of short-acting agents, such as albuterol.

Ipratropium (Atrovent) and tiotropium (Spiriva) are anticholinergic drugs. They are primarily used in patients with COPD. Both cause dryness in the mouth, throat, and eyes. These drugs are inhaled into the lungs and provide relief for shortness of breath. The brand Combivent combines ipratropium and albuterol.

Agents for Allergies

In allergies that involve the nose and lungs, neurotransmitters called histamines call forth a series of immune responses, such as itchiness, redness, nasal mucus or runny nose, swollen airways, and coughing. **Antihistamines** fight these histamine responses. Montelukast (Singulair)–available in tablet, chewable tablet, and granular forms–works in asthma and allergies to neutralize and prevent the release of chemicals that cause symptoms such as bronchoconstriction.

For less intense diseases and symptoms, physicians and pharmacists often recommend that the patient select OTC nonsedating antihistamines such as loratadine (Claritin) or fexofenadine (Allegra). Nasal sprays that provide intranasal steroids like fluticasone (Flonase) and mometasone (Nasonex) are used routinely to prevent seasonal allergy symptoms from developing. The intranasal steroids are now available without a prescription.

4.10 Gastrointestinal Agents

The **gastrointestinal (GI)** system comprises the esophagus, the stomach, and the small and large intestines. Table 4.15 lists some of the medications that are frequently prescribed for common GI ailments.

Patients often suffer from heartburn, ulcers (internal sores in the lining of the esophagus or stomach), and **gastroesophageal reflux disease (GERD)**—where stomach acid flows up through the esophagus. To resolve these conditions, the secretion of stomach acid must be reduced or stopped. The most often prescribed GI agents are the **proton pump inhibitors (PPIs)**, which work to prevent

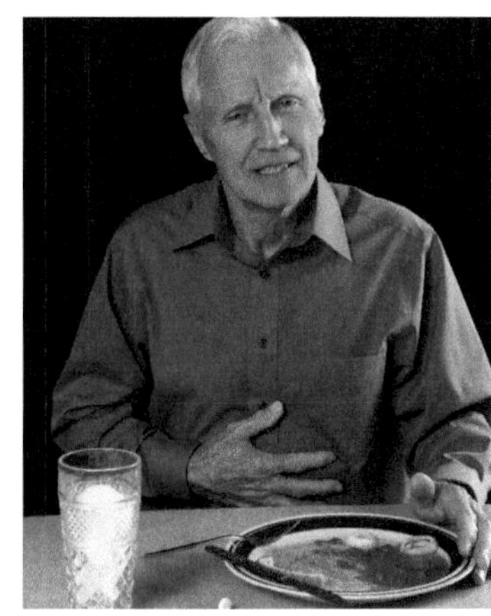

Millions of Americans suffer from various types of gastrointestinal (GI) ailments.

stomach acid production. These include esomeprazole (Nexium), lansoprazole (Prevacid), omeprazole (Prilosec), and pantoprazole (Protonix). The **histamine-2 antagonists**, such as famotidine (Pepcid), are a family of drugs taken before meals to reduce acid. They work to slow down the release of more acid in the stomach.

PPIs and histamine-2 antagonists are well tolerated, with only occasional reports of side effects such as headache and dizziness. However, PPIs can interfere with beneficial effects of the blood-clotting prevention drug clopidogrel (Plavix). These drugs should not be taken together, and there is concern even if they are taken 12 hours apart.

Long-term use of PPIs has been reported to decrease bone mineral density, especially in older women, so an OTC calcium supplement may be recommended to accompany these drugs. Some other gastrointestinal agents, such as promethazine, ondansetron, and metoclopramide, were previously listed in Table 4.6.

TABLE 4.15 Common Gastrointestinal Agents

Generic Name	Trade Name	Classification
esomeprazole	Nexium	Proton pump inhibitor
famotidine	Pepcid	Histamine-2 antagonist
lansoprazole	Prevacid	Proton pump inhibitor
omeprazole	Prilosec	Proton pump inhibitor
pantoprazole	Protonix	Proton pump inhibitor

4.11 Renal and Genitourinary Agents

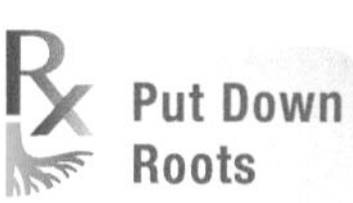

As seen in Table 4.15, proton pump inhibitors end in -prazole, and histamine-2 antagonists end in -tidine. The statins generally end in *–statin,* as in atorvastatin, lovastatin, and pravastatin.

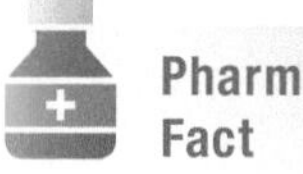

Male and female genitourinary systems each have unique qualities.

The renal system, or urinary system, includes the kidneys, bladder, ureters, and urethra. The **genitourinary** system includes both the genital reproductive system and the urinary tract. The most frequently prescribed renal and genitourinary agents are the diuretic drugs for all populations and the drugs to address erectile dysfunction (ED) and prostate problems for men (see Table 4.16).

Diuretics, sometimes called "water pills," work with the kidneys to eliminate excess salt and water from the body by dilating (widening) blood vessels. They are used to treat swelling from water retention, high blood pressure, and heart failure. Hydrochlorothiazide and furosemide (Lasix) act at different sites of the kidney, and their onset, duration of action, and potency differ. Diuretics should be taken in the morning or early evening. Most can cause a loss of potassium, which can cause muscle cramps or, in severe cases, irregular heart rates. Potassium loss can be offset by consuming potassium-rich foods, such as fresh citrus fruits and bananas, or taking potassium supplements. Diuretics that contain triamterene (Dyazide, Maxzide) or spironolactone (Aldactone) are considered potassium-sparing, meaning that they maintain healthier levels of potassium.

Many antihypertensive drugs previously listed in Table 4.7 are available in combination with a diuretic. However, patients taking ACE inhibitors, digoxin, and lithium must use diuretics with great caution. The pharmacy's computer system should flag any of these medications as a pharmacist needs to assess the potential for drug interactions.

TABLE 4.16 Renal and Genitourinary Agents

Generic Name	Trade Name	Classification
Diuretics		
finasteride	Proscar	Alpha blocker
furosemide	Lasix	Loop diuretic
hydrochlorothiazide	Esidrix, HydroDIURIL, Oretic	Thiazide diuretic
spironolactone	Aldactone	Potassium-sparing diuretic
tamsulosin	Flomax	Alpha blocker
triamterene-hydrochlorothiazide	Dyazide, Maxzide	Combination, potassium-sparing
Erectile Dysfunction, Prostate		
sildenafil	Viagra	Phosphodiesterase inhibitor
tadalafil	Cialis	Phosphodiesterase inhibitor
vardenafil	Levitra	Phosphodiesterase inhibitor

Erectile dysfunction drugs include the well-known and marketed brand drugs Viagra (generic sildenafil) and Cialis (generic tadalafil). These drugs vary by onset and duration of action. Rare side effects include changes in blue/green color vision and prolonged painful erections (priapism). *A life-threatening drop in blood pressure (hypotension) can occur if these agents are used with any nitrate.*

An enlarged prostate that is not due to cancer is treated with tamsulosin (Flomax) and finasteride (Proscar). These are part of a group of drugs called alpha blockers. Tamsulosin relaxes the prostate and bladder-neck muscles, making it easier to urinate.

Finasteride reduces the production of the sexual hormone that creates the enlarged state of the prostate. This reduction can cause hair loss but decrease sexual function. Some patients complain that the side effects last for a sustained period after ceasing use of the drug. In addition, the drug can pass in the semen and may harm a resulting fetus. It should not be used if a couple is trying to conceive, or if a man is sexually active without contraceptives with a woman of childbearing potential.

4.12 Hematologic Agents

Another system that often requires medication is the **hematologic** system, which involves blood. Hematologic drugs include those dealing with blood cell production, quality, and clotting.

Warfarin (Coumadin) is used both short- and long-term to prevent blood clots in high-risk patients. Warfarin works by inhibiting vitamin K-dependent clotting factors. Vitamins and diets that are high in vitamin K can impair the pharmacological effect of warfarin. The key is to maintain a stable intake of green vegetables without vitamins.

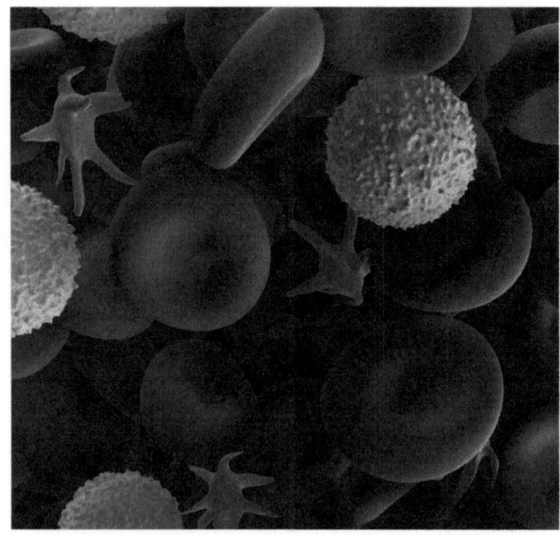
This illustration shows enlarged red blood cells and platelets.

Patients on warfarin are less likely to clot but more likely to bleed profusely. With blood thinners, toxic levels are not far from the therapeutic levels, so patients must be closely monitored on a routine basis with a blood test to measure the **international normalized ratio (INR)** to see how well the blood clots. The therapeutic level for warfarin is between 2.0 and 3.5.

Because blood thinners are so difficult to modulate at just the right levels, some prescribers write Coumadin as "brand necessary" (DAW). This drug (and other blood thinners) is *very susceptible* to drug interactions, such as with aspirin (a mild blood thinner) and many herbal drugs (such as ginger, gingko, and ginseng). When other drugs are added to the regimen or when dosages are adjusted, the pharmacist must assess the potential for serious interactions.

Table 4.17 lists other frequently prescribed hematologic medications. Newer agents have been introduced more recently to prevent clot formation, including dabigatran (Pradaxa) and rivaroxaban (Xarelto). They are faster acting and do not require regular blood testing. The disadvantages of these new agents are the high cost of antidotes for treating an overdose. Clopidogrel (Plavix) often works to further decrease the risk of blood clots by inhibiting production of blood platelets. When platelets clump together, a clot begins to form; clopidogrel (and aspirin) prevents the platelets from clumping together. Diet does not affect this drug, but the use of proton pump inhibitor drugs for the stomach can interfere with its therapeutic effect.

TABLE 4.17 Common Hematologic Agents to Prevent Blood Clots

Generic Name	Trade Name	Classification
clopidogrel	Plavix	Antiplatelet drug
dabigatran	Pradaxa	Thrombin inhibitor
enoxaparin	Lovenox	Thrombin inhibitor
heparin	generic only	Thrombin inhibitor
rivaroxaban	Xarelto	Factor Xa inhibitor
warfarin	Coumadin	Blood thinner

Heparin (generic only) is an anticlotting drug that is used intravenously (directly into the vein) and subcutaneously (under the skin) to treat and prevent blood clots. It is used especially in hospital settings for clots in lungs and legs. Frequent blood tests are required for IV heparin to prevent the major side effect—excessive bleeding. Enoxaparin (Lovenox) is used as an injection to prevent blood clots. It is particularly used in high-risk surgeries, or for "bridging." **Bridging therapy** provides short-term protection from blood clots after surgery before the slow-acting warfarin takes effect (usually in one week). Enoxaparin has been shown to be as effective as heparin, and it requires no blood tests and causes less bleeding.

IN THE REAL WORLD

There are FDA-mandated boxed warning statements for several injectable biotechnology drugs, including etanercept (Enbrel), infliximab (Remicade), and adalimumab (Humira). These drugs work by suppressing the immune system, thus increasing patient susceptibility to rare but serious bacterial and fungal infections.

4.13 Biotechnology Drugs

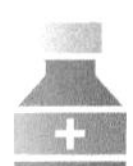

Pharm Fact

Infliximab (Remicade, Remsima, Inflectra) is an intravenous biologic drug used for treating autoimmune and inflammatory diseases such as Crohn's disease and rheumatoid arthritis.

Numerous drugs developed through biotechnology are used in the hospital or outpatient clinic for a variety of medical conditions: (1) to treat anemia from chronic kidney disease or cancer chemotherapy; (2) to boost white and red blood cell count for patients at risk of an infection or experiencing severe fatigue; and (3) to treat inflammatory diseases. The most common biotechnology drugs are shown in Table 4.18.

With the exception of adalimumab (Humira) and etanercept (Enbrel), the technician working in a community pharmacy will not be exposed to these costly and potent agents, though hospital technicians most likely will. Technicians working in a hospital or servicing a cancer or dialysis clinic need to be familiar with them. They are lifesaving drugs for patients, but there is a long list of short-term side effects, including serious allergic reactions and depression of the immune system. Long-term adverse effects are currently unknown. Adalimumab and etanercept have a wide spectrum of uses, from severe rheumatoid arthritis to GI inflammatory diseases like Crohn's, to severe psoriasis that is unresponsive to conventional therapy.

Biotechnology drugs are also available to stimulate the production of white blood cells (WBCs), which are needed to boost immunity, and red blood cells (RBCs) to carry oxygen. Cancer, chemotherapy, and radiation therapy can all cause damaging effects on white blood cells, red blood cells, or both. Low WBCs increase the risk of infections, and low RBCs increase the risk of fatigue.

TABLE 4.18 Biological and Immunological Agents

Biological Name	Trade Name	Classification	Indication
adalimumab	Humira	Inhibits inflammation	Inflammatory disorders
darbepoetin alfa	Aranesp	Stimulates bone marrow	Anemia from kidney failure
epoetin alfa	Procrit	Stimulates bone marrow	Anemia from kidney failure
etanercept	Enbrel	Inhibits inflammation	Inflammatory disorders
filgrastim	Neupogen	Stimulates white blood cell production	Prevents infection
pegfilgrastim	Neulasta	Stimulates more white blood cell production	Prevents infection

4.14 Miscellaneous Drugs

Other common prescription drugs fit in less anatomically based areas. A sample is offered in Table 4.19. Skin conditions such as eczema, psoriasis, and allergic reaction from bug bites or dermatitis from poison ivy are often treated with corticosteroids that can be applied topically, or on the skin.

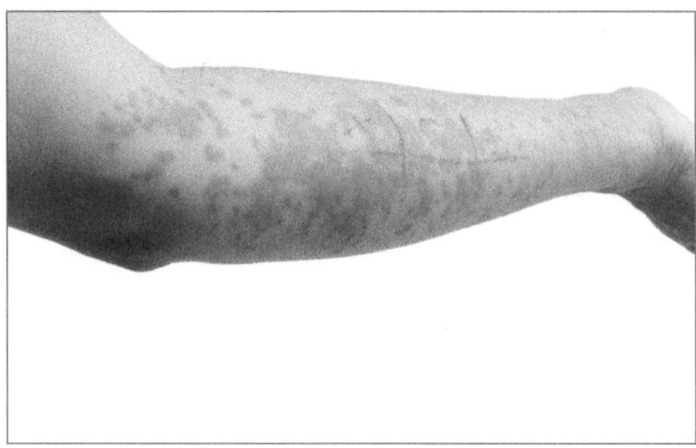

Rashes are often caused by allergic reactions and can be dealt with by OTC medications. If they persist or are severe, a prescription may be needed from a physician.

Triamcinolone is a corticosteroid and is the most frequently prescribed topical drug, available in different strengths in both a cream and an ointment form. Triamcinolone is more potent than the OTC drug hydrocortisone.

Since many diuretics can lower blood potassium levels, which increases the risk of toxicity from the heart drug digoxin, prescription-strength levels of potassium are needed. Potassium chloride (K-Dur, Klor-Con) can be prescribed alongside these drugs as one or two daily doses in tablet, capsule, or liquid form. This medication should be taken with food and a glass of water so that it does not irritate the esophagus.

TABLE 4.19 Miscellaneous Agents

Generic Name	Trade Name	Classification	Indication
cholecalciferol (vitamin D)	Many	Fat-soluble vitamin	Vitamin D, calcium, and phosphate deficiency, osteoporosis
folic acid	Many	B vitamin	Heart disease, with MTX
potassium chloride	K-Dur, Klor-con	Mineral	Potassium replacement
triamcinolone	Kenalog	Topical steroid	Inflammatory skin disease, eczema

Vitamin D and folic acid are commonly prescribed vitamins. Both are available over the counter, though the higher dosages must be carefully prescribed and monitored. For example, vitamin D is available as an OTC agent in dosages of 400 to 2,000 international units (IU) per day; a common prescription dose is 50,000 IU once a week. Vitamin D improves the absorption of calcium and is usually prescribed or recommended for patients who have or are at risk for osteoporosis.

The potent drug methotrexate (MTX) is commonly prescribed for rheumatoid arthritis. Folic acid may reduce some of this drug's toxicity. Folic acid is also recommended for patients who are or may become pregnant to decrease the risk of spina bifida (a birth deformity) in the child. High doses of folic acid are found in all prenatal vitamins. Some cardiologists recommend taking folic acid to reduce blood levels of homocysteine, which is thought to be a risk factor for heart disease.

4.15 Information for Pharmacy Personnel

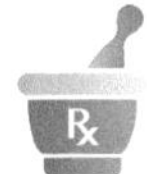

Practice Tip

The PI is an information resource for the pharmacist and pharmacy technician, not for the patient. Pharmacy technicians should expand their knowledge of new drugs by reading the PI documents when an opportunity arises in their workday.

Since technicians and pharmacists can't be expected to remember everything about every drug, the FDA requires that manufacturers provide scientific information for pharmacy personnel with each drug. This information is contained in the FDA label information otherwise known as the **package insert (PI)** or prescribing information insert, which accompanies the stock sent from the wholesaler. Package inserts are attached to or placed inside stock bottles. The information on the insert is provided in a specific order (see Table 4.20). These inserts provide key information, including indications, contraindications, warnings, side effects, and dosage, along with how to handle and store the medications. It includes the date of the most recent labeling revision.

Additional Pharmacy Drug Reference Guides

In addition to the FDA Orange Book and *Drug Facts and Comparisons,* there are other key pharmaceutical references. Many come in online versions, which are easier to keep up to date.

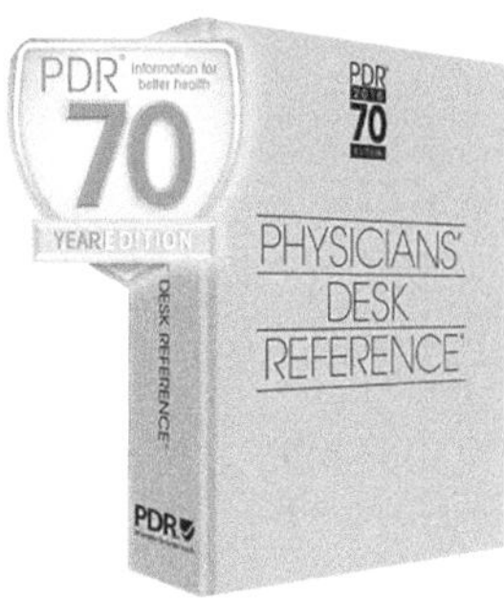

The *PDR* is available for consumer purchase in most bookstores.

General Drug References

Prescribers' Digital Reference This is a publication with reprints of PPIs from pharmaceutical manufacturers of most drugs. This digital resource is also useful for identifying unknown drugs by color, shape, and coding, and for alerting pharmacists and pharmacy technicians to boxed warnings. Pharmacy technicians can learn more about the drugs that they are dispensing by studying the *PDR* and reading PPIs during any free or slow times in the pharmacy. This resource can be accessed as an ebook at pdr.net and via *PDR* phone apps.

Drug Information Handbook This is a commonly used reference in most pharmacies (both community and institutional). Published by LexiComp, this handbook lists brand and generic drug names for all FDA-approved medications in a dictionary style format. It includes all pertinent pharmaceutical information (composition, strength, dosage, form, packaging, schedule, and usage) for over 1,700 drugs in the USP formulary.

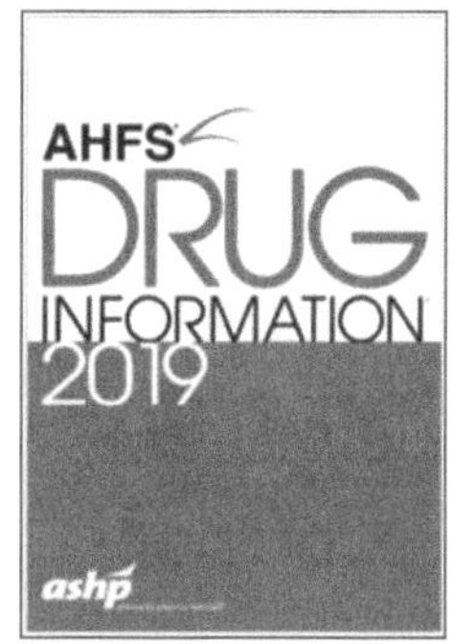

Numerous pharmacy references can help technicians learn more about the drugs they work with or compound.

TABLE 4.20 Organization of the Package Insert (PI)

• Description	• Adverse reactions
• Clinical studies	• Drug abuse and overdosage
• Indications and usage	• Dosage and administration
• Contraindications	• How supplied/preparation
• Warnings and precautions	• Stability/storage and handling

AHFS Drug Information This is a joint publishing effort between the American Society of Health-System Pharmacists (ASHP) and the American Hospital Formulary Service (AHFS). It is an excellent source of information, especially on parenteral drugs commonly used in hospital, long-term care, or home healthcare settings. Published by a professional and a scientific society, it offers an unbiased, comprehensive, evidence-based reference for drug information. The numerical structure of the pharmacologic-therapeutic classification is the basis for many hospital drug formularies. These references are commonly utilized by the pharmacist in hard copy or online to research a drug-related question from a patient or a prescriber. Subscribers receive electronic updates.

Thomson Reuters Micromedex This is an online computerized database that features monographs on more than 1,400 FDA-approved drugs, including dosing, adverse reactions, and drug-drug interactions. This reference also includes expanded, unbiased, evidence-based medicine ratings of drug indications.

Pharmacy Practice References

Remington: The Science and Practice of Pharmacy This is an extensive text especially for use in a compounding pharmacy where determinations of drug stability and compatibility are important. This reference covers the integration of scientific principles into clinical practice.

Trissel's Stability of Compounded Formulations This is an excellent reference for the pharmacy technician, used to check IV drug incompatibilities in the hospital or specialty compounding pharmacy. The book provides important stability and storage information through monographs on many compounded drug formulations (injectable, oral, enteral, topical, ophthalmic) in accordance with documented standards.

Manufacturing Pharmacy References

US Pharmacopeial Convention (USP) reference guides These are revised every five years with periodic online updated supplements. The first two reference works are also printed in a combined edition known as the *US Pharmacopeia–National Formulary (USP–NF)*. These detailed compendia of drug standards are utilized by all pharmaceutical companies when submitting a new drug application to the FDA:

- *US Pharmacopeia* describes drug substances and dosage forms.
- *USP National Formulary* describes pharmaceutical ingredients.
- *USP Dietary Supplements Compendium (DSC)* contains listings of supplements, including photographs and diagrams, reference tables, and safety and use studies. It also guides the industry in the best practices of manufacturing the supplements. The vitamin or mineral is defined and described with its chemical structures and delineations of scientific studies on use, effectiveness, dosage, forms, and safety warnings.

Homeopathic Pharmacopeia of the United States (HPUS) This is a compilation of standards for the source, composition, and preparation of homeopathic medications that may be sold in a community pharmacy. The *HPUS* is compiled by the Homeopathic Pharmacopoeia Convention of the United States (HPCUS).

Nonprescription Drug References

Handbook of Nonprescription Drugs This is published by the American Pharmacists Association and provides a good background text reference for OTC agents.

Natural Medicines Comprehensive Database This is a resource for dietary supplements, natural medicines, and complementary and alternative therapies. It is available online.

The Review of Natural Products This provides objective, scientific monographs on more than 350 herbal medications. It is available in an electronic edition.

4.16 Applying Pharmacology as a Technician

It is hard to remember the generic and trade names of all drugs and their indications and side effects, which is why the labels, pharmacy software alerts, product inserts, and online and book sources are so important. Pharmacy technicians can stay informed and up to date in many ways. Focusing on the most frequently prescribed drugs in the community and hospital pharmacy settings will provide a good start. Almost 90% of all prescriptions will be dispensed under the generic drug names due to insurance coverage and lower cost.

Working technicians will be able to put this knowledge to use daily as they check medication records, fill prescriptions, and ask questions about things that don't match up with what is known about a drug. Drugs prone to interactions with other drugs require even closer scrutiny to prevent problems. Technicians work as part of the team, referring patients to the pharmacist for counseling and alerting the pharmacist to patient needs that arise, always with the end goal of offering the best possible standard of care.

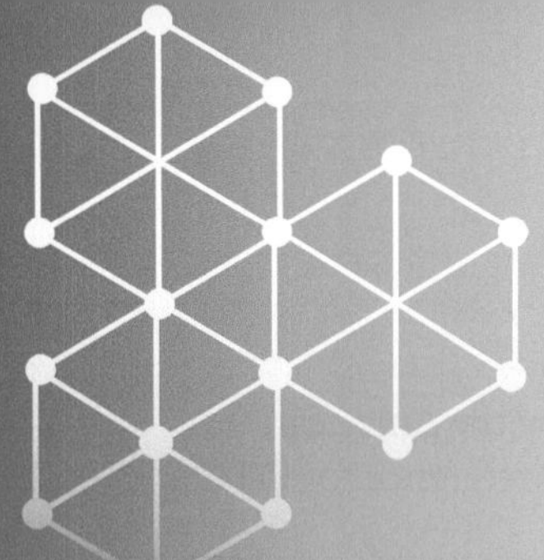

Review and Assessment

CHAPTER SUMMARY

- The study of pharmacology (drugs and their interactions) is related to other pharmaceutical areas, including therapeutics (appropriate uses or indications for drugs), pharmacodynamics (actions of the active ingredients and how they work), toxicology (poisonous effects and harmful side effects), pharmaceutics (release characteristics of dosages), pharmacokinetics (absorption, distribution, metabolism, and elimination), and pharmacognosy (medications from natural sources).
- A pharmacy technician should be able to understand and differentiate the terms *pharmaceutical equivalent, therapeutic equivalent, therapeutic alternative, biosimilar*, and *interchangeable* in the substitution of drug products.
- The online FDA Orange Book is the reference source for pharmacy personnel to check on which generic drugs can be safely substituted for brand name products.
- The online FDA Purple Book is the reference for the lists of licensed biological drug products and biotechnical or bioengineered drug products. The FDA also publishes the *Green Book: FDA Approved Animal Drug Products* for veterinary-oriented substances.
- A working knowledge of the generic and brand names of common drugs and their indications is important in the day-to-day work of the pharmacy technician; the *Drug Facts and Comparisons (F&C)* resource is used for this.
- Drugs are organized in the *F&C* by organ systems and mechanisms of action.
- Learning the varying classes of common drugs and their indications can be especially important in filling prescriptions effectively and safely. To remember the drugs in these classes, pay attention to their common suffixes.
- It is important to learn to be focused on details of spelling, dosages, interactions, and medications listed on a patient medication profile—and to double-check all your computer entries. Watch intently for all boxed warnings, flagged information, alerts, contraindications, harmful side effects, and other danger signals on the computer and in product package inserts, FDA information, labels, and drug references online and in books.
- Common central nervous system drugs include analgesics (narcotics, opiates, opioids) and anti-inflammatories (steroids and NSAIDs), anticonvulsants, antipsychotics, and antidepressives (including SSRIs). There are also drugs for ADHD, Alzheimer's disease, and muscle spasms and pain.
- Cardiovascular drugs are used to treat high blood pressure and/or heart failure and to lower "bad cholesterol." They include the antihypertensives, beta blockers, calcium channel blockers, ACE inhibitors, AR blockers (ARBs), statins, and diuretics.

- Many antibiotics (including penicillins, cephalosporins, tetracyclines, and sulfa drugs) are used to treat a wide variety of infections for short-term use in both the community and hospital pharmacy.
- Common hormone agents that help manage the endocrine system include drugs to treat diabetes (including the natural and synthetic insulins), thyroid disorders, osteoporosis (bisphosphonates), allergies, and chronic inflammatory diseases such as rheumatoid arthritis, Crohn's disease, and gout (corticosteroids).
- Respiratory drugs used to treat acute and chronic lung diseases include some of the antihistamines and bronchodilators, like fast-acting albuterol.
- Most of the drugs used to treat heartburn, such as the proton pump inhibitors and histamine-2 antagonists, are available as both prescription and OTC drugs.
- Hematologic drugs include both oral and injectable blood-thinning agents.
- Bridging therapy is common after surgery. Enoxaparin (Lovenox) is often used to prevent blood clots in transition before warfarin (Coumadin) begins working.
- Some needed vitamins come in prescription-level doses; they must be carefully matched with the medication profile because some vitamins, such as K combinations, interact poorly with other drugs.

CHECK YOUR UNDERSTANDING

To ensure that you recall and understand the key chapter concepts, please read the question or statement and select the appropriate lettered option.

1. The absorption, distribution, metabolism and elimination of drugs in the body comprise the scientific study of
   a. pharmacology.
   b. pharmacokinetics.
   c. pharmacognosy.
   d. pharmaceutics.
2. A harmful response to a drug or resulting from an extended use of a drug is defined as a(n)
   a. drug interaction.
   b. side effect.
   c. adverse drug event.
   d. contraindication.
3. To be considered pharmaceutically equivalent to a brand name, a generic drug must have the same
   a. active ingredient.
   b. inert ingredients.
   c. shape and color.
   d. expiration dating.

4. A pharmacy technician receives a prescription for the brand name Prinivil, an antihypertensive drug. The DAW box was not checked. The generic in stock is both pharmaceutically and therapeutically equivalent to Prinivil. The technician should
   a. contact the prescriber to see if the lower cost generic can be substituted.
   b. substitute the generic without prescriber approval.
   c. check to see if the brand name Prinivil is in stock.
   d. contact the insurance provider to determine if the brand name drug will be covered.

5. You receive a prescription for hydroxyzine hydrochloride 10 mg. You have on the pharmacy shelf a drug with the same active ingredient but a different salt form: hydroxyzine pamoate. These drugs are considered
   a. generic equivalents.
   b. pharmaceutical equivalents.
   c. biosimilars.
   d. pharmaceutical alternatives.

6. Identify the *correct statement* on biosimilars as compared to innovator products.
   a. a generic equivalent
   b. exactly the same biologically
   c. bioequivalent
   d. cannot be substituted without permission of prescriber

MAKE CONNECTIONS

Take a moment to consider what you have learned in this chapter and respond thoughtfully to the following prompts. Note that some of these activities will require internet access.

1. Whether or not a pharmacist may substitute a biosimilar product without prescriber authorization varies from state to state. Research the arguments for and against unilaterally requiring prescriber authorization on biosimilar products. Argue which side you are for.
2. Reviewing a patient's profile for conflicting medications is a responsibility shared by the pharmacist and the technician. Using the FDA Orange and Purple Books, create a short list of medications that would conflict with the following drugs: atorvastatin, metformin, albuterol, and losartan.

The online course includes additional review and assessment resources.

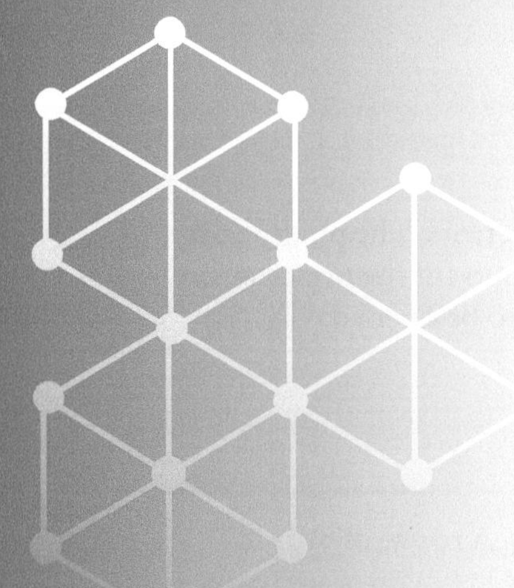

5 Routes of Drug Administration and Dosage Formulations

Learning Objectives

1. Differentiate between the terms *route of administration*, *dosage form*, and *drug delivery system*. (Section 5.1)
2. Identify different inactive and inert ingredients and various tablet coatings and their functions. (Section 5.2)
3. Explain the properties of oral, transmucosal, topical (dermal and transdermal), inhalation (intrarespiratory), and parenteral routes of administration and their dosage forms. (Sections 5.3–5.7)
4. Explain the advantages and disadvantages of the varying routes of administration to better understand and remember prescription and OTC directions. (Sections 5.3–5.7)
5. Explain the advantages and disadvantages of the varying drug formulations and their indications. (Sections 5.3–5.7)
6. Demonstrate correct techniques for administration of topicals, transmucosal agents, inhalers, and various parenteral injections (subq, IM, IV, and ID). (Sections 5.3–5.7)
7. Contrast the advantages and disadvantages of insulin administration from syringes versus pens, and discuss the importance of syringe and needle selection. (Sections 5.3–5.7)
8. Understand the common drug delivery systems that delay, extend, or target delivery and their prescriptive notations. (Section 5.8)

ASHP/ACPE Accreditation Standards
To view the *ASHP/ACPE Accreditation Standards* addressed in this chapter, refer to Appendix B.

Healthcare providers have many pharmacological agents at their disposal and a wide variety of dosage forms with which to customize patient treatment. Before selecting the appropriate medications for their patients, however, providers must have a good understanding of two scientific areas in addition to pharmacology: **pharmacokinetics** (how drugs are absorbed, circulated, metabolized, and eliminated) and **pharmaceutics** (how drugs release their active agents in specific forms).

A thorough study of these scientific areas is well beyond the scope of this text, but a pharmacy technician student must gain an appreciation of the advantages and disadvantages of various routes of administration and drug formulations that are used in everyday pharmacy practice. A favorable patient outcome may well depend on selecting not only the most appropriate medication, but also the most appropriate route of administration and formulation to meet the patient's needs and reduce the risk of preventable medication errors. The pharmacist will make the selection, but technicians must be aware enough to fill the prescription correctly and notice when something is problematic or needs to be queried.

5.1 Routes of Administration

Medications can be introduced into the body by several routes. A **route of administration** is a way to get a drug into or onto the body, and there are many ways to do this—through the mouth, by swallowing, as with tablets; through the skin with ointments or patches; through the inner linings of the mouth, rectal, or genital areas; through injections, as in shots or IV solutions; or through surgical implants. Drugs are aimed at two kinds of therapeutic effects—either a **systemic effect**, where the drug gets into the bloodstream to affect the whole body or a bodily system; or a **localized effect**, where the drug is meant to exert its therapeutic action at or near the site of administration (for example, an ear drop in the ear).

A **dosage form** is the physical manifestation of a drug—such as a tablet, capsule, suspension, ointment, cream, patch, or injection—that is designed to deliver the medication by a specific route of administration. The dosage form selected is the one best suited to produce the desired systemic or localized effect in either an immediate or time-delayed manner. The suitability of the various common dosages for both systemic and localized routes of administration will be explained later in this chapter, along with their advantages and disadvantages. Table 5.1 outlines their categories.

Pharm Fact

A localized drug can sometimes have a systemic side effect, and a systemic drug can sometimes have a localized side effect.

As you can see, dosage forms are adapted to different routes of administration, depending on their intended uses. Furthermore, many drugs, such as nitroglycerin, can be delivered to the body via different routes of administration: orally as a tablet or capsule; transdermally (through mucus linings) as a patch; sublingually as a tablet (under the tongue); translingually (across the tongue) as a spray; topically as an ointment; via inhalation as an aerosol spray; or intravenously as an IV solution.

Effects, however, are not always so clear-cut. It is important to understand that some medications used for localized effects can also have unintended systemic effects. For example, inhaler solutions used to open airways in patients with asthma can also have some systemic absorption that results in tremors, dizziness, nervousness, and other side effects. Pharmacists need to keep unintended systemic effects in mind as well as any possible interactions with systemic drugs. A drug with a systemic route of administration can also produce a localized side effect at the area of the administration site, such as numbness at the injection site of a systemic painkiller.

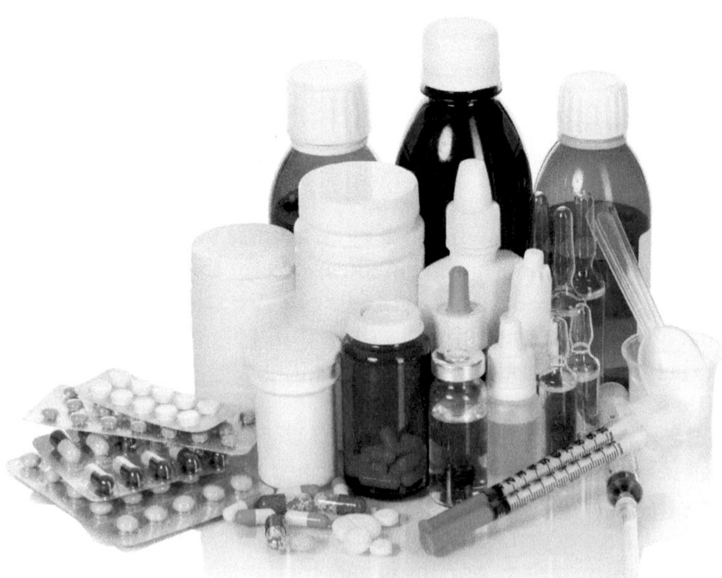

Medications are available in many dosage forms that can be given by several routes of administration.

TABLE 5.1 Common Routes of Administration and Corresponding Dosage Forms

Route of Administration	Common Dosage Forms
Systemic Effects	
Oral enteral (into mouth and swallowed)	Tablets, capsules, syrups, suspensions
Transmucosal (through mucous of inner linings):	
• Oral buccal (absorbed between cheek and gums)	• Lozenges, sprays, troche tablets (dissolving), effervescent tablets
• Oral sublingual (absorbed under tongue)	• Tablets (melting), drops, sprays, lozenges, effervescent tablets
Topical transdermal (absorbed through the skin)	Creams, ointments, pastes, patches, plasters
Inhalation/intrarespiratory (breathed in)	Dry powder inhalers, metered-dose inhalers, nebulizer solutions
Parenteral/injection (injected into muscle, skin, or under the skin)	Injection shots, injectable pen solutions, IV solutions
Rectal and vaginal (transdermal and transmucosal)	Rings, suppositories, solutions (these are less frequently systemic)
Implants	Pumps, radiation seeds, stents, wound dressings
Localized Effects	
Topical dermal (on or in the skin)	Creams, lotions, ointments, powders, solutions
Inhalation (breathed in)	Dry powder inhalers, metered-dose inhalers, nebulizer solutions
Transmucosal (through mucous membranes):	
• Intranasal (through inside of the nose)	• Sprays, solutions
• Ophthalmic (through eyes)	• Sprays, solutions
• Otic (through ears)	• Solutions, suspensions
Vaginal and rectal (transdermal and transmucosal)	Suppositories, solutions, creams, gels, ointments

5.2 Active Versus Inactive Drug Ingredients

Safety Alert

The designer street drugs named "bath salts"are addictive and extremely dangerous, producing paranoia, hallucinations, suicidal thinking, and extreme agitation. They are disguised to look like common Epsom or soaking salts.

Oral drug compounds contain one or more active ingredients along with inert, or inactive, ingredients. There are many reasons for the addition of **inert ingredients**. They fulfill functions of the compound that are not directly related to the medicinal purpose.

For example, one inert ingredient may be a **diluent**, a filler substance that creates a usable size of tablet or liquid from a small amount of a high-potency active ingredient. Other purposes for inert ingredients may be to bind the compound together, stabilize the ingredients, preserve them, put them in a solution, or give the tablet an appealing color. Common types of inert ingredients used in tablets and their functions are listed in Table 5.2. Patients may be allergic to inert ingredients. All inert ingredients must be listed in the manufacturer product insert that accompanies the prescription product. For over-the-counter (OTC) products, the inert ingredients must be listed for the consumer on the product labeling.

The active drug ingredients in many tablets, capsules, and suspensions are often powders or granules (small particles). At times the active ingredient can be combined with a mineral to form a tightly bonded crystal granule form, or ionized salt, to extend the shelf life of the drug or affect the characteristics of how the drug is released into the bloodstream. Different salt forms are not the same and cannot be substituted

TABLE 5.2 Common Inert Tablet Ingredients and Their Uses

Ingredient	Use	Example
Binder	Promotes adhesion of the materials in the tablet	Methylcellulose
Coating	Assists the patient's swallowing of the tablet; improves the flavor of the tablet; protects the stomach lining from the side effects of the drug; delays the release of the medication once it has been consumed	Saccharine
Coloring	Provides tablet identification	FDA-approved coloring agents and dyes
Diluent	Allows for appropriate concentration of the medication in the tablet; provides bulk and cohesion	Lactose
Disintegrant	Helps break up the ingredients once the tablet has been consumed	Starch
Lubricating agent	Gives the tablet a slippery sheen; aids in the manufacturing process	Talc
Solubilizer	Maintains the ingredients in solution; helps ingredients pass into solution in the body	Cyclodextrin

without physician direction or approval. For example, diclofenac tablets exist in two salt forms: diclofenac potassium and diclofenac sodium. They have different chemical makeup and crystalline sizes. At equivalent doses, their therapeutic effect would be similar but not the same, and neither the pharmacy technician nor the pharmacist can substitute one for the other without contacting the prescriber.

Drug compounds can be formulated to have the active ingredients directly released or to have delayed-release characteristics to allow for less frequent dosing and/or fewer side effects. The different ingredients and salt or non-salt forms help determine this. Also, the same chemical salt can have different crystalline sizes, which influences how fast the active drug ingredients are released. For example, a Macrodantin 100 mg capsule contains 75 mg of mononitrate salt and 25 mg of a controlled-release macrocrystalline (large crystal) mononitrate salt. This formulation offers better absorption (particularly when taken with food), less nausea and GI upset, and a longer duration of action when compared with a generic drug that contains only 100 mg of the mononitrate salt.

Some drugs have salts for different dosage forms. For example, hydroxyzine 50 mg is available as a hydrochloride salt tablet formulation and as a pamoate salt capsule. In this case, the two different dosage forms are considered therapeutically equivalent. Therefore, if the pharmacy is out of stock of one dosage form, the other dosage form could be safely substituted—*but only with the approval of the pharmacist and/or prescriber*.

However, this substitution process for dosage form (e.g., capsule versus tablet) is not always possible. For example, Zanaflex 4 mg capsules and Zanaflex 4 mg tablets are *not considered therapeutically equivalent* and, consequently, cannot be substituted. In many cases, prescribers may not be familiar with which dosage forms are available or the subtle differences in bioavailability or release characteristics among drug products. Pharmacist review of the medication substitution, therefore, is critical.

5.3 Oral Routes of Administration

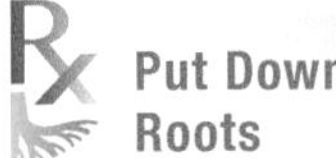

Put Down Roots

The term *enteral* comes from the Greek word *enteron*, which means "intestine."

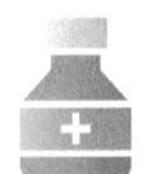

Pharm Fact

The absorption rate of different oral medications is determined by many factors, such as the type of drug, the presence of food in the digestive tract, and any digestive disorders.

Safety Alert

The oral route of administration is not appropriate for patients who are experiencing nausea or vomiting.

Any medication administration that passes through the gastrointestinal (GI) tract for systemic circulation (such as through the mouth or a feeding tube) is referred to as an **enteral route of administration**. Enteral administration by drinking, swallowing whole, or chewing and swallowing is also known as the **oral route of administration**. However, the term *oral* can also refer to a medication applied topically to the mouth (as in the localized treatment of a cold sore) or to other dosage forms that are put into the mouth cavity, so the term can be confusing. Physicians use the prescription abbreviation *po* (from the Latin term *per os*, meaning "by mouth") to indicate the swallowing route of medication administration.

Oral (enteral) dosage forms proceed through a series of discrete steps: passing through the mouth and throat into the stomach; dissolving and absorbing in the stomach or small intestine; **metabolizing** (the transformation of food into energy) in the liver; distributing to the tissue or target organ; and eliminating the remnants from the body, often via the kidneys. Because of these many progressive steps, oral tablets, capsules, and liquids generally all have a delayed systemic effect of at least 30 minutes or longer.

Some drugs are administered in the mouth but not swallowed. These oral drug forms are absorbed by the inner linings of the mouth through the mucous layers. Any drugs absorbed by the mucus layers are called **transmucosal**. The two oral transmucosal routes of administration are the **sublingual route of administration**, where a medication is dissolved and absorbed under the tongue, and the **buccal route of administration**, where a medication is dissolved and absorbed between the cheek and gums. These transmucosal drug forms are considered different from the general oral dosage forms because the medications are absorbed directly in the mouth rather than going through the digestive system; they will be explained in more detail later.

Tablets, capsules, solutions, suspensions, syrups, and elixirs are all common oral (enteral) dosage forms that are swallowed. In general, oral dosage forms offer convenience, safety, and ease of use. However, these medications also have disadvantages associated with their passing through the digestive tract, which include delayed onset and absorption, and destruction of some of the medicinal power of the drug by digestive fluids. Each dosage form has a unique set of benefits and drawbacks that pharmacy technicians must know to provide safe and effective care.

Tablets

Tablets are one of the most common forms of oral administration. The **tablet** is a solid dosage form produced by compressing dry drug ingredients of either powder or granules (small particles or crystals). Tablets are available in a wide variety of shapes, sizes, surface markings, and coatings. Most tablets are imprinted with a distinctive letter and/or numerical code as well as coloring from their manufacturers for drug identification purposes. Drugs may come in a variety of salt and tablet dosage forms.

Tablets are easier and less costly to produce in bulk than other forms, so they are often cheaper. For patients, tablets offer low cost, more precise dosing, and increased usability due to specialized coatings. They offer high physical, chemical, and antimicrobial stability so that they can have a long shelf life in the pharmacy and at home.

Tablets have some major disadvantages:

- delayed onset of action because the dosage form must disintegrate in the stomach and small intestine before being absorbed

- destruction of the drug by GI fluids
- local GI side effects in the stomach, such as nausea, heartburn, or ulcers
- delayed absorption of the medication because food is present in the stomach
- ineffectiveness for patients who are experiencing nausea or vomiting or who are comatose, sedated, or otherwise unable to swallow

All oral distribution forms that involve swallowing include these disadvantages to a lesser extent. **Delayed-release (DR) formulation** tablets address some of these concerns (to be explained in more detail later in this chapter). Because the release is slower and more gradual, the longer duration of action usually produces fewer side effects and requires a reduced dosing schedule. Consequently, the DR tablet form improves patient adherence and patient outcomes. DR tablets, though, also have several disadvantages. They have a slower onset of action, cannot usually be split or crushed, can have prolonged side effects, and are more expensive. (See Table 5.3 for examples of DR tablets.)

TABLE 5.3 Common Brand Names of Delayed-Release Tablets and Capsules*

Adalat CC (nifedipine ER)	Glucotrol XL	Sinemet CR (carbidopa-levodopa ER)
Adderall XR	Glucophage XR (metformin ER)	Taztia XT
Ambien CR	Inderal XL (propranolol ER)	Toprol XL (metoprolol succinate ER)
Augmentin XR	Indocin SR	Uniphyl (theophylline ER)
Calan SR (verapamil ER)	Klor-Con (potassium chloride)	Voltaren XR (diclofenac ER)
Concerta	Lamictal XR	Wellbutrin SR/XL (budeprion SR/XR)
Depakote ER (divalproex DR/ER)	MS Contin	Xanax XR (alprazolam ER)
Diltia XT (diltiazem SR/XT)	Niacin SR	
Ditropan XL	OxyContin	
Effexor XR	Ritalin LA	
Glipizide XL	Seroquel XR	

* Do not split tablets or open up capsules.

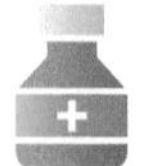

Pharm Fact

A common chewable adult tablet is 81 mg of aspirin.

Tablet Types

Tablets can be designed to be easily swallowed, mask a drug taste, or exert an immediate pharmacological response. The different intentions result in different types of tablets.

Compression Tablets Large pharmaceutical manufacturers use heavy tool and die machinery to make **compression tablets** by several methods. In the direct compression process, the powder or granular ingredients are compressed to produce a tablet as the end product. Standard one-pass compression tablets are the most inexpensive and common dosage form used today. Acetaminophen (Tylenol) is an example of a compression tablet.

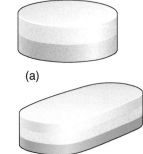

FIGURE 5.1 Multiple Compression Tablets

(a) Two layers or compressions
(b) Three layers or compressions

(a)

(b)

Multiple Compression Tablets A **multiple compression tablet (MCT)** is produced by multiple compression cycles and is, in effect, either a tablet on top of a tablet or a tablet within a tablet. An MCT may contain a core and one or two outer shells (or two or three different layers, as shown in Figure 5.1), each containing a separate medication and colored differently. MCTs are created for appearance alone or to combine incompatible substances into a single medication. The Ambien CR (zolpidem tartrate) brand is an example of an MCT.

Chewable Tablets A **chewable tablet** contains a base that is flavored and/or colored. The dosage form is designed to be **masticated** (chewed) and absorbed quickly for a slightly faster onset of action. Chewing is preferred for antacids, antiflatulents, commercial vitamins, and tablets designed for children. They can be prescribed for small children in lieu of other dosage forms. For example, the drug montelukast (Singulair), used to control asthma symptoms, and the drug amoxicillin, used to treat infections, are both available in a children's chewable tablet form.

Oral Disintegrating Tablets An **oral disintegrating tablet (ODT)** is designed to melt in your mouth. ODTs are useful for pediatric and geriatric patients who have difficulty swallowing or for patients with nausea and vomiting. Examples include rizatriptan (Maxalt) for the treatment of migraine headaches, donepezil (Aricept) for the treatment of Alzheimer's disease, and ondansetron (Zofran) for the treatment of nausea and vomiting.

Caplets Some pharmaceutical companies manufacture an oblong tablet called a caplet. The **caplet** is simply a tablet shaped and sometimes coated to look like a capsule. The inside of the caplet is solid rather than filled with powder or granular material like the inside of a capsule. Caplets have many beneficial properties. They are easier to swallow than large tablets, have a longer shelf life, and—unlike capsules—are tamper-proof. Caplet formulations on the market include the OTC drug brand naproxen (Aleve) and the prescription drug brand oxaprozin (Daypro).

Tablet Coatings and Additives

Most compression tablets are uncoated, but some tablet dosage forms are covered by a special outside layer that dissolves or ruptures in the stomach or small intestine. Coatings on tablets can be used to improve appearance, flavor, or ease of swallowing. Common tablet coatings include sugar or a film coating.

A **sugar-coated tablet (SCT)** contains an outside layer of sugar that protects the medication and improves both appearance and flavor. Sugar coating masks the bitter taste of some drugs (such as ibuprofen) and increases the stability of the drug. The major disadvantage of a sugar coating is that it makes the tablets much larger, heavier, and more difficult to swallow. An SCT could be crushed, but the bitterness of the drug would no longer be masked. Most multivitamins contain a sugar coating to mask the bitter smell and taste of the vitamins, especially prenatal vitamins.

A **film-coated tablet (FCT)** contains a thin outer layer of a polymer (a substance containing very large molecules) that can be either soluble or insoluble in water. Film coatings are thinner, lighter in weight, and more efficient and less expensive to manufacture than sugar coatings. They are colored to provide an attractive appearance and, at times, to protect the stomach lining or delay the release of the drug. An enteric coating is a special coating designed to resist destruction by gastric fluids. This film barrier also protects the drug from being digested and released too quickly. (For more discussion on enteric coatings, see the section titled "Drug Delivery Systems" later in this chapter.) Certain dosage forms of the antibiotics erythromycin (Erythrocin) and metronidazole (Flagyl) have enteric coatings to prevent serious GI side effects that commonly occur with these drugs. An FCT can be crushed, but doing so may lose its taste-masking benefit.

A **buffered tablet**, as in "buffered aspirin," is a tablet in which an antacid, such as calcium carbonate, is added to the medication to reduce the stomach acids that can cause both abdominal distress and damage to the stomach lining.

Capsules

The active ingredient(s) of a **capsule** are commonly in the form of a granular powder or liquid gel that is enclosed by a **gelatin shell**. Gelatin is a protein substance obtained from vegetable matter and/or from the skin, connective tissue, and bones of animals. The gelatin shell of the capsule can be hard or soft, and it may be transparent, semitransparent, or opaque. It may be colored or marked with a code to facilitate identification. The "body" is the longer portion that is filled, and the "cap" covers it. In commercial manufacturing, the body and the cap are usually sealed to protect the integrity of the drug within and to prevent tampering. Because a capsule encloses the drug components, flavorings are not common for this dosage form.

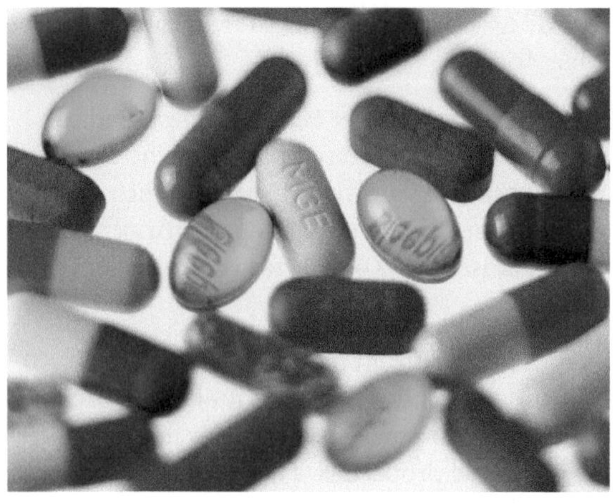

Capsules and tablets are manufactured in a variety of sizes, shapes, and colors to help patients identify their different drugs.

Compared with tablets, capsules are typically easier to swallow, have a more rapid dissolution, and have a faster onset of action. Capsules, though, do not allow as much dosage manipulation as tablets or liquid formulations. The contents of most immediate-release capsules, however, can be mixed with water and administered to a child or to a patient with an enteral or a nasogastric feeding tube. Some capsules are used to compound specific oral solutions.

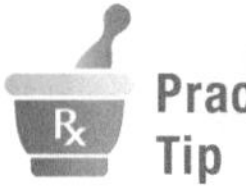

Practice Tip

Some patients, for personal or religious purposes, might avoid certain animal products. Be aware that gelatin in capsules is often from cows or pigs. Patients may prefer vegetarian sources for capsules.

Liquid Dosage Forms

Most medicinal liquids are commercially available as solutions (such as syrups and elixirs), suspensions, emulsions, and colloids for oral administration, each of which will be explained later in this section. Liquids consist of one or more active ingredients in a liquid vehicle. Liquids have several advantages as a dosage form, including a faster onset of action than oral tablets or capsules, easy administration, and individualized dosing according to a patient's body weight.

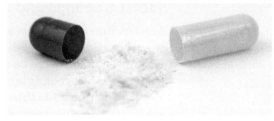

A capsule includes a cap (red) and a body (gold) that is filled with medication.

Liquid medications are also ideal for certain age groups. For young children, liquids have easier dosage adjustments. For example, a flavored antibiotic liquid or suspension can be accurately dosed based on a patient's body weight and may be preferable to a tablet or capsule. For geriatric patients, liquid medications are easier to swallow, especially for those patients with swallowing difficulties due to Parkinson's disease or cancer. For patients who have to swallow large tablets, such as potassium chloride, prescribers can order a liquid formulation that offers the same dose and has the added benefit of less GI upset.

Liquids also have a few disadvantages. Liquid dosage forms are often less stable than their solid dosage tablet and capsule counterparts. Consequently, pharmacy personnel should monitor proper storage conditions of liquid medications, rotating and checking stock for expiration dates.

Solutions

A **solution** is a liquid in which the active ingredients are completely dissolved in a liquid vehicle so that they appear transparent (as opposed to murky). Each solution has the drug agent dissolved in a liquid base that composes most of the solution called a **solvent**. Solutions are often classified by their liquid base: **aqueous solutions** are water-based; **alcoholic solutions** are alcohol-based; and **hydroalcoholic solutions** are water-based and alcohol-based. The ingredient dissolved in the solution is known as the **solute**. Promethazine hydrochloride (Phenergan) is an example of a prescription drug for nausea that is available as a solution (also as a tablet and a suppository).

Most liquid formulations for children are syrups or elixirs flavored to mask the taste and ease the swallowing of the medication. Syrups (as in cough medicines) are preferred because they do not contain alcohol.

Practice Tip

Patients need to be reminded to shake suspensions before each use. For a patient who has difficulty with this, another dosage form might be best, as recommended by the pharmacist. Following the directions for refrigeration or storage at room temperature is also important.

Syrups A **syrup** is an aqueous solution thickened with a large amount of sugar—generally sucrose—or a sugar substitute, such as sorbitol or propylene glycol. Syrups are classified as medicated and nonmedicated. Examples of medicated syrups include lithium citrate (Phenergan) for bipolar depression, ranitidine hydrochloride (Xantac) for heartburn, or cetirizine hydrochloride (Zyrtec) for allergies.

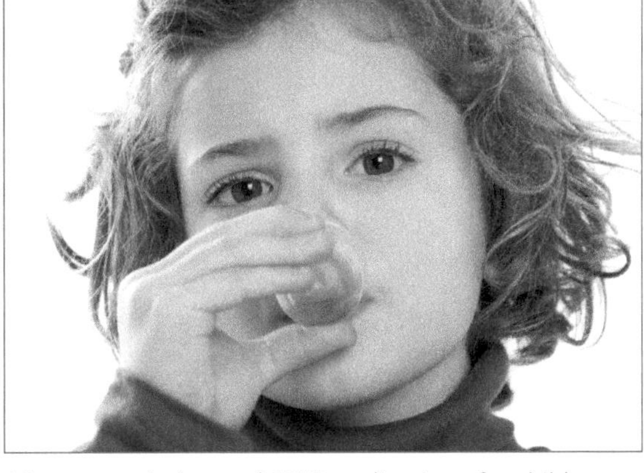

Many prescription and OTC medications for children come in flavored syrup formulations with high sugar or corn syrup content.

Syrups usually contain additional flavorings, colorings, or aromatic agents. Codeine and guaifenesin Cheratussin AC is a medicated prescription cough medicine that contains more than 10 inactive ingredients, including several flavoring agents. Common nonmedicated syrups include fruits or cocoa syrups used to make flavored drinks.

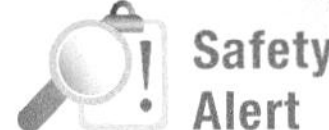

Safety Alert

Because of their high sugar content, syrups should be used cautiously in patients with diabetes, especially children.

The higher sugar content of syrups can pose problems for patients with diabetes. Therefore, pharmacists generally recommend sugar-free OTC products for this patient population. In contrast, some less sugary suspensions, such as amoxicillin/clavulanate (Augmentin) and clindamycin (Cleocin), have the disadvantage of unpleasant taste. Although the taste of medication can be masked by various flavorings to promote adherence, certain flavorings may be physically incompatible with components of the suspension. With that in mind, pharmacy technicians must follow proven "recipes" when selecting the proper flavoring agent. (The role of the pharmacy technician in flavoring suspensions is further discussed in Chapter 7.) The fact that suspensions have to be shaken by the patient before every use can be another disadvantage.

Elixirs An **elixir** is a clear, sweetened, flavored solution containing ethanol with the water base (hydroalcoholic). An example of a drug in this dosage form is phenobarbital elixir, which contains phenobarbital, orange oil, propylene glycol, sorbitol solution, color, alcohol, and purified water. This elixir is used to treat anxiety and seizures.

Less Common Solutions Other available solutions include aromatic water, fluidextracts, solid extracts, tinctures, and spirits:

- An **aromatic water** is a solution of water containing oils or other substances that have a pungent and usually pleasing smell and are volatile (i.e., easily released into the air). Rose water is an example.
- A fluidextract is a liquid dosage form, such as an oil or sap, extracted from plant sources and commonly used in the formulation of syrups. Vanilla extract is an example of a fluidextract.
- A solid extract is a potent dosage form derived from animal or plant sources from which most or all of the liquid has been evaporated to produce a powder, an ointment-like form, or solid matter. Some extracts are reduced down from fluidextracts and used in the formulation of medications. Dried herbal leaves are examples of a solid extract.
- A tincture is made by combining a fluid- or solid extract with an alcoholic or hydroalcoholic solution. Examples include iodine and belladonna tinctures, and some herbal dietary supplements.
- A spirit is an alcoholic or hydroalcoholic solution containing aromatic ingredients that can easily enter the air as gases, so they are less stable. Examples include camphor and peppermint spirit, both of which can be used as medicines or flavorings.

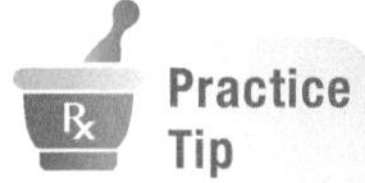

Practice Tip

Pharmacy technicians should always "shake well" a stock bottle of an oral suspension before transferring the medication to a smaller, labeled prescription bottle.

Suspensions

Unlike a solution, a **suspension** is a liquid medication in which the solid particles of the substance remain *undissolved* in the liquid even after mixing, so the medication appears murky or cloudy. The solid drug ingredient particles can be from powders or granulated crystals. A suspension is considered a **dispersion** because the medication is simply mixed to have the particles evenly dispersed, or distributed, throughout the liquid base. As noted, they have to be mixed again, often by shaking by the patient, to keep them combined.

Like solutions, suspensions often contain many inactive ingredients, including colorings, coatings, and flavorings, such as the cherry-mint Nystatin oral suspension (an antifungal treatment). Some suspensions are commercially available over the counter, such as Mylanta (both a combination of aluminum hydroxide, magnesium hydroxide, and simethicone) and Motrin and Advil (or ibuprofen) oral suspensions. Others come in the form of dry powders or granules that are mixed or reconstituted by the pharmacist or pharmacy technician with purified distilled water prior to dispensing to the patient.

Antibiotic suspensions are often mixed by adding sterile water to irregular-shaped granules, which are not as likely as powders to float on the surface of a liquid. These suspensions have excellent flow characteristics and are more stable than those mixed from powders. A well-prepared suspension pours easily and settles slowly but can be redispersed quickly by gentle shaking.

Most antibiotic suspensions have a limited shelf life. In fact, the expiration date for most reconstituted antibiotic suspensions or those mixed with water is 7 to 10 days at room temperature and 14 days if stored in the refrigerator. Pharmacy technicians should also be aware that some antibiotics, such as cefdinir and azithromycin, are best stored at room temperature after reconstitution and *should not be placed in the refrigerator*. Consequently, it is key that technicians address medication storage requirements with patients during pickup.

Emulsions

Another type of dispersion is known as an emulsion. An **emulsion** is a mixture of two unblendable substances, such as an oil-and-vinegar salad dressing. It must be shaken well to mix it evenly before use. Medicated emulsions often contain an **emulsifying agent** that makes the liquid more stable and less prone to separation by binding the two ingredients together. Pediacare Gas Relief Drops is a commercially available oral emulsion of simethicone. Many skin care products on the market are emulsions.

Colloids

A **colloid** is a mixture having physical properties between those of a solution and a fine suspension. A **magma**, or milk-like liquid, is an example of a dispersion containing ultrafine colloidal particles in a suspension. An example of a magma is Milk of Magnesia, which contains magnesium hydroxide and is used to neutralize gastric acid. Another type of colloidal dispersion is the **microemulsion**, or a liquid that is dispersed in another liquid. Unlike other emulsions, however, it is clear because of the extremely fine size of the droplets of the dispersed phase. An example of a microemulsion is Haley's M-O (magnesium and mineral oil).

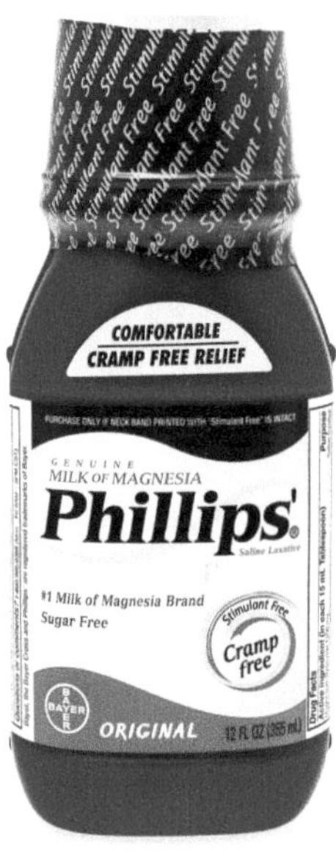

Milk of magnesia, which helps with stomach distress, is an example of a colloid mixture.

Powders and Effervescent Salts

Other oral dosage forms like powders and effervescent salt mixtures that patients add to water are less frequently prescribed. They are often OTC medications and home-style remedies. Still, these dosage forms offer some advantages over tablets and capsules for those who have difficulty swallowing tablets or capsules.

Powders

A **powder** is a preparation in the form of fine particles. Commonly requested OTC powders include Goody's (acetaminophen, aspirin, and caffeine) and BC (aspirin and caffeine) headache powders, brewer's yeast, and fiber laxatives (such as Metamucil). The headache powders take less time to dissolve than tablets and are thought to work more quickly than tablets in relieving a headache. In large-scale commercial manufacturing, as well as in compounding pharmacies, powders are milled and pulverized by machines and placed into gelatin capsules. Some patients simply drop a teaspoon of baking soda into a glass of water as a home remedy for stomach distress.

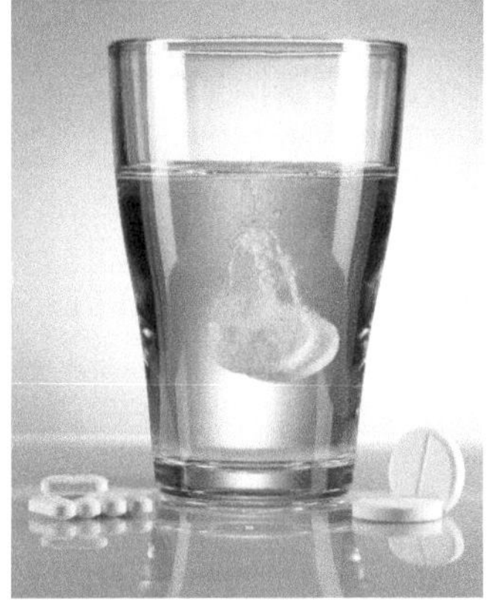

Effervescent salts release carbon dioxide gas when added to water.

Effervescent Salts

An **effervescent salt** is a mixture of granules or coarse powders that contains one or more medicinal agents (such as an analgesic) as well as some combination of sodium bicarbonate with citric acid, tartaric acid, or sodium biphosphate. When dissolved in water, the effervescent salts release carbon dioxide gas, causing a distinctive bubbly or fizzy appearance and sound. Most people are familiar with effervescent tablets, such as the common OTC immunity builder Airborne (a dietary supplement) or the Alka-Seltzer line of products that are used to relieve headaches, hangovers, or indigestion. Alka-Seltzer once had the marketing tagline "Plop plop, fizz fizz, oh what a relief it is!" that makes it easy to remember what an effervescent salt is.

Patient Administration of Oral Dosage Forms

When patients receive a new oral medication, it is important for technicians to guide them to the pharmacist for counsel before they leave the store. The pharmacist should discuss with the patient what drinks and foods to take with the medications as well as which consumables to avoid. For most medications, water is preferred to coffee, tea, juices, or carbonated drinks as an aid in swallowing. In fact, some beverages—such as milk, coffee, and tea—may inactivate certain antibiotics and osteoporosis medications.

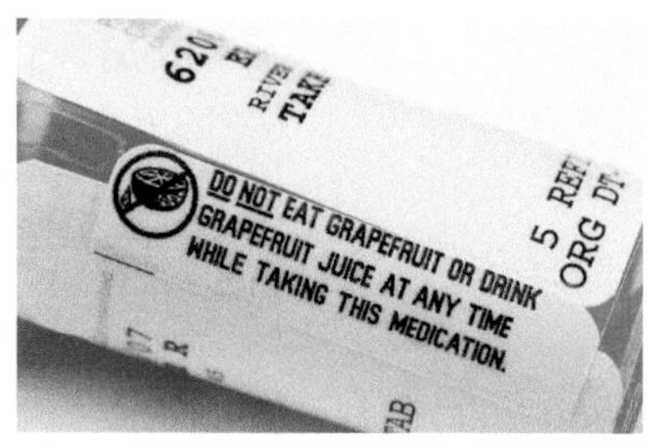

Pharmacists may direct technicians to apply auxiliary labels to prescription containers to aid patient use.

Pharmacists also need to counsel patients as to behaviors to avoid while taking medications. Some of these curtailed behaviors include alcohol consumption, sun exposure, and driving. To remind patients of these medication restrictions, as explained in the previous chapter, you can affix auxiliary labels to the drug containers.

It is also usually up to the pharmacy technician to explain to patients how to properly store their oral medications. In addition, specific oral dosage forms have their unique dispensing and administration guidelines, as discussed below.

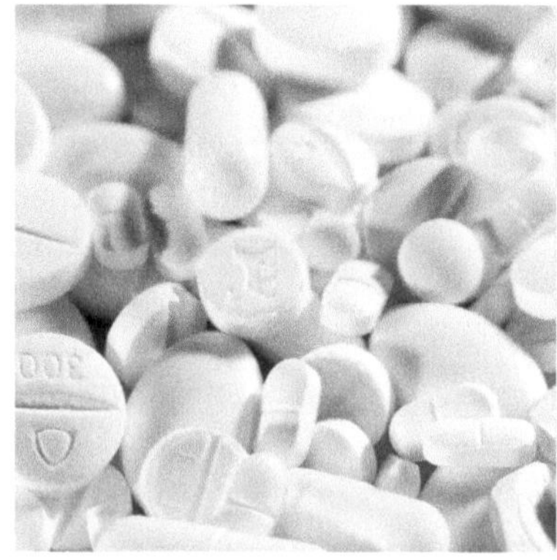
Tablets that are meant to be split have a prepressed scoring line for easy breakage in halves or fourths.

Tablet Administration

Practice Tip

It is important to make patients aware that, although careful tablet splitting may reduce medication costs, it is not recommended for all drugs.

Patients who have difficulty swallowing solids should be instructed to place the tablet on the back of the tongue and tilt the head backward, which will stimulate swallowing. Patients should also be reminded not to crush (or split) tablets that are intended to be swallowed whole, such as any delayed-release or enteric-coated drug.

For traditional tablets that are not delayed-release, a patient can take a portion of a tablet, one tablet, or several tablets as the prescribed dose or as personal adjustment requires. Many tablets are scored once or twice by the manufacturer to facilitate ease of breakage into portions for half (or even

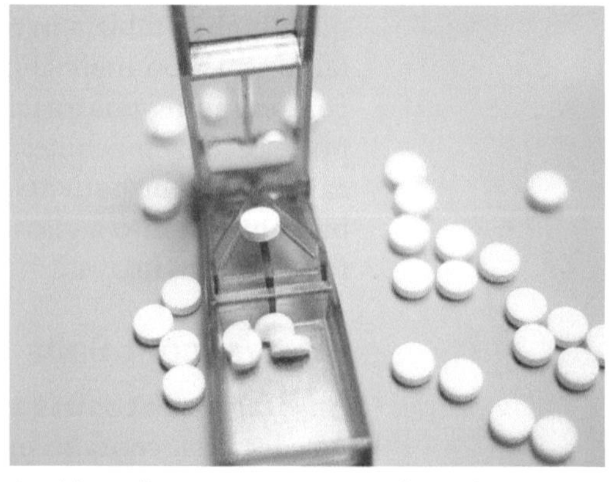
A tablet splitter can save money for patients taking high-cost medications, especially for chronic medical conditions.

quarter) doses. The **scoring**, or indenting, of a tablet is designed to (almost) equally divide the dose in each section or quadrant.

Due to rising drug costs, patients commonly use a tablet splitter to break both scored and unscored tablets when treating chronic conditions, such as high blood pressure. Under a healthcare provider's oversight, a patient can use a tablet that is twice the strength of their intended dose and only ingest half a tablet per dose. Splitting medications can save up to double the price for patients, and limited studies suggest that this practice with select medications does not appreciably affect the control of the disease state. Patients should keep in mind that not all tablets can be split in equal doses even with the use of a tablet splitter. For example, odd-shaped tablets such as valsartan (Diovan) or tadalafil (Cialis) are particularly difficult to cut.

If a tablet is not scored, it is generally recommended that it should not be split because the dose may not be equal in each piece. Based on results of scientific studies, the Food and Drug Administration (FDA) has approved a limited number of prescription drugs for tablet splitting.

Capsule Administration

As with tablets, patients who have difficulty swallowing solids should place the capsule on the back of the tongue and tilt the head backward to ease the process. Some formulations, such as Theo-Dur Sprinkles (theophylline) and divalproex sprinkle capsules, are suitable to be opened up and sprinkled on food when swallowing proves difficult for a child or an adult with asthma or seizures. Again, patients should be reminded not to open capsules that are intended to be swallowed whole, such as any delayed-release drug.

To reduce errors in medications, it is recommended to provide metric dosing cups, spoons, and oral syringes to patients instead of relying on household teaspoons and tablespoons for measurement.

Liquid Administration

It is also important to remind patients that liquid medication doses should be accurately measured in a medication cup or measuring spoon. Common household utensils are often inaccurate measurements of a "teaspoonful" (5 mL) or "tablespoonful" (15 mL). Oral and **tuberculin syringes**, measuring spoons, medication cups, and droppers are commonly dispensed in the hospital and community pharmacy settings to administer doses ranging from 0.1 mL to 30 mL. Specific information on some of these pharmacy measurement devices is discussed below.

Oral Syringes An **oral syringe** is used to measure and deliver oral liquid medications to pediatric patients. This type of syringe is a calibrated device consisting of a plunger and a cannula, or barrel, and is used without a needle to administer precise amounts of medication by mouth. Oral syringes may be used to slowly administer liquid medications to not only pediatric patients, but patients who cannot open their mouths. For very small doses (less than 1 mL) for an infant, a 1 mL tuberculin syringe (again, without the needle) may be provided.

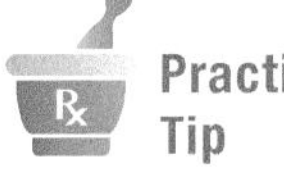

Pharmacy technicians should be aware that the abbreviation "gtt" (from the Latin *guttae* meaning "drops") is used as a measurement for droppers as well as for IV infusions.

Medication Cups Most manufacturers provide a medication cup for OTC liquids that are used to treat fever, cough, cold, and the like. These plastic cups contain specific dose demarcations in different units of measurement, such as 1 teaspoonful (5 mL), 2 teaspoonfuls (10 mL), and 1 tablespoonful (15 mL). Parents or caregivers should be directed to check the OTC package label for the specific dose appropriate for their child's age and weight or to ask the pharmacist. Measuring cups that also list fluid drams (an apothecary measurement equal to approximately 3.7 mL) should be disposed of to avoid accidental mistakes in dosing, which have happened even in hospitals.

Droppers **Droppers** are critically important for delivering the correct dosage of smaller volumes of medication to infants and children. A dropper contains a small, squeezable bulb at one end and a hollow glass or plastic tube with a tapering point on the other end. Squeezing the bulb creates a vacuum for drawing up a liquid. A dropper is commonly calibrated to deliver 1.25 mL (one-fourth teaspoon) to 2.5 mL (one-half teaspoon). Because different medicines may each have a different **viscosity** (fluid thickness and flow characteristics), the size of a drop varies considerably among different suspensions and solutions. In light of that, droppers that are packaged with medications can only be used to measure those specific medications.

Safety Alert

Reconstituted products are less stable than other products. Pharmacy technicians should always point out the manufacturer's recommendations for storage and the expiration dates.

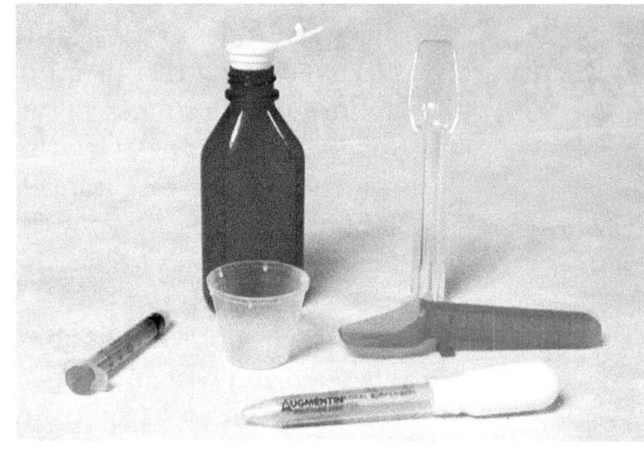

Parents can offer their infants or young children more accurate dosing of liquid medications when they are administered with one of these devices (syringe, cup, dropper, or measuring spoon).

5.4 Transmucosal Routes of Administration

Some of the disadvantages of oral drugs can be avoided if the medication can be more quickly available to the body by not going through the digestive tract. A transmucosal route of administration circumvents these disadvantages by allowing a drug to be absorbed through or across the sieve-like or permeable mucous membranes of the mouth, eyes, ears, nose, rectum, vagina, and urethra. These routes offer a more rapid and reliable onset of action and increased effectiveness coupled with a lower incidence of unpleasant side effects.

Transmucosal dosage forms are generally prescribed for patients who need immediate relief of symptoms. A disadvantage of these dosage forms is the difficulty in reversing the effects of a drug that is rapidly absorbed in the bloodstream. For example, if a patient experiences an adverse drug reaction, it would be difficult to quickly reverse the medication's effects.

Put Down Roots

Sub is a prefix meaning "under." *Lingual* is from the Latin *lingua*, meaning "tongue." That's why *sublingual* means "under the tongue." *Bucca* is Latin for "cheek."

Oral Transmucosal Forms

These forms include tablets, gum, and lozenges that are administered via the sublingual (under the tongue) route or the buccal (by the cheek) route of administration. These alternative dosage forms are able to bypass absorption delays in the stomach and proceed directly to the bloodstream to exert their beneficial therapeutic effect.

Sublingual Transmucosals

When a sublingual tablet is placed under the tongue, it is rapidly absorbed by blood vessels. One common medication administered via the sublingual route is the lifesaving drug nitroglycerin. Patients who are experiencing chest pain are instructed to place one nitroglycerin tablet under the tongue every five minutes until the pain is relieved or until three tablets have been administered. The sublingual route provides a rapid onset of action (less than 5 minutes) that is critical for immediate relief. The swift onset is the result of the medication entering the bloodstream directly without passage through the stomach or breakdown in the liver. A disadvantage of sublingual tablets is their short duration of action (less than 30 to 60 minutes), making this route of administration inappropriate for routine delivery of medication.

Buccal Transmucosals

Similar to the sublingual medications, a buccal drug form is absorbed by the blood vessels in the cheek. Common examples of buccal drugs are OTC nicotine gum (to counter nicotine addiction) or a lollipop-like lozenge, such as the narcotic fentanyl citrate. A **lozenge**, also known as a *troche*, is a solid dosage form containing active ingredients and flavorings, such as sweeteners. It is dissolved in the mouth as the lozenge is sucked or resting. Lozenges generally have local therapeutic effects.

Commercial OTC lozenges for the relief of sore throats are quite common, although many other drugs, including such prescription drugs as nystatin or clotrimazole, are also available in a lozenge form. Compounding pharmacies may prepare lozenge formulations for specific indications in special-needs pediatric or geriatric patients.

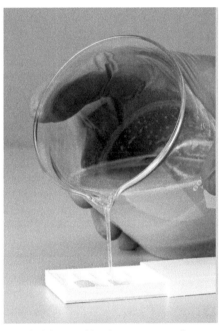

A technician working in a compounding pharmacy may prepare lozenge formulations by pouring a compounded solution into a lozenge mold.

The advantages of buccal medications include a faster onset of action than oral medications and, perhaps, fewer side effects. General disadvantages of the buccal route are an unpleasant taste and local mouth irritation, as in the case of nicotine gum. Another disadvantage of this route is that eating, drinking, and smoking can have an effect on absorption of the medication. It is also not advised for patients who have open sores in the mouth. If a patient does not follow the medication directions by redosing too often, an excessive amount of drug will be absorbed in a short period of time, which some refer to as "dose dumping."

Ophthalmic, Otic, and Nasal Transmucosal Forms

Transmucosal routes of administration are almost always prescribed for their fast onset of action and localized therapeutic effects to treat conditions of the eye, ear, nose, or sinuses.

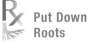

Put Down Roots

The Greek term *ophthalmikos* means things "pertaining to the eyes." The Latin word for "eye" is *occulus*.

Ophthalmic Transmucosals

Medications for transmucosal administration in the eye, or the **ocular route of administration**, are manufactured as solutions, suspensions, or ointment formulations—all of which must be sterile. These formulations are called **ophthalmics** because they pertain to the eye. Solutions have a more rapid onset of action, but suspensions have a longer duration. Pharmacy technicians should be aware that these two dosage forms should *not* be interchanged without the permission of the pharmacist and/or prescriber. For instance, Betoptic (betaxolol hydrochloride) is a solution and Betoptic S is a suspension. The suspension should be gently shaken prior to use.

IN THE REAL WORLD

The narcotic Actiq (fentanyl citrate) is a pain medication that comes in the form of a lozenge, a form commonly used for sore throats in both prescription and OTC medications for localized treatment and relief. (It also comes as a lollipop.) Actiq is a strong opioid designed particularly for cancer treatment. Because it is for pain and comes in the lozenge form, physicians have occasionally mistakenly prescribed it for sore throats. Patients who are suffering from a cold and sore throat and have a prescription for this medication should be referred to the pharmacist, and a call should be made to the physician to double-check the prescription.

Ophthalmics are available as both prescription drugs and OTC medications (for example, Sulamyd or sodium sulfacetamide for conjunctivitis, or "pink eye," and Visine for red eye irritation). The eye is more prone to infection than most areas of the body, so only sterile ophthalmic solutions, suspensions, or ointments should be used. Ophthalmic medications that are used repeatedly must contain a preservative to maintain antimicrobial sterility; examples of preservatives include methylparaben, propylparaben, thimerosal, and benzalkonium chloride.

Medications for eyes are often for localized effect. For instance, the ophthalmic solution ketorolac tromethamine (Acular LS) is a nonsteroidal anti-inflammatory drug that is prescribed to relieve pain and discomfort after eye surgery. However, some medications prescribed for the eye have a systemic effect and can adversely affect blood pressure (in patients with hypertension) and breathing (in patients with lung disease). Pharmacy personnel should recommend that patients carefully read the labeled instructions and precautions on all OTC ophthalmics and seek out proper counseling from their pharmacist if questions arise.

Another example of an ophthalmic solution is timolol maleate, a glaucoma medication that is available as both a solution and a longer-acting gel-forming solution (GFS). These two products cannot be substituted for each other without the permission of the prescriber. Pharmacy technicians must be extremely careful in selecting the right products from the shelf and comparing NDC numbers.

Remind patients that ear drops can never be used in the eye, though eye drops can be used in the ear.

Exercise caution when selecting ophthalmic and otic (ear) medications. Some products such as Neosporin are available as both, but the otic product must *not be dispensed or used* in the treatment of an eye disorder even if it contains the same dose, drugs, and concentration because an otic drug is not sterile. However, ophthalmic drugs may be administered in the ear.

Otic Transmucosals

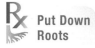

The Greek term *ōtikos* means "of the ear" as *ōt* means "ear."

Nonsterile drug solutions or suspensions that are administered into one or both ears through the ear canal(s) are using the **otic route of administration**. Like ophthalmics, otic products as a solution or a suspension should not be interchanged without the permission of the pharmacist and/or prescriber. Analgesic otic solutions can provide almost immediate pain relief to pediatric patients suffering from ear infections. The analgesic otic antipyrine/benzocaine contains anhydrous glycerin and oxyquinolone sulfate as inactive ingredients. Be aware that these inactive ingredients can occasionally cause allergic reactions.

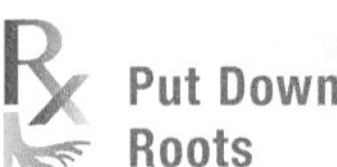

The Latin term *nasus* means "nose," and the French term *nasal* means "of the nose."

Nasal Transmucosals

The **intranasal route of administration** is the application of a drug into the nose or nasal passages. Sprays are often used for OTC nasal decongestants. A **spray** is a dosage form that consists of a container with a valve assembly unit that, when activated, emits a fine dispersion of liquid. Examples of nasal sprays include oxymetazoline (Afrin) for nasal congestion, intranasal steroids such as fluticasone and mometasone (Flonase and Nasonex, respectively) for the prevention of allergy symptoms, nitroglycerin for the relief of chest pain, and Imitrex for the treatment of migraine headaches.

Sprays for inhalation through the nose may be prescribed for either their local or their systemic pharmacological effects. Proper dosing administration and frequency are crucial to therapeutic success, especially if patients are self-medicating with OTC medications. Overuse of certain OTC nasal spray and solution decongestants for more than three days can lead to an adverse side effect known as chronic rebound congestion, the worsening of nasal congestion secondary to nasal spray use.

Antihistamine nasal sprays, such as Astelin and Astepro (azelastine), offer relief of allergy symptoms without the disabling drowsiness that accompanies most potent oral antihistamines such as Benadryl (diphenhydramine). However, some nasal medications have systemic side effects, and precautions are advised for patients with certain medical conditions. Pharmacy personnel should recommend that patients carefully read the labeled instructions on OTC antihistamine nasal sprays and, if questions arise, seek out proper counseling from their pharmacist.

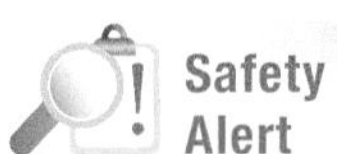

Some suppository ingredients, such as phenylephrine (used to shrink hemorrhoids), must be used with caution in patients with hypertension and other diseases. Refer patients to the pharmacist for OTC product selection.

Rectal, Vaginal, and Urethral Transmucosal Forms

The types of dosage forms suited for these lower body cavities and canals come in suppositories, solutions, creams, foams, and ointments. A **suppository** is a semisolid dosage created from a soft inactive base ingredient (such as cocoa butter or glycerin) that is formulated to melt at body temperature and release an active drug. Suppositories are designed for insertion into body orifices, such as the rectum, vagina, or, less commonly, the urethra. These medications vary in size and shape according to their site of administration and the patient's age and sex. Some suppositories are meant for systemic action while others are for localized treatment. This dosage form is often formulated in a compounding pharmacy if products are not commercially available.

Rectal Transmucosals

The **rectal route of administration** is used to deliver drugs into the **rectum**, or the final section of the intestines ending in the anus. Because of the rich supply of blood and lymphatic vessels in the rectum, suppositories, solutions, ointments, creams, and foams are used for both localized and systemic actions, such as in the treatment of internal hemorrhoids (swollen clumps of veins in the rectum) and ulcerative colitis (sores in the large intestine). Rectal dosage forms, including suppositories and solutions, are used primarily to deliver systemic drugs if:

- an oral drug might be destroyed or diluted by acidic fluids in the stomach
- an oral drug might be too readily metabolized by the liver and eliminated from the body
- a patient is unconscious and needs medication
- a patient may be unable to take oral drugs because of nausea and vomiting or because of severe acute disorders of the GI tract

Other rectal transmucosal medications are designed for more localized action, as in the treatment of external hemorrhoids. Very often, rectal suppositories, solutions, or enemas are used for cleansing the bowels; for laxative or cathartic action that pushes the bowels to empty themselves; for reducing the swelling, pain, or itching of hemorrhoids; or for drug administration in colon diseases.

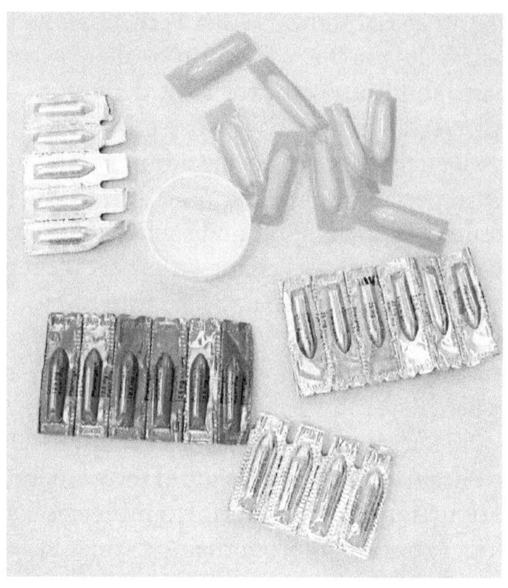

The site of of a suppository administration determines its size and shape.

Because rectal doses do not transverse the digestive system for absorption, these dosage forms can be used in both young children and adults in appropriate dosages. For infants and young children, OTC glycerin suppositories are available for the safe treatment of mild constipation. Acetaminophen suppositories are also administered to young children who have a high fever but who will not or cannot take oral formulations of the medication. For adults, promethazine suppositories are prescribed for severe nausea and vomiting from the flu or side effects of chemotherapy.

Disadvantages of rectal formulations include patient inconvenience and discomfort, premature expulsion of the suppository or solution, and erratic and irregular drug absorption.

Enemas An **enema** is an example of a water-based solution administered rectally for cleansing or evacuating the bowel before a GI procedure, as a treatment for constipation, or for delivering an active drug. An evacuation enema, such as Fleet, is often administered to cleanse the bowels in preparation for a colonoscopy. A retention enema, such as Cortenema, is administered to deliver medication locally or systemically in the case of acute inflammatory bowel disease. Hospital pharmacy technicians will also compound patient-specific enemas of Epsom salts, glycerin, and sterile water.

Vaginal Transmucosals

The **vaginal route of administration** is the application of any drug within the vagina. Common dosage forms include vaginal tablets, suppositories, and creams but may also include emulsion foams, inserts, ointments, rings, solutions, and sponges. Typically, this route of administration is used for its localized therapeutic effects, such as cleansing (douches), contraception, hormone replacement therapy, or treatment of common bacterial or yeast infections.

A variety of OTC vaginal suppositories are available for self-treatment of yeast infections that often occur as a side effect of oral antibiotic treatment. The pharmacist can assist with proper product selection.

Urethral Transmucosals

The **urethral route of administration** is the application of a drug within the urethra, the duct that conveys urine out of the body. Dosage forms include implants, tablets, and suppositories. Drugs delivered by this route may be effective in treating cancer, incontinence, or impotence in men.

Patient Administration of Transmucosal Dosage Forms

Due to their unique design characteristics, transmucosal medications have certain dispensing and administration guidelines.

Sublingual Administration

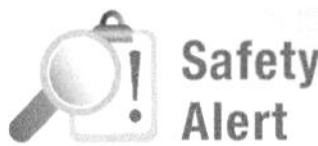

Sublingual nitroglycerin tablets are sensitive to air and light and, consequently, will lose potency over a certain period of time. These tablets should be kept in their original container and replaced every six months.

Sublingual medications are placed directly under the tongue and are not swallowed. Instead, sublingual medications are allowed to dissolve and are rapidly absorbed via the blood vessels under the tongue. Sublingual medications can be beneficial when rapid onset of action is needed or when swallowing is impractical. Nitroglycerin, a common sublingual medication, has specific storage requirements to safeguard the potency of the tablets. Because this medication is relatively unstable, pharmacy technicians must instruct patients to store the nitroglycerin tablets in their original brown bottle to shield the medication from sunlight, which degrades its potency. Technicians should also remind patients to tightly secure the lid of the container to avoid the introduction of air—another factor that lessens the potency of the medication. Physicians usually advise patients to refill their nitroglycerin with a fresh bottle every three to six months.

Buccal Administration

Safety Alert

Technicians need to caution patients that, if nicotine gum is chewed vigorously, too much nicotine can be released, causing unpleasant side effects.

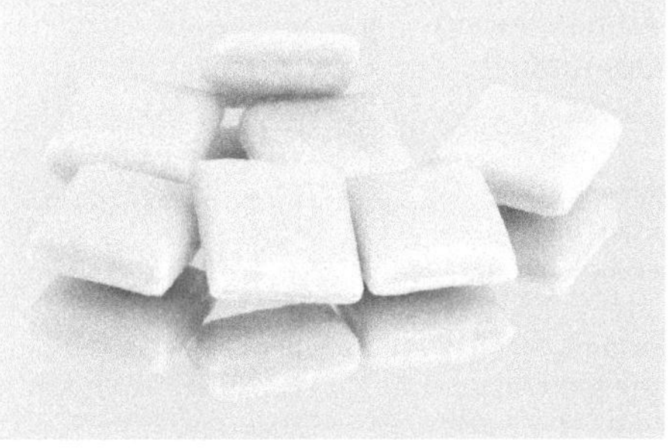

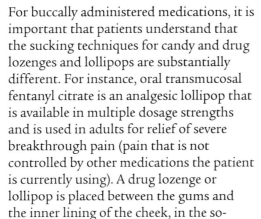

Because OTC nicotine gum looks so much like candy gum, it is especially important for technicians to remind patients that it is a drug, and proper use techniques must be followed to avoid side effects.

For buccally administered medications, it is important that patients understand that the sucking techniques for candy and drug lozenges and lollipops are substantially different. For instance, oral transmucosal fentanyl citrate is an analgesic lollipop that is available in multiple dosage strengths and is used in adults for relief of severe breakthrough pain (pain that is not controlled by other medications the patient is currently using). A drug lozenge or lollipop is placed between the gums and the inner lining of the cheek, in the so-called buccal pouch, and is sucked slowly until it is dissolved in the mouth (over approximately 15 minutes). Drug lozenges are to be used similarly.

There are also differences in technique for chewing regular gum and for chewing nicotine gum. If the nicotine gum is chewed vigorously, too much nicotine will be released, causing unpleasant side effects such as nausea and vomiting. Proper administration allows the gum to release the nicotine slowly, decreasing cravings. Counseling on the proper technique for administration of the nicotine gum is provided in Table 5.4.

Ophthalmic Administration

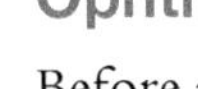

Before administering an ophthamlic preparation, patients should be advised to wash their hands to prevent contamination at the application site or of the medication. Unless otherwise specified, drugs should be at or near room temperature before application. When applying the ophthalmic medication, patients should be careful to not let the tube or the dropper touch the infected site. Any inadvertent contact between the container and the application site could contaminate the medication.

TABLE 5.4 Proper Technique for Administration of Nicotine Gum

1. Chew the gum slowly, and stop chewing when you notice a tingling sensation in the mouth.
2. Park the gum between the cheek and gum, and leave it there until the taste or tingling sensation is almost gone.
3. Resume slowly chewing a few more times until the taste or sensation returns.
4. Park the gum again in a different place in the mouth.
5. Continue this chewing and parking process until the taste or tingle no longer returns when the gum is chewed (usually after 30 minutes).
6. Do not eat or drink for 15 minutes before or while using the gum.

To instill eye drops or apply ophthalmic ointment, the patient's head should be tilted back, and the medication should be administered to the outer surface of the eye or to the lower eyelid conjunctival sac, respectively (see Figure 5.2). Placing a small dab in this lower eyelid lining is usually the easiest route of self-administration for the patient to achieve a higher concentration of drug at the site. Blinking will help distribute the medication to the upper lid area.

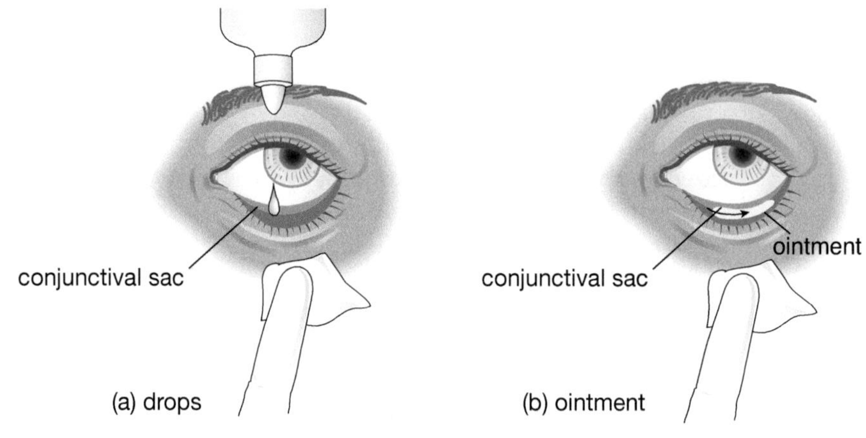

FIGURE 5.2 Administering Ophthalmic Medication

After gently lowering the lower eyelid and instilling the drop (a) or ointment (b), the patient should blink to disperse it. The lids are some of the body's most delicate skin areas and must be handled very carefully.

Once the medication is administered, it is important for the patient to place a finger in the corner of the affected eye next to the nose to gently close the tear duct, thus preventing loss of medication. The patient should also keep the eye closed for one or two minutes after application.

When multiple drops of more than one medication are to be administered, the patient should be advised to wait five minutes between different medications lest the first medication be washed away. If an ointment and a drop are to be used together, the patient should instill the drops first and then wait 10 minutes before applying the ointment. Previously applied medications should be cleaned away as should any drainage from the eye. Cotton balls work well for this purpose.

Ophthalmic ointments are generally applied at night, before sleep, and are the formulation of choice when extended contact with the medication is desired because tears wash them out less easily. The patient should be reminded that they might experience some temporary blurring of vision after application.

All medications should be stored according to the package insert to reduce bacterial growth and to ensure drug stability. Some ophthalmics—such as travoprost (Travatan), trifluridine (Viroptic), azithromycin (AzaSite), and latanoprost (Xalatan)—require refrigeration and should be stored appropriately in the pharmacy before the patient picks up the prescription. During pickup, the pharmacy technician should remind the patient about proper storage at home.

Some OTC and prescription sterile eye medications are dispensed in single unit-of-use packages for one-time use only. This type of packaging does not require a preservative but is typically more costly. After each use, the product is discarded. Restasis (cyclosporine), a medication for the treatment of chronic dry eye syndrome, is an example of a single unit-of-use eye product.

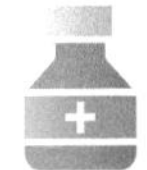

Pharm Fact

Otic products must be stored at room temperature. Heated drops may cause a rupturing of the tympanic membrane (eardrum) whereas cold drops can cause vertigo and discomfort.

Otic Administration

Otic suspensions usually have no or low acohol content while otic solutions have high alcohol content. Certain ear conditions dictate the type of otic medication prescribed. For example, a patient with a ruptured eardrum would be treated with a suspension containing no alcohol—a substance that would create more pain and a burning sensation in the ear. A patient who has suspected eardrum damage would most likely be prescribed a low-alcohol-content otic solution or suspension.

Patients should be instructed in the proper technique for administering otic medications. This technique varies between children and adults (see Figure 5.3). To administer an otic medication to children under the age of three, parents or caregivers should tilt the child's head to the side with the ear facing up, pull the earlobe *down and back*, and place the product in the ear. This technique takes into account the child's inner ear anatomy and allows the medication to reach the desired site. For patients over the age of three, the same procedure should be followed with the exception that the earlobe for this age group should be pulled *up and back* to accommodate the inner ear anatomy.

After administration of the otic medication, the patient's head should remain tilted for two to five minutes. Cotton plugs placed in the ear after administration of ear drops will prevent excess medication from dripping out of the ear. The plugs will not reduce the amount of drug that is absorbed.

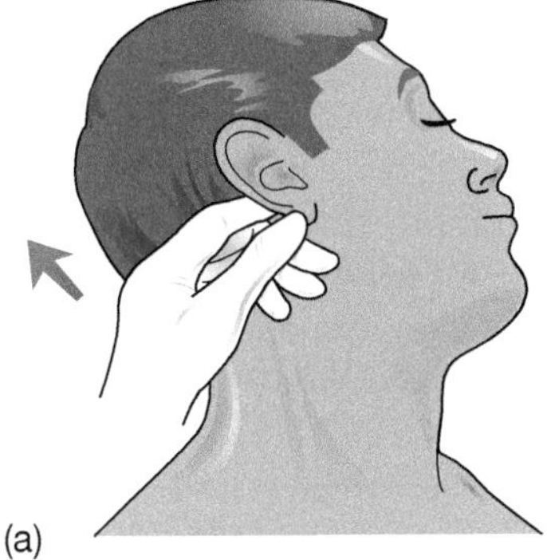

(a)

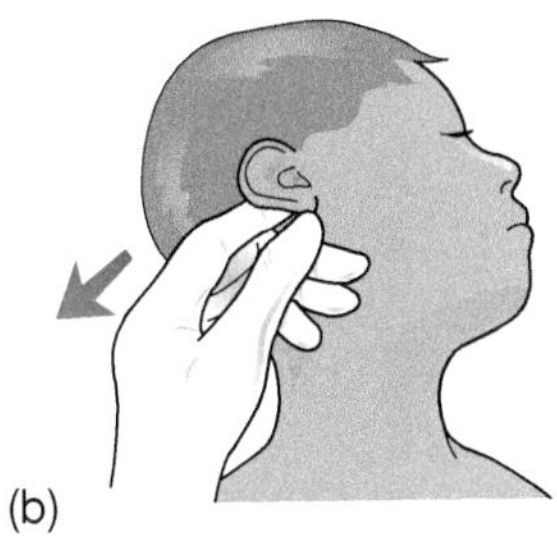

(b)

FIGURE 5.3
Administering Otic Medications

a) Adults and children over the age of three should have their ear pulled up and back when administering the medication.

b) Children under the age of three should have their ear pulled down and back.

Nasal Administration

Nasal medications are applied by **instillation** (drops), sprays, or aerosols. Application may be for relief of nasal congestion or prevention of allergy symptoms. The patient should be instructed to tilt the head back; insert the dropper, spray, or aerosol tip into the nostril; point it toward the eyes; and apply the prescribed number of drops or sprays (repeating the process in the other nostril if indicated). Patients may experience postnasal drip and taste the nasally administered medication. Breathing should be through the mouth to avoid sniffing the medication into the sinuses.

Nasal sprays and solutions are commonly prescribed for administration in both nostrils. Some medications, however, are to be administered in only one nostril daily, alternating nostrils, to reduce irritation. The osteoporosis drug Miacalcin (calcitonin), for example, is administered using this alternating pattern. The dosage for nasal sprays differs as well. For example, in children, the dose of steroid intranasal sprays is one spray. For adults, it is two sprays. Pharmacy technicians need to be aware of this dosage distinction when entering the dosage and patient instructions into the computer. Entering incorrect information could result in a twofold overdose in a pediatric patient.

Eye, Ear, and Nose Irrigating Solutions

An **irrigating solution** may be administrated for cleansing or bathing the eyes (OTC sterile saline or eye washes), nose (such as OTC saline or homemade salt-water solution), and ears (such as OTC acetic acid solution). The eye saline solutions *must be sterile* and kept that way. Eye lubricants or irrigating solutions are not meant for medication absorption (unless they contain some transmucosal agents). They are not considered to be transmucosal drug forms, but they do offer key medicinal benefits to fight infection or other issues. It is important for technicians to know the differences between irrigating solutions and transmucosal medications. The irrigating solutions can be purchased as OTC medical supplies. They are administered in the same ways as already described for medicated solutions for the eyes, ears, and nose.

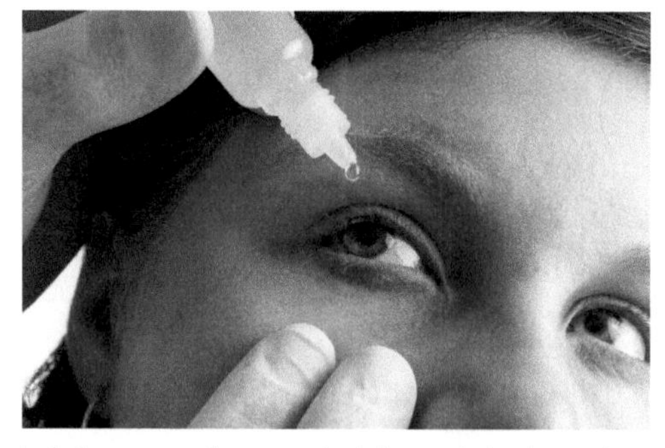

Lubricant eye drops—administered via the ophthalmic route—relieve dry, irritated eyes.

Practice Tip

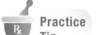

Refrigeration is necessary to store most rectal suppository medications.

Rectal Administration

Instructing patients or caregivers how to administer rectal suppositories should be straightforward. First, wash hands, put on gloves, and then unwrap the suppository. Allow the suppository to reach room temperature for a few minutes and lubricate it with a small amount of petroleum jelly. (Lubrication is especially important for infants and children to ease the pain and difficulty of insertion.) Insert the small, tapered end into the rectum using the index finger and gently press in for the full length of the finger.

Rectal enemas should be used after a bowel movement. The patient should be instructed to lie on their left side with the left knee bent toward the chest. Next, the patient or caregiver should shake the enema container, unwrap it, and gently insert the nozzle of the container into the rectum. The bottle should then be firmly squeezed to release the entire drug into the rectum (unless otherwise directed). After administration of the medication, the patient should continue to lie on the left side, retaining the medicine in the rectum for as long as possible before evacuating the bowels.

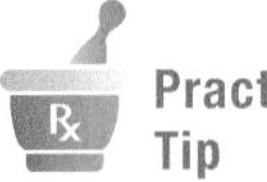

Practice Tip

Pharmacy personnel should remind patients who are using suppositories to remove the packaging prior to insertion.

Vaginal Administration

Patients whose treatment includes a vaginal medication should be instructed to use the medication for the prescribed period to ensure effective treatment. Many vaginal creams are delivered to the site with the use of an applicator tube; the medication is dissolved and absorbed through the vaginal mucosa. Miconazole (Monistat) is an example of an OTC vaginal cream used to treat yeast infections. If the medication is to be applied with an applicator, the application should follow the steps outlined in Table 5.5. Vaginal tablets may be less messy than cream formulations although absorption of the active drug is less predictable.

TABLE 5.5 Proper Technique for Administration of Vaginal Medications

1. Empty the bladder and wash the hands.
2. Open the container and place the dose in the applicator.
3. Lubricate the applicator with a water-soluble lubricant if it is not prelubricated.
4. Lie down, spread the legs, and open the labia with one hand. With the other hand, insert the applicator about two inches into the vagina. (An alternative method is to insert the applicator and medication while standing up, and placing one foot on the edge of a bathtub.)
5. Release the labia; use the free hand to push the applicator plunger, releasing the medication.
6. Withdraw the applicator and wash the hands. Wash the applicator and dry it if it will be reused.

5.5 Topical Routes of Administration

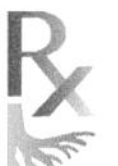

Put Down Roots

Topical comes from the Greek word *topos,* meaning a specific "place."

The **topical route of administration** typically refers to applying a drug directly to a specific area on the skin surface. There are two routes of topical administration: dermal and transdermal. **Dermal routes of administration** refer to those topical applications that provide a localized effect on the skin layers. The **transdermal routes of administration** refer to drugs applied to a specific place on the skin and absorbed through both the dermal and muscle layers into the bloodstream (a little like transmucosals). Generally, topical drug forms refer to the dermal forms even though transdermal forms are also applied topically on the skin. In the community pharmacy, you will see many topical prescriptions available and sold as OTC medications. The dermal medications tend to be sold over the counter for localized therapeutic effects while the transdermal medications tend to be prescribed for more systemic purposes.

Transdermal medications also have slower action than dermal medications, because of the longer time to reach the bloodstream. Transdermals, though, usually have longer-lasting effects.

Topical medications of both dermal and transdermal administration routes include creams, ointments, lotions, and gels, which vary in **viscosity**. Other topical medications include sprays and aerosols, such as OTC local anesthetics to treat sunburn, antiseptics to clean wounds, and antifungals (such as clotrimazole) to treat athlete's foot. Caution is advised if certain topical medications are administered to broken skin. There are also medicated skin patches (square-shaped) and disks (round).

Patients may be familiar with common types of topical forms because they often purchase OTC ointments, pastes, plasters, gels, jellies, and lotions. Technicians need to be aware of the differences in properties, function, appearances, and consistencies of the different topical forms, via both prescription and over the counter, due to their differing base ingredients and routes of administration.

Put Down Roots

The term *dermal* comes from the Ancient Greek *dérma*, meaning "skin" or "hide." The prefix *trans* comes from the Latin word that means "across," "beyond," "through."

Dermal Dosage Forms

The major advantage of topical dermal formulations is that they have a fast onset of action with relatively few wide-ranging systemic side effects due to their localized therapeutic application and action. For example, most mild cases of poison ivy may be treated locally by applying an OTC topical formulation, such as hydrocortisone cream. However, if the equivalent dose of prednisone tablets were administered to treat this skin rash, the risk of GI side effects would be greater, especially if used on a long-term basis.

Numerous dermal medications can be found in many drug categories, including anesthetics, analgesics, anti-inflammatories, antibiotics, antifungals, antiseptics, astringents, moisturizers, pediculicides (for killing lice), protectants (for sun protection), and scabicides (for killing mites).

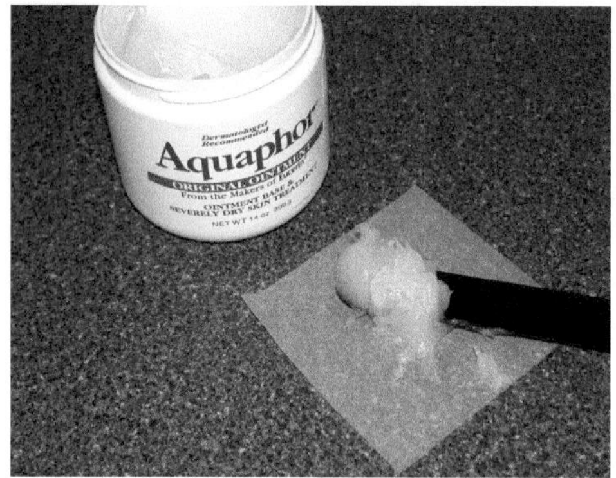

An ointment is referred to as a water-in-oil (W/O) preparation, and is often yellow or opaque in appearance. An ointment is easily applied but typically makes the skin feel oily or greasy.

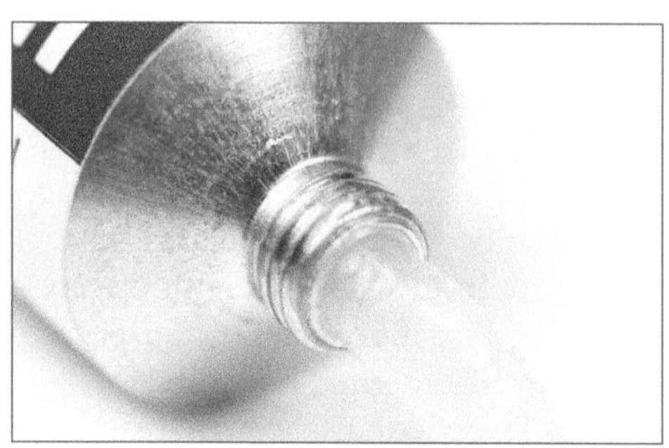
Ointments are often dispensed in tubes because of their greasy consistency, which works well for specific purposes.

Ointments

An **ointment** is a dosage form that is a water-in-oil emulsion. A **water-in-oil (W/O) emulsion** is a formulation that contains a small amount of water dispersed in oil. Many cortisone-like medications and topical antibiotics are available in both an ointment and a cream formulation. Ointments may be more therapeutically effective due to their skin adherence, but they are not as cosmetically acceptable as creams.

Ointments may be nonmedicated or medicated, prescription or OTC. They often contain various kinds of bases:

- bases made from hydrocarbons, such as mineral oil or petroleum jelly (as used in liniments for rubbing on the skin for pain relief—like Bengay)
- water-in-oil emulsions, such as lanolin or cold cream
- water-soluble or greaseless base ointments, such as polyethylene glycol ointment (used in the topical antibiotic mupirocin)

Ointments are especially good for extremely dry areas of the skin where moisture needs to be retained as well as for areas prone to friction from clothing or other body parts. Because they generally have a longer contact time with the skin, ointments have a longer duration of action than creams, lotions, and gels. However, the disadvantages of ointments include a longer time to absorption and often a greasy residue on the skin.

Pastes

A **paste** is a water-in-oil (W/O) emulsion containing more solid material than an ointment, creating a denser consistency. This consistency makes the application of a paste thicker than that of an ointment. Examples include zinc oxide paste, which is used as an astringent and a sunscreen, and triamcinolone acetonide paste, which is an anti-inflammatory dental preparation.

Plasters

A **plaster** is a solid or semisolid medicated substance that adheres to the body and contains a backing material, such as paper, cotton, linen, silk, moleskin, or plastic. Plasters can be either medicated or nonmedicated preparations. An example is the OTC salicylic acid plaster used to remove corns. A corn is a painful thickening of the skin that typically occurs in areas of excessive pressure, such as the toes.

Creams, Lotions, and Gels

Creams, lotions, and gels apply more smoothly to the skin and leave a very thin film. They are also more readily absorbed and are more cosmetically acceptable for most patients. Topical vaginal medications are often prescribed because they treat a local infection and are less likely to be absorbed systemically and cause side effects.

Creams Pharmaceutical **creams** are emulsions of oil and water. Some are water-in-oil (W/O) emulsions because they contain a small amount of water dispersed in an oil base, which are moisturizing. Others are **oil-in-water emulsions (O/W)**, which are less greasy. Most creams are considered "vanishing," which means they are invisible once applied and rubbed into the skin. This quality makes creams cosmetically acceptable to most patients.

A variety of OTC creams are available for the self-treatment of vaginal yeast infections that often occur as a side effect of oral antibiotic treatment. The major disadvantage of vaginally administered medications is the messiness of the creams.

Like topical vaginal medications, topical hormone creams provide localized treatment and are less likely to cause systemic side effects. This dosage form also has seen increased use in light of recent studies that have shown a connection between long-term use of oral hormone medications and hormonal cancers. Compounding pharmacies can prepare individualized bioidentical hormone cream formulations based on saliva and blood tests; bioidentical hormones in a topical cream formulation provide individualized dosing, thus minimizing systemic absorption and the risk of side effects.

Lotions A lotion is another O/W emulsion for topical application. Containing insoluble dispersed solids or immiscible liquids, lotions are easily absorbed and can cover large areas of the skin. This topical treatment is especially effective for hairy areas of the body, such as the scalp. Examples of lotions include calamine lotion, used for relief of itching, and benzoyl peroxide lotion, used to control acne.

Gels Much like a suspension, a gel contains solid particles in a liquid, but the particles are fine or ultrafine. Topically, gels apply evenly and leave a dry coat of the medication in contact with the area. One example of a gel is the prescription drug diclofenac (Voltaren), a topical medication used to treat arthritis. This anti-inflammatory drug can provide relief to an aching knee without the risk of GI effects associated with the oral formulation. Another marketed gel is the anti-infective Metrogel, which is available in two different strengths: for vaginal use (0.75%) and for adult acne or rosacea (1%). Wart removal gels are also popular as OTC medications. Ultrafine gel dispersion dosage forms include jellies and glycerogelatins:

- A **jelly** is a gel that contains a higher proportion of water in combination with a drug substance and a thickening agent. Jellies are present in many antiseptic, antifungal, contraceptive, and lubricant medications. Lubricants are commonly used in pelvic and rectal examinations of body orifices. Lubricants are also used as an aid in sexual intercourse in postmenopausal women who experience vaginal dryness from an age-related hormone deficiency. Because of their high water content, jellies are subject to contamination and usually contain preservatives.

- A **glycerogelatin** is a topical gel preparation made with gelatin, glycerin, water, and medicinal substances. The hard substance is melted and brushed onto the skin where it hardens again and is generally covered with a bandage. An example is zinc gelatin (Unna boot), used as a pressure bandage to treat varicose ulcers.

Colloids and Collodions

As mentioned earlier in this chapter, a colloid is a mixture with physical properties that fall between those of a solution and a fine suspension. A colloidal dispersion is a mixture in which ultrafine particles of one substance are evenly distributed throughout another substance. Aveeno Bath Treatments are made with natural colloidal oatmeal milled into an ultrafine powder. When dispersed in water, this powder forms a soothing milky bath. It moisturizes and relieves dry, itchy, irritated skin caused by rashes, eczema, poison ivy, oak, sumac, and insect bites.

Collodions are syrupy solutions in which a thick liquid medication is dissolved into a mixture of alcohol and ether. After application, the alcohol and ether solvent vaporizes, leaving a medicated film coating on the skin. The OTC product Compound W One-Step Wart Remover consists of acetic acid and salicylic acid in an acetone collodion base and is used to remove corns or warts.

Solutions for Antiseptic Washing and Irrigation

An irrigating solution, known as a *douche*, is introduced into the vaginal cavity for local cleansing. Douche medications are often reconstituted from a powder and flushed with a dispenser into the vagina. Irrigating solutions are also used in the hospital postoperative setting to bathe the abdominal cavity after surgery. Irrigating powders, such as polymyxin B sulfate (Neosporin) and bacitracin zinc, are used topically to prevent bacterial infections. Domeboro effervescent tablets are an OTC product that contains aluminum acetate and is used topically on the skin as a soak or compress for minor "weeping" skin irritations, such as those caused by poison ivy.

Patient Administration of Dermal Dosage Forms

Depending on the dosage form, certain topical medications have specific application and handling guidelines that pharmacy personnel must relay to patients.

Ointment Administration

Pharmacy personnel should be aware that topical corticosteroid products are not all the same. For example, the topical corticosteroid betamethasone is commercially available as a valerate and dipropionate salt and in a regular and "augmented" ointment (and cream) formulation. The potency of each of these products differs. The pharmacy technician must be careful to select the correct product during preparation and filling of the prescription. The overuse or inappropriate use of potent topical corticosteroids, such as the augmented formulations, can lead to serious local and systemic side effects.

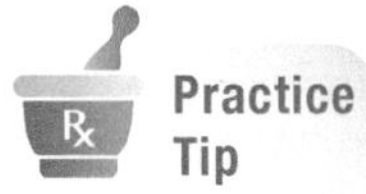

Practice Tip

Remind patients that they need to wear gloves when applying any topical medication that has any toxicity or systematic effects to avoid skin damage or overdosing, respectively.

Cream, Lotion, and Gel Administration

Like ointments, certain cream, lotion, and gel formulations also have specific precautions that patients should follow during application. Menthol or camphor creams, lotions, or gels can be rubbed on aching areas for some cooling relief. Products such as

Vicks VapoRub and generic counterparts have also been found, when rubbed on the chest, to help cold sufferers have some breathing and coughing relief. Gloves need to be worn when applying any topical medication of any toxicity, such as those for wart or corn removal.

Transdermal Dosage Forms

Pharmacy technicians must keep in mind, however, that transdermal topical products have the disadvantage of being absorbed systemically, resulting in potential systemic side effects. For example, OTC hydrocortisone and similar cortisone-like products—if used over large areas of the body for extended periods of time—can cause systemic side effects. Topical dosage forms can also cause a hypersensitivity reaction in some patients. As with toxic dermal applications, topical transdermal applications also require gloves. For instance, one can experience side effects or accidentally overdose with a nitroglycerin ointment if one doesn't wear protection when applying it.

Transdermal Patches and Disks

The transdermal patch (square) or disk (round) consists of an adhesive fabric backing holding a drug reservoir with a rate-controlling membrane. Once the protective strip for the adhesive is removed, the fabric is attached. The chemicals in the patch or disk force the drug across the membranes of the skin and into the deepest layer of skin and fat where optimal absorption into the bloodstream will occur. Transdermal skin adhesives provide a slow-release, steady level of drug in the system. In some patches/disks, the membrane controls the rate of drug delivery, but, in others, the skin itself controls the rate. This mechanism of action is similar to controlled-release tablets or capsules but produces fewer side effects as less drug is released. Although the skin presents a barrier, absorption does occur slowly and is affected by patient-specific factors such as skin thickness and blood flow, both of which vary with age.

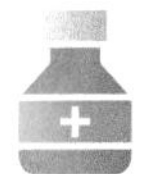

Pharm Fact

Investigational helminthic therapies, which involve small doses of parasitic worms to help direct the immune system, are administered through transdermal patches.

Therapeutic effects may last from 24 hours to one week. Common transdermal patches for systemic effects include the following:

- nicotine for cessation of smoking
- nitroglycerin for relieving chest pain
- narcotic analgesics for relieving chronic pain
- clonidine for lowering blood pressure
- scopolamine for prevention of motion sickness
- estrogen/progestin for birth control
- estrogen and testosterone for female and male hormone replacement, respectively

For instance, an estradiol transdermal patch (Vivelle-Dot) is administered twice a week and is indicated for the topical treatment of postmenopausal symptoms with less risk of systemic side effects than an oral tablet formulation such as Premarin.

There are some localized treatments as well. For example, the nonsteroidal anti-inflammatory drug diclofenac (similar to ibuprofen) is available as a transdermal patch. This patch can deliver the medication directly to an injury site (strain, sprain, or contusion) for short-term treatment without the risk of the severe adverse GI effects of its oral counterpart.

Transdermal Gels, Emulsion Lotions, and Sprays

Some transdermal medications are also administered through topical gels, emulsion lotions, and sprays. These medications operate in some similar ways to their topical counterparts, but they are more powerful and require more care and caution in their use because they work through the skin down into the blood (see Figure 5.4). They have less of a time-release mechanism than patches and disks, and they can be washed off. The response time is more immediate but less long-lasting. There could also be more danger for long-term use because of the continual application to the localized skin cells. Patients are often advised to rotate places on the skin for the adhesion of the transdermal medications. (Scientific studies are ongoing to measure effects of different administrations.)

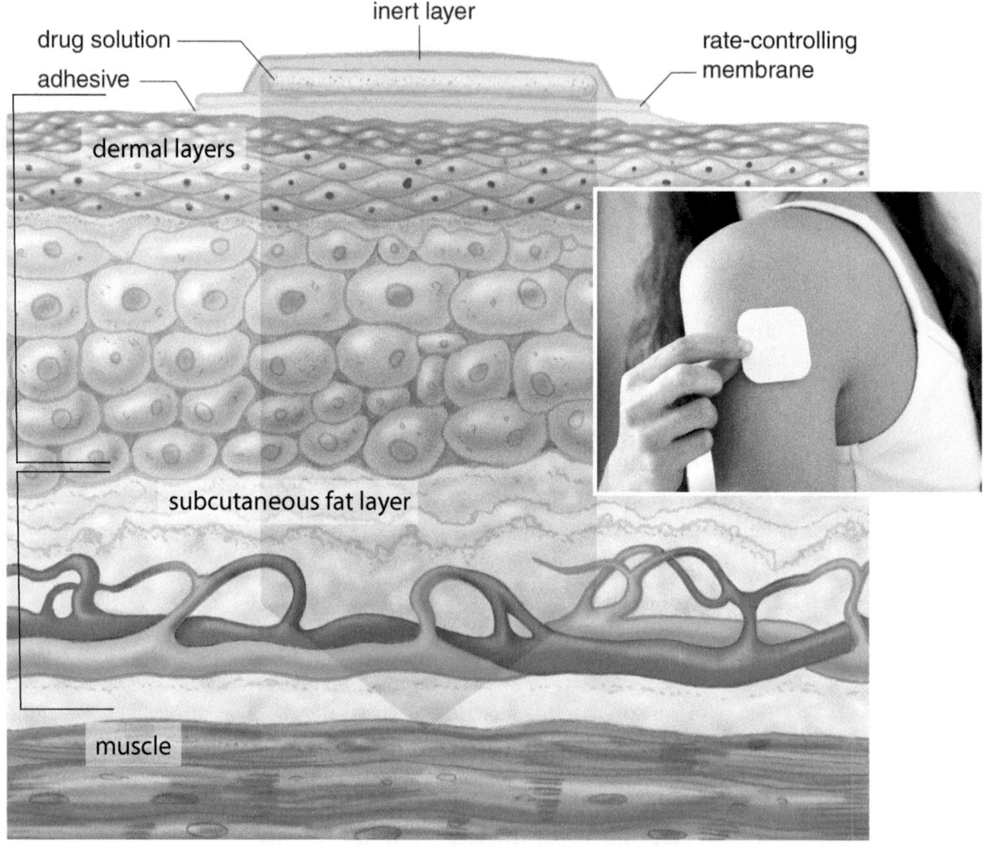

FIGURE 5.4 **Transdermal Patch**

Transdermal patches (squares) and disks (round) have become popular among patients who find it difficult to remember to take an oral medication every day. The convenience enhances their ability to adhere to therapy. The drug is absorbed through the layers of skin and muscle into the blood vessels.

AndroGel, a product used to treat adult males with low testosterone, is available as individual gel packets as well as a pump. The pump must be carefully primed three times prior to initial use. Each pump thereafter delivers a specified amount of medication. The gel is applied by hand to shoulders, upper arms, or stomach area. Once applied, the patient should not shower or swim for five hours.

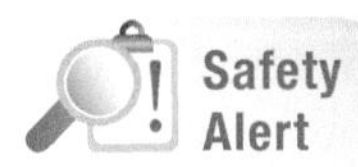

Transdermal patches administered to infants and young children may result in toxicity and are generally not recommended.

Certain products, such as nitroglycerin ointment, require the patient or caregiver to wear gloves during application to avoid absorbing excessive amounts of the drug, which could cause headaches. A risk of increased absorption is also an issue in the application of topical potent corticosteroid ointments. Many of these ointments should be applied sparingly to affected areas of the body for short periods and—unless directed by a physician—should not be covered with bandages or other occlusive dressings (including diapers). Doing so can increase the absorption of the medication and the risk of side effects. Increased absorption of the product can also occur when select topical corticosteroids are applied to the face, underarms, or groin area. Pharmacy personnel should instruct patients to read medication instructions carefully when applying these topical medications.

An OTC transdermal cream containing capsaicin (active ingredient in hot chili peppers) must also be applied with gloves because severe irritation can occur if the cream is inadvertently rubbed into the eyes. Capsaicin is available in both regular-potency and high-potency formulas and is used for treating arthritis symptoms. OTC hydrocortisone creams and lotions should be applied sparingly and for short periods.

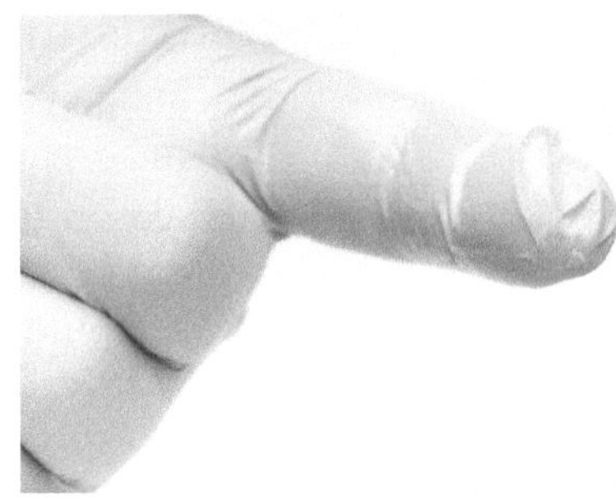
OTC capsaicin (consisting of ground up chili peppers) is used to treat patients with arthritis and must be applied with gloves.

Transdermal prescriptions for pets are often in the form of gels or lotions. If not commercially available, many transdermal cream and lotion formulations, such as hormonal creams, are commonly prepared in a compounding pharmacy (see Chapter 10).

Patient Administration of Transdermal Dosage Forms

Because transdermal medications will work through any skin, patients must be advised to be very careful when applying the patches, disks, gels, sprays, and lotions, as the skin on one's fingers can be affected. Patients who have skin cancer or allergic skin reactions should avoid such products. Sun exposure should also be avoided when using transdermal products. Women of childbearing potential who are pregnant, trying to get pregnant, or could accidentally become pregnant should also avoid certain transdermal products, as they can be harmful to the development of the growing child.

Patch and Disk Administration

Safety Alert

Patients should be advised to carefully discard their used patches. The nicotine or narcotic patches, for example, can cause serious side effects or death when used or ingested by children or pets.

The site of administration for transdermal patches and disks should be relatively hair-free (usually the upper arm). These skin adhesives should not be placed over an area of scar tissue or damaged skin, which may increase or decrease the release of the drug. Some skin adhesives are replaced every day, but others maintain their therapeutic effect for 3 to 7 days and are replaced appropriately. The site of application should be rotated to minimize localized skin reactions.

One type of transdermal patch—a Lidoderm (lidocaine) and nitroglycerin patch—provides 24 hours of relief from a 12-hour application. Most physicians advise their patients to remove the nitroglycerin and lidocaine patch at bedtime to prevent the development of drug tolerance. Drug tolerance occurs when the body requires higher drug doses to produce the same therapeutic effect (explained more in Chapter 14).

Patches and disks are often applied to the upper arms or wrists, but they may be applied in other areas, depending on the prescriptive directions. For instance, estradiol hormonal patches for menopausal symptom relief may be applied below the belly button on the hip or buttock region.

Another transdermal patch delivers fentanyl, a potent Schedule II opiate analgesic. This drug is slowly absorbed through the skin into the bloodstream and can relieve chronic pain for up to three days with a single patch application. Sun exposure should be avoided, and heating pads, electric blankets, heat lamps, saunas, hot tubs, or heated water beds cannot be used with this drug. Localized heat speeds up the movement of fentanyl from the patch into the body. If the patch is damaged, then increased absorption of the active drug can occur. Both situations create a higher risk for a serious drug overdose.

Transdermal Gel, Lotion, and Spray Administration

Transdermal gels and lotions come in various containers, including traditional tubs and tubes. They also come in measured pump dosage dispensers. Lotions are packaged in single-dose pouches too, while sprays often come in propellant (pressurized gas) canisters. To begin the process and prime the pump or spray, the pump or nozzle should be directed toward the garbage can, pressed down once, and covered to be kept from children and pets. Patients should wash and dry the application area, pump or spray one dose, and spread it around. The pouch can also be torn open, and the contents squeezed onto the skin. Common application areas include the upper arms, wrists, inner thighs (for female hormonal medications), and specific areas of pain. The medication should be spread very thinly over the area.

If patients do not have protective gloves for application, Saran Wrap (do not substitute another plastic wrap as this one is the only one with a full plastic barrier) on the hands can be used. In all cases, patients should thoroughly wash their hands with soap and water after each application. The application area should be allowed to dry before putting on clothes. Afterwards, patients should avoid showers, baths, hot tubs, and saunas for a number of hours to allow the medication to work—the package insert will give the precise instructions, and technicians need to remind patients to read them carefully.

5.6 Inhalation Route of Administration

The **inhalation route of administration**, also known as the **intrarespiratory route of administration**, is defined as the application of a drug through inhalation, or breathing, into the lungs, typically through the mouth or the nose. Because the lung tissues are designed for the transmission of oxygen from the air into the bloodstream, the lungs serve as an excellent site for the absorption of medications. The drugs are also absorbed through the mucosal layers of the mouth and/or nose and into the blood capillaries. The inhalation route is primarily used to deliver bronchodilators and anti-inflammatory agents to asthma or allergy sufferers or for those with chronic lung diseases. This route can be used to treat systemic conditions (there is even an inhalable insulin!) or to relieve localized breathing conditions.

Inhalation Dosage Forms

Inhalation dosage forms are primarily aerosols and sprays intended to be inhaled by simple unaided breathing. However, sterile solutions, volatile medications, and micronized powders require special inhalation devices to be properly delivered.

Aerosols and Metered-Dose Inhalers

An **aerosol** is a pressurized container that dispels a mist or spray. A **metered-dose inhaler (MDI)** is a handheld, aerosol-driven device that dispels a single "puff" dose of a drug into the patient's mouth to be breathed in. MDIs are commonly used by patients who have been diagnosed with asthma, severe allergies, or chronic lung disease. An MDI can come preloaded with the prescription drug or have drug cartridges loaded into it. Each drug is premixed with the aerosol propellant gas, which is usually hydrofluoroalkane, or HFA.

Ventolin HFA, Proventil HFA, and ProAir HFA are all aerosol solutions of the drug albuterol that MDIs deliver to relieve shortness of breath in acute asthma.

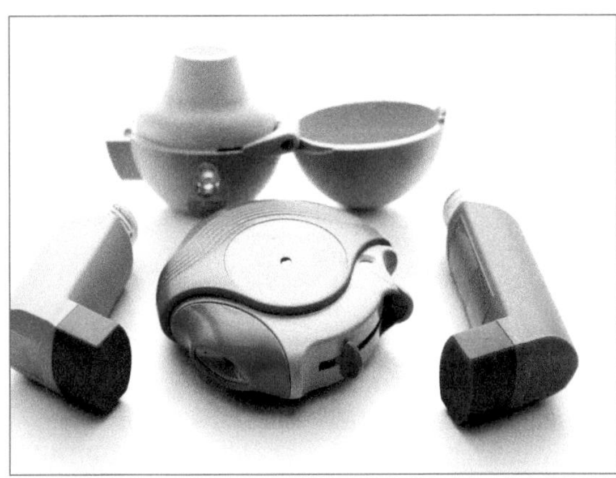

Several types of inhalers are used in delivering both aerosol (MDIs) and powdered medications (discus and bulb shaped).

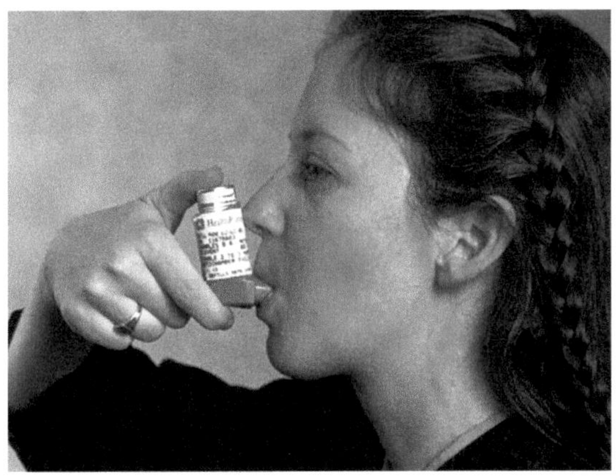

A metered-dose inhaler (MDI) is a common device used to administer a drug through inhalation into the lungs.

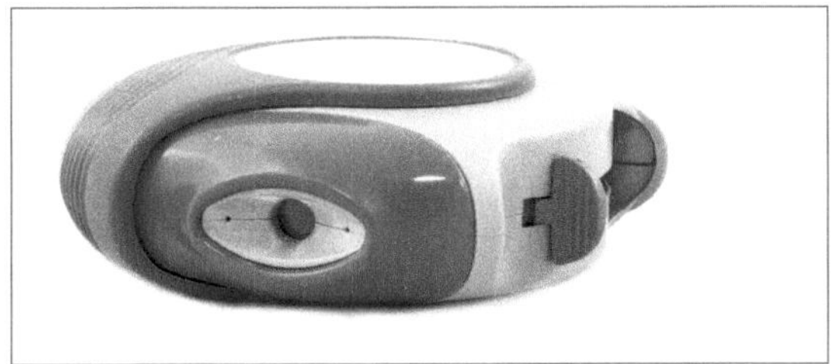

One type of dry powder inhaler looks like a small handheld discus and is activated by breathing deeply at the opening.

Budesonide/formoterol (Symbicort HFA) and fluticasone/salmeterol (Advair HFA) contain two active drugs in an aerosol form to reduce incidents of asthmatic attacks. Depending on the formulation of the product and on the design of the valve, an aerosol may commonly emit a fine mist or a coarse liquid spray.

Micronized Powders and Nonaerosolized Inhalers

Some manufacturers use a nonaerosolized, breath-activated powder for inhalation to avoid propellants. This newer dosage form uses a non-gas mechanism to administer a higher concentration of the drug into the lungs as a micronized powder. The result may be a controlled release of active ingredients for the prevention of recurring symptoms, with potentially fewer side effects. Some of the dry powder, breath-activated inhalers come in interesting shapes and names: Accuhaler, Turbohaler, Diskhaler. Advair Diskus and Spiriva HandiHaler are examples of inhalants used for the prevention and long-term treatment of asthma or chronic lung disease symptoms. Patient counseling by the pharmacist is critical for proper use of these nonaerosolized inhalers.

Patients need to breathe deeply and strongly to pull the powder into their mouth and lungs. The prescription powder comes in small capsules or foil packets that are opened by the dry powder inhaler as the patient presses the dosage lever.

Inhalation Solutions and Nebulizers

Inhalation drugs are also delivered via a **nebulizer**, which transforms sterile liquid drug solutions into a mist to be breathed through a mouthpiece or a face mask. The nebulizer blasts compressed air or oxygen through a dose of prescribed solution to break the liquid into misted particles. The prescription medications come premixed or must be mixed with sterile saline water and filled into the medicine cup of the nebulizer. An example of a nebulizing solution is the "rescue" medication albuterol, which is available in different concentrations. Albuterol is often prescribed for the relief of bronchial spasms and wheezing in infants and children.

Nebulizing machines come in the electric tabletop or portable battery-powered models, which can use disposable or rechargeable batteries. Some nebulizers can be plugged into car batteries. Some models are as small as a deck of cards so that they can be carried easily anywhere. The different models and their features affect the price of the device. The tubing, masks, and spacers are medical supplies often purchased in the community pharmacy.

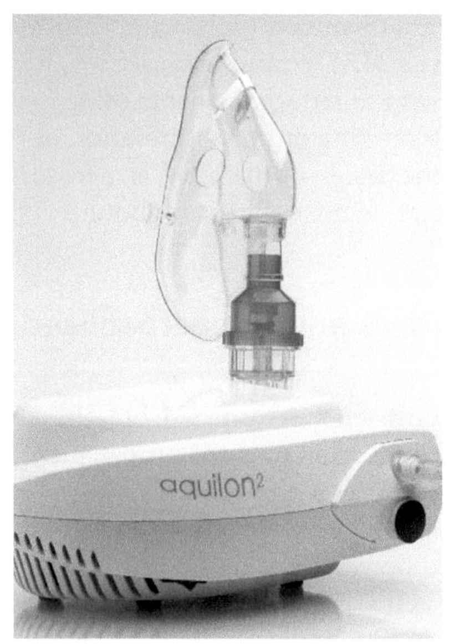

A jet nebulizer, once called an atomizing machine, is effective for vaporizing a drug and delivering it through tubing to a mask for breathing.

The advantage of a nebulizer is that, for patients who need more than one inhalation drug, multiple medications can be mixed in the nebulizer to be administered at the same time. Also, there is no need to hold onto something at one's mouth while trying to breathe deeply and administer the correct dose. For those who don't have great power of inhalation, it works better than breath-activated, dry inhalers.

Volatile Medications and Vaporizers

Vaporizers and humidifiers are other mechanical devices commonly used to deliver moisture to the air for relief of cold symptoms. Volatile medications, such as Vicks VapoSteam, can be used with some vaporizers to help relieve problems with breathing.

Patient Administration of Inhalation Forms

Patients must be instructed in the proper administration of aerosolized medications to control or relieve their respiratory symptoms. Following the correct inhalation technique ensures that the medication reaches the lungs. Spacer devices are often recommended for use in pediatric and older adult patients who use MDIs.

With a **spacer device**, the medication is released into a "storage chamber" where it can be more easily inhaled by the patient. Use of this device allows the patient to inhale a higher concentration of medication, thus providing better relief of symptoms. Spacer devices may be packaged with the medication or dispensed separately and are available in small, medium, and large sizes for infants, children, and adults.

Breathing deeply and slowly and not exhaling too quickly are key requirements for all inhalation drugs. Also, keeping all parts of the inhalers and nebulizers clean and sanitized is important. Washing hands before use is essential.

Metered-Dose Inhaler Administration

Hand-eye coordination and timing of inhalation are critical for optimum drug delivery with an MDI that requires a pump for administration. Table 5.6 lists steps patients should follow when administering MDIs. After MDI administration of a cortisone-like drug, a patient should rinse the mouth thoroughly to prevent an oral fungal infection. The mouthpiece of the MDI device itself should also be washed with soap and water at least once weekly.

TABLE 5.6 Proper Technique for Administration of an MDI

1. Shake the canister well (otherwise, only the propellant may be administered).
2. Prime the canister by pressing down and activating a practice dose. (Check priming instructions for each product as they vary, depending on the manufacturer and active ingredient.)
3. Prepare the MDI by inserting the canister into a mouthpiece or spacer to reduce the amount of drug deposited on the back of the throat. (This is especially helpful for young children or older adults who may have difficulty with hand-eye coordination.)
4. Breathe out and hold the spacer between the lips, making a seal.
5. Activate the MDI and take a deep, slow inhalation at the same time.
6. Hold the breath briefly, and slowly exhale through the nose or pursed lips.

Patients who are taking more than one drug via MDI should administer the more immediate-acting drug first followed by the second drug 5 to 10 minutes later. The pharmacist can review the drugs prescribed and assist the patient in suggesting a prioritized order of drug administration.

A spacer device improves the delivery of inhaled medications, especially in children and older adults.

Nebulizer Administration

Before using the nebulizer, the medicine cup must be filled with the properly measured dosage of the prescribed medicine. If more than one inhalation drug is needed, there is a possibility that they can be mixed but only if the pharmacist says so. Also, some medications come in concentrated forms and must be diluted with a sterile saline solution when added to the medicine cup of the nebulizer. These things must be explained to the patient.

The nebulizer and its parts must be fully cleaned after each use and disinfected at least three times a week. Patients can soak it in diluted white vinegar or a suitable nebulizer disinfectant.

5.7 Parenteral Routes of Administration

A **parenteral route of administration** is one that uses injection to reach its destination in the bloodstream, muscle, skin, or intestine. A sterile, or microbial-free, solution (with or without medication) is administered by means of a hollow needle or catheter inserted through one or more layers of the skin.

Parenteral Dosage Forms

Parenteral dosage forms are commonly administered through four paths:

- subcutaneous (subq), under the skin
- intramuscular (IM), into a muscle
- intravenous (IV), into a vein
- intradermal (ID), into the skin

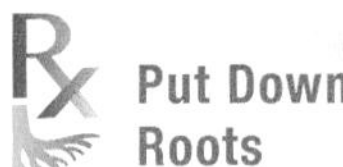

Put Down Roots

The term *parenteral* comes from the Greek roots *para*, meaning "beside," and *enteron*, meaning "intestine." Parenteral administration bypasses—or goes "beside" rather than through—the digestive tract.

Parenteral solutions—prepared for injections, especially intravenous (IV) bolus and infusions—have an *immediate* systemic effect, since they bypass the stomach and are rapidly absorbed and distributed into the bloodstream. The parenteral route is often used for medications whose molecules are too unstable or large to be absorbed or for medications that are broken down so quickly in the stomach or liver that they cannot be taken orally.

Because the body is primarily an aqueous, (water-containing) vehicle, the ingredients of most parenteral preparations are dissolved or reconstituted in sterile solutions, such as dextrose in water or normal saline. Even immunizations and insulin medications are premixed in solutions. Some parenteral medications are available in single-use vials or ampules that contain no preservative; others may be available in a multi-dose vial of lyophilized powder with preservatives. Preparation and administration of parenteral solutions deserve special attention because of the complexity, widespread use, and potential for both therapeutic benefit and danger. All parenteral injections—whether administered via subq, IM, IV, or ID routes—must be sterile because they introduce medication directly into the body. (This is covered more in Chapter 13.)

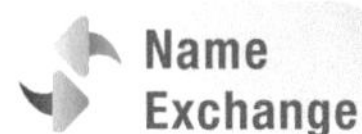

Subcutaneous injections are abbreviated as SUBCUT, Subcut, SUBC, SUBQ, SC, SQ. SC and SQ are discouraged because they get mixed up with SL.

Subcutaneous Route

The **subcutaneous (subq) route of administration** injects medication into the fat layer, or subcutaneous tissue, just under the skin. Common subq medications include the following:

- insulin (to treat diabetes)
- heparin and enoxaparin (to prevent blood clots)
- sumatriptan (to treat migraines)
- certain immunizations (such as measles, mumps, rubella, and others)
- epinephrine/adrenaline (to treat emergency asthma attacks or allergic reactions)

Intramuscular Route

The **intramuscular (IM) route of administration** involves injecting the drug directly into the muscle. The IM route offers a quick, convenient way to deliver injectable medications for longer-lasting effects than some other parenteral methods. The route is used to administer several immunizations, including the influenza (flu) immunization, that are offered in many community pharmacies. IM injections are also commonly used for antibiotics, narcotics, medications for migraine headaches, male and female hormones, antipsychotic medications, vitamins, and minerals. For example, vitamin B12 and testosterone medications are commercially available as a single-dose vial and a multiple-dose vial in the community pharmacy.

Testosterone injections are available as a cypionate salt (suspended in cottonseed oil) or as an enanthate salt (suspended in sesame oil). Though not interchangeable without prescriber permission, both of these salts deliver a similar amount of medication over a 10- to 14-day period.

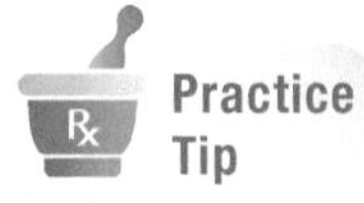

Insulin is never administered intramuscularly.

The IM route is also used to deliver lifesaving medications, such as epinephrine, in an emergency. An EpiPen, a single-dose autoinjector device, delivers intramuscularly as well as subcutaneously, and it comes in different doses for adults and children. The medication device is required to be dispensed in a two-pack. It can be used for repeated injections—one can be on hand at home and the other at school. Several states allow school personnel to legally administer epinephrine in emergency situations, such as a hypersensitivity to insect stings or a severe allergic reaction to peanut butter.

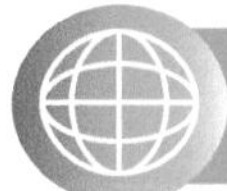

IN THE REAL WORLD

Almost all insulins and insulin-like products for diabetes are administered by the subcutaneous route. Insulins vary in their onset and duration of action. Most of these medications work within 30 to 60 minutes, and some of these products may lower blood glucose levels for up to 24 hours. Insulins are also available as mixtures of rapid-acting and long-acting products, typically in a 75/25, 70/30, or 50/50 concentration. In the hospital or in the emergency room, regular or fast-acting insulin can also be administered via the IV route.

Although the response time to a medication is slower than with the IV route, the duration of action for an IM injection is much longer, making it more practical for use outside the hospital setting. In fact, some IM injections may exert a therapeutic effect for a period ranging from two weeks to three months. Still, a drawback of the IM route is its unpredictable absorption rate. For this reason, the IM route is not recommended for use on patients who are unconscious or in a shock-like state.

In an emergency situation, such as after a bee sting, an EpiPen can be administered into the muscle through clothing.

In addition to the flu immunization, the most common IM immunizations are those for tetanus, diphtheria (Td) or tetanus, diphtheria, pertussis (Tdap), meningitis, pneumonia, hepatitis A and B, and human papillomavirus. Certain drugs must be given via the IM route because they are known to irritate veins and cause phlebitis if given by the IV route. Many narcotic pain medications are administered by IM injection in the hospital and nursing home.

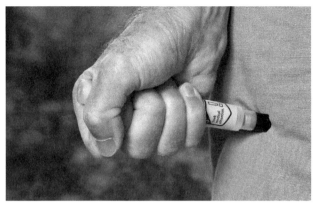

Intravenous Route

One of the more common parenteral routes of drug and fluid administration in hospitals and skilled nursing facilities is the **IV route of administration**, which means to inject directly into a vein. This allows immediate bodily access to large amounts of medicated or nutritional fluids that can be dispensed either quickly or over a longer time period. Critical care medications, antibiotics, chemotherapy, and nutrition are commonly administered in this fashion. IV medications act rapidly to control and treat symptoms and can be administered via any vein in the body.

These medications are administered using two different methods: IV bolus and IV infusion.

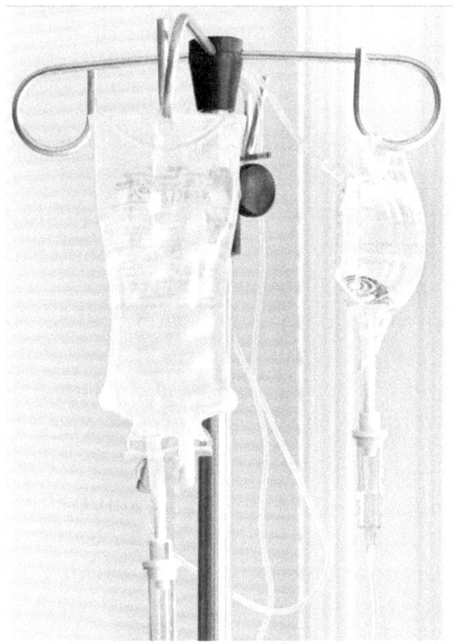

Both IV fluids and medications can be administered via infusions in the hospital.

IV Bolus Injections With an **IV bolus injection**, also referred to as IV push, the drug is administered all at once into the vein, such as in the use of epinephrine or adrenaline in the case of a cardiac arrest, or in the use of glucagon when the blood glucose level of a patient with diabetes is dangerously low. (These drugs can also be administered by the IM and subq routes.) The IV route is the preferred route of administration to deliver medications in an emergency situation.

IV Infusions An **IV infusion** is a method for delivering a large amount of fluid and/or a high concentration of medication directly into the bloodstream over a prolonged period and at a slow, steady rate. The ordered medications are infused into a saline or dextrose solution and hung by the bed in an IV infusion bag that uses gravity or an IV pump to gradually infuse the fluids through a tube and the needle into the vein. This method can provide a continuous amount of needed medication over a given period of time. The medication may be slowly infused over time (8 hours) in the IV solution, or it may be administered over 20 to 30 minutes in a smaller "minibag" connected to the IV solution.

The advantage of an infusion is that there is less fluctuation in drug blood levels than is experienced with other routes of administration. The infusion rate can be adjusted to provide more or less medication as the situation dictates: a higher infusion rate for pain relief or a slower infusion rate if the patient experiences side effects such as shortness of breath. If patients are dehydrated, they may receive IV solutions such as normal saline or dextrose with water (with or without added medication) to keep them hydrated.

Total parenteral nutrition (TPN) is an IV infusion therapy that supplies a patient with all the nutrition and/or fluids that they need. Total parental nutrition is suited for patients whose medical conditions do not allow them to ingest anything by mouth (referred to as NPO patients, from the Latin term *nil per os*). They may be sustained on the nutrient-containing solutions of TPN. Olimel is an example of a TPN solution that is administered intravenously.

Put Down Roots

The word *hypodermic* comes from the Greek root words *hypo*, meaning "under or beneath," and *derma*, meaning "skin."

Intradermal Route

The **intradermal (ID) route of administration** is typically used for diagnostic and allergy skin testing, local anesthesia, various diagnostic tests, and immunizations. For allergy skin testing, small amounts of various allergens are administered (usually on the surface of the back or arm) to detect allergies before beginning desensitization allergy shots. For diagnostic testing, such as for tuberculosis (TB), injections are given in the upper forearm, below where IV injections are given. If a patient is allergic or has been exposed to an allergen similar to TB, the patient may experience a severe local reaction.

Administration of Parenteral Dosage Forms

All parenteral injections are administered into the body with the use of a syringe and/or needle. A **syringe** is a calibrated device used to accurately draw up, measure, and deliver medication to a patient through a needle. Two types of syringes are commonly used for injections: glass and plastic. Glass syringes are fairly expensive and must be carefully sterilized between uses. Some drugs may require a glass syringe due to an incompatibility with plastic material. Plastic syringes are easier to store, handle, and dispose of after use; these syringes come from their manufacturers in sterile packaging. Disposable plastic is clearly preferred medically and used both in and out of the hospital setting for most medications. For example, the blood thinner enoxaparin (Lovenox) is available in a prefilled plastic syringe in doses ranging from 30 mg per 0.3 mL to 100 mg per 1 mL. Proper disposal of plastic syringes and needles (and medications) is both a health and environmental concern. Sharps containers are recommended for home and pharmacy use to safely dispose of used syringes and needles (this will be addressed in Chapter 14 on medical safety).

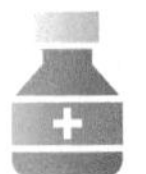

Pharm Fact

The shingles vaccine must be stored in a freezer, and, once reconstituted with sterile water, the vaccine must be administered subcutaneously within 30 minutes.

Only trained professionals and healthcare providers are legally allowed to give parenteral injections. In recent years, however, home health nurses and pharmacists have taught patients (and their spouses or caregivers) how to administer injections or start infusions at home. In the pharmacy setting, many pharmacists are becoming increasingly involved in immunization administration programs after completion of training and certification, which includes cardiopulmonary resuscitation (CPR) in case of a radical immunization reaction. Pharmacy technicians, however, must check their state regulations to determine whether they are allowed to draw up or prepare injections for a final check by the pharmacist. To better assist pharmacy and hospital personnel, pharmacy technicians must have a basic understanding of various syringe and needle sizes.

Parenteral administrations all need needles and often syringes. Common types of syringes include the following:

- the insulin syringe, which measures in units, from 30 units to 100 units (equivalent to 0.3 mL to 1 mL), and has a longer needle than the tuberculin syringe; comes in sizes of 30 units or less (3/10 mL half units marked), 31 to 50 units (1/2 mL), and 51 to 100 units (1 mL)
- the tuberculin syringe, with a cannula (hollow area inside the syringe needle) ranging from 0.1 mL to 1 mL
- the larger hypodermic syringe, with a cannula ranging from 3 mL to 60 mL

Great care must be taken not to mix up the syringes and consequently have incorrect dosages administered. Insulin syringes are used by diabetic patients to administer insulin. Tuberculin syringes are used for skin tests and for drawing up very small volumes of solution. Hypodermic syringes are used with hypodermic needles to inject parenteral drugs into the body or to remove blood from the body (see Figure 5.5). These syringes may be glass or—more commonly—disposable plastic with clear demarcations for accurate dosing. Hypodermic syringes (without a needle) are often used to more easily administer oral liquids to infants, children, and pets.

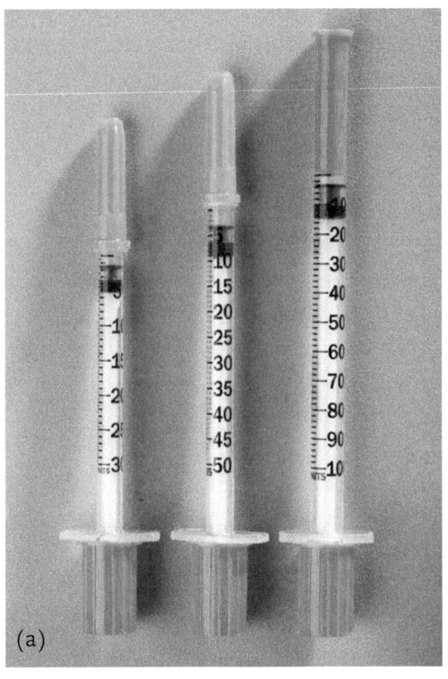

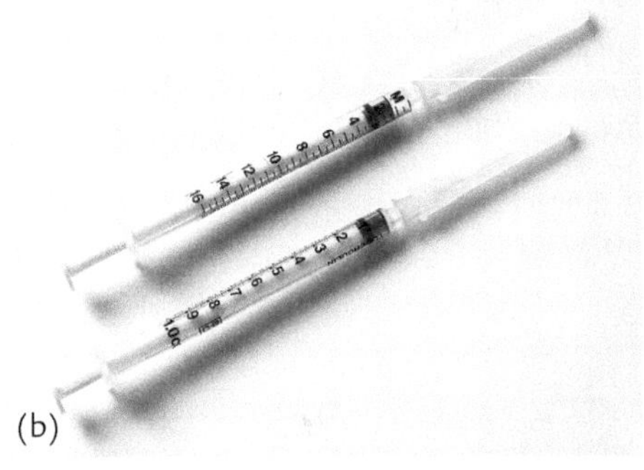

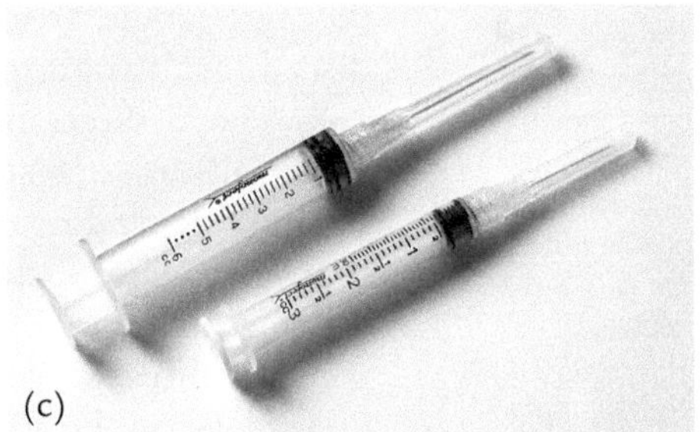

FIGURE 5.5
Common Types of Syringes

(a) Insulin syringes in 30 unit, 50 unit, and 100 unit sizes
(b) Tuberculin syringes marked with metric measures
(c) Hypodermic syringes in 6 mL and 3 mL sizes

A needle is attached to the tip of a syringe to either draw fluid into the syringe or push fluid out. Needles come in various lengths and sizes. Needle length and size depend on the route of administration, patient factors such as body size, and drug formulation characteristics. Needles commonly range from 18 gauge to 32 gauge, with 32 being the thinner, finer needle. The size of the gauge corresponds conversely to the size of the needle's lumen (hollow inner core): the larger the gauge number, the thinner the needle and the smaller the needle's lumen.

Different states have different regulations on the sale of syringes and needles without prescriptions because of their potential diversion for the injection of illegal drugs. Some states (or pharmacies) may require a prescription or that syringes be kept behind the prescription counter to control access to their sale. Some pharmacies will

IN THE REAL WORLD

Knowing and paying attention to the differences in syringe sizes can save or prevent harm to a life. In cases reported in Pennsylvania, tuberculin syringes were accidentally used to administer low-dose insulin. The tuberculin syringe, which was packaged similarly to an insulin syringe, is calibrated in milliliters (mL) from 0.1 to 1, while the insulin syringe is in units. In these cases, 0.4 mL, 0.6 mL, and 0.9 mL doses of insulin were delivered instead of the 4 units (0.04 mL), 6 units (0.06 mL), and 9 units (0.09mL) that were prescribed. So in each case, a tenfold overdose occurred—40 units, 60 units, and 90 units.

not sell syringes directly to the public unless buyers can provide proof of medical necessity. The final decision may be at the discretion of the pharmacist.

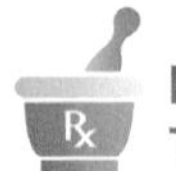

Practice Tip

Storing insulin needles separately from tuberculin needles helps to prevent confusing them.

Subcutaneous Parenteral Administration

Subcutaneous injections are typically administered on the outside of the upper arm, the top of the thigh, or the lower portion of either side of the abdomen. These injections should not be made into grossly fattened, hardened, inflamed, or swollen tissue.

The needle used for subcutaneous injections is typically $\frac{3}{8}$ to $\frac{5}{8}$ of an inch in length, with a needle gauge in the range of 25 to 32. The gauge used by patients with diabetes may vary from 28 to 32, with short, fine, or ultrafine needles. The correct length of the needle is determined by a skin pinch in the injection area. The proper needle length will be one-half the thickness of the pinch.

Subcutaneous injections are usually given just beneath the pinched skin with the syringe held at a 45-degree angle (see Figure 5.6). In lean older patients with less tissue and in obese patients with more tissue, the syringe should be held nearer to a 90-degree angle. To avoid pressure on sensory nerves, which may cause pain and discomfort, a volume of 1 mL or less is injected.

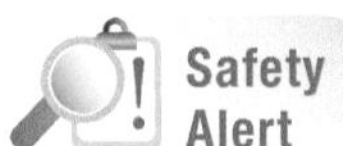

Safety Alert

The patient or patient's caregiver should be reminded never to touch the needle but only the cap and connecting plastic. The needle must be kept sterile.

The medication most commonly administered subcutaneously is insulin. Insulin is typically injected several times a day, with timing generally around mealtimes and bedtime, depending on the type of insulin. Several types are available, including immediate, short-acting, intermediate-acting, and long-acting. These medications differ in onset and duration.

Insulin absorption varies, depending on the administration site and patient activity. The patient should be properly counseled regarding the role that insulin therapy will play in meal planning and exercise so as to gain the best advantage of the medication and avoid the chances of hypoglycemia (low blood glucose levels). The pharmacist should also instruct the patient with diabetes or the parent of the patient to rotate the administration site from the abdomen, to

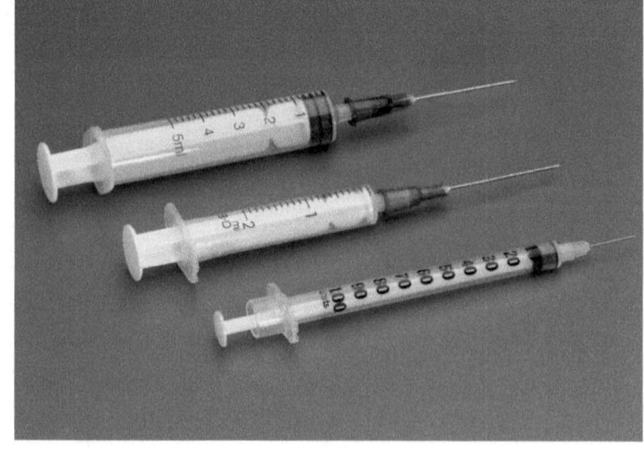

Disposable syringes use different sized needles, depending on the medication, the thickness of the skin, and whether it is a subq, IM, or ID administration.

FIGURE 5.6
Subcutaneous Injection

Subcutaneous injections usually are administered just below the skin at a 45-degree angle.

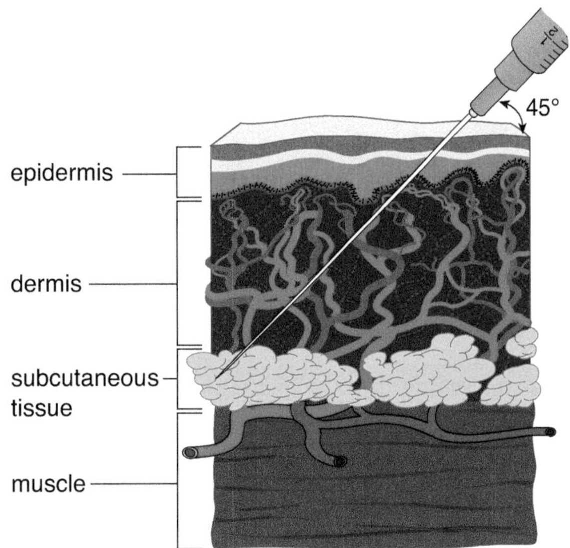

each leg (upper thigh), and then to the arm to avoid or minimize local skin reactions and scarring.

Syringe size, needle length, and needle gauge are critical factors in insulin product selection. A higher-gauge, smaller needle is used due to multiple daily injections. As noted, insulin dosage is prescribed in units rather than in milliliters. The concentration is usually 100 units per 1 mL. However, there is a concentrated insulin that is 500 units per 1 mL. The insulin expiration date should always be checked before administration.

Practice Tip

Remind patients that insulin vials should never be shaken.

Insulin Vials Insulin comes in glass multi-dose vials with rubber stoppers. The proper size insulin syringe should be selected from several volume sizes, such as 0.3 mL, 0.5 mL, and 1 mL, and is determined by the dose needed. When preparing the insulin vial for administration, the vial should be gently agitated and warmed by rolling it between the hands. Then the vial's rubber stopper should be cleaned with an alcohol wipe before inserting the syringe.

To fill the syringe, the same amount of air as the desired insulin dose should first be drawn into the syringe and then injected into the vial through the rubber stopper at an angle. Holding the vial upright and the syringe in a 90-degree position, the correct amount of insulin should be withdrawn. To remove air bubbles from the syringe, the patient should hold the syringe needle up, tap the syringe lightly, and gently push the plunger to expel the air. If air bubbles remain, the insulin should be injected back into the container, and the process started again until the insulin in the syringe has no bubbles. Then, the injection can be performed.

Some patients require the use of two different insulins simultaneously. In order to avoid two different injections, patients may need to mix a cloudy and clear insulin from two different vials. The proper amount of air must be injected into the syringe with cloudy insulin before beginning. Because the process is complicated, the patient should always seek the assistance of a pharmacist or, if in an institutional care facility, the nurse. For more specific information on the process, see the description on the WebMD website: https://PharmPractice7e.ParadigmEducation.com/WebMD.

Insulin Pens An **insulin pen** is a portable device in which the prescribed dose of medication is "dialed up" to administer the proper amount of insulin. There are two kinds: reusable pens that use replaceable insulin cartridges, and prefilled disposable pens designed for single use. An insulin pen can deliver anywhere from 1 unit to 160 units of a prescribed insulin (see Figure 5.7). First, the patient should prime their insulin pen by dialing up two to three units (there is an audible click per dial) and shooting them in the air. Priming removes air bubbles from the pen and ensures that the pen is working appropriately. Next, the patient dials up the correct number of units and injects the medication.

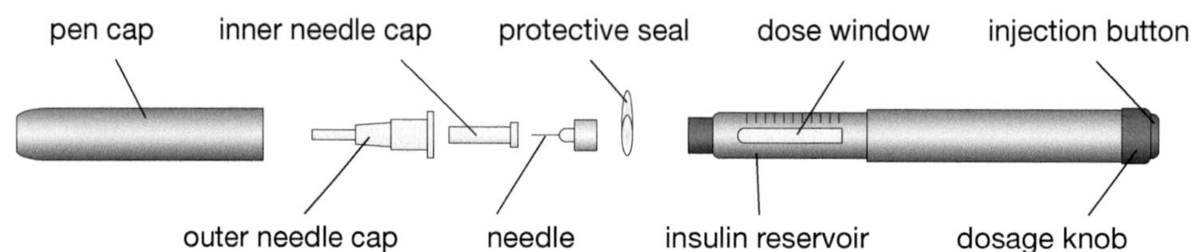

FIGURE 5.7
Components of an Insulin Pen

The insulin pen is easy to learn, simple to use, and convenient to carry.

Insulin pens have many advantages for patients. The pens:

- are more convenient and easier to transport than traditional vials and syringes
- can last for nearly a month (28 days) without being refrigerated
- do not require the additional purchase of syringes
- deliver more accurate dosages
- are easier to use for those with fine motor skill or visual impairments (such as a child or an older adult patient)
- cause less injection pain (as polished and coated needles are not dulled by insertion into a vial of insulin before a second insertion into the skin)
- retain a memory of past injections
- are disposable

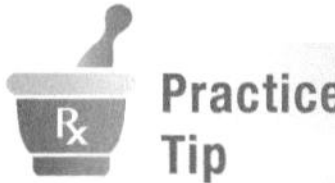
Practice Tip

Some insulin therapies involve a pen for one kind of insulin and a syringe for another, or two insulin pens for two different insulin types.

The major disadvantage of the pens is their cost. Some but not all drug insurance plans cover them as they do syringes and needles. Most insulin pen companies also offer coupons. Common insulin pens include Humalog KwikPens, NovoLog, Levemir FlexPens, Apidra, Lantus Solostar, and Toujeo. Byetta and Victoza are insulin-like products that are also available in a prefilled pen.

Pharmacy personnel should be aware that insulin pens can also come in different mixes, such as the Humalog KwikPen, which is available in a 75/25 and a 50/50 mixture of immediate and long-acting insulin. Most disposable insulin devices are packaged in five-packs, with each pen or cartridge containing 300 units. For lower-dosage insulin, there are reusable pens that come in half-unit dialing increments.

Storage of Insulin All insulin must be protected from temperature extremes. Patients should be instructed to keep insulin refrigerated and to check expiration dates frequently. Opened vials or insulin pens can be stored at room temperature and should generally be discarded after one month, because the insulin can lose a portion of its potency even if stored under ideal conditions. Unopened vials or insulin pens should be refrigerated to maintain their potency until their time of expiration. If the insulin cartridges or prefilled pens have not been refrigerated for 28 days or more, they should be discarded.

Safety Alert

In the past, insulin pens all contained standard concentration insulin (100 units per 1 mL). Now insulin pens are also available with concentrated insulin (300 units per 1 mL).

Insurance Coverage for Insulin Supplies Insurance companies, including Medicare, require a prescription for coverage of syringes, needles, and other diabetic supplies, such as lancets, blood glucose monitors, and test strips. For patients over age 65, Medicare may cover some of the cost of diabetic supplies if proper paperwork is completed. Assisting patients with diabetes is a very important role for the pharmacy technician in the community pharmacy.

Intramuscular Parenteral Administration

In adults, IM injections are generally given into the muscular portion of the upper or the outer portion of the gluteus maximus (the large muscle of the buttocks). Another common site, especially for immunizations, is the lower portion of the deltoid muscles (at the top of the shoulders). Care must be taken during deep IM injections to avoid hitting a vein, artery, nerve, or even bone. Figure 5.8 shows the needle angle and injection depth for an IM injection. The volume of IM injections is usually limited to less than 2 mL.

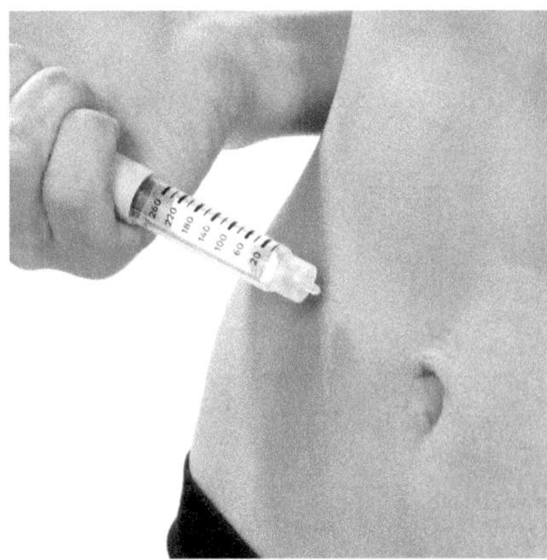

Some diabetes patients use a subcutaneous injection.

FIGURE 5.8
Intramuscular Injection

Intramuscular (IM) injections are administered at a 90-degree angle.

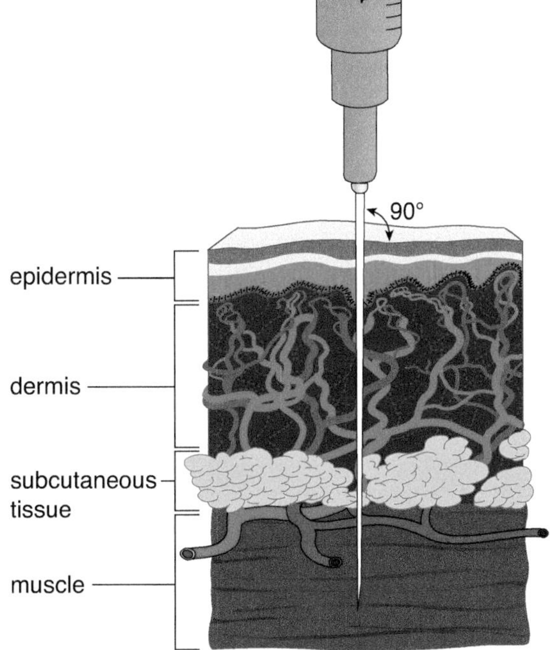

Practice Tip

Remember: the larger the needle's gauge number, the smaller the lumen and the smaller the hole the needle makes. Conversely, the smaller the gauge, the larger the lumen and the larger the hole.

IM injections typically are administered using a 22- to 25-gauge, $^{5}/_{8}$ to 1.0 inch long needle. The needle must be sufficiently long to inject the drug through the dermal or skin layers into the muscle. The needle length for an IM injection may also be dependent on the patient's fat content versus lean muscle at the injection site. A smaller-size needle can be used in a lean patient with average or smaller arm size or skin thickness. Though a large gauge (smaller needle) is always preferable for patient comfort, some medications, due to their viscosity (such as hormone injections), may require a small gauge (thicker needle) to withdraw the medication from the vial and inject the drug into the muscle.

As explained earlier, some emergency medications, such as epinephrine, are administered intramuscularly by EpiPens or other specialized devices. The Twinject auto-injector is a device designed to administer a first dose of epinephrine in an emergency into the thigh muscle through clothing. The auto-injector must be held against the skin for 10 seconds for the medication to be released. A second dose may be administered into the muscle if needed. An IM injection does not work as fast as an IV injection (or infusion), but the pharmacological effect will last longer.

Intravenous Parenteral Administration

IV bolus injections and infusions are usually administered into visible major veins, most often the vein of the arm inside the elbow although other sites are used as well. These injections are given at a 15- to 20-degree angle (see Figure 5.9).

FIGURE 5.9
Intravenous Injection

Intravenous (IV) injections are administered at a 15- to 20-degree angle.

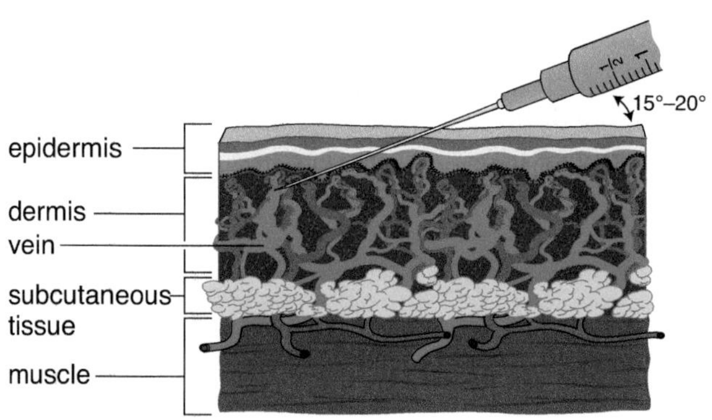

Before administration of the IV solution, the nurse must inspect the solution for precipitates, swab the IV site with an alcohol wipe, and select the correct syringe and needle for the procedure. During administration of the IV product, the nurse must ensure that the solution is free of particulate matter and air bubbles—both of which may lead to **embolism** (blockage of a vessel) or **phlebitis** (a severe painful reaction at the injection site).

The IV route does have associated inherent dangers. A major disadvantage is the potential for introducing toxic agents, microbes, or **pyrogens** (fever-producing by-products of microbial metabolism) straight into the vein, resulting in their dispersal throughout the body. Consequently, to minimize infection, IV products are prepared by pharmacy technicians in an isolated cleanroom environment using special techniques and equipment to ensure sterility, which will be explained in depth in Chapters 12 and 13. After preparation of each IV product, the technician as well as a pharmacist must inspect the solution for contaminants as well as salt precipitates, which are evidence of incompatibility.

Failure to follow protocol for IV products may result in serious adverse effects for the patient. (To learn more about germ theory and the importance of aseptic technique, see Chapter 12.)

Infusion pumps are primarily used in the inpatient hospital setting to deliver IV infusions. They continuously deliver medication 24/7 to regulate the amount, rate,

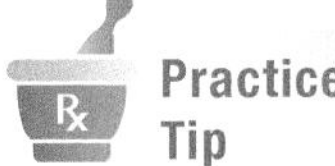

Practice Tip

Pharmacy personnel should be aware that PCA pumps are patient-controlled. Patients push a handheld controller to self-administer a dose of pain medication intravenously.

and/or timing of infused fluid or medication. Examples of infusion pumps include the following:

- a patient-controlled analgesia (PCA) pump, which is a programmable machine that delivers small doses of painkillers on patient demand
- a jet injector, such as for epinephrine, which uses pressure rather than a needle to deliver the medication in an emergency
- an ambulatory injection device, such as an insulin pump, that the patient can wear while moving about and maintaining a normal lifestyle

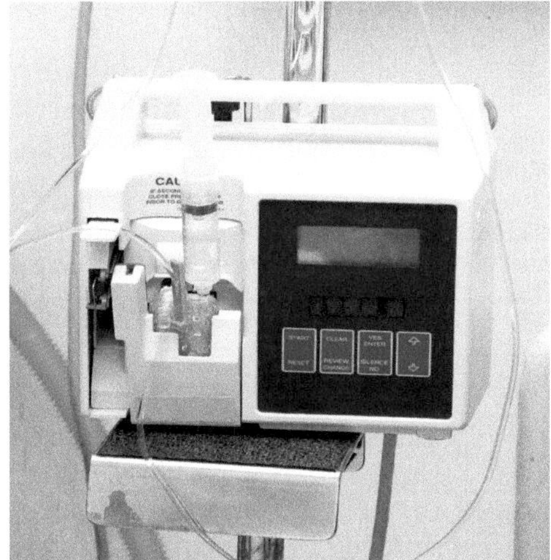

Infusion pumps are commonly used in the hospital to accurately regulate the rate of IV infusions.

Because infusion pumps are electronic, they need to be tested between patients to make sure that they are working properly and infusing accurately.

Intradermal Parenteral Administration

ID injections are given into the capillary-rich skin layer just below the epidermis (see Figure 5.10). A small amount of medication is injected into the dermal layer of skin to form a wheal, or small raised reddened mark. It is used for allergy and TB tests.

FIGURE 5.10
Intradermal Injection

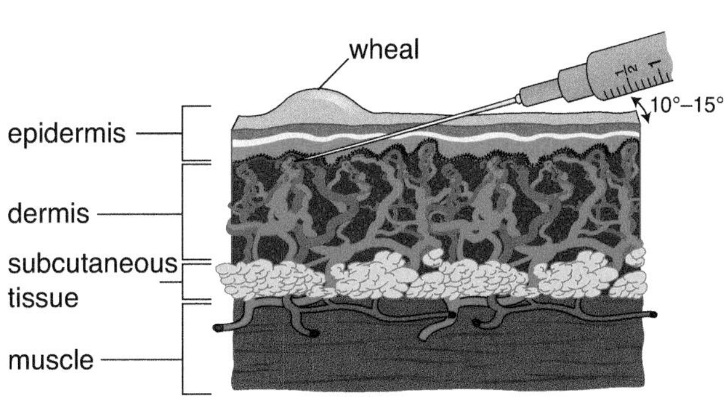

Intradermal injections pierce the skin at a 10- to 15-degree angle. A small amount of medication (0.1 mL) is injected slowly into the dermal layer to form a wheal.

5.8 Drug Delivery Systems

A **drug delivery system** is an engineered technology used to target the delivery and/or timing of a drug to be most therapeutic. It takes into consideration the absorption, distribution, and elimination of the drug from the body. Drug delivery systems can be part of a design feature of the drug's ingredients and/or form or a delivery device.

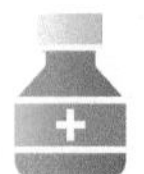

Pharm Fact

Quillichew ER (methylphenidate hydrochloride) is a medication for patients 6 years and above with ADHD. These cherry-flavored chewable tablets are comprised of tiny coated spheres of medication that dissolve at different rates, with 30% immediate release and 70% delayed release. It is a Schedule II drug.

Oral Dosage Forms with Drug Delivery Systems

Oral dosage forms with specialized drug delivery systems include the disintegrating tablet, the sublingual tablet, and the buccal lozenge. These products have modified absorption and distribution phases in order to enhance their therapeutic effects. Other tablets and capsules have been formulated with an enteric coating to delay their release and protect the stomach or extend their release (SR, XR, XL) over a 12- to 24-hour period. These extended-release medications have a less frequent dosing schedule, which improves patient convenience and adherence and, ultimately, provides better disease control.

Delayed-Release Tablets and Capsules

Most tablet and capsule formulations are immediate-release; that is, the medication is designed to be activated or released shortly after the drug is taken. When treating an infection, immediate-release formulations are desirable to initiate a fast onset of action. However, when treating certain conditions, such as hypertension or hyperglycemia, immediate-release formulations would require a long-term, frequent dosage schedule, which may be an inconvenience to patients. For these patients, a medication designed to control blood pressure or blood glucose levels for 24 hours would be preferable.

Many tablets and capsules are available in a confusing alphabet of release formulations: DR, CR, CD, XR, SR, XT, and XL (see Table 5.7). The abbreviations DR (delayed release), CR (controlled release), and CD (controlled delivery) all refer to drug formulations that have some form of delaying the onset of the drug delivery and/or delaying and then incrementally delivering the drug. The abbreviations LA (long action), TR (timed release), SR (sustained release), XT (extended time release) and XL (extended length/release) have some immediate delivery but extend the effects by incrementally releasing more medication or having longer-lasting ingredients.

TABLE 5.7 Drug Delivery Abbreviations

Abbreviation	Meaning
CD	Controlled delivery
CR	Controlled release
DR	Delayed release
LA	Long acting
SR	Sustained release
TR	Timed release
XL	Extended length/release
XT	Extended time release

Safety Alert

Never substitute a different release formula of the same drug without direction from the pharmacist to do so as it may cause great harm to the patient.

Pharmaceutical manufacturers market different release formulations to serve patients but also to extend their existing product lines, lengthen patent protections, and improve bottom-line profits. For example, Depakote—a medication commonly used for seizures—is available as both a DR enteric-coated drug and an ER or extended-release drug. Many other medications are also designated with release formulations. For example, the antihypertensive drug diltiazem and the antidepressant drug bupropion (Wellbutrin) have multiple immediate-release and extended-release products from several drug manufacturers. *However, these drugs are not interchangeable, and their inadvertent substitution could lead to toxicity, patient injury, or, possibly, patient death.*

The pharmacy technician must be aware of the many versions of common drug products on the pharmacy shelf—enteric-coated, delayed-release, sustained-release, extended-release, and so on. Many medications with special drug release characteristics do not have a generic equivalent.

In light of that, you must exercise caution when filling prescription medications and pay special attention to these initials at the end of medication names to avoid medication errors. (For more information on medication safety, refer to Chapter 14.) Technicians also need to be aware that many of these delayed-release and extended-release formulations come with a higher cost or copayment for consumers, and some are paid for by insurance while others are not. Some of the ways these different delays and extensions have been designed into the drugs have already been mentioned, but they could use a little more explanation.

Enteric-Coated Tablets As mentioned earlier, delayed-release tablets have a special enteric coating that prevents immediate release until after digestion so that the drug is not released in the stomach itself. Because the enteric coating resists breakdown by acidic gastric fluids, the side effects of nausea and stomach upset are theoretically minimized. **Enteric-coated tablets (ECTs)** include aspirin, naproxen, and potassium chloride—all drugs that can be irritating to the stomach. Unlike an ECT, a sugar coating on a tablet makes the drug more palatable but does not affect or delay the release characteristics of the drug in the bloodstream.

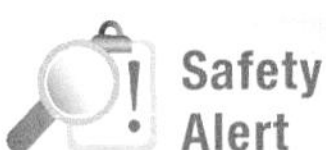

Safety Alert

Beware: a sustained-release (SR) dosage form is *not* the same as an extended-release (XL) dosage form of the same drug. They are often confused by technicians.

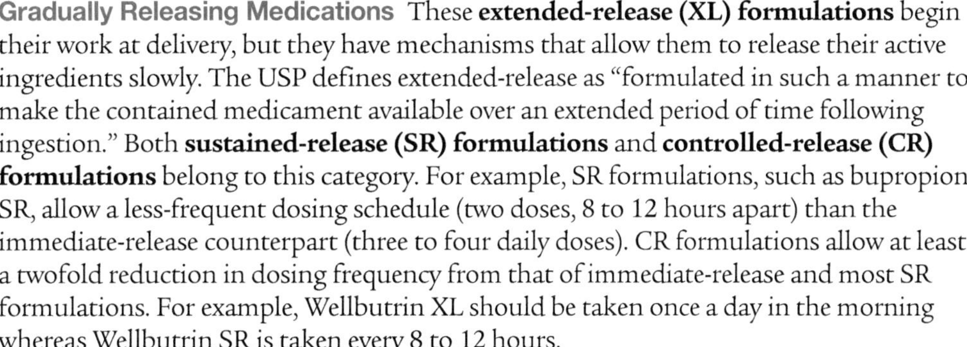

Gradually Releasing Medications These **extended-release (XL) formulations** begin their work at delivery, but they have mechanisms that allow them to release their active ingredients slowly. The USP defines extended-release as "formulated in such a manner to make the contained medicament available over an extended period of time following ingestion." Both **sustained-release (SR) formulations** and **controlled-release (CR) formulations** belong to this category. For example, SR formulations, such as bupropion SR, allow a less-frequent dosing schedule (two doses, 8 to 12 hours apart) than the immediate-release counterpart (three to four daily doses). CR formulations allow at least a twofold reduction in dosing frequency from that of immediate-release and most SR formulations. For example, Wellbutrin XL should be taken once a day in the morning whereas Wellbutrin SR is taken every 8 to 12 hours.

Extended-Release Tablets and Capsules

There are different ways to accomplish extension of drug availability within a system. Several options offer different formulations that attain these extended drug deliveries.

Differing Drug Salts Differing delivery effects can be achieved by altering the drug salts that are mixed with the active ingredients. The oral nitrate tablet isosorbide 30 mg is available as a mononitrate salt (with once-daily dosing) and a dinitrate salt (twice-daily dosing) to prevent chest pain. Another example is the antihypertensive drug metoprolol. It is available as an immediate-release tartrate salt and also as an extended-release succinate salt in doses of 25 mg, 50 mg, and 100 mg. Though the active ingredients are exactly the same, these drugs are not interchangeable—even at identical doses—and the pharmacy technician must take care and precaution to select the correct stock bottle.

Wax Matrix Delivery Systems In **wax matrix systems**, the drug is embedded in an inner chamber surrounded by a waxy substance, and a portion of the drug is partitioned in the inner core of the tablet by the waxy matrix (material surrounding it) for later release. As the outer drug portion is digested, the inner portion is sustained until the wax substance is dissolved or eroded, at which point the encapsulated drug ingredients are released. The narcotic drug OxyContin is an example of a matrix-controlled release (CR) formulation in which the medication is slowly released over a period of 12 hours.

Ion-Exchange Resin Capsules of hydrocodone/chlorpheniramine (Tussionex), an extended-release (XR) narcotic cough medication, are imbedded in a special substance that encourages slow exchanges of the drug ingredients through a permeable resin coating that diffuses the release of the drug. This drug design permits a gradual release of the active ingredients over 12 hours. In addition to an increase in the duration of action, this formulation has a resin coating that can mask taste, prevent tablet disintegration, and improve the chemical stability of the active ingredient.

Osmotic Pressure Release Formulations The **osmotic pressure system** uses the power of water to equalize pressure and salinity between the inside and outer regions of the formulation. The tablets have a rigid coating that has microscopic laser-created holes. As the watery fluids from the digestive system push in, they slowly push the medicine out of the tablets into the digestive system, and into the bloodstream. This drug delivery system has several therapeutic uses for a 24-hour drug delivery:

- to maintain a constant drug plasma concentration for behavioral control—methylphenidate (Concerta), amphetamine/dextroamphetamine (Adderall XR)
- to regulate blood glucose levels—glipizide (Glucotrol XL)
- to manage depression—venlafaxine (Effexor XR)
- to treat hypertension—nifedipine (Procardia XL)

Other Innovative Extended and Targeted Drug Delivery Systems

Other recent drug delivery systems employ biotechnologic delivery processes to produce long-term therapeutic effects. The transdermal patches have already been described. They are formulated to release their medication slowly over 12 hours, 24 hours, 72 hours, or one week. Drugs can also be injected into a kind of internal pool or reservoir so that the surrounding tissue can gradually absorb the pool. This is called a **depot injection**. Other innovative systems include targeted drug delivery systems and surgical implants.

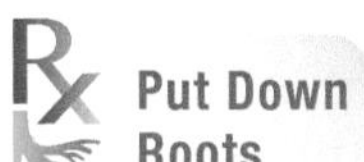

Lipo in Greek means "fat," and *soma* means "body," so liposomes are sometimes known as fat bodies.

Targeted Drug Delivery Systems

Targeted drug delivery systems deliver the medication directly to the targeted internal body location. This intensifies and prolongs the therapeutic action, as the effects of the medication are not diluted by being dispersed throughout the whole bodily system. The drug is injected directly into a tumor or affected area or "carried" by a specific substance to the correct area. The most common current carrier is a **liposome**. It is a bubble-like sphere made of organic cell membrane-like material (often of natural fat or lipid material) generally holding a watery fluid sac. The active drug ingredients are inserted into the fluid of the sac (see Figure 5.11). The liposome is covered with a protective coating. Attached to the covering are "homing" molecules designed to be attracted to the target site—for instance, a cancerous site. The liposomes often have a "head" molecule that is attracted to water and a "tail" that is not; this has the effect of naturally propelling the liposome forward. This liposome drug delivery system is commonly formulated for chemotherapeutic drugs, targeting only the cancerous organ.

Employing this method avoids the adverse effects associated with other chemotherapies, such as decreased blood counts, alopecia (hair loss), and severe GI disturbances that occur when the toxic agents are distributed systemically.

FIGURE 5.11
Liposome

Using a liposome to deliver drugs to specific cells increases the drug's effectiveness and reduces toxic side effects.

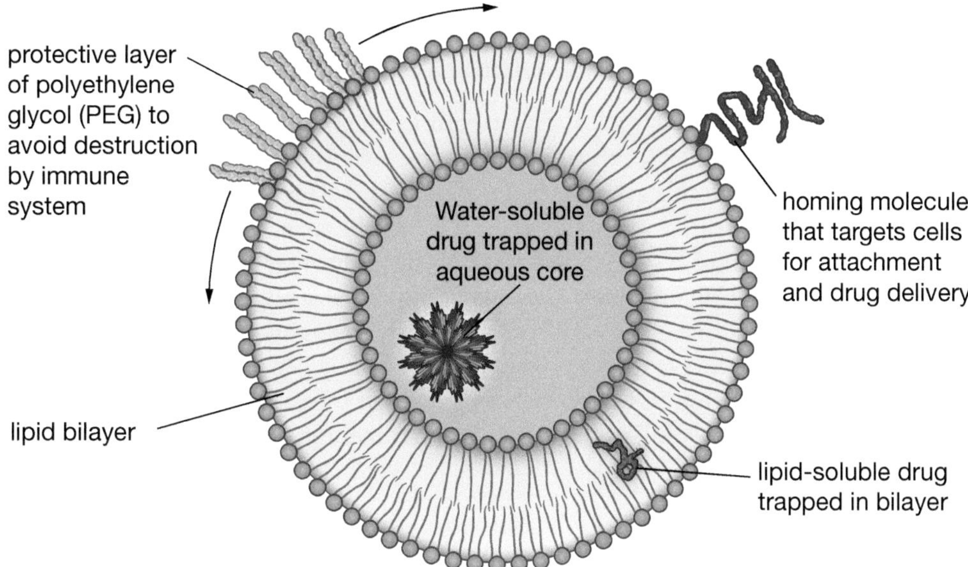

Internal devices can also target the drug delivery. Vaginal rings and hormonal intrauterine devices are inserted vaginally to prevent pregnancy. These contraceptive devices provide a slow release of hormones when placed in contact with the mucosa of the reproductive tract (so they utilize the transmucosal route of administration).

NuvaRing is an example of a vaginal-ring delivery system used to prevent conception. The ring is two inches in diameter and is made of a flexible plastic that is inserted vaginally once a month. Once in contact with the vaginal mucosa, estrogen and progestin hormones are released and slowly absorbed and distributed into the bloodstream. This steady, consistent release of medication may result in fewer hormonal variations than when using other hormonal methods. NuvaRing is as effective in preventing conception as oral contraceptives. In fact, a patient may be more adherent to therapy with a once-monthly ring rather than the daily ingestion of an oral contraceptive. It is recommended that the contraceptive ring be refrigerated before being dispensed.

An **intrauterine device (IUD)** is a t-shaped plastic device that is nonsurgically fitted into the uterus through the vagina by a physician as a drug delivery form to prevent pregnancy. IUDs come wrapped in copper (such as Paragard) or contain a hormonal drug that damages or kills sperm, discouraging conception. Hormonal IUDs contain a progestin-only hormone that is slowly released and localized primarily in the uterus, thus decreasing the risk of long-term adverse effects. This device provides a higher degree of contraceptive protection with a lower failure rate than tablets, patches, and contraceptive vaginal rings.

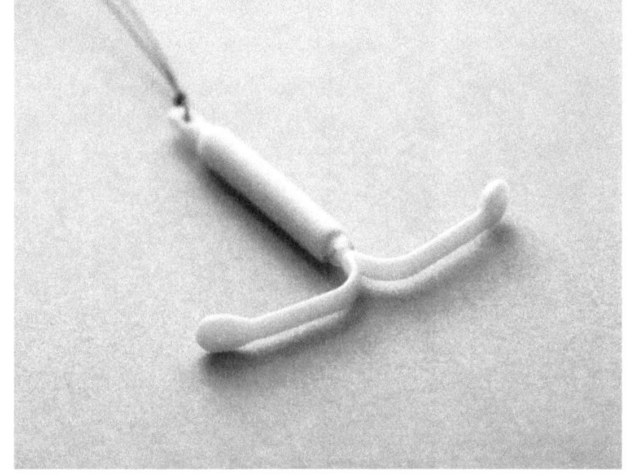
An IUD like this releases a progestin-only hormone within the uterus that prevents conception.

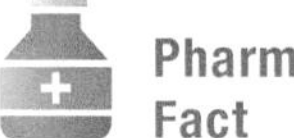
Pharm Fact

Because IUDs do not have to be changed for 3 to 10 years, it can help with therapy adherence, especially for women who forget to take oral forms. An IUD may also be less expensive. However, it can shift position, which can cause mild to severe difficulties.

IN THE REAL WORLD

Scientists are always experimenting with more efficient ways to release drugs and have them keep releasing over time. A new form called **hydrogels** is an injectable gel drug that is pliable and offers extended release of the drug. Researchers see this as ideal for filling a cavity left after the removal of a cancer tumor. The hydrogel form of the chemotherapy could help the area heal by taking up pliable space while slowly releasing cancer-fighting components. The hydrogel form will also work to help stop macular degeneration, a deterioration of the eye that is presently addressed by periodic injections in the eyes. This hydrogel form of drug could cut the injection rate from six to one. This delivery form is still in the stages of experimentation, but you can watch for it to be available soon!

Surgical Implants

Other innovations in drug delivery systems include surgically implanted catheters (thin flexible tubes) and drug pumps, which can provide medication either through the catheter to an external pump or to an internal pump. This has been used, for instance, with pain drugs administered to the spinal cord. Eyes have been implanted with various devices for drug delivery that are made of organic and inorganic materials. Radioactive "seeds" have been implanted in prostates to provide ongoing targeted chemoradiation to the cancerous area. Because these implants and approaches are not commonly seen by pharmacy technicians, they will not be described, but it is good to be aware of how vast and innovative the full field of drug delivery systems is.

5.9 Leading the Way

As you can see, being a pharmacy technician puts you on the leading edge of medical developments: new drugs being constantly designed along with new methods and forms of delivery. It is a field that will never be static or boring.

It is also a field where ongoing learning is a must. This is both the delight and the challenge. That is why growing in practice and experience makes such a difference. Understanding the differences in routes of administration and their various dosage forms will help you know what to watch for on prescriptions to fill them most accurately. This knowledge can also help you avoid medication errors because you will be aware of how the medications work and why they are named the way they are.

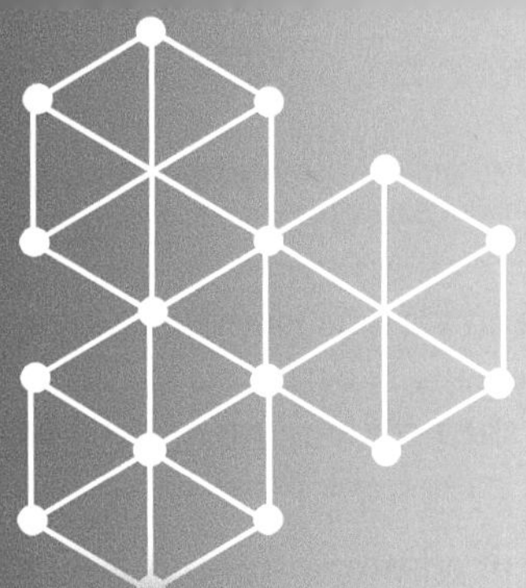

Review and Assessment

CHAPTER SUMMARY

- Drugs are administered in many dosage forms. Factors influencing the decision on the route of administration include ease of administration; site, onset, and duration of action; quantity to be administered; drug metabolism by the liver or excretion by the kidneys; and drug toxicity.
- Common routes of administration include oral, transmucosal, topical (dermal and transdermal), inhalation, and parenteral.
- The oral route of administration allows medications to be swallowed and travel through the digestive tract where they are absorbed for distribution, unless they have a delayed-release coating.
- Oral dosage forms include tablets, capsules, liquids, powders, and effervescent salts, with each dosage form offering convenience, safety, and ease of use for patients.
- Measuring spoons, oral syringes, medication cups, and droppers are critical for accurate dosing of liquid medication in infant and pediatric patients.
- The transmucosal routes of administration offer a fast onset of action by introducing active ingredients to be absorbed through mucous membranes of the linings of the mouth, eyes, ears, nose, rectum, vagina, and urethra.
- Transmucosal routes of medication administration include the oral (sublingual and buccal), ocular, otic, intranasal, vaginal, urethral, and rectal.
- Topical drug applications include two routes of administration—dermal (into the skin for localized action) and transdermal (through the skin to the blood vessels below). Commonly “topical” and “dermal” are used to mean the same thing.
- Topical application forms include ointments, pastes, plasters, creams, lotions, gels, patches, disks, emulsion lotions, sprays, and irrigating solutions. Dermal dosage forms typically have a fast onset of action and minimal systemic side effects due to their localized therapeutic action. Transdermal topical agents have more systemic effects and are slower in their therapeutic action.
- The inhalation, or intrarespiratory, route of administration allows medication to be inhaled through the oral respiratory route.
- Aerosols and sprays are common inhalation dosage forms and offer a rapid onset of action.
- MDIs, nebulizers, vaporizers, and humidifiers are devices used to deliver inhalation therapy.
- The parenteral route of administration includes the injection of any drug or fluid into the bloodstream, muscle, or skin.

- Parenteral administration commonly includes subcutaneous (subq), intramuscular (IM), intravenous (IV), and intradermal (ID) injections.
- Insulin is a common medication administered via the subcutaneous route.
- Medications administered by IM injection include antibiotics, narcotics, vitamins, hormones, and immunizations.
- IV injections and infusions are injected directly into the bloodstream. Special precautions must be taken in their preparation and administration to maintain sterility and to prevent air embolisms and phlebitis.
- IV medications can be given by an IV bolus injection (when the entire drug is administered at once) or by IV infusion (when a drug is administered slowly over a designated period of time).
- IV infusions are given for a variety of purposes, including the delivery of fluids, electrolytes, nutrients, and drugs.
- Common types of syringes include the insulin syringe, the tuberculin syringe, and the hypodermic syringe.
- Needles come in various lengths and sizes; the size of the gauge corresponds conversely to the size of the needle's lumen. As a result, the larger the gauge, the thinner the needle.
- The ID route of administration is typically used for drug and allergy tests, local anesthesia, and various immunizations.
- Drug delivery systems are dosage forms whose design affects the delivery of the drug.
- Common drug delivery systems include delayed-release and extended-release tablets and capsules, matrix-controlled release formulations, osmotic pressure release formulations, and targeted drug delivery systems. It is important to distinguish between and memorize the different abbreviations indicating the different forms to avoid mixing them up when filling prescriptions.
- Certain methods of contraception, such as the vaginal ring and the IUD, use drug delivery systems to release hormones and prevent pregnancy.To ensure that you recall and understand the key chapter concepts, please read the question or statement and select the appropriate lettered option.

CHECK YOUR UNDERSTANDING

1. Which of the following inert ingredients may improve the flavor of a tablet?
   a. lactose.
   b. starch.
   c. methylcellulose.
   d. saccharine.
2. One of the most common and economical drug dosage forms is a(n)
   a. compression tablet.
   b. extended-release capsule.
   c. transdermal patch.
   d. inhalation aerosol.
3. Which of the following indications is commonly treated with a chewable tablet formulation?
   a. conjunctivitis
   b. cancer
   c. heart arrhythmia
   d. flatulence
4. Many patients purchase a tablet splitter to save on the cost of prescription medications. Which one of the following medication tablets can safely be split?
   a. Promethazine hydrochloride.
   b. Aspirin EC.
   c. Wellbutrin XL.
   d. Concerta ER.

5. The primary function of a film-coated tablet is to
   a. improve taste.
   b. provide a faster onset of action.
   c. protect the stomach lining.
   d. rapidly dissolve in stomach acid.

6. Once reconstituted with water, antibiotic granules become a(n)
   a. suspension.
   b. tincture.
   c. syrup.
   d. elixir.

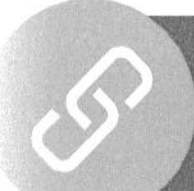

MAKE CONNECTIONS

Take a moment to consider what you have learned in this chapter and respond thoughtfully to the following prompts. Note that some of these activities will require internet access.

1. Research the following drugs: diazepam, losartan, acetaminophen. What are all the ways each can be administered? For those with multiple routes, why would a physician choose one route over another? What are the pros and cons of each route of administration?
2. A six-month-old infant with eczema on the cheeks has been prescribed a steroid cream (0.25%). The mother states that she has a similar high potency drug at home in an ointment formulation (1%) and wants to know whether she can use what she has at home because the prescribed steroid cream is expensive. How should the pharmacy technician respond to this question? What should the pharmacist tell this mother about the differences between these two products?

The online course includes additional review and assessment resources.

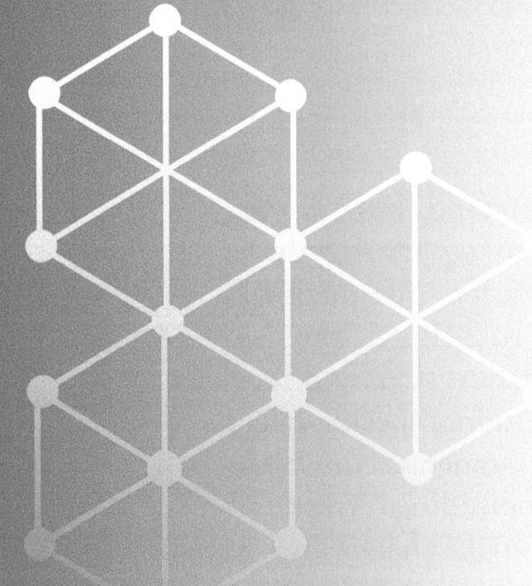

6 Pharmacy Measurements and Calculations

Learning Objectives

1. Convert Roman numerals to Arabic numerals (Section 6.1).
2. Convert percentages to and from fractions and to and from decimals and perform basic operations with ratios and proportions, including finding an unknown quantity in a proportion. (Sections 6.2, 6.3)
3. Convert standard time to 24-hour time and temperatures to and from Fahrenheit and Celsius. (Section 6.4)
4. Describe the different systems of measurement (avoirdupois, imperial, apothecary, household, and metric) that have been used in pharmacy. (Section 6.5)
5. Explain why the metric system is the official pharmaceutical system, and describe the meanings of the prefixes most commonly used. (Section 6.6)
6. Convert from one metric unit to another (e.g., grams to milligrams, liters to milliliters). (Section 6.6)
7. Convert units to the metric system using equal proportion equations and dimensional analysis (unit cancellations). (Section 6.7)
8. Calculate dosages from weight-in-weight, volume-in-volume, and weight-in-volume concentration ratios. (Section 6.8)
9. Perform dosage calculations using body weight and body surface area. (Section 6.8)
10. Determine volume-in-volume powder measurements and administration volumes to reconstitute powdered medications. (Section 6.9)
11. Solve compounding problems involving powder volume in solutions and dilutions. (Section 6.9)
12. Apply the alligation alternate method to prepare solutions and topical products. (Section 6.9)
13. Calculate the specific gravity of a liquid and use milliequivalents. (Section 6.9)

ASHP/ACPE Accreditation Standards
To view the *ASHP/ACPE Accreditation Standards* addressed in this chapter, refer to Appendix B.

Pharmacy technicians use exact measurements in their daily work. When you measure liquids for reconstituting solutions or calculate the amount of ingredients for compounding drugs and preparing parenteral intravenous solutions, the measurements and calculations must be precise. A mistake can have severe consequences, such as drug side effects, toxicity, or even death. Consider this comparison: achieving 90% on your pharmacy calculations test might be an exemplary grade of an A, while achieving a 90% rate of error-free medication preparations would definitely be a failing grade and could cause terrible harm.

Therefore, it is essential for pharmacy technicians to understand the basic measurement systems, mathematical calculations, and formulas used in pharmacy and other healthcare fields. A knowledge of the fundamentals is critical to minimizing medication errors involving dosage, flow rates, and concentrations. This chapter is merely an introduction to lay the foundation for these mathematical skills and provides an overview of the kinds of calculation skills you will need. Additional specific calculations used in compounding are covered in Chapter 10, "Extemporaneous Nonsterile Compounding," and Chapter 13, "Sterile and Hazardous Compounding." The retail math concepts of how to calculate markups and discounts and make change are covered in Chapter 9, "The Business of Community Pharmacy."

6.1 Numerical Systems

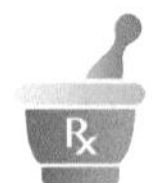

Practice Tip

Rule of thumb for Roman numerals: if a small value comes before a larger value, subtract the smaller value. If the larger value comes before the smaller value, add. And there cannot be more than three of the same numerals in sequence.

Two familiar numerical systems are used in pharmaceutical calculations: Arabic and Roman. Each serves as a kind of numerical abbreviation system for amounts, just as abbreviations are used in texting for words like *lol, idk, cya,* and others. The **Arabic numeral system** includes numbers, fractions, and decimals that we use every day (*1, 2, 3* $^1/_8$, $^1/_4$, $^1/_3$; *10.5, 2.75, 3.25; $10.50, $2.75, $3.25*). In the **Roman numeral system**, numerical values are expressed in capital letters or lowercase letters (*I* or *i* equals 1; *V* or *v equals 5*; and *X* or *x* equals 10). See Table 6.1 for common Roman numerals and Arabic values.

You may see clock faces and *Star Wars* movie episode titles using Roman numerals. Similarly, the official number of the Super Bowl has always been marketed in Roman numerals.

Roman numerals are read from left to right like our standard Arabic numbers, starting from the largest number place to the smaller one: *I, II, III* or *i, ii, iii*. However, to avoid repeating the same Roman numeral more than three times, there is a different way of noting numbers related to four. You put the numeral for one before the five, subtracting the "i" from "v" to get the value of 4 (or 1 subtracted from 5). So you end up counting, *i, ii, iii, iv, v, vi, vii*....The same thing happens with the value of nine. You put the numeral for one before the ten, subtracting the "i" from "x" to get the value of 9 (or 1 subtracted from 10). So you end up counting *vi, vii, viii, ix, x, xi, xii, xiii, xiv, xv, xvi, xvii, xviii,* and *ixx*.

IN THE REAL WORLD

Many students feel stress and anxiety at the thought of math. Remember that attitude counts! Studies show that students of equal ability who look at learning something different as an important challenge they want to take on as opposed to an intimidating obstacle they have to suffer through do far, far better than those who do not.

Ashanti La Roche was afraid of math and had always failed at it. Then she decided to become a pharmacy technician. She had a very good teacher, asked many questions, and completed every problem in her textbook to build her math skills. She came to learn math and now even teaches math in a pharmacy technician certification program! "Learning math is like building a house; you identify the pieces and their uses," she says, "but you have to actually do the work and practice to master the skills!"

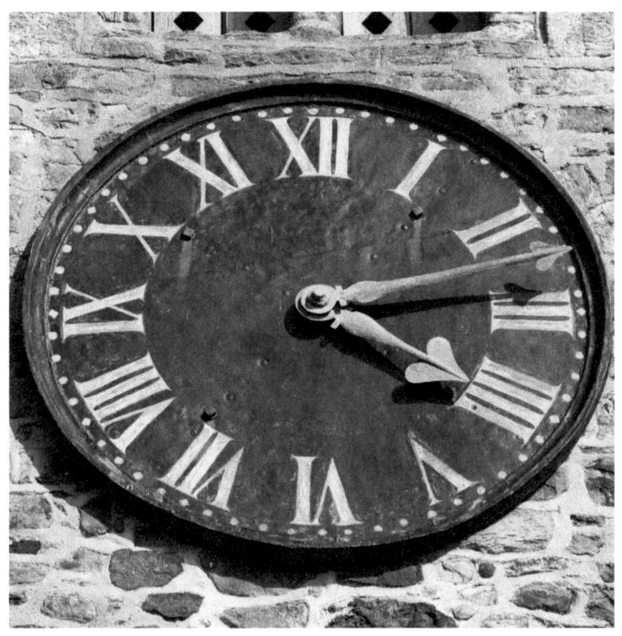

Some clock faces use Roman numerals, giving them an old-fashioned feel.

A similar process occurs for all values related to four and nine, such as forty (*xl* or *XL*, because *L* = 50), four hundred (*CD* or *cd*, because *c* = 100 and *d* = 500), ninety (*XC* or *xc*), or nine hundred (*CM* or *cm*, because *M* = 1,000). Refer again to Table 6.1 and note the derivatives of one, five, and ten as compared to the derivatives of four and nine.

The general principle is if there is a smaller value before a larger one, as in *iv*, you subtract the one from the other. If a smaller value comes after, you add it. If you are translating a Roman numeral and are confused about whether to add or subtract a numeral, as in *MCM*, move from the right and subtract first. *MCM* equals 1,900 because *CM* equals 900 (1,000–100), and when you add 900 to the front *M*, it equals 1,900.

Each level of number (tens, hundreds, thousands) is added or subtracted separately so you get long strings of letters. For instance, 99 ends up as *XCIX* (90 [*XC*] + 9 [*IX*]), never just *IC*; 999 is *CMXCIX* (900 [*CM*] + 90 [*XC*] + 9 [*IX*]), not *IM*. Remember, there are no shortcuts in Roman numerals—you have to use all those letters—but thankfully you will not be using them much in pharmacy practice.

The most frequently used Roman numerals in pharmacy practice are the uppercase letters *I*, *V*, and *X*, which represent the Arabic numbers 1, 5, and 10, respectively. For example, tablet quantities of a narcotic prescription are often written in uppercase letters, such as *XXX*, indicating 30 tablets. Because they can be confusing, however, pharmacy practice is moving away from them to the standard Arabic numerals.

Safety Alert

New safety guidelines discourage the use of Roman numerals in pharmacy practice. Prescribers of controlled substances may use them as a safety precaution to avoid having someone change the 30 tablets to 80 by completing the curves of the 3s, so the prescriber may write XXX tablets or 30 (XXX).

TABLE 6.1 Roman Numeral Symbols and Arabic Values

Roman Numeral	Arabic Value	Roman Numeral	Arabic Value
ss	½	XL (xl)	40
I (i)	1	XLI (xli)	41
II (ii)	2	XLIX (xlix)	49
III (iii)	3	L (l)	50
IV (iv)	4	LI (li)	51
V (v)	5	LIV (liv)	54
VI (vi)	6	LXXXIX (lxxxix)	89
VII (vii)	7	XC (xc)	90
VIII (viii)	8	XCI (xci)	91
IX (ix)	9	XCIX (xcix)	99
X (x)	10	C (c)	100
XI (xi)	11	CD (cd)	400
XII (xii)	12	CDXCIX (cdxcix)	499
IXX (ixx)	19	D (d)	500
XX (xx)	20	DI (di)	501
XXIX (xxix)	29	CMXCIX (cmxcix)	999
XXXIV (xxxiv)	34	M (m)	1,000
XXXIX (xxxix)	39	MI (mi)	1,001

The lowercase Roman numerals *i*, *ii*, and *iii* are also occasionally used in pharmacy practice. These numerals are commonly seen on prescriptions using apothecary measures, and they follow—rather than precede—the unit of measurement. For example, "aspirin gr vi" means "six grains of aspirin." Lowercase Roman numerals are also sometimes used to express other quantities, such as volume ("tbsp iii", meaning three tablespoons). However, errors have occurred so often that Roman numerals are discouraged. If they are used, *i*, *ii*, and *iii* are often written with a line above the letters ($\bar{i}$, $\bar{ii}$, $\bar{iii}$). The fractions in Roman numerals follow a different notation system (*ss* means ½), which is part of the reason that Roman numerals are being phased out of pharmacy practice.

6.2 Basic Mathematical Principles Used in Pharmacy Practice

Pharmacy work often requires performing basic mathematical operations involving fractions, decimals, and percentages. A brief review of these basic mathematical operations is needed to understand the differing measuring systems and their conversions as well as pharmaceutical calculations.

Fractions

When something is divided into parts, each part is considered a **fraction** of the whole. For example, a pie might be divided into eight slices—each one is a fraction or ⅛ of the whole pie. A simple fraction consists of two numbers: a **numerator**—the number on the top or the left of the fraction—and a **denominator**—the number on the bottom or the right of the fraction. The denominator represents the number of equal pieces the whole pie is broken into (eight, in the case of the pie) and the numerator represents the number of those pieces which are selected (one of the pieces) (see Figure 6.1).

numerator ⟶ 1
denominator ⟶ 8

$$\frac{1}{8}$$

A fraction is also a convenient way of writing a division equation. For example, the fraction 6/3 is a shorthand way of writing $6 \div 3 = 2$. Fractions can also be a way of writing a **ratio**, the comparable relationship of one element to another and the whole, such as six parts of an ingredient to three parts of the diluting substance (6:3), which will be addressed in more detail in the pharmaceutical measuring section to come.

FIGURE 6.1 Fractional Proportions of the Whole Pie

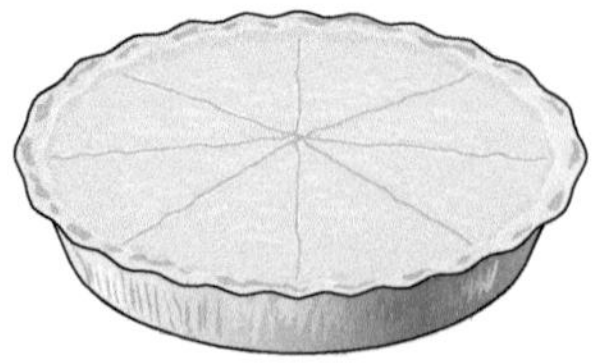

8 slices = 1 whole pie = $\frac{8}{8}$ of the whole pie

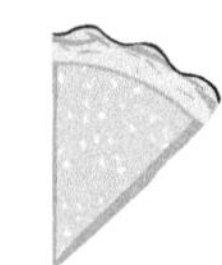

1 slice = $\frac{1}{8}$ of the whole pie

Adding and Subtracting Fractions

To add or subtract fractions, the numbers must have the same denominator, referred to as a common denominator. When fractions share a common denominator, they are easy to add together. For example: $^1/_4 + ^2/_4 = ^3/_4$. If the fractions don't share a denominator, you need to convert them to a common denominator first. For example, to add $^1/_8$ to $^3/_{15}$, you need to find a number that both 8 and 15 can be divided into as a denominator. (To subtract $^1/_8$ from $^3/_{15}$, you have to do the same). Here is how you do it:

Put Down Roots

The term *numerator* comes from Medieval Latin, and means "counter" or "number." *Denominator* comes from Latin, and means "namer" and signifies the namer of the total amount.

Step 1 Find a common denominator for $^1/_8$ and $^3/_{15}$. A quick way to determine a possible common denominator is to multiply the denominators.

$$(8 \times 15 = 120)$$

Thus, 120 will be the common denominator for the two fractions.

Step 2 Convert each fraction to the common denominator. Creating a common denominator requires transforming each fraction by multiplying it by a fraction that is equal to 1. Multiplying a number by 1 does not change the value of the number ($5 \times 1 = 5$). Therefore, if you multiply a fraction by a fraction that equals 1 (such as $^{15}/_{15}$), you do not change the value of the fraction.

First, we will convert $^1/_8$ to the common denominator of 120. This can be achieved by multiplying $^1/_8$ by $^{15}/_{15}$.

$$\frac{1}{8} \times \frac{15}{15} = \frac{15}{120}$$

Next, we will convert $^3/_{15}$ to the common denominator of 120. This can be achieved by multiplying $^3/_{15}$ by $^8/_8$.

$$\frac{3}{15} \times \frac{8}{8} = \frac{24}{120}$$

Now both fractions have a common denominator.

Step 3 Add or subtract the fractions with common denominators.

$$\frac{15}{120} + \frac{24}{120} = \frac{39}{120}$$

Simplifying Fractions

There are cases when a fraction needs to be reduced, or simplified. This requires finding numbers that are divisible by both the numerator and denominator (also called a common factor). Consider the example of simplifying the fraction $^3/_{27}$.

The common factor of 3 and 27 is 3. Therefore:

$$\frac{3}{27} = \frac{1 \times 3}{9 \times 3} = \frac{1}{9} \times \frac{3}{3} = \frac{1}{9}$$

Another way to simplify $^3/_{27}$ is to divide both the numerator and denominator by a common factor (in this case 3).

$$\frac{3}{27} = \frac{3 \div 3}{27 \div 3} = \frac{1}{9}$$

Now simplify the fraction $^2/_{12}$. The common factor of 2 and 12 is 2.

$$\frac{2}{12} = \frac{1 \times 2}{6 \times 2} = \frac{1}{6} \times \frac{2}{2} = \frac{1}{6}$$

Another way to simplify $^2/_{12}$ is to divide both the numerator and denominator by a common factor (in this case 2).

$$\frac{2}{12} = \frac{2 \div 2}{12 \div 2} = \frac{1}{6}$$

Expanding Fractions

You can also make a fraction more complex by multiplying the numerator and denominator equally by a fraction that equals one, such as $^2/_2$, $^3/_3$, or $^{10}/_{10}$. You would do this if you were trying to get two fractions with the same denominator.

For instance, say you had two fractions $^6/_{10}$ and $^5/_{56}$, and you wanted to work with them together to find out which one was larger or smaller. You could multiply:

$$\frac{6}{10} \times \frac{56}{56} = \frac{336}{550} \text{ and } \frac{5}{56} \times \frac{10}{10} = \frac{50}{560} \text{ to come up with } \frac{336}{560} \text{ and } \frac{50}{560}$$

Now you could subtract or add them since they *share the same denominator* (or have a common denominator).

Multiplying Fractions

To multiply fractions, multiply numerators by numerators and denominators by denominators. Another way to think of this is to use the fractional line as a floor. You multiply the numbers of the upper story or top level and the basement or bottom level separately. Then you simplify the fraction as a whole, two-story unit (which will be explained next).

Say you want 24 of $^1/_4$ tablets, and you want to know what the total would be. Make the whole number 24 into a fraction by placing it over the denominator 1. Multiply this fraction by $^1/_4$, multiplying each level separately.

$$\frac{24}{1} \times \frac{1}{4} = \frac{24 \times 1}{1 \times 4} = \frac{24}{4}$$

Simplify the fraction by dividing 24 by 4, and you end up with 6 tablets.

To multiply two fractions, you simply line them up and multiply the levels separately.

$$\frac{1}{4} \times \frac{2}{5} = \frac{2}{20}$$

This is simplified to $\frac{1}{10}$.

Dividing Fractions

To divide by a fraction, change the division sign to a multiplication sign, and invert the number to the right of the operation sign. (The inverted number is called the reciprocal.) Then multiply the fractions and reduce as necessary. You can also think of this using the floor analogy. To divide a fraction thinking of floors, invert the second fraction and then multiply the upper and basement levels as before.

Consider the following example. Divide $^1/_2$ by $^2/_3$.

$$\frac{1}{2} \div \frac{2}{3}$$

Step 1 Invert the fraction to the right of the operation sign and change the operation sign from "÷" to "×."

$$\frac{1}{2} \times \frac{3}{2}$$

Step 2 Multiply the numerators by the numerators and the denominators by the denominators.

$$\frac{1 \times 3}{2 \times 2} = \frac{3}{4}$$

Another example is to divide the fraction $^7/_{16}$ by 2. This requires that you make the whole number 2 into a fraction first.

$$\frac{7}{16} \div 2$$

Step 1 Convert any whole numbers to fractions.

$$\frac{7}{16} \div \frac{2}{1}$$

Step 2 Invert the fraction to the right of the operation sign and change the operation sign from "÷" to "×."

$$\frac{7}{16} \times \frac{1}{2}$$

Step 3 Multiply the numerators by the numerators and the denominators by the denominators.

$$\frac{7 \times 1}{16 \times 2} = \frac{7}{32}$$

IN THE REAL WORLD

A physician prescribed ".5 mg" of IV morphine in the hospital for a 9-month-old infant for the management of postoperative pain. However, a unit secretary in the hospital did not see the decimal point and transcribed the order by hand onto a medication administration record (MAR) as "5 mg." An experienced nurse followed the directions without question and gave the baby 5 mg of IV morphine initially and another 5 mg dose two hours later. The two doses administered were each ten times the prescribed dose. Sadly, about four hours after the second dose, the baby stopped breathing, suffered a cardiac arrest, and died. If the order had been written as "0.5 mg" or "X.5 mg," it is likely that this child would still be alive.

Decimals

The US money system is based on dividing things into fractions of 10 or 100. There are ten pennies in a dime ($^{1}/_{10}$) or one hundred pennies in a dollar ($^{1}/_{100}$). These amounts are commonly written as decimals ($ 0.01). Understanding decimals is crucial to understanding money as well as to preparing and compounding prescriptions.

A **decimal** is a number written out in proportion to fractions of "tenths" or multiples of ten. In a decimal, everything to the left of the decimal point is a whole number, and everything to the right is a portion of a whole number in powers of ten, such as three one-hundredths—0.03. You can see this relationship clearly in terms of US money, since one dollar ($1.00) is equal to 100 cents (100 × 0.01). The amount of five dollars and twenty cents is written as the decimal $5.20, which is equal to five full dollar units and $^{20}/_{100}$ called twenty cents (or two dimes that are each worth $^{1}/_{10}$ of a $1.00 bill).

In prescriptions, you often go into decimals with fractions of 1,000 or 10,000 because you need to deal with very small drug quantities. The decimal 0.056 means 56 one-thousandths or $^{56}/_{1,000}$ while 0.0184 would be 184 ten-thousandths or $^{184}/_{10,000}$ (see Figure 6.2). Most prescriptions and hospital medication orders are written using decimals as shown below:

℞ **Digoxin 0.125 mg #30. Take 1 tablet every day to control heart rate.**

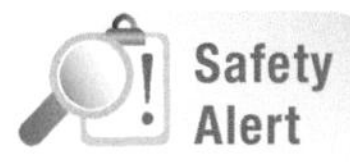

Always watch for decimal points! When transcribing or inputting a decimal value less than one, always use a leading X or zero to prevent errors.

If a decimal number is less than one, place a zero (0) before the decimal point, as in 0.36. This zero is called a **leading zero** and is used to prevent confusion and potential medication errors when reading decimals. For example, the decimal 0.131313 is less than one and has a leading zero placed to the left of the decimal point. When the calculations are done, this leading zero should be changed to an X when writing down the final answer, prescription, or compounded amount. This ensures that the correct decimal place is seen: X.131313.

FIGURE 6.2 Decimal Units and Values

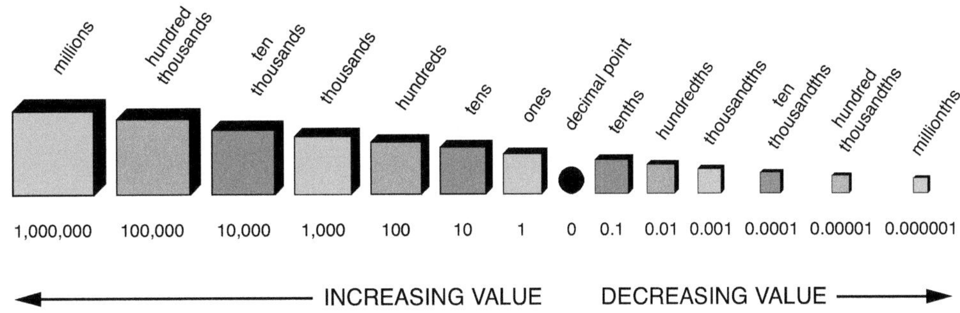

Converting Decimals to Fractions

Any decimal number can be expressed as a fraction by using the appropriate power of 10 as the denominator. To do this, remove the decimal point and use the resulting number as the numerator. Then count the number of places to the right of the decimal point in the original decimal number to designate the correct power of 10, with 10 for one place, 100 for two places, and so on. For instance, $0.24 = {}^{24}/_{100}$. Use Table 6.2 to find the corresponding power of 10 to put in the denominator.

$$2.33 = \frac{233}{100}$$

$$0.1234 = \frac{1,234}{10,000}$$

$$0.00367 = \frac{367}{100,000}$$

TABLE 6.2 Decimals and Equivalent Decimal Fractions

$1 = \frac{1}{1}$	$0.01 = \frac{1}{100}$	$0.0001 = \frac{1}{10,000}$
$0.1 = \frac{1}{10}$	$0.001 = \frac{1}{1,000}$	$0.00001 = \frac{1}{100,000}$

Example 1

The heart drug digoxin is available as a 0.25 mg tablet. Convert 0.25 to a fraction.

$$0.25 = \frac{25}{100}$$

Simplifying Decimal Fractions

Some fractions use decimals. When this happens, you will want to simplify them to get rid of the decimals in the fractions. You do this by multiplying the fraction by the sufficient power of ten to transform the decimal into a whole number. This is the same as moving the decimal point to the right the same number of zeros you add to the denominator. Consider the following examples with ${}^{0.2}/_{10}$, which becomes ${}^{2}/_{100}$.

$$\frac{0.2}{10} \times \frac{10}{10} = \frac{2.0}{100} \text{ which simplifies to } \frac{1}{50} \text{ So } \frac{0.2}{10} \text{ is the same as } \frac{1}{50}$$

Here's another example with $^{0.45}/_{90}$ equals $^{45}/_{9,000}$, or $^{1}/_{200}$:

$$\frac{0.45}{90} \times \frac{100}{100} = \frac{45}{9{,}000} = \frac{1}{200}$$

Converting Fractions to Decimals

To do pharmaceutical measurements, you often have to convert a fraction to a decimal. Doing this can be a little trickier if the denominators are not in tenths, hundredths, or thousandths. To find the correct decimal number, divide the denominator into the numerator. For instance, the fraction $^{7}/_{8}$ is 7 divided by 8, which equals the decimal value 0.875. Here are some other examples:

$$\frac{1}{2} = 1 \div 2 = 0.5$$

$$\frac{1}{3} = 1 \div 3 = 0.33333$$

$$\frac{438}{64} = 438 \div 64 = 6.84375$$

Example 2

A patient receives the following prescription.

℞ **Amoxicillin, ¾ tsp, three times daily.**

What is the decimal amount equivalent to a $^{3}/_{4}$ tsp? (Assume 1 tsp = 5 mL; so what is $^{3}/_{4}$ of it?)

Step 1 Convert $^{3}/_{4}$ into a decimal: $3 \div 4 = 0.75$.

Step 2 0.75×5 mL $= 3.75$ mL, which is equivalent to $^{3}/_{4}$ tsp.

Rounding Off Decimals

When decimal numbers get too long, with too small fractional amounts at the end, the end amounts need to be "**rounded off**," or simplified. To do this, simplify to the nearest tenth place by either adding a little or taking a little away. For instance, if you have a number that goes into the nearest hundredth, like 2.68, and you want a simpler number, you round to the nearest tenth, which would be 2.7. You do this by checking the number in the hundredths place (the "8" in this case). If the number in place is 5 or greater, add 1 to the tenths-place number. If the number in the hundredths place is less than 5, simply drop off the digit in the hundredths place (2.64 to 2.6). Here are some other examples:

5.65 becomes 5.7 (you added 0.05 to the 5.65)

4.24 becomes 4.2 (you dropped 0.04)

The same procedure may be used when rounding to the nearest hundredths or thousandths place.

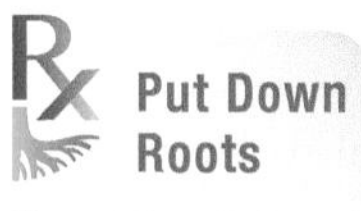

The abbreviation *gtt* comes from the Latin word *guttae* meaning "drops."

3.8421 is rounded down to 3.84 (hundredths place)

41.2674 is rounded up to 41.27 (hundredths place)

0.3928 is rounded up to 0.393 (thousandths place)

4.1111 is rounded down to 4.111 (thousandths place)

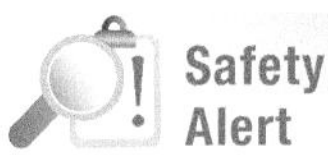

When rounding calculations of IV fluid drops per minute (gtt/min), generally round partial drops *down*.

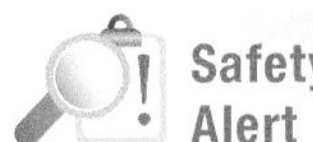

Unless told differently for a specific prescription, round down in dosages for infants and children.

Rounding down or up, however, can depend on the requirements of the measuring device and the situation. For example, scales all have different degrees of measurement where rounding is required, and the more powerful or toxic the substance, the greater the degree of exactitude you need.

The calculated dose needed is 0.08752 g

Rounded to nearest tenth: 0.1 g

Rounded to nearest hundredth: 0.09 g

Rounded to nearest thousandth: 0.088 g

Rounding to the nearest tenth place is typical in dosages for adults. However, with large amounts, this rounding off can make huge differences. For instance, you will see 1 pint listed as 473 mL but also rounded up as 480 mL. Also, when you are dealing with especially vulnerable populations, such as people with low body weight, you may tend to round down rather than up, even if the numeral in the rounding place is 5 or more.

Because children are so much smaller than adults, not just in weight but in bone density, and because their organs and muscles are not fully formed, you always want to lean towards caution. It is better to underdose than overdose, as you can always administer more if needed. That is why in doses for children, rounding to the nearest hundredth or thousandth may be more appropriate, and you almost *always round down for children, especially for premature babies and infants.*

Example 3

You need to convert from fluid ounces to milliliters to figure out a days' supply for an otic solution. One fluid ounce is 29.57 mL. How would you round this to the nearest tenth of a milliliter? How would you round this to the nearest milliliter?

Since 7 is greater than 5, 29.57 would be rounded to the nearest tenth of a milliliter to 29.6. Since the tenths digit is 5 or greater, 29.57 would be rounded up to 30 mL.

Example 4

A newborn is prescribed ampicillin for severe meningitis, and the calculation for the correct amount based on the baby's body weight is 45.8 mg. How would you round this dose to the nearest milligram?

Normally since 0.8 is over 0.5, you would round it up to 46 mg. However, since this is a neonate, you will round it down to 45 mg.

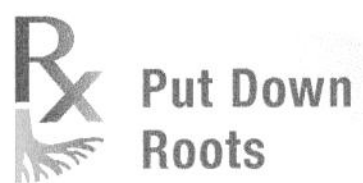

The word *percent* comes from the Latin phrase *per centum*, meaning "in one hundred."

Calculating Percents

A **percentage** is a specific portion related to a whole of 100 units. For instance, 3% means 3 out of 100. So if 12 patients out of 100 request to speak with the pharmacist, that would mean 12% of the patients seek counseling.

Percentages are very important for mixing dilutions and compounds. Percents are often used to communicate the portion, or percentage, of the active ingredient in the whole drug product. The whole drug product is considered to be 100%, and every ingredient in it has a lower percentage of this whole. Percentages of an active ingredient are usually expressed as the specific weight or volume of the ingredient as compared to the weight or volume of the whole of 100 units, such as 1% hydrocortisone cream. Percents can be expressed in many ways, and all of the following expressions are equivalent:

- a percent (e.g., 3%, or 3 percent)
- a fraction with 100 as the denominator (e.g., 3/100)
- a decimal (e.g., 0.03)
- a ratio (e.g., 3:100, or 3 to 100)

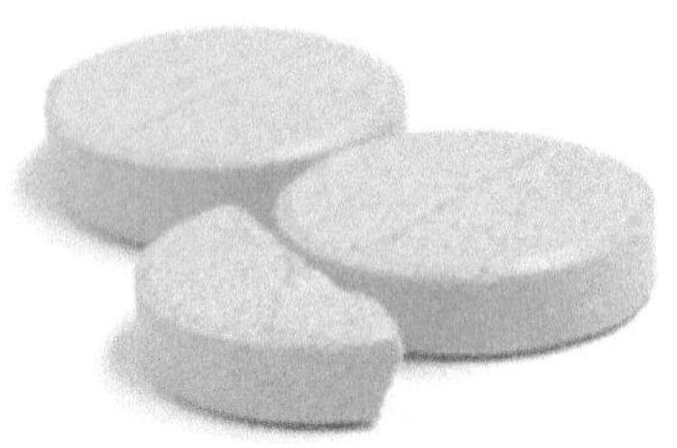

A pharmacy technician must be able to describe a piece of a tablet as a ratio (1:2), a fraction ($^1/_2$), and a percentage (50%).

Converting Percents to Decimals

Since 3% equals $^3/_{100}$, it can easily be written as a decimal (0.03) as shown above. To convert any percent to a decimal, simply drop the percent symbol and divide the number by 100. Dividing a number by 100 is equivalent to moving the decimal two places to the left and inserting zeros if necessary.

$$200\% = 200 \div 100 = 2.00$$

$$4\% = 4 \div 100 = 0.04$$

$$0.75\% = 0.75 \div 100 = 0.0075$$

Example 5

You have a request for 0.9% of an IV of isotonic normal saline. How would you write that as a decimal?

$$0.9\% = \frac{0.9}{100} = 0.9 \div 100 = 0.009$$

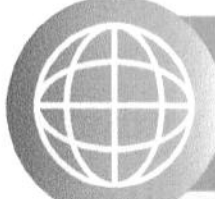

IN THE REAL WORLD

Jaden Williams was born prematurely and weighed only slightly more than 4 pounds. At one month, he was diagnosed with meningitis, a serious infection. He was prescribed the antiviral medication acyclovir IV. The medical order stated that he was to receive 28 mg in the IV solution every 6 hours, or a maximum total daily dose of 168 mg over a 24-hour period.

Due to an error of one decimal place in the compounding of the sterile IV liquid, Jaden received 280 mg IV in one dose, ten times the amount. This put the baby into cardiac arrest and caused his brain to swell. The hospital in southern California was able to resuscitate Jaden, but, sadly, he has been forced to live on a ventilator with less brain function and extensive costly hospitalization, radically affecting his life and that of his family.

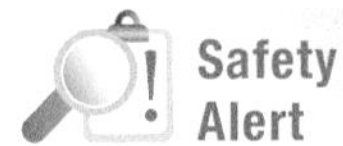

Safety Alert

If you move decimal places to change a decimal to a percent, always double-check by multiplying by 100.

Converting Decimals to Percents

To change a decimal to a percent, multiply by 100 or move the decimal point two places to the right, and add a percent symbol.

$$0.015 = 0.015 \times 100 = 1.5\%$$
$$0.25 = 0.25 \times 100 = 25\%$$
$$1.35 = 1.35 \times 100 = 135\%$$

Example 6

A medication order is for 0.05 dextrose in a sterile water IV. What percent is dextrose?

$$0.05 \times 100 = 5\%$$

This solution can be abbreviated $\mathbf{D_5W}$, meaning a solution of 5% dextrose in water.

6.3 Figuring Ratios and Proportions

Ratios, proportions, and equations are perhaps the most frequently used mathematical equations in pharmacy practice. They are used in determining dosages and in compounding formulas

Ratios

A ratio is a way to demonstrate how two amounts of similar elements compare to each other in a whole. For example, if a beaker contains two parts water and three parts alcohol for a total of five parts, then the ratio of water to alcohol in the beaker can be expressed as the fractions $^2/_5$ to $^3/_5$ or as the ratio 2:3. The ratio is read not as an equation (2 ÷ 3), but as the expression "a ratio of two parts to three parts."

Another common use of ratios is to express the number of parts of one substance contained in another substance of known parts. For example, suppose that there are 3 mL of an ophthalmic solution dissolved in a total 60 mL sterile saline solution. Thus it would be expressed as the ratio $^3/_{60}$, which reduces to $^1/_{20}$. In other words, the ratio of the active ingredient to the sterile saline solution is 1 to 20, or 1 part in 20 parts.

Converting a Ratio to a Percent

To express a ratio as a percent, designate the first number of the ratio as the numerator and the second number as the denominator. Multiply the fraction by 100 ($^{100}/_1$), and add a percent sign after the product.

$$5{:}1 = \frac{5}{1} \times \frac{100}{1} = \frac{5 \times 100}{1} = 500\%$$

$$1{:}5 = \frac{1}{5} \times \frac{100}{1} = \frac{100}{5} = 100 \div 5 = 20\%$$

$$1{:}2 = \frac{1}{2} \times \frac{100}{1} = \frac{100}{2} = 100 \div 2 = 50\%$$

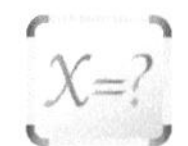

Math Morsel

Any time you have an element that is equally proportioned on the top or bottom of a fraction, such as in powers of ten, you can cross them out to simplify the equation or fraction, as they negate each other.

Consider:

$^{20}/_{200} = {}^{2}/_{20}$ simplified to $^{1}/_{10}$.

Example 7

If the ratio of dexamethasone is 1:3 in a 100 mL oral suspension, what is the percent?

$$1{:}3 = \frac{1}{3} \times \frac{100}{1} = 100 \div 3 = 33\%$$

Converting a Percent to a Ratio

To convert a percent to a ratio, change it to a fraction by dividing it by 100 (and if needed, reduce the fraction to its lowest terms). Express the fraction as a ratio by making the numerator the first number and the denominator the second number.

$$2\% = 2 \div 100 = \frac{2}{100}; = 2{:}100$$

Then simplify by dividing both numerator and denominator by 2 (the common factor).

$$\frac{1}{50} = 1{:}50$$

Now use the same process for the following conversions:

$$10\% = 10 \div 100 = \frac{1\not{0}}{10\not{0}}; \text{ reduced to } \frac{1}{10} = 1{:}10$$

$$75\% = 75 \div 100 = \frac{75}{100}; \frac{75 \div 25}{100 \div 25} \text{ is reduced to } \frac{3}{4} = 3{:}4$$

$$0.50\% = 0.50 \div 100 = \frac{.50}{100}; \text{ increase by multiplying by } \frac{2}{2} \text{ (which equals 1)}$$

$$\frac{1.00}{200} = 1{:}200$$

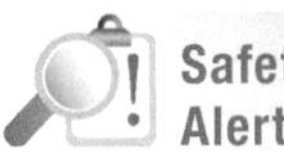

Safety Alert

Pharmacy technicians should always double-check the units in a proportion, the setup of their ratio equations, and their calculations. The pharmacist needs to check them as well.

Example 8

The pharmacy receives the following prescription.

℞ **100 mL IV bag of 4% lidocaine to treat arrhythmia**

The active ingredient of lidocaine comes in grams. What is the ratio?

$$4\% = 4 \div 100 = \frac{4}{100} \text{ means 4 g of the medication in 100 mL.}$$

The $^{4}/_{100}$ simplifies to $^{1}/_{25}$ or 1:25 ratio, or 1 g to 25 mL. So a 50 mL bag will have 2 g of lidocaine, and a 250 mL bag will have 10 g of lidocaine.

Equivalent Ratios

Two ratios that have the same value when simplified are different ways of saying the same ratio, such as $^{1}/_{2}$ and $^{4}/_{8}$. They are called **equivalent ratios**. A pair of equivalent ratios together is called a **proportion.** The proportion can be expressed in three different ways:

$$a/b = c/d \quad \text{example: } \frac{1}{2} = \frac{4}{8}$$

$$a{:}b = c{:}d \quad \text{example: } 1{:}2 = 4{:}8$$

$$a{:}b :: c{:}d \quad \text{example: } 1{:}2 :: 4{:}8$$

Because the ratios are equivalent, you can multiply the numerator of the first ratio with the denominator of the second ratio and then multiply the denominator of the first ratio with the numerator of the second ratio. The two resulting amounts should be equal.

The first and fourth numbers, or outside numbers, are called the **extremes**, and the second and third numbers, or inside numbers, are called the **means**.

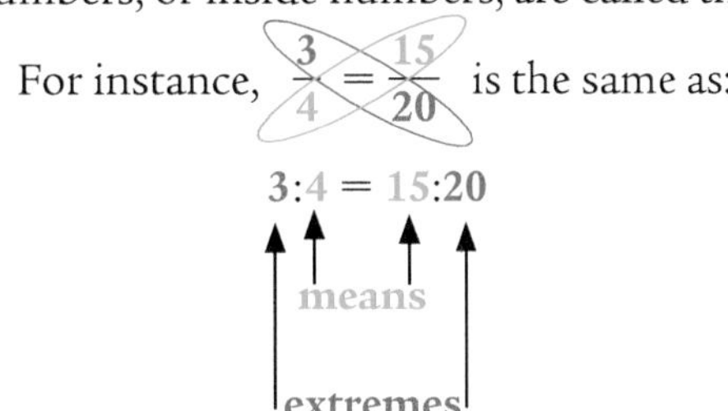

$$3 \times 20 = 60 \text{ and } 4 \times 15 = 60; \text{ or } 3 \times 20 = 4 \times 15$$

When you see it with the colors above, you can see why some people call this cross multiplication the "butterfly technique" or butterfly multiplying.

This cross multiplying can be stated as a rule:

$$\text{If } \frac{a}{b} = \frac{c}{d}, \text{ then } a \times d = b \times c$$

the product of the *extremes* = the product of the *means*

As you have seen, the numerator of the first fraction times the denominator of the second is equal to the denominator of the first fraction times the numerator of the second. In other words, the multiplied extremes equal the multiplied means.

Here's another example:

$$\text{If } 4:12 = 8:24, \text{ or } \frac{4}{12} = \frac{8}{24}; \text{ then } 4 \times 24 = 12 \times 8, \text{ or } 96 = 96.$$

Example 9

A patient is prescribed the following order.

℞ **8 mL of a drug in a 120 mL sterile saline IV solution**

You have a solution with a concentration of 10 mL drug in 150 mL solution. Is this the same ratio as the prescribed drug (8 mL of drug in 120 mL of solution)?

Step 1 The desired drug ratio would be expressed as $\frac{8 \text{ mL}}{120 \text{ mL}}$ or 8:120.

Step 2 This can be simplified by dividing the numerator and denominator by a common factor.

$$\frac{8 \text{ mL} \div 8}{120 \text{ mL} \div 8} = \frac{1}{15}$$

In other words, the ratio of the active ingredient to the sterile solution is 1 mL to 15 mL, or 1 part to 15 parts.

Step 3 The ratio of the solution on hand would be expressed as $\frac{10\text{ mL}}{150\text{ mL}}$.

You can cancel the end zeros, and you find $\frac{1}{15}$ or 1:15, the same ratio.

Step 4 Since 8 mL/120 mL and 10 mL/150 mL are equivalent ratios, you could dispense 120 mL of the 150 mL solution. To be sure, you can do the butterfly multiplying.

$$\frac{8}{120} = \frac{10}{150} \text{ would be } 8 \times 150 = 120 \times 10 \text{ where both } = 1{,}200.$$

A Reciprocal Ratio

A **reciprocal ratio** is the inverse ratio, or the switching of the numerators with the denominators of *both* fractions. This gives you the mirrored ratio, which should also be equivalent, or proportional, though not equal to the originals.

$$\text{If } 1{:}20 = 3{:}60, \text{ or } \frac{1}{20} = \frac{3}{60}; \text{ then } 1 \times 60 = 20 \times 3 = 60$$

$$\text{Inversely if } 20{:}1 = 60{:}3; \text{ or } \frac{20}{1} = \frac{60}{3}; \text{ then } 20 \times 3 = 60 \times 1 = 60$$

These ratios are proportionally mirrored and also equivalent ratios though they are different in real value from the original ratios and fractions.

Another example:

$$\text{If } 3{:}2 = 9{:}6, \text{ or } \frac{3}{2} = \frac{9}{6}, \text{ then } 3 \times 6 = 2 \times 9 = 18$$

then 2:3 will be an equivalent ratio to 6:9 though.

Using Equal Ratios and Proportional Equations of Extremes and Means

Pairs of equivalent ratios are useful in making conversions from one measurement system to another. Because they are proportionally equal, they can be used together with the butterfly technique to discover missing information and solve pharmaceutical conversions.

In mathematics, it is common to express unknown quantities by using letters from the lower end of the alphabet to represent them, especially x, y, and z.

Because x can get mixed up with the × for the multiplication sign, we will primarily use y and z. In our first example, the missing information has been named y, and you use the butterfly technique to figure out what y is.

$$\text{Say } 3{:}4 = 15{:}y \quad \text{or } \frac{3}{4} = \frac{15}{y}. \quad \text{Then } 3 \times y = 4 \times 15. \quad \text{This is } 3y = 60.$$

Then you just have to divide both sides of the equation by 3. Dividing by 3 is the same as multiplying by $^1/_3$ as seen below:

$$\left(\frac{1}{3}\right) 3y = 60\left(\frac{1}{3}\right) \text{ or } \frac{3y}{3} = \frac{60}{3} \text{ to come up with } y = 60 \div 3 \text{ or } y = 20$$

Whenever you have an equation where you have a specified number of y that equals another number, as in the $3y = 60$, all you have to do is take the number accompanying the y and divide each side of the equation by that number, as in: $y = 60 \div 3$.

Consider the equation $66y = 5{,}280$. Solve for y by dividing each side of the equation by 66.

$$\frac{66y}{66} = \frac{5{,}280}{66}$$

Now we are left with:

$$y = \frac{5{,}280}{66} = 80$$

Another way to approach this process is to multiply each equation by $^1/_{66}$.

$$66y = 5{,}280$$

$$\frac{1}{\not{66}} \times \not{66}y = \frac{1}{66} \times 5{,}280$$

We arrive at the same conclusion utilizing this method:

$$y = \frac{1}{66} \times \frac{5{,}280}{1} = \frac{5{,}280}{66} = 80$$

Here's another example of a proportion with missing numbers. You need to make 35 mL of a distilled water solution with a concentration of 2 g sodium chloride (salt) to each 7 mL of distilled water (or 2 g : 7 mL). How many grams of sodium chloride are needed?

$$\frac{y}{35} = \frac{2}{7}$$

By the proportional rule, $2 \times 35 = 7y$, which equals $7y = 70$. That means that y alone is equal to 70 divided by 7 or $y = 70 \div 7$ or $y = 10$. Another way to think of this is to divide both sides by 7.

$$\frac{\not{7}y}{\not{7}} = \frac{70}{7}$$

You can then cancel out the same multiplying factor on the top and the bottom of an equation and then divide 70 by 7 to equal 10. So this would leave $y = 10$ g of sodium chloride.

The following example shows how the ratio and proportion method is essential in both the community and hospital pharmacy settings for converting from one measurement system to another.

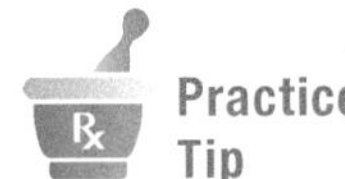

It is important to know that 2.2 lb is considered as the equivalent of 1 kg.

Example 10

A patient weighs 44 pounds (lb). What is the patient's weight in kilograms?

You are seeking to find out: 44 lbs $= y$ kg. The conversion rate is: 1 kg = 2.2 lb.

Step 1 Convert the problem into fractions: $\frac{y}{44\text{ lb}}$ and $\frac{1\text{ kg}}{2.2\text{ lb}}$.

Step 2 Since these two amounts are equivalent, they both equal 1 whole or $\frac{1}{1}$, so set up the proportional ratio equation.

$$\frac{y\text{ kg}}{44\text{ lb}} = \frac{1\text{ kg}}{2.2\text{ lb}}$$

$$y\text{ kg} = \frac{(44\not{\text{lb}})\ 1\text{ kg}}{2.2\not{\text{lb}}}$$

$$y\text{ kg} = \frac{44\text{ kg}}{2.2} = 20\text{ kg}$$

The patient weighs 20 kg.

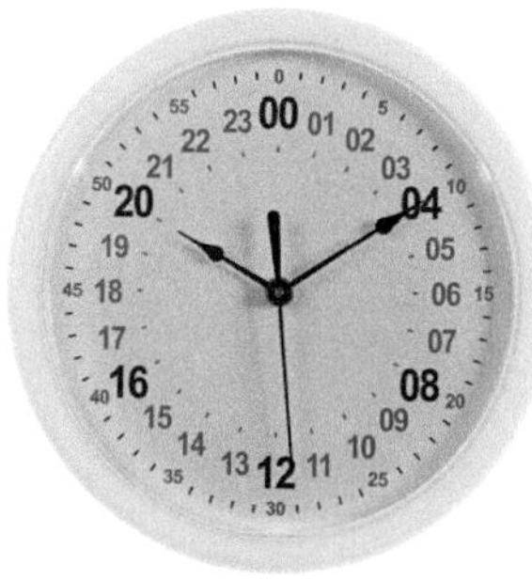

Twenty-four-hour clocks begin at midnight each day, and the first twelve hours until noon are similar to the normal clock. From noon to midnight, the counting continues after 12 instead of starting to count again.

6.4 Systems for Measuring Time and Temperature

Now that you understand basic mathematical principles, you can begin to apply them to pharmaceutical measurements, conversions, and calculations. In life and in pharmacy practice, different dimensions are measured—the dimensions of time, temperature, weight (liquid, solid, or gas), and volume (for each). The dimensions of distance (length), width, and speed are less used. There are several systems to measure the varied dimensions used in pharmacy practice, sometimes with differing systems used in other parts of the world than in the United States.

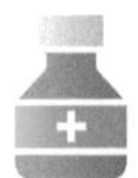

Pharm Fact

The 24-hour format for time originated as early as the Eleventh Dynasty in Egypt around 2100 BCE.

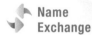

Name Exchange

The 24-hour clock used in healthcare settings is also known as *military time* because the military uses the same system.

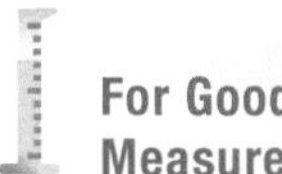

For Good Measure

The standard international notation for time uses the 24-hour clock and colons between hours, minutes, and seconds—*hh:mm:ss*—as in 02:30:00, which would be 2:30 a.m. Healthcare settings usually drop the colons and the seconds.

Time

In the hospital setting, medication orders are commonly written with a 24-hour clock rather than the common 12-hour clock based on **Greenwich mean time**. Because medical care is around the clock, dosage administration schedules consider that 0000 is midnight and noon is the 1200 hour. The first two digits are the time in hours, and the second two digits are the time in minutes. The 24-hour clock, which is also known as **military time**, creates less confusion in pharmacies, hospitals, and other healthcare facilities because there is no need for a.m. or p.m.

To switch from the 12-hour to the 24-hour clock, cut the 12 in 12:00 a.m. to 00 and start counting minutes and hours from there, dropping the colon and the a.m. or p.m., as seen in Table 6.3. After 12:59 p.m., just add 1200 to the 12-hour time until you get to 2359 and then start over.

To convert military time to regular time, simply take the time after midnight (or 0000) and substitute the first 00s with 12, adding a colon and a.m. up until 0059 military. From 0100 to 1259, simply add the colon and a.m. after the first two numbers and the p.m. from 1201 to 1259. From 1300 on, subtract 1200, adding the colon and the p.m. at the end (see Table 6.3).

TABLE 6.3 Military Time Versus Greenwich Mean Time

24-Hour Clock	12-Hour Clock
0000	Midnight–12:00 a.m.
0030	12:30 a.m.
0100 (the first hour)	1:00 a.m.
0230	2:30 a.m.
0600 (the 6th hour)	6:00 a.m.
0845	8:45 a.m.
1200 (the 12th hour)	Noon–12:00 p.m.
1645	4:45 p.m.
1800 (the 18th hour)	6:00 p.m.
2130	9:30 p.m.
2300 (the 23rd hour)	11:00 p.m.

Example 11

At 0125, you receive the following order.

℞ **Gentamicin 80 mg IV every 8 hours, administer at 0200, 1000, and 1800**

Put Down Roots

The Romans used a 12-hour clock, and the Latin words *ante meridiem* (before midday) and *post meridiem* (after midday) became abbreviated as a.m. and p.m.

The order was received at 1:25 a.m. according to the 12-hour clock. When should doses be delivered to the patient care unit by the same clock?

Using Table 6.3 and the conversion process, the first dose is to be immediately prepared and sent to the patient care unit to be given at 2:00 a.m. A follow-up dose is scheduled for 10:00 a.m. The final dose is scheduled for 1800. To convert any amounts over 1200, subtract 12 hours and add p.m.

$$1800 - 1200 = 600, \text{ or } 600 \text{ p.m.}$$

So 6:00 p.m. will be the last dose before more medication will be delivered to the patient care unit.

For Good Measure

Depending on whether you are converting from standard time to military time or vice versa, you will either add 12 hours in the p.m. or subtract them. For practice, try setting your phone to international time to get used to the 24-hour clock!

Temperature

The United States is one of the few countries in the world that commonly uses Fahrenheit as its temperature scale. The **Fahrenheit temperature scale** assigns 32 °F as the temperature at which water freezes to ice and 212 °F as the temperature at which water boils, with the difference between these two extremes of 180 °F.

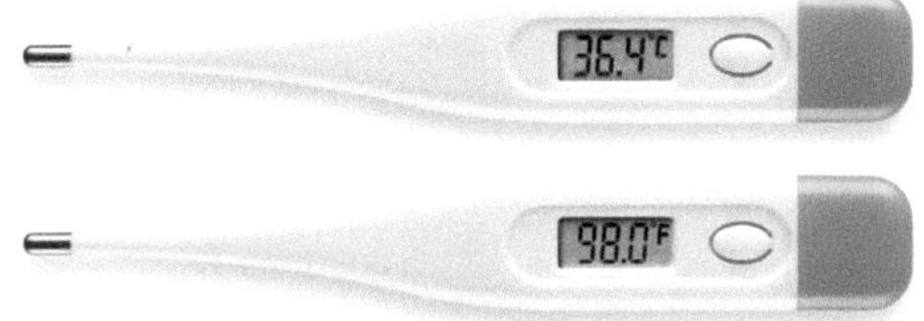

Pharmacy technicians may be asked to help patients convert between temperature readings in degrees Celsius and Fahrenheit. This calculation must be done carefully. Some thermometers display both.

In contrast, the **Celsius temperature scale** is commonly used in Europe and internationally in science. In 1742, the Swedish astronomer Anders Celsius proposed a thermometer scale with a difference of 100 degrees between freezing and boiling. He designated the freezing point of pure water at sea level to be zero degrees (0 °C), the boiling point to be 100 °C, and all things to be measured in 100 equal increments within that temperature span, and in equal increments above and below it. Celsius is the scale generally used in pharmacy and medicine. Many thermometers show both Celsius and Fahrenheit.

For Good Measure

The conversion from Celsius to Fahrenheit uses multiplication and addition. The Fahrenheit to Celsius equation uses division and subtraction.

An understanding of the Fahrenheit and Celsius temperature scales is important to the proper storage of medications. Maintaining refrigerator and freezer equipment at their appropriate temperatures is an important responsibility. Technicians monitor the refrigerators and document the temperatures once or twice daily, depending on their pharmacy's protocol. Most refrigerators in the pharmacy need to maintain a temperature of 2 °C to 8 °C. Technicians can find the storage temperature requirements for each drug in Celsius on the manufacturers' drug package inserts. In addition, technicians have the responsibility of monitoring and documenting the temperature conditions of the freezer medications. In the hospital, they may need to also monitor the refrigerated medications on each nursing unit.

A temperature log documents the refrigerator and freezer temperatures on a daily basis. Currently, the temperature logs in most pharmacies document to the tenth place for accuracy. If the log does not require a decimal, the temperature should be rounded off.

As a pharmacy technician, you must be able to perform conversions between the Celsius and the Fahrenheit scales. Table 6.4 shows the temperature equivalencies between these two scales. As you can see, every 5 °C change in temperature is equivalent to a 9 °F change.

In addition to using this chart, there are several mathematical methods of converting from Fahrenheit to Celsius and vice versa. If you begin with a Fahrenheit measurement and are converting to a Celsius measurement, you can use the following equation.

$$(°F - 32°) \div 1.8 = y°C$$

If you begin with a Celsius reading and are converting to Fahrenheit, use the following equation.

$$(°C \times 1.8) + 32° = z°F$$

TABLE 6.4 Temperature Equivalencies between Celsius and Fahrenheit

Celsius	Fahrenheit
0°C	32°F
5°C	41°F
10°C	50°F
15°C	59°F
20°C	68°F

Example 12

Convert 70°F to degrees Celsius using this equation: (°F – 32°) ÷ 1.8 = z°C.

Step 1 $(70°F - 32°) \div 1.8 = z°C$

Step 2 $38° \div 1.8 = 21.1°C$

Step 3 21.1°C, rounded down to 21°C, so 70°F = approximately 21°C.

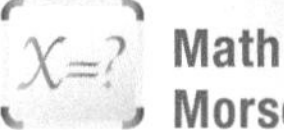

Math Morsel

An alternative method of conversion between Fahrenheit and Celsius uses the following algebraic equation: $°F \times 5 = °C \times 9 + 160$.

Example 13

Convert 30°C to degrees Fahrenheit using this equation: (°C × 1.8) + 32° = z°F.

Step 1 $(30°C \times 1.8) + 32° = z°F$

Step 2 $54° + 32° = 86°F$, so 30°C = 86°F.

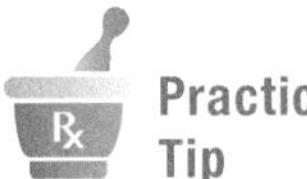

Practice Tip

Be sure to become proficient at temperature conversions. It is almost guaranteed that there will be at least one question on the certification exam! Remember the refrigerated temperature of 2–8° C is equal to 36–46° F—the storage of many medications including insulin.

Example 14

According to the Enbrel package insert, the manufacturer requires that a syringe of this expensive biotechnology drug must be stored at a temperature of 2° to 8°C. What should the range of the Fahrenheit temperature setting be on the thermostat in the refrigerator?

Step 1 Convert the degrees Celsius at the low end of the range using this equation: $(°C \times 1.8) + 32° = z°F$.

$$(2°C \times 1.8) + 32° = z°F$$
$$3.6° + 32° = 35.6°F$$
$$2°C = 35.6°F\text{, rounded up to } 36°F.$$

Step 2 Convert the degrees Celsius at the high end of the range using this equation: $(°C \times 1.8) + 32° = z°F$.

$$(8°C \times 1.8) + 32° = z°F$$
$$14.4° + 32° = 46.4°F$$
$$8°C = 46.4°F\text{, rounded down to } 46°F \text{ (depending on the device).}$$

The pharmacy technician should be sure that the thermostat setting in the refrigerator is between 36° and 46°F.

Example 15

An anxious parent telephones the pharmacy on a Saturday night. Their six-month-old child has a fever. The only thermometer they have records a temperature of 38.5°C. Their pediatrician told them to call if the child's temperature reached 101°F. What is the child's temperature in degrees Fahrenheit? Should the parent call the pediatrician?

Step 1 Use this equation: $(°C \times 1.8) + 32° = z°F$
$(38.5°C \times 1.8) + 32° = z°F$

Step 2 $69.3° + 32° = 101.3°F$; $38.5°C = 101.3°F$, rounded down to 101°F. Therefore, the parent should call the child's pediatrician.

6.5 Traditional Systems for Measuring Distance, Weight, and Volume

Three common measurement systems used to be applied in pharmacy—the avoirdupois system, the apothecary system, and the household system. However, because of safety issues, they have been replaced by the more scientific and universal metric system. It is, however, important to know about the other systems and how they relate to the metric system—the official pharmacy measurement system.

Grain and gram can be easily mixed up, resulting in medication errors. So be careful with medication orders with these abbreviations! *Metric should be used instead of alternates.*

The US Systems: Avoirdupois and Imperial Systems

Like languages, measurement systems often evolve by folk processes. For example, a foot as a measurement was originally equal to the length of an average man's foot. It grew out of traditions in France and is known as the **avoirdupois system**. This system, still used in the United States, has 12 inches to 1 foot and 3 feet to 1 yard. The changing set of proportions from 12 to 1, then to 3 to 1 makes it difficult to convert different measurements as they go up or down in amount. The British used part of the avoirdupois system along with nautical miles, fluid ounces, drams, pints, quarts, and gallons, plus grains, pounds, stones, and tons. They called their combined system the **imperial system** (or the British imperial system). This system, for the most part, was used in the pharmacies of the American colonies but is no longer used.

The Apothecary System

Another system the British imperial and American systems used was the **apothecary system.** One of the oldest systems of measurement, it is based on the Roman systems of weights. Stones, seeds, and grains were used as reference points for the weights; filled gourds and other containers were utilized for volume (evolving into grains, pounds, and ounces). The system also included the fluid dram (approximately equivalent to 3.75 mL) and the scruple (roughly equivalent to 1.3 g). The apothecary system has been generally replaced by the metric system.

One unit in the apothecary system still sometimes used in pharmacy is the **grain (gr)**, a dry weight measure. A common example can be seen in aspirin and acetaminophen products, which are sometimes labeled as 5 gr, an amount approximately equivalent to 325 mg (since 1 gr = 65 mg).

To confuse matters, 1 gr could also be equal to 60 mg (as in codeine) and 64.8 mg (as in phenobarbital). Often the differences depend on whether the drug is synthetic, is semisynthetic, or comes from a natural source. Some drug stock labels will reflect both units of measurement (see phenobarbital to the left). Because of such confusion, the grain is not a safe measurement to use.

Other units of measurement established by the apothecary system include the pint, quart, gallon, ounce, and pound—all of which have survived over the centuries (with changes to their equivalencies). However, with very few exceptions, these measurements are not used in general pharmacy practice today and can also lead to medication errors if put into practice. (See Table 6.9 in the conversion section to see how some of these measurements compare to the metric system.)

NDC 0603-5166-32
Tablets / 32.4 mg (1/2 gr)

Phenobarbital

1,000 Tablets

Rx only

Because the size of a grain can vary from drug to drug, avoid using it in measurements.

The Household System

The **household system** of measurement is based on the apothecary system and was established to help patients take their medications at home: the drop, teaspoon, tablespoon, and cup. Like the apothecary and avoirdupois systems, this system includes the quart, ounce, and pound but also several liquid units (see Table 6.5). As some OTC medications still use the household system of teaspoons and tablespoons for dosages, it's important to be aware before dispensing if a medication is using the household system or the more common metric system. (See Table 6.8 later in this chapter for an overview of the metric measurements.)

TABLE 6.5 Common Household English (US) Measurements

Weights	Liquid Volumes
1 pound = 16 ounces	1 gallon = 4 quarts 1 quart = 2 pints 1 pint = 2 cups 1 cup = 8 fluid ounces 1 tablespoon = 3 teaspoons 2 tablespoons = 1 fluid ounce

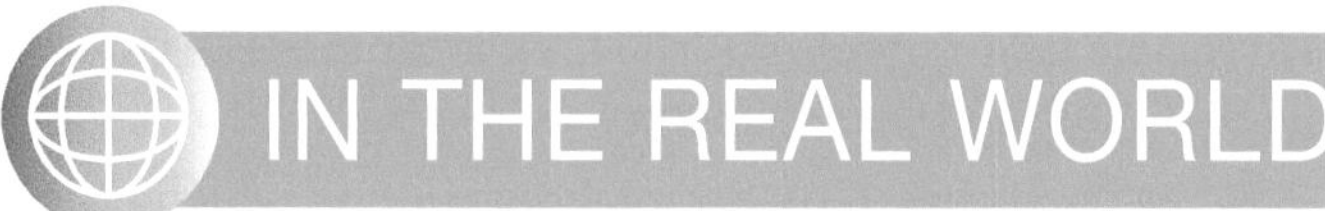

For years, most dosing cups listed fluid ounces on one side and drams on the other. Numerous errors occurred as nurses assumed that the dram measurement lines were for milliliters, because the writing on the cups was difficult to read. In one case reported to the National Medication Errors Reporting System, the nurse offered a hospice patient 1 fluid dram of a 100 mg/5 mL morphine sulfate medication instead of the 1 mL in the prescription. The dose was more than three-and-a-half times the correct amount. In another case, a nurse gave 5 fluid drams of a 100 mg/1 mL solution of acetaminophen, thinking that it was 5 mL or 500 mg. The dose turned out to be 18.45 mL, or 1,845 g, almost four times the correct amount!

Because of errors like these, in June 2015 a call for the elimination of all dosage cups with drams and a complete use of the metric system was requested from numerous health and pharmacy organizations–including the Institute for Safe Medication Practices, American Academy of Pediatrics, American Society of Health-System Pharmacists, Centers for Disease Control and Prevention, Consumer Healthcare Products Association, American Pharmacists Association, US Pharmacopeial Convention, and National Council for Prescription Drug Programs.

6.6 Pharmaceutical Measuring: The Metric System

Safety Alert

An error of a single decimal place is an error by a factor of 10 and can have tragic results if not noticed.

All those early common measurement systems were inconsistent and imprecise. Depending on which system was being used, practitioners were dispensing widely differing doses. For example, a pound in the apothecary system is equivalent to 12 ounces, whereas a pound in the avoirdupois and household systems is equivalent to 16 ounces. An apothecary ounce is 31.1 g, but an avoirdupois ounce is 28.35 g. These discrepancies led to many medication errors.

Consequently, a standardized system was needed. The metric system was developed in France in the 1700s, and, by 1893, the United States designated it as the legal standard of pharmacy measurement. It is the international measuring system in pharmacy and other sciences, as it is the safest, most standard, most accurate, and easiest for conversions.

The **metric system** is based on multiples of ten, one hundred, and one thousand. Three basic units in the metric system are the meter (length and cubic volume), liter (fluid volume), and gram (mass/weight) as seen in Table 6.6.

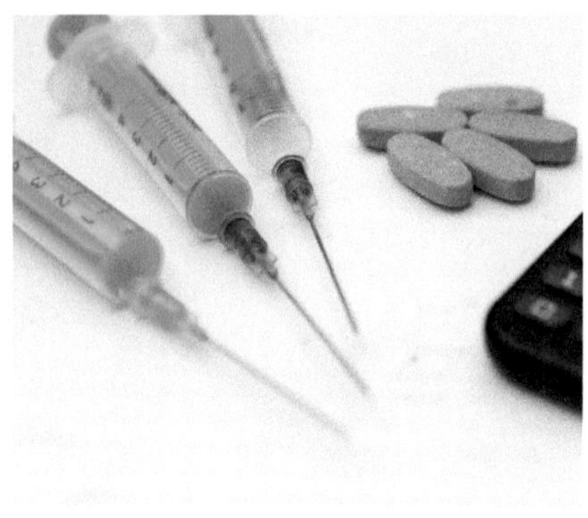

Injectable drugs in the hospital or oral dosage forms in the community pharmacy are prepared using the metric system. Calculators are used by technicians for accurate preparations, dosages, and conversions.

The Benefits of the Metric System

The metric system has several distinct advantages over other measurement systems.

- The metric system contains clear proportional correlations among the differing units of measurement of length, volume, and weight, which simplifies calculations. For example, the standard metric unit for volume, the liter, is almost exactly equivalent to 1,000 cubic centimeters, as seen in Table 6.6.
- The metric system is based on decimal notation in which units are described as multiples of 10 (0.001, 0.01, 0.1, 1, 10, 100, 1,000). This decimal notation also makes calculations easier.
- With slight variations in notation, the metric system is used worldwide, especially in scientific measurement, and therefore, like music notation, can be considered a "universal language."

TABLE 6.6 Common Metric Units

Measurement Unit	Equivalent
Length: Meter	
1 meter (m)	100 centimeters (cm)
1 centimeter (cm)	0.01 meter (m); 10 millimeters (mm)
1 millimeter (mm)	0.001 meter (m); 1,000 micrometers or microns (mcm)
Volume: Liter	
1 liter (L)	1,000 milliliters (mL); 1,000 cubic centimeters (cc)
1 milliliter (mL)	0.001 liter (L); 1,000 microliters (mcL)
Weight: Gram	
1 gram (g)	1,000 milligrams (mg)
1 milligram (mg)	0.001 grams (g); 1,000 micrograms (mcg)
1 kilogram (kg)	1,000 grams (g)

Applying Metric Units

The most commonly used metric units for pharmacy are applied to measuring liquid volumes in liters and mass/weight in grams. Meters are rarely used, but it is important to understand how they relate to the rest of the metric system. (Outside of the pharmacy, the common metric measurements used are a meter for length/distance as in kilometers for a running race; liters for measuring liquids as in 2 L bottles of juice or soda; grams for the weight of bags of sugar or flour.)

For Good Measure

The cubic centimeter (cc) is the one metric measurement being phased out in pharmacy practice because it can cause confusion and errors; sometimes it looks like two extra zeros. It is being replaced by liter measurements: 1 cc of volume is approximately equal to 1 mL of liquid volume, which is one-thousandth of a liter.

Meters

The **meter** is used not only in measuring distance, but also area and volume. Distance is measured by a single length, whereas area is two-dimensional flat space measured by two lengths multiplied (length and width); and volume, which is three-dimensional space, is measured by three lengths multiplied (length, height, depth—or width—resulting in cubic meters and cubic centimeters [abbreviated as cc]).

Liters

The **liter** (L) is the base unit of measurement for the volume of liquid medications for oral and parenteral solutions. It is often broken down into smaller units: the milliliter (mL), or one thousandth of a liter, and microliter (mcL), or one millionth of a liter. For example, you may fill a prescription for an antibiotic for administration of 4 mL by mouth every 12 hours for 10 days. In the hospital or home healthcare setting, you could prepare a solution of 1 g antibiotic cefazolin in a 50 mL sterile saline IV solution to be administered over 30 minutes.

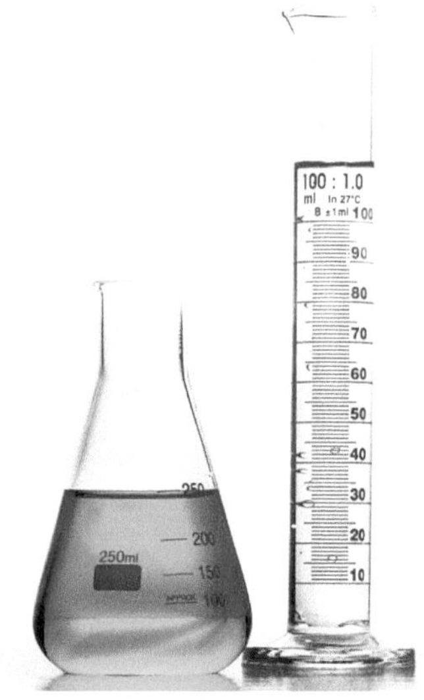

Pharmaceutical volumes are usually expressed in milliliters. To measure nonsterile liquids, volumetric flasks of varying sizes are used, such as those pictured here.

Grams

The **gram** is the weight of 1 cubic centimeter of water at 4 °C. It used in pharmacy for:

- measuring the weight of the amount of medication in a solid dosage form
- indicating the amount of solid medication in a solution
- expressing the weight of a patient or in a counterbalance measuring weight

Pharmaceutical dosages are commonly expressed in grams (g) or milligrams (mg). For example, you may fill a prescription for 1 g tablet per day of the anti-ulcer medication sucralfate or prepare a 600 mg antibiotic suspension of amoxicillin/clavulanate to be reconstituted or mixed with 5 mL sterile water.

For Good Measure

Some students remember the order of metric prefixes by remembering the first letters of the phrase: *King Henry Died By Drinking Chocolate Milk, MOOOOOO*!

Standard Proportional Prefixes

As explained, these different metric units of measurement come in powers of ten. Prefixes, or syllables placed at the beginnings of words, are added to the names of the basic metric units to specify a particular size of unit measure, such that *milli-* (meaning 1,000) can be added to *liter* to form a new unit milliliter or one-thousandth of a liter.

The set of standardized metric prefixes based on powers of 10 is called the Système International (SI)—(see Table 6.7). Each of these metric units has its own abbreviation, which is the same for both single and plural measurements (for example, 1 mL, 3 mL; 1 g, 3 g). Each prefix is affixed to a basic unit of measurement, such as a liter, meter, or gram. In contemporary pharmacy, the prefixes *centi-*, *deca-*, *deci-*, and *hecto-* are rarely *if ever* used. (You can see how the abbreviations for *deca* and *deci* could easily be mixed up, resulting in a difference of a 100 times!) In prescriptions with metric numbers, decimals are used rather than fractions.

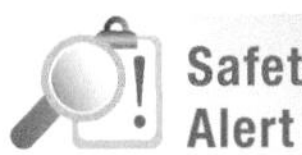

Safety Alert

To avoid dangerous mixups, *deca-* and *deci-* are prefixes not being used in pharmacy practice. *Hecto-* is rare too.

TABLE 6.7 **Système International Prefixes**

Prefix	Symbol	Meaning
kilo-	k	one thousand times (basic unit × 103, or unit × 1,000)
*hecto-**	h	one hundred times (basic unit × 102, or unit × 100)
*deca-**	da	ten times (basic unit × 10)
no prefix (*liter, gram,* or *meter*)	L, g, or m	base unit
*deci-**	d	one-tenth (basic unit × 10–1, or unit × 0.1)
*centi-**	c	one-hundredth (basic unit × 10–2, or unit × 0.01)
milli-	m	one-thousandth (basic unit × 10–3, or unit × 0.001)
micro-	mc or μ	one-millionth (basic unit × 10–6, or unit × 0.000001)

* These units are generally not used in pharmacy.

Practice Tip

See the link below for a video with easy-to-learn stair-step conversions of kilograms, grams, milligrams, and micrograms: https://PharmPractice7e.ParadigmEducation.com/MetricConversion.

Converting to Proportionally Larger or Smaller Units

The most common calculations in pharmacy involve conversions up to higher proportional amounts and down to lower ones using milligrams, grams, and kilograms, or milliliters and liters. Multiplying or dividing by 1,000 takes you up and down the unit steps. After properly doing your calculations, you end up moving the decimal point positions to the left to convert to larger units or to the right to convert to smaller units. Figure 6.3 and Table 6.8 show how these conversions work. To double-check your calculated conversions, count the correct decimal places to the right or left.

Note that an error of a single decimal place is an error by a factor of 10. Therefore, you must exercise due diligence when recording, interpreting, transcribing, and measuring medication dosages containing metric decimals, because even minor errors can lead to serious medication errors. As noted earlier, for numbers less than one (1), a leading x or a zero (0) must be placed before the decimal point to prevent misreading, as in digoxin X .25 or 0.25 mg.

FIGURE 6.3 **Steps Worth a Thousand**

Metric units of measurement go up and down by steps of 1,000. Remember each step is separated by three decimal places, by a power of one thousand. To go to smaller measurements, move from left to right. For larger ones, move from right to left.

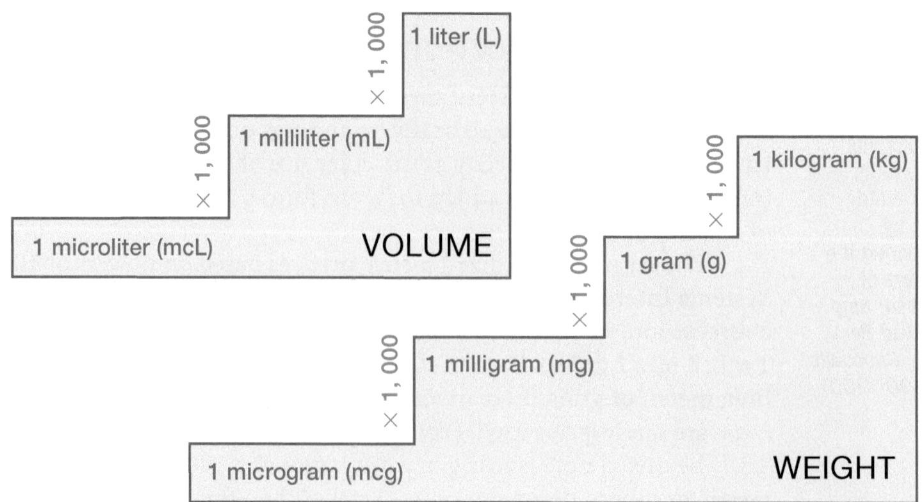

TABLE 6.8 **Common Metric Conversions**

Conversion	Instruction	Example
kilograms (kg) to grams (g)	multiply by 1,000 (*move decimal point three places to the right*)	6.25 kg = 6,250 g
grams (g) to milligrams (mg)	multiply by 1,000 (*move decimal point three places to the right*)	3.56 g = 3,560 mg
milligrams (mg) to grams (g)	multiply by 0.001 (*move decimal point three places to the left*)	120 mg = 0.120 g
liters (L) to milliliters (mL)	multiply by 1,000 (*move decimal point three places to the right*)	2.5 L = 2,500 mL
milliliters (mL) to liters (L)	multiply by 0.001 (*move decimal point three places to the left*)	238 mL = 0.238 L
microliters (μL or mcL) to milliliters (mL)	multiply by 1,000 (*move decimal point three places to the left*)	1,000 μL or mcL = 1 mL

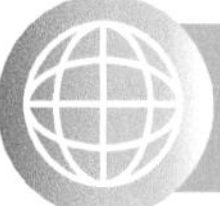

IN THE REAL WORLD

A 42-year-old patient with breast cancer in Florida was given a good prognosis as she was responding well to chemotherapy. Her doctor prescribed warfarin, a blood thinner, due to a high risk of blood clots. The uncertified technician typed in 10 mg instead of 1 mg. Unfortunately, the inaccurate prescription (with a tenfold dosage error) was filled and dispensed, and the mother of three experienced a brain bleed; she suffered a stroke and fell into a coma after 23 days of treatment.

Once out of the coma, she had to relearn to eat, talk, walk, and do other tasks. Sadly, she was too weak to continue her cancer treatments, and she died four-and-a-half years after taking her prescription. The civil court decision required the pharmacy to pay $25.8 million dollars to the bereaved family. The chain pharmacy appealed and lost the case, with the court awarding the family $33 million.

6.7 Converting Other Systems to Metrics

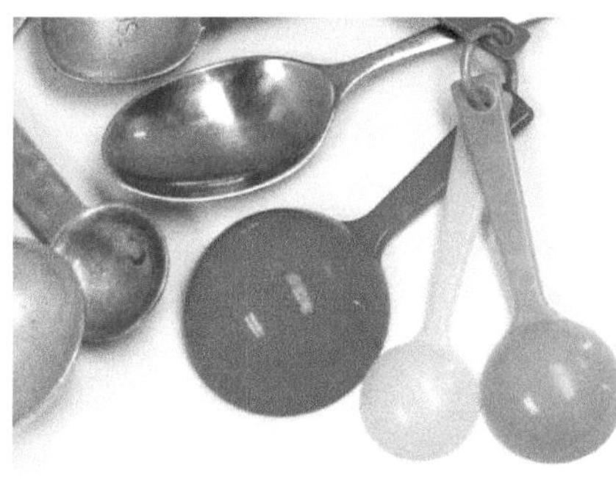

The volume held by a household teaspoon may vary, which is why it is not used for pharmaceutical measurements, but a true teaspoon equals 5 mL.

Due to safety reasons, the avoirdupois and apothecary systems have been almost completely phased out. However, occcasionally home dosage or medication orders are written in the household system. To convert any other system to metrics, first convert the units into decimals, and then apply the conversion amounts listed in Table 6.9.

Rounding Off Decimal Conversions

To simplify and standardize conversions, pharmacy practice rounds the conversion rates up or down. For example, when converting from fluid ounces to milliliters, it is common practice to round 29.57 mL to 30 mL, as has been explained earlier. But remember, the discrepancy becomes much larger when measuring large amounts of fluid ounces and rounding them off.

Consider the situation when converting a household pint (16 fl oz). When you multiply the rounded-off 30 mL by 16, it equals 480 mL. This calculation becomes problematic because the more exact 29.57 mL multiplied by 16 is equal to only 473.12 mL—a difference of almost 7 mL! However, bottled solutions are often put in 8 or 16 fl oz containers and usually dosed out in 30 mL increments. So you may use the rounded 30 mL value for a fluid ounce and the rounded 480 mL for a pint when performing pharmacy calculations for this chapter.

Another calculation problem can occur with the ounce. The apothecary ounce is a weight measure and not a liquid measure. The ounce unit has been rounded down (from 31.1 g to 30 g) in the apothecary system and rounded up (from 28.35 g to 30 g) in the avoirdupois system, so they both use 30 g. Today, some physicians still occasionally write prescription orders for liquid dosage forms in ounces.

As explained earlier, the grain unit also poses accuracy and safety problems and has different conversion rates. Most pharmacists consider 1 gr to be equal to 65 mg, but manufacturers often use a 60 mg conversion for 1 gr. In most cases, this difference in measurement is not clinically significant. However, for premature infants and neonates, precise calculations and uniform measurements must be used.

While slight differences in metric conversions do exist, the use of standardized metric equivalents aid greatly in accurate medication dosing and safe patient care. Pharmacy technicians should confer with the pharmacist if in doubt about any conversions to metric equivalents to ensure that the correct conversion rate is selected.

TABLE 6.9 Household and Avoirdupois/Apothecary Measurements

Measurement Unit		Equivalent within System	Metric Equivalent
Avoirdupois System			
	1 gr (grain)	–	65 mg
	1 oz (ounce)	437.5 gr	30 g (28.35 g)*
	1 lb (pound)	16 oz or 7,000 gr	454 g
Household System			
Volume	1 tsp (teaspoon)	–	5 mL
	1 tbsp (tablespoon)	3 tsp	15 mL
	1 fl oz (fluid ounce)	2 tbsp	30 mL (29.57 mL)**
	1 cup	8 fl oz	240 mL
	1 pt (pint)	2 cups	480 mL
	1 qt (quart)	2 pt	960 mL
	1 gal (gallon)	4 qt	3,840 mL
Weight	1 oz (ounce)	–	30 g
	1 lb (pound)	–	454 g
	2.2 lb	–	1 kg

* An avoirdupois ounce actually contains 28.34952 g; however, that number is usually rounded up to 30 g. It is common practice to use 454 g as the equivalent for a pound.

** In reality, 1 fl oz (household measure) contains less than 30 mL; however, 30 mL is usually used. When packaging a pint, companies will typically present 473 mL rather than the full 480 mL, thus saving money over time.

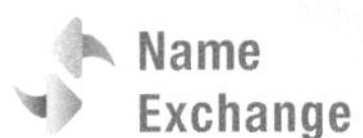

Name Exchange

Dimensional analysis calculation is also known as *unit cancellation* because it cancels out the measuring units of the known dimensions. The method is also called calculation by cancellation, unit label method, or factor label method.

Using Unit Cancellation to Calculate Conversions

When converting to measurement units of different dimensions (time, temperature, volume), you will often use a process known as **dimensional analysis calculation**. This is a very intimidating name for a very simple process that uses techniques *you already know*: multiplying by fractions of one and canceling elements out that balance each other. In fact, dimensional analysis is often considered an accurate shortcut, cutting out extra steps to get to the same end.

You already know that if you multiply anything by 1, the amount stays the same. So if you are trying to convert pounds into kilograms, you multiply the pounds by a fraction that represents one as the single unit of 1 kg/2.2 lbs.

In dimensional analysis, you must set up the problems so that the starting units cancel one another out and you are left with the desired units. This is why dimensional analysis is also called "unit cancellation" or calculation by cancellation.

$$\text{starting units} \times \frac{\text{desired units}}{\text{starting units}} = \text{desired units}$$

Using dimensional analysis, calculate the number of minutes in one hour. The desired units (the units you want to find) are minutes and the starting units (the units you are given) are hours.

$$1\ \cancel{\text{hour}} \times \frac{60\ \text{minutes}}{1\ \cancel{\text{hour}}} = 60\ \text{minutes}$$

The starting units of hours are canceled out and leave the desired units as minutes.

Example 16

Consider you have the following prescription.

℞ Acetaminophen 400 mg

However, the stock bottle measures the drug only in grains. How many grains of acetaminophen are prescribed?

Step 1 Look up the conversion rate for grains to milligrams. Table 6.9 shows the conversion rate is 1 gr = 65 mg. Set up your equation so that the starting units cancel out (in this example, milligrams).

$$400\ \cancel{\text{mg}} \times \frac{1\ \text{gr}}{65\ \cancel{\text{mg}}} = 6.1538\ \text{gr}$$

Step 2 Round this down to the nearest whole number as grains cannot be split. This means 6 gr should be measured and used in the prescription. If you have tablets of 3 gr each, you will need two tablets per dose.

The conversion above could also have been done as a ratio and proportion equation using the butterfly technique of multiplying the means and extremes and then cancelling measurement units to come up with the same answer. You could have written the first equation as a proportion and gone from there:

$$\frac{y\ \text{gr}}{400\ \text{mg}} = \frac{1\ \text{gr}}{65\ \text{mg}};\ \text{so}\ y\ \text{gr} \times 65\ \text{mg} = 400\ \text{mg} \times 1\ \text{gr}$$

$$y \text{ gr} = \frac{400 \cancel{\text{mg}} \times 1 \text{ gr}}{65 \cancel{\text{mg}}} = 6.1538 \text{ gr; rounded to } 6 \text{ gr}$$

In conversions, you can use the ratio and proportion approach to check the dimensional analysis answer and vice versa.

Practice Tip

The oral dosage forms for nitroglycerin often come in proportions of $^1/_{200}$ gr, $^1/_{150}$ gr, and $^1/_{100}$ gr.

Example 17

You are to dispense 300 mL of a liquid preparation. If the medication amount (the dose) is 2 tsp, how many doses will there be in the final preparation?

Step 1 Begin setting up this problem with all the known information and the conversion value in Table 6.9, which is 1 tsp = 5 mL.

$$1 \text{ dose} = 2 \text{ tsp} \times \frac{5 \text{ mL}}{1 \text{ tsp}} = 10 \text{ mL}$$

Step 2 In simple math, you ask how many times does 10 mL go into 300 mL? Take 300 mL and divide by 10 mL per dose for y doses to come up with 30 doses.

You can also complete this calculation using dimensional analysis, either in one step or multiple steps. Both examples are shown below.

One-step method:

$$300 \text{ mL} \times \frac{1 \text{ tsp}}{5 \text{ mL}} \times \frac{1 \text{ dose}}{2 \text{ tsp}} = 30 \text{ doses}$$

Multiple-step method:

Step 1 Calculate the number of milliliters per dose.

$$\frac{2 \text{ tsp}}{1 \text{ dose}} \times \frac{5 \text{ mL}}{1 \text{ tsp}} = \frac{10 \text{ mL}}{1 \text{ dose}}$$

Step 2 Calculate the number of doses in 300 mL.

$$300 \text{ mL} \times \frac{1 \text{ dose}}{10 \text{ mL}} = 30 \text{ doses}$$

Example 18

A patient receives the following prescription.

℞ **60 mL of medication in prefilled hypodermic syringes**

There are 3 L of the solution available. How many hypodermic syringes can be filled with the available solution?

You can figure this out using dimensional analysis in either one or multiple steps.

One-step method:

$$3\,\cancel{L} \times \frac{1{,}000\,\cancel{mL}}{1\,\cancel{L}} \times \frac{1\text{ syringe}}{60\,\cancel{mL}} = 50\text{ syringes}$$

Multiple-step method:

Step 1 Convert 3 L to milliliters.

$$3\,\cancel{L} \times \frac{1{,}000\text{ mL}}{1\,\cancel{L}} = 3{,}000\text{ mL}$$

Step 2 Use the calculated volume to determine the number of doses.

$$3{,}000\,\cancel{mL} \times \frac{1\text{ syringe}}{60\,\cancel{mL}} = 50\text{ syringes}$$

Example 19

A physician prescribes the following order.

℞ **0.8 mg of nitroglycerin**

The available supply has tablets containing 1/150 gr nitroglycerin. How many tablets should be given to the patient?

You can figure this out using dimensional analysis in either one or multiple steps. Table 6.9 says 1 gr = 65 mg. Remember we are told that 1 tablet = $^1/_{150}$ gr. It is easiest to approach this problem by calculating $^1/_{150}$ gr.

$$1\text{ tablet} = \frac{1}{150}\text{ gr} = 0.0067\text{ gr}$$

One-step method:

$$0.8\,\cancel{mg} \times \frac{1\,\cancel{gr}}{65\,\cancel{mg}} \times \frac{1\text{ tablet}}{0.0067\,\cancel{gr}} = 1.83\text{ tablets, rounded up to 2 tablets}$$

Multiple-step method:

Step 1 Calculate the number of grains in 0.8 mg.

$$0.8\,\cancel{mg} \times \frac{1\text{ gr}}{65\,\cancel{mg}} = 0.0123\text{ gr}$$

Step 2 Convert 0.0123 gr to tablets.

$$0.0123\,\cancel{gr} \times \frac{1\text{ tablet}}{0.0067\,\cancel{gr}} = 1.84\text{ tablets, rounded up to 2 tablets}$$

Remember, when multiplying with equivalent ratio fractions to solve medication-dosing problems, both numerators must be in the same units and both denominators must be in the same units. For example, in oral medications, the active ingredient is usually expressed in milligrams (mg), and the solution is expressed in milliliters (mL).

Incorrect: $\frac{1.5 \text{ g}}{100 \text{ mL}} = \frac{400 \text{ mg}}{y \text{ mL}}$

Correct: Convert the grams to milligrams: 1.5 g × 1,000 = 1,500 mg and then simplify.

$\frac{\textbf{1500 mg}}{\textbf{100 mL}} = \frac{\textbf{400 mg}}{y \textbf{ mL}}$ You can then use the butterfly technique.

$15y \textbf{ mL} = \textbf{400 mL}$; then $y \text{ mL} = \frac{400}{15} = 26.666...$ rounded to 26.7 mL

6.8 Calculating Dosages Using Equal Proportion Equations

As has been explained, multiplying of extremes and means in equal proportion equations can be used to discover missing pharmaceutical information and answer questions. Now that you have a firm sense of metrics and pharmaceutical measurement systems and conversions for time, temperature, weight, and volume, you can apply these skills on even more pharmaceutical examples (see Table 6.10).

TABLE 6.10 Rules to Remember for Equal Proportion Equations

- Three of the four values must be known.
- The numerators must have the same unit of measurement.
- The denominators must also have the same unit of measurement.

One of the most common calculations in pharmacy practice is that of determining the correct dosages to provide when using the specific drug concentrations of available stock. Setting up the equation correctly is essential to getting the correct answer. The term **ratio strength** in pharmacy refers to the concentration level of an active ingredient to the completed product or to the substance that holds it. In concentration ratios, the first number is the number of parts (numerator) of active ingredient compared to the whole total, which is the second number (denominator). The concentrations come in different formulations:

- A liquid solution or suspension with a dissolved ingredient (solute) is usually expressed as a concentration of solute weight to volume (w/v) of the dissolving liquid (solvent) of the final product. The w/v is usually expressed in grams/per milliliters (g/mL) or milligrams/per milliters (mg/mL).
- Liquid solutes are expressed as volume to volume (v/v)—the volume of the drug ingredient to the volume of the final solution with all ingredients. The v/v is usually expressed in milliliters/per milliliters (mL/mL) or microliters/per milliliters (mcL/mL).

- Solid or semisolid concentrations are expressed as weight to weight (w/w)—the weight of the drug ingredient compared to the weight of the total solid with all ingredients added. You will usually see grams/per grams (g/g).
- Solid drug products may be also divided into "units," which are like units of dosage or like "servings" of food.

Remembering these ratio rules of thumb will help you when you are looking at a prescription or medical order and are trying to decide how to set up your calculation ratios and fractions. Also, follow the drug directions for use. The available stock is usually labeled with the concentration ratio of an active ingredient in the w/v, v/v, or w/w ratios described earlier, which refers to the following:

$$\frac{\text{active ingredient (weight or volume)}}{\text{final product (weight or volume)}}$$

Practice Tip

If you are unsure how to set up an equation for filling a prescription or medical order, or for compounding, the directions on the label or package insert (PI) usually offer directions.

Calculating Dosages with Weight-in-Volume Concentration Ratios

In prescriptions with **weight-in-volume** concentrations, the final weight of the active ingredient to be administered in the dosage will be provided. The unknown quantity to be calculated is the amount of the correct concentration of stock drug product to achieve this desired dose.

$$\frac{\text{active ingredient (prescribed)}}{\text{final product volume (needed for administration)}}$$

To calculate the amount of stock solution/suspension needed, you must set the two ratios into a proportion equation:

$$\frac{\text{active ingredient (prescribed)}}{y\text{ product volume (needed)}} = \frac{\text{active ingredient weight (stock)}}{\text{solution volume (stock)}}$$

Or you can flip both sides to put the unknown on top, but it can be confusing, as it does not represent the units as stated in common pharmacy problems. It is better to have mg/mL than mL/mg even if the unknown y is in the denominator.

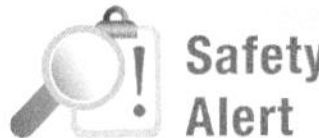

Safety Alert

Whenever you are calculating dosages with ratios, always make sure that the numerators have similar units of measurement, and the denominators have similar units. If not, first do the conversions, and then do your calculations.

Example 20

A prescription for a sick child is received from the emergency room on Saturday night.

℞ Amoxicillin/clavulanate 600 mg/5 mL for 4 mL po twice daily

No other pharmacies are open in town. The pharmacy technician discovers that the pharmacy is out of stock on the 600 mg/5 mL concentration of the prescribed suspension, but the 400 mg/5 mL concentration is in stock. The prescribed concentration could be ordered, but the child would be without medication until Monday at noon. Since the child needs 4 mL of the 600 mg/5 mL concentration, what is the amount of amoxicillin/clavulanate per dose?

How much of the 400 mg/5 mL stock concentration would be needed to make this individual dose?

Step 1 Calculate the original prescribed dose for the child.

$$y \text{ mg}/4 \text{ mL} = 600 \text{ mg}/5 \text{ mL} \quad \text{or} \quad \frac{y \text{ mg}}{4 \text{ mL}} = \frac{600 \text{ mg}}{5 \text{ mL}}$$

$$y \text{ mg} = \frac{600 \text{ mg} \times 4 \cancel{\text{mL}}}{5 \cancel{\text{mL}}} = 2{,}400 \text{ mg} \div 5 = 480 \text{ mg}$$

The amount of prescribed amoxicillin needed to be taken two times each day is 480 mg. How much would that be of a 400 mg/5 mL suspension?

Remember, if you are calculating the drug volume for an injectable or IV medication, do not include the volume (in milliliters [mL] or liters [L]) or strength (in percent [%]) of the stock base in equations. Select the correct base solution from the medical order but do not add its numbers to your equations.

Step 2 Calculate the volume (mL) of the available concentration of 400 mg/5 mL.

$$\frac{480 \text{ mg (prescribed)}}{y \text{ mL}} = \frac{400 \text{ mg (stock)}}{5 \text{ mL}}$$

$$400y \text{ mL} = 480 \text{ mg} \times 5 \text{ mL}$$

Step 3 Find the value of y by dividing each side by 400.

$$\frac{\cancel{400}y \text{ mg}}{\cancel{400} \text{ mg}} = \frac{480 \text{ g} \times 5 \text{ mL}}{400 \text{ mg}}$$

$$y \text{ mL} = \frac{2{,}400 \text{ mL}}{400} = 24 \text{ mL} \div 4 = 6 \text{ mL}$$

You can also solve this problem using dimensional analysis.

The calculated 6 mL dosage of the stock 400 mg/5 mL concentration of amoxicillin/clavulanate suspension is equal to the prescribed 4 mL dosage of the 600 mg/5 mL suspension. Consequently, the pharmacy fills the prescription and allows the sick child to begin treatment right away. The child will take this 6 mL twice a day.

Calculating Dosages with Volume-in-Volume Percent Ratios

Volume-in-volume (v/v) concentrations are usually expressed as a percentage of the active ingredient in milliliters (mL) per 100 mL. For example, the common disinfectant used in the hospital is 70% isopropyl alcohol (IPA), which is 70 mL of IPA for every 100 mL of sterile water solution—as seen below, which is a v/v equation.

Example 21

How many milliliters of isopropyl alcohol (IPA) are contained in an 8 fl oz bottle of 70% IPA?

Step 1 Rewrite 70% IPA as a volume-in-volume equivalent.

$$70\% \text{ IPA} = \frac{70 \text{ mL alcohol}}{100 \text{ mL solution}}$$

This means that 70% IPA is 70 mL alcohol in 100 mL of solution (70 mL alcohol/100 mL).

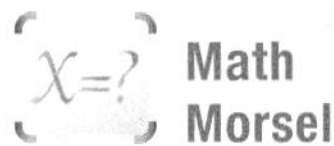

Remember that if a multiplier is on one side of an equation, you can keep the same values by transferring it to the other side by dividing and vice versa. You transfer a denominator from one side of an equation and turn it into a multiplier on the other.

Step 2 Set up a ratio and proportion to calculate the unknown amount of milliliters of IPA (y) in 8 fl oz of the 70% solution by using the conversion rate from Table 6.9 of 8 fl oz to 240 mL.

$$\frac{y \text{ mL alcohol}}{240 \text{ mL solution}} = \frac{70 \text{ mL alcohol}}{100 \text{ mL solution}}$$

Step 3 Use the butterfly technique of multiplying extremes and means.

$$100y \text{ mL} = 70 \text{ mL} \times 240$$
$$100y \text{ mL} = 16{,}800 \text{ mL}$$

Step 4 Solve for the value of y by transferring the multiplier of y to the other side of the equation as a denominator (to divide that side proportionally).

$$y \text{ mL} = \frac{16{,}800 \text{ mL}}{100} = 168 \text{ mL alcohol, the volume of IPA in 8 fl oz of solution.}$$

You can also solve this problem using dimensional analysis.

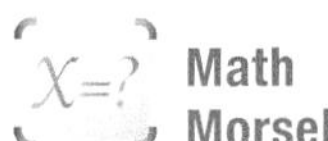

Many neonatal physicians and pharmacists are deeply concerned about adult therapeutic dosages calculated proportionally down directly for premature babies, newborns, and children without more adaptation and studies. To improve safety and reduce the number of calculations needed, a table that lists recommended neonatal doses for common drugs was published in the *Journal of Pediatric Pharmacology and Therapeutics* in 2014. It can be accessed at https://PharmPractice7e.ParadigmEducation.com.

Calculating Dosages with Weight-in-Weight Concentration Ratios

Ointments and creams commonly use a percentage **weight-in-weight (w/w)** concentration, which is defined as the weight of the active ingredient per 100 grams of the final drug formulation (cream or ointment). For example, a 2.5% hydrocortisone cream is equal to 2.5 grams of active ingredient (hydrocortisone) per 100 grams of cream.

Example 22

What would be the weight (in grams) of zinc oxide in 240 g of 40% zinc oxide ointment?

Step 1 Rewrite 40% zinc oxide as a weight-in-weight ratio.

$$40\% \text{ zinc oxide} = \frac{40 \text{ g zinc oxide}}{100 \text{ g ointment}}$$

Step 2 Set up a ratio and proportion to calculate the unknown value of zinc oxide (y) in 240 grams of the ointment.

$$\frac{y \text{ g zinc oxide}}{240 \text{ g ointment}} = \frac{40 \text{ g zinc oxide}}{100 \text{ g ointment}}$$

Step 4 Use the butterfly technique of multiplying extremes and means.

$$100y \text{ g} = 40 \text{ g} \times 240 \quad 100y \text{ g} = 9{,}600 \text{ g} \quad y \text{ g} = \frac{9600 \text{ g}}{100} = 96 \text{ g}$$

The weight of zinc oxide in 240 grams of ointment is 96 g.

You can also solve this problem using dimensional analysis.

Calculating Dosage Concentrations Based on Patient Weight

Dosages are often based on the patient's body weight in kilograms. Before determining the correct dosage of the existing concentrations, you must first convert the patient's weight from pounds to metric kilograms. As has been emphasized, most calculation dosage errors happen to neonates, infants, and children, so question the pharmacist or the prescriber about any prescription that would be in the normal range for adults but would not be in a safe range for children.

Example 23

For a serious infection in an 11-pound, 2-month-old infant, the hospital physician put in the following antibiotic order.

℞ **Ceftazidime, 50 mg IV per 1 kg of patient weight every 8 hours**

What is the total daily dose of IV ceftazidime for an 11-pound, 2-month-old infant?

Step 1 Convert pounds to kilograms. You can do this by dimensional analysis or ratio and proportion with butterfly multiplication, and both answers will be the same. The ratio and proportion method will be used in this example.

$$\frac{y \text{ kg}}{11 \text{ lb}} = \frac{1 \text{ kg}}{2.2 \text{ lb}}; \text{ then } 2.2y \text{ kg} = 11 \text{ k}$$

$$y \text{ kg} = 11 \text{ kg} \div 2.2 = 5 \text{ kg}$$

The patient weighs 5 kg.

Pharmacy personnel should remind parents or caregivers to use only the oral syringe provided with their child's product to administer the medication.

Step 2 Calculate the dose of the antibiotic based on the patient's weight using the ratio and proportion method. Please note this could also be solved using dimensional analysis.

$$\frac{y \text{ mg}}{5 \text{ kg}} = \frac{50 \text{ mg}}{1 \text{ kg}} \qquad y \text{ mg} = 5 \times 50 \text{ mg} = 250 \text{ mg per dose}$$

Step 3 Calculate the total daily dose. Since ceftazidime is given every 8 hours, which makes 3 doses in a 24-hour period (24 ÷ 8 = 3), the total daily dose is as follows:

3 doses per day × 250 mg per dose = 750 mg per day

Example 24

A parent visits your pharmacy on a Saturday night with a prescription for Infants' Tylenol for their 3-month-old daughter, who weighs 15 lb. The dose recommended is 10 mg/kg. The concentration of Infants' Tylenol is 160 mg/5 mL. What is the correct dose in milligrams (mg) and volume in milliliters (mL) that the mother should administer to their child?

This problem can be solved using the ratio and proportion method or dimensional analysis. Dimensional analysis will be used in this example. The one-step and multiple-step methods will be shown.

One-step method:

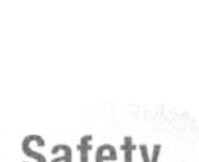
Safety Alert

Medication doses for premature infants, neonates, and pediatric patients may use two decimal places rather than just one if they are not rounded down.

Solve for the correct dose in milligrams.

$$15 \text{ lb} \times \frac{1 \text{ kg}}{2.2 \text{ lb}} \times \frac{10 \text{ mg}}{\text{kg}} = 68 \text{ mg}$$

Now solve for the correct dose in milliliters.

$$15 \text{ lb} \times \frac{1 \text{ kg}}{2.2 \text{ lb}} \times \frac{10 \text{ mg}}{1 \text{ kg}} \times \frac{5 \text{ mL}}{160 \text{ mg}} = 2.1 \text{ mL, rounded down to 2 mL}$$

Multiple-step method:

Step 1 Convert the patient's weight from pounds to kilograms.

$$15 \text{ lb} \times \frac{1 \text{ kg}}{2.2 \text{ lb}} = 6.8 \text{ kg}$$

Step 2 Using the patient's weight in kilograms, calculate the dose of Infants' Tylenol needed in milligrams.

$$6.8 \text{ kg} \times \frac{10 \text{ mg}}{1 \text{ kg}} = 68 \text{ mg}$$

Step 3 Convert the dose in milligrams to milliliters.

$$68 \text{ mg} \times \frac{5 \text{ mL}}{160 \text{ mg}} = 2.1 \text{ mL, rounded down to 2 mL}$$

The dose is 68 mg or 2 mL.

6.9 Advanced Calculations Used in Pharmacy Practice

As you will see, some pharmaceutical problems entail many complex steps or more advanced calculating concepts and skills. For instance, as a pharmacy technician, you may be asked to **compound** new solutions by combining measured amounts of different solutions of concentrated ingredients. This section will present some of these types of complex calculations. Other types of compounding require additional specialized knowledge or training and may be addressed in other chapters.

All require calculations practice, and this section is just an introductory overview to familiarize you with what you need to know before taking a course for further study. Because you need to understand both dimensional analysis and ratio and proportion, both techniques will be used for the advanced calculations, sometimes showing both options. This is not to confuse you, but to show that there are two options, and you can use one to double-check the other. Also, by knowing both, you understand the deeper principles of why they work.

Calculating Concentrations Based on Body Surface Area

For greater precision with particularly potent or toxic drugs, some dosages are based on body surface area instead of just weight. **Body surface area (BSA)** is a formulation of a patient's weight and height expressed as meters squared (m^2). (There are different medical formulas for arriving at the BSA.) Dosage prescriptions are then written as mg/m^2.

Many medications have a wide range for recommended dosages, because patients' body shapes, sizes, bodily responses, and adverse reactions vary extensively, even among adults. That is why physicians prescribing cancer chemotherapy drugs particularly use BSA. Typical BSA averages used in US pharmacy are male adult, 1.9 m^2; female adult, 1.6 m^2; 12–13 years, 1.33 m^2; 10 years, 1.14 m^2; 9 years, 1.07 m^2; 2 years, 0.5 m^2; newborn, 0.25 m^2. As is clear, these are very general averages, not entailing differences in the age of the adults or the gender of the youth.

An equal proportion formula for calculating a specific dosage by BSA is this:

$$\frac{y \text{ mg}}{\text{patient's m}^2} = \frac{\text{dose mg}}{1 \text{ m}^2}$$

Example 25

To treat the breast cancer of a patient with a BSA of 1.6 m^2, the oncologist writes the following prescription for.

℞ **Doxorubicin at a dose of 60 mg/m^2**

Doxorubicin is toxic to the blood cells and heart in excessive doses. What is the proper dose?

$$y \text{ mg}/1.6 \text{ m}^2 = 60 \text{ mg}/1 \text{ m}^2$$

$$\frac{y \text{ mg}}{1.6 \text{ m}^2} = \frac{60 \text{ mg}}{1 \cancel{\text{m}^2}}; \quad y \text{ mg} = 60 \text{ mg} \times 1.6$$

$$y \text{ mg} = 96 \text{ mg}$$

The prescribed dose of doxorubicin is thus 96 mg.

Most pediatric prescribers favor those medications that have been particularly formulated for pediatric doses. However, there are times when a medical order comes in for calculating a child's portion of an adult-use drug, so it is safer to prescribe using BSA instead of just weight. Remember to round down the dosage rather than up in pediatric patients for safety reasons.

Example 26

An adult patient with a BSA of 1.72 m^2 requires a dose of 12 mg of a given medication. The same medication needs to be given to a child in a smaller pediatric-size dose. The child has a BSA of 0.60 m^2. If the pediatric dose were proportionally smaller than this adult patient's dose, what would be this pediatric patient's dosage? Round off the final answer.

As noted, children's doses are often estimated with different proportional equations than adult dosages. However, if the child's dose is to be directly proportional, it is possible to use a simple ratio and proportion equation to answer this question:

$$\frac{\text{child's dose}}{\text{child's BSA}} = \frac{\text{adult dose}}{\text{adult BSA}}$$

$$\frac{y \text{ mg}}{0.6 \text{ m}^2} = \frac{12 \text{ mg}}{1.72 \text{ m}^2}$$

$$y \text{ mg} \times 1.72 = 0.6 \times 12 \text{ mg} \qquad 1.72y \text{ mg} = 7.2 \text{ mg} \qquad y \text{ mg} = \frac{7.2 \text{ mg}}{1.72 \text{ mg}}$$

$$y \text{ mg} = 4.186 \text{ mg, rounded to } 4 \text{ mg}$$

Because this dose is for a child, it is appropriate for safety reasons to round the dosage down to 4 mg rather than up to 4.2 mg.

Working with Dilutions

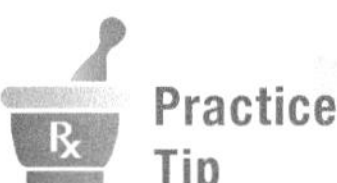

Practice Tip

Many medical scientists are finding that different age groups, especially in childhood ages, have different metabolism rates and organ effects. Some pediatric practices call for calculating dosages through additional formulas. That is why pediatric compounding is becoming a specialty for pharmacists and technicians.

Medications may be diluted for several reasons. They are sometimes diluted prior to administration to infants, children, and older adults to meet dosage requirements. Medications may also be diluted so that they can be measured more accurately and easily. For example, volumes less than 0.1 mL are usually considered too small to measure accurately. Therefore, they must be diluted first. Many pharmacies have a policy for tuberculin syringes that the injection should have a volume greater than 0.1 mL and less than 1 mL.

The pharmacist usually calculates the dilution amounts. However, the technicians double-check the answers to ensure accuracy. If there is a discrepancy, the technician brings the different answer to the pharmacist for the pharmacist to recalculate.

The following example demonstrates the method for solving typical dilution problems. The first step is to determine the sufficient volume of the final product needed to attain the prescribed drug strength. One must first establish the ratio of diluted solution strength to the desired strength. The second step is to determine the amount of diluent needed by subtracting the original amount of the solution from the total volume of the final diluted product. (Both of these small volumes are approximate because they depend on the calibration and accuracy of the measuring devices used.)

Although the second step uses subtraction to determine the amount of diluent needed, the diluent will actually be added to the original concentration. The abbreviation QS for "sufficient quantity" is used to describe the process of adding enough of the ingredient to reach the desired volume for sufficient active drug strength.

For Good Measure

An injected dose in a tuberculin syringe generally measures a volume greater than 0.1 mL but less than 1 mL.

Example 27

Dexamethasone sodium phosphate is available as a 4 mg/mL sterile preparation for injection. An infant is to receive 0.35 mg. The volume needed would be a miniscule 0.08 mL of the 4 mg/mL solution, which is very difficult to accurately measure. Prepare a dilution in a syringe or vial for a final concentration of 1 mg/mL.

How much sterile water diluent will you need to add? How much of the newly diluted solution will you need to draw into the syringe (or vial) for an accurate measurement of the 0.35 mg prescription?

Step 1 Determine the volume needed (in milliliters) of the final diluted product that will be mixed in a vial or syringe. The strength of the dexamethasone is currently 4 mg/mL, which means that every 1 mL has 4 mg of the drug. You want a final concentration of 1 mg/mL, so to have 4 mg of the medication at a 1:1 ratio, you will need to have 4 mg/4 mL. (This is a common pharmaceutical dilution concentration goal, since it makes it easy to determine the volume needed because of the

1:1 ratio.) This means that you will need 4 mL total volume of the final product, as shown below, using the ratio and proportion method.

Prescribed drug strength Desired concentration

$$\frac{y \text{ mL}}{4 \text{ mg}} = \frac{1 \text{ mL}}{1 \text{ mg}}$$

$$y \text{ mL} = \frac{4 \cancel{\text{mg}} \times 1 \text{ mL}}{1 \cancel{\text{mg}}} = 4 \text{ mL}$$

For Good Measure

When calculating dilutions for sterile compounding, check for the amount of "overfill" on the label. Manufacturers of IV solutions overfill them by a certain percentage to allow for evaporation. This will affect your dilutions. Different cleanrooms have different ways of handling overfill. This will be addressed in Chapter 13.

Step 2 Take the required volume (4 mL) and subtract from it the volume (1 mL) of the original 4 mg/mL prescribed solution to determine the volume of sterile water needed.

$$4 \text{ mL} - 1 \text{ mL} = 3 \text{ mL}$$

Therefore, an additional 3 mL of sterile water is needed to dilute the original 1 mL of the preparation to arrive at a final concentration of 1 mg/mL.

Step 3 Set up a dimension analysis equation to determine the volume of medication to be prepared from the diluted medication.

$$y \text{ mL} = 0.35 \cancel{\text{mg}} \times \frac{1 \text{ mL}}{1 \cancel{\text{mg}}}$$

$$y \text{ mL} = 0.35 \text{ mL}$$

This volume of 0.35 mL can be more accurately compared to original 0.08 mL, yet the same 0.35 mg drug strength will be administered.

IN THE REAL WORLD

In the neonatal intensive care unit of a major hospital, a microdilution of insulin was ordered for a newborn. The desired insulin was to be 1 mL per unit. The insulin required two dilutions to get into micro-dilutions, moving from:

$$\frac{100 \text{ units}}{1 \text{ mL}} + \text{dilution} = \frac{10 \text{ units}}{1 \text{ mL}} + \text{dilution} = \frac{1 \text{ unit}}{1 \text{ mL}}$$

The technician successfully did the first dilution but unfortunately either stopped there or mixed up the dilutions and drew the wrong solution for the patient's final dose. The pharmacist did not catch the error, and the patient received a tenfold dose of insulin. This resulted in serious complications for the infant.

Calculating Percent Weight-in-Volume for Dilution Levels

Injectable drugs and IV solutions are available in concentrations expressed in various percentages, and many IV solutions may be medically ordered as a percentage of active ingredient weight based on solution volume. **Weight-in-volume** is usually expressed as grams of the active ingredient per 100 milliliters of solution, as expressed by the following formula:

$$1\% = 1 \text{ g per } 100 \text{ mL}$$

Percent weight-in-volume is most commonly used in pharmacy practice. Premade preservative-free lidocaine, for instance, is available in 1% and 2% concentrations for intravenous use. To calculate dilution levels, you need to convert from percentages to fractions and from grams to milligrams of actual ingredient in a concentration. For instance:

Step 1 Convert from grams to milligrams.

$$1 \cancel{g} \times \frac{1{,}000 \text{ mg}}{1 \cancel{g}} = 1{,}000 \text{ mg}$$

$$1\% = 1{,}000 \text{ mg per } 100 \text{ mL}$$

Step 2 Simplify the proportion, eliminating powers of ten or equal numbers of zeros at the end of the numerator and the denominator.

$$\frac{1{,}0\cancel{00} \text{ mg}}{1\cancel{00} \text{ mL}} = 10 \text{ mg per } 1 \text{ mL}$$

Example 28

How much potassium chloride (in grams) is needed to prepare a 2% solution in 1 Liter of normal saline? Both the ratio and proportion method and dimensional analysis will be shown.

Using the ratio and proportion method:

Step 1: Rewrite 2% potassium chloride with the units of grams per milliliter. By definition, 2% potassium chloride is 2 g of potassium chloride per 100 mL of solution. Written as a fraction,

$$2\% \text{ potassium chloride} = \frac{2 \text{ g potassium chloride}}{100 \text{ mL solution}}$$

Step 2: To ensure the units in the numerator and denominator of both proportions are the same, convert 1 L to milliliters.

$$1 \text{ liter} = 1{,}000 \text{ mL}$$

Step 3: Set up the two equivalent ratios and solve for the unknown grams of potassium chloride and solve for the unknown grams per potassium chloride.

$$\frac{y \text{ g potassium chloride}}{1{,}000 \text{ mL solution}} = \frac{2 \text{ g potassium chloride}}{100 \text{ mL solution}}$$

$$y \text{ g potassium chloride} = 2 \text{ g potassium chloride} \times \frac{1{,}000 \text{ mL}}{100 \text{ mL}}$$

$$y \text{ g potassium chloride} = 20 \text{ g potassium chloride}$$

Dimensional analysis method:

$$1{,}000 \text{ mL solution} \times \frac{2 \text{ g potassium chloride}}{100 \text{ mL solution}} = 20 \text{ g}$$

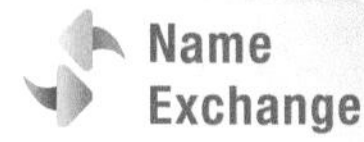

Name Exchange

Total volume (tv) can also be known as final volume (fv); diluent (dv) is also abbreviated (Dil).

Mixing Dry Powders and Dilution Rates

At times, you will need to do calculations with dry powdered forms of active ingredients. For example, parenteral products are often reconstituted by adding a diluent to a lyophilized or freeze-dried powder to prepare an IV solution. The product is commercially manufactured in powder form because of the instability of the drug in a solution over a long period. The active ingredient (the powder) is expressed in terms of weight, but it also occupies a certain amount of space, or volume. This space is referred to as **powder volume (pv)**. It is equal to the difference between the **total volume (tv)** of the final product and the volume of the diluting ingredient, or the **diluent volume (dv)**, as expressed in the following equations:

$$\text{total volume} = \text{powder volume} + \text{diluent volume} \quad [tv = pv + dv]$$

or

$$\text{powder volume} = \text{total volume} - \text{diluent volume} \quad [pv = tv - dv]$$

or

$$\text{diluent volume} = \text{total volume} - \text{powder volume} \; [dv = tv - pv]$$

Trying to keep the different aspects involved in a powder-reconstitution equation straight can be very confusing. It is important to break the information into pieces and use the form in Figure 6.4 to help you do the calculations correctly.

The weight of the powder drug is the amount that shall be added for the solution concentration. The space that the active drug will take up in the final solution is what is not taken up by the diluent. So if you consider the final drug as a couple's closet, the powder volume is the amount of room one partner gets to use versus the other (and that it is rarely equal!). The space each takes up is different from the weight of the shoes and clothes stored in that part of the closet.

FIGURE 6.4 Drug Dilution Calculation Form

Active Drug Weight (usually expressed only in weight: mg)	**Concentration** (proportional amount of drug per given solution volume)	**Powder Volume** (mL)	**Diluent Volume** (mL)	**Total Volume of Final Drug Solution** (mL)	**How much to administer?**

Example 29

A dry powder antibiotic must be reconstituted for use. The label states that the dry powder occupies 0.5 mL. Using the formula provided, determine the diluent volume (with the amount of solvent added). You are given the total volume for three different examples with the same powder volume but different diluent volumes and resulting concentrations.

$$\text{tv} - \text{pv} = \text{dv}$$

Total Volume		Powder Volume	Diluent
(1) 2 mL	–	0.5 mL	= 1.5 mL
(2) 5 mL	–	0.5 mL	= 4.5 mL
(3) 10 mL	–	0.5 mL	= 9.5 mL

Example 30

You are to reconstitute 1 g of dry powder. The label states that you are to add 9.3 mL of diluent to make a final solution of 100 mg/mL. What is the powder volume?

If the patient's medical order is for 50 mg of the drug, how much must be drawn from the vial into the syringe?

Active Drug Weight (usually expressed only in weight: gm, mg)	Concentration (proportional amount of drug per given solution volume)	Powder Volume (ml)	Diluent Volume (mL)	Total Volume of Final Drug Solution (mL)	How much to administer?
1 g (1,000 mg)	100 mg /1 mL		9.3 mL		

Step 1 Calculate the total volume using the ratio and proportion method. The strength of the final solution must be 100 mg/mL, so you need to convert the grams of active ingredient into milligrams. Since you start with 1 g = 1,000 mg of powder, for a total volume y mL of the solution, it will have a strength of 1,000 mg/y mL.

$$\frac{100 \text{ mg}}{1 \text{ mL}} = \frac{1{,}000 \text{ mg}}{y \text{ mL}}$$

$$100 \text{ mg} \times y \text{ mL} = 1 \text{ mL} \times 1{,}000 \text{ mg}$$

$$y \text{ mL} = \frac{1{,}000 \cancel{\text{mg}} \times 1 \text{ mL}}{100 \cancel{\text{mg}}} = 10 \text{ mL}$$

Step 2 Using the calculated total volume of the final product and the given diluent volume, calculate the powder volume.

$$tv - dv = pv$$

$$10 \text{ mL} - 9.3 \text{ mL} = 0.7 \text{ mL}$$

Step 3 You have a final drug solution of 100 mg per 1 mL, or 1 mL containing 100 mg of the drug. You must have only 50 mg in the syringe. So how much drug volume should be put into the syringe?

$$50 \cancel{\text{mg}} \times \frac{1 \text{ mL}}{100 \cancel{\text{mg}}} = \frac{50 \text{ mL}}{100} = 0.5 \text{ mL}$$

So now you can finish filling in the chart, and load the syringe with 0.5 mL of the drug solution.

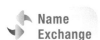

Name Exchange

Because of the grid used in the alligation alternate method, it has been nicknamed "Tic-Tac-Toe Math."

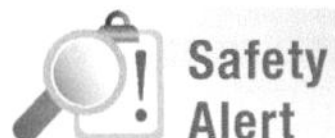

Safety Alert

Pharmacy technicians should always have the pharmacist verify their calculations and double-check those of the pharmacist.

Using Alligation to Combine More than One Concentration Level

Physicians often prescribe concentrations of medications that are not commercially available, and these prescriptions must be compounded, or prepared by an integration of ingredients, at the pharmacy. When a prescribed concentration is not commercially available, it may be necessary to combine two products of different concentrated strengths to reach the prescribed concentration. This process is called an alligation. The resulting concentration will be greater than the weaker strength but less than the stronger strength.

For example, a 1% and a 5% hydrocortisone ointment may be combined to provide a 3% ointment. An alligation calculation method is used when the two quantities to be combined are both relatively large. (To learn more about the techniques for combining topical creams of different strengths, refer to Chapter 10.)

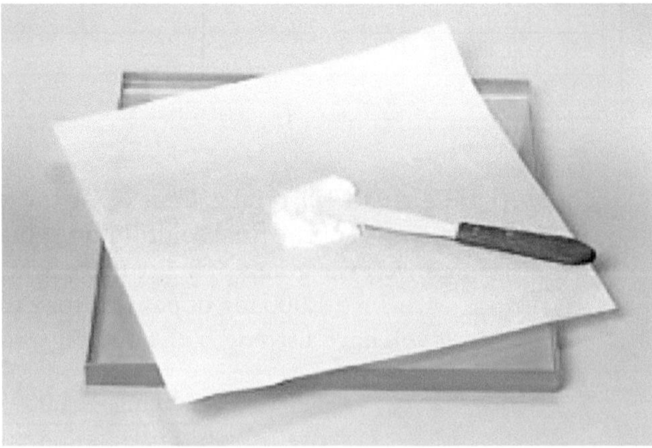

When the desired concentration of a cream (ointment or solution) is not available, the technician can use alligation to calculate how much cream of each concentration should be mixed together to compound the prescription.

There are two alligation methods: alligation medial and alligation alternate. The amount of each stock product ingredient to be added together is calculated by using what is known as the **alligation alternate method**. It is a very visual form of calculation, where you create a kind of tic-tac-toe grid to calculate the different percentages.

The first step is to make the familiar tic-tac-toe grid and place the highest ingredient percentage concentration in the top left-hand corner box. The lowest concentration is placed in the lower left corner box. Your target concentration, logically, is placed in the middle box. Then you need to figure out the "steps" in between each corner amount and the middle. You do this by subtracting the middle amount from the top left number (i.e., the smaller from the larger) and placing the answer in the lower right corner. This makes a diagonal line going from top to bottom (see Figure 6.5).

Now subtract the lower left number from the center number (i.e., the smaller from the larger) and put it at the upper right corner. This gives you another diagonal line going from bottom to top.

At this point, you have two percentages in the first column of the grid. Across from them in the facing corners, you have the number of parts of that percentage needed for the full solution. You will apply the number of parts to the percentage in each row going across. Then you add up the number of parts (or proportional items) you need to create your whole.

Once you know the total parts, you can divide that into the desired volume of the completed product to find out how much each part is worth, or its volume. Once you know that, then you can put it together like a recipe, mixing in the correct number of parts of each. It will make more sense when you follow the examples below.

FIGURE 6.5
Alligation Grid

The tic-tac-toe grid pattern of alligation helps one calculate how many parts of each strength are needed. The reason it crosses from top to bottom and bottom to top that you always want fewer parts of the high strength to go with more parts of the low strength to balance out to the mid strength.

A (higher %)		D (parts of higher %; the difference of B − C)
	B (desired %)	
C (lower %)		E (parts of lower %; the difference of A − B)

KEY
A = higher concentration or strength (stated as a percent [%])
B = desired concentration or strength (stated as a percent [%])
C = lower concentration or strength (stated as a percent [%])

Example 31

Prepare 250 mL of dextrose 7.5% weight-in-volume (w/v)—or 250 mL of $D_{7.5}W$. Combine the stock products of dextrose 5% (D_5W) w/v and dextrose 50% ($D_{50}W$) w/v. How many milliliters of each will be needed?

Step 1 Identify the variables by determining the component concentrations. B% is the desired concentration. The higher concentration (A%) and lower concentration (C%) are determined by the stock IV base solution strengths on hand in your pharmacy. In this case, the desired concentration is 7.5%, the higher concentration is 50%, and the lower concentration is 5%.

Step 2 Using the alligation grid from Figure 6.5, fill in the concentration strengths (given as percentages) in the key section below the tic-tac-toe grid. Place the same strengths in their designated squares on the grid.

A (higher %) 50		D (parts of higher %; the difference of B − C)
	B (desired %) 7.5	
C (lower %) 5		E (parts of lower %; the difference of A − B)

KEY
A% =50
B% = 7.5
C% = 5
D (Parts of 50% solution)
E (Parts of 5% solution)

Step 3 Determine the number of parts of each component (higher % and lower %).

a. To find the value of D in the upper right-hand square, set up the equation $B - C = D$.

   Fill in the values for B and C (found in Step 2) in the equation, as shown below:

   $7.5 - 5 = D$

   $D = 2.5$ (or the number of parts of 50% dextrose)

   Record the number 2.5 in the key and in the upper right-hand square.

b. To find the value of E in the lower right-hand square, set up the equation $A - B = E$.

   Then fill in the values for A and B (found in Step 2) in the equation, as shown below:

   $50 - 7.5 = E$

   $E = 42.5$ (or the number of parts of 5% dextrose)

   Record the number 42.5 in the key and in the lower right-hand square.

Check that your completed grid now matches the grid shown below:

A (higher %) 50		D (parts of higher % ; the difference of B − C) 2.5
	B (desired %) 7.5	
C (lower %) 5		E (parts of lower % ; the difference of A − B) 42.5

KEY
A% = 50
B% = 7.5
C% = 5
D (Parts of 50% solution) = 2.5
E (Parts of 5% solution) = 42.5

Step 4 Set up a ratio using the values of D and E as shown in the right-hand column of your completed grid.

$$\frac{D}{E} = \frac{2.5}{42.5}$$

This ratio indicates that to prepare the desired concentration (in this case, a $D_{7.5}W$ solution), dextrose 50% ($D_{50}W$) and dextrose 5% (D_5W) must be mixed in a 2.5:42.5 ratio: 2.5 parts of D50% and 42.5 parts of D5%.

Step 5 Using the ratio from Step 4, add D and E to obtain the total number of E (Parts of 5% solution) = 42.5 parts (tp).

$$D + E = tp$$
$$2.5 + 42.5 = tp$$
$$45 = tp$$

Step 6 Determine the volume of each component.

a. Determine the volume of dextrose 50% ($D_{50}W$) needed:
total volume (tv) of desired concentration = 250 mL
parts of $D_{50}W$ (D) = 2.5
total number of parts (tp) = 45

$$\frac{D}{tp} = \frac{x}{tv}$$

$$\frac{2.5}{45} = \frac{x}{250 \text{ mL}}$$

$$x = 13.9 \text{ mL of } D_{50}W$$

b. Determine the volume of dextrose 5% (D_5W) needed:
total volume (tv) of desired concentration = 250 mL
parts of D_5W (E) = 42.5
total number of parts (tp) = 45

$$\frac{E}{tp} = \frac{x}{tv}$$

$$\frac{42.5}{45} = \frac{x}{250 \text{ mL}}$$

$$x = 236.1 \text{ mL of } D_5W$$

Therefore, to make D7.5% ($D_{7.5}W$) 250 mL, mix 13.9 mL of dextrose 50% ($D_{50}W$) with 236.1 mL of dextrose 5% (D_5W).

Step 7 Verify your answer. The volume of each component (determined in Steps 6a and 6b) when added together should equal the total volume of the desired concentration.

$$\text{volume of } D_{50}W = 13.9 \text{ mL}$$
$$\text{volume of } D_5W = 236.1 \text{ mL}$$
$$13.9 \text{ mL} + 236.1 \text{ mL} = 250 \text{ mL}$$

Example 32

You are instructed to make 454 g of 3% zinc oxide cream. You have in stock 10% and 1% zinc oxide cream. How much of each percent will you use?

Step 1 Identify the variables by determining the component concentrations. The desired concentration (B%) is what you are asked to prepare. The higher concentration (A%) and lower concentration (C%) are determined by the stock strengths on hand in your pharmacy. In this case, the desired concentration is 3%, the higher concentration is 10%, and the lower concentration is 1%.

Step 2 Using the alligation grid from Figure 6.5, fill in the concentration strengths (given as percentages) in the key section below the tic-tac-toe grid. Place the same strengths in their designated squares on the grid.

A (higher %) 10		D (parts of higher %; the difference of B − C)
	B (desired %) 3	
C (lower %) 1		E (parts of lower %; the difference of A − B)

KEY
A% = 10
B% = 3
C% = 1
D (parts of 10% cream)
E (parts of 1% cream)

Step 3 Determine the number of parts of each component (higher % and lower %).

a. To find the value of D in the upper right-hand square, set up the equation B - C = D.

Fill in the values for B and C (found in Step 2) in the equation, as shown below:

$3 - 1 = D$

$D = 2$ (or the number of parts of 10% zinc oxide cream)

Record the number 2 in the key and in the upper right-hand square.

b. To find the value of E in the lower right-hand square, set up the equation A - B = E.

Fill in the values for A and B (found in Step 2) in the equation, as shown below:

$10 - 3 = E$

$E = 7$ (or the number of parts of 1% zinc oxide cream)

Record the number 7 in the key and in the lower right-hand square.

Check that your completed grid now matches the grid shown below:

A (parts of higher %; the difference of B – C) 10		D (parts of higher %; the difference of B – C) 2
	B (desired %) 3	
C (lower %) 1		E (parts of lower %; the difference of A – B) 7

KEY

A% = 10

B% = 3

C% = 1

D (parts of 10% cream) = 2

E (parts of 1% cream) = 7

Step 4 Set up a ratio using the values of D and E as shown in the right-hand column of your completed grid.

$$\frac{D}{E} = \frac{2}{7}$$

This ratio indicates that to prepare the desired concentration (in this case, a 3% cream), zinc oxide cream 10% and zinc oxide cream 1% must be mixed in a 2:7 ratio: 2 parts of zinc oxide cream 10% and 7 parts of zinc oxide cream 1%.

Step 5 Using the ratio from Step 4, add D and E to obtain the total number of parts (tp).

$$D + E = tp$$
$$2 + 7 = tp$$
$$9 = tp$$

Step 6 Determine the volume of each component.

a. Determine the amount of zinc oxide cream 10% needed.

total amount (ta) of desired concentration = 454 g
parts of zinc oxide cream 10% (D) = 2
total number of parts (tp) = 9

$$\frac{D}{tp} = \frac{x}{ta}$$

$$\frac{2}{9} = \frac{x}{454\text{ g}}$$

$$x = 100.9\text{ g of zinc oxide cream 10\%}$$

b. Determine the amount of zinc oxide cream 1% needed.

total amount (ta) of desired concentration = 454 g
parts of zinc oxide cream 1% (E) = 7
total number of parts (tp) = 9

$$\frac{E}{tp} = \frac{x}{ta}$$

$$\frac{7}{9} = \frac{x}{454\text{ g}}$$

$$x = 353.1\text{ g of zinc oxide cream 1\%}$$

Therefore, to make zinc oxide cream 3% 454 g, mix 100.9 g of zinc oxide cream 10% with 353.1 g of zinc oxide cream 1%.

Step 7 Verify your answer. The volume of each component (determined in Steps 6a and 6b) when added together should equal the total volume of the desired concentration.

amount of zinc oxide cream 10% = 100.9 g
amount of zinc oxide cream 1% = 353.1

$$100.9\text{ g} + 353.1\text{ g} = 454\text{ g}$$

Calculating Specific Gravity

In precision compounding, it is important to understand that each substance has its own specific gravity due to its particular density or molecular structure. This determines how well various elements mix in solutions, suspensions, and emulsions. For instance, oil is less dense than water or has a lower specific gravity, so oil floats.

Specific gravity is the weight of a substance compared in a ratio to the standard weight of an equal volume of water when both are the same temperature at sea level. Water is the standard because 1 mL of water at sea level and room temperature weighs approximately 1 gram (it is 1.0 gram precisely at 39.2°F/4.0°C).

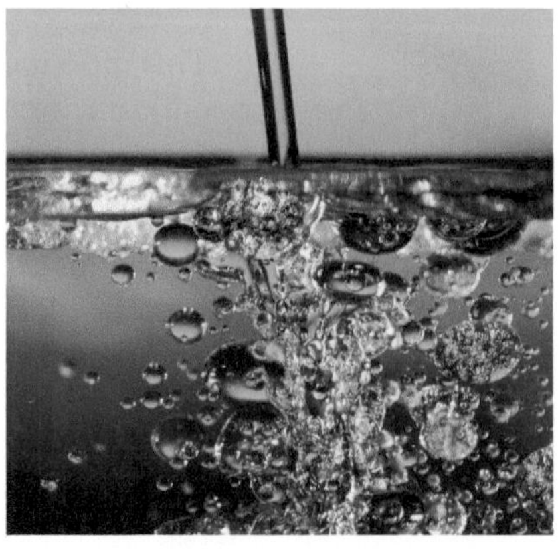

Water and oil have different specific gravity ratings.

$$1 \text{ mL volume of water} = 1 \text{ g weight of water}$$

$$\text{Specific gravity of water} = 1.0$$

Specific gravity measurements are always calculated from the weight of the substance in grams compared to an equal volume of water in grams. The resulting number is a rating against the standard of 1. The formula for a specific gravity rating is as follows:

$$\text{specific gravity rating} = \frac{\text{weight of a substance (g)}}{\text{weight of an equal volume of water (mL)}}$$

$$\text{or mL} = \frac{\text{weight (g)}}{\text{specific gravity}}$$

$$\text{or g} = \text{mL} \times \text{specific gravity}$$

The formulas above can be used to calculate the unknown value of specific gravity, or the ratio and proportion method can be utilized. When the specific gravity is known, certain assumptions can be made regarding the physical properties of a liquid. Solutions that are thick (or viscous) often have specific gravities higher than one (1), meaning that they are heavier than water. Solutions that contain volatile chemicals (or something prone to quick evaporation, such as alcohol) often have a specific gravity lower than one (1), meaning that they are lighter or less dense than water. If the specific gravity is known, you can determine the weight of a liquid volume by reversing the equations or by using equal proportion equations (see Table 6.11).

TABLE 6.11 Specific Gravity Ratings for Different Liquids

Liquid	≈ Specific Gravity Rating at Sea Level
Alcohol—isopropyl	0.79
Ammonia	0.662
Beer	1.01
Butane	0.584
Corn oil	0.924
Glucose	1.35
Mercury	13.6
Molasses (blackstrap)	1.49
Seawater	1.02

Example 33

If the weight of 100 mL of dextrose solution is 117 g, what is the specific gravity of the dextrose solution?

$$\text{specific gravity rating} = \frac{\text{weight of a substance}}{\text{weight of an equal volume of water}}$$

$$y = \frac{117 \text{ g}}{100 \text{ mL}} = 1.17.$$ This solution is heavier than water.

Example 34

If 500 mL of glycerin weighs 275 g, what is the specific gravity?

$$y = \frac{275\text{ g}}{500\text{ mL}} = 0.55.\text{ This solution is lighter than water.}$$

Example 35

If a liquid has a specific gravity of 0.85, how much does 125 mL of it weigh?

Because the specific gravity of the liquid is 0.85,

$$0.85 = \frac{85\text{ g}}{100\text{ mL}}$$

Now, use the ratio and proportion method to find the weight of 125 mL.

$$\frac{y\text{ g}}{125\text{ mL}} = \frac{85\text{g}}{100\text{ mL}}$$

$$100y\text{ g} = 125 \times 85\text{ g} \qquad y\text{ g} = \frac{10{,}625\text{ g}}{100} = 106.26\text{ g}$$

So, 125 mL of the liquid weighs 106.25 g.

Calculating Milliequivalents

This section is challenging and may require some basic chemistry knowledge as well as mathematical prowess. It is designed for pharmacy technicians who will be compounding sterile products in a hospital or home healthcare IV facility or nonsterile products in a community pharmacy setting. Even so, a basic understanding of electrolytes and milliequivalents (mEq) will enhance the expertise of any pharmacy technician and may minimize calculation errors. Because of this, technician programs must teach these calculations, and these calculations could be included in the Pharmacy Technician Certification Board (PTCB) certification examination.

Calculating Atomic and Molecular Weights

Most electrolyte solutions in the hospital pharmacy are measured by milliequivalents (mEq), which are related to molecular weight. Molecular weights are calculated using the established atomic weight of each of the common chemical elements. You may recall from high school chemistry class the periodic table of elements on the wall. On it was listed the **atomic weight** of each element—the weight of a single atom as compared to the weight of one atom of hydrogen, which is the standard. For instance, the atomic weight of H (hydrogen) is 1; C (carbon) is 12.01 rounded off to 12; and Na (sodium) is 22.9898, rounded off to 23.

The **molecular weight** of a compound is the sum of the atomic weights of all the atoms in one molecule of the compound. The molecular weight of sodium bicarbonate ($NaHCO_3$) is 23 +1 + 12 + 48 (see Table 6.12).

TABLE 6.12 Valences and Atomic Weights of Common Elements

Element	Valence	Atomic Weight	Rounded-off Value
Hydrogen (H)	1	1.008 g	1 g
Carbon (C)	2, 4	12.011 g	12 g
Nitrogen (N)	3, 5	14.007 g	14 g
Oxygen (O)	2	15.999 g	16 g
Sodium (Na)	1	22.9898 g	23 g
Magnesium (Mg)	2	24.305 g	24.31g
Sulfur (S)	2, 4, 6	32.065 g	32.1 g
Chlorine (Cl)	1, 3, 5, 7	35.453 g	35.5 g
Potassium (K)	1	39.102 g	39.1 g
Calcium (Ca)	2	40.08 g	40.1 g

A **mole (mol)** is a unit of measurement based on the number of particles in a given substance. The mass of one mole of a substance is its molecular weight expressed in grams. The number of grams in one mole differs between substances. For example, a mole of potassium (K+) is 39.10 grams and a mole of chlorine (Cl-) is 35.45 grams. A **millimole (mmol)** is one-thousandth of a mole, or the molecular weight expressed in milligrams. One millimole of potassium (K+) is 39.19 mg and one millimole of chlorine (Cl-) is 35.45 mg.

atomic weight of sodium (23 g) + atomic weight of chlorine (35.5 g) = 58.5 g

Compounds are also measured in moles. For example, 1 mole of salt (or sodium chloride, NaCl) would equal the total of the atomic weights of the two components in grams, which is as follows:

As another example, 1 mole of calcium chloride ($CaCl_2$) would be:

1 mole of calcium (40) + 2 moles of chlorine (71) = approximately 111 g

As stated earlier, 1 mM is the molecular weight of one millimole expressed in milligrams.

1 mM of sodium chloride = 58.5 mg

1 mM of calcium chloride = 111 mg

Understanding the Dissolving Capacity of Solutes

Besides atomic weights, each element is described by its ability to form bonds with other elements. In chemistry, the **valence** is a positive or negative number that represents its rated capacity to combine with other atomic substances to form a molecule of a stable compound. The valence is based on the number and typical activities of the outer electrons of the element to bind or repel electrons in other atoms. An element can exist in various forms, and the valence can vary depending on the molecular form and compound. In pharmacy, the valence is used to determine the number of grams of solute that have the capacity to fully dissolve in 1 mL of solution.

Table 6.12 lists the atomic weights and valences of common elements. For pharmaceutical calculations, atomic weights are usually rounded to the nearest tenth, as shown in the fourth column of the table.

An **equivalent (Eq)** weight is a unit that takes into account both moles and valence. In pharmacy, you are often trying to find out the equivalent weight of the amount of solute substance that is fully able to dissolve in 1 mL. The equivalent (Eq) weight is equal to 1 mole of the molecule divided by its valence, or the number of grams of solute that could dissolve in 1 mL of solution as shown in the following formula:

$$\text{equivalent (Eq) weight} = \frac{\text{1 M's molecular weight (in grams)}}{\text{valence}}$$

$$\text{Eq} = \frac{\text{1 M g}}{\text{valence}}$$

A **milliequivalent (mEq)** weight is equal to 1 mM divided by its valence.

$$\text{milliequivalent (mEq) weight} = \frac{\text{1 mM's molecular weight (in milligrams)}}{\text{valence}}$$

$$\text{mEq} = \frac{\text{1 mM (in mg)}}{\text{valence}}$$

Further, 1 Eq equals 1,000 mEq.

Determining the Milliequivalents of Compounds

The first step in determining the number of milliequivalents of a compound is to identify the formula of the compound. The next step is to separate the formula into the atomic weight of each element. The atomic weight of an individual atom of each element is then multiplied by the number of those atoms. Then the products are added together, and that sum is substituted into the formula for atomic weight.

Example 36

The molecular weight of magnesium sulfate (Mg + SO_4) is 120 g. This comes from Mg + S + O_4 = 24.306 g + 32.064 g + 15.999 g (× 4) = 120 g. Its valence is 2. How many milligrams does 1 mEq of magnesium sulfate weigh?

$$1 \text{ mEq} = \frac{120 \text{ mg}}{2} = 60 \text{ mg}$$

Example 37

Magnesium has an atomic weight for a mole of 24 g. What is the weight of 1 mM?

To solve this problem, you must recall metric prefixes. The prefix *milli-* means 1,000. Therefore, 1 M = 1,000 mM. Now we will use dimensional analysis to calculate the number of grams in 1 mM.

$$\frac{24 \text{ g}}{1 \text{ M}} \times \frac{1 \text{ M}}{1{,}000 \text{ mM}} = 0.024 \text{ g per mM} = 24 \text{ mg per mM}$$

Converting between Milligrams and Milliequivalents

To convert back and forth between the weight of a substance in milligrams and its dissolving weight in milliequivalents, use the following formula:

$$\text{number of milliequivalents} = \frac{\text{weight of substance (in milligrams)}}{\text{milliequivalent weight}}$$

This equation will be demonstrated in the following example.

Example 38

Sodium has an atomic weight of 23 mg and a valence of 1. How many milliequivalents are in 92 mg of sodium?

Step 1 Determine the weight of 1 milliequivalent of sodium by dividing the molecular weight (from the atomic weight) by the valence.

$$1 \text{ mEq} = \frac{\text{molecular weight}}{\text{valence}} = \frac{23 \text{ mg}}{1} = 23 \text{ mg}$$

Step 2 Determine the number of milliequivalents in 92 mg of sodium.

$$y \text{ mEq} = \frac{\text{weight of sodium in solution}}{\text{weight of 1 mEq of sodum}} = \frac{92 \text{ mg}}{23 \text{ mg}} = 4 \text{ mEq}$$

Measuring Electrolytes

Many IV fluids used in hospital pharmacy practice contain dissolved mineral salts; such a fluid is known as an **electrolyte solution**. These fluids are so named because they conduct an electrical charge through the solution when connected to electrodes. For example, the compound potassium chloride (abbreviated KCl) breaks down to K^+ and C^{1-} ions in solution.

Milliequivalents (and sometimes millimoles) are used to measure electrolytes in the bloodstream and/or in an IV preparation. For these you need to figure out the milliequivalents able to dissolve in the solution to reach the proper concentration.

Example 39

You are requested to make a sterile preparation in the IV room by adding 44 mEq of sodium chloride (NaCl) to an IV bag. Sodium chloride is available as a 4 mEq/mL solution. How many milliliters will you need to add to the IV bag?

Set up a ratio and proportion, comparing the solution you will need to create to the available solution, and solve for the unknown y.

$$\frac{4\ \cancel{\text{mEq}}}{1\ \text{mL}} = \frac{44\ \cancel{\text{mEq}}}{y\ \text{mL}}$$

$$y\ \text{mL} \times 4 = 44 \times 1\ \text{mL}$$

$$y\ \text{mL} = \frac{44 \times 1\ \text{mL}}{4}$$

$$y\ \text{mL} = 11\ \text{mL}$$

You can also solve this problem using dimensional analysis.

Determining IV Administration Flow Rates

In sterile compounding, pharmacy technicians are often called upon to calculate IV drip rates, drop factors, and the IV quantity for the prescribed period based on infusion rates prescribed by the physician. Because these rates are in part determined by the size and nature of the tubing, these calculations will be addressed in Chapter 13 after the IV tubing and sets have been described. The calculation of overfill volumes is also handled in Chapter 13 on sterile and hazardous compounding procedures.

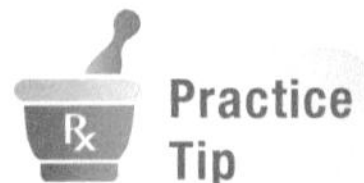

A beyond-use date is a term that applies to both sterile and nonsterile compounded preparations, whereas an expiration date is a term that applies to manufactured products.

Beyond-Use Dating

When compounding together two different manufactured drug products, each comes with its own properties of **stability**, or ability to maintain its potency and essential properties and active ingredients over time in proper storage and temperature conditions. Stability includes physical properties (appearance, taste, uniformity, dissolution, and suspendability) and chemical properties (potency). Based on this, an expiration date, or date of last recommended use, has been assigned by the manufacturer. Each ingredient in the alligated or compounded product has a different expiration date.

From these dates, the pharmacist needs to calculate a date for last recommended use, called **beyond-use date (BUD)** for the product, and the technician serves to double-check the calculation. The pharmacist considers the expiration dates and the stability of the new compound's ingredients and then calculates a BUD from them.

The US Pharmacopeial Convention has established beyond-use-dating guidelines for alligation and compounded nonsterile drug products in *USP* General Chapter <795> (rev. 2019) and for sterile products in *USP* <797>. Since nonsterile and sterile products have different BUD dating guidelines, the way to calculate them will be addressed in Chapter 10 and Chapter 13.

6.10 Commitment to Calculating with Confidence

Though calculations should always be checked by the pharmacist, the technician must take personal ownership of his or her work. Never guess on your calculations. Check and double-check your work! You must strive to be 100% right 100% of the time. Remember, the pharmacist is always there to verify your reasoning and your mathematical calculations, and you are there to double-check those of the pharmacist.

As is clear in the "In the Real World" examples, calculations performed in the pharmacy can truly be a life or death issue. Of particular concern is treating very sick or vulnerable patients, including tiny premature infants and older adult patients, with potent lifesaving drugs. A missed decimal place or similar careless calculation error could result in tenfold or more levels of overdoses and fatal consequences.

With classroom and laboratory training and experiences in the field, as well as a focus on detail and diligence in your profession, you will gradually gain the necessary skills to do calculations confidently in any pharmacy environment. Additional examples and additional calculating skills will be introduced in upcoming chapters relating to nonsterile and sterile compounding (Chapters 10, 12, and 13) and on business and insurance calculations in Chapter 9. Remember that working in the pharmacy profession is a lifelong learning commitment–you really do learn something new each day! And it all takes practice.

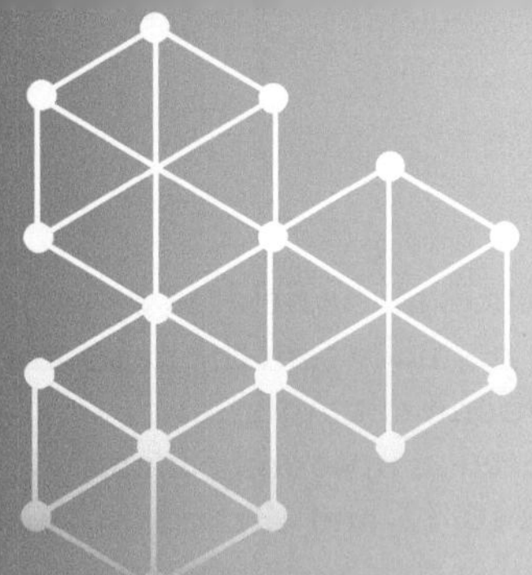

Review and Assessment

CHAPTER SUMMARY

- Arabic and Roman are the basic numerical systems.
- Understanding fractions, decimals, percents, and their conversions is essential to pharmacy calculations.
- Pharmacy technicians working in hospital pharmacies must be comfortable working with 24-hour time (also called military time or international time).
- Technicians must be able to convert temperatures to and from Fahrenheit and Celsius.
- The metric system is preferred worldwide for making accurate, standard scientific measurements, including pharmacy calculations.
- The metric system of measurement makes use of decimal units, including the basic units of the gram (for weight) and the liter (for volume).
- The most widely used units of measure in pharmacy include milligrams, grams, kilograms, milliliters, and liters.
- Pharmacy technicians should be familiar with the standard prefixes for abbreviating metric quantities and with the basic mathematical principles used to calculate and convert doses using dimensional analysis and equal ratio and proportion equations.
- Pharmacy professionals should be able to convert between the different systems including metric, apothecary, and household measures.
- Technicians should be able to find an unknown quantity in a proportion when three elements of the proportion are known using the ratio and proportion methodology.
- Drug dosage calculations can be based on body weight in kilograms (kg) or body surface area (BSA).
- Correctly calculating powder volume and dilutions is an important skill to learn in compounding preparations.
- Technicians should also be able to use the alligation alternate method to compound a sterile and nonsterile product from products having different concentrations.
- Technicians should understand the concepts of powder ingredient volumes in a solution and specific gravity.
- In dilutions and compounding, the technician must learn how to calculate and convert atomic weights, equivalents, and milliequivalents. They are essential for judging the number of electrolytes to add to a solution.

✓ CHECK YOUR UNDERSTANDING

To ensure that you recall and understand the key chapter concepts, please read the question or statement and select the appropriate lettered option.

1. A decimal converted to a fraction has as its denominator a power of
   a. 2.
   b. 5.
   c. 10.
   d. 25.

2. A patient weighs 176 pounds. The dose of medication is written in mg per kg. How many kilograms does this patient weigh?
   a. 60 kg
   b. 70 kg
   c. 75 kg
   d. 80 kg

3. An IV medication order is received in the hospital with the first dose to be started at 2200 hours. What is the Greenwich Mean Time equivalent?
   a. 10:00 a.m.
   b. 10:00 p.m.
   c. 2:00 a.m.
   d. 2:00 p.m.

4. What is the temperature range allowed for an item requiring refrigeration?
   a. 36°F to 46°F
   b. −50°C to −15°C
   c. 25°C to 35°C
   d. −58°F to 5°F

5. The only unit of measure that is shared between the apothecary system and avoirdupois system is the
   a. grain.
   b. gram.
   c. liter.
   d. ounce.

6. The set of standardized metric prefixes based on powers of 10 is called the
   a. avoirdupois system.
   b. Système International (SI).
   c. household system.
   d. apothecary system.

MAKE CONNECTIONS

Take a moment to consider what you have learned in this chapter and respond thoughtfully to the following prompts. Note that some of these activities will require internet access.

1. The patient has received a bottle containing 240 mL of a liquid medication. The patient is to take 4 tsp of the medication per day. How many days will the bottle last?
2. An unopened bottle of Latanoprost ophthalmic solution should be stored in a refrigerator (2–8° C) per the product package insert. Once opened, the medication is stable for six weeks at 25° C. What is the equivalent temperature in degrees Fahrenheit?

 The online course includes additional review and assessment resources.

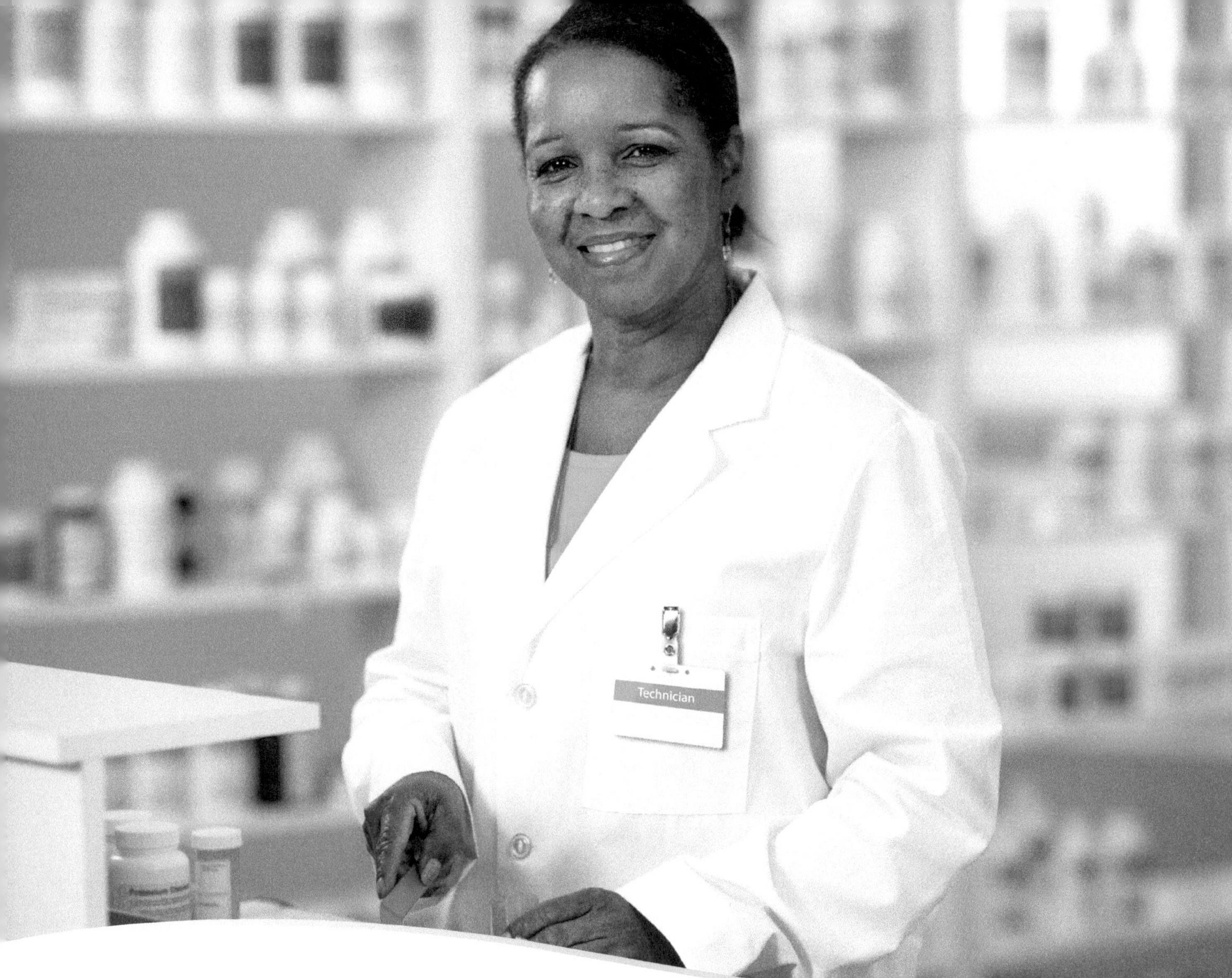

UNIT 3 Community Pharmacy Practice

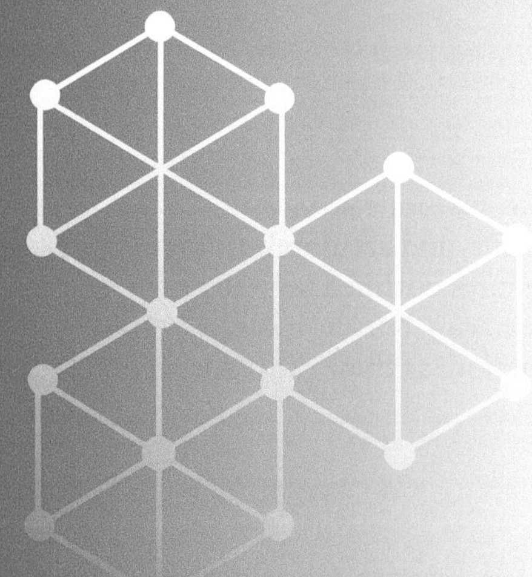

7 Community Pharmacy Dispensing

Learning Objectives

1. Outline the overall processes of community dispensing and a pharmacy technician's general responsibilities within them. (Sections 7.1, 7.2)
2. Identify the parts of a prescription. (Section 7.3)
3. Summarize the various types of prescriptions and the step-by-step procedures to fill them. (Section 7.3)
4. Translate the most commonly used pharmacy abbreviations. (Section 7.4)
5. Describe how the pharmacy data management system interfaces online with an external health information network and databases, and with internal software for varied pharmacy and business functions. (Section 7.4)
6. Paraphrase how to build a patient profile, and discuss the importance of updating current information about drug and supplement use, allergies, adverse drug reactions, and insurance for medication reconciliation and following HIPAA-mandated guidelines. (Section 7.5)
7. Describe the process and importance of the Drug Utilization Review. (Section 7.6)
8. Identify the parts of a stock drug label, and know the importance of comparing National Drug Code numbers in medication selection and filling. (Section 7.7)
9. Discuss how automation is utilized along with a final check and verification by the pharmacist to minimize medication errors. (Section 7.7)
10. Identify three different NDC checks that help reduce the risk of medication errors. (Section 7.8)
11. Outline the different ways to educate a patient about their prescription using labels and medication guides. (Section 7.9)
12. Describe the steps a pharmacist will take when doing a final check on a prescription. (Section 7.10)
13. Summarize the aspects of patient prescription dispensing, including pre-pickup storage and pickup options. (Section 7.11)
14. Describe medication therapy management (MTM), Point-of-care testing, and other health services provided in a community pharmacy setting. (Section 7.12)

ASHP/ACPE Accreditation Standards
To view the *ASHP/ACPE Accreditation Standards* addressed in this chapter, refer to Appendix B.

According to the most recent data, almost three-quarters of pharmacy technicians practice in a retail pharmacy (sometimes called a community pharmacy) setting (over 200,000 of the 285,000 positions in the United States). Ideally, the retail pharmacy is and has been a place where local citizens come in and get their prescriptions filled by people they know and trust.

This chapter covers the critical role of the technician—in customer service, updating patient profiles, entering prescriptions into the profile, and accurately filling and dispensing new and refill prescriptions. The exact procedures outlined (as well as the pharmacy software) will vary between specific retail pharmacies, but the basic tasks are similar. You must learn these steps and this information, as these procedures will take up the majority of time as a pharmacy technician.

7.1 Retail Pharmacy Facilities

More than 4.4 billion prescriptions were dispensed by chain, independent, and grocery retail stores along with mail-order warehouse pharmacies in 2016. The number has grown since then, and most pharmacy technicians work in one of these nonhospital settings.

Most community pharmacies are divided into two store areas: an unrestricted retail front area that houses over-the-counter (OTC) drugs, medical supplies, dietary supplements, and other merchandise; and a back area restricted to pharmacy personnel only. The back area is where the prescription medications are stored and prepared for dispensing, and it is secured and off-limits to the public (no family or friends are allowed). The pharmacy counter and a transparent shield often separate these two areas.

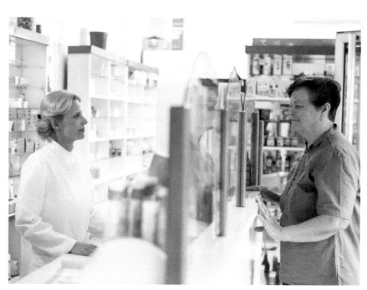

Most community retail pharmacies are divided into a restricted, secure prescription area offering prescription merchandise and related items, and an open retail area in front offering OTC drugs, dietary supplements, medical supplies, and other merchandise.

If there is no pharmacist on duty (even if a technician is present), this glassed-off section must be closed and locked according to most state laws. The remainder of the store may remain open to sell any other merchandise or products, including OTC drugs and dietary supplements.

Patient convenience is important. Community pharmacies, especially chain store pharmacies, have hours of operation that accommodate working families, shift workers, and patients recently discharged from emergency rooms and hospitals. Many offer a drive-through area for prescription drop-off and pickup. Drive-through pharmacies are especially convenient for parents with children, the elderly, and those with physical limitations or disabilities. Community pharmacies may also partner with home healthcare or hospice services to dispense (and deliver) narcotic pain-relieving medications to terminal patients in their care. Numerous independent pharmacies also offer free delivery for homebound patients without transportation.

7.2 The Roles of a Retail Pharmacy Technician

The ratio of pharmacy technicians to pharmacists allowed per shift differs in each state (depending on the laws of each state's board of pharmacy), and so do the exact roles and experiences of the technicians. In smaller community pharmacies, technicians often engage in prescription filling as well as clerical and retail activities. Pharmacy sales clerks without technician training, certification, and experience may be limited to customer contact, cashiering, and inventory control functions.

The certified pharmacy technician has varied days and may spend time directly with customers, entering new and refill prescriptions into the computer, filling and labeling prescription orders, reconciling insurance claims, stocking drugs, or checking inventory levels and drug expiration dates. Typically, the technician is juggling several different tasks at once, with each task requiring due diligence to ensure accuracy. The variety of different jobs helps sharpen one's mental acuity, and it may minimize the risk of serious medication errors if technicians can focus well and shift from one task to the next without being distracted.

A pharmacy technician may also be involved in simple **nonsterile compounding** (also known as *extemporaneous compounding*), in which the technician prepares non-injectable, not-commercially-available medications specifically for a patient's immediate need. These tasks may be as simple as mixing three or four commercially available ingredients into a prescribed mouthwash. Or they may involve more sophistication, training, and equipment to compound a cream or ointment.

A list of a technician's general tasks can be seen in Table 7.1, but these duties fluctuate, depending on a facility's approved policies and procedures.

In addition to assisting in customer service and prescription filling, the pharmacy technician is involved in the business operations of the community pharmacy, including handling insurance processing and charge-backs; selling nonprescription products, dietary supplements, and supplies; ordering and receiving the drug inventory; and organizing and stocking shelves. The processing of prescription claims through insurance will be covered in Chapter 8, and the inventory control responsibilities will be discussed in Chapter 9. Lastly, the pharmacy technician is expected to help maintain a clean work environment by vacuuming the pharmacy restricted area, cleaning counters and counting trays, bundling and removing trash, and securing the disposal of patient-specific information. Counters also need to be sanitized.

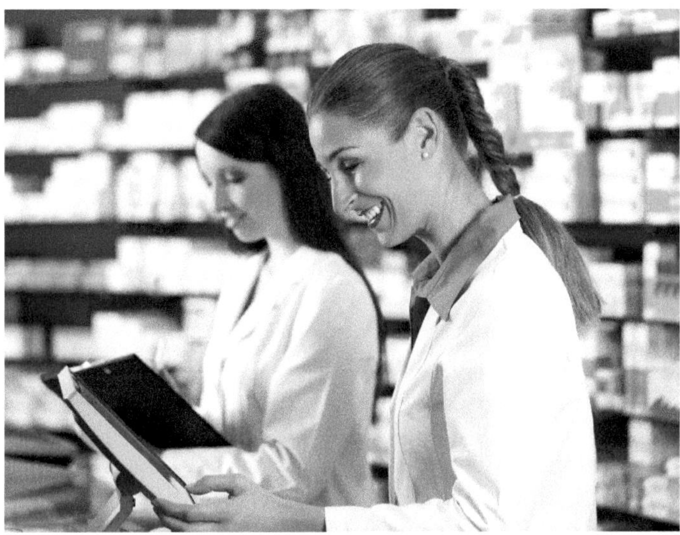

The pharmacist and technician work together as a team to provide customer service as well as efficient and safe dispensing of medications.

A community pharmacy's regulations are typically explained during an on-the-job training program for new pharmacy technicians and in a written policies and procedures manual. The training program or manual not only reflects the requirements of the pharmacy's own guidelines, but also relevant state laws and regulations for a safe and effective operation. It is important for the pharmacy technician to understand and learn well these policies, procedures, and laws for various types of prescriptions.

TABLE 7.1 Key Dispensing Duties in the Community Pharmacy

- Greet customers at the pharmacy counter or drive-through window, and receive written new or refill prescriptions
- Answer the telephone and refer call-in new or refill prescriptions or transfers to the pharmacist
- Update patient profiles, including patient demographics, drug use, allergies, and health conditions
- Clarify and resolve questions about a prescription (name, directions, and so on) with the prescriber's office
- Scan and/or enter new prescriptions (or refill requests) into the patient profile
- Enter and/or update billing information for third-party reimbursements
- Submit prescription claims online for medication reconciliation and insurance adjudication (see Chapter 8)
- Refer to a pharmacist any medication contraindications, and drug and allergy interactions
- Resolve eligibility or prescription processing issues
- Calculate prescription quantity and days' supply for accurate billing
- Retrieve and count drug products from restricted storage for prescription filling
- Reconstitute, package, and/or repackage products as needed for prescriptions
- Prepare extemporaneous, nonsterile compounds when necessary
- Select medication containers and affix labels
- Seek final verification by the pharmacist
- Store completed prescriptions for future patient pickup
- Return stock bottles to their proper storage locations
- Retrieve medications for patient pickup
- Offer a medication counseling opportunity with the pharmacist to the patient
- Distribute labeled medications with reminders of label directions
- Accept and process payments and copayments for the prescription(s) and in some cases for OTC drugs, supplements, and retail items
- Handle cash register, change, and credit processing responsibilities
- Resolve refused insurance payments
- Stock shelves
- Assist in inventory management
- Assist in technology management
- Assist in business functions
- Help keep the prescription filling area clean, organized, and tidy

7.3 Overview of Prescription Processing

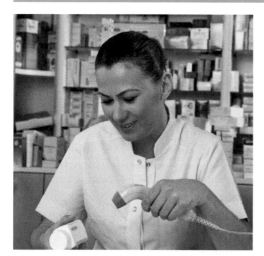

Before filling the prescription, the technician should scan the stock bottle to ensure that the correct drug with the proper NDC number has been selected from the inventory.

Most people go to a community pharmacy to fill, refill, or pick up a prescription. A **prescription** (**script** for short) is defined as a patient medication order issued by a legally authorized physician or a qualified licensed practitioner for a valid medical condition to be filled by authorized pharmacy personnel. On prescription drug labels and packaging there is the recognizable "Rx only" designation, which means that the product cannot be sold without a prescription.

Processing a prescription is a complex procedure, with many skills being gained only through experience. No matter what type of prescription is ordered, it follows a similar critical path as described below. However, some prescriptions require additional elements or documentation. For instance, high-cost medications or drugs not on a patient's insurance formulary require **prior authorization (PA)**, or documented approval, from a prescriber (which will be described in Chapter 8). Dispensing controlled substances and drugs that require a specific risk evaluation and mitigation strategy (REMS) also entail special safety steps and documentation. For instance, unique patient education processes must accompany the dispensing of fentanyl (Actiq), an immediate-release narcotic for severe pain, and dofetilide (Tikosyn) for irregular heartbeats. Buprenorphine hydrochloride (Subutex) for opioid dependence also has a REMS to follow. These will be addressed in Chapter 14.

In all situations, the filling process must be accurate and efficient, which requires teamwork and communication between the pharmacy technician and the pharmacist. Each step will be explained in some depth.

The Prescription Components

Put Down Roots

Some think that Rx comes from an abbreviation of the Latin command *recipere*, which means "take." Many recipe directions started with "Take this [ingredient]…" The *R* in recipe may have been combined with part of the Egyptian Eye of Horus, a symbol of good health and power.

All prescriptions must include the same information, so you must be familiar with the basic components. Rx is the official symbol of a prescription. After the pharmacy technician checks that each prescription is complete and accurate—whether on computer, handwritten, or via phone or fax—then the pharmacist double-checks the technician's work. Each Rx must have the components listed in Table 7.2.

TABLE 7.2 Parts of a Prescription

Part	Description
Prescriber's information	Name, address, telephone number, and other information identifying the prescriber; NPI and DEA numbers; and, sometimes, the state license number
Date	Date on which the prescription was written; this date may differ from the date on which the prescription was received
Patient's information	Full name, address, telephone number, and date of birth of the patient
℞	Symbol ℞, from the Latin verb *recipere* meaning "to take"
Inscription	Medication prescribed, including generic or brand name, strength, and amount
Subscription	Instructions to the pharmacist on dispensing the medication
Signa	Directions for the patient to follow (commonly called the *sig*)
Additional instructions	Any additional instructions that the prescriber deems necessary
Signature	Signature of the prescriber

Prescriber's Information

Prescriber Contact Information The name, address, telephone, and fax number are required for verification on all controlled substances and in case of follow-up questions.

Prescriber's DEA Number The Drug Enforcement Administration (DEA) issues a number authorizing a prescriber to be able to medically order controlled substances. The **DEA number** is essential on all prescriptions for controlled substances. In some states, it functions as an ID number to identify the prescriber. For security reasons and to prevent forgeries, the DEA number of the prescribing physician may not be preprinted on the prescription form but must be specifically written or entered in. Most pharmacies have a database containing local prescribers' DEA numbers. A formula can be used to check the accuracy of DEA numbers. This information is found in Chapter 14.

Practice Tip

The NPI number may be identified online at the website of the National Plan and Provider Enumeration System (NPPES) at https://PharmPractice7e.ParadigmEducation.com/NPPES.

National Provider Identifier Number The **National Provider Identifier (NPI)** is necessary for each healthcare provider to get reimbursed for services provided (though not essential for the prescription to be filled). Physicians, physician assistants, nurse practitioners, dentists, and pharmacists are all eligible for an NPI. The NPI number does not replace the DEA number or state license number.

State License Number Some states also require prescribers to include this. Know your state's rules.

Patient's Information

Patient's Name This should be given in full, including first and last names. Initials alone are not acceptable. If the writing is illegible on a paper form, the technician should verify the spelling of the patient's name and rewrite it in full above the name on the prescription.

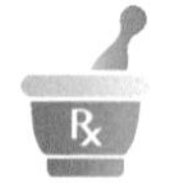

Practice Tip

The terms *sex* and *gender* are not interchangeable. *Sex* is defined as the classification of people as male, female, or intersex based on physical anatomy at birth. *Gender identity* is defined as one's internal sense of being male or female. For many people, their sex and gender identity are the same. For others, their sex and gender identity are not the same.

Patient's Birth Date and Sex This additional identifying information is often required for third-party insurance billing and for correct identification with patients of the same name. Preprinted prescriptions often contain spaces for the birth date. If this space is not filled in, then the technician must request it from the patient or person presenting the prescription. Knowing the patient's age and sex (many names can be male or female) helps the pharmacist evaluate the appropriateness of the drug, its quantity, and the dosage form prescribed, thus minimizing medication errors.

Patient's Address, Telephone Number(s) A home and/or cell phone number is/are needed for patient records. An email address is also preferred but optional. A home address is important for billing and insurance purposes. Requesting this information aids patient identification and minimizes dispensing errors. Asking for a secondary phone number (cell or business) assists in following up with patients. For controlled substances, federal law requires a verifiable physical address (not a post office box).

Medication Information

Date the Physician Wrote the Prescription For controlled drugs, the date must be present to have the prescription filled. If no date is included online or written on the prescription, then the technician should call the provider to verify the date. If the undated prescription is for an antibiotic, then the pharmacist should verify with the physician that the patient is still under his or her current care and find out when the antibiotic was issued. The antibiotic may no longer be necessary and, in fact, could be harmful.

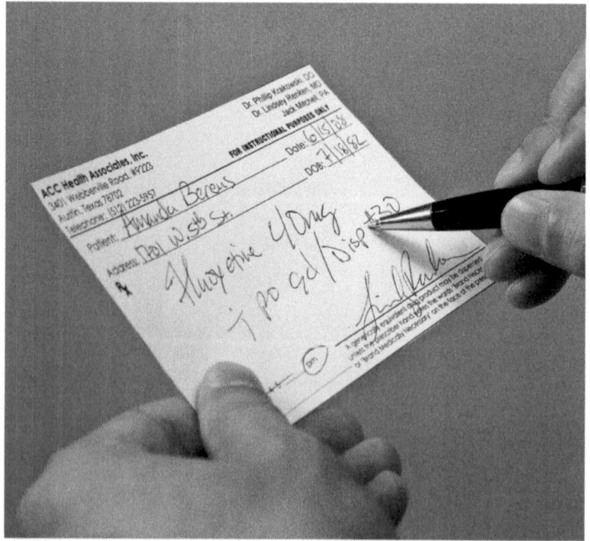

Reviewing a prescription for completeness and accuracy in whatever form it is delivered is essential.

Inscription The medication's name (brand or generic), strength, and amount are listed in the **inscription**. A drug may be marketed under various brand and generic forms. Most times, the bioequivalent generic drugs are automatically substituted for the brands by the pharmacy software unless the brand is specified as necessary by the prescriber (see "Subscription" below). If the prescription is filled with a generic equivalent, then the name, strength, and manufacturer of the generic drug will be printed on the dispensed medication container label—so remember, the label will not always exactly match the original prescription. That is why a technician needs to know the generic substitutions of the most common brand name drugs prescribed, as discussed in Chapter 4.

> **Put Down Roots**
>
> PRN comes from the Latin *pro re nata*, meaning "for the occasion of need."

Signa A **signa (sig)** is the prescriber's directions about how a prescription should be taken or used. This information is transferred from the prescription by the pharmacist or technician into the pharmacy software's patient profile, which prints it onto the medication container label for patient use. Technicians need to spend time checking the many abbreviations used in the signa—which will be covered in a section to follow. (For a full list of signa abbreviations, see Appendix A.)

Subscription The **subscription** is the part that lists the prescriber's instructions to the pharmacist about filling the inscribed medication, including refill information, compounding and labeling instructions, and notes about dispensing drug equivalents. The prescriber may note **dispense as written (DAW)** or "brand name medically necessary," which is sometimes shortened to "brand necessary," if a prescriber wishes that only the inscribed brand name product be dispensed. This is entered into the computer and billed to insurance as DAW1, required by provider. At times, a patient may request a brand name to be dispensed in lieu of a generic drug, abbreviated as DAW2. When billed to insurance, DAW2 often results in an increase in patient copayment, as noted in earlier chapters.

The prescriber fills in a number (or circles one on a preprinted form) to delineate how often the medication can be filled without requiring a new order. If left blank, then the prescription cannot be refilled. The words *no refill* (or *NR*) will appear on the medication container label, and *no refill* or *no refills* will be entered into the patient's computer record. If the prescription indicates *as needed*, or **prn** (or p.r.n.), then it can be filled up to a limited number of times, as set by state or federal laws. Most pharmacies and state laws require at least yearly updates on prn, or as needed, prescriptions.

Prescriber's Signature The prescriber's signature must appear online as an electronic signature or at the bottom of the paper prescription form in ink. It should be legible and recognizable by both the pharmacy technician and the pharmacist to detect possible forged prescriptions. Signatures by rubber stamps or by nurses and other office personnel are not valid. Faxed prescriptions must also be hand-signed before transmission. E-prescriptions must all be sent through a pharmacy security system approved by the state board of pharmacy. A phoned-in new prescription can come from the provider or provider's assistant—unless it is a C-II (Schedule II) drug. In some states, two blank signature lines are required at the bottom of the preprinted paper prescription: one next to *dispense as written* and the other next to the *substitution permitted*. If the former line is signed, the substitution of a generic equivalent is not permitted (see Figure 7.1). Other states require only one signature line—then *brand-necessary* directions must be specifically written out as part of the subscription.

If there are any doubts about the authenticity or completeness of a prescription, the pharmacy technician should alert the pharmacist immediately. A telephone call from the pharmacy technician or the pharmacist to the prescriber's office might be necessary to clarify an order. The technician may be allowed to clarify a prescription in some states, but all changes must be documented on the prescription (and/or in the patient profile). The changes must be accompanied by the name of the provider representative who clarified the issues, the date, and the initials of the technician and pharmacist who made the changes.

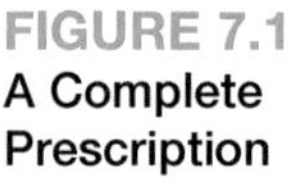

FIGURE 7.1 A Complete Prescription

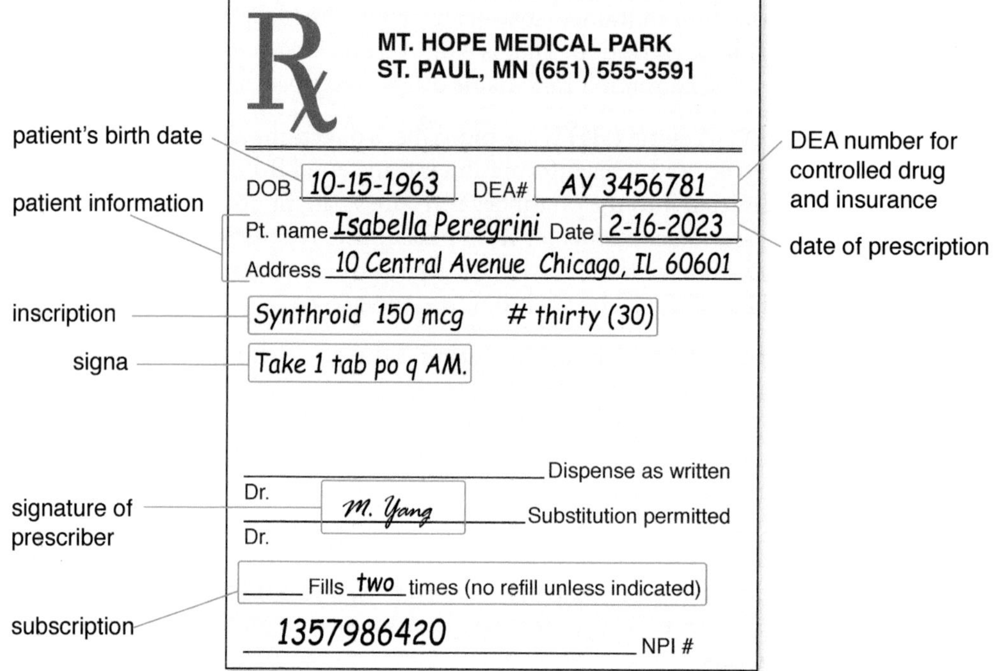

TABLE 7.3 The Critical Path of a New Prescription

1. No matter the type of prescription, make certain that it is complete, authentic, and legible. Electronic prescriptions may be printed out to be reviewed for completeness and potential errors. Phone-in orders must be transcribed onto paper.

2. Update the patient information in the patient profile, inform the patient of HIPAA privacy rights, and have them sign the form as required. If the patient is not in the pharmacy database, ask the patient for the necessary demographic, health, drug and supplement use, allergy, and insurance information.

3. Enter (type or scan) the prescription into the patient profile, and process the prescription for billing to the insurance company (Pharmacy Benefit Manager, or PBM). If approved, the amount of the patient's copay or coinsurance percentage payment will appear on-screen. If not, error messages will appear (more on this in Chapter 8.

4. Show the prescription (now in the profile) to the pharmacist for review against the original prescription and approval. The pharmacist then generates the medication container label. (Some pharmacies have the pharmacist do the checks of the prescription entry and the filling in the final verification step instead of in two separate steps.)

5. Perform a drug utilization review (DUR) with the pharmacy software to check on compatibility of the prescribed medication with medical and drug history, allergies, other prescriptions, OTC drugs, and supplements the patient is taking. Alert the pharmacist of anything you notice or that the computer flags or alerts. The pharmacist then checks the DUR and signs off on it. If the DUR is rejected because of the flag "refill too soon," contact the patient and provide the date the prescription can be filled.

continues

6. Select the appropriate medication, and match the National Drug Code (NDC) number barcoded on the stock drug bottle against the computer-generated medication label. (Some pharmacies have automatic dispensing machines that do some of these steps automatically, and you will have to double-check the work of the dispenser.)
7. Prepare the medication (the prescribed number of tablets or capsules are counted or the prescribed amount of liquid measured). Add flavorings if appropriate. Controlled drugs are often double-counted and initialed by both the pharmacy technician and the pharmacist.
8. Package the medication in the appropriate size and type of container (child-resistant or not).
9. Affix (or have the pharmacist affix, depending on state law) the computer-generated medication label and any auxiliary labels to the prescription container.
10. Assemble the prescription process elements (including the original prescription, stock drug bottle, medication container and label, and patient information, including a Medication Guide if required) for the pharmacist to complete a final verification.
11. The pharmacist checks the prescription and may initial the label and file the prescription in the pharmacy with a duplicate label.
12. Bag the approved prescription(s) for patient sale, inserting any medication information sheets (and a Medication Guide if required) about indications, interactions, and possible side effects (in some pharmacies and/or states, the pharmacist does this).
13. Return the stock drug bottle to the inventory shelf, and deliver the packaged prescription to the cash register area for patient pickup or to temperature-controlled refrigerated or frozen storage.
14. At pickup, verify that the correct patient is receiving the prescription by asking for address and/or birth date verification. Ask if counseling is needed or desired, and direct the patient to the pharmacist if appropriate. If someone other than the patient is picking up a controlled drug prescription, check the profile for any permission, and perhaps ask for a photo ID or birth date to establish the relationship to the patient (depending on state laws and pharmacy policies). You may need to document this on the prescription in the profile.
15. If payment is due, accept cash, credit card, or check. Some insurance providers require the patient to sign a printed or computer form verifying that the prescription was picked up.

Processing Time Expectations

The prescription filling process, which begins with the receipt and review of the prescription and ends with the dispensing to the patient, ideally takes about 5 to 10 minutes per prescription—without interruptions, such as phone calls, other patients dropping off prescriptions, insurance issues, questions to the pharmacist, and so on. Most likely, though, there will be many interruptions during a pharmacy shift, so at times it may take 15 to 20 minutes or more to process a prescription. If there are insurance issues (see Chapter 8), a longer time delay can be expected.

7.4 Computer Communications and Efficiencies

To process prescriptions and accomplish the other pharmacy functions, almost all community pharmacies are now equipped with a specially designed pharmacy software and **database management system (DBMS)**. It is a pharmacy-oriented computerized information system that integrates and interfaces (communicates) with the many different software programs needed for pharmacy operations and online transmissions and networking.

Pharmacy Software Interoperability

The ability to exchange and process information between various internal and external databases, software, and technology is called **interoperability**, and it creates the possibility of working together between different pharmacy functions and out-of-pharmacy stakeholders (like the prescriber and insurance representatives) for the best care of the patient. It also provides the most economical and time-efficient community pharmacy practices.

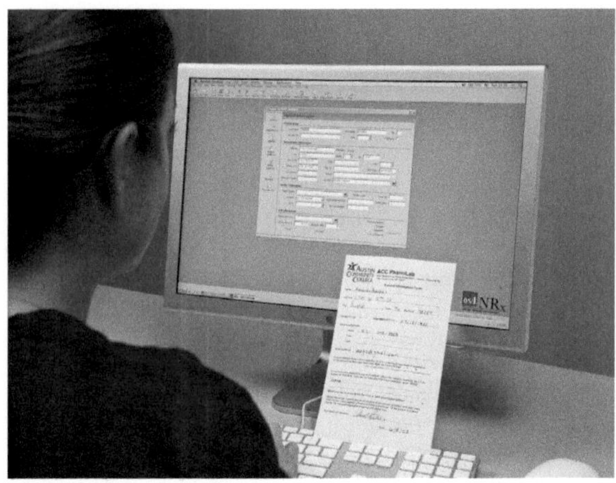

A technician must carefully input the hard copy prescription and insurance information into the patient's computer profile to begin the internal and online processing through the pharmacy's interfacing DBMS.

Prescribers also depend upon interoperability within their clinics and hospital networks for medical information and to transmit e-prescriptions. (see Figure 7.2).

FIGURE 7.2 Interoperability and E-Prescription Flow

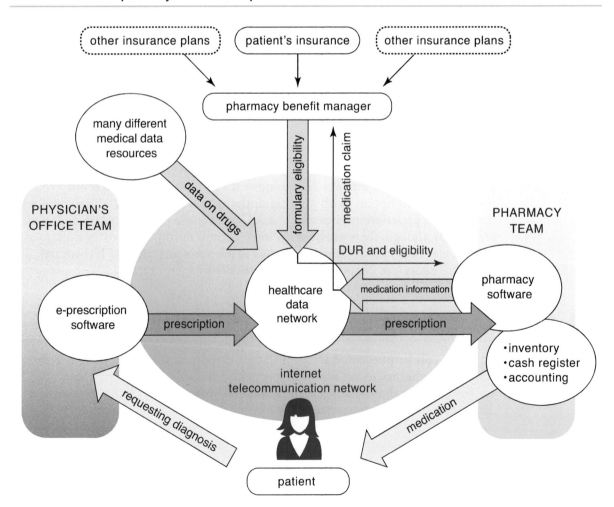

other insurance plans
patient's insurance
other insurance plans
pharmacy benefit manager
many different medical data resources
formulary eligibility
medication claim
data on drugs
PHYSICIAN'S OFFICE TEAM
PHARMACY TEAM
DUR and eligibility
healthcare data network
medication information
pharmacy software
e-prescription software
prescription
prescription
•inventory
•cash register
•accounting
internet telecommunication network
requesting diagnosis
medication
patient

Usually the DBMS software is menu-driven or Windows-based, allowing the technician to choose fields or functions easily from a menu of options on the screen by typing a single keystroke or function key on the keyboard. The pharmacy database typically contains the patient profile, physician database, pharmacy drug inventory, and a directory of prescribers and insurance plans. The software usually allows the technician to scan a written prescription and enter new prescription information or retrieve refill information. The fields of information can be sorted or queried to the patient's name, address, phone number, and date of birth; the prescription's number, drug name, National Drug Code (NDC) number, dosage and quantity of the drug, and number of refills; and the prescriber's name, address, phone number, and DEA number. As part of the drug utilization review (DUR), the systems provide automatic warnings about possible allergic or other adverse reactions. Some software applications even provide a picture or description of the medication to avoid errors.

Most of these pharmacy database systems also are capable of tracking expenses and inventory reports, generating reports concerning controlled substances or patient insurance, performing special dosing calculations, and retrieving medical and pharmacy literature. (More will be presented on the pharmacy DBMS and online insurance processing in Chapter 8 and overall pharmacy informatics, or information systems, in Chapter 10.)

Some examples of pharmacy software management systems include Rx30 Pharmacy System, SRS Pharmacy Systems, Epic's NCPDP Script Interface, and Prodigy's PROscript 2000. Some interface with bar code scanning technology and other automation, billing, retail accounting, purchasing, inventory, quality control, and productivity information. The DBMS also interfaces with electronic health records, medical databases, and insurance processing company systems. These interoperability functions are growing with the push of universal electronic health records shared among appropriate healthcare professionals.

Because of this computer integration, computer availability for technicians affects workload and efficiency. Some computers are intelligent or **smart terminals** that contain their own storage and processing capabilities. Others are **dumb terminals**, computer devices with a monitor and keyboard that do not contain storage and processing capabilities. The dumb terminal is connected to a **remote computer**—often a minicomputer or a mainframe at the main pharmacy, company headquarters, or home office—that stores and processes the data, such as patient information, prescription history, and insurance coverage. This computer communication involves the transmission of data signals through cables or the air via transmitters, receivers, and satellites. Some chain pharmacies have a terminal dedicated for each pharmacist and pharmacy technician. In independent pharmacies, both pharmacists and technicians may work at one or more computers throughout the pharmacy during a shift. Technicians sign on with their user names and passwords for each computer they will be working on; pharmacists must do likewise.

Types of Prescriptions

Before being able to process a prescription properly, a technician must understand the different requirements for the varying kinds of prescriptions:

- an electronic prescription
- a written hard copy on a prescriber's form from the patient
- a telephone or fax order from a prescriber
- a verbal order transcribed by a pharmacist

- a prescription on the profile
- a transfer prescription from another pharmacy
- a patient refill request
- a partial fill
- an emergency fill with prescriptions allowing no refills by the pharmacist
- a prescription transferred to and from another pharmacy

It is important to learn how to handle the different kinds of prescriptions because you will encounter them all in a community pharmacy.

E-Prescriptions

Nearly 70% of prescriptions are communicated from the prescriber to the pharmacy digitally via the internet through an examination room computer, a personal digital assistant a (PDA), tablet, or even a smart phone. These electronic or **e-prescriptions** (e-Rxs or e-scripts) are transmitted from the prescribers to the computers of the pharmacist or technician through a **healthcare interface network**, which offers online prescription processing that accesses national health and drug information systems to check the order and communicate it to the pharmacy (refer to Figure 7.2 and see Figure 7.3). Pharmacy online networks also work with the insurance processors. The most commonly used pharmaceutical healthcare networks are Surescripts and RxHub.

The direct nature of e-prescribing offers overall speed, accuracy, and improved billing. It minimizes the risk of medication errors due to illegible prescriber's handwriting, misinterpretation of abbreviations, and difficult-to-read faxes.

For patients, e-prescribing may decrease wait times. In fact, because e-prescriptions are forwarded from the prescriber's office directly to the pharmacy, the prescriptions are typically filled and ready to be dispensed to patients upon their arrival at the pharmacy. If a paper and an electronic transmission are both received at a pharmacy, one should be voided.

Electronic Prescriptions for Controlled Substances In addition, e-prescriptions for controlled substances are considered safer from forgeries than the handwritten prescriptions because the prescribers have to go through numerous steps to initiate the prescription.

As with handwritten prescriptions, e-prescriptions must have the DEA number and state eligibility for prescribing these substances, but they must also have a controlled-substance identity authentication and a protection software program and/or a private cryptographic key that encrypts, or puts into secret code, the prescriber's information to protect it from web theft. The prescriber's identity must be authenticated and double-protected by at least two of the following:

- a password or response to a security question
- a biometric, such as a fingerprint or eye scan
- a hard token that serves as a cryptographic or one-time password device

This does not mean that forgeries cannot happen through hacking, the carelessness of a prescriber, or the spying of an assisting associate, but forgeries are far less likely than with handwritten prescriptions.

FIGURE 7.3 E-Prescription

SAFFIRE, WILLIAM (DOB: 12/1/1955; ID: 1030) 64 year old man

ePrescribing ▾ epocrates online ▾ Settings

Current Allergies

codeine, sulfa drug (Updated by JONATHAN on 12/09/2009 06:10 AM)

Current Medications

Active ▾ Add New

nitroglycerin 0.4 mg subl...	Take 1 pill by m...
Viagra 25 mg oral tablet	Take 1 pill by m...

Viagra 25 mg oral tablet
Sig: Take 1 pill by mouth QD X 1 Month (30d)
Disp#: 30
Refills: 1
Prescribed By: Jonathan Bertman, MD
Last Filled: 12/09/09 (0 days ago)

INTERACTIONS:
- nitroglycerin 0.4 mg sublingual tablet and Viagra 25 mg oral tablet
- Viagra 25 mg oral tablet and nitroglycerin 0.4 mg sublingual tablet

Search the med database, then select the correct choice from within the list.

Only medications found in this list are eligible for interaction checking and electronic transmission.

Quick Script Writer

Open Quick Script Writer automatically.

Include State ID on script

Include DEA on script

Omit Signature

Dispense As Written

Comments:

1. Prepare Script

Inactivate History Refill All

Interactions

	Severity	Interaction	Type
✖	High	nitroglycerin 0.4 mg sublingual tablet and Via...	Drug/Drug
✖	High	Viagra 25 mg oral tablet and nitroglycerin 0.4 ...	Drug/Drug

Pending Medications

Check Interactions Double-click the interaction for details. Remove Pending Med 2. PRESCRIBE

2 interactions found

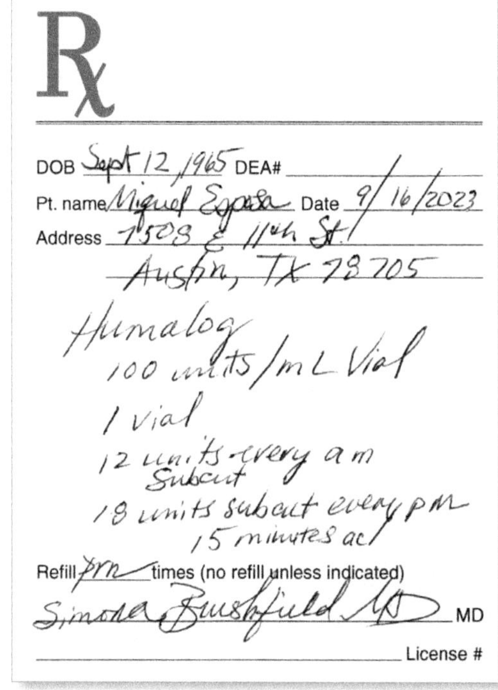

Rx

DOB Sept 12 1965 DEA#

Pt. name Miguel Espana Date 9/16/2023

Address 1508 E 11th St

Austin, TX 78705

Humalog
100 units/mL Vial
1 vial
12 units every am Subcut
18 units subcut every pm
15 minutes ac

Refill prn times (no refill unless indicated)

Simona Bushfield MD MD

License #

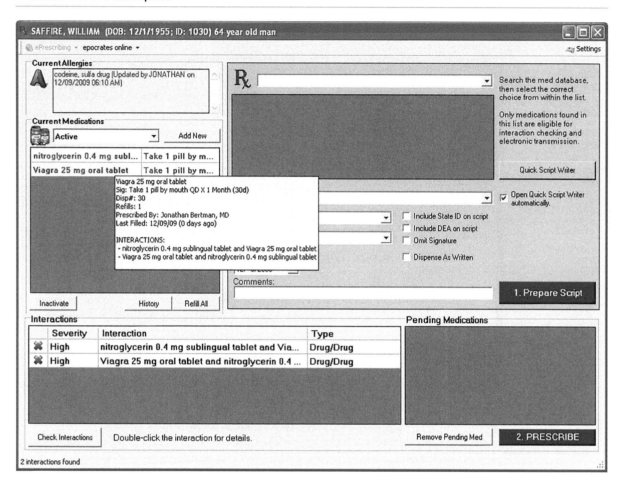

FIGURE 7.4 Handwritten Humalog Prescription

The prescription should be legible and contain all the information needed for the technician and the pharmacist to fill it accurately.

Written Prescriptions

The traditional written prescription (Rx) on a preprinted form is typically dropped off at the pharmacy counter or at the drive through window (see Figure 7.4). If the pharmacist is unclear on any component of the prescription, the technician or the pharmacist should call the prescriber's office for clarification; the name of the physician's representative along with the clarification should be entered onto the hard copy of the prescription and into the computerized patient profile.

In most pharmacies, the hard copy is scanned and recorded permanently into the electronic patient profile (see Figure 7.5). Prescriber information, the NDC number of the dispensed drug, and a photo of the drug are all recorded to minimize the chance of the wrong drug being entered into the computer or being dispensed. If the pharmacist or the technician misses entering the refills on the original prescription, the scanned prescription can be accessed to confirm the error.

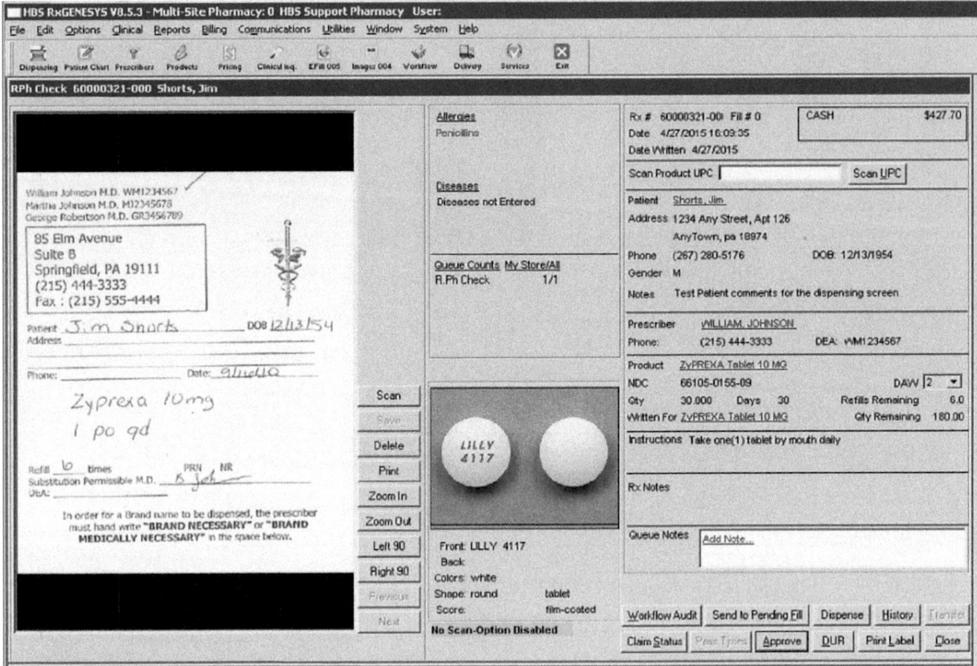

FIGURE 7.5 Written Prescription Processing

A written prescription can be scanned into a patient-specific electronic profile by the technician or the pharmacist.

Medicaid Prescriptions and Tamper-Resistant Prescriptions Medicare and Medicaid encourage secure e-prescriptions. If handwritten, prescriptions for Medicaid patients have distinct requirements. The Centers for Medicare and Medicaid Services (CMS) in cooperation with each state board of pharmacy requires that all prescriptions for Medicaid patients be written on a tamper-resistant prescription pad. A **tamper-resistant prescription (TRP)** is specifically designed to prevent copying, erasing, or alteration. Each state establishes its own acceptable characteristics for a TRP. Examples include some combination of chemical-protected paper, heat-sensitive image or other security features, and pantographs indicating "void" or "illegal" if copied. In Georgia, for example, the prescription for a Medicaid patient must possess one or more of the following requirements:

- a gray security background—the word "VOID" appears when script is photocopied
- an identifier production batch number in the margin on the front of the sheet
- a consecutive number in the upper left-hand corner of the sheet
- erasure protection—a white mark appears when erased with an ink eraser
- a security watermark on the back of the sheet—hold up to the light at a 45-degree angle to view (when duplicated, the artificial watermark is not visible on the copy)
- a coin-activated security mark on the back of the script—rub with a coin to validate the script

If an audit reveals that prescriptions for Medicaid patients were not written on TRP paper or authenticated by pharmacy personnel, claims for reimbursement may be denied. A prescription for a controlled substance not written on a TRP paper should particularly cause closer scrutiny by both the technician and the pharmacist.

IN THE REAL WORLD

Surescripts, an information technology company that monitors e-prescriptions between healthcare organizations and pharmacies, reviewed more than 40 million of its prescription records in a study to compare the effectiveness of e-prescriptions versus paper prescriptions on first-fill medication adherence (the picking up of new prescriptions by patients). First-fill pickups on e-prescriptions improved by 10% over traditional written, verbal, and faxed prescriptions.

Problems, however, can still occur in electronic systems. In 2014, Surescripts discovered that one of its data sources contained glitches with special characters corrupting the decimal points in its listing of medication dispensing levels. For instance, what should have been "ramipril 2.5 mg capsules" was being transmitted as "ramipril 25 mg capsules." Surescripts alerted pharmacies and pulled this source from its database until the problem could be resolved. The Institute for Safe Medication Practices (ISMP) reminds technicians, pharmacists, and other healthcare professionals to question and verify any medication dosages reported in medication histories or data that seem strange or out of the normal ranges.

Telephone

Telephone prescriptions must generally be taken by a pharmacist, though in some states such as South Carolina, a certified pharmacy technician may take a verbal prescription over the telephone (as well as handle transfers in or out of the pharmacy). Generally, the pharmacist transcribes the telephone order onto a prescription pad and verifies its accuracy. Then the technician can enter the information into the patient profile and initiate the dispensing process. The pharmacist then checks the prescription a second time after technician order entry or during the final verification step.

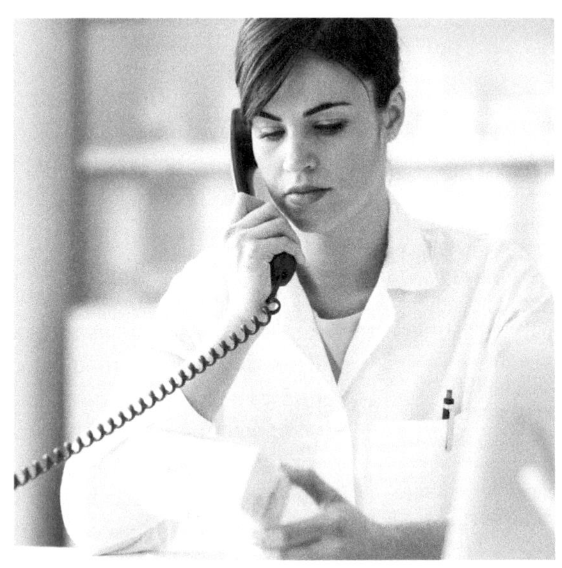

In most states, only the pharmacist may take verbal prescriptions over the phone.

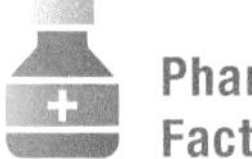

Pharm Fact

As e-prescriptions are on the rise, fax prescriptions are being phased out by many healthcare prescribers.

Fax Orders

Medical offices that are not yet equipped to send e-prescriptions may elect to fax new or refill medication orders to a dedicated fax line in the pharmacy. Fax orders contain all the necessary patient demographic, prescriber, and medication information to fill the prescription. Faxed prescriptions are scanned and/or entered into the patient profile by the technician (or the pharmacist) and verified by the pharmacist before being filled. With very few exceptions, C-II controlled prescriptions cannot be faxed and require a hard copy and signature from an authorized prescriber registered with the DEA. If a fax number is not available for the prescriber, the pharmacist may need to call the medical office for refill authorization.

Prescriptions Not Yet Due

Not all prescriptions are filled and delivered on the same day as they are received. Often a patient may present a new written prescription that does not need to be (or cannot be) filled until a future date. The pharmacy may also receive a similar verbal, faxed, or electronic prescription. This type of prescription is referred to as placing a **prescription on profile**, and it may be on hold for a variety of reasons. For example, the patient may have sufficient medication at home, especially if the dose was lowered. Or the prescription may be held because the patient does not have the cash on hand to pay for all the prescribed medications. A prescription may also be held due to lack of insurance coverage until a future date. With the exception of controlled drugs, prescriptions are valid to be filled from one year of the original date written.

If a handwritten prescription to be held is for a C-II drug, it is typically stored in an alphabetized file box and listed on the patient profile for easy retrieval at a later date, not to exceed six months. Some state boards of pharmacy—as well as the policies of individual pharmacies—may not permit the storage of C-II prescriptions, and these prescriptions must be returned to the patient. Check with your pharmacy to see its policy on profiled C-II prescriptions.

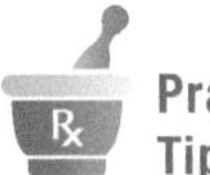

Practice Tip

Many insurance groups are opening their own mail-order pharmacies and putting restrictions on three-month supplies to encourage patients to use their pharmacies instead of local pharmacies. Knowing customers' names and faces encourages them to return.

Refill Requests

Refill requests in person or over the phone are relatively easy to process if the patient has the prescription container or can tell you over the phone the prescription number on the label. Some pharmacy software systems have the capability to prepare automatic refills when their time is due if patients desire it. Since the prescription information for refills has already been previously entered into the patient profile and verified by the pharmacist, the dispensing time is shorter. The technician first verifies that a refill is allowed and not early for the medication (based on the inscription and days' supply calculation) and then forwards the request for pharmacist review.

Most pharmacies and insurance plans allow medications to be refilled approximately five days prior to the next scheduled refill date. For example, a patient may request that a three-month supply of medication be filled to save on copayments or to avoid traveling to the pharmacy each month. If a prescriber writes a prescription for a 3-month (90-day) supply, and the insurance company approves it, there is no problem. However, if the prescription was written for a 30-day supply with two refills, the pharmacy technician or pharmacist must sometimes call the prescriber's office to get approval for the full 90-day supply at one time. If the prescription is filled without documentation of prescriber approval, then some state boards may consider this an overstepping of the pharmacist's role into that of the physician—and possible legal ramifications may ensue.

No Refills Under certain circumstances, no refills are permitted—*despite what the medication label indicates*. Prescriptions that may not be refilled include those that are:

- more than 12 months old,
- for a C-II drug where no refills are allowed without a new prescription,
- for a controlled drug (C-III–IV) written more than six months ago or already refilled five times,

- for a controlled drug that has been previously transferred to another pharmacy,
- from a hospital emergency room (ER), commonly only for short-term use with no refills,
- hospital discharge prescriptions (most allow no refills).

In any of these situations, pharmacy technicians should explain the common protocol to patients. They need to contact their primary care physicians to refill any prescription originating from the ER or a hospital discharge.

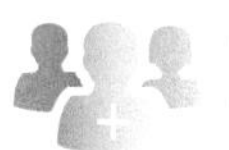

Work Wise

Just before holidays and vacation seasons, many customers may ask for early refills or need reminders not to count on getting refills in foreign countries. To refill prescriptions early, technicians have to ask the patients' insurance companies for vacation overrides.

Partial Refills At times, a pharmacy will not have enough drugs in its inventory to completely fill or refill a prescription, so it will dispense a **partial fill** or a two- to five-day supply to hold the patient over until new drug inventory is received. For example, a patient may present a prescription for a 3-month, or 90-day, supply of gabapentin, but the technician discovers that the inventory has stock containing a total of only 150 capsules.

Common practice is to issue a five-day supply (in this case, 15 capsules) and order the remaining medication for the next business day. The five-day supply hopefully will cover the weekends or holidays and not inconvenience the patient. The remaining 135 capsules in inventory can be used for other prescriptions for gabapentin received later that day. Obviously, the technician must explain the reason for the partial fill to the patient and say when the remainder of the prescription can be picked up. The patient may be billed only for the amount of drug dispensed at that time or for the entire amount when picked up later, depending on store policy.

Early Refills A patient may ask for an early refill due to special circumstances, such as an upcoming vacation or a lost prescription. Insurance companies often will reject an early refill automatically. The pharmacy technician may offer to call the insurance provider to try to get approval for a "one time" override for an early refill. If not granted, the patient may need to pay for the medication until insurance covers the next refill.

If a refill request is made too early (more than five days before the refill date), then the request will definitely be rejected by a third-party insurance company. For example, suppose that a patient requests a refill of Motrin (ibuprofen) 600 mg #90, 1 tab tid prn for 30 days. The patient's profile indicates that the prescription was filled on April 1. Because this is a 30-day supply, the refill is then due May 1, which means that the technician can initiate the refill request on or after April 25. Each pharmacy and insurance provider has its own policy outlining the procedure for handling early refills, especially for controlled substances. When needed, the technician should explain the pharmacy's policy and reasons for it to the patient.

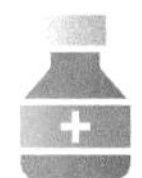

Pharm Fact

In most states and pharmacies, birth control medications are not considered eligible for an "emergency fill," though it may feel like an emergency to many patients. Technicians have to explain the policies.

Emergency Refills An emergency fill is for a short-term emergency supply of a needed medication for a chronic condition, such as high blood pressure, diabetes, high cholesterol, or epilepsy. Patients with these or related conditions typically have prescriptions with limited refills, requiring them to schedule follow-up visits with their primary care physician for monitoring and blood work. Even so, they may need a refill to bridge the gap at night or on weekends when refill authorization is not feasible. Most states allow pharmacists to use their best professional judgment to provide a short-term emergency supply (usually two to three days) of an essential medication until refill authorization can be obtained.

Typically, there is no patient charge for this temporary emergency fill. When the prescriber renews the prescription, the amount of medication "loaned" to the patient is subtracted from the refill. For example, if three tablets of amlodipine 10 mg are loaned and a new prescription is received the next day for #90, then 87 tablets will be

Remember that controlled substance prescriptions can be transferred only once in the lifetime of the prescription unless the transferring pharmacies share an online, real-time database. Then they can transfer as many times as there are allowed refills. However, C-II substances cannot be transferred. A written prescription is always necessary for C-II substances, except in an emergency if verified by the prescriber.

dispensed, but 90 tablets will be billed to the insurance company. Emergency fills of controlled drugs are seldom permitted except under extremely unusual circumstances or for pain relief for terminally ill patients.

Transfer Prescriptions

At a patient's request, prescriptions can be legally transferred from one pharmacy to another. Common transfer reasons may be insurance coverage and customer service issues, including the pharmacy's hours of operation or location. According to the law in most states, only a licensed pharmacist can transfer or copy a prescription from (or to) another pharmacy, and the new pharmacist must personally talk to the pharmacist at the originating pharmacy.

Transfer Out A **transfer out** is a prescription refill in which the pharmacist, at the request of a patient, transfers the refill to a new pharmacy. Controlled prescription drugs, with the exception of C-II drugs, cannot be transferred to be refilled "early" and can be transferred only one time. If the prescription was already filled at your pharmacy but not yet picked up by the patient, then it must be retrieved from the storage bin and returned to inventory. The medication charges must then be reversed with the insurance provider.

Transfer In When a previously filled prescription arrives at a new pharmacy, it is called a **transfer in** prescription. After the phone discussion between the two pharmacists, the originating pharmacy provides over the phone, fax, or electronic transmission all the relevant information (including any remaining refills on the prescription) to the transfer pharmacy. The originating pharmacy must agree to "close" the prescription to any remaining refills.

Transfer-in prescriptions require additional time to find the phone number and make the telephone call, wait on the phone to connect one pharmacist to the other, transcribe the prescription information, and enter the prescription into the patient profile. The transfer process is easier if the patient presents to the new pharmacy the medication vial containing the medication's name, dosage, prescription number, and the originating pharmacy's name and telephone number. However, the transfer can also be made if the patient supplies their name and birth date, the name and phone number of the originating pharmacy, and the name of the medication to be transferred. Figure 7.6 shows an example of a form that may be used to document information that must be received for each transfer prescription.

FIGURE 7.6 Information Needed for a Transfer Prescription

A form like this on paper or online must be filled in by the transfer-out pharmacy and must be received by the transfer-in pharmacy.

The Corner Drug Store — **Transferred Rx**

Patient Name ____________ Date ____________
Address ____________
Phone Number ____________ Birth Date ____________
Allergies/Health Conditions ____________ Hold ☐ DAW ☐
Pharmacy Phone # ____________ Pharmacy ____________
RPh ____________
Rx # ____________
Last Fill ____________
Original Date ____________
Remaining Refills ____________
Prescriber ____________
Prescriber Phone # ____________
MD DEA ____________ Pharmacist initials ______
Pharmacy DEA (if controlled substance) ____________

If the prescription is for a new patient, then more time is needed to get necessary demographic, allergy, health and medication history, and insurance information to complete the patient profile. If the transfer prescription has no remaining refills or if the original date is beyond one year or, in some cases, six months, the technician or pharmacist must call the physician's office to request a new prescription.

Many chain pharmacies have a shared database of patient profiles, which allows transfers without the need of a telephone call and verification of patient and medication information. An affiliated pharmacy in Alabama would typically send an electronic message to the pharmacy in Georgia to notify personnel of the transfer. By law, the transfer of controlled substances still requires a telephone call in most states.

Mail-Order Prescriptions

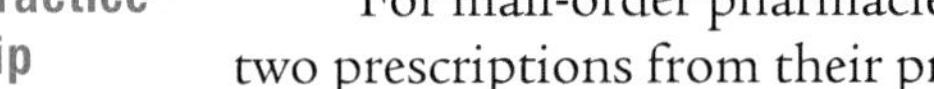

Practice Tip

Many abbreviations are particularly easy to mix up. To access the ISMP's List of Error-Prone Abbreviations, Symbols, and Dose Designations, pharmacy technicians should visit https://PharmPractice7e.ParadigmEducation.com/ISMP-abbreve.

For mail-order pharmacies, new patients for long-term medications generally get two prescriptions from their prescribers—one sent online to a community pharmacy for immediate filling of a 30-day supply, and a second one in paper handed to them for a 90-day supply. The patients fill out an online survey for their patient profile and then print out and send in the order form along with their paper prescription. Once received, the technicians and pharmacists verify and check the prescription in the same way as a regular community pharmacy. If there are problems, they call the patient or the prescriber for more information before filling the prescription. Refills are done through phone calls or by checking the refill box online.

Signa and Subscription Abbreviations

To translate any prescription for filling, one must know the common abbreviations used in the signa and subscription. (Examples are shown in Table 7.4 and a more complete listing in Appendix B.) This knowledge is essential to avoid any misinterpretation of prescription abbreviations, which may result in a serious medication error due to entering the wrong drug, wrong dose, or wrong directions.

The Institute for Safe Medication Practices (ISMP) has called for the complete elimination of handwritten prescriptions to avoid problems from illegible or confusing handwriting and for the elimination of some that are easily confused or misread, such as *qid* (four times daily) and *q6h* (every six hours), in favor of using the appropriate words.

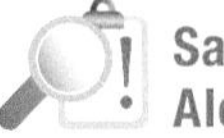

Safety Alert

Show all prescriptions with questionable authenticity or illegible handwriting to the pharmacist before entering them into the computer database.

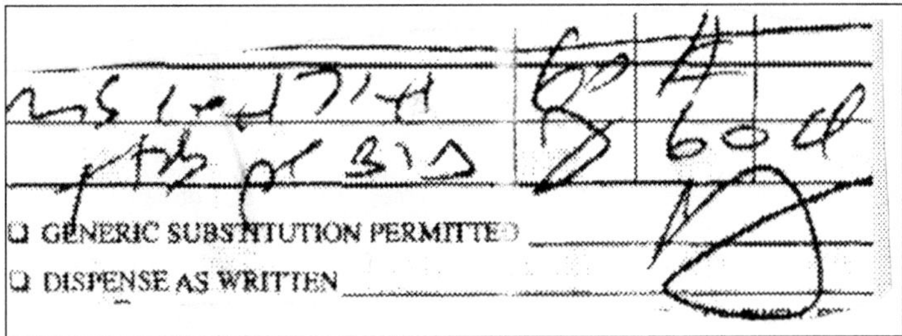

This prescription for morphine sulfate 60 mg is indecipherable in many ways. A follow-up call to the prescriber's office is necessary.

TABLE 7.4 Common Prescription Abbreviations

Category	Abbreviation	Meaning
Amount	cc*	cubic centimeter (mL)
	g	gram
	gr	grain
	gtt	drop
	mg	milligram
	mL	milliliter
	qs	a sufficient quantity
	tbsp	tablespoonful
	tsp	teaspoonful
Dosage form	cap	capsule
	MDI	metered-dose inhaler
	sol	solution
	supp	suppository
	susp	suspension
	tab	tablet
	ung	ointment
Time of administration	ac	before meals
	am	morning, before noon
	bid	twice a day
	hs*	at bedtime
	pc	after meals
Time of administration	pm	evening, after noon
	prn	as needed
	q6h	every 6 hrs.
	qid	4 times a day
	tid	3 times a day
	tiw	3 times a week
Site of administration	ad*	right ear
	as*	left ear
	au*	both ears
	od*	right eye
	os*	left eye
	ou*	both eyes
	po	oral, by mouth
	pr	rectally
	sl	sublingual (under the tongue)
	top	topical (skin)
	vag	vaginally

*These abbreviations, although commonly utilized by practitioners, are easily misread. Consequently, the abbreviations have been designated as dangerous by the Institute for Safe Medication Practices (ISMP).

7.5 Working with the Patient Profile Database

To process any prescription, a patient profile must be created or updated. The **patient profile** is the *confidential* data file in the pharmacy software that contains the customer's demographic and insurance information. The profile lists all of the prescriptions that have been dispensed at that pharmacy for that individual by any prescriber.

Creating a New Patient Profile

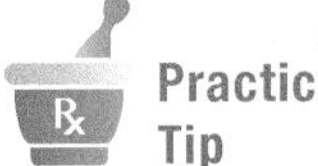

Practice Tip

It is helpful to ask patients if they have had prescriptions filled at other pharmacies and explain that this information is important for the safe dispensing of their new prescription.

When new customers come in with a prescription, the pharmacy technician needs to have them answer questions or have them complete a written patient profile questionnaire. Every pharmacy patient must have a current, updated profile to have a prescription filled. (See a sample profile form in Figure 7.7.) Components of the essential information include patient demographics (name, birth date, address, phone numbers, email address); insurance and billing information (covered in Chapters 8 and 9); medical, allergy, and prescription histories; and prescription preferences, such as no child-proof caps, large-print medication sheets, foreign language specifications, and so on. For an explanation of each of these components, see Table 7.5.

It is also good if the patient questions and profile cover OTC drug and alcohol use, homeopathies, and dietary supplements (including vitamins and nutritional substances).

TABLE 7.5 **Components of the Patient Profile**

Component	Content
Identifying information	Patient's full name including middle initial in some cases, street address, telephone number, birth date, and sex (Increasingly, some programs are entering email addresses so that refill notifications and other communications can be made.)
Insurance and billing information	Information necessary for billing (More information on insurance billing is discussed in Chapter 8.)
Medical and allergy history	Information concerning existing conditions; for example, diabetes or heart disease, known allergies, and adverse drug reactions the patient has experienced (The pharmacy software reviews the medical history for the pharmacist to make sure that the prescription is safe to fill for a given patient.)
Medication and prescription history	Any prescriptions filled at this pharmacy location; some software includes OTC medications and supplements (The pharmacy software reviews this information for the pharmacist to make sure that the prescription will not cause adverse drug interactions [i.e., negative consequences] because of the combined effects of drugs and/or other drugs or foods.)
Prescription preferences	Patient preferences as they apply to prescriptions; for example, child-resistant or non-child-resistant containers, generic substitutions, large-print labels, foreign language preference, and so on
HIPAA confidentiality	Each new patient is required by law to receive and sign a statement of patient confidentiality, which is then documented and stored on the patient profile (This statement is for the protection of the pharmacy.)

FIGURE 7.7
Written Patient Profile Form

PATIENT PROFILE

Patient Name

Last ______ First ______ Middle Initial ______

Street or PO Box

City ______ State ______ ZIP ______

Phone ( ) ___ ___

Date of Birth ______ Month Day Year

□ Male
□ Female

Social Security No. ___ ___ ___

□ Yes, I would like medication dispensed in a child-resistant container.
□ No, I do not want medication dispensed in a child-resistant container.

Medication Insurance	Cardholder Name ______		
□ Yes	□ Cardholder	□ Child	□ Disabled Dependent
□ No	□ Spouse	□ Dependent Parent	□ Full-Time Student

MEDICAL HISTORY

HEALTH		ALLERGIES AND DRUG REACTIONS
□ Anemia	□ Epilepsy	□ No known drug allergies or reactions
□ Angina	□ Glaucoma	□ Aspirin
□ Arthritis	□ Heart condition	□ Cephalosporins
□ Asthma	□ Kidney disease	□ Codeine
□ Blood-clotting disorders	□ Liver disease	□ Erythromycin
□ High blood pressure	□ Lung disease	□ Penicillin
□ Breast-feeding	□ Parkinson's disease	□ Sulfa drugs
□ Cancer	□ Pregnancy	□ Tetracyclines
□ Diabetes	□ Ulcers	□ Xanthines
Other conditions ______		□ Other allergies/reactions ______

Prescription Medication(s) Being Taken ______

OTC Medication(s) Currently Being Taken ______

Would you like generic medication when possible? □ Yes □ No

Comments ______

Health information changes periodically. Please notify the pharmacy of any new medications, allergies, drug reactions, or health conditions.

______ Signature ______ Date □ I do not wish to provide this information.

Technicians need to make patients comfortable and encourage them to write down everything about their drug and supplement history.

Finally, it is important to know if the patient gets prescriptions filled at more than one pharmacy, as this makes the potential for drug interactions more possible. If so, the pharmacist may want to talk with the patient more before filling the prescription.

HIPAA Requirements

In addition to completing the profile, the patient must also be given a copy of the pharmacy's personal information privacy policies to comply with the Health Insurance Portability and Accountability Act (HIPAA). Patients have to sign off that they have received this notice, and proof is commonly scanned and saved in the computerized

Practice Tip

For questions about HIPAA rules, go to the Frequently Asked Questions section of HIPAA at https://PharmPractice7e.ParadigmEducation.com/HIPAA.

patient profile. If someone other than the patient is picking up the prescription, the signature on the HIPAA form may need to be deferred to a later date. It is extremely important that the confidentiality of patient medical information be maintained at all times. (For more information on patient confidentiality protocol, see Chapter 15.)

Pharmacist Verification of New Profile

Once all the prescription information has been entered into the patient profile, it is verified by the pharmacist before or after the prescription is filled. The pharmacist will check that the correct date, patient, drug, dose, directions, refills, and prescriber were entered without typos or other errors.

Updating Current Customer Profile

If a patient profile already exists, the pharmacy technician finds the record and double-checks it, matching the patient name with the correct address. This step is critical, as more than one patient often has the same name (Bob Anderson) or a similar name (Michael versus Michelle Courier). Also, there may be more than one address listed in the patient profile. Patients may also be known by and entered under their middle name, for example as R. Karen Lee instead of the legal name of Roberta K. Lee.

Changed or hyphenated names can also be tricky. Those who have recently married or divorced may have a new last name, but only their earlier name may be recognized by an insurance company.

As a safeguard, a second patient identifier is usually used for verification just as with prescriptions. This identifier is commonly the date of birth (see Figure 7.8). Failure to verify the identifiers may result in a serious medication error—a prescription entered into the wrong patient profile and thus filled for the wrong patient.

FIGURE 7.8
Computerized Patient Profile Sample

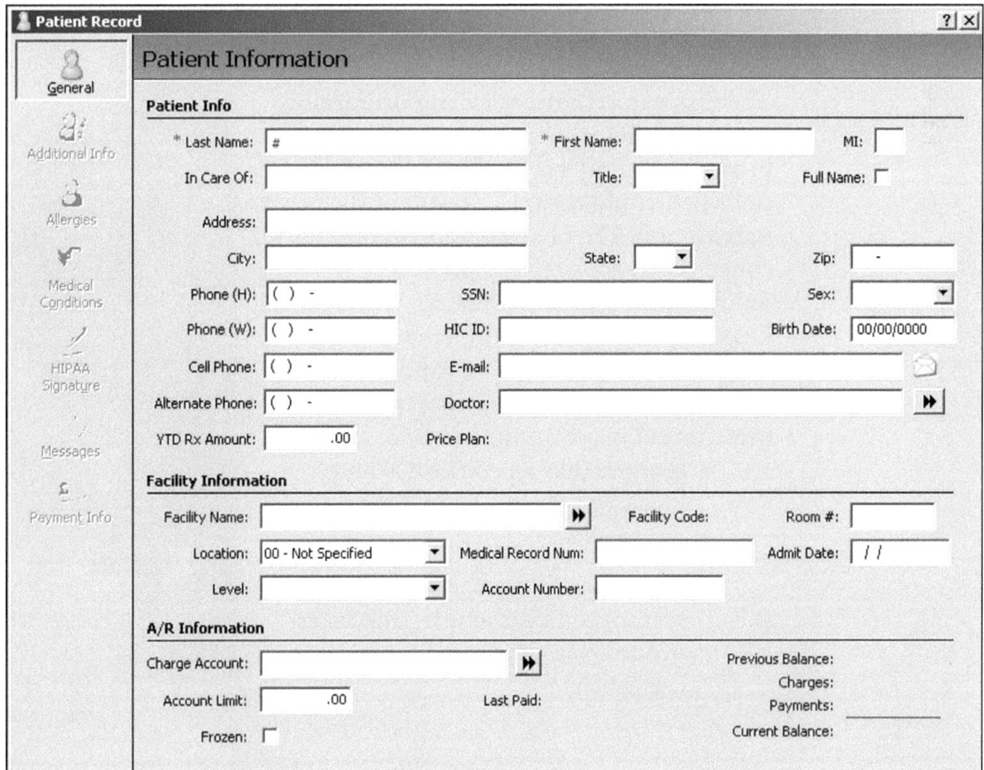

The pharmacy technician also needs to verify that the name, address, and phone number of the prescriber have not changed and match the information in the patient profile. Many prescribers practice at more than one medical office. If an incorrect phone number is entered, refill requests will be faxed or telephoned to the wrong medical office.

The patient's medication and prescription history section will contain the information on all the prescriptions filled by this pharmacy (and all the pharmacies of the same chain), including the drug names, prescription numbers (automatically assigned by the computer at each prescription filling), dosage forms, quantities, numbers of refills authorized (if any), prescriber's name and identifiers, and patient cost or copayment for the prescriptions. Patients often have many different prescribers.

All new information entered must also be verified by the pharmacist.

7.6 The Medication Reconciliation Process

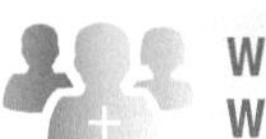

If prescription problems arise, the technician should ask the patient whether he or she prefers to wait for the prescription to be filled and, based on workload and staffing, provide a good estimate for the waiting time to allow the patient to elect to wait, shop, or run errands.

After an initial review of the prescription and completing or updating the patient profile, the technician enters the new prescription into the profile via inputting or scanning. The correct entry of the prescription is so critical because many drugs have similar names, and the incorrect drug or dose can be easily chosen from the drop-down menus in the computer database.

Also, any written comments by the prescriber must be included in the database and on the medication label. For example, a narcotic prescription may include "may cause sedation," "do not fill until [date]," or "refill no sooner than every 30 days." Likewise, a prescription for an antibiotic may include "take for 10 days" or "take with food." All of these instructions must appear on the medication container label for the patient. Once the pharmacist has approved the profile and the entered prescription, the medication reconciliation process can begin.

The Drug Utilization Review

The first step is to run the **drug utilization review (DUR)**, which scans the patient profile to identify any problematic interactions that could occur as a result of the new prescription. The pharmacy software will concurrently transmit the prescription online for insurance processing. When the DUR detects potential problematic reactions, it offers warning alerts and action steps. There are many reasons a new prescription may be problematic:

- allergies (like a penicillin allergy)
- a complicating medical condition (like diabetes or asthma)
- duplicate of a similar drug already prescribed (for example, two different drugs or narcotics for migraine headaches)

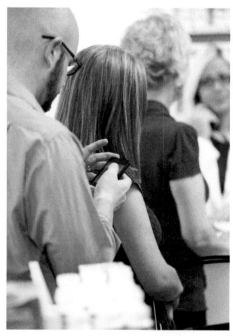

While no one likes to wait, accurately and safely processing a prescription has to take priority over rushing to keep someone from waiting.

- it has been prescribed in doses too low subtherapeutic or too high (toxic) for the patient (as with pediatric or geriatric patients)
- it may not be safe or should be used only with caution for the patient because of being part of a vulnerable patient population (for example, women of child-bearing age or who are pregnant or breast-feeding)

The DUR always offers an onscreen alert or alert code for any potential **adverse drug reactions (ADRs)**, which are negative consequences from taking a particular drug or mix of drugs. The harmful responses can range from skin reactions and breathing problems to temporary injury, permanent disability, or death. An ADR can also create an **allergy** (hypersensitivity reaction) if that drug or a similar drug is taken again. Different pharmacy software programs, online networks, and insurance companies use different DUR codes, abbreviations, and messages, but all offer alerts (see Table 7.6).

TABLE 7.6 Sample of Drug Utilization Review Screen Codes

Administrative	Dosing/Limits	Drug Conflict	Disease Management	Precautionary
AN - Prescription Authentication	ER - Overuse	AT - Additive Toxicity	AD - Additional Drug Needed	DF - Drug-Food Interaction
CH - Call Help Desk	EX - Excessive Quantity	DA - Drug-Allergy	AR - Adverse Drug Reaction	DL - Drug-Lab Conflict
MS - Missing Information/ Clarification	MX - Excessive Duration	DC - Drug-Disease (inferred)	CS - Patient Complaint/ Symptom	DS - Tobacco Use
NA - Drug Not Available	HD - High Dose	DD - Drug-Drug Interaction	DM - Apparent Drug Misuse	OH - Alcohol Conflict
NC - Non-Covered Drug Purchase	LD - Low Dose	DI - Drug Incompatibility	ED - Patient Education/ Instruction	SE - Side Effect
NF - Non-Formulary Drug	LR - Underuse	IC - **Iatrogenic Condition**	ND - New Disease/ Diagnosis	
NP - New Patient Processing	MN - Insufficient Duration	ID - Ingredient Duplication	NN - Unnecessary Drug	
PS - Product Selection Opportunity	NS - Insufficient Quantity	MC - Drug-Disease (reported)	PC - Patient Question/ Concern	
P - Plan Protocol	SF - Suboptimal Dosage Form	NR - Lactation/ Nursing Interaction	PN - Prescriber Consultation	
TP - Payer/Processor Question	SR - Suboptimal Regimen	PA - Drug-Age	RF - Health Provider Referral	
		PG - Drug-Pregnancy	SD - Suboptimal Drug/ Indication	
		PR - Prior Adverse Reaction	TN - Laboratory Test Needed	
		SX - Drug-Sex		
		TD - Therapeutic Duplication		

Safety Alert

As a technician, never perform or acknowledge a DUR. Once it has been acknowledged, the system thinks that it has been addressed, and the pharmacist's opportunity to decide a course of action or counsel the patient is lost. All software actions related to a DUR pertaining to drug interactions should be executed by a pharmacist for safety.

Safety Alert

The technician must not rely just on the software but must also be on the lookout for any possible problems and let the pharmacist know.

Once a DUR message appears, the technician *must show it to the pharmacist,* who will then guide and help the technician to review and resolve the problem. The technician also needs to explain to the patient that a potential medication problem exists that must be resolved prior to dispensing. For example, if hydrocodone, a codeine derivative, is prescribed to patients whose profile indicates that they are allergic to codeine, then a precautionary message or code, such as *DA*, meaning *Drug Allergy*, will pop up. The pharmacist will check the patient profile for prior use of the drug and/or ask patients whether they remember taking hydrocodone without an allergic reaction. Similarly, if a patient is allergic to penicillin, the computer will generate a red flag if cephalexin (Keflex), a related antibiotic, is prescribed.

The technician cannot override DUR flags without pharmacist review, but the technician generally does prioritize the alerts for the pharmacist in terms of urgency. The DUR is an extremely important shared responsibility of the technician and the pharmacist. A missed drug allergy or serious drug interaction can cause great patient harm or even death and could also trigger a major negligence lawsuit.

The insurance response often comes back during the DUR. It provides additional alerts and action steps, some of which the technician can directly handle, such as notifying the patient that there is an "early refill" rejection. (Insurance processing will be covered in Chapter 8.) The technician, however, can notify the patient that there is an "early refill" rejection by the insurance provider.

The DUR and insurance processing steps are specifically designed to provide an additional level of protection to catch problems before they can occur. The processes address two real-world pharmacy practice issues: (1) no pharmacist (or prescriber) can remember all doses, adverse effects, and drug interactions for all medications, especially while juggling a typically busy medical office or pharmacy workload; and (2) a complete centralized medication profile usually does not exist, because patients often go to more than one pharmacy or more than one physician.

The pharmacy software catches issues from the patient profile, while the insurance software often catches problems with medications received at other pharmacies, among other issues. However, when a patient is taking unlisted OTC medications and supplements or using alcohol or other substances, it is not possible to assess the full potential of drug issues. That is why it is a "best practice" for the pharmacy technician to ask for additional information about these uses to enter them into the patient profile, or have the pharmacist discuss all of this with the patient in conversation or a medication therapy counseling appointment.

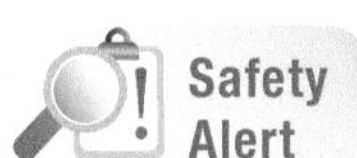
Safety Alert

Technicians and pharmacists have to fight alert fatigue, or getting so used to common alerts that they are not taken seriously. Some computer systems lock up after alerts until the pharmacist resolves the issues and unlocks the system.

Pharmacist Responses to Drug Utilization Review Alerts

Most DUR notifications are categorized by their potential severity: mild, moderate, or severe (see Figure 7.9). Generally, the pharmacist must document the actions taken on moderate and severe alerts. Sometimes the needed response is listed on-screen. The pharmacist must use professional judgment to review the profile and assess the significance. Then the pharmacist must determine what type of action, if any, is necessary. Options include the following:

- contacting the prescribing physician for more information or options
- counseling the patient on potential issues prior to dispensing
- overriding the DUR and filling the prescription

The pharmacy technician will not be able to proceed to fill the prescription for the patient until the pharmacist resolves the DUR alert(s). Often the pharmacist will write a reminder note that the patient needs counseling about the drug's use and potential effects. When the patient arrives to pick up the medication, the technician will tell the pharmacist so that this conversation can happen.

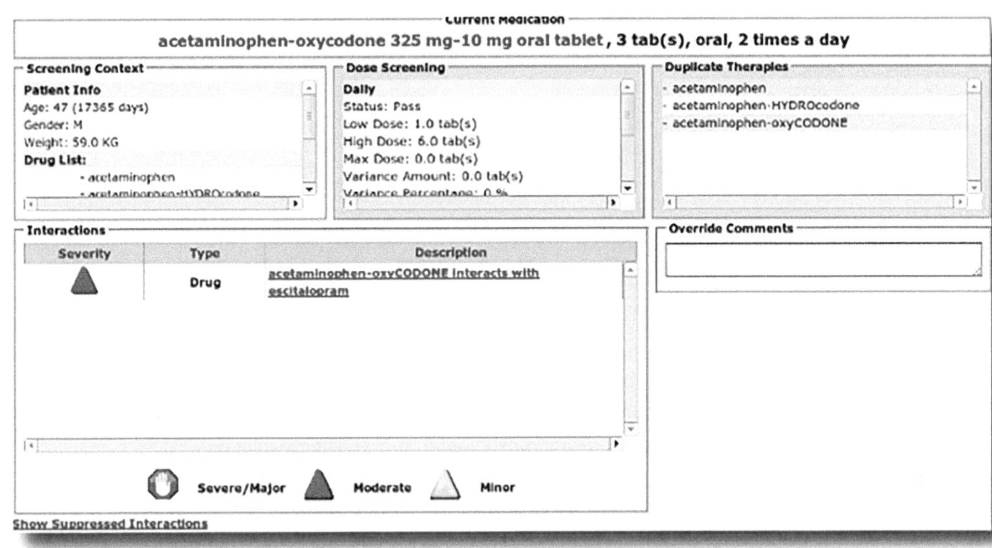

FIGURE 7.9
Sample DUR Alert

When pharmacy software detects a potentially serious drug interaction, the technician must alert the pharmacist to have it resolved before filling and dispensing.

7.7 Stock Selection and Medication Preparation

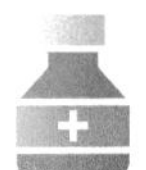

Pharm Fact

One in four filling errors is due to a confusion of names, which is why NDC checks are essential.

Once the prescription's entry into the computer has passed through the DUR and been approved for insurance, the pharmacist approves it and prints a medication container label (and any required medication information) to initiate the filling process. This label includes patient demographics, insurance billing information and copayments, the name of drug being dispensed (name, strength, form, and quantity), the National Drug Code, and the potential for refills on the prescription.

To identify the exact manufacturer, drug, dose, and package size, the technician uses the NDC number to (1) retrieve the correct manufacturer's **stock bottle**, or bulk inventory container, from the storage by matching the NDC numbers of the label and the stock bottle; (2) select the proper size medication container based on the quantity prescribed; and (3) fill the prescription with the required number of dosage units (such as tablets or capsules) from the stock. The stock drug bottle should be returned to its correct location on the inventory shelf. One label is affixed to the container, and the other is filed with the original prescription. See Figure 7.10 for a sample stock drug bottle label.

Care, of course, must be taken with stock bottle selection. A common error is the selection of the wrong stock drug bottle, dose, or package size, because different products can look-alike (similar labeling), sound-alike, or have different formulations available (SR, XL, XR, DR). Almost all community pharmacies now use bar coding to enhance accuracy. The manufacturers affix a bar code that corresponds to the product's National Drug Code (NDC) to the stock bottles and prepackaged units. The NDC drug bar code may pull up a screen recommendation–for example, that the 250 mg of cephalexin prescribed should contain red and gray capsules with certain markings. If 500 mg of cephalexin of a different color were to be selected, the error could be identified.

FIGURE 7.10 Parts of a Stock Drug Bottle Label

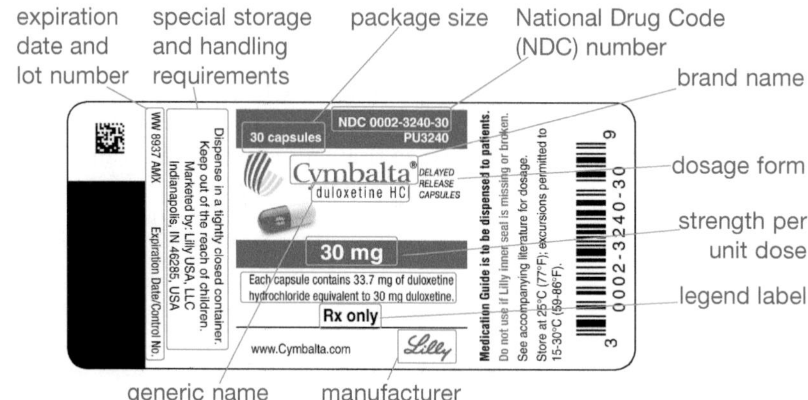

Safety Alert

Because of the frequency of severe patient allergies, counting equipment should be cleaned immediately after counting sulfa, penicillin, or aspirin products.

Tablets and Capsules

The most commonly dispensed drug form in a community pharmacy is the tablet or capsule. Figure 7.11 shows the equipment and procedure for manually counting tablets and capsules. A special counting tray is used that has a trough on one side to hold counted tablets or capsules and a spout on the opposite side to pour unused medication back into the stock bottle.

Pharmacy technicians should minimize any direct finger contact with the oral dose forms of medications. The tablets and capsules should always be counted with a clean spatula and picked up with forceps if dropped on the counter. The spatula, tray, and forceps should be cleaned often throughout the workday with 70% isopropyl alcohol, and these items should always be cleaned after counting a product that leaves a powder residue or is known to cause allergic reactions.

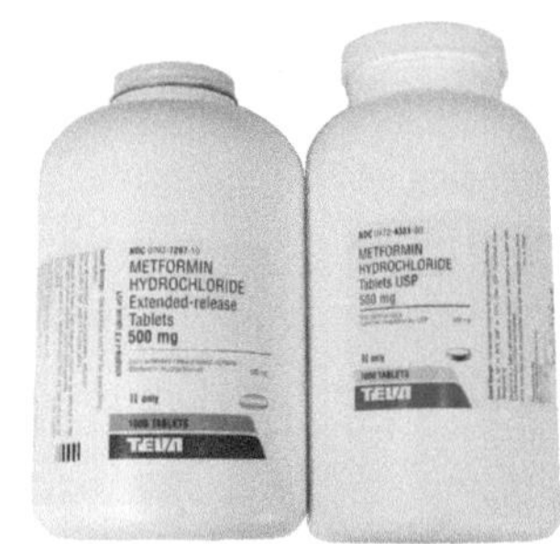

Both of these drugs are metformin 500 mg, but one bottle is immediate release and the other is extended release. Selecting the wrong bottle could result in a grave medication error and patient harm. Matching the NDC assists in accuracy.

FIGURE 7.11 Counting Tablets

(a) Tablets should be counted by fives and moved to the trough with a spatula. (b) The unneeded tablets should be returned to the stock container by pouring them from the spout. (c) The counted tablets should then be poured into the appropriately sized container.

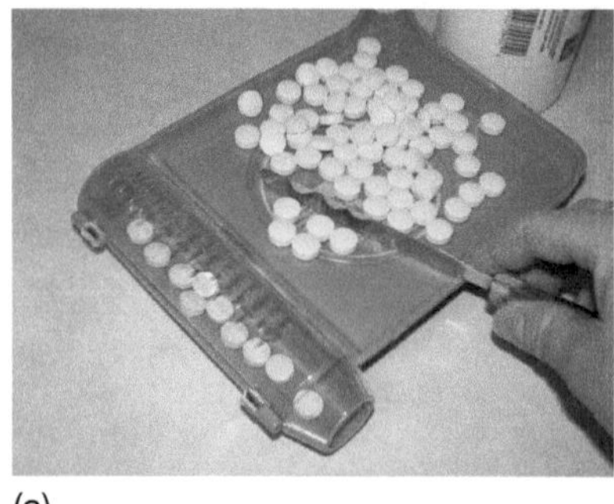
(a)

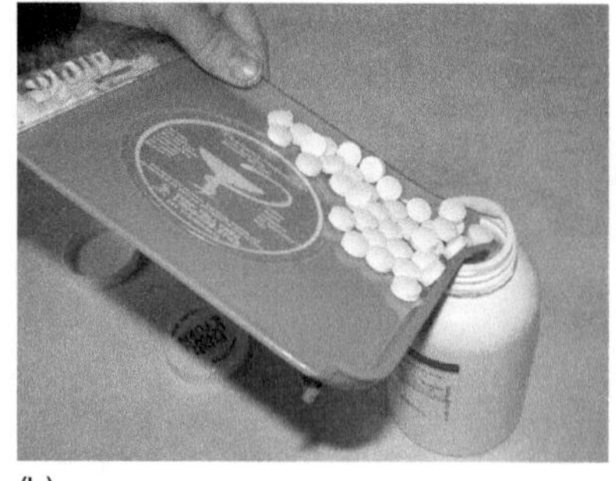
(b)

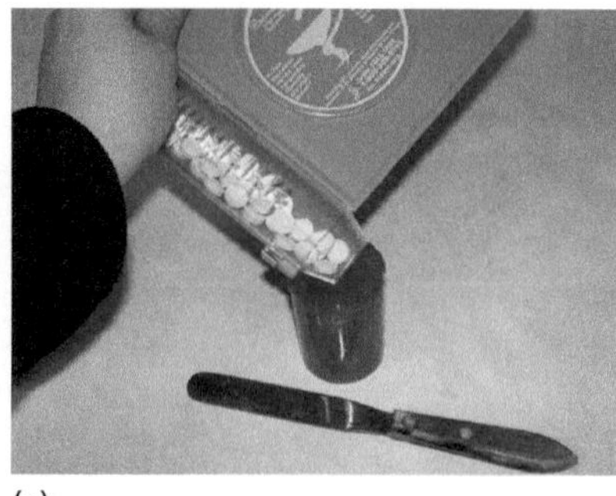
(c)

Liquid Formulations

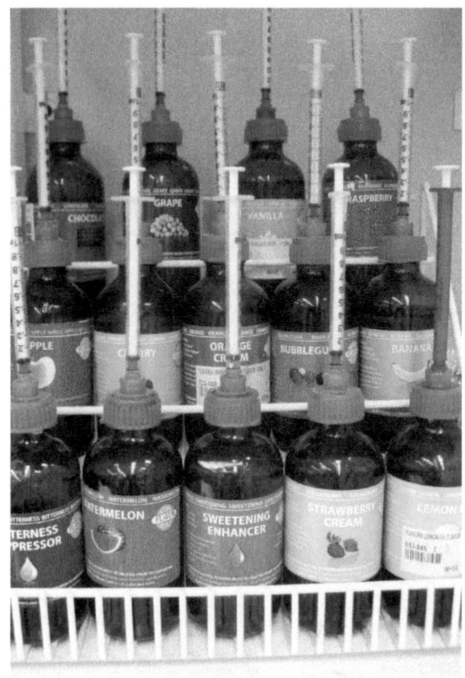

Flavor formulas to improve the taste of liquid drugs are available and a great customer service.

Liquid products (such as pediatric cough and cold syrups and antibiotic suspensions) are sometimes dispensed in their original packaging. They are also commonly poured from a stock bottle directly into an appropriately sized dispensing bottle (from 2 fl. oz. to 16 fl. oz.). Antibiotics are commonly **reconstituted**, or mixed with liquid, by adding distilled water to a dried antibiotic powder. In most cases, due to a short expiration period, the antibiotic suspension should not be prepared by the pharmacist or the technician (adding the distilled water) until the patient (or parent) picks up the medication. These medications should always be dispensed with an appropriate measuring device and an appropriate auxiliary label(s) such as "Shake well before using," "Refrigerate," or "Protect medication from exposure to light." (These will be explained later in greater detail.) The expiration date is commonly 14 days after reconstitution and should be added to the labeling. Because antibiotics and other liquid medications taste bad, flavorings are often added.

It may be easier for children to adhere to drug therapy if flavor is added to their prescribed medication. Manufacturers have created appropriate flavors for pediatric liquids. In most cases, the amount of distilled water to be added to the antibiotic powder is adjusted slightly to account for the small volume added from the liquid flavoring agents.

The correct flavoring formulas for each drug and dose are provided in the computer database. For several "unpleasant tasting" drugs, such as amoxicillin/clavulanate and clindamycin, pharmacy technicians often flavor the medications without an additional charge. In many cases, the medication taste may still be unacceptable to the child. Some pharmacies have the capability to add additional flavorings upon request from a patient or a parent at a minimal additional charge.

Flavoring agents have sweetening enhancers as well as bitterness suppressors and come in many flavors: apple, banana, bubble gum, cherry, chocolate, grape, lemon oil, orange cream, raspberry, strawberry cream, vanilla, and watermelon. Formulas for flavoring agents often combine one or more agents to result in the desired flavor. They are drawn up in an oral syringe and added to the liquid suspension. Although some flavors are incompatible with a specific medication, most flavors will not interfere with active ingredient(s) of drugs. Flavors are free from dyes and sugar and are hypoallergenic, so they are safe to use for those with allergies or diabetes, or even those who are gluten or casein (milk protein) sensitive.

Flavoring drugs is a patient service that can improve customer loyalty and, therefore, customer retention. More importantly, this service improves patient compliance with the prescribed medication regimen, resulting in a happy child, a happy parent, and a happy prescriber.

Choosing Medication Containers

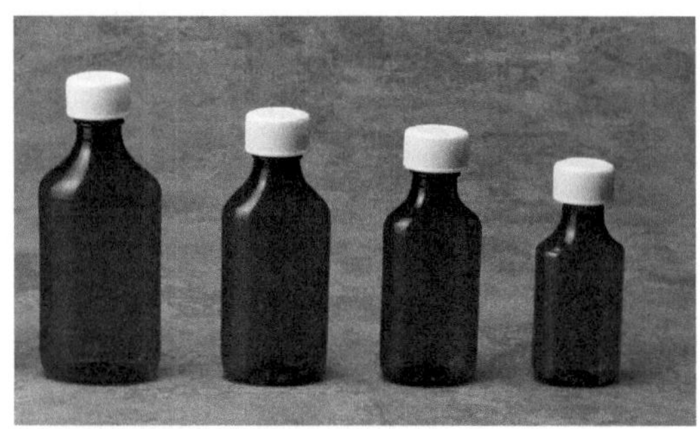

Amber-colored containers protect medications from UV light exposure.

A wide variety of plastic vial sizes are available for tablets and capsules in various dram sizes—from 10 to 60 drams. (This is one of the few times an older apothecary unit is still utilized without difficulties.) Selecting the proper vial size is a skill that becomes easy with experience. The pharmacy software printout on the patient medication information sheet may even recommend a vial size. Liquid containers are available in various sizes, from 2 oz. to 16 oz. Most pharmacy containers are amber-colored to prevent ultraviolet (UV) light exposure, which can degrade the medication.

All medications must be dispensed in child-resistant containers designed to be difficult for children to open. The Poison Prevention Packaging Act of 1970 requires (with some exceptions, such as sublingual nitroglycerin tablets, unit-of-use, and unit dose packages) that all prescription drugs be packaged in child-resistant containers. A container without a child-resistant top may be used if the patient requests it. For example, many older patients, especially those with arthritis, may request an exemption because they have difficulty opening child-resistant containers.

Some states require patients to sign such a request for each prescription, while others allow it to be added to the patients' profiles for future reference. Certain OTC drugs and supplements, such as aspirin and iron, are packaged in child-resistant containers due to their potential toxicity in accidental overdoses in children.

Handling Prepackaged Drugs

Manufacturer prepackaging is provided for prescription products such as otics, ophthalmics, suppositories, creams, ointments, respiratory and nebulizer drugs, syringes, metered-dose inhalers (MDIs), and oral contraceptives. The prescription label is attached directly to the product or the box. These medications are commercially available in **unit-dose** (single dose) or **unit-of-use** (fixed number of common use doses) prepackaging, as described below. They simplify the filling process by eliminating the counting step: the technician retrieves the drug from inventory by matching the correct name, manufacturer, quantity, and strength with the prescription and verifying them with the bar code scanner. Even though these medications are prepackaged, the pharmacist must still check and approve the medication label, ensuring that the proper drug, dosage form, and amount were chosen for dispensing to the correct patient.

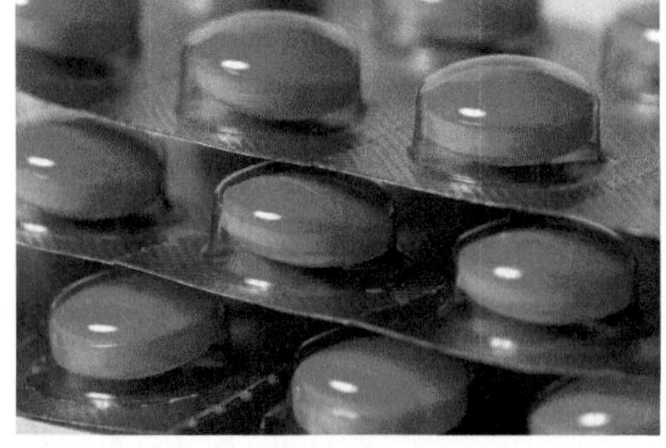

Several medications are available in unit-dose blister packs, with each unit having a scored perimeter for easy tear-off. Some blister packs come in boxed packages that contain a month's dosage supply.

Unit-Dose Packaging

Each unit dose of a tablet or capsule is a single dosage that is individually packaged in sealed foil and is considered tamper-proof. For unit-dose drugs that are individually packaged, a label is commonly affixed to a resealable plastic bag. The packaging label must include the manufacturer's name, lot number, and expiration date in addition to the drug's name and strength. For example, a prescription of ondansetron 8 mg ODT #8 for nausea and vomiting requires that eight individually packaged unit doses be placed in a medication container or plastic bag with a medication label. Other medications commonly available in unit doses include suppositories and migraine medications. Unopened unit doses may be legally returned to pharmacy stock. (For information on unit-dose packaging, see Chapter 11.)

Unit-of-Use Packaging

A unit-of-use package is a fixed number of dosage units sealed together in prepackaging. Examples include birth control, topical ointments and creams, nasal sprays, metered dose inhalers (MDIs), eye drops, and ear drops. Unit-of-use packaging consists of a month's supply, which is often 30, 60, or 90 tablets or capsules, a tube of cream or ointment, or a bottle of nasal spray, MDI, eye drops, or ear drops. Filling a prescription with unit-of-use packaging amounts to little more than locating the correct drug in the correct strength, verifying the NDC number, and affixing the correct medication container label.

Automated Filling Technology

To meet the demands of the increasing numbers of prescriptions, many high-volume community pharmacies, especially chain and mail-order pharmacies, have adopted automation technology to dispense with greater speed and accuracy. For example, the automated system Parata Max labels, fills, caps, sorts, and stores 188 drugs by NDC number and up to 232 prescriptions, processing up to 60% of total prescription volume of a specific community pharmacy with near 100% accuracy. Automation reduces the number of manual fills by pharmacy staff, helping to lower the cost per prescription. It also reduces the time in counting, labeling, sorting, and capping, and adds to medication safety by integrating the bar code technologies used for other retail products.

In addition to bar code scanners, some higher-volume pharmacies use automated scales for liquids and powders and liquid-filling machines. For large quantities (usually greater than 100) of tablets or capsules for medication orders, automated counting machines help reduce errors. Some counting machines have internal scales that take into account the weight per unit of an individual tablet or capsule based on 10 dosage units. However, these machines are not 100% accurate and should not be used to count prescription doses for controlled drugs. Each counting machine must be calibrated and documented daily by the pharmacy technician; a measuring weight (for example, 200 g) is placed on the balance, and the device is recalibrated if needed.

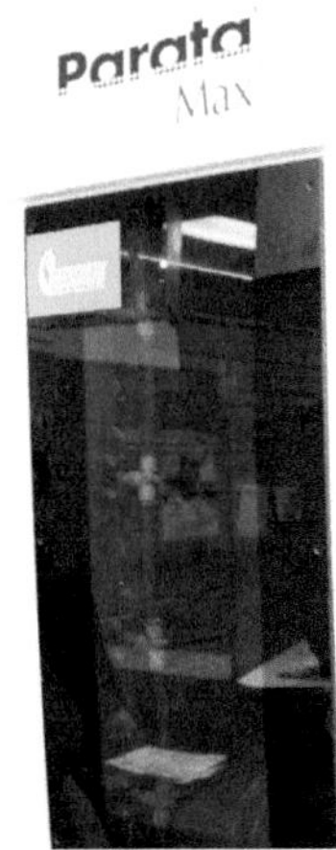

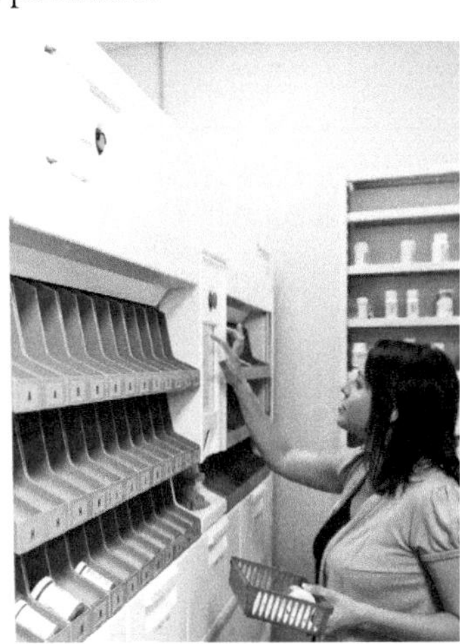

Parata Max is one of many different kinds of high-speed, high-accuracy automated dispensing systems.

Another option is the visual-precision counting equipment from Eyecon. This technology is 99.99% accurate; it documents the quantity of each prescription using scanner technology. It eliminates underfills (too little of the medication) and overfills (too much) accurately and consistently enough to use with C-II prescriptions.

Automated dispensing machines are linked to the pharmacy's DBMS. The software can send filling orders directly to the automated dispensing device that then fills, caps, labels, sorts, and stores the prescriptions for retrieval by the technician and approval by the pharmacist.

Most chain and mail-order pharmacies utilize a conveyor belt to improve the efficiency of moving a prescription through its various steps, with different technicians doing different tasks and the pharmacist checking all technician work in the end. One technician may be entering prescriptions into the computer while another is filling the medication orders for each patient. As each medication order is filled, the labeled medication, the original prescription (if available), and printed medication information are all placed in a plastic bin and then placed onto a conveyor belt—like a mini-assembly line—for the pharmacist's final check.

7.8 Technician and Accuracy Checks

Exercise caution when selecting insulin from the refrigerator. Insulin mix-ups are a common medication error.

Throughout the filling process, the technician must continue to check the prescription, the printed label, the NDC provided by the pharmacy software, and the stock drug container. Since the prescribed brand is different from the filled generic, the prescription and the label will not match for the drug name, and the NDC of the prescribed medication will not appear on either. Instead, the pharmacy software will provide the new NDC number and communicate it to the bar code scanner. Technicians must check both. Though a generic drug may have been substituted, the patient instructions on the label must read exactly as indicated on the original prescription's signa (see Figure 7.12).

FIGURE 7.12 Prescription and Label Comparison

The original prescription (a) contains precise instructions, or signa, for the patient that must appear on the label (b).

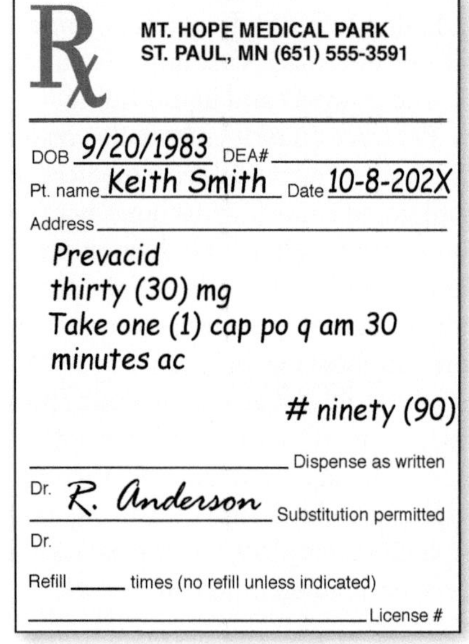

(a)

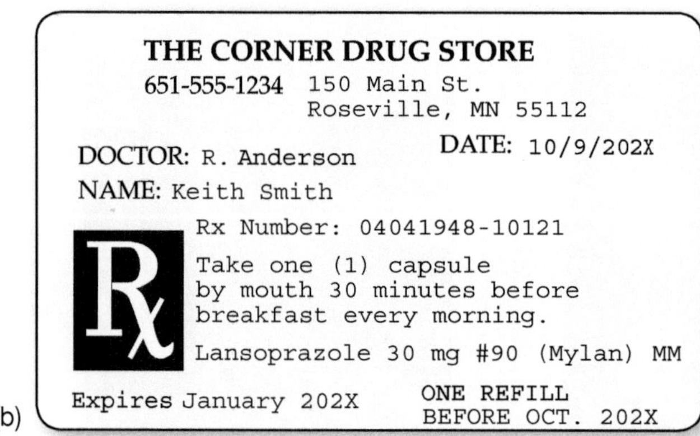

(b)

IN THE REAL WORLD

If prescriptions filled on a given day in the United States were only 99% correct, then the average pharmacy filling 200 prescriptions daily would have 2 incorrect prescriptions each day. This is unacceptable. According to a study in the *Journal of the American Medical Association*, more than 100,000 Americans die each year of adverse drug reactions. This means that harmful drug responses are the sixth leading cause of death in the United States. (Some estimates are higher, making medication errors the third leading cause of death.)

Part of the problem is consumer expectations for quick prescription filling, but also responsible are long hours without enough breaks for technicians and pharmacists, insufficient training and certification for technicians, understaffing, multitasking, and distractions.

The Minnesota Board of Pharmacy began taking public comments in 2015 about a new law for mandatory breaks for pharmacy personnel to prevent fatigue-induced medication errors. One pharmacist wrote about being distracted due to feeling lightheaded and shaky from hunger as she was given no breaks to eat. Pharmacies that have been cutting staff and lengthening shifts have been magnifying the problem. Various pharmacy boards are starting to address these issues.

Before completion, a final bar code scan of the stock NDC and comparison with the label is an essential safety check to avoid accidentally having selected a similar looking but incorrect bottle. For instance, selecting the wrong insulin from the refrigerator is one of the most common medication errors. As noted earlier, the names of several types of insulin manufactured by Eli Lilly are quite similar: Humulin R, Humulin N, Humalog, Humalog mix 50/50, Humulin mix 70/30, and Humalog mix 75/25. Some types of insulin are available in 10 mL vials; other insulin is administered through the use of prefilled pens. It is easy to inadvertently select the incorrect insulin from the refrigerator, but bar code scanning will detect the error.

Although speed is important, 100% accuracy is most important—a life-or-death matter, many times. Precise work habits need to become ingrained in technicians, including carefully avoiding drug retrieval based just on drug manufacturer label design (i.e., two different drugs from the same generic manufacturer stored in close proximity to one another) but instead utilizing bar code technology and carefully reading and comparing the stock drug label with prescriptions and printed labels.

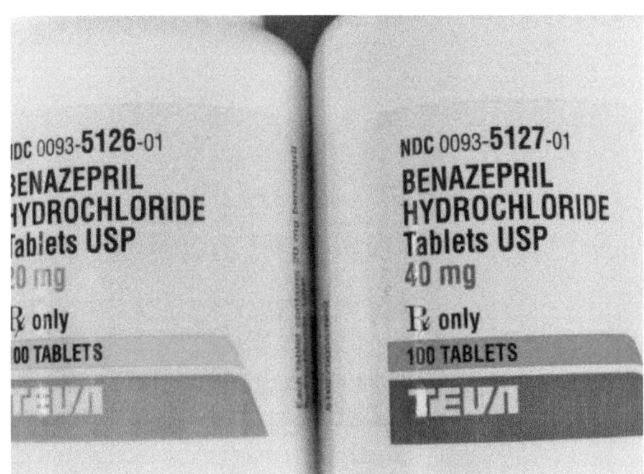

These bottles show the same drug, manufacturer, and package size, but the dosages are different. Scanning the NDC bar code helps ensure that the technician selects the right bottle, even when feeling rushed.

You must integrate three separate NDC checks as habits to prevent errors: (1) when the product is initially being pulled from the inventory shelf; (2) at the time of preparation; and (3) when the stock product is returned to the shelf. Do these same checks when filling any automatic dispensing machines. (For more information on medication safety practices, see Chapter 14.)

7.9 Preparing Customer Education Resources

Another key way to prevent errors is to provide each patient with sufficient information to correctly take the prescribed medication. You do this through the medication container label, auxiliary labels, and medication information sheets (including the FDA-mandated Medication Guide for some high-risk drugs).

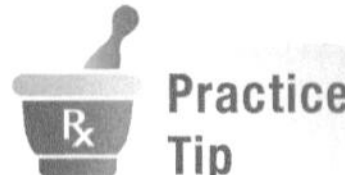

Practice Tip

In some states, the law requires the pharmacist to affix the medication container label to the container after the final check.

Medication Container Label

Medication container labels reinforce the dosing instructions of the prescriber. However, some prescription orders simply state "Take as directed." If that is the case, the pharmacy technician must verify that the prescriber gave the patient sufficient directions and match them with usual directions for medications, or call the prescriber's office for a more specific signa. To avoid insurance rejections during an audit, any prescriptions that are clarified with the prescriber's office should be documented on the prescription and/or in the patient profile. If left with "Take as directed," the technician might also request that the pharmacist counsel the patient on appropriate use (refer to Table 7.7).

TABLE 7.7 Patient Container Label Information

- Prescription's serial number
- Pharmacy's name, address, and telephone number
- Patient's name
- Prescriber's name
- All directions for use given on the prescription
- All necessary auxiliary labels containing patient precautions
- Medication strength
- Drug manufacturer's name
- Drug quantity
- Drug expiration date or date after which drug should not be used because of possible loss of potency or efficacy
- Initials of the licensed pharmacist
- Number of refills allowed, or the phrase "No Refills"

Colored Auxiliary Labels for Cautionary Directions

Label instructions for containers and packaging are limited, so additional details may be given in the form of colored auxiliary sticker labels. Some medication may be labeled with one or more auxiliary labels as you saw in Chapter 4 that highlight special cautions provided by the pharmacist (see Figure 7.13). Some pharmacy software may automatically print drug-specific auxiliary labels when the medication container label is printed. The technician often affixes all computer-generated auxiliary labels but should have the pharmacist counsel on prioritization. If the technician is in doubt about the appropriateness of any auxiliary labels or any that may be missing, they should ask for counsel from the pharmacist.

FIGURE 7.13 Auxiliary Labels

Auxiliary labels like these are affixed to the medication container by the pharmacist or the pharmacy technician under their direct supervision.

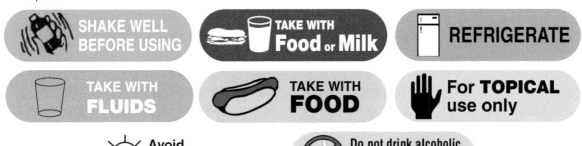

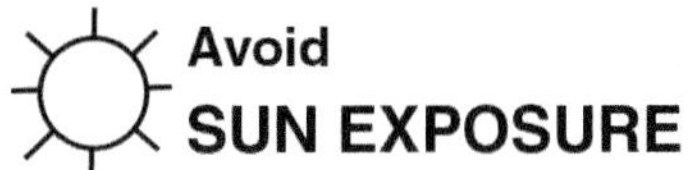

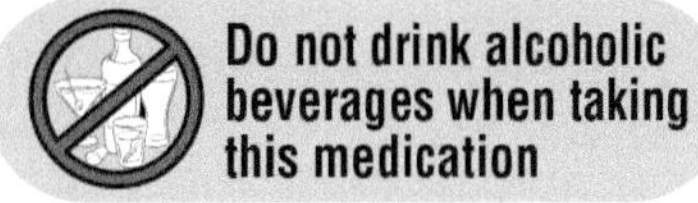

Container labels for C-II through C-V drugs must contain the transfer warning "Caution: Federal law prohibits the transfer of this drug to any person other than the patient for whom it was prescribed." It is common practice for this statement to be placed in small print on all medication container labels.

On any unit-of-use packaging, care should be exercised by the technician to not place the label over the drug name or expiration date because that makes the pharmacist's final check more difficult.

Medication Information Sheet

The technician also includes the **medication information sheet** in the customer's bag (or stapled to it). This preprinted sheet from the manufacturer or printout from the pharmacy software provides more extensive, easy-to-read information about how to safely take the medication and what to expect and watch for:

- Ingredient Name
- Common Uses
- Before Using This Medication
- How to Use This Medication
- Cautions
- Possible Side Effects
- Overuse
- Additional Information

The medication sheet may also contain a section called Product Identification, which includes the shape, color, and any markings on the tablet or capsule. This information allows patients to compare the product identifiers with the medications contained in the bottles, providing an added verification check that the correct drug was dispensed.

Occasionally, the NDC number of the prescription order will not match that on the stock drug bottle. The pharmacy (or the wholesaler) may have changed the package size or generic manufacturer source of a drug product since the patient's last refill. Thus, a patient may receive tablets or capsules with a different color or shape because of this "change of manufacturer." The pharmacist must double-check the differences in the old and current NDC and approve it. If so, the technician (or the pharmacist) will need to update the patient profile with the currently available drug with the new NDC. It is also important to explain to the patient at the time of pickup why the appearance of the medication changed.

Medication Guides and Risk Evaluation and Mitigation Strategies

As discussed in Chapter 3, for select high-risk drugs, the FDA mandates specific extra precautions from the manufacturers and pharmacists beyond the norm through the use of Medication Guides and Risk Evaluation and Mitigation Strategies (REMS).

Medication Guides

Medication Guides are enlarged FDA boxed warnings that advise consumers of a potential adverse reaction or of the proper use of a medication with a special dosage formulation, such as the inhaled pulmonary drugs fluticasone (Advair) or albuterol (Combivent). A Medication Guide goes into more depth than the information sheets. It may be printed with the medication label, or after the final pharmacist check and approval, and inserted in or stapled to the bag. Birth control drug manufacturers publish their own FDA-approved Medication Guides to be dispensed with the medication.

If the required Medication Guides are not distributed, the pharmacy may be subject to fines during an audit or inspection. The pharmacy technician should encourage the consumer to read this information at home, especially for all new prescriptions, and to ask or call the pharmacist with any questions or concerns. Common drugs that require an FDA-mandated Medication Guide are at the FDA website and can be found at https://PharmPractice7e.ParadigmEducation.com/FDA-Common.

Targeted Risk Evaluation and Mitigation Strategies

As noted earlier, a subset of the FDA's Medication Guides list is certain drugs that are particularly dangerous for certain populations. The FDA requires the manufacturer to develop extra strategies to ensure that the benefits of the drugs outweigh the risks—these are called **Risk Evaluation and Mitigation Strategies (REMS)**. Common REMS drugs include isotretinoin (Accutane), exenatide (Bydureon), buprenorphine-naloxone (Suboxone), and dofetilide (Tikosyn). Life-threatening risks include severe infections or allergic reactions, liver damage, or birth defects. For safety reasons, these high-risk drugs require additional verbal and written communication and monitoring. In the past, the FDA would not have approved or kept these drugs on the market. Patients, prescribers, and pharmacies must be registered or certified in order to receive, prescribe, or dispense the drugs. The specific procedures will be discussed in more detail in Chapter 14.

Dispensing Drugs to Women with Childbearing Potential Drugs also need to be carefully dispensed to all women of childbearing age who are sexually active, pregnant, or breast-feeding. Many of the REMS are aimed at this population. Non-REMS drugs also have cautions for these patients. There are over 6 million pregnancies in the United States each year, and more and more women are taking advantage of the health benefits of breast-feeding their children. Pregnant and nursing women take an average of three to five prescription drugs, which need to be carefully considered and monitored for the safety of the child who ingests the drugs in the womb or via breast milk. Pharmacists may need to offer medication counseling for these mothers. Safety checks that technicians need to know are also addressed in the Chapter 14.

7.10 The Pharmacist's Final Check

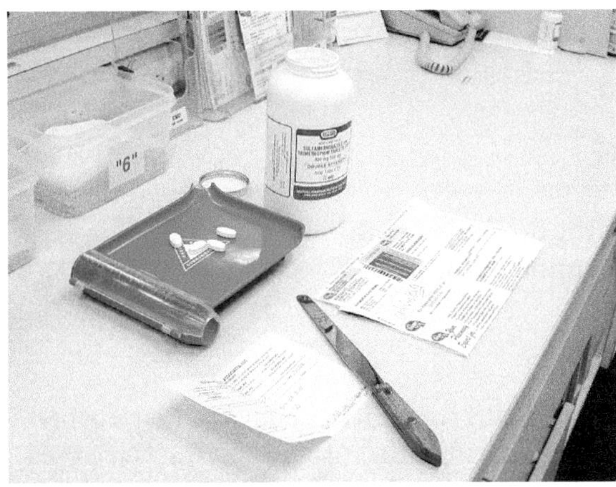

The technician must lay out all the elements of a prescription for checking.

It is extremely important—and required by law—that the pharmacist checks every prescription before it is dispensed to the patient to verify and approve its accuracy. Typically, the pharmacy technician will present the printed electronic, fax, or handwritten prescription and the labeled container with the prescribed medication, NDC number, and drug stock bottle for this final check. The stock bottle of tablets, capsules, or liquid must be provided to check the medication source and its NDC number.

The pharmacist compares the prescription with the patient profile, confirms that the medication label that has been affixed to the container is accurate, and confirms that the drug selected by the technician is correct. Some experienced pharmacists can identify the characteristic smells and scents of liquids. If there are no preprinted auxiliary labels, the pharmacist may choose or ask the technician to refer the patient to counseling at pickup. Medication Guides and medication information sheets that are attached to (or inserted in) the paper bag containing the prescription are also checked.

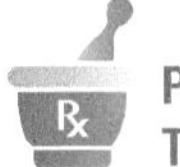

Practice Tip

The pharmacist must check all drugs prepared by the pharmacy technician and assume legal responsibility for them.

Additionally, the pharmacist may look over the insurance and billing situation to make sure that the prescribed drug is covered or billed to the correct insurance plan, especially if more than one plan is available. (See Chapter 8.)

After this review, the pharmacist commonly initials the medication container label and/or the original prescription. In doing so, the pharmacist assumes legal responsibility for the correctness of the prescription. However, the pharmacist does not necessarily assume sole responsibility. Technicians have been held legally responsible for dispensing and labeling mistakes, especially in situations in which the dispensing error was the result of negligence on their part or not following established policies and procedures. Most commonly, a wrong dose of medication was retrieved from storage.

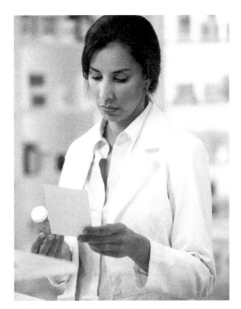

Before dispensing, the pharmacist will perform a visual check comparing the original prescription with the labeled instructions and the stock bottle for approval.

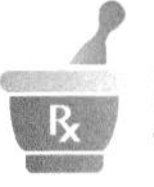

Practice Tip

Technicians must remember the tasks that are solely the pharmacist's responsibility: overriding computer DUR alerts, final auxiliary label choices, final approval, and patient medication advice or counseling.

A duplicate of the computer-generated patient container label is usually affixed to the back of the prescription by the pharmacist or the pharmacy technician to provide a paper trail of exactly which product (drug, dose and quantity, directions, and NDC number) was dispensed. It is not uncommon for the verifying pharmacist to initial this copy too, especially in the case of a controlled substance. The original prescription printout with documentation is filed numerically according to the prescription number (automatically assigned by the computer for each prescription). Prescription records must be stored (often in filing boxes or cabinets, with older ones moved to back storage or off-site). Those from the most current months and years must be readily retrievable for potential review and audit. Controlled substances have even more specific documentation and filing rules that are explained in Chapter 14.

7.11 Dispensing to the Patient

After the final verification and filing of the original prescription, the medication is available for immediate or future distribution to the patient.

Pre-Pickup Storage

Completed prescriptions are stored alphabetically for patient pickup. Patients generally have seven days to pick up the prescription before the insurance claim is reversed, and the drug is returned to stock. Patients may elect to have the prescription status sent to an email address or to a cell phone via a text message.

Some medications–in particular, insulins, injections, and some eye drops and suppositories–should be stored in the refrigerator once the final verification by the pharmacist is completed until patient pickup. If you cannot find a customer's medication, make sure that you check the refrigerator or freezer. It could have been placed in one of these places correctly or by mistake.

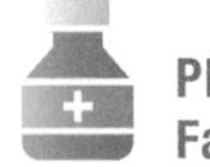

Pharm Fact

Medical errors often occur at pickup, when patients are presented with the wrong prescription package, so be careful!

Patient Pickup Options

Customers may pick up their medications at the pharmacy window inside the store or, in some cases, at a drive-through window. Before presenting the medication, check the patient address and/or birth date. This ensures that the right patient is receiving the prescription. Many independent pharmacies request that the person picking up the medication sign a receipt (which is filed by date) or a computerized signature pad. A signature is absolutely required for controlled substances, especially C-II drugs, along with a government issued ID for address and photo validation. If the person picking them up is not the patient, a verifying phone call must occur. (These procedures are addressed more in Chapter 14.)

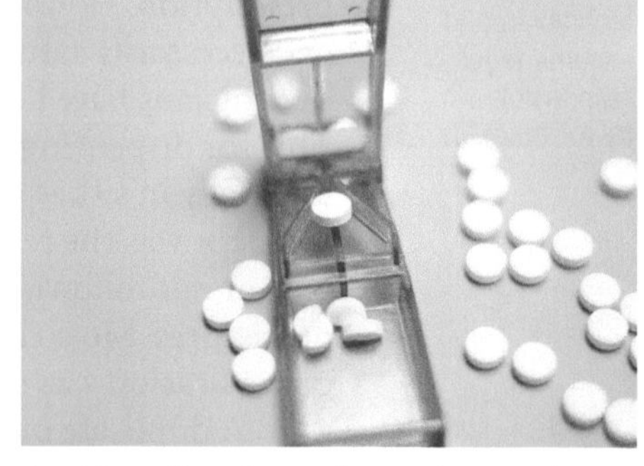

A tablet splitter is a safety and convenience device for prescribed half-tablet doses.

In the cases of a "partial fill" or a "change of manufacturer," you must relay this information to the patient along with the reasons. For a partial fill, provide the patient with a promised time for pickup of the remainder. If half-tablets have been prescribed, you may recommend that the customer purchase a **tablet splitter** to more easily divide the tablets, especially if the tablets are not scored.

When handing the prescription to the patient, make sure to ask if they understand how to take the medication correctly. Point out the labeled information (including auxiliary labeling) and any accompanying patient information inserts, including the Medication Guide. Politely ask, "Do you have any other questions? Would you like to talk to a pharmacist?" The technician must legally (by OBRA-90 law) offer the

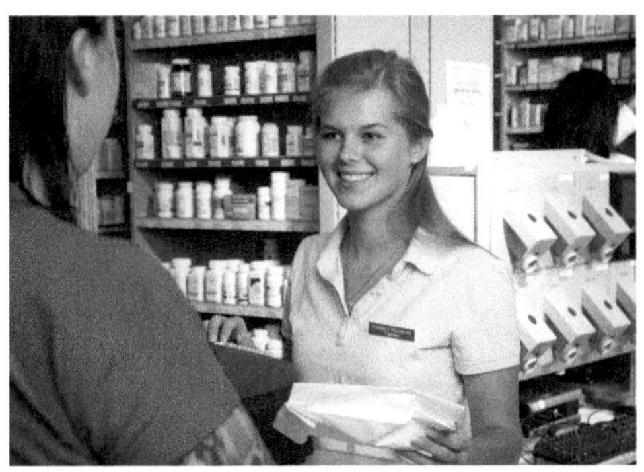

When a technician provides a prescription to the patient, they must be warm and pleasant, and provide all the drug information needed, asking if there are any questions for the pharmacist.

individual the opportunity to talk to the pharmacist about the drug to make sure that all the use instructions and potential side effects or drug interactions are understood. You may have to have the patient sign an electronic prompt screen or a receipt to indicate that they had been given the invitation to talk to the pharmacist (see Table 7.8).

Counseling is especially important for all new prescriptions. Most pharmacists try to make an extra effort to talk to these patients and be available for any questions on refill medications. The packaging or the look of the drug may have changed, prompting questions. If there is a change in dose, schedule, or a possible allergy or interaction, the pharmacist often will take the initiative to approach the patient. The pharmacist will also commonly ask to talk to the patient if there is a duplicate therapy, potential side effect, or a drug-drug interaction warning that appeared during the prescription filling process. Sometimes a computer reminder for mandatory counseling may be prompted from a DUR.

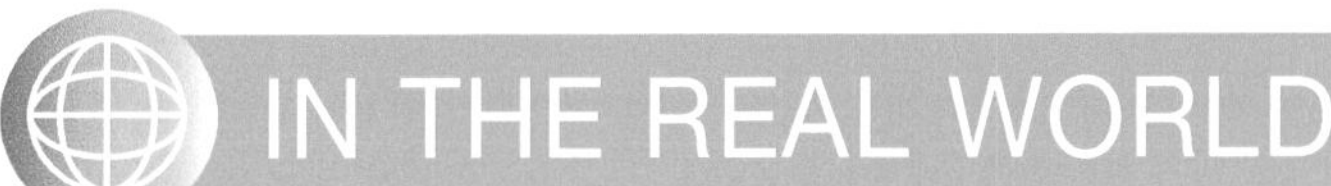

IN THE REAL WORLD

In Gallup polls over the years, the pharmacist is commonly named as either the number 1 or number 2 most trusted healthcare practitioner among patients. The pharmacist is much more accessible than most other healthcare providers, does not generally require an appointment, and provides accurate information on medications at no charge! Pharmacists will also assist patients with medication-related questions over the phone—again, at no charge. Many patients also seek the counsel of the pharmacist on the proper selection of an OTC drug, vitamin, dietary and herbal supplement, or homeopathic drug for themselves or a family member. Because technicians assist in filling prescriptions, pharmacists are able to provide information or counseling on the following issues:

- name and type of the medication or supplement and how it works on the body or mind
- best form of administration and proper dose
- duration of drug therapy
- action to take after a missed dose
- common severe side effects or adverse effects
- interactions and therapeutic contraindications, including preventive steps and actions to be taken if they occur
- methods for self-monitoring of the drug therapy
- proper storage and refill information
- special directions and precautions for preparation, administration, and use of the drug by the patient

TABLE 7.8 General Tips for Reducing Medication Errors

Tips for Technicians	• Verify information with the patient or caregiver when the prescription is received at the pharmacy and when the filled prescription is sent out of the pharmacy. • Observe, listen to, and report to the pharmacist pertinent information that may affect the safety or effectiveness of drug therapy. • Always keep the prescription and the label together during the filling process. • Know the common look-alike and sound-alike drugs and keep them stored in different areas. • Keep dangerous or high-alert medications in a separate storage area of the pharmacy. • Always question illegible handwriting. • Check that prescriptions and medication orders contain accurate information, including the correctly spelled drug name, strength, appropriate dosing, quantity or duration of therapy, dosage form, and route. Obtain any missing information from the prescriber. • Use the metric system. A leading X or 0 (zero) should always be present in decimal values less than one (e.g., 0.3). • Question prescriptions and orders that use uncommon abbreviations. Avoid using abbreviations that have more than one meaning, and verify with the pharmacist or the prescriber any abbreviations of which you are unsure. • Be aware of insulin mistakes. Insulin brands should be clearly separated from one another while stored in the refrigerator. Always educate patients about the described proper use of various insulin products at the time of purchase. • Keep the work area clean and uncluttered. Keep only those drugs that are needed for immediate use close at hand. • Always verify information at each step of the prescription-filling process. • Be sure that at least two people compare the label with the original prescription and NDC number. • Regularly review work habits and actively look for actions to take that improve safe and accurate prescription filling.
Tips for Pharmacists	• Take all DUR alerts seriously and respond with cautionary actions • Check the original prescription, the NDC number, and the drug stock bottle. • Cross-reference prescription information with other validating sources. • Encourage documentation of all medication use, including OTC medications and dietary supplements, in patient profiles. • Document all clarifications on orders. • Inspect the product in the bottle before initialing the prescription and the container. • Maintain open lines of communication with patients, healthcare providers, and caregivers.

Most state boards of pharmacy now require that the pharmacist engage in an education interchange with the patient at the prescription pickup, most particularly for Medicaid. Unfortunately, no additional Medicaid reimbursements are provided for this mandatory counseling. In fact, as state Medicaid programs attempt to balance budgets in challenging economic times, reimbursements to pharmacists have not kept pace with inflation. This adds additional challenges to pharmacies, requiring pharmacists to depend even more on technicians.

7.12 Additional Health Services in a Community Pharmacy

More and more, community pharmacy staff fulfills other services besides just providing prescriptions and retail services. Here are some other services that customers or insurance providers are seeking from pharmacists.

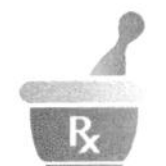

Practice Tip

The CDC has posted on its website the recommended vaccine schedules for the most common vaccines. You can access them at https://PharmPractice7e.ParadigmEducation.com/Vaccines.

Medication Therapy Management Services

Pharmacists are increasingly receiving requests from pharmacy benefit managers (health insurance claims management companies) to counsel patients on the proper medications or to investigate perceived medication problems. For example, the patient may be prescribed two similar cholesterol medications and the insurance company asks the pharmacist to check on this overlap, or a patient may be seemingly noncompliant on chronic disease medications. The technician can assist by raising questions when looking at the prescription or computer alerts and documenting outcomes for insurance companies. In terms of monitoring drug therapies, the technician can alert the pharmacist to a patient who is "late" in requesting refills. The pharmacist can try to identify reasons for noncompliance to drug therapy (cost, side effects, the patient forgot, etc.) and offer counsel or suggestions to resolve the issue.

Vaccinations

Some community pharmacies are now offering vaccine administration for patients over the age of 12 (age may vary depending on the state). Common vaccines include flu, pneumonia, and shingles; there are also vaccines for diphtheria/tetanus, typhoid, and other diseases. Pharmacists must complete specialized vaccine and basic life support (BLS) training in order to provide this service.

The role of the technician is to prepare the paperwork (including a signed consent form) and billing, and in some states to prepare the vaccine for administration. The pharmacist then counsels the patient, administers the vaccine, and completes the paperwork. The technician then notifies the primary care physician that a vaccine has been administered at the pharmacy. In the future, it is projected that certified technicians who have received specialty training may be able to legally administer vaccines.

Blood Pressure Checks

A prescriber often requests the pharmacist to check a patient's blood pressure in association with a high blood pressure prescription or is asked by a patient for this service. Over 30,000 pharmacies also offer self-testing, automatic blood pressure monitors as a customer service to patients. In some locations, the American Heart Association offers its "Check. Change. Control." program for Heart Health. To check for a program near you, visit https://PharmPractice7e.ParadigmEducation.com/BPMonitor.

In pharmacies without an automated monitor, the pharmacists can check the patient's blood pressure. Regular blood pressure checks can help educate patients on their own bodies and how best to control their hypertension. The pharmacist and physician can offer dietary and lifestyle recommendations and suggest better administration times for taking blood pressure medications. This service may be provided free or at a cost to the patient.

Glucose and Cholesterol Screenings

The American Diabetes Association (ADA) recommends that every three years people with normal levels and few risk factors should get a full-panel blood glucose test. Those who are overweight and/or over the age of 45 may be recommended by physicians to have the test more often. According to the ADA, over one-fourth of seniors have diabetes, and childhood diabetes is skyrocketing. Diabetes has been the seventh leading cause of death in the United States. That is why pharmacy screenings are so helpful. Many chain stores, such as Walgreens, offer these screenings for individuals over the age of 18 at their locations where the state allows it. If pharmacists are allowed to do finger-stick blood testing, the cost of the service is borne by the patient; insurance will not cover these costs. The pharmacist can counsel on nutrition and lifestyle choices as well as medications if blood sugars are too high or too low.

Glucose and cholesterol levels can be checked in the same test. The full-panel cholesterol findings include the LDL ("bad cholesterol"), HDL ("good cholesterol"), triglycerides, and total cholesterol. This information can help the pharmacist in offering the proper medication, nutrition, and lifestyle counseling to help prevent heart attacks, stroke, chronic high blood pressure, vascular disease, and diabetes. Technicians assist in scheduling, collecting screening supplies, and documentation.

Point-of-Care Testing

Point-of-care testing (POCT)—diagnostic testing completed at or near the time and place of patient care is an example where the roles of the pharmacist and the pharmacy technician are expanding beyond medication dispensing. In pharmacy POCT, patients typically provide a blood sample (often from a finger prick), and a pharmacist or a pharmacy technician operates portable analyzers that provide laboratory-caliber test results quickly. Examples of commonly used POCT include blood glucose and hemoglobin A1c (for patients with diabetes), cholesterol profiles (for patients with high cholesterol), and anticoagulation measurements (for patients at increased risk for blood clots).

A main benefit of POCT is the timeliness of test results. For example, a hemoglobin A1c measurement can be obtained within minutes utilizing point-of-care analyzers. The same test measurement may take hours to be returned utilizing traditional blood draws and laboratories. Quick results enable healthcare providers to make rapid treatment decisions. This can be especially convenient for patients who can complete blood work and receive care based upon their results at the same visit. Another benefit is that POCT usually requires only a small blood sample from the finger; venipuncture is not typically used.

POCT is different from glucose and cholesterol screening (discussed previously). Glucose and cholesterol screening is a tool used to assess a patient's blood sugar and cholesterol. Screening is not meant to be diagnostic. Because POCT is considered diagnostic and is used to influence decisions regarding a patient's care, it requires more oversight than screenings. Most sites that perform POCT must receive a waiver from the Centers for Medicare and Medicaid Services. Furthermore, pharmacists and pharmacy technicians who perform POCT have additional Occupational Safety and Health Administration (OSHA) training requirements. The OSHA Bloodborne Pathogens standard is an example of an additional training requirement.

Smoking Cessation Programs

Some pharmacists have been trained to work with patients on smoking cessation programs, with some success. If a pharmacist has shown and documented positive outcomes at smoking cessation, the pharmacy may be reimbursed from some insurance providers. Other pharmacies hire nurse practitioners to come in to offer this type of health care and other prevention education programs.

Nursing Homes, Home Care, and Hospice Pharmaceutical Services

Many community pharmacies are contracted to provide drug therapy services for nursing homes (long-term care facilities, or LTCFs), home healthcare services, and hospice facilities. When working with nursing homes, pharmacies are required by law to provide and document online monthly profile reviews for all patients, which are commonly conducted by a board-certified consultant pharmacist. A critical role of that pharmacist is to ensure rational, appropriate, and safe medication use through the review of a patient's medication therapy and patient history for potential adverse drug reactions. The monthly profile review is critical, as these patients are often prescribed multiple drugs and have age-related physiological changes in organ function (such as the kidney) with minimum physician oversight. Home care and hospice facilities contract the services that best fit them, often working with the nurses and nurse practitioners assigned to the patient cases.

7.13 Becoming a Community Pharmacy Technician

As you can see, the role of the pharmacy technician is not only key to the community pharmacy, but it is as complex and varied as the functions of the pharmacy itself. You need to strive to be versatile, customer oriented, comfortable with people, able to focus, and detail oriented. The job is not boring, as it is ever changing and filled with many different kinds of tasks. Your role as pharmacy technician is important because it contributes to the health and well-being of every single patient for whom you fill a prescription. By supporting the pharmacist in so many different duties, you free the pharmacist to spend more time resolving medication-related problems and reaching out to patients who can then use the in-person advice about medications to help improve their health. In the community pharmacy, a pharmacy technician assumes a number of responsibilities related to prescription drugs; these depend on federal and state laws and regulations.

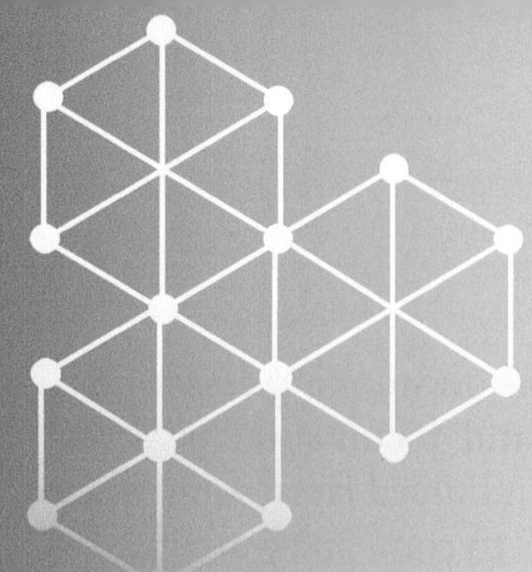

Review and Assessment

CHAPTER SUMMARY

- The pharmacy depends upon computers and a pharmacy database management system (DBMS) that communicate online with external healthcare network servers for e-prescriptions, medication reconciliation, and insurance claims processing.
- The DBMS has designed interoperability so that the software interfaces with the various internal programs for the pharmacy's accounting, purchasing, ordering, and inventory work. The DBMS also communicates with the external programs of the insurance companies and prescribers.
- The technician assists in building the patient profile, entering updates and prescriptions into it, reconciling medications and filing insurance claims, filling and labeling prescriptions, and dispensing to the patients.
- Prescriptions arrive at the pharmacy in different forms, including e-prescriptions, paper forms, telephone calls, and fax prescriptions.
- Prescriptions come in different types of new and refill prescriptions that involve slightly different steps, such as new patient prescriptions, emergency fills and refills, standing orders, and transfer refills.
- Filling prescriptions commonly involves retrieving stock bottles of drugs, counting the prescribed quantity of medications, placing the medication in the appropriate containers, and affixing medication container and auxiliary labels.
- The technician can legally take written prescriptions from walk-in customers but cannot, in most states, take new or transfer prescriptions by telephone and transcribe them.
- The parts of a prescription include prescriber information, the date, patient information, the symbol Rx, the inscription (the medication or medications prescribed and their amounts), the subscription (the instructions to the pharmacist), the signa (directions to the patient), additional instructions, and the prescriber's signature.
- The pharmacy technician is often responsible for entering the new prescription orders and creating or updating the computerized patient profile, including identifying information, medical history, medication/prescription history, drug allergy information, insurance/billing information, and prescription preferences.
- The pharmacy technician must become familiar with common abbreviations that are needed to interpret prescriptions and enter information into the patient profile database.

- Patients receive medication information by way of drug and auxiliary labeling on the medication containers, the medication information sheets for each drug dispensed, Medication Guides for higher-risk drugs, and counseling by the pharmacist.
- Medication container labels must contain a unique prescription number, the name of the patient, the date of the prescription, directions for use, strength and name of the medication and its manufacturer, drug quantity, expiration date, pharmacist initials, and number of refills. Auxiliary labels may also be affixed to the container at the discretion of the pharmacist. The name, address, and phone number of the pharmacy must also be on the label.
- The pharmacist is responsible for the final check of the original prescription and for reviewing the patient profile, the accuracy of the drug and the quantity dispensed, and the medication container label.
- With the support of the pharmacy technician, the pharmacist is able to resolve DUR issues; counsel patients and provide various MTM services; perform vaccinations, blood pressure checks, glucose and cholesterol screenings, and POCT; and engage in pharmaceutical outreach services to nursing homes, home health care, and hospices.

CHECK YOUR UNDERSTANDING

Take a moment to reflect on what you have learned in this section and answer the following questions.

1. Which of the following is not a function of the pharmacy technician?
   a. processing insurance claims
   b. providing customer service
   c. performing non-sterile compounding
   d. counseling patients
2. In a prescription, the subscription is the
   a. signature of the prescriber.
   b. initials of the pharmacist.
   c. directions for the patient to follow.
   d. instructions to the pharmacist on dispensing the medication.
3. The term *DAW2* means
   a. a prescriber requires a brand name medication to be dispensed.
   b. a patient requests a brand name to be dispensed.
   c. a patient requests a generic drug to be dispensed.
   d. a pharmacist is permitted to substitute a therapeutic equivalent drug.
4. Identify the incorrect statement about the dispensing of Schedule II drugs.
   a. Schedule II drugs cannot be routinely phoned in or faxed to the pharmacist or technician.
   b. Schedule II drug refills are limited to five times in six months.
   c. Schedule II drugs require the signature and DEA of an authorized prescriber.
   d. Schedule II drug prescriptions must be written on TRP paper.

5. In most states, a pharmacy technician can process all the following prescriptions with the exception of a(n)
   a. e-Rx received over the computer.
   b. transfer prescription from another pharmacy.
   c. faxed prescription from a prescriber's office.
   d. prescription on profile.

6. The ability to exchange and process information between various internal and external databases, software, and technology such as insurance and health care providers is called
   a. interoperability.
   b. national drug code.
   c. prior authorization.
   d. national provider identifier.

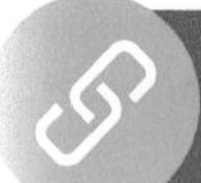

MAKE CONNECTIONS

Take a moment to consider what you have learned in this chapter and respond thoughtfully to the following prompts. Note that some of these activities will require internet access.

1. An important function of the pharmacy technician is to assist a new patient in creating an accurate patient profile for prescription entry into the computer database. Write a short essay that addresses the following questions:
   a. What are the essential components of a patient profile?
   b. Discuss the importance of each.
   c. How and when should the profile be updated? Why?
   d. Why should OTC drugs and dietary supplements be included in the profile?
   e. What are HIPAA requirements in the retail pharmacy?
2. Conduct internet research and answer the following questions about the changing roles for pharmacists and pharmacy technicians:
   a. Identify three examples of expanded roles for a community pharmacist.
   b. How can a pharmacy technician assist in each of these roles?
   c. In the future, can a certified and trained technician assume some of these roles? Why or why not?

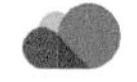
The online course includes additional review and assessment resources.

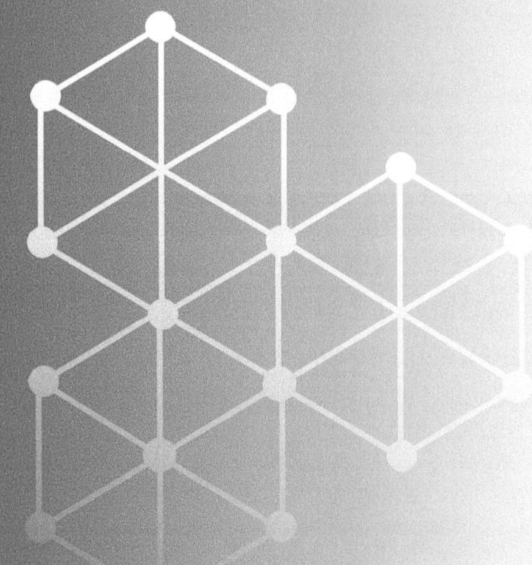

8 Prescription Drug Insurance in Health Care

Learning Objectives

1. Describe the importance of insurance to address rising prescription drug costs. (Section 8.1)
2. Identify components of health insurance, and define common terms and concepts associated with health insurance. (Section 8.2)
3. Define key terms, such as *average wholesale price*, *monthly premium*, *insurance policy*, *benefits*, *deductible*, *copayment*, *coinsurance*, *tiered copay*, *in-network providers*, *out-of-network providers*, *prior authorization*, *pharmacy benefit manager*, *coordination of benefits*, and *online adjudication*. (Sections 8.1–8.6)
4. Explain the concept of tiered copayments for private commercial drug insurance programs. (Section 8.2)
5. Identify various aspects of commercial insurance and how it works. (Section 8.3)
6. Describe the multiple forms of government insurance, such as Medicare, Medicaid, and others. (Section 8.4)
7. Summarize the role of pharmacy benefit managers and the role of the technician in explaining to patients the costs and options related to insurance drug coverage. (Section 8.5)
8. Identify the necessary information on a prescription insurance card to process claims online for various types of insurance and workers' compensation claims, and paraphrase the role of technicians in identifying medication assistance and patient advocacy. (Section 8.6)
9. Paraphrase the role of technicians in identifying and resolving errors in online adjudication. (Section 8.6)
10. Explain how to prepare a drug claim for online processing including entering specific information about each prescription filled, including the medication quantity and days' supply of medication. (Section 8.7)
11. Summarize the role of technicians in explaining insurance drug coverage to patients. (Section 8.8)
12. Identify steps to resolve problems with audits and charge-backs. (Section 8.9)
13. Discuss how to assist financially struggling patients through medication assistance advocacy. (Section 8.10)

ASHP/ACPE Accreditation Standards
To view the *ASHP/ACPE Accreditation Standards* addressed in this chapter, refer to Appendix B.

Almost 90% of Americans have some type of private or government insurance for hospital, medical, and prescription drug benefits or a combination of healthcare coverage plans. Every insurance plan has its own unique eligibility and payout criteria based on deductibles and copayments.

You will need a working knowledge of all of these various health insurance programs because, in a retail or mail-order pharmacy, you will spend 20%–25% of your time entering, updating, and processing insurance-related information as well as resolving issues and educating patients.

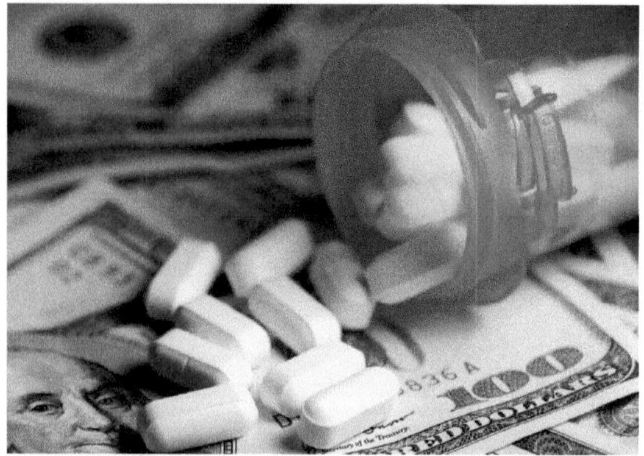
With rising prescription costs, informed technicians can help patients through effective insurance claims processing, medication access counseling, and advocacy.

The job requires a thorough understanding of the terminology utilized and the steps in processing and reconciling claims. Though this may at times seem like burdensome administrative detail, it helps patients receive the care they deeply need. Insurance coverage can mean the difference between access or no access to lifesaving drug therapies, to affordability or crippling debt. Knowing how to process insurance claims can make a real difference in people's lives.

8.1 Rising Costs of Health Care

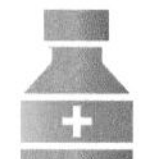
Pharm Fact

Over 1,000 new genetically engineered, targeted cancer drugs are in development. A monthly course of Votrient (pazopanib), 120 capsules, for renal cancer costs almost $14,000.

The cost of health care, especially prescription drugs, is far outpacing the rate of inflation. In 2017, spending on prescriptions in the United States was $456 billion. Costs have continued to rise. The reasons include (1) an increase in innovative and expensive new drugs; (2) manufacturers boosting the **average wholesale prices (AWPs)** of brand name drugs *and* generic brands; and (3) fewer brand name drugs coming off patent. The AWP is the average price that pharmacies, hospitals, and other healthcare facilities pay for stock of a specific drug. The AWP serves as the benchmark from which insurance companies estimate the percentage of pharmacy reimbursement. The pharmacies then use the AWP to determine the retail price for patients. Most of the current research and development (R&D) pharmaceutical costs are going into creating new and more expensive innovator drugs. The high AWPs of specialty drugs now account for about 33% of all drug spending, and this is projected to reach 50% in the near future (see Figure 8.1).

On the positive side, more biosimilar and interchangeable drugs will be FDA-approved within the next 5 to 10 years. Some of these drugs will be able to be substituted for the expensive, patented biotechnology drugs, which will help bring down the prices for such expensive medications. This may neutralize some of the swelling research costs of the vast array of new biotechnology drugs being developed.

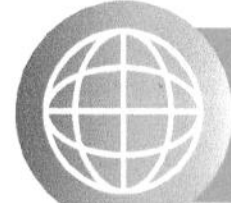

IN THE REAL WORLD

In 2019, the FDA approved a new biotechnology drug called atezolizumab (Tecentriq) for the treatment of certain cancers. This injectable drug is currently approved for cancers of the breast, lung, and urinary system. The drug is infused every three weeks. The cost is $12,500 per month.

FIGURE 8.1
US Prescription Drug Insurance Coverage

Source: Centers for Medicare and Medicaid Services 2017

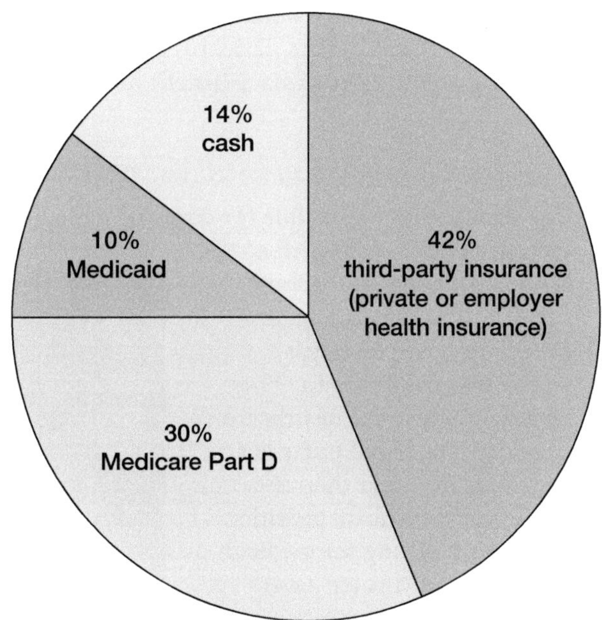

8.2 Health Insurance Components

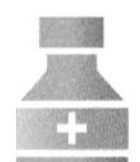

Pharm Fact

In 1990, 1.47 billion prescriptions were dispensed at an average cost of $6.62. In 2014, over 4 billion prescriptions were dispensed at an average cost of $77.20!

Various countries handle medical costs differently. In the United States, every person must enroll in some form of health insurance coverage. **Health insurance** helps patients cover incurred medical costs for such items as pharmaceuticals, physician visits, laboratory costs, and hospitalization. In Canada, health care is funded and administered by each province and territory. The Canadian government ensures that coverage is made available to every Canadian citizen. Insurance in Canada is used for out-of-system services and expenditures.

Healthcare coverage in the United States may be provided by commercial insurance paid by the individuals, or through their employers (with shared premium costs), or by one of the state or federal programs:

- Medicare (Parts A, B, C, and D) for those over 64 or disabled, administered through the US Department of Health and Human Services and contracted private insurers
- Medicaid for low-income patients and their dependents, administered by individual states
- Children's Health Insurance Programs (CHIPs) and affordable care health exchanges, primarily administered by individual states
- Tricare for active military (including National Guard and Reserves), veterans, and military dependents, administered through the Defense Health Agency

The components and payment structures of each health insurance plan are determined both by the type of insurance provider and the individual insurer.

Commonly, patients have only one **primary health insurance plan**, which pays up to its coverage limits. Some patients also have a **secondary health insurance plan**, which pays what the primary does not—if the service is covered under the secondary plan. The patient may still have out-of-pocket costs even with two insurance plans. Some patients who have excessive drug needs have to combine more than one healthcare insurance program with a specific prescription drug insurance policy.

There are several important concepts and terms the pharmacy technician must understand related to insurance coverage. These include responsible payment parties, coinsurance, copayments, catastrophic insurance, health savings accounts, flexible spending accounts, pharmacy benefit managers, and insurance billing codes.

Responsible Payment Parties

The **first party** responsible for covering a medical bill is typically the person who directly receives the benefits, services, or product. In some cases, a parent, guardian, or other responsible party is considered the first part. The **second party** is the healthcare provider. The **third party** is an organization other than the patient or healthcare provider involved in paying for medical expenses. Third party payers include insurance companies, government agencies, or individual employers.

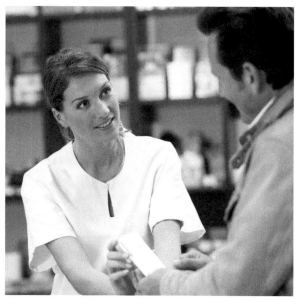

Pharmacy technicians need to understand insurance terms and types of policies so that they can answer patients' questions intelligibly.

To receive health insurance coverage, the patient pays a **monthly premium**, or enrollment fee. This fee may be paid directly to the insurer or more commonly is deducted from one's paycheck to be paid by the employer to the insurance company along with an employer subsidy (offered as an employee benefit).

The monthly premium allows the patient access to the health services and products outlined in the specific **insurance policy**, or plan. These specific health services and products are called **benefits**. The policy describes the specific circumstances under which the policy will cover these expenses. The plan includes the processes, rates, rules, and restrictions. Many policies, especially with Medicare, cover preventive office visits, such as annual physicals and well-baby checks without additional costs above the premium.

Most health insurance plans include some combination of individual and/or family annual deductible levels. The **deductible** is the designated amount of annual medical costs that must be paid by the patient *before* the full coverage by the insurance company kicks in. So in that sense, this amount is *deducted* from coverage benefits. For instance, if a plan designates a $5,000 deductible for an individual, the patient must pay for a large portion or all of the medical costs up to $5,000 before the insurance company will consider paying the full or majority portion of each expense. In this high deductible plan, the patient may have numerous office visits and tests done and perhaps an emergency room visit before the insurance company will cover much or anything at all.

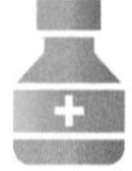

Pharm Fact

Costs toward a prescription drug insurance deductible usually start accruing with the first day of the calendar year.

The higher the deductible, the lower the monthly premium because the patient is assuming much of the risk. Lower deductible plans often start at a $250 or $500 annual deductible with higher monthly premiums. The designated annual deductible levels and monthly premiums are reviewed annually and often change year by year to meet rising costs (like the collision insurance on your car).

IN THE REAL WORLD

In a high-profile case in 2015, Turing Pharmaceuticals purchased the patent rights to the antiparasitic drug tablet pyrimethamine (Daraprim). It is the only treatment currently approved for toxoplasmosis, which is a parasitic condition commonly associated with deer ticks in the United States. Also used to fight malaria, the drug is on the World Health Organization's List of Essential Medicines. Martin Shkreli, the former hedge fund manager who became Turing's CEO, decided to turn a profit on the drug. In one day in September, he raised the price of Daraprim by 5,000%, from $13.50 to $750, causing outrage from citizens and government officials alike. Because of the outrage, Shkreli reduced the price somewhat, but his actions illustrated the reality of drug price gouging and profiteering. It also highlighted the fact that many patients struggle to pay for their prescriptions (even when they have insurance) because of high coinsurance payments and deductibles.

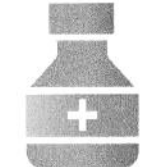

Pharm Fact

As the number of manufacturers of the heart drug digoxin decreased from eight to three over the past decade, the cost of the drug increased by over 600%!

Patient Coinsurance Payments

For some policies, when patients receive a medical service or drug product, they must immediately pay a certain percentage of the cost, or **coinsurance** payment, with any potential further billing to come later. Coinsurance payments and percentages vary with the service provided and the insurance policy. Coinsurance payments remain an element of Medicare Part A but are less common today in other government and private insurance programs.

Patient Copayments

A different shared approach is the **copayment (copay)**. It is a flat out-of-pocket fee that the patient is required to pay for each health visit, service, or product at the time of delivery. For instance, a copay could be $20 per office visit and $10 per generic prescription. The remaining costs would either be covered by the insurance company or by the patient until the annual deductible level is reached, when the insurance will pay a higher percentage. Copays vary by insurance company, as outlined in the policy of each company. Plans with higher premiums often have no copayments or a lower copayment and deductible.

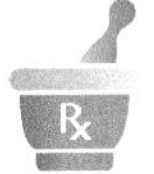

Practice Tip

In a tiered copay, the patient might pay $5 for generic, $25 for brand, and $100 for nonpreferred.

Healthcare plans may have a **tiered copayment** system, such as $20 per non-emergency office visit and $200 per emergency room visit. Prescription drug insurance companies also often establish a **dual copay** with one flat fee for generic drugs versus another fee for brand name drugs. There can also be a three- or four-tiered copay program, having different copays for generics, preferred brands, nonpreferred brands, and specialty drugs.

Catastrophic Insurance

Catastrophic insurance is an insurance plan that is used only when a person has experienced a severe accident or unexpected debilitating illness or disease. It has very low monthly premium payments but a very high deductible (e.g. $5,000-$10,000) and few preventive services. It also generally has no copayments or coinsurance payments, putting the full weight upon the patient for every medical expense until the annual high deductible level is reached. Young, healthy people who rarely visit the doctor often rely on this kind of insurance. It's considered a "safety net" for people who don't *expect* to have many medical bills but want coverage in case a "catastrophe" strikes.

Health Savings Accounts

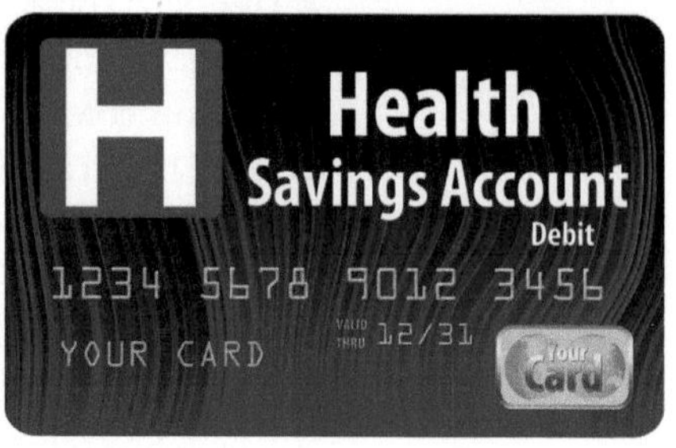

To assist people in putting money away for healthcare costs not covered in high-deductible insurance plans, there are **Health Savings Accounts (HSAs)**. These are savings accounts that can be started by patients or their employers to set aside tax-deferred money specifically for healthcare costs not covered by insurance. The money is deposited before taxes and can be used only for legitimate health bills. HSAs are particularly helpful for individuals with high-deductible insurance plans or enormous annual health costs that go beyond the maximum levels paid by the insurance company in a year. The unused deposits in the HSA may accumulate from one year to the next.

Flexible Spending Accounts

In **flexible spending accounts (FSAs)**, patients, through their employer, can also place pretax dollars aside for medical expenses *and* child and dependent care. However, these dollars must be carefully predicted and spent within the year (though under certain circumstances, $500 a year may be carried over).

Pharmacy Benefit Managers

Nearly all insurance companies and plans that handle prescriptions work with a **pharmacy benefit manager (PBM)**, a division of the insurance company or a separate company that processes patient prescription claims (explained in more detail in a later section).

Insurance Billing Codes

Insurance companies all use established coding systems for billing claims so that the computers can speak to each other and the electronic health records (EHRs) can be consistently communicated across providers and insurance plans. These coding systems use combinations of numbers to designate the diagnoses and the associated prescription claims. Three kinds of billing code systems are used for different kinds of billing:

- **ICD-10** (International Classification of Diseases, 10th edition), to record diagnoses and disorders
- **HCPCS** (Healthcare Common Procedure Coding System–Level II), to record supplies, equipment, and devices supplied for medical purposes
- **CPT** (Current Procedural Terminology), to record procedures and services

The pharmacy software will translate and check the coding. As a pharmacy technician, you will make sure that the HCPCS coding from the physician is present to bill Medicare Part B for all diabetes test supplies, including blood glucose monitors, test strips, lancets, and syringes as well as respiratory solutions and nebulizer equipment and tubing. If the coding is not present, you will have to call the physician's office for it. Also, if a pharmacy has a Medicare Part B contract (contracts will be explained later in this chapter) for supplying large **durable medical equipment (DME)**—such as hospital beds, wheelchairs, and walkers—the technician will need the HCPCS supply code plus an ICD-10 diagnostic code from the physician. These coding systems are also necessary in the claims processing for the DME and specified pharmacy services of Medicare Part D patients.

Technicians may be involved in using the CPT coding system to bill PBMs for the medication therapy management (MTM) and patient care services provided by the pharmacist. These billing procedures are processed separately from the on-the-spot online processing of drug prescriptions.

8.3 Commercial Health Insurance

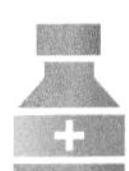

Pharm Fact

Many employers are increasing premium costs and/or reducing healthcare benefits, encouraging their employees to use Health Savings Accounts and retirees to enroll in a Medicare program.

Most patients have **commercial insurance**—or nongovernmental, private insurance—that they pay for on their own or that is subsidized by their employers as a benefit to employees and retirees. The employer contracts with the insurance company or companies to offer certain plans. While the workers are employed, the employer pays a portion of the monthly premium, and the remaining cost is deducted from the wage earners' pay prior to taxes; during retirement years, the retirees usually must pay the full portion and a higher premium depending on their age and health status. Common private insurers include Blue Cross/Blue Shield, Aetna, United Health, Humana, and others.

The Affordable Care Act (ACA) of 2010 sought to extend coverage to more Americans who were **uninsured** (without any insurance) or **underinsured** (insufficiently covered). Healthcare costs rise through higher hospital costs or taxes when individuals who cannot afford ongoing or preventive care are forced to go to emergency rooms, fall into poverty because of medical costs and loss of work, or have a parent die from illness. The ACA mandated that all businesses with more than 50 full-time employees offer a health insurance option. Private insurance comes in three types: health maintenance organizations (HMOs), which have their own staff of providers or a network of preferred providers; preferred provider organizations (PPOs), that encourage patients to use contracted providers; and traditional healthcare insurers, which allow patients to seek out their own providers.

Managed Care Organizations and Network Providers

Many insurance and healthcare companies are seeking ways to cut costs by limiting patient health choices to those considered or contracted to be the most cost-efficient and effective for the most people. These **managed care organizations (MCOs)** utilize preferred drug formularies and providers. Managed care insurance plans come generally in two types: HMO or PPO.

Health Maintenance Organizations

Health maintenance organizations (HMOs) require members to get services and products only through their staff or contracted providers and facilities. As described in Chapter 1, HMOs put an emphasis on preventive care and have their own employed or contracted providers, clinics, hospitals, and in-house pharmacies. Patients select or are designated a primary physician within the system who acts as a gatekeeper for the rest of the services provided within the HMO provider network. The system offers incentives and coaching to encourage patients to eat well, exercise, and take time for annual exams, immunizations, and certain screenings to prevent problems, which the system offers at no extra charge.

For specialized services that the system and primary care physician cannot provide, patients need a **referral**, or an official approved consent from the primary physician for additional services. If a patient has a severe accident or develops a complex medical condition, a case manager is often assigned to help coordinate the many different kinds of services needed.

Pharm Fact

Employers usually choose an insurer that uses some choice reductions for cost-containment strategies.

Patients in an HMO system generally have no copayments, coinsurances, or deductibles along with lower monthly premiums as compared to most traditional health insurance plans. In return for these cost benefits, there is little to no choice in their doctors, hospitals, pharmacies, and other providers. HMOs have a restricted drug formulary with a strong emphasis on lower-cost generic drugs.

Preferred Provider Organizations

Preferred provider organizations (PPOs) have some elements of the HMO model but with more choice. PPOs have tiered copay rates or coinsurance percentages that favor preferred **in-network providers** (those with whom the insurance company has a working contract) over **out-of-network providers** (those who have no contract with the insurance company). The insurance companies charge patients less for the services or products from a PPO member provider because the insurance company has already negotiated a group discount rate. These discounted rates do not apply to out-of-network providers.

Health Insurance Companies

Traditionally, private health insurance coverage was primarily limited to hospitalizations and emergency room (ER) visits with a 20% deductible. That is, the insurance would cover 80% of the hospital or ER costs, and the patient would be responsible for the remaining 20%. A patient had to pay cash for each physician visit and for each prescription. These insurance companies generally had no free preventive services, such as annual exams, but there was free choice of provider, clinic, hospital, and pharmacy because there were no in-network or out-of-network providers or restricted drug formularies.

Many traditional insurance companies, however, have now taken on some of the managed care cost containment and preventive medicine strategies of HMOs and PPOs. Many commercial plans (except catastrophic plans) in the marketplace now cover the preventive care of annual exams, immunizations, and certain screenings, and favor specific drug formularies and negotiated contract preferred providers.

Many health insurance companies have integrated preventive medicine managed care strategies, such as paying for well-baby checks and annual physicals, and have preferred drug formularies.

Supplemental Health Insurance

Some patients have supplemental, secondary insurance in addition to their primary insurance coverage to address uncovered services. Individuals with personal or parental histories of debilitating diseases or cancers may choose to get this additional coverage in anticipation of future health problems. For example, patients with chronic health issues and high annual medical and prescription drug costs who have primary coverage through a government insurance program such as Medicare may also have insurance provided through their employer as a supplemental insurance to lower their out-of-pocket costs.

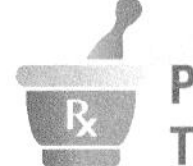

Practice Tip

It is helpful to get to know the laws and procedures of your state's workers' compensation program, because each program differs from state to state.

Other Forms of Insurance

Another form of health insurance comes through the employer that is separate from general healthcare insurance. This is **workers' compensation** insurance (commonly referred to as "workers' comp") to cover illness or injuries caused by or related to one's job, and it varies in its structure per each state's laws. Employers purchase a private disability insurance plan for their employees through a state-sponsored insurance plan with a deductible, or they insure their employees themselves. Employers generally pay a commercial insurance carrier or PBM specializing in workers' comp claims to administer the program. (The states determine whether or not the coverage is from a state-established provider or a private insurance company.)

This form of insurance offers ill or injured employees some medical and prescription drug benefits and some wage replacement in exchange for a waiver of the employee's right to sue the employer for the work-related health problem. Employees do not receive a workers' comp insurance card but commonly have an 800 number to call. The pharmacy technician receives the billing information from the assigned caseworker and the PBM or commercial insurance carrier. The pharmacy is then reimbursed directly through it.

The workers' comp coverage for a specific injury generally has an expiration date determined by the type and extent of the injury. If the employee is killed through the injury, dependents receive death benefits.

For those with a business-sponsored insurance who have lost or left their jobs, employers are required to allow former employees to stay on the employee insurance plans at full premium cost for 18 to 36 months. This is called **COBRA insurance**—named after the Consolidated Omnibus Budget Reconciliation Act (COBRA) that mandated that an employer must retain its former employees in its coverage plans to allow transition to their next jobs without loss of health insurance.

8.4 Government Insurance Health Programs

Presently, most patients ages 65 and over have some form of Medicare, while many low-income patients and families of any age have state-funded Medicaid coverage.

Up until 1965, over 50% of citizens over the age of 65 years had no health insurance at all! Through the Social Security Amendments of 1965, Medicare and Medicaid were approved, providing government-assisted health insurance coverage for seniors, people with disabilities, and the financially vulnerable. (However, there was no prescription coverage for seniors until the Medicare Modernization Act in 2006.) Medicare programs are administered by the federal government, whereas Medicaid programs are administered by state governments. The Children's Health Insurance Program (CHIP) was established in 1997 through the Balanced Budget Act of 1997.

The ACA established the Affordable Care insurance exchanges in 2014. These are both administered by individual states.

Medicare

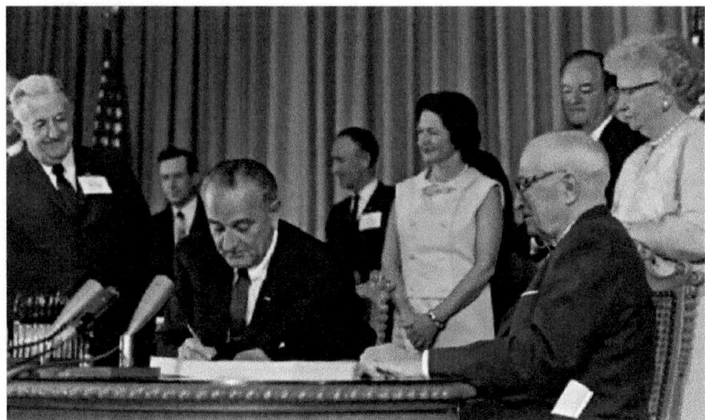

Medicare became the first federally funded health insurance program when President Lyndon B. Johnson signed it into law on July 30, 1965.

In 2018, over 59 million persons were enrolled in one or more Medicare programs. Once a patient is 65 years old, he or she is eligible for the **Medicare** programs. Other Medicare participants include those with a chronic kidney disease or those who have received Social Security disability insurance (SSDI) for 24 months. Because of the debilitating nature of the disease, patients with ALS (amyotrophic lateral sclerosis, or Lou Gehrig's disease) are able to receive coverage from the first month of their Social Security disability coverage.

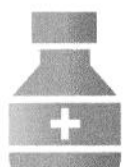

Pharm Fact

The Medicare Parts Open Enrollment Period goes from mid-October to the first week in December each year.

If a person becomes eligible for Medicare while still working, it is recommended by most health insurance consultants that they elect to continue current employer coverage too, because the Medicare programs cover only a portion of incurred medical costs. The employer may in part subsidize the monthly insurance premiums of enrolled employees or retirees. However, there is no penalty for delaying Medicare benefits—a patient may wish to remain insured through the employer plan if the insurance is comprehensive and affordable so that there is no need for a secondary insurance.

Medicare funding is drawn from a monthly premium automatically deducted from the patient's monthly Social Security check during retirement. One's Social Security account has the accumulated amount from payroll deductions during one's working years. If the patient is not yet receiving Social Security, they must pay a quarterly or monthly premium to the Center for Medicare and Medicaid Services (CMS).

Four different Medicare programs provide various types and levels of healthcare insurance, and it is important for the pharmacy technician to know the basics of each plan (Parts A, B, D, and comprehensive C), as only some cover some prescription drug costs or pharmacist services. Medicare can often be used when patients are away from home and seek medical attention out of their home state.

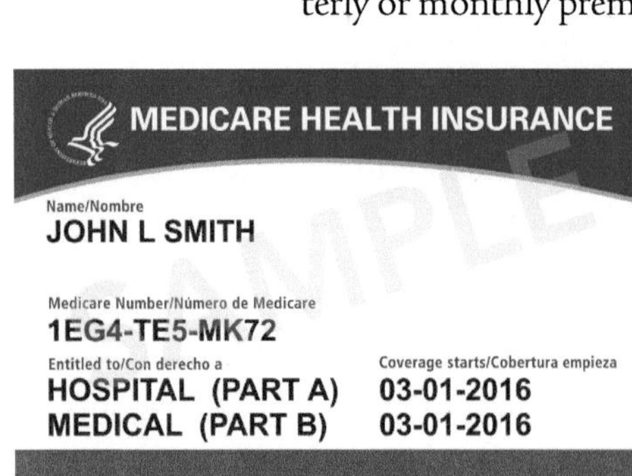

MEDICARE HEALTH INSURANCE
Name/Nombre
JOHN L SMITH
Medicare Number/Número de Medicare
1EG4-TE5-MK72
Entitled to/Con derecho a
Coverage starts/Cobertura empieza
HOSPITAL (PART A) 03-01-2016
MEDICAL (PART B) 03-01-2016
SAMPLE

The familiar red, white, and blue Medicare coverage card covers only Medicare Parts A and B. The insurance cards for Medicare Parts D and C are similar to commercial insurance plans, as they are through contracted providers and PBMs.

Medicare Part A

Medicare Part A typically covers 80% of the cost of hospital stays as well as limited coverage of skilled nursing and physical rehabilitation facilities, and home health care. (A community pharmacy cannot bill for *any* drugs or services under Medicare Part A.) Any person who reaches age 65 and submits an application automatically qualifies for this health coverage. The monthly premiums are the same for all participants, regardless of income or assets.

Medicare Part B

Medicare Part B is designed to go with Part A and covers 80% of the cost of doctor visits to diagnose and treat an illness after a low deductible is met. Again, the monthly premiums are the same for all participants, regardless of income or assets. (The 2019 monthly premium was $135.50 with a $185 deductible). It does not cover any prescriptions either, but it does fully cover some preventive medicine, such as vaccines and screening tests. If these services are provided through a pharmacy, the technician will ask for the red, white, and blue card for insurance processing.

This Medicare program may also cover a portion of the costs of some medical devices, known as durable medical equipment (DME), when these are deemed "medically necessary" by the healthcare provider. For some DMEs, a **certificate of medical necessity (CMN)** form must be completed online or on paper with an ICD-10 diagnosis code, and it must be signed by the patient and the pharmacist (see Figure 8.2). If the community pharmacy has been awarded a contract with the Center for Medicare and Medicaid Services as a provider of DME, it may bill for equipment (such as wheelchairs and hospital beds) and services directly to Medicare Part B.

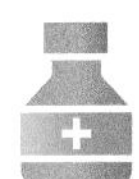

Pharm Fact

Though Medicare Parts A and B don't generally cover drugs, Part B will cover the total cost of the administration of the annual flu vaccine and the pneumonia vaccine every five years.

In addition, some disposable medical supplies may be covered by Medicare Part B, but these do not require a CMN form to be completed—though they do require other documentation of medical necessity by the prescriber, such as a Written Order/Prescription Prior to Delivery (WOPD). Included are diabetes supplies such as syringes, needles, pen needles, lancets, blood glucose monitors, and test strips. The prescription must include the correct ICD-10 diagnostic code for diabetes and the necessary frequency of daily insulin injections and blood glucose testing (see Figure 8.3).

Medicare Part B also requires a prescription for coverage of a nebulizer and solutions, with a new nebulizer allowed and required every five years. To fill a nebulizer solution prescription, such as for albuterol, the pharmacy must have documentation that a nebulizer has been purchased within the past five years. In addition, Medicare cannot be billed until the patient (or patient's guardian) personally picks up the diabetes supplies or nebulizer and/or solution. Other drug insurance plans often cover the nebulizer solutions but not the nebulizer machine itself.

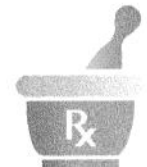

Practice Tip

Medicare Part B will cover some disposable and durable medical equipment, but technicians must have the proper documentation to file claims.

To be reimbursed for medication therapy management services, the pharmacist must be contracted for them by a Medicare-approved health center or clinic. The billing would then be submitted to Medicare via the contracting center, which would then pay the community pharmacy.

Medigap Insurance Plans

Since Medicare Parts A and B cover only some medical services, some patients also opt to purchase a supplemental **Medigap insurance** plan from a private health insurance provider (such as Blue Cross/Blue Shield) to cover the additional costs of outpatient physician visits as well as laboratory and x-ray costs, vision, hearing, and dental products and services. Medigap policies also typically do not cover the cost of any prescription drugs.

Medicare Part D

As has been established, Part A, Part B, and Medigap insurance plans do not cover prescription drugs. However, the Medicare Prescription Drug, Improvement, and Modernization Act (MMA) of 2003 established the option of **Medicare Part D**—a **prescription drug insurance** targeted at helping patients pay for medication costs. Enrollees can add this program to their existing Medicare A/B health coverage with an additional monthly charge to their current Medicare premium. Medicare Part D

FIGURE 8.2 Certificate of Medical Necessity for Oxygen

This is a sample of a DME form that must be filled out by the provider to allow for some insurance reimbursement.

DEPARTMENT OF HEALTH AND HUMAN SERVICES
CENTERS FOR MEDICARE & MEDICAID SERVICES

Form Approved
OMB No. 0938-0534

CERTIFICATE OF MEDICAL NECESSITY
CMS-484 — OXYGEN

DME 484.3

SECTION A: Certification Type/Date: INITIAL ___ / ___ / ____ REVISED ___ / ___ / ____ RECERTIFICATION ___ / ___ / ____

PATIENT NAME, ADDRESS, TELEPHONE and HICN

(___) ___-____ HICN ________

SUPPLIER NAME, ADDRESS, TELEPHONE and NSC or NPI #

(___) ___-____ NSC or NPI # ________

PLACE OF SERVICE

SUPPLY ITEM/SERVICE PROCEDURE CODE(S)

PT DOB ___ / ___ / ____ Sex ___ (M/F) Ht. ___ (in) Wt. ___

NAME and ADDRESS of FACILITY if applicable (see reverse)

PHYSICIAN NAME, ADDRESS, TELEPHONE and UPIN or NPI #

(___) ___-____ UPIN or NPI # ________

SECTION B: Information in this Section May Not Be Completed by the Supplier of the Items/Supplies.

EST. LENGTH OF NEED (# OF MONTHS): ____ 1–99 (99=LIFETIME)

DIAGNOSIS CODES: ____ ____ ____ ____

ANSWERS	ANSWER QUESTIONS 1–9. (Check Y for Yes, N for No, or D for Does Not Apply, unless otherwise noted.)
a) ____ mm Hg b) ____ % c) ___ / ___ / ____	1. Enter the result of most recent test taken on or before the certification date listed in Section A. Enter (a) arterial blood gas PO2 and/or (b) oxygen saturation test; (c) date of test.
☐ 1 ☐ 2 ☐ 3	2. Was the test in Question 1 performed (1) with the patient in a chronic stable state as an outpatient, (2) within two days prior to discharge from an inpatient facility to home, or (3) under other circumstances?
☐ 1 ☐ 2 ☐ 3	3. Check the one number for the condition of the test in Question 1: (1) At Rest; (2) During Exercise; (3) During Sleep
☐ Y ☐ N ☐ D	4. If you are ordering portable oxygen, is the patient mobile within the home? If you are not ordering portable oxygen, check D.
____ LPM	5. Enter the highest oxygen flow rate ordered for this patient in liters per minute. If less than 1 LPM, enter an "X".
a) ____ mm Hg b) ____ % c) ___ / ___ / ____	6. If greater than 4 LPM is prescribed, enter results of most recent test taken on 4 LPM. This may be an (a) arterial blood gas PO2 and/or (b) oxygen saturation test with patient in a chronic stable state. Enter date of test (c).
ANSWER QUESTIONS 7–9 ONLY IF PO2 = 56–59 OR OXYGEN SATURATION = 89 IN QUESTION 1	
☐ Y ☐ N	7. Does the patient have dependent edema due to congestive heart failure?
☐ Y ☐ N	8. Does the patient have cor pulmonale or pulmonary hypertension documented by P pulmonale on an EKG or by an echocardiogram, gated blood pool scan or direct pulmonary artery pressure measurement?
☐ Y ☐ N	9. Does the patient have a hematocrit greater than 56%?

NAME OF PERSON ANSWERING SECTION B QUESTIONS, IF OTHER THAN PHYSICIAN (Please Print):

NAME ________ TITLE ________ EMPLOYER ________

SECTION C: Narrative Description of Equipment and Cost

(1) Narrative description of all items, accessories and options ordered; (2) Suppliers charge; and (3) Medicare Fee Schedule Allowance for each item, accessory, and option (see instructions on back)

SECTION D: PHYSICIAN Attestation and Signature/Date

I certify that I am the treating physician identified in Section A of this form. I have received Sections A, B and C of the Certificate of Medical Necessity (including charges for items ordered). Any statement on my letterhead attached hereto, has been reviewed and signed by me. I certify that the medical necessity information in Section B is true, accurate and complete, to the best of my knowledge, and I understand that any falsification, omission, or concealment of material fact in that section may subject me to civil or criminal liability.

PHYSICIAN'S SIGNATURE ________ DATE ___ / ___ / ____

Signature and Date Stamps Are Not Acceptable.

Form CMS-484 (11/11) 1

contracts with insurance companies or PBMs to offer approved prescription drug plans (PDPs). Patients can choose from several drug insurance plans that are available in each region, designated by zip code.

Medicare Part D is complex with many choices. Each contracted plan has its own advantages and disadvantages. Though a government program, it is funded in part by patient premiums and administered by private insurers such as Blue Cross/Blue Shield, Aetna, Humana, and United Health, or by PBMs such as Express Scripts

FIGURE 8.3
Form Used to Bill for Diabetes Supplies to Medicare Part B

Prescribed diabetes supplies will be covered by Medicare Part B if the physician writes the correct ICD-10 coding and the pharmacy technician completes the proper form with signatures from the pharmacist and the patient.

Patient Demographics	
Select Type of Diabetes n Type 1 IDDM, Insulin-Dependent n Type 2 NIDDM, Noninsulin-Dependent n Type 2 NIDDMIR, Requires Insulin	**Indicates Diabetes Diagnosis** ICD-10______________ ICD-10______________ Type 1 Diabetes, ICD-10 must end in odd number. Type 2 Diabetes, ICD-10 must end in even number.

	Required Supplies		
Number of Tests/Day	**Number of Test Strips**	**Number of Lancets**	**Healthcare Orders**
n 1			
n 2			
n 3			____ test strips
n 4			____ lancets
n 5			____ glucometer(s)
n 6			____ lancet skin piercing device(s)
n 7			____ bottle(s) of control solution
n 8			
n 9			
n 10			
n 11			
n 12			
Provider Demographics with Date and Signature of Patient and Pharmacist			

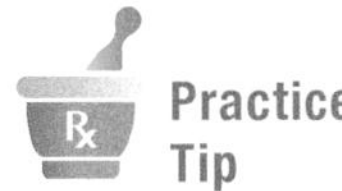

Practice Tip

Technicians can remind customers nearing age 65 that they are eligible for Medicare Part D and inform them of the benefits. They can find more information online at the Medicare website, which can be accessed at https://PharmPractice7e.ParadigmEducation.com/MedicareD.

International. Premium costs can vary widely, from approximately $20 per month to over $100 per month, depending on the deductible. In addition, there may be copayments with each prescription.

Medicare Part D has special provisions for low-income seniors and provides catastrophic coverage for all patients who develop serious medical conditions requiring expensive drug treatments. Information on the Medicare Part D insurance cards of eligible low-income members dictates their lower copayment costs. Almost 40 million patients who are eligible for Medicare have taken advantage of signing up for a Medicare Part D insurance program. If patients opt not to enroll when eligible at age 65, the monthly cost may be higher by the time they decide to join. Individuals must renew their enrollment annually during the open enrollment period (late October through the first week in December).

Every patient who enrolls in Medicare Part D can expect to save an average of 25% to 30% annually from the actual consumer costs of prescriptions. However, in some plans, a deductible of approximately $400 on prescription costs must be paid before patients are eligible for initial coverage benefits. After the deductible is met, patients pay an average of 25% of the cost for their new and refilled prescriptions (generic and brand names) for the first $2,960 of total drug costs (from both out-of-pocket and insurance).

Medicare Part C (Comprehensive)

If Medicare patients don't want three or more insurance plans to get full coverage, there is Medicare Advantage, or **Medicare Part C**. This program offers the full package of hospital, doctor visits, and prescription drug insurance. Like Part D, Medicare Advantage is administered by various private commercial insurance companies contracted by Medicare. They come in all kinds, such as HMOs, PPOs, fee-for-service plans, special needs plans (SNPs), and Medicare Medical Savings Account Plans. That is why Medicare C is complex and often confusing.

Approximately 30% of all Medicare-eligible patients opt for a Medicare Advantage program. If the community pharmacy has a contract with a Medicare Part C insurer, there may be coverage for DME equipment such as hospital beds, wheelchairs, walkers, and other supplies including nebulizers and blood pressure monitors, depending on the plan. Vision, hearing, and dental services are not typically covered by Medicare. However, some Medicare Advantage plans may offer some coverage. Some Medicare Advantage programs may restrict the choice of doctors, specialists, or hospitals, or charge additional costs for out-of-network doctors or hospitals.

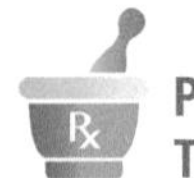

Practice Tip

When filling Medicaid prescriptions, check that the patient's card is from in-state. If not, let patients know that Medicaid will not cover their prescriptions. Out-of-state travelers and tourists may not realize this.

Medicaid

Medicaid is a healthcare insurance program run jointly by the federal and state governments. Medicaid subsidizes the cost of health care, including drugs, for eligible disabled, low-income, part-time, and unemployable state citizens of any age. (Some disabled older adults are "**dual eligible**" for both Medicare and Medicaid.) Each state designs its own state plan that has different eligibility requirements and benefits. There is no monthly premium, but patients may be charged an additional copay when they pick up their prescription(s). Pharmacy technicians should know their own state policies, procedures, and regulations on the reimbursement of prescription drugs for eligible Medicaid patients. Medicaid does not cover prescriptions that are filled in a state other than the state in which the patient resides. It also does not cover prescriptions from providers who are not in the state plan's network.

Eligibility is based on income and number of dependents, and it is frequently reviewed by the state. Patients may be covered by insurance with their employer but still need Medicaid to fill the gaps. To help all citizens get insured, the ACA provides financial incentives for states to extend their Medicaid eligibilities to cover more uninsured patients, so the eligibility ranges have expanded and they are variable according to state legislative decisions.

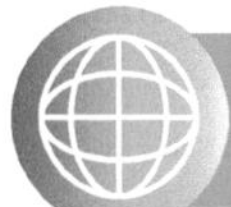

IN THE REAL WORLD

Medicare is prohibited from using its huge negotiating power (over 50 million members) with pharmaceutical manufacturers to lower drug costs on brand name and specialty drugs. This is one of the reasons why drugs are so much cheaper in many other countries, such as Canada. An amendment to this law would need to be approved in the future to control future drug price increases.

Children's Health Insurance Program

Like Medicaid, the **Children's Health Insurance Program (CHIP)** is a low-cost-to-free healthcare insurance program run jointly by the states and the federal government aimed at uninsured children from ages 0 to 19 whose parents (including pregnant women) earn over the federal poverty line but too little to cover healthcare insurance for their children. Most state CHIP plans do not have a deductible, but they do charge monthly premiums and copays.

Affordable Care Insurance Exchanges

Many people are not covered by either government-sponsored or employer insurance. Many small employers (fewer than 50 employees) have elected *not* to provide health insurance coverage as an employee benefit because it is too expensive. Their workers have to purchase health insurance on their own. Self-employed contractors and entrepreneurs also have to find insurance on their own. In addition, employees working part-time (less than 30 hours per week) or who are unemployed also need to find insurance.

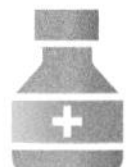

Pharm Fact

Recent polls by the Centers for Disease Control and Prevention indicate that the number of uninsured people in the United States has continued to decrease from 14% in 2013 to 8.8% in 2018.

To assist these individuals and families, the ACA established online affordable **healthcare exchanges** so that eligible individuals and families can comparison shop online for plans within their price range. These plans are lower cost than the regular market plans because of group discounts as well as governmental subsidies in many cases. This is a system of shared coverage among Medicaid, Children's Health Insurance Programs, and affordable care eligibility programs. Some of these exchanges are state run, some are federally run, and some are run in partnership. Each insurance plan must meet standards of financial accessibility for patients in order to offer the program through the exchanges.

Individuals or families pay a monthly premium on a sliding scale based on their income. Depending on how individual or family income compares to federal poverty levels, individuals and families can qualify for a subsidy or a discount on their monthly insurance premium. Of the citizens who qualify for government subsidies, 85% pay less than $100 per month.

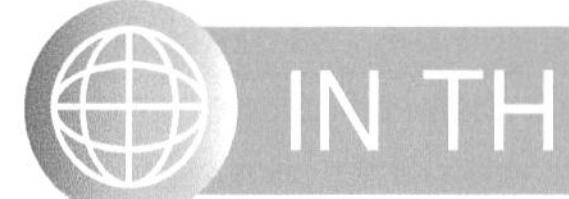

IN THE REAL WORLD

Back in 2013, 15% of US citizens, or 41.3 million people, were uninsured, with little affordable access to health care. About two-thirds of uninsured individuals had one person in the family working, but that employment situation offered no healthcare. Since the passage of the ACA, great progress in coverage has been made. In the first full year of implementation in 2014, 15.7 million previously uninsured persons received healthcare coverage either through healthcare exchanges or expansion of the state Medicaid programs. The rate of uninsured children decreased from 13.9% in 1997 to 4.6% in 2015.

However, 14 states in 2018 still had not expanded Medicaid eligibility or found ways to cover those in the zone of federal poverty level, and 8.8% of all Americans, or 28 million citizens (a large portion of whom are children), remain uninsured, according to the United States Census Bureau (September 2018). For an independent analysis on the effects of the ACA on the uninsured, visit the Kaiser Family Foundation website at https://PharmPractice7e.ParadigmEducation.com/KFF.

There are generally four plans available—bronze, silver, gold, and platinum—going from least expensive and least comprehensive to most. The bronze plan usually has a high deductible. After it is met, the bronze plan covers 60% of healthcare costs.

The silver plan typically covers 70%, and the gold plan 80%. The platinum plan that covers 90% has the highest monthly premium. For young, healthy patients, the bronze or silver plan is recommended due to its lower cost. Most insurance buyers (75%) favor the silver plan. All of the programs have a cap on the total annual out-of-pocket costs through in-network providers for an individual (approximately $6,500 in 2015) and for a family ($13,200). The programs, premiums, and coverage limits are annually renewable and adjustable. The enrollment period for healthcare exchanges is from November 1st through January 30th each year.

To offer lower patient costs for prescriptions, the various insurance providers in the healthcare exchanges and their PBMs negotiate reimbursement rates in contracts with pharmacies. Technicians need to understand that not all community pharmacies have contracts with all the insurers in their state's healthcare exchange due to low reimbursements. If your pharmacy does not have a contract with the PBM of the patient's ACA insurance provider, then you will not be able to process the prescription claim and must let the patient know this prior to filling the prescription.

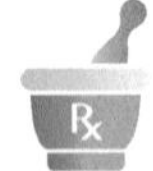

Practice Tip

Mail-order prescriptions can result in some delivery delays. If a prescription is needed before the mail-order arrival, the pharmacy with the prescription on file may call the provider and the PBM for an insurance overide to provide a small supply to bridge the time gap.

Military Health Insurance

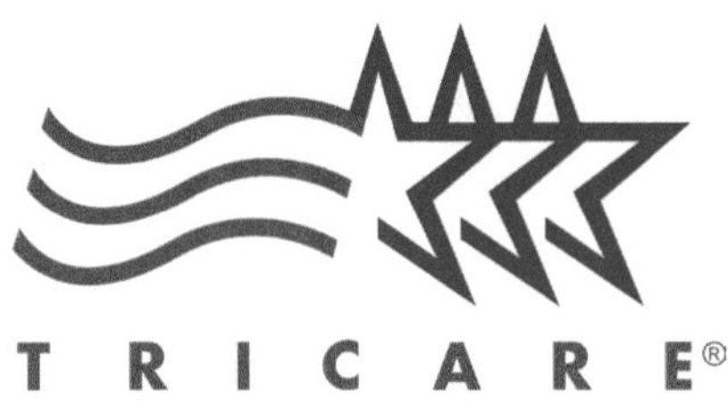

In 2018, Tricare Select replaced Tricare Standard and Extra.

The **Defense Health Agency (DHA)** administers **Tricare**, which is the four-part federal health and prescription drug insurance plan for active and retired members of the military and their families. For active duty members, their military photo IDs or military dependent IDs double as proof of insurance. Retirees and their family members generally pay a higher premium than active duty members.

The patients who come to community pharmacies generally have Tricare Select or Tricare for Life. Prescription copays or coinsurance payments may differ, depending on the patient's active or inactive status in the military. As with other insurance programs, the payment fees and the coinsurance proportions for prescription drugs have been increased—with little or no notice to military patients, their families, or retirees. Pharmacy technicians often have to explain why patients' copayments unexpectedly increased at the time of dispensing.

The VA has its own outpatient and inpatient pharmacies at hospital centers where many pharmacy technicians work. To avoid lines and save money, the VA encourages its members to use one of its seven highly automated mail-order pharmacies. Over 316,000 veterans receive a package of prescriptions in the mail every day. Convenience is the main reason that most members utilize the VA's mail-order service.

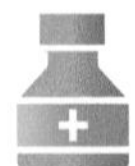

Pharm Fact

The seven VA mail-order pharmacies process almost 460,000 prescriptions per day—nearly 80% of all outpatient prescriptions.

Tricare Prime

Tricare Prime is a military service HMO, with assigned primary care physicians and in-network providers. It is the most cost-effective program, but a person needs to live near a military base and/or **Veterans Health Administration (VHA)** hospital and clinics to receive the generous coverage of hospital admissions, medical visits, and services with relatively low copays for prescribed drugs. There is an annual enrollment fee if the enrollee is not on active duty and small fees per visit, service, or product.

Tricare Select

Tricare Select offers the most choices, with open selection of providers and pharmacies, and it costs the most. It has an annual deductible and a coinsurance payment for what Tricare says the medical service or product should cost.

8.5 Insurance and Patient Responsibilities

Unlike most medical and dental offices, a pharmacy processes a claim *prior to* the patient receiving the service to check the claim's viability with the insurer's pharmacy benefit manager. Most commercial insurance, Medicare D plans, state Medicaid, and workers' comp programs outsource the administrative processing of prescription drug claims to a pharmacy benefit manager. Commonly known PBMs include Merck, Express Scripts International (ESI), CVS Caremark, and Medco.

Each PBM develops with the insurer its own **preferred drug list**, or formulary of medications that are fully covered or covered at a lower cost. Using the formulary and the insurance policy, the PBM processes insurance drug claims and pharmacy reimbursements.

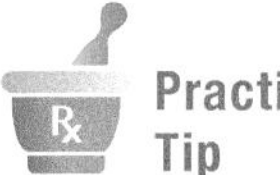

Practice Tip

If a pharmacy does not have a contract with a patient's insurance PBM, the technician may suggest that the patient visit another nearby pharmacy that might fill the prescription.

Practice Tip

If drug affordability becomes an issue, the technician can offer resources for price reduction, while the pharmacist can discuss therapy options with the patient, prescriber, and PBM.

Pharmacy Benefit Manager–Contracts and Reimbursements

In community pharmacy, the very same drug may be billed at different rates to patients, different insurance companies, and government programs. That is because each community pharmacy must have a drug-provider contract negotiated with each PBM it works with. Typically, pharmacies have annually renewable contracts with PBMs to provide prescription benefits at specified reimbursement rates to the insurance enrollees managed by that PBM. Larger PBMs that can promise more business can negotiate lower rates of reimbursement. The rates are generally based on **usual and customary (U&C) charges** for drugs plus a pharmacy dispensing fee. Technicians need to learn the different rate schedules. The U&Cs are based on the AWP for each drug. By law, the pharmacy cannot charge or negotiate a higher cost to the government programs than to a commercial user or PBM for the same prescription.

Community pharmacies usually have contracts with all the major PBMs, thus being able to provide drugs to the widest clientele possible. However, some independent or chain pharmacies will not enter into certain PBM contracts because those PBM reimbursements do not sufficiently cover direct and indirect pharmacy expenses. The very survival of a pharmacy depends on its ability to contain personnel and drug acquisition costs. To continue as a business, community pharmacies must avoid agreeing to unprofitable contracts with any PBM, whether representing a government or a private insurance program.

Pharmacy Benefit Manager-Based Patient Charges

In most cases, insurance companies and their pharmacy benefit managers pay only a portion of the prescription cost, so patients need to pay up front some portion through a coinsurance percentage or copay. The most common drug insurance plans use a tiered-level copay for less expensive to more expensive drugs. In this scenario, the patient pays a lower copay for the generic than the preferred brand drug and an even higher copay for a nonpreferred brand or specialty drug. A non-formulary drug is most likely not covered at all. Some PBMs have high-cost innovator or specialty drugs as a fourth-tier formulary option: the patient usually pays a percentage (coinsurance) of the drug cost rather than a fixed copay amount.

For example, a PBM may elect to cover the generic drug simvastatin for the treatment of high cholesterol, which incurs a $5 copay. However, simvastatin (the nonpreferred generic drug) may have a $10 copay, and Livalo (the nonpreferred brand name drug), a $60 copay.

Technicians can help patients understand these options. Patients also need to know that most insurance plans cover only a 30-day supply of a brand name medication in a community pharmacy. Sometimes a 90-day supply will be covered at a cost-saving copay if the PBM's mail-order pharmacy is used.

Even with drug insurance coverage, a patient who has high blood pressure, diabetes, and high cholesterol commonly pays five or six copays at the time of their medication refills if they all come due at the same time. The patient may need to pay $100 to $250 or more per month in out-of-pocket expenses–in addition to the monthly insurance premium expenses. That is where drug coupons can come in handy for patients on commercial insurance.

8.6 Processing Prescription Drug Claims

To work successfully in any community or mail-order pharmacy, technicians need to process drug claims on the spot with great efficiency–while the patient is watching and waiting. You will face all kinds of situations: new patients with new insurance, established patients with expired insurance, drug discount cards, workers' comp claims, patients with no insurance, and patients with multiple insurances. All the information must be accurately entered into the pharmacy's computer software to process the drug claim.

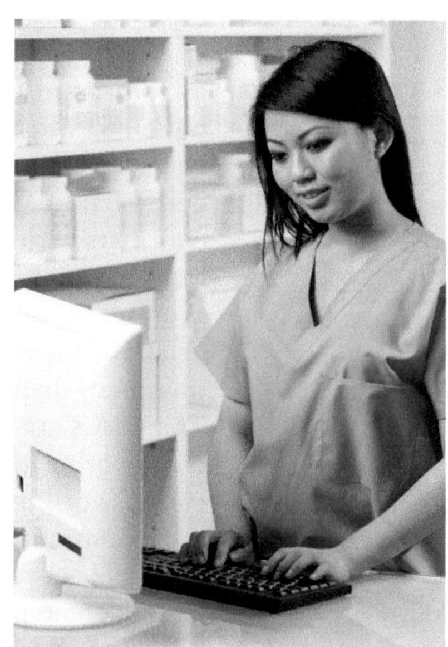
The pharmacy technician has to enter both the insurance information and the prescription into the computer for processing the claim and filling the prescription.

Pharmacy software differs, but, in almost all cases, billing involves direct online transactions between the pharmacy and the customer's insurance PBM. The procedures to bill online PBMs for commercial insurance, federal or state governments' plans, or workers' comp are similar but not identical. Learning the ins and outs of various insurance plans as well as their interfacing with the pharmacy's software package is a challenging task.

Technicians must be trained in the specific processes and procedures for each pharmacy and PBM to avoid insurance-claim problems. Pharmacies can receive stiff financial and civil penalties from the PBM for intentional or unintentional billing errors caught in a PBM audit. If the PBM challenges an incorrectly processed claim, the pharmacy can lose both the cost of the drug and any dispensing fee.

IN THE REAL WORLD

An estimated 3.2 million Americans are infected with hepatitis C. The specialty drug sofosbuvir (Sovaldi) is 90% effective in treating and preventing complications. A typical regimen for a 12-week course of therapy is $84,000. The average cost of such a prescription—without insurance—is over $16,000. A similar drug, ledipasvir (Harvoni), costs over $1,000 per tablet. Even with insurance, a 25%–33% coinsurance is beyond the means of most patients. Technicians can then direct the patient to try to qualify for assistance directly from the drug manufacturer to help defray the high copayment costs.

One patient remarked, "I just found out that I have hepatitis C and have had it for years, so the doctor told me I needed a particular drug. It was so expensive I couldn't possibly pay for it! The technician saved my life by telling me how to sign up for a special program from the manufacturer. I can't thank her enough."

Receiving and Entering Insurance Information in the Computer

To begin the process, you need to ask for the customer's insurance card to input the information into the computer (or double-check it with existing customers). The card usually includes the following information:

- name of the primary insured person (or name of family member with their person code)
- insurance carrier
- nine-digit **patient identification number (ID)**
- **group number** and/or employer
- **bank identification number (BIN)**, designating the pharmacy benefit manager
- **processor control number (PCN)**, designating the kind of plan and processing flow
- the date coverage became effective

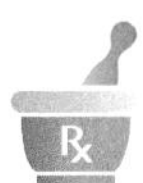

Practice Tip

Helping patients sort out their insurance cards and understand their copayments or coinsurance and formularies are elements of great customer service.

Additionally, some cards will show which family members are covered and the amount of copay for generic and brand name prescriptions. See Figure 8.4 for an example of how this information may be displayed on the insurance card. The BIN and PCN are needed to identify the PBM.

If the customer is not new, you must ask if any information has changed. If the information on the card (name of cardholder, patient identification number, etc.) is still current, make sure that the card hasn't expired. If the cardholder's employment status has changed recently, then the drug insurance on the profile will likely have changed. A patient may be dual eligible, having more than one insurer. If so, the information on both cards must be entered, designating which is the primary and which is the secondary insurer.

Collecting and entering insurance information can be a challenging task. First, the information is not standardized or always accurate. At times, the pharmacy technician may have to call the insurer to verify eligibility.

Some patients, such as those with Medicare Parts C or D and many commercial insurers, have unique medical/drug insurance cards apart from their regular medical insurance or their primary and secondary coverage. They may not know which is which. The patient's relationship to the cardholder (spouse, child) is represented by the **person code**, which is required for processing the online claim of a dependent.

You will have to be patient and spend time with customers who are confused or overwhelmed. They may have insurance cards for medical but not pharmacy claims or insurance cards for other members of the family but be missing their own.

Keep in mind that the claim must be successfully processed *before* the drug is released to the patient, and the patient often expects to receive their prescription(s) within 15–20 minutes or less. Consider all the time it takes to enter the insurance information into the computer, verify the PBM, enter the prescription, process the claim, fill the prescription, and have it checked by the pharmacist. Patience and efficiency have to work hand in hand!

FIGURE 8.4
Parts of an Insurance Identification Card

In this example, the mother is the primary insurance holder for her four children, the insurer is Central Healthcare, and the employer is UDrug. Not all insurance cards list each person covered, as this example does. Some insurance companies issue cards for each person insured.

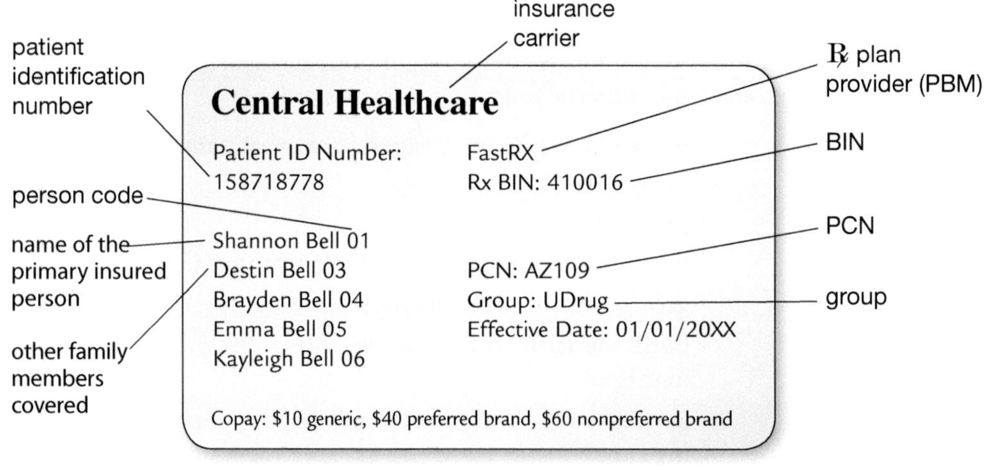

Practice Tip

It is a good idea to ask patients to offer their insurance information and any coupons when they drop off their prescriptions rather than waiting until the pickup. This helps reduce the waiting time for them later.

Verifying the Pharmacy Benefit Manager

Once the patient insurance profile is complete, you will use the BIN and PCN to identify the correct pharmacy benefit manager (PBM) and the internal processing code for this patient's plan. (Some insurance cards do not list a PCN, making the technician's job a little more difficult.) As insurance and Medicaid-funded programs may switch PBMs within the calendar year without patient notice or issuance of a new insurance card, PBM information must be identified and updated with each patient visit.

Since there are hundreds of healthcare plans with the same PBM, the group number is also needed to process the claim. The BIN, PCN, and group number designate the specific plan for the specific patient or family. Entering the combination of ID, BIN, PCN, and group number/employer pulls up the proper PBM for verification to establish eligibility to process the claim.

With patients who have dual eligibility, the primary insurance is always billed first online. The remaining amount or copayment may be covered by the secondary insurance. Drug coupons are processed like insurance and applied before the primary insurer is billed to reduce the price, with all pertinent information also entered into the patient database (see Figure 8.5).

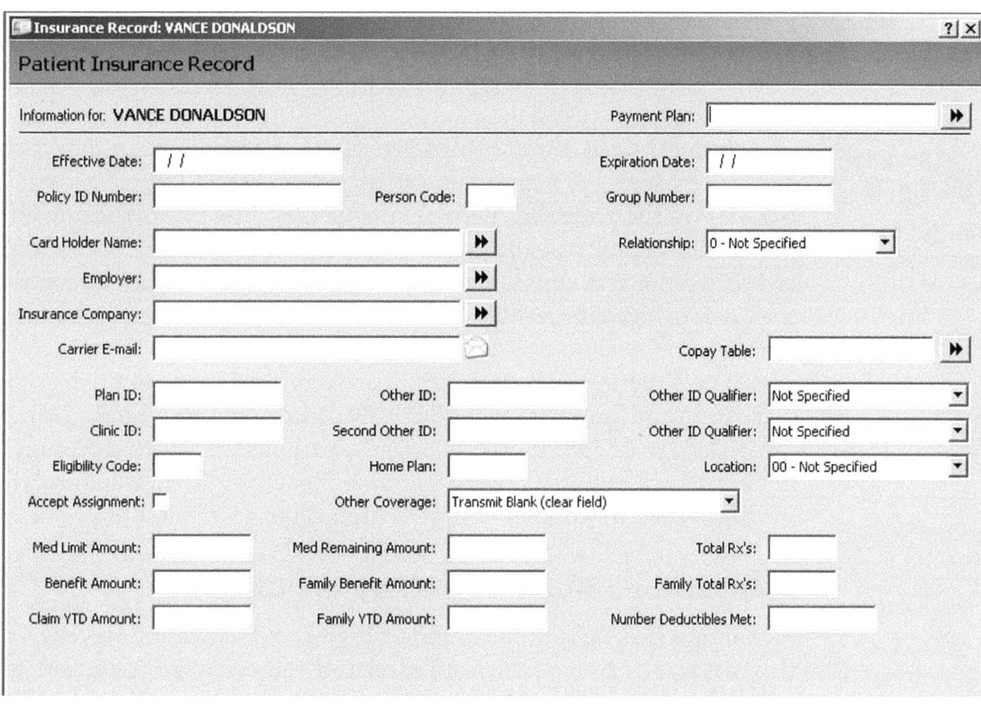

Insurance Record: VANCE DONALDSON

Patient Insurance Record

Information for: VANCE DONALDSON
Payment Plan:
Effective Date: / /
Expiration Date: / /
Policy ID Number:
Person Code:
Group Number:
Card Holder Name:
Relationship: 0 - Not Specified
Employer:
Insurance Company:
Carrier E-mail:
Copay Table:
Plan ID:
Other ID:
Other ID Qualifier: Not Specified
Clinic ID:
Second Other ID:
Other ID Qualifier: Not Specified
Eligibility Code:
Home Plan:
Location: 00 - Not Specified
Accept Assignment:
Other Coverage: Transmit Blank (clear field)
Med Limit Amount:
Med Remaining Amount:
Total Rx's:
Benefit Amount:
Family Benefit Amount:
Family Total Rx's:
Claim YTD Amount:
Family YTD Amount:
Number Deductibles Met:

FIGURE 8.5
Insurance Plan Database

An important responsibility of the technician is to update the prescription drug insurance information in the pharmacy database.

Pharmacy Benefit Manager's Prescription Processing

When entering and submitting prescriptions into the pharmacy software for the drug utilization review (DUR), technicians do not know off the top of their heads (nor do pharmacists and prescribers) which drugs are in the formulary of a specific PBM and which are not. PBM formulary selections are constantly changing, often without notice (with very few exceptions, OTC drugs are not covered). So the software or the technician also transmits the prescription online to the PBM to complete the crucial insurance adjudication step.

Practice Tip

Though DUR alerts regarding drug interactions, allergies, and other safety issues should not be handled or acknowledged by the technician, DUR notices dealing with DME diagnosis codes, some formulary issues (such as NDC not covered) or days' supply concerns *can* in many cases be handled by the technician.

Online Adjudication

Online adjudication refers to the process of electronically submitting prescription claims to the appropriate PBM for its judgment on whether or not it will provide reimbursement. It usually takes less than 30 seconds to receive a reply.

The best-case scenario is when the PBM approves the prescription right away—vthen the technician will be immediately notified onscreen of the patient's required copayment or coinsurance. You then inform the patient of the cost if it is an expensive copay to make sure that he or she is prepared to pay it. If the patient is surprised and unready, there are options. If the drug is already a generic but expensive, the pharmacist should be alerted to discuss with the prescriber less costly alternatives if available.

The PBM online response also states the proportion of pharmacy reimbursement amount compared to the AWP. Occasionally, the PBM will reimburse the pharmacy less than the AWP. In that case, you need to alert the pharmacist or supervisor, as it is likely that the pharmacy will not be able to fill that prescription.

Many insurance price printouts, which accompany the medication for dispensing, list the amount the patient saved through insurance coverage. It is a good service practice to highlight this amount to customers so that even if the amount they paid is higher than they like, they can walk away feeling a little better about their purchases, knowing that you and the community pharmacy care that they are receiving medication savings.

Always let the customer know if a generic drug is cheaper to pay out of pocket than the insurance copay.

In some cases, the cost for a generic drug without insurance is cheaper than the insurance copay. For instance, a patient copay was $10 for all generic drugs. However, the AWP of the prescribed generic anti-nausea drug promethazine was so low that the patient could purchase the generic drug without insurance for only $7.50. The technician made the customer aware of this so that the patient could save money and the time involved in the online insurance adjudication process by just paying out of pocket.

The patient may have multiple prescriptions that need to be processed for pick-up at one time. This will obviously complicate the adjudication process, as each drug needs to be adjudicated separately, perhaps with both a primary and secondary insurer, which requires a coordination of benefits (COB), which will be described later in the chapter. In workers' compensation claims, COB is almost always needed.

Medications Not Covered by Insurance

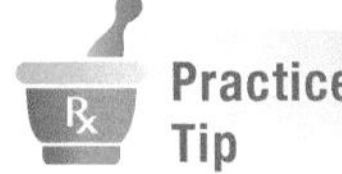

For a high-cost drug, remind patients to check online or in local papers for manufacturers' coupons (or do it for them) or enroll in the pharmacy's prescription savings plan if it is an often used medication.

A common message for any brand or high-cost medication is *NDC Not Covered.* When this message or *Not an Option* appears on the screen in adjudication, it means that this particular drug with its National Drug Code is not covered by the PBM formulary. You can then present the following options to the patient: (1) pay the out-of-pocket costs if not too exorbitant; (2) keep the prescription on file for a later date; (3) the patient can call the prescriber and request a less costly alternative if available; or (4) have the pharmacist discuss the situation with the patient and call the prescriber with recommendations for alternative options or prior authorization if that is needed.

Cases exist in which the medication selected by the physician is not covered by the insurance under any circumstances—not even with a prior approval! This lack of coverage often applies to new innovative drugs that are extremely expensive; drugs that promote weight loss or sleep; certain medications for anxiety or nervous disorders; certain cough syrups for adults; and drugs that have less costly alternatives or that are available as OTC drugs.

If such questions about coverage arise, then use the appropriate (toll-free) insurance contact phone number. If the insurer denies coverage, the patient has the right to appeal. This is not done by the technician or pharmacist but by the patient. However, you or the pharmacist must break this news to the patient. Most patients are unaware of this right, and they also need to know that the process requires the completion of a lot of paperwork and is exceedingly slow. In most cases, the patient pays cash or uses a discount card if eligible.

Other rejection messages can appear, and you will get to know them fairly quickly. They are often accompanied by a "reject code." Claims get rejected for many reasons, including problems with missing or mistyped information, wrong dosages, or special medications requiring prior authorization (PA). Each rejection message will require its own response action to resolve the problem.

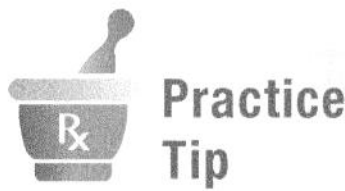

Practice Tip

Resolving insurance claims may be time-consuming for a technician, but it fosters patient trust and customer loyalty, which is often the difference between surviving and not surviving for a small independent pharmacy.

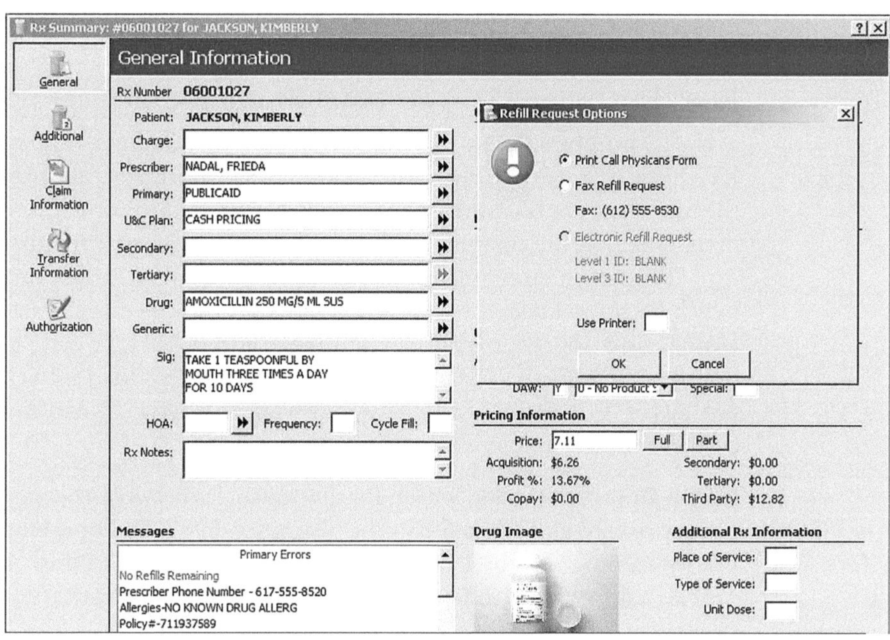

In this situation, Kimberly Jackson's prescription for amoxicillin 250 mg from Dr. Nadal was turned down for a refill as the number of refills had run out. The pharmacy software popped up the action window noting that a call to the physician was needed.

Practice Tip

It is often important to explain to customers that their copayments and drug coverage are determined by the insurance plan, not by the pharmacy.

Catching and Fixing Processing Errors

The goal is to have a safe and accurate prescription and **capture the claim**, or achieve reimbursement confirmation from the PBM. Yet many things can go wrong in filing a prescription claim, which results in claim denial or no reimbursement. Was an error made in entering the multiple insurance card numbers? Is the patient (or a family member) not eligible? Is the drug prescribed not covered, or does it require special authorization? Does the patient not have any insurance? An experienced technician will be able to resolve most of these questions in real time, as the patient is often waiting in the pharmacy or parked in the drive-through, watching the technician.

If a claim cannot be processed because of any unresolved issues, you can try calling the toll-free number on the back of the patient's insurance card for assistance to clear up the issue. Clearly, much can go wrong when a technician is processing a drug claim, and persistence is a plus.

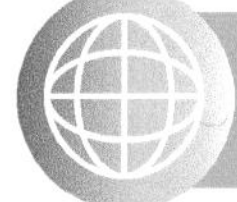

IN THE REAL WORLD

For 2019, the PBM Express Scripts International (ESI) will cover only Humulin (not Novolin) and Humalog (not NovoLog). CVS Caremark will cover just the opposite on their preferred drug formulary. Even though these drugs are "therapeutic equivalents," the pharmacist or technician needs to get approval from the prescriber to process the right insulin that fits both the patient and the insurer's PBM!

As a technician, you will need to be on the lookout for and know how to resolve the most common insurance problems described below.

ID Number Issues If the PBM cannot find a record of the patient, take another look at the ID numbers. Many plans may use letters preceding the ID number, e.g., XYZ1199A2883. Some insurance plans require the letters, but some do not. Letters in the middle of the ID number are usually required. If the error message still pops up, make sure that the customer did not accidentally give you an out-of-date card.

To make matters more complicated, the group number on the prescription card may be incorrect because it has changed, or it may be missing (some plans like Humana do not require a group number), and it will take time to track down the right number and enter it. The correct numbers are then added into the patient insurance profile for future processing. You may want to advise the cardholder to add the correct number in marker to the insurance card.

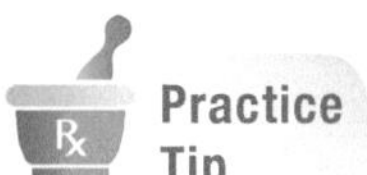

Practice Tip

Be aware that you may enter all the patient information correctly (such as date of birth, gender, address, relationship to cardholder), but the PBM may have it listed wrong in its system because of a typo or input error. You (or the patient) will need to call the PBM to resolve the issue.

Name Discrepancies Watch for discrepancies between the name on the patient's insurance card and the name in the insurance database. For example, Rick Smith may be in the insurance database under his legal name Charles R. Smith, and if you try to process a drug claim under Rick Smith, it will be denied with the error message *Unmatched Recipient.*

Birth Date Discrepancies If the pharmacy and the insurance company have differing information due to typos or mistakes, the error message *Check Birth Date* will pop up. Even if the pharmacy has the correct birth date but this does not match the PBM database, the claim will not be approved. To process the claim, call the PBM, verify the listed date of birth (DOB), and enter the incorrect date in the patient profile. The patient (or parent) must then call the insurance company (PBM) to correct the DOB in its system and then advise the pharmacy on his or her next visit to update the birth date correctly in the patient profile.

Person Code Discrepancies Some insurance plans (or pharmacy software) require a two-digit or three-digit person code to follow the ID number. For example, a husband may be there to pick up a prescription, but his wife is the primary insured person under her employee plan. His wife might have the 11-digit ID number 119922883-01 (or 001), whereas he would have the same first nine numbers but the person code of 02 (or 002) as the spouse. The numbers for their dependent children would end with 03 (003), 04 (004), 05 (005), and so on, generally in their birth order. (Most Medicare Part D and Medicaid programs have a patient-specific ID number, so there is no need for an additional person code.) Always double-check that the right person code was entered.

Prescribers' NPI Issues The correct **National Provider Identifier (NPI)** number is required for the prescriptions from each physician, physician's assistant, nurse practitioner, dentist, and pharmacist to be legitimate and processed. (Nurse practitioners or physician's assistants may use the NPI number of their supervising physician with approval.) These NPI numbers must always be carefully checked to ensure that they match up with the prescriber's name. In the case of controlled medication, the prescriber must also have a DEA (Drug Enforcement Agency) number on file in order for the claim to be processed and billed.

Out-of-Network Prescriber In rare cases, the claim can even be rejected because the prescriber is not contracted with the patient's insurance plan (as with Medicaid). This may happen with any new prescriber or with hospital prescribers whose practice is limited to inpatients. In that case, another prescriber or supervising physician in the network must be contacted by phone, and that prescriber must agree to put his or her name on the prescription (except for controlled substances) to process the claim. If the pharmacist or pharmacy technician can identify no alternative prescriber, the patient must pay cash for the prescriptions.

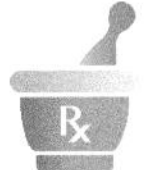

Practice Tip

If a prescriber's NPI number is not on file with that patient's insurance provider, the online claim will be rejected.

Drug Interactions and Combination Rejections There are also the DUR rejections where the PBM software compares the prescriptions with the patient's medication profile. The review may find that the patient is receiving more than one similar medication, such as two antibiotics at the same time, or it could be that the drug may interfere with another prescribed drug (a drug interaction) or produce an allergic reaction. In these cases, the technician must alert the pharmacist to carefully review the rejection. The pharmacist may choose to override the rejection with the computer software. If not, the PBM and/or prescriber must be notified.

Drugs Requiring Prior Authorization Some prescribed drugs require **prior authorization (PA)**, or prior approval. This can be because the drug is atypical for the patient's age, gender, or condition; because the drug is not on the PBM formulary; because the patient is already prescribed a similar drug; or the continued use of a drug exceeds the medication's short-term use recommendations. The pharmacist or technician is then responsible for electronically sending, telephoning, or faxing a PA request to the prescriber's office. The physician's representative will then contact the PBM to determine whether coverage can be approved (and for how long) or whether an alternative drug must be prescribed. Basically, both the doctor's office and the patient's insurance PBM must review the necessity of approving the prescribed drug versus a lower-cost alternative.

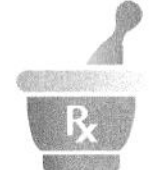

Practice Tip

PA rejections are very confusing to patients, especially if they previously recieved a drug without a PA. You will need to explain that the PBM wants to communicate with the prescriber to get more information about the ongoing need for a prescription.

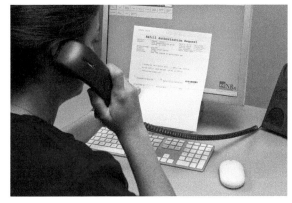

A pharmacy technician should alert the prescriber's office if the PBM requires a prior authorization to resolve the insurance claim rejection.

For example, if a patient's cholesterol cannot be controlled with lovastatin (a generic cholesterol drug) and the patient has suffered an adverse reaction to Crestor (the preferred brand cholesterol drug), the PBM would, in most cases, approve coverage for Livalo, providing Livalo with a copay more comparable to the Crestor than its usual copay.

In another example, rabeprozal (Aciphex) is prescribed for heartburn but not covered by insurance. The prescriber may elect to change the order to the generic omeprazole or pantoprazole rather than take the time to pursue PA. In this scenario, it is best that the pharmacist speak with the prescriber and counsel the patient about the best drug for the best outcome.

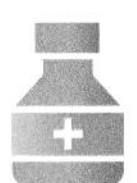

Pharm Fact

Since prior approvals can take days to process, the prescriber may have a back-up prescription option to use instead, or the patient may opt to pay cash, if affordable.

PA often takes 72 hours or longer to resolve, so technicians have to gently ask the customer to return later and explain why. The time needed depends on the efficiency of the doctor's office and the PBM. If other less costly medications have been unsuccessfully attempted, the drug will most likely be approved (for a limited duration of up to a year). Commonly, the PBM or the physician's office will notify the pharmacy when the PA goes through. You can then call the patient and proceed again with online adjudication and prescription filling.

If the PA is denied, the patient can decide to pay cash for the prescribed drug or request that an alternative drug be prescribed. The patient, technician, and prescriber are put into a difficult position if the PA is for a lifesaving drug, such as one of the newer innovative drugs for hepatitis, and the decision is delayed. Pending legislation in some states would allow the pharmacist to act on behalf of the prescriber and the patient in resolving PAs. This is another example of the expansion of the clinical role of the pharmacist into patient care.

Refill Too Soon Refills with most insurers can be processed within five to seven days of the end date of the current medication (based on days' supply), but some plans are more restrictive. Then you may get the *Refill Too Soon* message. You can then tell the patient the exact date the insurance claim can be processed—oftentimes it is only a day or two later from when the patient comes in.

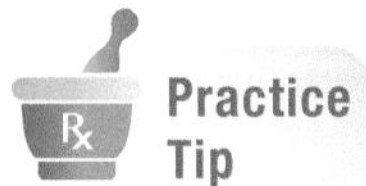

Practice Tip

It is helpful to keep a notebook to write down tips (especially on anything you had to look up, to avoid doing so again), shortcuts, and notes on the various insurance plans and PBMs.

If a refill involves a controlled substance, then the pharmacy's policy may not allow early refills even if insurance does. To monitor overuse and abuse, many pharmacies will not refill any Schedule III–V controlled substances until the prescription is within one to two days of the current prescriptions' completion date. For a 30-day supply of medication, the refill would be available 28 to 29 days later, per store policy.

Incorrect Days' Supply A rejection may also be due to an incorrect amount for days' supply—the amount of medication required to last for the duration of the prescription. If you make a mistake in calculating or inputting the days' supply, or if the PBM only permits a limited portion at a time, the claim will be rejected. For instance, the prescription may be for a 90-day supply of atorvastatin but only 30 days are covered by insurance. So you can adjust the medication history in the patient profile to note 30-day supply with two refills and have the patient come in every month to pick up the 30-day supply. How to calculate days' supply will be addressed later in the chapter.

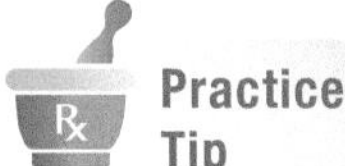

Practice Tip

Patience and empathy are definitely skills needed, as customers get more and more impatient, frustrated, confused, and sometimes desperate with the complex insurance adjudication process and high cost of medications.

Coordination of Benefits

When you have a patient with multiple insurance plans, adjudicate the claim to the primary insurer first, and if the primary insurer does not cover the claim or a deductible or copay exists, then adjudicate the remaining amount to the secondary insurer. (There may still be an amount left to be paid by the patient.) This filing with different insurance companies is called a **coordination of benefits (COB)**.

Here is how it works. Say the disabled patient has primary coverage from Medicare Part D and secondary coverage from Medicaid. Medicare Part D will not cover the anti-anxiety drug alprazolam (Xanax) or any of its alternatives. So you would process the claim to Medicaid as the secondary insurer and any other drugs to Medicare Part D.

COB also occurs when a patient presents a coupon from the medical office for a prescription. The coupon generally covers part or all of the copayment from the primary insurance. If the patient has no drug insurance, the coupon will reduce the cost by a set amount. In nearly all cases, the coupon is for an expensive brand name medication.

Practice Tip

To seek prior approval for a prescribed drug for a workers' comp case, the technician would call the caseworker or adjuster instead of a PBM.

For an authorized illness or injury, a workers' comp carrier is generally entered as the primary insurer (assuming that the patient has other drug insurance coverage). The coverage of the injury typically ranges from 3 to 12 months, based on the injury's extent and severity. Drug coverage is usually limited to the specific drug classes appropriate for that injury. For example, if back pain is the primary symptom, analgesic and back spasm medications would likely be covered, but antibiotics for a sinus infection would not. For approved drugs, the patient pays no copay.

To electronically process a workers' comp insurance claim, you must ask for additional information to enter into the patient profile. Besides the BIN, PCN, and group number, you will need the Social Security number, date of injury, and name of

IN THE REAL WORLD

Recently, a pharmacy technician received a prescription for topiramate 150 mg daily. The drug was available in 50 mg and 100 mg capsules. The technician entered 90 of the 50 mg capsules (total daily dose of 3 mg per day) for a 30-day supply—yet the PBM rejected the claim due to exceeding the number of dosage units per day.

With the patient's permission, the technician reentered 30 of the 50 mg capsules on one prescription and 30 of the 100 mg capsules on another prescription for a total daily dose of 150 mg. The PBM then accepted these claims as they fit the PBM's supply parameters. Without the quick thinking of the technician, there would be a delay in the patient receiving this drug to prevent migraine headaches. However, this is not always an acceptable solution since it can result in two copays for the patient.

compensating business. The initial data entry may take additional time because it generally requires a telephone call to a caseworker or adjuster to obtain or verify the information and drug coverage. The pharmacy may have a contract with more than one workers' comp PBM, each with its own team of caseworkers and adjusters.

Adding to the complication, the patient may have multiple claims to process at the same time—some drugs must be billed to worker's compensation while other selected drugs must be sent to the patient's normal primary insurer's PBM and, if there is unpaid cost, to the patient's original secondary insurance.

8.7 Calculating Medication Quantity and Days' Supply

Preparing a drug claim for online processing includes entering specific information about each prescription filled, including the medication quantity and days' supply of medication. **Days' supply** is the correct amount of medication to fit the prescription duration until refill or end of use. If the information submitted is incorrect, the claim may be denied, or—if audited—the costs of the medication and services may not be reimbursed. Thus, calculating days' supply of medication accurately is an important skill.

Certain drug formulations, such as ear (otic) and ophthalmic solutions and suspensions, are challenging to calculate when determining days' supply. Many are available in both a solution and a suspension formulation. When calculating drops for a *solution*, the standard measure is equivalent to 20 drops per mL. For example, suppose that a prescription was written for Cortisporin otic solution, 4 drops into affected ear 3 times a day for 7 days, or 12 drops daily for 7 days. That would equal 84 solution drops. The 5 mL package size (providing 100 drops) would be dispensed.

However, suspension drops, because they are thicker in density, have fewer drops per mL than solutions. In the past, the measure was 16 drops of suspension to 1 mL, but since IV drops go in rates of 10, 15, and 20 gtt (drops) per minute, there has been a movement toward standardization to round down the measurement to 15 drops of suspension per mL rather than up to 16. The suspension drop rate now depends on individual pharmacy and insurance reimbursement policies.

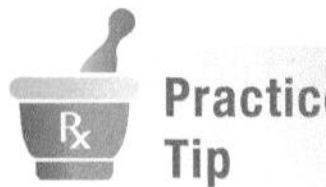

Practice Tip

The standard measurement for solutions is 20 gtt (drops) to 1 mL. A suspension, which is a thicker liquid, is calculated as 15 or 16 drops to 1 mL (depending upon store or PBM policy).

You could receive a prescription for loteprednol (Lotemax) suspension with the sig "Place two drops in each (OU) eye four times a day for 10 days with one refill." So two drops times four is eight drops a day. For 10 days, this prescription would need 80 drops. If you go by 16 gtt/mL, a 10 mL bottle would be estimated to contain 160 drops, and a 5 mL bottle estimated to contain 80 drops.

However, if 15 drops per mL were used for estimation, the 5 mL bottle would be calculated to have 75 drops, which would be insufficient for a 10 days' supply. The 10 mL bottle would be needed. If the technician provided the 15 mL package size pictured, or entered a 7 days' supply amount instead of 10 days' supply, then the claim could be rejected or challenged in an audit.

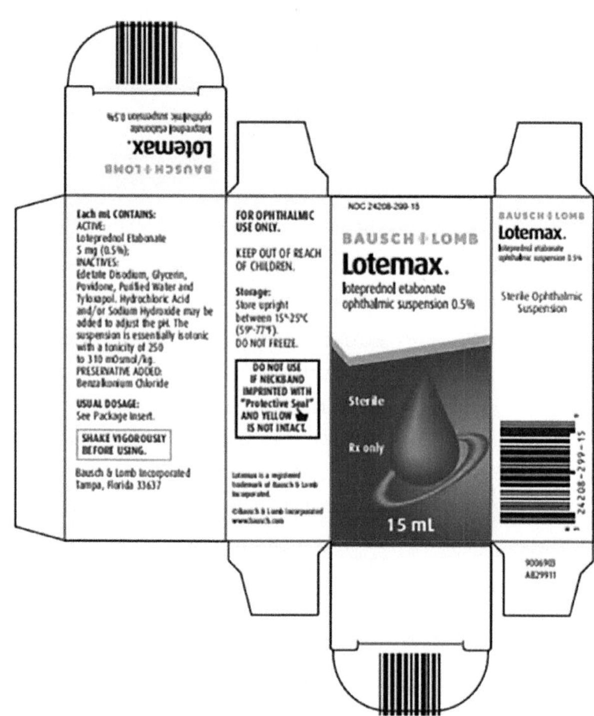

Technicians find that it can often be tricky to calculate the days' supply of prescribed suspension drops for eyes and ears. One needs to apply the formulation of the specific pharmacy or PBM for suspension drops per milliliter (gtt/mL).

For some prescriptions, dispensing the exact days' supply is not practical. A pharmacy may receive a prescription for cefdinir (Omnicef) antibiotic suspension with a sig "Give 1 teaspoonful daily for 10 days." The total volume is 50 mL (5 mL/day × 10 days), but the smallest bottle of cefdinir suspension is 60 mL. Insurance plans recognize that there will be 10 mL of wastage and will approve the claim. In this circumstance, the technician should add the statement "Discard remainder after 10 days" to the medication container label.

The following examples show how to calculate medication amounts and days' supply for actual prescriptions.

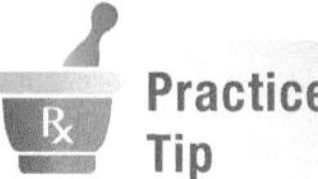

Practice Tip

When a # sign comes before a number in a prescription, it means that this is the total quantity to be prescribed or in the packaging. For instance, #90 means 90 units (such as tablets, capsules, patches, and other forms).

Example 1

A prescription is received for:

 **Ciprofloxacin 500 mg**
Take 1 tablet twice daily for 2 weeks.

How many tablets are needed for the 2 weeks' supply?

1 week = 7 days × 2 weeks = 14 days
2 tablets/day × 14 days = 28.
Days' supply is 28 tablets.

Example 2

How many days will the following medication last?

> ℞ Hydrocodone/APAP in a strength of 5 mg/325 mg #90
> Take 1 tablet every 4 to 6 hours prn for pain.

Step 1 Calculate the maximum number of tablets taken each day. If the patient takes 1 tablet every 4 hours, divide 24 (representing the total number of hours in a day) by 4 (24 ÷ 4) = 6. This means a maximum of 6 tablets could be taken in a day.

Step 2 Assuming the patient takes all 6 tablets per day, calculate the days' supply for the 90 tablets dispensed.

$$\frac{90\ \cancel{\text{tablets}}}{6\ \cancel{\text{tablets}}/\text{day}} = 15\ \text{days}$$

$$\text{or}\quad \frac{90\ \cancel{\text{tablets}}}{1} \times \frac{1\ \text{day}}{6\ \cancel{\text{tablets}}} = 15\ \text{days}$$

This means that a new prescription cannot be filled—or the claim processed—prior to 15 days from the date of initial dispensing.

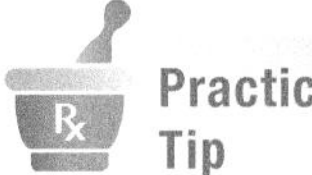

Practice Tip

Most computer systems only allow for a full day when calculating the days' supply. For instance, if 8.4 days is calculated, many pharmacies will round down to 8 full days, or up to 9 days if 8.5 or over.

Example 3

A prescription is received for:

> ℞ Augmentin 600 mg/5 mL
> Give $^3/_4$ teaspoon twice daily for 10 days.

Augmentin is a brand suspension available as a generic suspension of amoxicillin and clavulanate potassium in quantities of 75 mL, 100 mL, and 150 mL. What is the days' supply? What size bottle should be used? How much dispensed product will be unused?

Step 1 Calculate the volume prescribed for each dose remembering the conversion that 1 tsp = 5 mL.

This can be done using the ratio and proportion method as follows.

$$\frac{1\ \text{tsp}}{5\ \text{mL}} = \frac{0.75\ \text{tsp}}{x\ mL}$$

Then cross multiply.

$$\frac{(1\ \text{tsp})(x\ mL)}{(1\ \text{tsp})} = \frac{(0.75\ \text{tsp})(5\ \text{mL})}{(1\ \text{tsp})}$$

Divide each side of the equation by 1 tsp to solve for x mL.

$$\frac{(1\,\cancel{tsp})(x\,mL)}{1\,\cancel{tsp}} = \frac{(0.75\,\cancel{tsp})(5\text{ mL})}{(1\,\cancel{tsp})}$$

$$x\text{ mL} = 3.75\text{ mL}$$

The volume prescribed can also be calculated using dimensional analysis.

$$\frac{0.75\text{ tsp}}{1\ dose} \times \frac{5\text{ mL}}{1\,\cancel{tsp}} = 3.75\text{ mL/dose}$$

Each dose is 3.75 mL.

Step 2 Calculate the volume of drug to be given each day.

$$\frac{2\ \cancel{doses}}{\text{day}} \times \frac{3.75\text{ mL}}{dose} = 7.5\text{ mL/day}$$

Step 3 Calculate the total volume needed for a 10 days.

$$\frac{7.5\text{ mL}}{\cancel{\text{day}}} \times 10\ \cancel{\text{days}} = 75\text{ mL}$$

Step 4 Select the most appropriate bottle size from the available stock and determine how much product will remain after the patient takes the prescribed amount.

You are told amoxicillin/clavulanate comes in 75 mL, 100 mL, and 150 mL bottles. The 75 mL bottle should be selected. Because the volume needed is the same as the supplied bottle, no medication will be leftover.

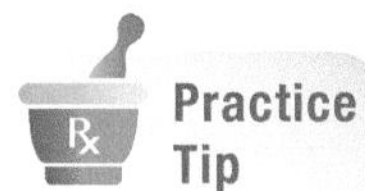

Practice Tip

Most computer systems only allow for a full day when calculating the days' supply. For instance, if 8.4 days is calculated, many pharmacies will round down to 8 full days, or up to 9 days if 8.5 or over.

Example 4

Insulin is available in 10 mL vials (1,000 units per 10 mL). How many days will the prescribed medication last?

> ℞ **Novolin N, 2 vials, inject 40 units under the skin in the morning and 25 units in the evening, prn refills**

Step 1 Calculate the total daily dose of insulin by adding the units in the two doses.

$$40\text{ units/am} + 25\text{ units/pm} = 65\text{ units/day}$$

Practice Tip

Multi-use insulin vials are good for only 28 days once they have been opened. So a single vial cannot have days' supply longer than 28 days.

Step 2 Calculate the number of days that two vials will satisfy. Each vial contains 1,000 units of insulin.

$$2\ \cancel{\text{vials}} \times \frac{1{,}000\text{ units}}{\cancel{\text{vial}}} = 2{,}000\text{ units}$$

Step 3: Now determine the number of days two vials of insulin will last.

$2{,}000\ \cancel{\text{units}} \times 1\text{ day}/65\ \cancel{\text{units}} = 30.769$ days, or approximately a 30 days' supply

If you mistakenly input a 56-day supply in the prescription (28 days for each vial instead of 2 vials for 30 days) for insurance processing, the initial claim will be processed; however, the patient will not be able to get a needed refill after 30 days without calling the insurance provider to change and correct the original prescription claim.

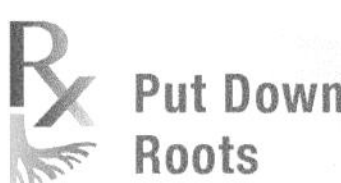

The sig *tid* comes from the Latin *ter in die,* which means three times in a day.

Example 5

The pharmacy receives a the following.

℞ **Augmentin 400 mg/5 mL, give 1 tsp tid for 7 days**

Medicaid insurance does not cover this strength but will cover Augmentin 600 mg/5 mL. Augmentin suspensions are available in 50 mL, 75 mL, and 100 mL bottles. If the substitution to the insured strength is made with prescriber approval, which bottle will be dispensed, what will the new dosing instructions be, and how much should remain after seven days?

Step 1 Determine how many milligrams of Augmentin are prescribed for each dose. Recall that 1 tsp = 5 mL.

$$\frac{1\ \cancel{\text{tsp}}}{1\ \text{dose}} \times \frac{5\ \cancel{\text{mL}}}{1\ \cancel{\text{tsp}}} \times \frac{400\ \text{mg}}{5\ \cancel{\text{mL}}} = 400\ \text{mg/1 dose}$$

Step 2 Determine the volume of Augmentin 600 mg/5 mL is needed to provide the prescribed 400 mg per dose.

$$\frac{5\ \text{mL}}{600\ \cancel{\text{mg}}} \times \frac{400\ \cancel{\text{mg}}}{1\ \textit{dose}} = 3.33\ \text{mL/per dose}$$

The new instructions should say "Take 3.33 mL three times day for seven days."

Step 3 Calculate the volume of Augmentin 600 mg/5 mL needed for one day.

$$\frac{3.33\ \text{mL}}{\cancel{\textit{dose}}} \times \frac{3\ \cancel{\text{doses}}}{\text{day}} = 9.99\ \text{mL/day, rounded to 10 mL/day}$$

Step 4 Determine the volume of Augmentin 600 mg/5 mL needed for the prescribed 7-day course.

$$\frac{10\ \text{mL}}{\cancel{\text{day}}} \times 7\ \cancel{\text{days}} = 70\ \text{mL}$$

Step 5 Select the most appropriate bottle size from the available stock and determine how much product will remain after the patient takes the prescribed amount.

You are told amoxicillin/clavulanate comes in 50 mL, 75 mL, and 100 mL bottles. The 75 mL bottle should be selected.

$$75\ \text{mL} - 70\ \text{mL} = 5\ \text{mL}$$

Approximately 5 mL will remain after 7 days and should be discarded. As the prescribed dose is 3.33 mL, a measuring device should be dispensed with the prescription. In most practice settings, the 3.33 mL dose would be rounded to 3.3 mL.

8.8 Helping with Insurance Issues

As you can imagine, patients (and pharmacy staff) are often confused by the myriad insurance issues. Here are some common insurance questions that a technician may encounter in the community pharmacy:

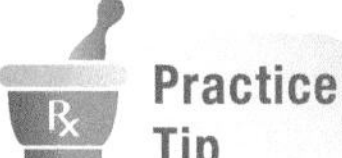

Practice Tip

Be careful not to share any personal information about a client to third-party payers beyond what is necessary for the claim or resolution of a claim. Any other information would be an infringement on privacy and HIPAA regulations.

- Why isn't this drug covered by my insurance?
- What do you mean, my insurance is expired?
- Why isn't my new baby covered on my insurance?
- What do you mean, my insurance plan has changed?
- Why is my copay $60 for this antibiotic prescription instead of $20?
- How come my medication costs more this month than last?
- What is a prior authorization, and why do I need it?
- Why do you have to call the physician to clarify my prescription? I am in a hurry!
- What do you mean you cannot fill my narcotic prescription today?
- Why did you give me a 30-day supply when my physician wrote a prescription for a 90-day supply of my medication?
- What do you mean, you do not have my medication in stock?
- Why have you filled my prescription with only a five-day supply?
- Why can't I use the coupon I received from my doctor's office?
- If I am on Medicare Part D, why can't I use a store or drug discount card?
- I am out of my heart medication and the physician's office is closed. What can I do?
- I forgot my medication and I am on vacation from out of state. Can you help me?

As a technician, you will need to be a problem solver and also a great communicator to help your customers with these questions and concerns. This list can serve as a great review for you. Go through each question and consider one possible answer for each based on what you have learned. In some of these cases, you will have to imagine the circumstances in which it could happen and how you would respond.

8.9 Resolving Claim Issues

There are times when a claim is approved online and the prescription is filled and picked up by the patient, but later the PBM refuses to pay the claim. The technician is often involved in resolving these "post-claim" functions: charge-backs and audits.

Charge-backs

A **charge-back** is a post-claim rejection of a prescription claim by a PBM or insurance provider that must be investigated and, if possible, resolved by the pharmacy technician. If the PBM representative feels that it has overpaid or paid something in error, it may charge back or deduct this amount from what it owes the pharmacy in reimbursement. A charge-back could occur for a number of reasons:

- The certificate of medical necessity for diabetes supplies was not completed properly (often missing a diagnostic code or frequency direction, as for blood sugar testing strips), or a signed renewal from the doctor was not obtained for a Medicare Part B claim.
- Online processing was not functioning due to an internet malfunction, and it was determined later that the patient was ineligible for drug insurance benefits.
- The primary insurer of a dual eligible patient was not billed or was billed second instead of first.
- A prescription was also filled at another pharmacy. (If this is the case, then the patient may need to be billed, and a flag put on his or her patient file to avoid repetition.)

In each case, to challenge or resolve the charge-back, the technician must verify the details of the original prescription and supplemental documentation, patient profile, and adjudication process. You must also find documentation on whether or not the patient actually received the prescription (by written or computer receipt) to figure out the inconsistences and perhaps fix the errors. If the charge-back is not resolved in a timely manner, then the pharmacy loses that money. If the prescription was dispensed several years ago, it may take hours to locate the prescription and resolve the issue to the PBM's satisfaction.

Since investigating charge-backs is so time-consuming and potentially frustrating, it is important to make sure that you are very accurate in inputting the prescription and insurance information in the computer when processing the claims.

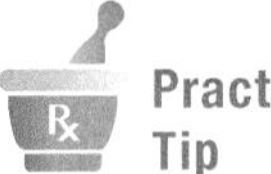

Practice Tip

If the label on a medication does not match the contents (brand versus generic, or generic versus brand, or a different medication altogether), it is illegal misbranding. This can cause problems with charge-backs and claims of insurance fraud.

Medication Audits

If there are a number of charge-backs or unresolved claims, the PBM might initiate an **audit**, or a checking of the pharmacy's prescription records to challenge problems (as is done by the IRS in a tax audit). These challenges can be from prescriptions that were processed three to six months earlier, or even two to three years ago. A community (or mail-order) pharmacy is also subject to periodic PBM medication audits. The audit challenge is commonly conducted via the mail, but occasionally a PBM representative will personally investigate past claims on-site. The technician may need to print out the prescription records of the patients listed on the audit.

Audits are intended to reduce fraud and waste. Correct billing and documentation of prescriptions are critical in overcoming the audit challenge. The following are examples of potential audit challenges:

- A patient was "not eligible" for prescription coverage on the date of the claim.
- The days' supply of the tablets, capsules, ear drops/eye drops, or antibiotic suspension was entered incorrectly; for example, a prescription for the migraine drug sumatriptan (Imitrex) 100 mg #9 should be entered as a 30-day supply, not as a 9-day supply.
- Initials were missing from the pharmacist's documentation of a phone prescription or from a transfer prescription; or the signature of the patient (or a representative) was missing.

- The pharmacy cannot prove the patient received the prescription. (The patient "attestation" signature is considered proof that the prescription was dispensed and must be present or sought out from the patient. Medicaid requires signatures on computer files or hard copies to be kept on file for audits.)
- On an "as directed" prescription, the frequency of the insulin dose or blood glucose check was not determined by a call to the prescriber's office. Therefore, the days' supply of medication might have been incorrect.
- Documentation was not provided on the original prescription of the reasons that a larger than normal quantity was dispensed.
- Problems occured with the DAW (dispense as written) designation. If a patient (not a prescriber) requests a brand name medication, then the order must be accompanied by DAW-2 (the patient is designated by the 2). If it is the prescriber who specifies "brand necessary," the order must be entered as a DAW-1.

The pharmacy technician investigates the validity of these and other claim challenges and must resolve the issues within two weeks of receipt of the challenge. If the audit challenges are not resolved in a timely manner, then the pharmacy forfeits all reimbursement to those claims, resulting in a revenue loss.

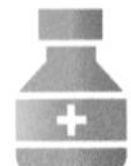

Pharm Fact

In 2015, a pharmacist in California was ordered to pay $644,000 in restitution for fraudulent billing of Medicare Part D claims.

Insurance Fraud

Challenges about false claims also need to be investigated and resolved. Filing a false claim is considered **insurance fraud**. It is subject to civil and criminal penalties if it is confirmed, as well as employment termination. For example, a pharmacy technician cannot dispense a medication to a patient and then post or bill the insurance three days later when the prescription refill is allowed. Instead, you must direct the patient to return in three days' time to pick up the medication after the insurance approves it. If it is an emergency and the patient has (or will) run out of medication (lost, spilled, or on vacation) before the current prescription duration runs out, you may request an override from the PBM or the patient can pay cash for the medication.

8.10 Assisting Uninsured Patients

Despite the passage of the ACA, approximately 10% of people in the United States still do not have any type of health or drug insurance. Many are the "working poor." Some could qualify for subsidized coverage for healthcare exchanges under the ACA, but they are not aware of this option, they don't know how to apply, or their states have not expanded coverage to include them. The first step to helping those struggling with healthcare insurance is to encourage them to check out the healthcare exchange for shopping online for an affordable program. They may also be eligible for their state's Medicaid or state-run healthcare assistance programs.

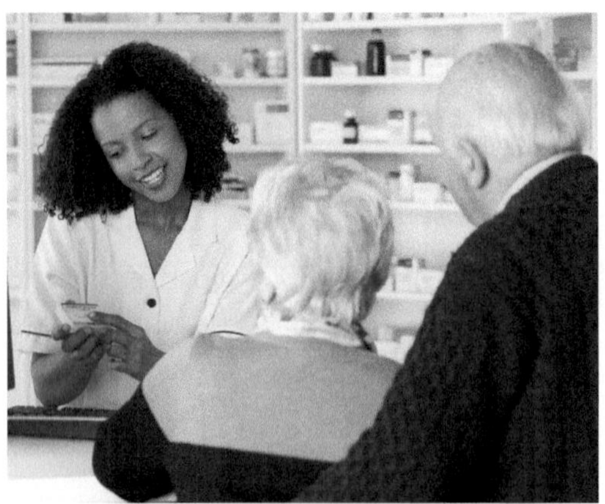

A pharmacy technician can make a real difference in the life of an uninsured or underinsured patient by helping him or her find the resources or coupons needed to afford a necessary medication.

IN THE REAL WORLD

In one community pharmacy, an uninsured patient came in requiring an antibiotic for a severe sinus infection resistant to the lower-cost antibiotics. The AWP of the needed antibiotic was $106. The pharmacy technician notified the pharmacist, who looked up the actual cost to the pharmacy for the antibiotic and decided to reduce the price to $30, which the patient could pay.

Another uninsured patient with diabetes brought in a prescription for Janumet, a marketed brand name that combines two drugs. The cost for a one-month supply was over $300! The pharmacy technician suggested that it might be cheaper to pay for the two drugs (sitagliptin and metformin) separately if the prescriber approved. Unfortunately, the cost was still very high. So the technician looked up Janumet on the manufacturer drug coupon site and found a drug manufacturer discount card that provided a free 30-day supply and discounts on the next 12 refills, which made the remaining drug affordable. This act of customer service made an immense difference in this customer's quality of life. This useful website can be accessed at https://PharmPractice7e.ParadigmEducation.com/ManufacturerCoupon.

As a technician, there are steps to take specifically when patients come in with prescriptions that they can't afford. Some technicians in large chain pharmacies even find themselves specializing in this area. You can suggest various options to patients to make their prescription or drug therapy more affordable.

Generic Drug Recommendations

You will almost always dispense a generic drug if one is available, but prescribers often forget that not all drugs have generic equivalents, so a call to the prescriber may sensitize them to the situation and have them consider a lower-cost, therapeutically equivalent drug. Also, not all generics are low-cost, as generic manufacturers are raising prices. Plus, if a patient is prescribed multiple generic drugs, this can become costly for them. So, generics can't always fix the problem, but they are a good start.

Free or Lower-Cost Prescriptions

Some pharmacies may advertise a list of "free" or low-cost ($4) prescriptions, usually for short-term antibiotic therapy. These medications are known within the trade as "loss leaders"—the community pharmacy chooses to lose or break even on these drug costs at the lowered prices to entice consumers to visit the store and buy more groceries or merchandise. Technicians can watch for these loss leaders and inform their customers.

Drug Discount Coupons and Cards

Sometimes drug companies offer discount coupons for their products to prescribers or providers. Pharmacy technicians, patients, or their family members can check at their store or online as well as call the provider's office to see if they have any available. Many high-cost brand name drugs have "patient assistance" discount programs online to cover all or a portion of the drug cost, often in combination with the primary insurer. This is a real world example of a coordination of benefits.

As a benefit to customers who pay for prescriptions on their own, some pharmacies offer a prescription savings club card for individuals and families (including pets). Many prescription **discount cards** are available in the mail or distributed as a charity fundraiser. Many of these cards do not reimburse the pharmacy sufficiently to cover expenses, so they may not be accepted, depending on store policy. The conditions for the discount card or coupon (including expiration date, amount of drug allowed, and so on) must be carefully reviewed by the pharmacy technician. Some cards need to be activated by the patient prior to use.

Drug discount and prescription club cards typically offer more savings for the patient when used for the more expensive brand name drugs as opposed to the less expensive generic medications. The drug discount cards are commonly used around the time that new drugs come on the market, as is seen in Figure 8.6, or if the brand name drug is scheduled soon to go off patent. Oftentimes, though, the technician should tell the patient that it may be still cheaper to purchase the generic drug at a discounted cash price rather than the "discounted" brand name drug.

Patients with government drug programs like Medicare Part D, Tricare, or

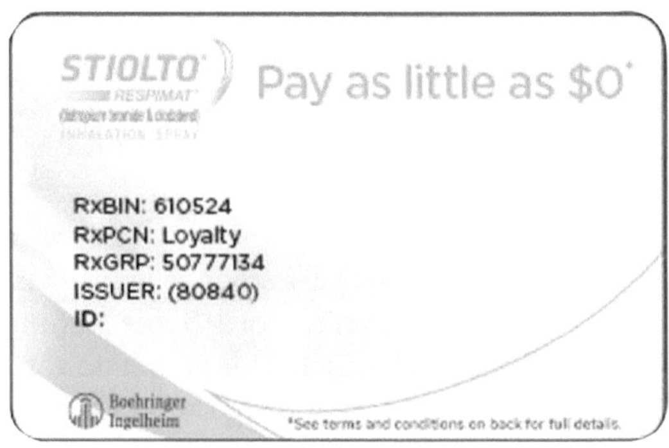

FIGURE 8.6 Sample of a New Drug Manufacturer Discount Card

Notice that the BIN, PCN, ID, and group numbers are similar to drug insurance cards. The patient must activate the card before it can be used to process the prescription in the pharmacy.

Medicaid are *not* eligible for a coupon or drug discount card reimbursement because of federal kickback laws. By law, discount cards can be used only for Medicare (and Medicaid) enrollees *if their primary Medicare Part C or D insurance is not billed* and the patient is personally paying for her or his medication.

Low-Fee and Charity Clinics

Technicians may also refer patients to free or low-cost charity clinics voluntarily staffed by doctors, nurses, dentists, and pharmacists, offering medical, dental, or even pharmacy services. These health professionals typically offer their services at no charge. In some cases, lay volunteers help process requests to manufacturer assistance programs on behalf of patients. If the community health center does have a pharmacy, the patient could qualify to get prescription drugs at government pricing through the federally funded 340B Drug Discount Program. Some clinics also have drugs and services available for free or at low cost because of donor and grant support. The pharmacy technician can make the patient aware of the location and hours of operation of these clinics and encourage patients to see if they qualify for assistance.

8.11 Becoming Confident with Pharmacy Insurance Practices

The more you understand the complex world of insurance, the better you can serve customers and help them get the care they need. In working in any community or mail-order pharmacy, you will be expected to understand, enter, process, and reconcile any issues revolving around the online adjudication of a prescription claim. Patients often come with questions, confusion, and frustration, and you will have the power and experience to help sort things out.

One-third of patients are not taking their required medications to control their diseases. Is this due in part to the high cost of medications? If patients stop refilling their prescriptions due to high costs, they may be jeopardizing not only their own health, but the financial effectiveness of the healthcare system. Uncontrolled high blood pressure, diabetes, or high cholesterol can increase the risk of heart disease and complications like heart attack and stroke, leading to costly hospitalizations. This leads to higher premiums and higher copays for all.

You may be able help some individuals who cannot afford to take care of their health with the prescribed drug therapy by processing their insurance claims and finding feasible ways for them to pay for the drugs they need. Your expertise will also help the pharmacist identify and counsel all patients to better control their disease as they will be able to access the therapies they need.

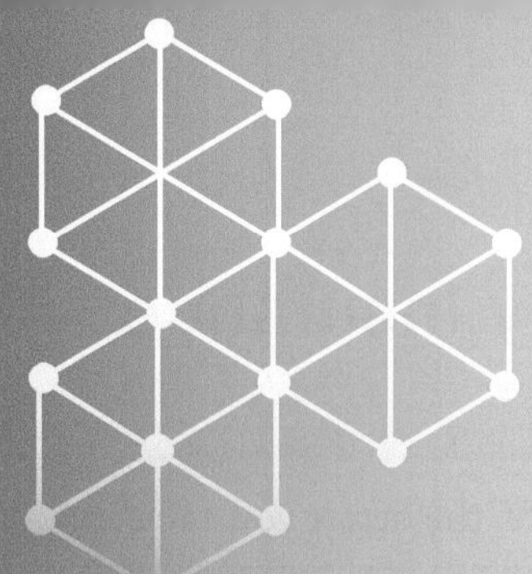

Review and Assessment

CHAPTER SUMMARY

- There are multiple commercial and governmental health and prescription insurance programs, and they are structured differently—health maintenance organizations (HMOs), preferred provider organizations (PPOs), traditional insurance, and government-subsidized programs.
- It is important to fully understand and be able to explain key terms, such as average wholesale price, monthly premium, insurance policy, benefits, deductible, copayment, coinsurance, tiered copay, in-network providers, out-of-network providers, prior authorization, pharmacy benefit manager, coordination of benefits, adjudication, and charge-backs.
- A patient who is hurt on the job may qualify for workers' compensation, but this insurance is a supplemental insurance that is targeted only for the drugs, medical services, and supplies necessitated by the injury or job-evoked illness. They require approval by the caseworker.
- Patients over the age of 65 years and many who are disabled qualify for Medicare coverage.
- The health and prescription insurance coverage differs for the various Medicare insurance programs—Part A (hospitalizations and emergency care), Part B (healthcare visits and clinics), Part D (drugs), and Part C (comprehensive), which is also known as Medicare Advantage (a combination of all three).
- Part C and Part D are offered through private companies with proportional government reimbursements.
- Part D offers prescription drug insurance coverage for patients over 65 years of age or those with disabilities.
- The passage of the Affordable Care Act has decreased the number of uninsured people in the United States and increased the prescription volume in the pharmacy.
- Low-income patients in each state may qualify for Medicaid coverage and subsidies from healthcare exchanges.
- Active and retired military and their dependents qualify for government insurance coverage through Tricare's different programs: Prime, Select, and For Life.
- All prescription drug claims are processed electronically online in real time while customers are waiting, so technicians need to become efficient in working with PBMs and online adjudication.
- Reviewing and entering the BIN, PCN, ID, and group numbers on an insurance card are needed to successfully process a prescription and capture a claim.
- If a patient has more than one insurance (or discount) card, a coordination of benefits (COB) between insurers must be sequenced and processed.

- There are many reasons why a prescription claim cannot be processed; the technician must identify and resolve the issue or call the PBM.
- Properly calculating the days' supply of a prescribed medication is critical to accurately processing a prescription claim.
- A prior authorization (PA) requires the prescriber to justify the need for a high-cost drug to the PBM; if not approved, then other options need to be discussed by the pharmacist, physician, and patient.
- PBMs may challenge the reimbursements to a pharmacy via charge-backs and audits that can be handled effectively by pharmacy technicians.
- Insurance fraud is a serious civil and criminal offense.
- Technicians can assist uninsured and underinsured patients with access to medications by medication advocacy, offering them several options to assist in paying for their medications or receiving them through a community clinic.

CHECK YOUR UNDERSTANDING

Take a moment to review what you have learned in this chapter and answer the following questions.

1. Which of the following is not a reason why drug costs continue to escalate?
   a. fewer brand name drugs coming off patent
   b. increase in innovative and expensive drugs
   c. increase in pharmacy technician salaries
   d. manufacturers boosting AWPs of brand and generic drugs
2. Most of the prescription costs in the US are covered by
   a. cash.
   b. Medicaid.
   c. Medicare Part D.
   d. third-party health insurance.
3. The healthcare insurance program run jointly by the government to subsidize the cost for eligible disabled, low-income, part-time, and unemployable state citizens of any age is called
   a. Medicare Part C.
   b. Medicare Part D.
   c. Medicaid.
   d. Workers' Compensation.
4. A copayment is best defined as a(n)
   a. flat out-of-pocket fee for each service provided.
   b. set percentage of the total cost of any service provided.
   c. out-of-pocket payment for office visits only.
   d. monthly premium for drug insurance coverage.
5. A PBM is best described as a(n)
   a. employer.
   b. processor of claims.
   c. drug wholesaler.
   d. military insurance plan.
6. The average price that PBM's reimburse a pharmacy is called the
   a. AWP.
   b. usual and customary charge.
   c. markup price.
   d. discount price.

MAKE CONNECTIONS

Take a moment to consider what you have learned in this chapter and respond thoughtfully to the following prompts. Note that some of these activities will require internet access.

1. Gerard ter Horst is a regular customer at your pharmacy and is very confused upon hearing that you cannot fill his prescription for Dexilant due to the need for a "prior authorization." Write a short essay of approximately 250 words on how you would handle the situation and include the following information:
   a. Describe a "prior authorization" in terms that the patient can understand.
   b. What is the technician role and process for resolving a PA?
   c. What other drugs are therapeutically equivalent to Dexilant?
   d. What else can be done to resolve the problem?
2. James Rodriguez, a 39-year-old male who is a new patient, presents prescriptions for Tramadol, Xanax, and amlodipine. He says he should be covered by Workers' Comp, but he also presents to the pharmacy a drug insurance card to process his prescriptions.
   Write a short essay of approximately 250 words on how you would handle the situation and include the following information:
   a. What is workers' compensation?
   b. What are the most likely indications for Mr. Rodriguez's prescriptions?
   c. Which of these drugs will be covered by Workers' Comp and which will not be covered? How is this determined?
   d. How would this be similar to processing a drug insurance claim?
   e. How would it differ from processing a drug insurance claim?

 The online course includes additional review and assessment resources.

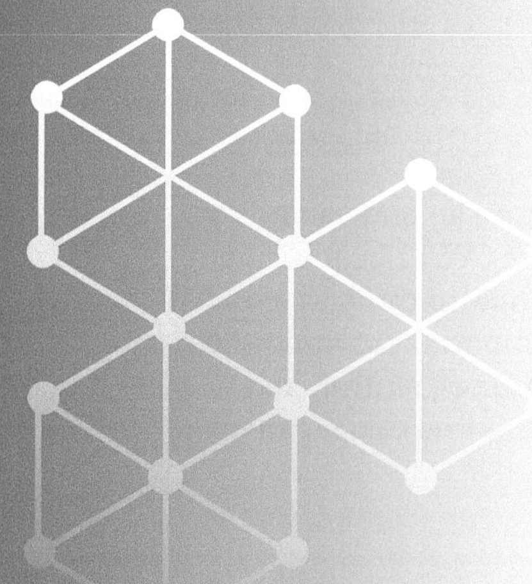

9 The Business of Community Pharmacy

Learning Objectives

1. Describe the roles, responsibilities, and limitations of the pharmacy technician in the sale of over-the-counter (OTC) drugs, supplements, and retail items. (Section 9.1)
2. Paraphrase how to accurately process restricted OTC drug sales, such as Schedule V cough syrups and decongestants containing pseudoephedrine. (Section 9.1)
3. Identify the advantages and disadvantages of alternative medicine products and various dietary supplements such as herbs, vitamins, and minerals, and list the differences in regulatory control and labeling requirements from prescription drugs. (Section 9.2)
4. Describe how to address customer needs for medical and home health supplies and durable medical equipment. (Section 9.3)
5. State necessary cash register functions for bar code scanning, taxable, and nontaxable items. (Section 9.4)
6. Describe how to change register receipt paper and ink toner, and how to provide correct change. (Section 9.4)
7. Calculate markups, discounts, and average wholesale prices. (Section 9.5)
8. Explain the technician's role in handling inventory—purchasing, receiving, posting, and returning stock for credit (including controlled substances). (Section 9.6)
9. Describe the importance of computer management and pharmacy informatics for generating business reports. (Section 9.7)
10. State the significance of pharmacy productivity and profits for ensuring a pharmacy's sustainability as a business. (Section 9.7)

ASHP/ACPE Accreditation Standards
To view the *ASHP/ACPE Accreditation Standards* addressed in this chapter, refer to Appendix B.

Each community pharmacy runs to serve customers and to make a profit so that it can survive as a business. Aside from assisting in prescription drug dispensing, pharmacy technicians are responsible for performing several business tasks vital to the daily operations and profitability of the community pharmacy. This chapter provides an overview of these business functions, including assisting customers in the purchase of OTC drugs, dietary supplements, and medical supplies; operating the cash register and retail computer system (including a bar code scanner); taking payments and providing change; overseeing computer information systems; and managing inventory.

To effectively complete these tasks, technicians need to have an understanding of retail concepts, such as taxable items, average wholesale price (AWP), acquisition costs, markup, and discounts. Technicians also need to know how to think in terms of business systems, such as how productivity is measured. It is important to understand how assessment, inventory counting, tracking, purchasing, postings, returns, and reorder levels all work together for business success. Gaining this knowledge can open up opportunities for advancement.

9.1 Nonprescription Retail Sales

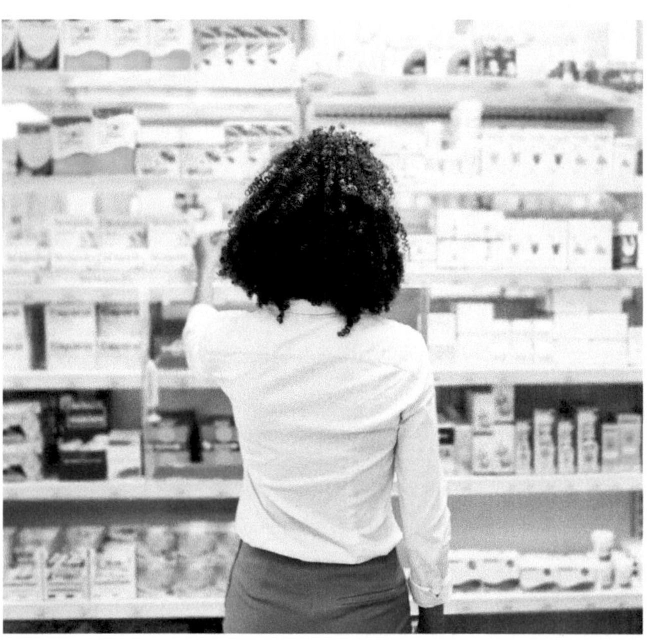

OTC medications are generally stocked according to their medical purpose such as pain relief, antacids, and so on.

The front retail space of community pharmacies offers not only many brand name and generic OTC drugs but also complementary and alternative holistic health treatments for patients. These alternative remedies include homeopathic products, vitamins, minerals, herbs, and dietary supplements. They are arranged on shelves to let customers choose what they want from a variety of package sizes and formulations. Also displayed are other health and medical supplies and non-healthcare products such as cosmetics and toiletries, candy, snacks, drinks, gifts and gift cards, and impulse merchandise.

Customer service remains paramount to the success of a community pharmacy. As a pharmacy technician, you will play a major role in assisting customers in locating the retail products they are seeking and processing their payments.

Over-the-Counter Drugs

Customers are purchasing OTC drugs for self-administration at an ever-increasing rate because of the increased cost and inconvenience of physician visits, the rising cost of prescription medications, the lack of adequate health insurance, and the high drug insurance deductibles. This self-medication practice, however, requires paying close attention to the product labeling, which not all customers do.

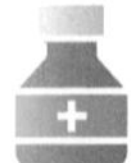

Pharm Fact

Displaying nonprescription products on shelves for customers to locate for themselves was popularized by Walgreens in 1960, with other retailers following shortly thereafter.

OTC drugs have been determined to be generally recognized by the Food and Drug Administration (FDA) as *safe and effective* for the approved indication when taken according to label directions. OTC drugs are usually arranged in the store by drug class or by indication, such as pain relievers, fever reducers, allergy medicine, contraceptive products (condoms, jellies), first-aid care, antacids, laxatives, foot-care products, and so on.

Commonly requested OTC drugs are listed in Table 9.1. Many popular OTC drugs, such as hydrocortisone and ibuprofen, once required a prescription. The active ingredients are the same as those found in the higher-strength prescription formulations but are simply present in lower strengths and dosages. For example, OTC ibuprofen is available in a strength of 200 mg, whereas the prescription strengths are 400 mg, 600 mg, and 800 mg.

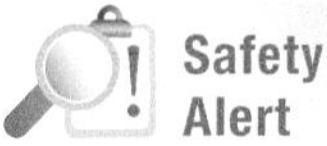

Safety Alert

Taking more than one OTC medication at once, such as cold and pain medications, can be dangerous. Teenagers particularly tend to self-medicate and mix medicines. Technicians can help all patients read labels and check ingredients. Acetaminophen products should not be taken with other OTC or prescription drugs containing acetaminophen.

Pharmacy technicians should also be aware that a few significant OTC drugs are located in the refrigerated area of the pharmacy—in particular, fast-acting regular insulins such as Novolin and Humulin. These insulins can be sold to a patient with or without a prescription. Requests for nonprescription insulin often occur when a patient is traveling and needs more insulin. Longer-acting insulins (e.g., Lantus, Levemir) or mixtures of immediate and extended-action insulins (Humulin 70/30, Novolin 70/30) always require a prescription.

TABLE 9.1 Common OTC Drugs and Their Indications

Generic Name	Brand Name	Indication(s)
ibuprofen	Advil/Motrin	Headache, pain
oxymetazoline	Afrin	Nasal decongestant
naproxen	Aleve	Headache, pain
fexofenadine	Allegra	Allergy
diphenhydramine	Benadryl	Allergy
loratadine	Claritin	Allergy
hydrocortisone	Cortizone-10	Itching, inflammation
esomeprazole	Nexium	Heartburn
famotidine	Pepcid	Heartburn
fluticasone	Flonase	Allergy
loperamide	Imodium	Diarrhea, irritable bowel syndrome
clotrimazole	Lotrimin	Topical antifungal
miconazole	Monistat	Vaginal antifungal
guaifenesin	Mucinex	Expectorant
triple antibiotic	Neosporin	Topical anti-infective
lansoprazole	Prevacid	Heartburn
omeprazole	Prilosec	Heartburn
triamcinolone	Nasacort	Allergy
cetirizine	Zyrtec	Allergy

Role of the Pharmacist

Customers often seek counsel to help them select the appropriate OTC product for a special condition. Consider a mother asking for a cough syrup for her diabetic son; a pregnant woman on prenatal vitamin and iron supplements seeking the right laxative; or an elderly man with high blood pressure looking for an appropriate nasal decongestant. These patients would have medical difficulties if they took the usual OTC medications, so you need to direct them to a pharmacist's counsel. Pharmacists are the only ones who can legally address questions about the right medication for a medical purpose or indication, the right dosage and administration, expected therapeutic effects, side effects, contraindications, and interactions—even for OTC vitamins.

Role of the Pharmacy Technician

You, however, can and should help customers find the brands and types of medications they are looking for. Who knows the store better than the person who has been stocking the shelves and putting the products in their places?

Technicians should also help customers understand the OTC product labels, which include the following:

- product name and therapeutic purpose
- directions for dosage and frequency of administration for different age groups
- active and inactive ingredients (such as dyes)
- any precautions or warnings
- any special storage requirements and expiration date

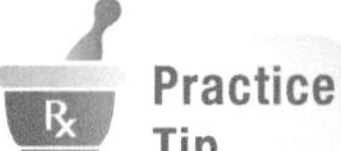

Be sure to remind customers that most OTC drugs should typically be used for only seven days or less.

Technicians are trained to understand this information and can go over labels with customers. Also, point out that manufacturers typically provide a toll-free number in case consumers have additional questions or concerns when they get home. If customers have questions about whether or not a certain product is a good therapeutic idea for them or about a patient use not covered on the label, simply refer the customers to the pharmacist.

Technicians can remind consumers that no drug, not even an OTC product, is completely safe or without side effects or adverse reactions. If the dosages recommended by the manufacturer are exceeded, OTC medications can be very dangerous. For instance, products that contain the cough suppressant dextromethorphan (DM) can cause auditory and visual hallucinations in high doses. Because DM products have a history of abuse among adolescents, consumers must be age 18 or older and must present an ID to purchase them.

In addition, *the FDA discourages giving any child under the age of six OTC cough and cold products* because the risk of adverse reactions is greater than the potential benefits.

Technicians can also remind consumers that OTC drugs should be used for a restricted period—usually less than seven days—for a short-term illness or condition unless otherwise directed by a physician. (For example, a physician may direct an adult patient to take a baby aspirin on a long-term daily basis in order to lower the risk of heart disease.) If a patient has self-medicated with an OTC drug for seven or more days without resolution, the patient should be referred by the pharmacist to the appropriate healthcare professional.

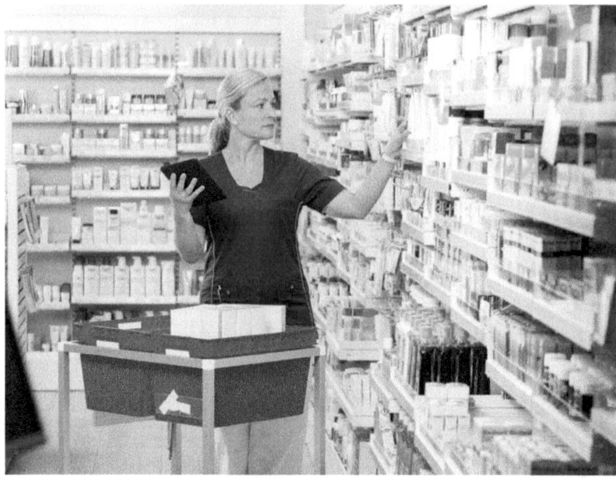

Technicians often know best where specific OTC products are because they stock the shelves and periodically check expiration dates.

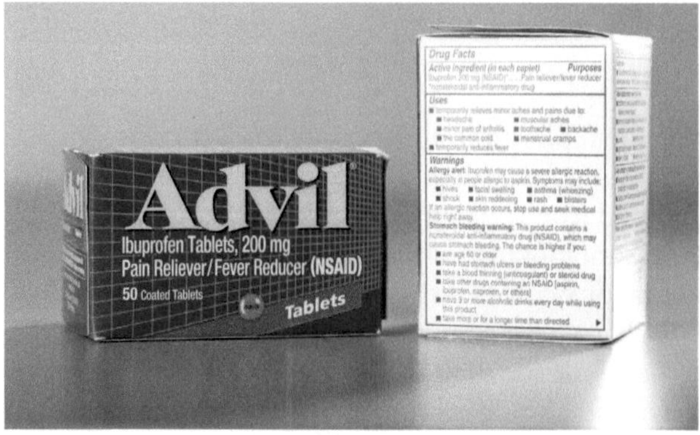

The FDA requires complete OTC labeling for safe and effective self-medication.

Safety Alert

OTC cough and cold products are generally not suitable for children under age six.

Restricted Sale of Certain OTC Products

As noted in earlier chapters, certain OTC products have specific restrictions and procedures that must be followed during consumer purchases. These products include **Schedule V drugs**, such as those containing pseudoephedrine and ephedrine.

An OTC Schedule V drug is restricted at the lowest level of controlled substances because it has some potential for abuse or creating physical or psychological dependence—though the potential is low. A common example of a Schedule V OTC medication is a cough medication containing codeine. There are federal restrictions and requirements for its sale:

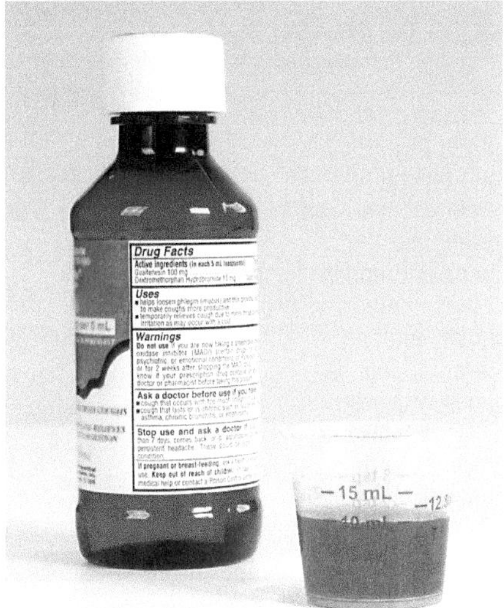

Most codeine-containing cough syrups are classified as Schedule V drugs and are stored behind the counter. But some state laws have them scheduled as more restricted drugs, with greater limits and requiring more documentation or even a prescription.

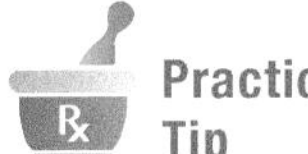

Practice Tip

Some states (and all drug insurance providers) require a signed or e-Rx prescription in order to dispense a Schedule V OTC drug. The pharmacy technician must get to know and follow the appropriate state laws and specific pharmacy protocols, which often differ.

- The drug must be stored behind the counter, in the prescription area.
- The amount of cough syrup sold to a single customer is generally limited to a specific volume (such as 120 mL or 4 fl. oz.) within a 48-hour period.
- Only a pharmacist (or the pharmacy technician under direct supervision) can make the sale.
- The purchaser must be 18 years of age and have proof of identity.

Schedule V Documentation To sell an OTC drug that is Schedule V, the pharmacy technician or the pharmacist must record the sale on the computer or in a logbook. This record must include the following information:

- name and address of the purchaser
- date of birth of the purchaser
- date of purchase
- name and quantity of the Schedule V drug sold
- initials of the pharmacist handling or approving the sale

OTC Drugs with Pseudoephedrine and Ephedrine Sales of OTC products that contain pseudoephedrine and ephedrine are closely monitored because of their use in the illegal creation of methamphetamine (meth)—the intensely addictive white crystalline street drug made in home labs. All products containing pseudoephedrine and ephedrine must be stocked behind the counter. These restricted OTC products include cold and sinus medications, ephedrine-containing tablets, and metered-dose inhalers (MDIs) for the treatment of asthma. Some states limit the purchase of these products to "prescription only," and several states require that only pharmacists conduct the sales. The federal limits for pseudoephedrine are 3.6 grams maximum purchase in one day *and* 9 grams maximum purchase in a month (30 days). State laws may be more stringent. Violations of the state or federal laws may result in the loss of the pharmacist's license or the pharmacy's business license.

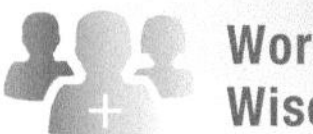

Work Wise

Looking customers in the eyes and talking to them will help you remember their faces and notice if they come in again. You can welcome familiar faces with warmth while noticing buying trends that may or may not be good.

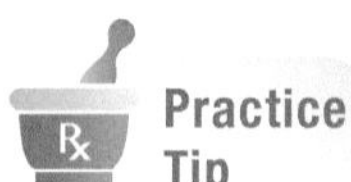

Practice Tip

Become familiar with the Combat Methamphetamine Epidemic Act of 2005 and the protocols to follow regarding OTC drugs that contain pseudoephedrine and ephedrine.

Technicians must legally document the purchases and purchasers of pseudoephedrine or ephedrine in a software program or manual logbook similar to that for Schedule V drugs (see Figure 9.1) and have the individuals sign for the purchases. This documentation must be kept for a minimum of two years to allow for Drug Enforcement Agency (DEA) and FDA tracking.

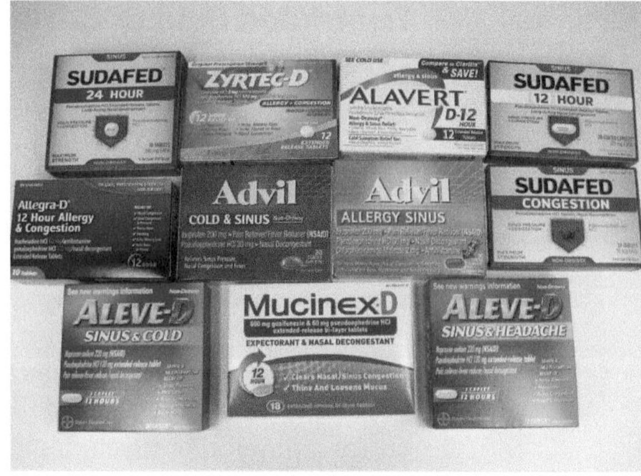

OTC products that contain pseudoephedrine must be stored in the prescription area, and certain conditions must be met for a sale.

In addition, to continue offering these drugs for sale, all pharmacies must electronically submit an annual self-certification to the DEA. This certification confirms the following:

- All employees have been trained in how to handle these products.
- Training records are being maintained.
- Sales limits are being enforced (for example, 3.6 grams per day/week, 9 grams per 30 days).
- Products are being stored behind the counter or in a locked cabinet.
- An electronic or written logbook is being maintained.

Beware of Smurfing! Technicians must be on the lookout for a practice called **smurfing**—when meth producers pay a number of other individuals to purchase the maximum allowable amount (3.6 grams) of the restricted OTC drug on their behalf so the meth producers will not get noticed buying enough ingredients for a new batch. If three or four patients come into the pharmacy in a short period of time to purchase such products, be suspicious! You or the pharmacist may elect to refuse the sales.

FIGURE 9.1
Form for Recording Sales of Restricted Products Containing Pseudoephedrine

Pseudoephedrine Products Dispensing Record

Purchaser's Name	Driver's License Number	Purchaser's Address	Date of Purchase	Product Name	Quantity Purchased	Dispensed by (Initials)	Purchaser's Signature

IN THE REAL WORLD

Women of all ages (formerly restricted ages) can now purchase an OTC emergency contraceptive without federal restrictions. Plan B One-Step and the generic Next Choice One Dose are common examples. These one-dose drugs should be taken within 72 hours of unprotected sexual intercourse—the sooner taken, the more effective they are, at 75% to 90%. But some nausea can be expected with these high-dose hormone tablets. Technicians may want to direct buyers, especially teenagers, to the list of side effects listed on the packaging, especially if they are on any other medications or have any health complications. If the patients have any questions, direct them to the pharmacist.

Some pharmacies keep the products close to or behind the counter to be requested to encourage counseling and prevent shoplifting. Patients may wonder how they work. They do not abort an already implanted fertilized egg but instead prevent a fertilized egg from implanting and growing into a fetus. Some pharmacists object to selling drugs for emergency contraception on religious grounds. Each state has laws governing actions for this moral and ethical dilemma.

9.2 Complementary and Alternative Medicine

For a variety of reasons, some patients will seek treatments outside the scope of conventional medicine. It's important for pharmacy technicians to have a base understanding of how these alternate remedies work. **Complementary medicine** is a nonconventional treatment that is used together with conventional medicine. **Alternative medicine** is a nonconventional treatment that is used in place of conventional medicine. And **integrative health** is the practice of coordinating conventional and complementary approaches in a holistic manner that can include mental, emotional, spiritual, social, and functional aspects of a patient's life.

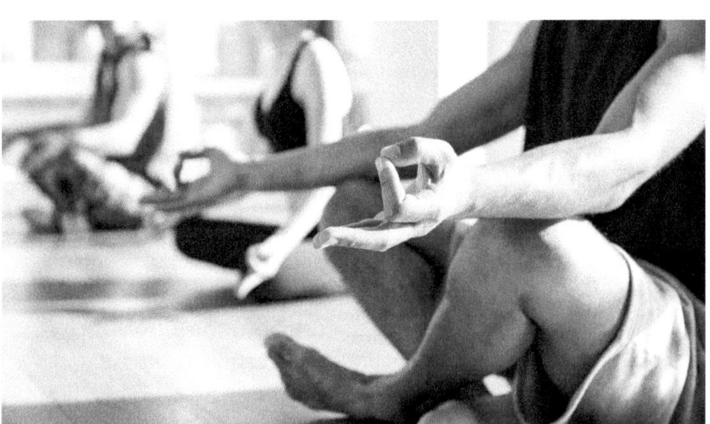

Meditation and guided breathing exercises are gaining credibility in the conventional medical community as complementary remedies.

Nonconventional treatments include natural products (homeopathic remedies, herbals, vitamins, minerals, and other dietary supplements), specialized diets, acupuncture, deep breathing and relaxation techniques, guided imagery, exercise movements such as yoga and Pilates, meditation, massage therapy, and chiropractic manipulations. The science behind the effectiveness of these treatments varies. But more and more primary care providers are incorporating both conventional and alternative treatments into their practices.

Dietary Supplements

A **dietary supplement** can be a vitamin, a mineral, or an herbal product that is considered useful for healthy nutrition, the prevention of an illness, or the alleviation or reduction of the symptoms of an illness. A large proportion of the population eat diets that are low in fresh vegetables and fruits and high in fast foods or processed snacks and mixes. Therefore, they do not receive the full range of vitamins and minerals needed for healthy nutrition. This is especially true for children, who particularly need vitamins and minerals for their growing bodies, so vitamins and supplements are often recommended. The typical uses, or indications, for some common dietary supplements are listed in Table 9.2.

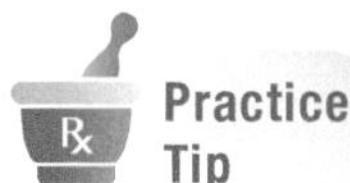

Most consumers do not realize that dietary supplements, including vitamins and minerals, are not regulated by the FDA in the same manner as are OTC drugs.

TABLE 9.2 Uses for Common Dietary Supplements

Dietary Supplement	Use(s)
calcium and vitamin D	Improves bone strength
echinacea	Boosts the immune system
garlic	Antibacterial and antiviral action; maintains healthy cholesterol
ginger	Relieves nausea, motion sickness, and morning sickness
ginkgo	Improves memory; treats tinnitus and peripheral vascular disease
glucosamine/chondroitin	Lessens joint pain
lactobacillus (a bacterium)	Improves digestion, helps prevent diarrhea
lutein	Maintains eye health
melatonin	Relieves insomnia, especially in shift workers or time-zone travelers
omega-3 fatty acid (fish oil)	Lowers triglyceride levels
policosanol	Maintains healthy cholesterol levels
red yeast rice	Maintains healthy cholesterol levels
saw palmetto	Treats benign prostatic hypertrophy (BPH)
zinc	Boosts the immune system; helps in the treatment of the common cold and wound healing

Safety and Oversight

The Dietary Supplement Health and Education Act (DSHEA) states that supplements must be *safe and accurately labeled.* As with other food products, the label of a supplement indicates the recommended "serving size" rather than a dose. The label provides far less product information than an OTC drug label. In addition, the amount of active ingredient on the label may not match what is actually in the supplement because of inconsistencies in quality control or product contamination. Scientific studies on the effectiveness of most supplements are usually quite limited.

Steering consumers toward products with the seal of *USP Verified* on them is usually safe. (For more information on this seal, return to Chapter 3.) Manufacturers of these products have voluntarily submitted the products to USP's stringent testing and auditing criteria for dietary supplements for quality, purity, and potency. This adds a layer of safety (and sometimes cost) to the product quality.

If a label contains a promise of a medical cure or effective treatment, the FDA can act to remove the drug from the market for false advertising since no proof of the label's claims has been submitted to the FDA. The FDA can also remove any dietary supplement that is deemed dangerous, which has occurred in the past with several "diet pills." The pharmacy technician should, of course, not counsel customers regarding the therapeutic uses of dietary supplements but refer patients to the pharmacist.

As many as 50% of consumers use one or more of these practices, often without their prescriber's knowledge. Some consumers associate "natural" with "safe," yet many of these products, especially herbal drugs and dietary supplements, have side effects or problematic interactions with prescription drugs even when used appropriately. It is good for technicians to urge customers to list these alternative medicine products and dietary supplements in their medication profile.

Technicians can also help customers understand that the safety and effectiveness of natural products are less assured than with OTC or prescription drugs because of the different federal oversight and level of required scientific studies. Patients should always consult with their physicians when choosing these various types of products for illnesses or conditions that last longer than seven days.

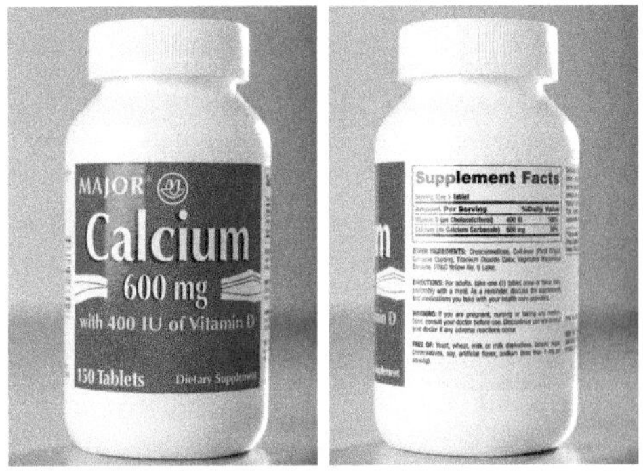

All vitamins and minerals are considered dietary supplements, so less information is legally required on their labels than for OTC drugs.

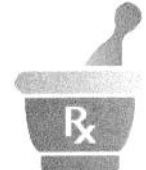
Practice Tip

Most vitamins lose potency when exposed to heat and light. Advise customers to keep their vitamins on dimly lit, cool shelves.

Vitamins and Minerals

There are many vitamin and mineral products on the market that range from multivitamins to doses of specific minerals and vitamins like the B complex, A, C, D, and E. Listed on the label of each is the proportion of active substance contained as compared to the **daily value (DV)**. The daily value is the recommended level of intake of a certain vitamin or mineral.

The use of a daily multivitamin is not considered alternative medicine. Children or adults may need a daily multivitamin just to reach the minimum daily value standards. Pregnant women are encouraged to consume a daily prenatal vitamin with folic acid (prescription or OTC) to promote the health of their unborn child and prevent birth defects. A technician can be helpful in directing patients to both brand name and generic vitamins, including those in chewable, gummy, and liquid formulations for children and elderly consumers.

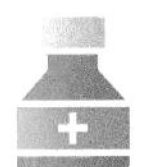
Pharm Fact

Vitamin E is not just one vitamin. It is actually a collection of eight fat-soluble vitamins with specific antioxidant properties.

Some consumers take short-term high doses of individual vitamins for different indications, such as vitamin C to build one's immunity and fight the common cold, vitamin E for heart health, and lutein for eye health. However, research has found that habitual megadoses of certain vitamins can be harmful to health. For instance, doses of vitamin E in excess of 800 IU per day may interfere with blood clotting or may increase the risk of heart disease. High supplement doses of vitamin A and other vitamins absorbed by fat can build up in the body and cause toxicity, liver damage, birth defects, and problems in the central nervous system.

Popular mineral supplements include iron and calcium. In many cases, these may be prescribed or recommended by the physician. Vegans and vegetarians, menstruating and pregnant females, and postsurgical patients may require extra iron to prevent anemia. Calcium combined with magnesium and vitamin D is recommended to keep bones strong and prevent osteoporosis (a weakening of the bones). Since the salt combinations of iron and calcium in different products contain variable amounts of "active minerals," questions should be referred to the pharmacist for proper product selection. The National Center for Complementary and Integrative Health provides counsel on dietary supplements at its website: https://PharmPractice7e.ParadigmEducation.com/Supplements.

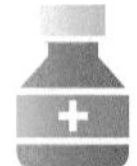

Pharm Fact

The International Unit (IU) is used to measure the amount of a substance. It is often used to quantify fat soluble vitamins (such as Vitamin A, D, and E.) The volume that makes up a single international unit depends on the substance being measured. For example:

1 mg of Vitamin E= approximately 1.21IU

Herbal and Medicinal Plants

Though considered "natural," **herbals** are also regulated as dietary supplements rather than as drugs by the FDA. The most popular herbals are echinacea, ginger, garlic, ginkgo, St. John's wort, and soy. Their common uses were listed in Table 9.2. Herbals are also dosed in serving sizes.

Herbals have powerful components that are metabolized by the liver, just as other drug substances are. That is why they *can cause drug interactions* or affect the absorption, distribution, and elimination of prescription and OTC drugs and other supplements. Like OTC drugs, herbal medications *do have side effects and can cause allergic reactions*—not just the first time they are used but even after sustained use. Some herbal substances can accumulate in the body or cause an immune response to build up gradually.

St. John's wort has a high potential for herb-drug interactions. St. John's wort should not be used with a wide range of prescription drugs, such as antidepressants, birth control medications, antiseizure drugs, cyclosporine (an organ-rejection prevention drug), digoxin (a heart medication), warfarin (an anticoagulant), and other anticoagulants. Goldenseal is another herbal with potentially dangerous drug interactions. Concentrated and prolonged ingestion of ginger, garlic, and ginkgo should not occur with blood thinners and must be discontinued a week prior to surgery.

There are other elements to consider. Because herbals and medicinal plants are grown and harvested, pesticides and other contaminants can be introduced to the body in the herbal compound, causing reactions.

Safety Alert

Remind patients who are buying herbal supplements to carefully watch for any allergic reactions, such as rashes, itchiness, difficulty breathing, watery eyes, or difficulty swallowing. If these symptoms occur, they should discontinue use immediately.

Herbal Medicine Resources The NCCIH offers a list of the common herbs and their best uses on its website—along with allergic reactions and potential drug interactions. This list serves as an excellent source for pharmacy technicians and pharmacists: https://PharmPractice7e.ParadigmEducation.com/HerbsataGlance.

Another excellent resource is the American Botanical Council (ABC). The mission of this nonprofit organization is to help the public live healthier lives through the safe use of medicinal plants based on science and traditional wisdom. It publishes research that is peer reviewed. This information can be found at https://PharmPractice7e.ParadigmEducation.com/HerbAlgram.

Finally, the **American Herbal Pharmacopoeia (AHP)** is a nonprofit organization of botanists, chemists, herbalists, physicians, pharmacists, pharmacologists, university professors, researchers, and regulators dedicated to researching, collating, and distributing information on herbals. The information includes the chemical and botanical descriptions, growing and processing procedures, purity standards, dosages, side effects, contraindications, and drug interactions. This organization seeks quality controls and scientific standards. Working with the University of Vienna and the American Herbal Products Association, the AHP publishes a textbook of botanical microscopy. It has 800 pages describing 140 medicinal plants and common adulterated ingredients to provide resources for testing laboratories on the purity of powdered herbal substances. This volume is accompanied by another textbook on herbal macroscopy (or characteristics viewable by the naked eye) of 125 of the most popular botanical substances. The AHP website can be found at https://PharmPractice7e.ParadigmEducation.com/AHPHerbal.

As with other supplements, if patients are wondering what to purchase for their health, the pharmacist should counsel them on product selection, dosage, indication, and proper, safe use.

Protein Shakes and Nutritional Supplements

Practice Tip

Protein is needed by the body, but too much protein can stress the kidneys and cause some calcium loss. Some studies suggest that individuals should not consume more than 2 to 2.5 grams of protein per kg of body weight per day.

Patients who do not eat well and are losing weight (such as seniors or patients undergoing cancer treatments) or athletes who need to replenish or build up their systems after vigorous workouts may be candidates for protein shakes and nutritional supplements. Sources of protein can be animal based (such as casein, milk, and whey) or plant based (pea, rice, and soy). Some processed supplements are high in sugar, so caution must be exercised with patients with diabetes or prediabetes. Ensure is a brand of nutritional supplement that is available in various flavors. Like other brands, it supplies needed calories containing protein, minerals, and vitamins without fat, and it can be used as a meal supplement or replacement. Thick-It is a supplement requested by many older adult customers. When added to water, juices, tea, milk, or protein shakes, Thick-It assists in swallowing and digestion.

Probiotics

Probiotics work to build up the "good" or "friendly" microorganisms in one's body, especially the positive-acting bacteria in the digestive system. Since antibiotics often destroy the bacteria causing the infection as well as the positive bacteria in the gastrointestinal (GI) tract (stomach and intestines), common side effects of antibiotic therapy include diarrhea and vaginal yeast infections. Physicians often advise patients taking antibiotics to eat yogurt that contains live bacteria cultures of *Lactobacillus acidophilus* or ingest a probiotic sold in the pharmacy. Patients who are lactose (milk sugar) intolerant often use probiotic supplements in order to combat digestive issues when they drink milk or eat cheese and other dairy products.

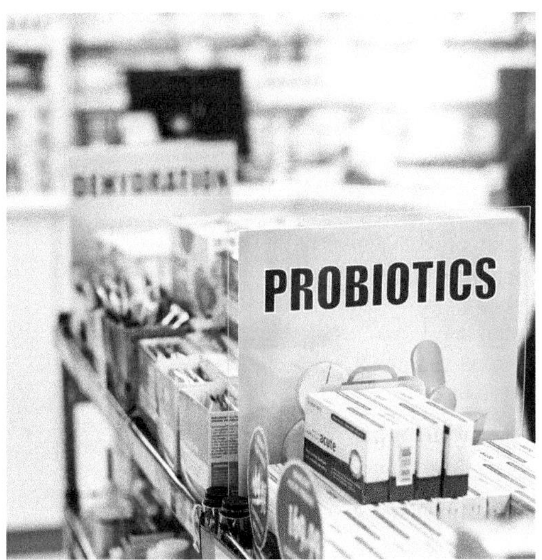

Depending on the individual product, probiotics may be stored without refrigeration (as pictured) or in a special refrigerated section.

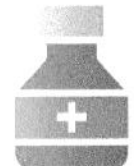

Pharm Fact

Some pioneering scientific studies are finding that having the right bacteria in one's digestive system to absorb the right nutrients may improve mood and energy.

Common probiotics contain various strains of *Lactobacillus* and *Bifidobacterium*, which can restore the balance of microorganisms in the GI tract. Some brand name probiotics include Culturelle, Align, and Lactinex (the latter is found in the refrigerator). Probiotics may also be used to treat the abdominal pain, cramping, and bloating of irritable bowel syndrome. Some scientific research is now finding that probiotics can help heal skin conditions, such as eczema, prevent allergies and colds, improve oral health, and assist with mood disorders.

9.3 Medical and Home Health Supplies and Equipment

Community pharmacies also sell the everyday first-aid and health supplies needed by customers. General health supplies and equipment include the usual bandages, tape, wound dressings, thermometers, heating pads, splints, braces, vaporizers, bathroom accessories, and adult/child diapers. These are all elements that do not need a prescription, and technicians can help patients find these stocked items.

Parents will often come into the pharmacy worried about a child with a high fever, looking for the right thermometer. Technicians need to become acquainted with the range available. Different types have different features, and it is helpful for a technician to be able to explain the differences to concerned parents. There are electronic/digital, infrared, and mercury thermometers for use in the mouth, armpit, rectum, ear, forehead, and vein areas. (Mercury thermometers are being phased out.) Oral thermometers are for those who can hold them under the tongue, which is often difficult for children or seniors. Rectal thermometers are generally used for infants. If customers have specific questions about the best type for detecting a specific illness or for a patient who is difficult to care for, the pharmacist should help them.

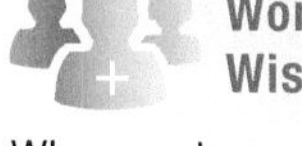

Work Wise

When customers are looking to find a certain test kit, it is important to be particularly courteous, as some conditions can make them feel uncomfortable, ashamed, vulnerable, or scared for the future.

Pharmacies also have specialized supplies suited for aging patients and specific chronic conditions, such as heart disease, respiratory diseases, and diabetes. Disposable medical supplies include such items as test kits, needles, and sterilizing wipes. **Durable medical equipment (DME)** and supplies are reusable and long-lasting for ongoing needs. DME includes canes, wheelchairs, walkers, crutches, blood pressure monitors, blood sugar monitors, nebulizers, and oxygen equipment, among other typical items. These are often prescribed by physicians.

It is helpful to be familiar with some of the key medical supplies and equipment sold in a community pharmacy.

Test Kits

People often want to diagnose and treat themselves, so they buy test kits to help them discern their conditions. Some of the most common test kits requested by patients include the following:

- pregnancy
- ovulation cycle
- bladder infection
- high cholesterol
- illegal drug use
- human immunodeficiency virus (HIV) infection

Practice Tip

An adult's normal temperature range is generally one degree above or below 98.6°F (37°C) taken orally and 99.6°F (37.5°C) rectally. However, a baby's normal temperature can range from 97.5°–99.3°F (36.5°–37.4°C) taken under the arm and up to 100.3°F (37.9°C) rectally, which is more accurate. An ear thermometer should not be used from newborn to six months.

Occasionally, the pharmacy may need to special order a less-requested test kit for a customer. The pharmacy technician can help customers select a test kit and understand the test instructions and outcomes. Patients will want to confirm the test finding with a doctor. Letting patients know where community clinics are in the area can be helpful.

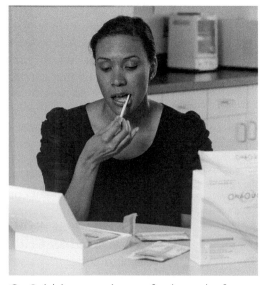

OraQuick is a screening test for those who fear that they may have contracted HIV.

IN THE REAL WORLD

An estimated 200,000 individuals are unaware that they are infected with HIV, but a test kit, OraQuick, can help reduce this number. This kit is designed for home screening for those age 17 or older. The FDA-approved OraQuick can detect the presence or absence of the virus in one's saliva. After the mouth is swabbed, results come within 20 minutes.

Consumers, however, need to understand that the results are not 100% accurate, and technicians should mention this. A positive test result is rarely wrong, but a negative test result may be. This means that if the test recognizes the presence of the HIV antibodies, it is most often correct, but it can miss 8 out of 96 patients who are HIV infected. Sufficient antibodies may not yet have developed. Patients who test positive on the OTC test should see their primary care providers soon for confirmatory testing. Those who test negative may still want to see their physician and should test again at a later date. The manufacturer also provides a toll-free phone number for individuals to call to discuss their results with a trained staff member or to get a referral to a local health center.

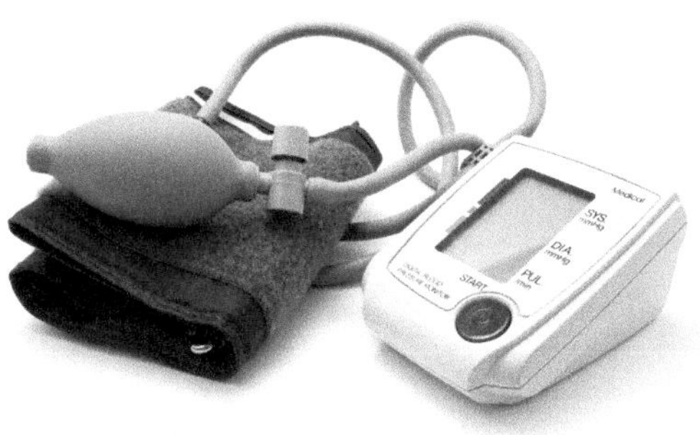

A digital blood pressure unit with a wrist cuff is easier to use for home use than an arm cuff.

Blood Pressure Monitors

Patients with high blood pressure often seek home monitors. They may want (or be urged by a prescriber) to purchase a type of **sphygmomanometer** for home use. A sphygmomanometer is a blood pressure gauge and cuff similar to that used in a physician's office. Many patients prefer to purchase a digital blood pressure cuff for their wrist as it is easier to use by oneself. Its results can be recorded and brought to the physician's office on the next visit.

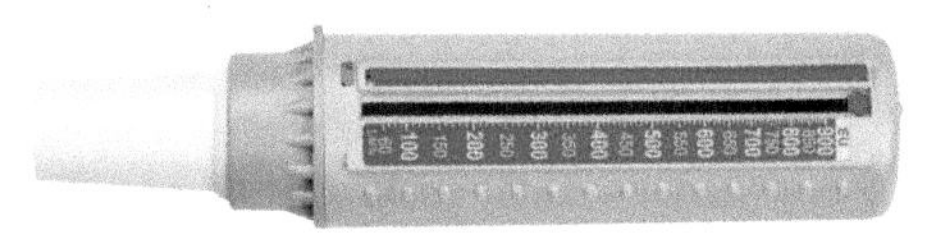

This is an example of a peak flow meter, which measures one's lung/breath capacity to monitor respiratory diseases such as asthma.

Respiratory Management Supplies—Inhalers and Nebulizers

Many children and adults suffer from asthma and other diseases that cause breathing issues, and they take prescribed medications through a **metered-dose inhaler (MDI)**. It is a small, pressurized canister of a prescribed medication that is pumped out in specific doses for inhaling. Some patients need a plastic **spacer device**, or extension tube, to deliver the medication more effectively. Spacers are particularly beneficial for the very young as well as elderly patients who may have difficulty with coordinating the movement needed for deep inhalation into the lungs. Spacers come in small, medium, and large sizes. If written as a prescription, the spacer will be covered on some drug insurance plans. Prescribers may also recommend that some respirator patients purchase an adjustable plastic **peak flow meter** to measure their breathing expirations to assess the severity of their asthma symptoms or the therapy benefits.

Occasionally, prescribers order medications in nebulizer form for patients with the acute wheezing or shortness of breath that accompanies chronic obstructive pulmonary disease (COPD). A **nebulizer** is a battery- or electric-powered machine that turns the asthma medicine into a fine mist that can be inhaled deep into the lungs to ease breathing difficulties. The pharmacy technician completes the processing for billing an insurance plan for the home nebulizers and medications. These both require prescriptions with diagnosis codes (ICD-10) for insurance coverage.

Practice Tip

To assist a patient needing insurance to pay for diabetic shoes, you will need to complete a foot assessment form and receive a diagnosis and ICD-10 code from the physician.

Diabetic Management Supplies

Nearly 10% of US citizens are affected by diabetes, and the percentage is growing. Community pharmacies offer a wide range of products to serve these patients. Even special therapeutic footwear for patients with diabetes, which helps prevent injury, may be prescribed or recommended by physicians and carried by some community pharmacies. Many pharmacists acquire specialty training and certifications in serving patients with diabetes and matching them with the particular drugs and supplies they need.

Pharmacy technicians can complete a special diabetes training, pass an examination, and become certified in patient education for patients with diabetes. Such skills are considered valuable within the pharmacy and may enhance hourly pay. Even without this specialty training, technicians in a community pharmacy are often called upon to assist patients in locating or selecting diabetes supplies, such as a glucometer, insulin syringes, pen needles, test strips, lancets, and alcohol wipes for skin cleansing.

Technicians are also key to helping patients work with the insurance companies to pay for their diabetes supplies and durable medical equipment. Insurance covers many of these items. Below is a sample of some of the varied diabetic supplies pharmacies carry.

Glucometers

To determine the level of glucose in one's body, and therefore how much insulin is needed, patients can use a **glucometer**, or blood sugar measuring device. Patients insert a test strip (explanation to follow) in the machine and add a drop of blood (most often from a fingertip). The glucometer then screens the blood to check the glucose levels.

Glucometers are available from several manufacturers in different sizes. They vary as to the amount of blood needed to make a reading, the time period necessary to provide the results, the memory capacity, and the ability to interface with a computer. Patients without insurance coverage for this equipment can often purchase glucometers with generous manufacturer rebates that negate the majority of the stated purchase prices. Companies frequently upgrade their glucometers, so it is essential for both the pharmacist and the technician to keep abreast of product changes.

Diabetes patients are often frequent customers, needing glucose tablets and gels, lancets, alcohol wipes, and different sizes and gauges of needles, among other supplies.

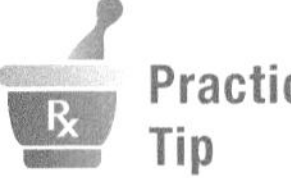

Practice Tip

Technicians can make patients aware that they can keep an online log of their glucose readings at https://PharmPractice7e.ParadigmEducation.com/Diabetes, sponsored by the American Diabetes Association.

Test Strips, Lancets, and Alcohol Wipes

Specialized disposable test strips are needed with each glucometer. The test strips are machine specific and must be matched for the glucometer type being used. Technicians can assist patients in product matching. Some bottles of test strips come with a computer chip that has a specified lot number that must be inserted in the glucometer. Failure to replace this glucometer chip when using a new bottle of test strips (with a different lot number) leads to errors in the blood glucose readings. Technicians always need to check the expiration dates of the strips as well. Since patients test their blood using new test strips from one to six times daily, strips are expensive if patients do not have insurance coverage. However, purchasing generic or store-brand test strips, especially with discount coupons, can result in up to a 50% patient savings.

In addition to the test strips, patients need alcohol wipes and lancets, or mini blades, to make the sterile pinpricks to access blood. Technicians can assist them in finding and purchasing these items.

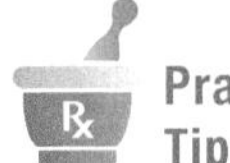

Practice Tip

Patients with diabetes also may struggle with high blood pressure and may benefit from blood pressure monitoring equipment.

Insulin Syringes and Needles

As explained in Chapter 5, insulin syringes and needles come in different sizes, and technicians can help patients select the correct length and gauge. Remind patients that the higher the gauge of the needle, the smaller the width, potentially resulting in less pain at the injection site. Insulin-pen needles have to be purchased separately and are available with gauges from 29 to 32. Pen-needle lengths are commercially available as original (12.7 mm, or 1/2 inch), short (8 mm, or 1/3 inch), mini (6 mm, or 1/4 inch; 5 mm, or 1/5 inch), and nano (4 mm, or 1/6 inch). The shortest pen needle, which usually causes the least pain, is the 4 mm, 32-gauge needle. States vary in their laws about selling syringes, concerned that they will be used for illegal drug administration. Some pharmacies have a policy that no insulin syringes can be sold unless the patient comes with a prescription or is a known customer of the pharmacy.

Large Durable Medical Equipment

In addition to the smaller DME, some independent community pharmacies with more storage or warehouse space also specialize in the sale or rental of larger DME, such as hospital beds, wheelchairs, prosthetics, orthotics, and so on. These pharmacies generally host a more limited inventory of standard retail merchandise (products that are nonhealth-related) to have more room for home healthcare supplies and equipment.

Community pharmacies that provide home healthcare supplies and equipment must meet quality standards and accreditation requirements set by the Centers for Medicare and Medicaid Services (CMS). CMS generally awards contracts to pharmacies or medical supply warehouses to provide DME that is directly reimbursable by Medicare Part B. Besides assisting customers in finding and completing the sales for medical supplies, technicians often help assemble the equipment, bill insurance, and restock items.

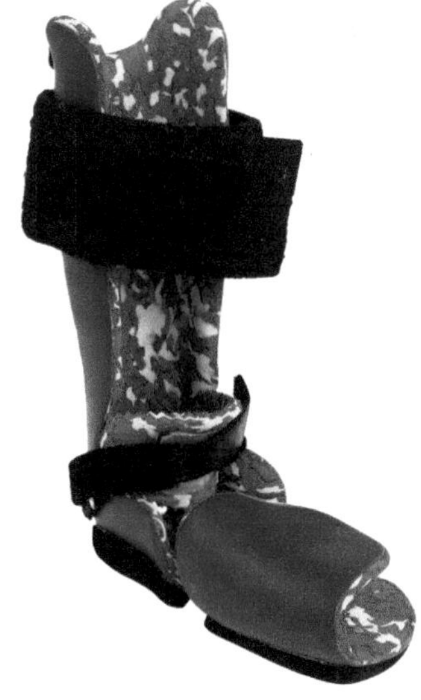

The orthopedic equipment to correct a clubfoot in a child or a foot boot for those who have undergone surgery are examples of DMEs that a pharmacy might sell.

9.4 Cash Register Management

As part of working in a retail pharmacy, you are responsible for collecting payments from customers. The price of each prescription, medical supply, OTC drug, supplement, and retail item is either scanned with a bar coder to pull the price into the **point-of-sale (POS) cash register** (an automated cash register system), or it is hand entered into a less automated one. Cash register procedures differ with each pharmacy and its technology.

There are separate buttons on the cash register for "Rx" (nontaxable prescription items) and other retail merchandise (taxable items). There are also separate buttons for cash, credit cards, and checks. The retail items, including OTC drug products and dietary supplements, will usually have bar codes for the cash register scanner for easy pricing. If an item is on sale, the sale price should be reflected on the bar code. Independent pharmacies often have sale price stickers attached to items that are then hand entered into the cash register.

When a prescription code is scanned, the computer system may automatically prompt the technician to offer the patient counseling by the pharmacist. (Also, the pharmacist often makes notes on the medication bag to indicate that the patient needs counseling.) Scanning particular OTC items—such as pseudoephedrine products and Schedule V cough syrups—may activate a prompt for you to ask for additional information from the patient, such as proof of age, identification, and a signature to comply with federal and state laws.

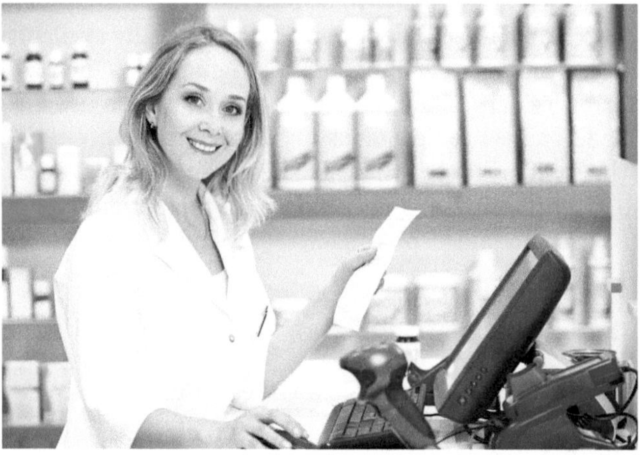
Pharmacy personnel must be able to handle the responsibilities of filling prescriptions while also working on the retail end of running the cash register for customer purchases.

The register has a drawer at the bottom with a removable tray that has separate compartments for various denominations of bills and coins. Checks, credit card receipts, and bills larger than $20 are generally kept in a separate compartment or underneath the money tray in the drawer. All credit card receipts (and coupons) are also placed under the change tray or in a separate, secure location for reconciliation at the end of the day (which will be explained in the end of this section).

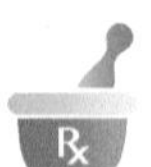
Practice Tip

If a prescriber writes a prescription for a medical supply or a piece of durable medical equipment, it is generally considered a medical necessity and is not taxable.

Taxable Versus Nontaxable

FDA-approved prescription drugs for humans (not animals) and certain medically necessary supplies are federally exempt from states adding any sales tax, so these are **nontaxable items**. Tax-exempt medical supplies include disposable or consumable medical items (such as glucose test strips and nutritional drinks for diabetic patients) and durable medical equipment (such as canes, walkers, crutches, orthopedic and diabetic shoes, but not hospital beds). Other nontaxable items include prescribed devices such as neck collars, ankle braces, slings, and wrist and arm braces.

States can choose to make many common health and first-aid items such as thermometers, adhesive bandages, medicated gum, OTC drugs, and dietary supplements **taxable items**. You will need to get to know your state laws since sales taxes are determined by the states. Generally, common retail merchandise items (such as magazines, cards, carbonated drinks, cosmetics, pet products, toys, gifts, snack foods, and tobacco) are all subject to taxes. Some states allow baby formulas, dietary supplements, herbs, foods, and bottled water to be exempt from taxes, while others tax them.

The states also determine the rate of the sales tax to be added—generally a small percentage of the purchase price. Each pharmacy's cash register is programmed to apply the state's tax laws, so that is why pressing the correct code button for the type of purchase is key—then the register will automatically do the tax math for you.

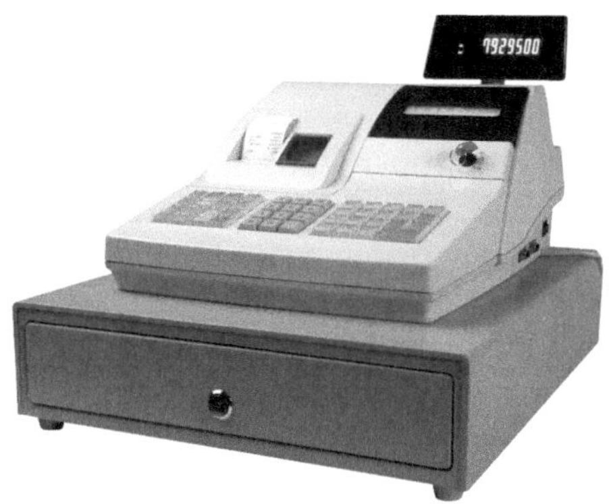
A cash register often requires replacement of the paper roll and/or ink toner to print a readable receipt for each patient transaction, so technicians need to get to know this key skill.

Payment Options

Customers often pay for their purchases using various cards (credit cards, debit cards, flex cards, and gift cards), cash, or checks. Each payment option has a unique processing method; these payment methods should be demonstrated in the pharmacy's training program. Regardless of the form of payment, the pharmacy technician should always present the customer a payment **receipt**, or proof-of-purchase printout.

Learning the ins and outs of your pharmacy's particular cash register and receipt system is important—even how to change the paper printout ribbon or the ink cartridge (see Table 9.3). Think of how frustrating it is for the customer if you don't know how to fix or refill these when they run out.

TABLE 9.3 Changing Paper and Ink

If the paper receipt is streaking red, it is time to replace the paper roll. Though each cash register will differ, with different release levers, the process generally follows in this order:

1. Remove the cover.
2. Take out the existing paper roll.
3. Insert the new paper roll so that it rolls from the bottom up (you will see the back of the paper) and feeds up through the correct slot.
4. Attach the paper stream onto the rolling spool of the printer so that it starts the automatic feed.
5. Verify that correct placement has occurred by tapping a transaction button.
6. Replace the cover.

If the receipt printout is faint, it is time to replace the ink roller. This small, plastic roller is located underneath the receipt paper exit. Remove the cover, slip out the roller, clip the replacement back in (cash register model-specific), and replace the cover. Check YouTube for a step-by-step video on the model of cash register in your pharmacy for more specific instructions. Newer cash registers often employ thermal printers, which typically require that you change the paper roll only.

Online Card Transactions

The various kinds of payment cards need to be verified with a card-swiping monitor or chip reader for online transaction approval (pharmacy gift cards need in-house approvals of card amounts). Though sometimes you will do the swiping, the most common technology has the customer swipe or insert any type of card and follow the prompts. The processing company will either approve or decline the amount needed. If the amount submitted is declined, you will have to ask for an alternative card or form of payment.

Credit and debit cards often allow customers the option to request cash back after the claim is processed. Cash-back options may be limited ($20 or less) or not available per store policy. Some chain pharmacies offer customers the **express pay option**, where the customer puts their credit card on file to be processed automatically at the time of prescription filling.

Any payment done with a credit card either must be paid off by the customer at the end of the month or it accrues interest as a finance charge. Depending on pharmacy policy, patients may or may not need to sign for a credit card expense of less than $50. In most independent pharmacies, patients will sign for every credit card transaction.

Debit Cards A debit card is also a form of online cash payment, but unlike a credit card loan, a debit card instantly deducts the purchase cost from the customer's bank account. A debit card purchase requires the customer to enter a PIN for account verification. Generally, if the PIN is used, these cards do not require a signature because the money is immediately transferred from the bank account. However, as with credit cards, the amount submitted is sometimes declined, and then you will have to ask for some other form of payment. A debit card can be processed as a credit card if it is inconvenient for the customer to enter a PIN, such as when picking up prescriptions at a drive-through pharmacy.

EMV Chips To decrease fraudulent use, most credit and debit cards have moved to **EMV chip** credit cards, or cards with an embedded computer chip. (The chip is named after the three major developers: Europay, Mastercard, and Visa). Instead of swiping the credit card, the card is inserted into a chip reader available at the cash register. Each time the card is used, a one-time-only code will be utilized to process the transaction.

Mass retailers and chain pharmacies have adopted chip readers. While it is not required to have a chip reader, without one, liability for fraud falls back onto the retailer rather than the credit card issuer. The customer must type in a confidential PIN or sign the transaction on screen or paper. This new technology has been nicknamed "chip and pin" or "chip and signature." This technology will eliminate duplicate or fraudulent cards, but it does not yet address added security for online sales. Pharmacies will have to handle both forms of credit cards for some time as the transition is in progress.

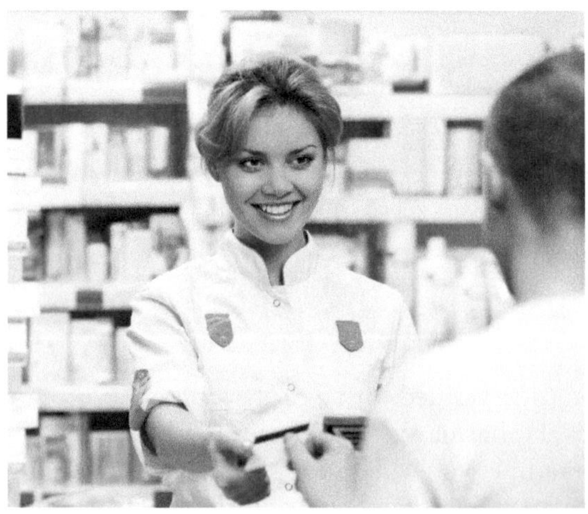

If a credit card, debit card, or check is refused for insufficient funds, a technician must politely return the payment and ask in a friendly manner for a new form of payment.

Flex Cards A **flex card** is a medical debit card for out-of-pocket "qualified medical expenses," according to the IRS. Such expenses include all prescriptions, insulins, and OTC items that are written as prescriptions. The flex credit card minimizes the need for submission of receipts, prevents delays in reimbursement, and offers tax advantages. It has an allotted amount of money on the card account, as in a debit card bank account, which is "rechargeable" by adding more money.

Gift Cards Unlike credit, debit, and flex cards, gift card charges are made against an account balance linked to the card's bar code. The bar code on the gift card is scanned or manually entered. With product or store coupons, as well as drug rebate forms, the technician must carefully review the requirements and expiration date before scanning.

Cash

Cash transactions are fairly straightforward. At the start of each business day, each cash register begins with a set number of bills and coins. Large bills, such as $50 and $100 bills, are usually placed under the change drawer to minimize mix-ups. *Always, always check the kind of bill offered to you by the customer* before putting it into the change drawer so that you don't assume that a $20 bill is a $10 dollar bill or vice versa. Scam artists can hand you a lower bill denomination and say that they gave you a higher one. They can also give you counterfeit money, so do a quick check as bills are put in your hands. To become proficient in identifying counterfeit bills, go to https://PharmPractice7e .Paradigmeducation.com/Counterfeit.

Most cash registers automatically display the change due for each transaction. Knowing how to count change is a key skill for excellent customer service and pharmacy accounting. You can easily practice at home, as there is an art to doing it confidently (see Table 9.4).

TABLE 9.4 Counting Change

Counting change out to a customer is essential for good service. The cash register's screen will tell you the amount to return if you have properly scanned and/or punched in all the numbers of the product price and money offered you. But you cannot just plop the change into the customer's hand. You need to count the cash as you hand it back to show that it is the correct amount. Say that a woman purchases a bottle of Tylenol and a bottle of vitamin C for the total purchase price of $10.73. She offers you a $50 bill. There are two ways to count her change:

Counting out the amount listed on the register

1. Confirm the amount of change to be received based on the amount listed on the register, which says $39.27. You can say, "You have *thirty-nine dollars and twenty-seven cents* in change coming." The customer can then tell you if there is a disagreement.
2. Then count the money into her hand, from the biggest to smallest coins and biggest to smallest bills—first a quarter and two pennies, then a $20 bill, a $10, a $5, then four $1 bills, saying, "*Twenty-five, twenty-six, twenty-seven cents, twenty dollars, thirty, thirty-five, thirty-six, thirty-seven, thirty-eight, thirty-nine, thirty-nine twenty-seven.*"

Counting change starting from the register total is the easiest for the technician, but it is not for the customer. Customers often do not know off the top of their heads how much change they should receive. They generally feel most comfortable having the change counted back to them starting at the purchase price and ending at the cash they gave you.

Counting from the purchase price

1. Take the amount of change needed, as noted on the register, from the cash drawer.
2. Begin at the purchase price, $10.73, count out the coins needed to reach the next bill. Count into the customer's hand two pennies ($0.02 to reach $10.75), then a quarter ($0.25) to make $11.00, counting "*Ten-seventy-four, ten seventy-five, eleven dollars.*"
3. Then, offer $1 bills to the point where you can use the next highest denomination, which would be a $5 bill counting, "*Twelve, thirteen, fourteen, fifteen dollars.*"
4. Then, you use the next highest bill denomination up until you reach the amount first given to you. So you can use a $5 dollar bill to reach $20 dollars, then a $10 bill to reach $30, and a $20 bill to reach $50, counting, "*Twenty, thirty, and fifty dollars.*"

Personal Checks

Some customers elect to pay for their pharmacy purchases with a personal check, though this is becoming less common and some businesses no longer accept checks. Procedures differ, depending on the pharmacy. Larger pharmacies usually have a check reader connected to the cash register. The signed check is fed into the reader and the bank account is immediately accessed. In some cases, the check reader prints the entire check, ready for customer signature. If the account shows insufficient funds, a prompt alerts you not to accept the check and to seek an alternate source of payment. If the check transaction is successfully processed, you can return the check to the customer along with a receipt.

For pharmacies without a check reader, if the patient is not recognized as a regular customer, you may need to ask for identification, such as a driver's license, and to transfer that information to the check. The amount of the check and the signature should always be verified. Checks written for a large amount (commonly greater than $100) may require approval of the store manager, since it is possible for the pharmacy to receive a check with insufficient funds to cover the bill. Most pharmacies have a policy of charging a high fee to rebill bad checks. In some cases, the pharmacy keeps a list of customers who are not allowed to pay with checks.

Personal Charge Accounts and Delayed Billing

Some independent pharmacies allow their most frequent customers to run a charge account and have the pharmacy bill them at the end of the month. This is a convenience for the customer but adds to operating expenses of the pharmacy, so it needs to be done with prudence, as decided by the owners.

Price Verification, Voided Sales, and Refunds

Cashiering includes some other functions that technicians need to know how to handle. Customers often ask to verify the price of store items or, in some cases, to modify them. You can scan the bar code on the item for price checking. If the advertised price is not accurately reflected, you will have to manually enter it into the register. If the pharmacy is out of stock on a *buy one, get one free* item, you may be allowed to adjust the price by 50%, depending on store policy.

Occasionally, completed sales need to be voided because a mistake has been made or the customer changes their mind. For instance, the drugs are not covered by insurance, the copays are too high, or the merchandise is not available at the price the customer thought. Following store policies, you will likely void the transaction on the cash register, initial the receipt, and document the reason for the void before storing it in the register. If a patient is due a refund from a prior purchase, you may need to obtain administrative approval from either the pharmacist or the store manager before proceeding with the refund.

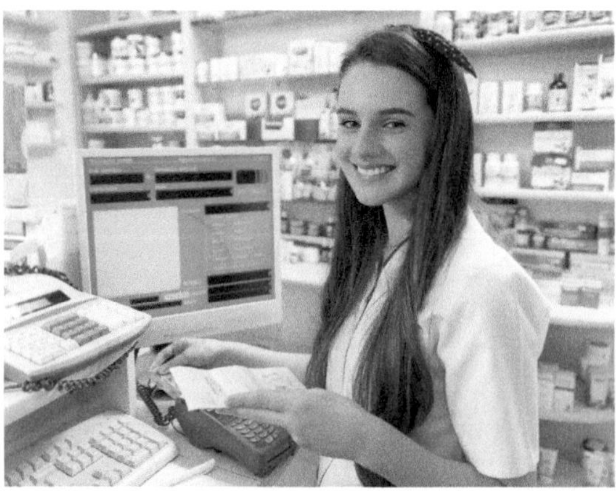
It is important for a technician to log off of the register when it is not in use.

At the end of the business day (or a shift), a pharmacy manager or a designated technician has the responsibility to **reconcile**, or match, the cash, credit card receipts, personal checks, coupons, rebates, voided sales, and patient charges (if allowed) with the printout from the cash register.

To do this, the bills, coins, and checks in the cash register drawer must be counted, and the amount of cash in the register when the day started must be subtracted. The amount left must equal the exact amount of cash-check transactions that occurred as tallied by the cash register. The credit and debit transaction receipts will also be counted to check against the register totals of credit-debit transactions. Voided transactions and discounts must also be subtracted.

Then these totals must be added to those of other registers to find the full amount of business for the day. The complete total will be checked against the total of the purchase prices of the prescriptions filled and merchandise sold according to the bar code scanners, minus the insurance reimbursements expected. It is complicated, but automation does a great deal of the work. The bar code scanning technology works in concert with the POS cash register. A POS cash register has the advantage of automatically reordering inventory at the end of each day.

In larger pharmacies with multiple technicians, pharmacists, and POS cash registers, it is not uncommon for each technician to have a sign-on and password code to enter when starting the shift on a certain register, to assist in tracking transactions and reconciling the receipts at the end of the day or shift. A technician is accountable for all customer receipts at their register during the shift. It is common to be off a few cents or dollars once in a while, but frequent or large discrepancies are brought to the attention of the pharmacist. Major cash discrepancies during a technician's shift, especially if there is a pattern of such discrepancies, will require explanation and should be discussed privately. Surveillance cameras are available in many pharmacies to protect the pharmacy from money loss or drug diversion by staff or customers.

9.5 Accounting, Pricing, and Retail Math

A community pharmacy operates under the same principles as any other business—it must make a **profit** to survive. In other words, it must have more income than expenses to continue to provide services. One of the responsibilities of the pharmacy technician is to help ensure that inventory turns over and that the insurance reimbursements and sales are greater than the expenses.

The technician is often responsible for marking up OTC products and other merchandise by a certain percentage over the acquisition cost and marking other products down by a percentage discount. To be successful, you need to master basic mathematical skills used in markup, discount, and average wholesale price. Understanding the terminology and mathematics used in community pharmacy is an important part of the pharmacy technician's job and can directly affect business profitability.

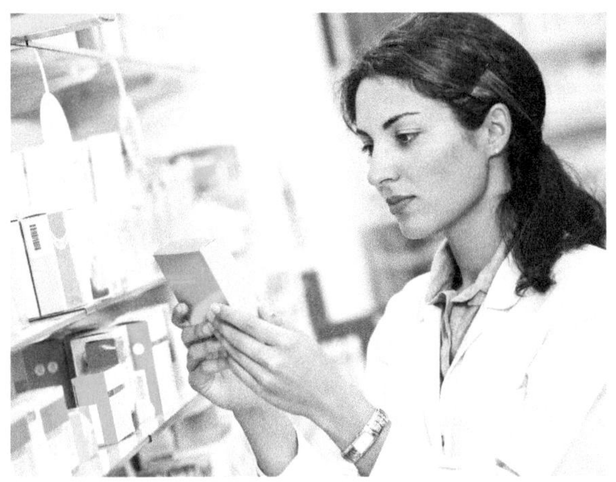

For pharmacies to offer prescription discounts to cash- or credit-paying patients, pharmacists and technicians need to be well aware of a drug's AWP, the negotiated acquisition price, and the pharmacy markup percentage.

Acquisition Costs and Pharmacy Reimbursements

Like all businesses, pharmacies purchase their products (in other words, drugs) at a generally lower-than-retail price from a wholesaler or supplier called the **acquisition cost**. The wholesaler is a company that purchases drugs, supplements, and supplies directly from manufacturers and then distributes them to pharmacies from a local or regional warehouse. When purchasing as a group, the purchasing agent for a number of independent pharmacies or for a pharmacy chain negotiates favorable contract terms and a discount for high-volume purchases. The state pharmacy association sometimes can act as a facilitator for group purchasing, contracting for its members as a benefit.

Average Wholesale Price Versus Acquisition Cost

The **average wholesale price (AWP)** of a drug is the *average* price that wholesalers charge pharmacies for a given drug, dose, and package size. AWP has been compared to the "sticker price" on an automobile. There is generally a difference between the AWP and the actual acquisition cost, because the AWP does not include discounts for the pharmacy's volume purchasing, prompt payment, or rebates from pharmaceutical manufacturers for brand name drugs.

Usually, the **pharmacy benefit managers (PBMs)** (which handle insurance company claims) and other third parties reimburse pharmacies a brand drug's AWP minus a third-party volume discount agreed upon in a negotiated contract, plus a pharmacy dispensing fee (in the range of $2.50 to $4.00 per prescription) for services rendered. The dispensing fee is supposed to cover the pharmacy's personnel costs.

Estimating Insurance Reimbursements

Insurance companies and their PBMs calculate a prescription reimbursement price with the following formula:

AWP × reimbursement percentage rate + dispensing fee = reimbursement amount

To maximize the pharmacy's income, it is essential to purchase a stock quantity from a wholesaler at less than AWP to make up for low reimbursement percentages. Consider the following examples.

Example 1

The drug pioglitazone (Actos) comes in a quantity of 90 tablets with an AWP of $150. The pharmacy has an agreement with the supplier to purchase the drug at the AWP minus 15% (converted to 0.15 discount rate). The insurer is willing to pay the AWP less 5% plus a $3 dispensing fee. A patient on this insurer's plan purchases 30 tablets. How much profit does the pharmacy make on this prescription?

Step 1 Begin by calculating the amount of the 15% discount.

$150.00 AWP × 0.15 discount rate = $22.50 discount

Step 2 Use the discount to calculate the purchase price of the drug by subtracting it from the AWP.

$150.00 AWP − $22.50 discount = $127.50 purchase price

Therefore, the pharmacy can purchase 90 tablets for the **discounted acquisition cost** of $127.50.

Step 3 The insurance company will pay the pharmacy the AWP less 5%. (Note: 5% = 0.05.)

$150.00 AWP × 0.05 reimbursement rate = $7.50

$150.00 − $7.50 = $142.50 insurance reimbursement for 90 tablets (without dispensing fee)

Step 4 Using the insurance reimbursement of $142.50 for 90 tablets, calculate the reimbursement for 30 tablets.

$$\$142.50 \div 3 = \$47.50$$

Add $3.00 dispensing fee: $47.50 + $3.00 = $50.50 insurance reimbursement (for 30 tablets)

Step 5 Compare this to the pharmacy's cost of 30 tablets.

$$\$127.50 \div 3 = \$42.50 \text{ acquisition cost for 30 tablets}$$

Step 6 To find out the profit, subtract the pharmacy acquisition cost from the insurance reimbursement.

$$\$50.50 - \$42.50 = \$8.00 \text{ gross profit}$$

Example 2

The drug amlodipine 10 mg comes in a quantity of 500 tablets and has an AWP of $80. The pharmacy has an agreement with the supplier to purchase the drug at the AWP minus 10%. The insurer is willing to pay the AWP less 5% plus a $2.50 dispensing fee. What does the insurer's plan pay for 30 tablets? How much profit does the pharmacy make on this prescription?

Step 1 Begin by calculating the amount of the 10% discount.

$$\$80.00 \times 0.10 = \$8.00$$

Step 2 Use the discount amount to calculate the acquisition cost of the drug.

$$\$80.00 - \$8.00 = \$72.00$$

Therefore, the pharmacy can purchase 500 tablets for $72.00.

Step 3 The PBM will pay the pharmacy the AWP less 5%. (Note: 5% = 0.05.)

$$\$80.00 \times 0.05 = \$4.00$$

$$\$80.00 - \$4.00 = \$76.00 \text{ insurance reimbursement (for 500 tablets)}$$

(plus $2.50 dispensing fee)

Step 4 Calculate the insurance reimbursement for 30 tablets.

$$\$76.00 \div 500 \text{ tablets} = \$0.152 \text{ per tablet}$$

$$\$0.152 \text{ per tablet} \times 30 \text{ tablets} = \$4.56 \text{ for 30 tablets}$$

$$\$4.56 + \$2.50 \text{ dispensing fee} = \$7.06 \text{ insurance reimbursement (for 30 tablets)}$$

Step 5 Compare this to the pharmacy's cost of 30 tablets.

$$\$72.00 \div 500 \text{ tablets} = \$0.144 \text{ per tablet}$$

$$\$0.144 \text{ per tablet} \times 30 \text{ tablets} = \$4.32 \text{ acquisition cost}$$

Step 6 Therefore, the pharmacy's profit on 30 tablets is:

$$\$7.06 - \$4.32 = \$2.74 \text{ gross profit with reimbursement}$$

As you can see, the lower the acquisition cost for the pharmacy, the more money there is to cover operating costs and, hopefully, generate a profit. To survive as a business, the pharmacy has to purchase each drug at a price as far below the AWP as possible. However, now the PBMs of the insurance companies are also seeking to reimburse at lower levels, so independent pharmacies with less volume in sales purchasing have less negotiating power and often struggle to survive.

Markup and Profits

Pharmacies also buy their nonprescription products from wholesalers and sell them at a higher price. Pricing of nonprescription items is primarily determined by competition in the marketplace and customer expectations.

The difference between the store acquisition cost and the customer price is called the **markup**.

$$\text{pharmacy acquisition cost} + \text{markup} = \text{retail selling price}$$

$$\text{retail selling price} - \text{acquisition cost} = \text{markup}$$

The accumulation of these sales markups adds up to the **gross profit** of the business. The gross profit must cover the overhead expenses, or operating costs, including facility rental or maintenance, technology, utilities, marketing, and other expenses. What is left over after all the expenses are paid is the **net profit**. The quantity of net profit from both prescription and nonprescription sales determines whether the pharmacy can stay in business. With independent stores, this money goes to the owners, and with chains, it goes to the company and its shareholders.

Getting the right amount of markup is key to the success of a community pharmacy. Too high a markup drives customers away. Too low a markup means that the pharmacy cannot meet its expenses and make enough profit to stay in business. To understand the business side of pharmacy and perhaps be promoted as a manager, you need to understand how estimating pricing and markups works.

Determining Customer Price

Each independent pharmacy or chain determines a percentage of each sale that must go toward the operation costs and profit. This percentage is called the **markup percentage**. To determine the exact markup to charge for a specific item, whether prescription or retail, start with the acquisition cost from the wholesaler (supplier price) and multiply it by the pharmacy's markup percentage. (Pharmacies may have different retail versus prescription drug markup percentages.)

To calculate, turn the markup percentage into a decimal by dividing it by 100 to find your **markup rate**. Then take the rate and multiply the acquisition cost by that number to find the individual markup price. Add that markup price to the acquisition cost to get the retail cash price. The equations are set up as follows:

$$\text{markup } \% \div 100 = \text{markup rate}$$

$$\text{markup rate} \times \text{acquisition cost} = \text{markup price}$$

$$\text{acquisition cost} + \text{markup price} = \text{cash price}$$

Example 3

One case (twelve bottles) of esomeprazole (Nexium) 20 mg capsules are acquired for $202.28, and there needs to be a 13.64% markup to determine the customer price. What will be the cash price for one bottle of esomeprazole (Nexium)?

Step 1 Convert 13.64% to a decimal by dividing by 100 to find the markup rate.

$$13.64 \div 100 = 0.1364 \quad \{\text{or } \frac{13.64}{100} = 0.1364\}$$

Step 2 Multiply the markup rate by the acquisition cost.

$$0.1364 \times \$202.28 = \$27.590992\text{, rounded to } \$27.59.$$

Step 3 Add the acquisition cost and the markup price to find the cash price.

$$\$202.28 + \$27.59 = \$229.87 \text{ (for 12 bottles)}$$

Step 4 Divide the cash price for 12 bottles by 12 to find the price of one bottle.

$$\frac{\$229.87}{12} = \$19.16 \text{ is the retail cash price for one bottle of Nexium.}$$

Example 4

One vial of Humulin regular insulin sells (as a nonprescription) at the pharmacy at the cash price of $100 and costs the pharmacy $70. What is the markup price, and what is the markup rate?

Step 1 Determine actual price markup from selling price by subtracting product expense from selling price.

$$\text{selling price} - \text{product expense} = \text{markup amount}$$

$$\$100.00 - \$70.00 = \$30.00 \text{ markup}$$

Step 2 Compute the markup percentage.

$$\text{markup} \div \text{acquisition cost} = \text{markup rate}$$

$$\$30.00 \div \$70.00 = 0.43$$

Step 3 Convert 0.43 rate to percentage by multiplying by 100.

$$43\% = \text{markup percentage}$$

This is the pharmacy's profit/operating expenses markup for this item.

Determining Customer Discounts

As stated earlier, the drug stock price a wholesaler offers to a pharmacy is not always the AWP. Reduced standard rates are often established for frequent pharmacy purchasers or pharmacy buying groups. Sometimes, a wholesaler offers a lower price than its standard price in exchange for prompt payment. The independent pharmacy can then pass on the savings to the patients in a discount price. Having this discount leeway is particularly helpful for customers who are paying cash because they lack insurance and the pharmacist or technician wants to adjust the price to pass on the discount savings. To do this discounting, you need to determine the actual pharmacy acquisition cost and then provide an adjusted cost to the customer that will still cover the pharmacy dispensing fee. The calculation equations look like this:

$$\text{usual negotiated wholesale price} \times \text{prompt payment discount rate} = \text{amount of discount}$$

$$\text{usual wholesaler price} - \text{discount} = \text{discounted acquisition cost}$$

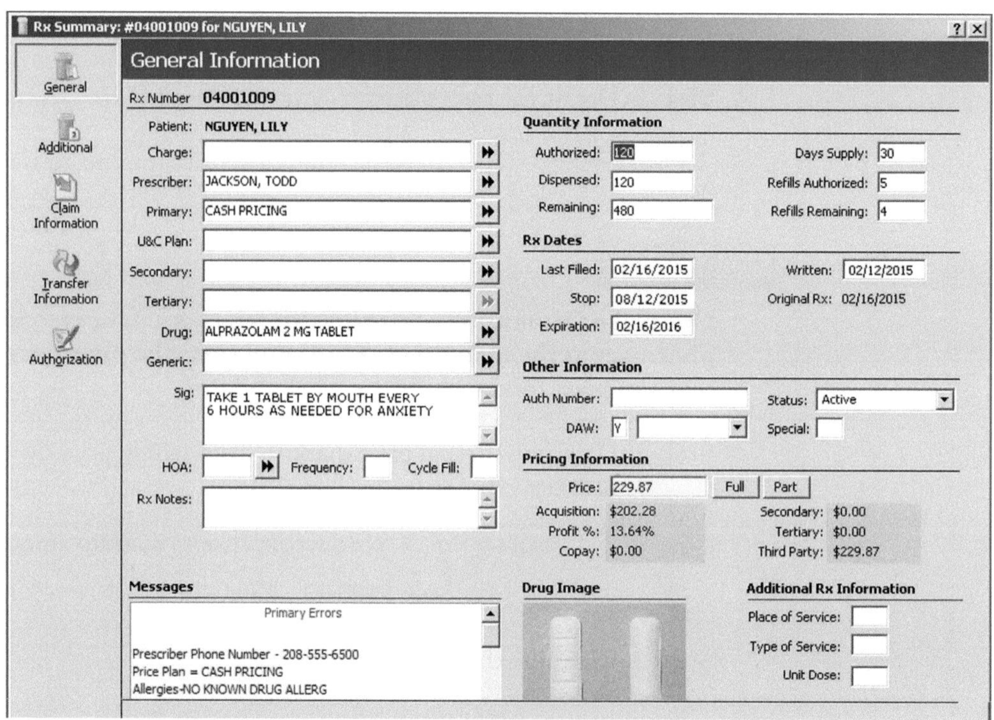

On this screen shot, the different pricing levels that are associated with a prescription price are visible: the acquisition cost, profit % (markup percentage), copay, and third-party fee.

Example 5

Assume that the pharmacy usually purchases five cases of hydrocortisone 1% cream at $100 per case. If the account is paid in full within 15 days, then the supplier (wholesaler) offers a 15% discount on the purchase. What is the discounted acquisition cost?

Step 1 Calculate the usual wholesale purchase price for quantity needed.

$$\text{quantity of product} \times \text{wholesale price per unit} = \text{typical acquisition cost}$$

$$\text{cases} \times \$100.00 \text{ per case} = \$500.00$$

Step 2 Calculate the 15% discount for payment within 15 days.

quantity acquisition cost × promptness discount rate = amount of discount

$$\$500.00 \times 0.15 = \$75.00$$

Step 3 To obtain the discounted acquisition cost, subtract the wholesaler discount amount from the original price.

total purchase price − discount = discounted acquisition cost

$$\$500.00 - \$75.00 = \$425.00$$

Step 4 To obtain the discounted price per case, divide the discounted acquisition cost by the number of cases.

$$\frac{\$425}{5} = \$85 \text{ per case}$$

Step 5 Finally, to calculate the discounted price per tube, divide the case price by the number of 1 ounce tubes in the case, which is 30.

$$\frac{\$85 \text{ per case}}{30 \text{ tubes}} = \$2.8333 \text{ per tube}$$

The pharmacy acquisition price is rounded to $2.83 per tube.

Step 6 If the pharmacy wants a markup percentage of 20% per tube, it would be as follows.

$$\$2.83 \times 0.20 = \$0.566 \text{ rounded to } \$0.57 \text{ cents}$$

So the pharmacy would be able to add up to $0.57 to the $2.83 cost for a $3.40 customer sales price.

Example 6

A bottle of 100 count zolpidem 10 mg has an AWP of $100, and the acquisition cost for the pharmacy is $40 for 100 tablets. A prescription for a month's supply of medication is 30 tablets. If the pharmacy charges the AWP for the prescription, what is the markup price for the prescription?

Step 1 Begin by calculating the wholesaler's standard cost per tablet by dividing the price by the quantity, and doing the same for the acquisition cost per tablet.

$$\$100 \div 100 = \$1.00 \text{ per tablet average wholesale price}$$

$$\$40 \div 100 = \$0.40 \text{ per tablet pharmacy acquisition cost}$$

Step 2 Then, calculate the wholesale costs for the quantity of tablets needed (30).

quantity × AWP per tablet = wholesale price for prescription

$$30 \text{ tablets} \times \$1.00 \text{ per tablet} = \$30.00$$

$$30 \text{ tablets} \times \$0.40 \text{ per tablet} = \$12.00$$

Step 3 Next, subtract the difference between the two: \$30 – \$12 = \$18. This \$18.00 is the markup from the actual acquisition cost and the profit leeway.

If insurance will not pay for the prescription, rather than charge the cash-paying patient the full \$30 AWP, the pharmacist could allow the technician to set the cash price lower, say to \$24, which is a \$6 discount from the average wholesaler price.

Step 4 To figure out what percentage discount you are offering at this price, divide the consumer discount amount by the original wholesale price.

$$\$6.00 \div \$30.00 \quad \text{or} \quad \frac{\$6.00}{\$30.00} = 0.20; \quad 0.20 \times 100 = 20\%$$

The pharmacy can offer a cash price of 20% price savings so that the customer pays \$24 instead of \$30. This deal is even lower than the wholesale price. The \$12 of markup adequately covers the operating costs and a pharmacy dispensing fee, while extending goodwill to the customer. Personnel working in independent pharmacies can make these cost adjustments, whereas personnel working in chain stores generally cannot.

Accounting Profitability and Productivity Reports

The daily functions of a pharmacy include running many different kinds of reports, often done by the pharmacy technician, including inventory orders, postings, pricing, accounts receivable, accounts payable, billing, third-party receipts, DEA prescribing, HIPAA compliance, controlled-substance compliance, and others. Knowing your way around these reports can lead to greater responsibilities and, at times, promotions.

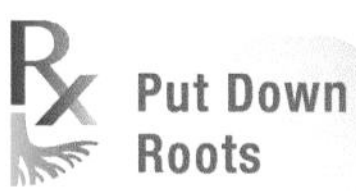

Put Down Roots

The inventory expression *par* in *par levels* came from an acronym for periodic automatic replenishment.

End-of-the-Day Report

At the end of each day, the pharmacist or technician prints out an **end-of-the-day report,** or daily **audit log**, from the pharmacy software. The report gives a thumbnail sketch of the profitability of the pharmacy based on that day's productivity. It documents the various computer logins by pharmacists and technicians, the prescriptions filled, costs accrued, and payments made.

The report lists not only the total number and drug names of all prescriptions dispensed per pharmacist, it also lists the AWPs, acquisition costs, selling prices, profit for each prescription sold, and each PBM billed. Categories of the report include a line-by-line breakdown description of the prescriptions/refills, a breakdown of the costs for these in each payment plan and the profit margins, and a daily cost analysis breakdown for each plan/payment system based on these lists. This report is signed and dated by the pharmacist to keep on file for future audit purposes and as proof that the billed drugs were dispensed to the patients. The pharmacy manager reviews all this information, which is helpful in negotiating annual renewals of the contracts with each PBM and wholesaler.

Cost-Benefit Analysis Spreadsheets

Technicians often generate the daily reports, and, from these reports, the computer can generate weekly, monthly, and yearly **cost-benefit analysis spreadsheets**. The itemized tables on these spreadsheets identify the costs invested, compared to the benefits or sales received and the present business net value and income. They tally direct expenses (such as cost of inventory and pharmacy personnel) and indirect overhead expenses (payroll and benefits, utilities, insurance, legal fees, rent, computers, etc.), as compared to sales income and third-party reimbursements. Technicians who become familiar with all these reports can build an in-depth knowledge that will allow them to move forward in business management.

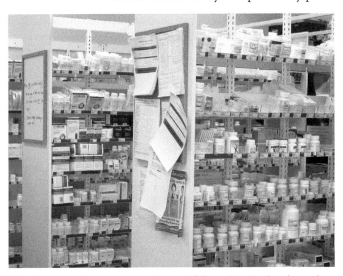

The pharmacy inventory must be carefully maintained to keep the costs down by having on hand what is needed without excessive extras.

One of the largest elements in the expense column is the cost of the drugs that need to be held as stock for prescriptions. The entire stock of pharmaceutical and retail products on hand is known as the **inventory** (which will be explained in more detail to come). Over time, these end-of-the-day reports, cost-benefit analysis spreadsheets, and itemized inventory reports can track trends useful for inventory investment and management, purchasing, and retail marketing.

9.6 Inventory Management

Community pharmacies must stock, or have ready access to, all drugs that may be desired by their customers or prescribers. Technicians assist in the everyday details of maintaining well-stocked but not overstocked shelves. They locate stock and label shelves; store products appropriately; restock, checking expiration dates and rotating products; and document reorder levels. Checking for expired vitamins and herbs is especially important because they can lose their labeled potency quickly. Technicians are also responsible for stocking the supplies they need for filling and processing prescriptions (various sizes of vials and bottles, medication and auxiliary labels, measuring devices, paper, and other supplies), making sure that they are reordered as needed.

Stock Levels and Inventory Value

Inventory value is defined as the total cost of the entire stock on a given day. The inventory includes prescription and OTC drugs, dietary supplements, medical and home health supplies and equipment, and front-end retail and impulse merchandise. Unlike some businesses, pharmacies must keep some slow-moving products on their shelves as a service to the few customers who will need them medically. If the pharmacy frequently runs out of needed supplies and medications, this causes great inconvenience to patients who will often just go to a different pharmacy. So pharmacies set **periodic automatic replenishment (PAR) levels** for each item, or minimum levels when each stock item needs automatic reordering.

Often, community pharmacies have $150,000 to $300,000 or more in inventory value on their shelves. Drug stock is generally the pharmacy's biggest expense. Pharmacies must absorb the costs of the drug inventory they purchase until the stock is sold and the insurance reimbursements are received, which can sometimes take four to eight weeks. That is why keeping track of inventory and specific drug turnover is very important. Returning unopened, unused extra stock is also key.

An excessive inventory ties up capital in the inventory, hinders the ability to invest in other areas, such as marketing and staffing, and incurs wastage due to product expirations. It also increases the likelihood of theft. Therefore, inventory levels must be kept adequate but not excessive, with a rapid turnover of drug stock on the shelf.

Purchasing Relationships and Contracts

As each drug prescription is filled, the pharmacy operations software automatically deducts the amount from the stock inventory. At the end of each day, a reorder list for the next business day is automatically generated, based on the PAR restock level for each individual drug set in software by the pharmacy. Many pharmacies use software that not only automatically generates the daily reorder lists, but also generates the specific drug orders with the established wholesalers.

Before any purchasing can happen, relationships with those who distribute, store, or manufacture specific drugs must be established. **Purchasing** is defined as acquiring products for use or sale. Purchasing contracts can be negotiated by an individual pharmacy or with other pharmacies as part of a group purchase contract.

Primary Wholesaler Purchasing

When pharmacies secure a contract with a wholesaler to be their primary supplier, they can receive the fastest moving products from a single source for the best negotiated price. This saves them from establishing contracts with multiple manufacturers or suppliers of brand name and generic pharmaceuticals. In most **primary wholesaler purchasing**, the pharmacy orders from a local or regional vendor that delivers the products to the pharmacy on a daily basis. The advantages include scheduled deliveries and ordering, automatic online ordering, reduced turnaround time for orders, lower inventory and lower associated costs, discounts, and reduced commitment of time and staff. The turnaround time for receipt of drug orders is usually the next business day, with the exception of weekends and holidays.

Disadvantages include higher purchase costs for individual stock items, occasional supply shortages (called *back orders*), and unavailability of some pharmaceuticals.

Prime Vendor Purchasing

In some situations, pharmacies need to work with more than one vendor, getting a large amount of stock from two or more suppliers. When pharmacy planning shows that a certain amount of money will for certain be spent on an established amount of drug products, the pharmacy may be able to set up a **prime vendor purchasing contract** with one of these vendors to secure a discount for high-volume purchasing. This is an exclusive agreement made with a wholesaler or warehouse to continually purchase a specified percentage or dollar amount toward different types of ordering and delivery methods. Prime vendor purchasing offers the advantages of lower acquisition costs, competitive service fees, electronic order entry, and emergency delivery services. Prime vendor purchasing is common in both retail and hospital pharmacies.

Just-in-Time Purchasing

To provide less outlay of funds at one time, pharmacies can also use just-in-time purchasing, which involves frequent purchasing in smaller quantities (often of less frequently requested items or for more expensive prices because of the convenience) that just meet supply needs until the next ordering time. **Just-in-time (JIT) purchasing** reduces the quantity of each product on the shelves and thus reduces the overall amount of money invested at one time in the inventory.

However, such a JIT system can be used only when supplies are readily available locally and pharmaceutical needs can be accurately predicted. Automation can enhance the accuracy of replacing needed inventory levels of drugs. In large chain pharmacies, a regional or centralized warehouse owned by the corporation generally provides the once-weekly purchasing. A local wholesaler is then used for any JIT brand name and **out-of-stock (OOS)** drugs needed on a day's notice. For independent pharmacies on a limited drug budget, JIT purchasing is more the norm.

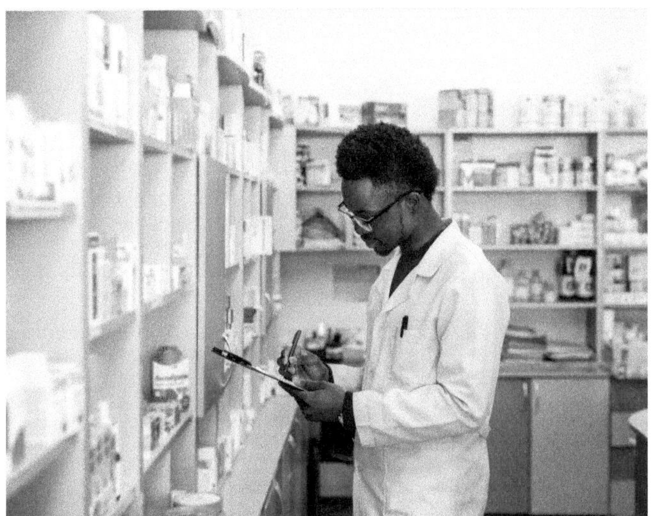

Technicians need to keep close track of the inventory, especially the most frequently purchased pharmaceuticals, to assist in deciding what needs to be purchased and how quickly.

Purchasing Orders

The technician reviews and verifies each of the drugs listed on the end-of-the-day reorder list and purchase orders to process them and alerts the pharmacist to the Schedule II drugs needing attention (generally only the pharmacist orders these). If the pharmacy is on a strict daily drug budget, you need to exercise good judgment and prioritize which drugs will be ordered for the next business day and which can wait. It is not uncommon for an independent pharmacy to wait to order an expensive drug rather than keep it in stock on the shelf.

When ordering next-day inventory, the technician assesses the predicted new prescriptions or refills for (1) OOS items; (2) partial fills; and (3) stock replenishment. Special orders for seldom-stocked high-cost injectable products often require additional delivery time directly from the manufacturer if they are not in the wholesaler's on-site inventory.

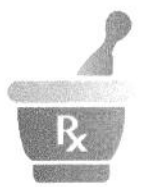

Practice Tip

When a patient does not pick up a prescription medication and it must be returned to stock, it needs to remain in the patient container to be placed back in the inventory with all patient information blacked out. The medication cannot be poured back into the stock bottle.

A small independent pharmacy often uses computer tracking or a manual logbook to record inventory that needs to be replaced. After a time, the technician will develop a good sense for how fast drug products move off the shelves and when they need to be reordered by watching the usage and seasonal patterns. For "fast movers," the purchase decision is often based on the most economical order quantity or best value (such as ordering capsules in a 1,000 count size rather than 100 count size or buying a case of antacid liquid rather than one or two bottles).

Each time wholesale drugs are purchased, the product, quantity, and price are entered into the computer database. Besides the PAR levels for each drug item, pharmacies usually have an **inventory range**—a maximum and a minimum number of units to have on hand. Orders are calculated from these levels.

Use this formula to calculate the minimum order amount:

$$\textit{minimum inventory} - \textit{present inventory} = \textit{minimum order amount}$$

Here are some examples of common stock dilemmas:

Example 7

The maximum inventory level for amoxicillin 500 mg capsules is 1,000 capsules. At the end of the day, the computer prints a list of items to be reordered. The list indicates a current inventory level of 225 amoxicillin capsules; the minimum quantity—and the point to reorder automatically—is set at 250 capsules. Has the automatic reorder level been reached? Each stock bottle contains 500 capsules. How many should be ordered?

250 capsules − 225 capsules = 25 capsules less than minimum level

Because the stock level has dropped under the minimum number needed to reorder, the automatic reorder or manual reorder will be processed for one bottle of 500 count 500 mg capsules.

Example 8

The maximum inventory level for cyclobenzaprine 10 mg tablets is 500 tablets and the minimum is 200. At the end of the day, the computer printout list indicates a current inventory level of 375 cyclobenzaprine tablets. Will the capsules be reordered?

200 tablets − 375 tablets = (−)175 tablets

Nothing needs to be reordered because 175 is the surplus above minimum levels.

Periodically, stock levels and ranges need to be modified or updated. For example, the software may indicate that there are 120 tablets of 300 mg ranitidine remaining in stock. If the minimum reorder level is 100 tablets, the drug will not be on the generated reorder list. However, if you retrieve the drug from the shelf and find only 25 tablets remaining, you will update the actual inventory count in the system so that the drug can be ordered for the next business day. (You and the pharmacist will need to try to figure out where the extra stock went.) Seasonal adjustments also need to be made, such as stocking more allergy products in the spring, sunscreen products in the summer, flu vaccine in the fall, and antibiotics in the winter. If a new medication is increasingly prescribed in your geographical area, its stock level will need to be increased.

Processing Order Deliveries

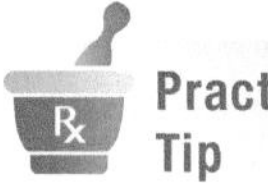

Practice Tip

When a medication is discontinued, or no longer manufactured, you will need to ask the pharmacist to discuss an alternative medication with the prescriber.

Once an order is delivered from a wholesaler, warehouse, or other pharmacy, the technician must go through a number of processes.

Receiving

When the wholesale delivery arrives, the process of **receiving** begins, which is a set of procedures to legally check in and accept the order. The pharmacist or the technician first must sign an invoice from the wholesale representative, verifying the receipt of the correct number and type of totes or boxes. **Totes** are the plastic containers that contain specialized medications, including those for refrigerated items (in cold packs) and controlled substances. These all come sealed. A separate invoice is usually required for the receipt of controlled substances. The pharmacist should check for and document intact seals and the contents of totes containing controlled substances.

Once checked by the pharmacist, you as the technician must then carefully match the pharmaceutical products received against the purchase invoice for the correct product items (matching names and bar codes), manufacturer, quantity, product strength, package size, and condition. In the case of a damaged or an incorrect shipment or an incorrectly shipped product (not stored properly), you should notify the wholesaler immediately for authorization to return the defective shipment and replace inventory as soon as possible.

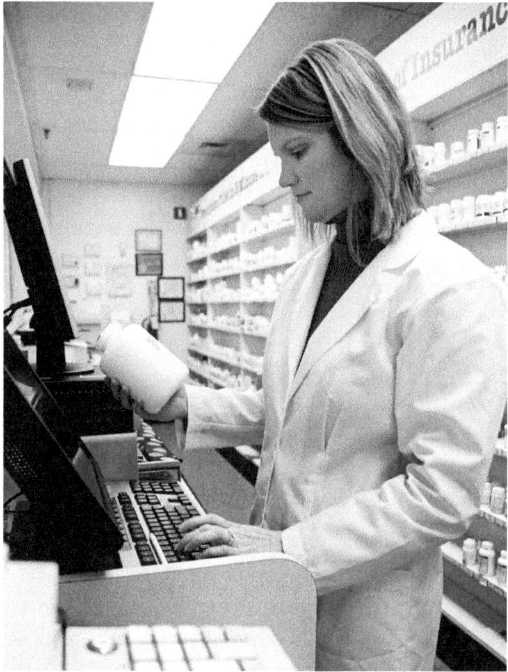

Shipment contents need to be carefully checked for their National Drug Code (NDC) numbers, price updates, and expiration dates, and then posted in the inventory software program so that everything lines up at the cash register.

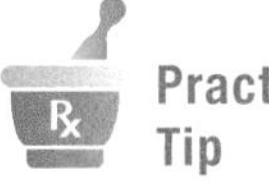

Practice Tip

When filling prescriptions for specially ordered, high-cost drugs, do not attach the patient medication label to the drug packaging. Attach it with a rubber band or place it with the packaging in a resealable plastic bag, so it can be returned to the warehouse if not picked up.

Occasionally, a pharmaceutical product is temporarily or permanently unavailable from a wholesaler. Drug shortages can be due to manufacturing quality control issues, FDA or voluntary drug recalls, expirations, or discontinuations. First determine the reason for the unavailability—for example, the drug is (1) on back order; (2) being recalled by the manufacturer; or (3) being discontinued. If the product is not expected to be received the next day, the pharmacist should then identify a therapeutically equivalent product with permission from the prescriber. Alternatively, the pharmacy could consider borrowing the drug from another local pharmacy or one in the corporate chain if a supply of the drug is available.

Posting

As the inventory order is checked and approved, it is important that the order is accurately posted. **Posting** is the process of updating inventory in the pharmacy software database and reconciling any differences between the new and current stock. This process includes checking the newly received drug inventory for NDC numbers, expiration dates, and drug cost updates.

Any large price increases should be brought to the attention of the pharmacist for verification. To highlight these differences, you can affix stickers to the received unit stock bottles to document the wholesaler's item number and pricing information. However, be careful where you stick them so that they do not harm the original label; if it looks worn or tampered with, the stock cannot someday be returned to the wholesaler for credit. Also, it is the recommended practice to avoid affixing medication labels to the original manufacturer packages for high-cost drugs in the event that the patient cannot afford them, and the drugs should be returned.

Once posted, the delivered drugs should immediately be appropriately stored—at room temperature, refrigerated, or frozen—depending on the requirements listed on the manufacturers' product package inserts.

All injectable vaccines (such as those for shingles and chicken pox) require refrigeration or freezing. Insulins and select eye drops are also required to be shipped and stored under refrigeration.

Shelf Maintenance and Rotating Stock

As the new products are added to the retail and storage shelves, check the expiration dates of the stock, and rearrange them for the oldest to be in the front (with shortest expiration dates) for quickest access and sale. This repositioning is known as **rotating the stock**. Products close to expiration dates need to be removed. Each pharmacy has a policy for an acceptable range of expiration dates. A typical requirement might be that products have expiration dates of at least 12 months from the date of wholesaler receipt, and products on the shelves must have a 4- to 6-month shelf life.

Handling Out-of-Stock and Partially Filled Medications

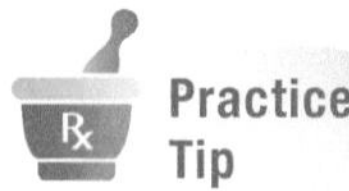

It is good customer service for technicians to call customers when the remainder of an out-of-stock or partial fill medication is available for pickup.

After receiving, posting, and shelving of the inventory is complete, it is important to initiate the prescription filling process for any OOS or **partial fill** prescriptions from the day before. A partial fill prescription is issued when the pharmacy doesn't have a full quantity of a specific drug on hand. They will supply patients with a limited amount—usually a few days' worth—until the drug is back in stock. The prescription order is then processed, verified, and filled so that it can be available for the patient to pick up later that same day, as promised. If possible, notify the patient when the prescription is ready for pickup. The completion of partial fill orders also takes priority after postings are complete. Insurance is commonly billed and the patient pays the copay for the entire amount at the time of the partial fill. When the order arrives and the prescription is filled for the remainder (less the partial fill quantity), the patient owes no additional payment.

Drug Recalls, Returns, and Credits

At times, drugs must be returned to the wholesaler for credit—in their original stock bottles or unit-of-use packaging and in their original condition. These returns can be because of pharmacy overstocks, patient decline of expensive medication pickup, soon-to-be-expired drugs, recalls by the manufacturer or FDA, reformulated drugs, drugs in out-of-date packaging, or drugs that are no longer manufactured. The different reasons for returns result in slightly different ways to handle them.

Drug Recalls

When an official alert for the drug occurs, known as a **drug recall**, the wholesaler typically emails or mails the drug recall information: drug name, dose, NDC, lot number, expiration date, etc., as well as the date and type of recall (voluntary, mandatory). Three classes of response levels of recalls exist, with Class I being the most urgent. The FDA staff determines the class that is appropriate based on manufacturer actions, the healthcare situation, and customer data from MedWatch and other sources. Table 9.5 describes the three levels of drug recalls.

For all drug recalls, the technician must check drug inventory and the retail shelves for each recalled item, pull it from inventory right away to protect the patient, and notify the pharmacist, who signs a recall form. This form is then returned to the wholesaler with any recalled drug stock items. The pharmacist should designate the appropriate plan to notify the patients who have received recalled drugs—notification in Class I is required; notifications for Class II and III are up to the pharmacist's/prescriber's judgment. Cash register and insurance transactions reports are essential for tracking down the customers who purchased the recalled items and talking to them about the recall. If they have specific questions about what to do to counteract any problems, the pharmacist should do the counseling.

TABLE 9.5 Recall Classes for Drugs

Class	Risk	Action Response
I	**Urgent, immediate danger**—A reasonable probability exists that the product will cause or lead to serious harm or even death.	All patients who have received or purchased this product should be notified.
II	**Moderate danger**—A probability exists that the product could cause adverse health events, but the events would be medically reversible or temporary.	Pharmacists and/or prescribers must decide the best practice about notifying patients.
III	**Least danger**—The product will probably not cause an adverse health event, but there is a product quality problem.	Pharmacists and/or prescribers must decide the best practice about notifying patients.

The role of the FDA is to monitor drug recalls and assess the adequacy of the manufacturers' actions. After a recall is completed, the FDA makes sure that the product is destroyed or suitably "reconditioned" (recategorized with new conditions for sale). It also investigates why the product was defective and the actions to take. The FDA posts weekly reports on drug recalls that pharmacists should read. These are posted at https://PharmPractice7e.ParadigmEducation.com/SafetyReport1.

In an effort to prevent problems even before drugs are officially classified, the FDA also posts two pages of drugs pending recall classification. One is for human drug product recalls pending classification at https://PharmPractice7e.ParadigmEducation .com/SafetyReport2. The other is non-blood product ongoing recalls, which can be accessed at https://PharmPractice7e.ParadigmEducation.com /SafetyReport3. These sites should also be checked regularly to keep patients informed.

At times, pharmacists and technicians may see that the drug has been recalled or is pending classification. The product should be pulled from the inventory. The manufacturer should be notified that a return and credit are desired. Consumers can also return a recalled drug for refund or credit, per pharmacy or drug wholesaler policy.

Return of Declined Medications

At times, patients do not pick up their filled medication within seven days, even after reminder calls and phone messages. Consequently, as the technician, you must "reverse" or cancel the online insurance billing, store the prescription order in the patient profile for possible future use, and return the stock to drug inventory. For example, if a patient declines to pick up the expensive diabetic drug dulaglutide (Trulicity), you can store it in the refrigerator and then return it to the wholesaler for credit, provided that the box is unopened, and that the prescription label (perhaps attached by rubber band) can be removed without altering the packaging label.

A return-for-credit form must be completed that lists the drug(s) and quantities to be returned for credit. You and the wholesale driver must verify the contents of the return totes or boxes, and sign for the credit. Your signature guarantees that the product was purchased directly from the wholesaler. Your signature also states, under penalty of perjury, that the drugs have been stored and handled in accordance with manufacturers' guidelines and all federal, state, and local laws. The containers are then sealed and returned to the wholesaler for credit. The signed form is filed for future reference if necessary.

Practice Tip

Prescription vials returned by the patient cannot be returned to stock once they leave the pharmacy premises, even if they are unopened.

Expired Medications

Pharmacy technicians must also check drug inventory (including OTC drugs and dietary supplements) for expired medications on a monthly basis, or per store policy. Remove all expired or near-expired (within three to six months) products from stock and return them to the wholesaler for partial credit. If a drug is past its expiration date, it can be returned to the wholesaler, but no credit will be issued. This process of drug returns and credits often involves a lot of paperwork and is time-consuming. However, it is another important part of inventory management and business profitability.

Wrongly Filled Prescriptions

At times, the wrong medication is filled in a prescription, which occasionally happens despite safety checks, especially when both generic and brand name drugs exist, and there is a mark of DAW1, or dispense as written, by the prescriber or DAW2, by the patient. Consider the following scenario: a patient or prescriber requests Synthroid (a brand name drug) to be dispensed, and the pharmacy inadvertently dispenses levothyroxine (the generic form of the drug). If the drug did not leave the pharmacy, the prescription can be corrected and the drug can be returned to stock.

However, if the patient left the pharmacy, discovered the mix-up, and then came back to the pharmacy later with the medication unopened, the generic drug can be returned for money back to the patient and the correct medication dispensed, but the generic must be discarded per law and pharmacy protocol. The pharmacy cannot recover the cost of the incorrect prescription.

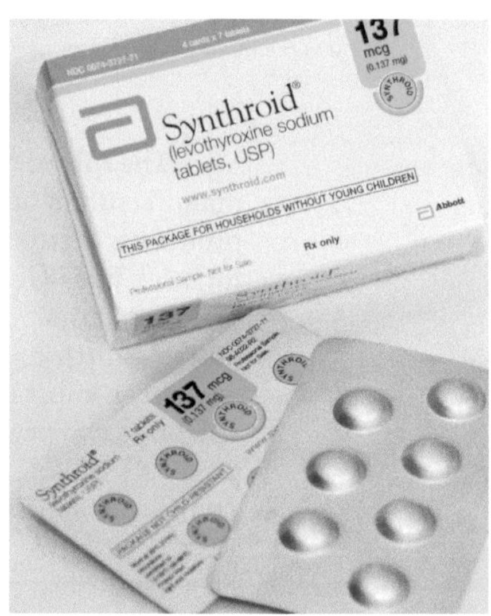

Synthesized thyroid hormone is available as an often-requested brand name drug (Synthroid) or as a generic drug (lexovthyroxine). Before dispensing the generic, make sure there are no DAW requests from the prescriber or patient so that the correct drug is dispensed.

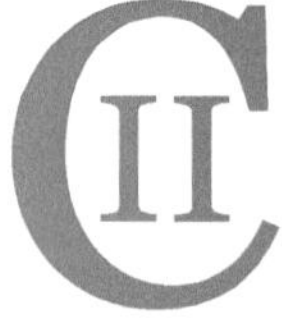

This symbol on the outside packaging quickly identifies that this is a Schedule C-II drug.

Handling Controlled Substances

Controlled substances demand special purchasing, receiving, and record keeping of inventory, according to the Controlled Substances Act. Each pharmacy must register with the DEA to purchase and dispense controlled substances, and the FDA requires that all controlled-substance containers be clearly marked with their "schedule" on the product label. In light of that, you should inspect containers for the schedule mark, which is an uppercase Roman numeral preceded by a C symbol (or not preceded by it): II or C-II; III or C-III; IV or C-IV; and V or C-V. The symbol C and/or the Roman numeral must be at least twice the size of the largest letters printed on the label. If a bottle is too small to display the symbol or numerals, the box and package insert must contain them. Symbols and/or numerals are not required on the patient containers.

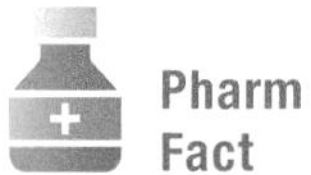

Pharm Fact

The DEA 222 form documents the ordering request to the manufacturer or wholesaler; the shipment receipt documents the pharmacy delivery; and the prescription receipt documents the dispensing to the patient.

Schedule III, IV, and V Drugs

In most pharmacies, the technician can order Schedule III–V medications. However, per store policy, the pharmacist may have to verify and sign for their receipt at delivery. After comparing the invoice with the ordered drug name, dosage, and quantity, the receipt can often be signed by the technician and verified by the pharmacist. These drugs can then be stored by the technician among the rest of the drug stock, usually alphabetically by generic drug name. All Schedule III, IV, and V prescriptions and records, including purchasing invoices, are commonly kept separate from other records and must also be kept in a readily retrievable form.

Schedule II Purchasing

Schedule II controlled substances follow stricter protocols per DEA law and regulations. Similar to other medications, PAR levels for most C-II drugs generate automated inventory alerts in the pharmacy software for reorders or special out-of-stock or partial-fill orders. However, purchase of Schedule II controlled substances must be specifically initiated and authorized by a pharmacist and executed on a DEA 222 form, either online or on paper (see Figure 9.2).

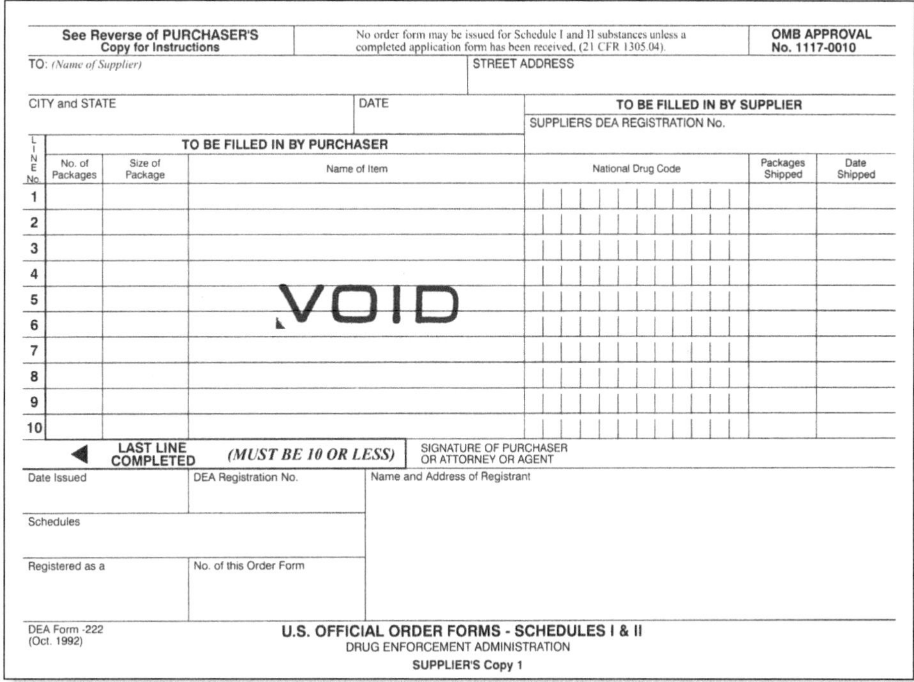

See Reverse of PURCHASER'S Copy for Instructions | No order form may be issued for Schedule I and II substances unless a completed application form has been received, (21 CFR 1305.04). | OMB APPROVAL No. 1117-0010

TO: *(Name of Supplier)* | STREET ADDRESS

CITY and STATE | DATE | TO BE FILLED IN BY SUPPLIER | SUPPLIERS DEA REGISTRATION No.

LINE No.	No. of Packages	Size of Package	Name of Item	National Drug Code	Packages Shipped	Date Shipped
1						
2						
3						
4						
5			VOID			
6						
7						
8						
9						
10						

◀ LAST LINE COMPLETED *(MUST BE 10 OR LESS)* | SIGNATURE OF PURCHASER OR ATTORNEY OR AGENT

Date Issued | DEA Registration No. | Name and Address of Registrant

Schedules

Registered as a | No. of this Order Form

DEA Form -222 (Oct. 1992)

U.S. OFFICIAL ORDER FORMS - SCHEDULES I & II
DRUG ENFORCEMENT ADMINISTRATION
SUPPLIER'S Copy 1

FIGURE 9.2
DEA 222 Form

The DEA form must be completed online or on paper by the pharmacist for Schedule II drug purchasing.

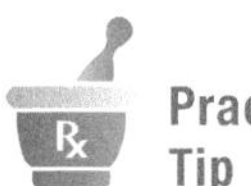

Practice Tip

The theft or loss of C-II drugs requires the pharmacist to complete a DEA 106 form and submit it to the DEA.

To order online, each pharmacy has a DEA registration number, and each of its pharmacists has a secure pharmacy user name and password protection. Online access to ordering allows next-day delivery in most cases. If Schedule II drugs are borrowed from another pharmacy, the pharmacist has to complete and sign a hard copy of a DEA 222 form.

Schedule II Receiving and Documentation When receiving the sealed totes of Schedule II drugs, the technician should check that the seal is not broken. The pharmacist must then personally break the seal on the tote and verify the contents with the invoice. After verification, the pharmacist must document the following information on the DEA 222 delivery receipt section: the date, the name and amount of Schedule II drugs received, and the corresponding NDC numbers. You, as the technician, can then post the Schedule II drug inventory to the database, including the NDC numbers, prices, and expiration dates.

Controlled Substance Disposal As Schedule II substances in the inventory expire or are defective (such as a case of broken tablets), they must be disposed of properly. Any controlled drug disposal must be itemized, recorded, witnessed, and signed by a second pharmacist. In most cases, Schedule II drugs are saved for destruction until the next visit of the state drug inspector, or they are returned to an authorized destruction depot after proper documentation has been completed and filed. (The proper disposal of other drugs, needles, and materials will be addressed in Chapter 14 on medication safety.)

The DEA also allows community pharmacies to conduct take-back programs as a customer service. These programs allow patients to bring in (or mail in) their unused, unwanted, or expired prescribed controlled substances (not illegal substances) to a pharmacy-maintained collection receptacle. (Take-back programs are also covered more in Chapter 14.) The receptacle must be stored in the locked portion of the pharmacy with the controlled substances, where an employee is always present. Community pharmacies may also maintain take-back control substance receptacles at long-term care facilities they service if there is a locked, staffed area.

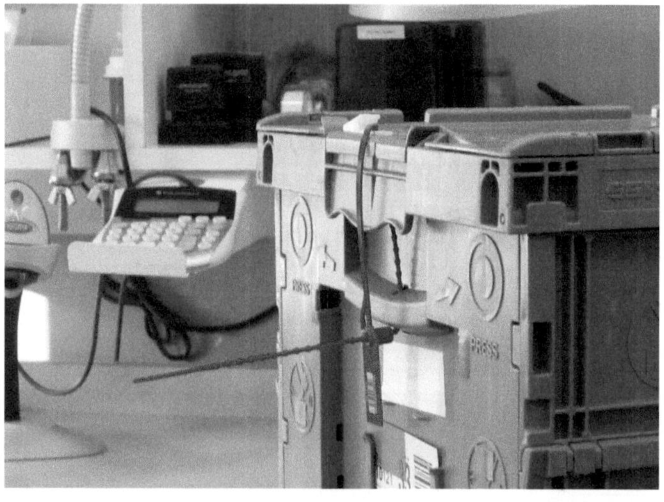
The seal on totes for controlled substances must arrive undisturbed and must be broken only by a pharmacist.

Schedule II Perpetual Inventory Record As you have seen, the inventory of controlled substances must be documented at every step in the process, from purchasing through storage, dispensing, and disposal. (Dispensing documentation will be explained in Chapter 14.) The precise count of each and every capsule, tablet, patch, liquid, injection, and other forms must be accounted for at all times. Because of this, there are special policies, procedures, and schedules for counting the inventory of controlled drug substances. Community pharmacies use automated or manual perpetual inventory to maintain inventory and close control of all Schedule II drug stock.

A **perpetual inventory record** is a method of accounting for all Schedule II medications on a tablet-by-tablet (or other dosage form) basis. Figure 9.3 shows an example of a printed perpetual inventory record, which documents each and every dosage of Schedule II drugs received and dispensed. This record includes product, dosage, quantity, date received or dispensed, prescription number, remaining inventory, and signature or initials of the pharmacist. Community pharmacies typically use an automated perpetual inventory system.

Biennial Inventory Count In addition, a biennial (every two years) inventory of Schedule II drugs must be taken. Some states (and pharmacies) have even more stringent requirements, such as a yearly inventory. These inventories should closely approximate the perpetual inventory record. For Schedules III, IV, and V substances, an estimated count and/or measure is permitted, unless a container holds more than 1,000 capsules or tablets. If the container has been opened, an exact count is required.

FIGURE 9.3
Perpetual Inventory Record

Some pharmacies use red ink pens for quantities removed from inventory for dispensing, and black ink pens for amounts of inventory received or maintained.

Drug and Dose	Oxycodone 5 mg/325 mg APAP
Record Starting Date	01/02/202X
Record Starting Quantity	500

Prescription Number	Dispensing Date	Quantity Dispensed	Cumulative Total	RPh Initials
246734	01/03/202X	40	460	RJA
247981	01/06/202X	16	444	RJA
248103	01/07/202X	120	324	RJA
DEA 001234988	01/10/202X	+500	824	RJA
249008	01/12/202X	60	764	RJA

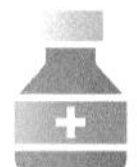

Pharm Fact

Whenever a pharmacy is in the process of being sold, an inventory count is required, and the value of the drug stock is included in the purchase price.

The Schedule II inventory count should not vary by more than four days from the biennial inventory date. The copy of the inventory must be sent online to the DEA, or the original hard copy must be sent by mail. Major deviations on Schedule II drug inventory must be investigated and reported if not resolved.

Additional tracking mechanisms exist by state and federal authorities to monitor the distribution of Schedule II drugs. If there is evidence of overprescribing by a physician, overdispensing by a pharmacy, or overselling of Schedule II drugs by a wholesaler, the DEA—after a thorough investigation—has the authority to temporarily or permanently revoke the DEA license of that physician, pharmacy, or wholesaler. A wholesaler can limit the monthly amount of controlled substances distributed to a community pharmacy if it deems that there has been excessive use.

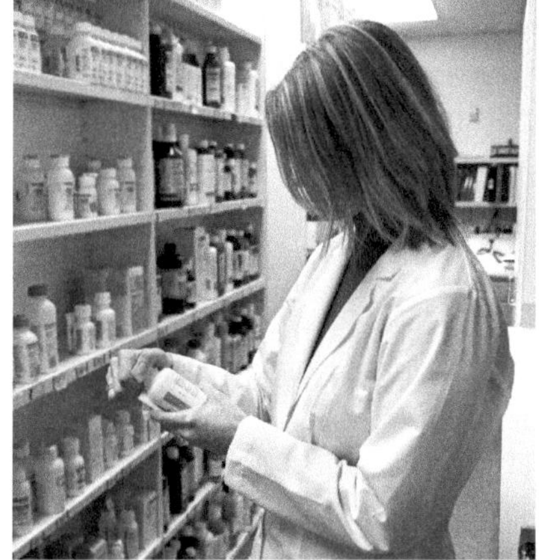

An experienced technician is responsible for ordering and stocking not only the drug product inventory, but necessary medical supplies and supplements as well.

Estimating Overall Drug Inventory Value and Turnover

Once each year, each item in stock must be counted, and the task is often assigned to a senior pharmacy technician, or it is outsourced. The inventory survey is used to determine the inventory value (cost) and turnover rate and to make any necessary adjustments in stock levels. Many pharmacies aim for an **inventory turnover rate** of approximately 10–12 times a year. If the inventory of a specific drug or product turns over every other month, the turnover rate is 6. If the inventory turns over every month, the rate is 12.

From the information gleaned from the inventory assessment, several important inventory decisions must be made:

1. How much of each drug and product should be maintained?
2. When should inventory levels be adjusted?
3. Where should inventory be stored?

Factors that need to be considered for these decisions encompass the individual pharmacy's track record of product turnover, the new drugs being released that will need to be added, floor space allocation, design and arrangement of shelves, and demands on available refrigerator or freezer space. Adjustments may include returning a portion of the drug stock to a wholesaler, selling or transferring stock to another pharmacy, and lowering automatic restock levels.

Because inventory information takes time to get to know well, technicians need experience working with the various aspects of inventory management before they move into positions of such responsibility. By watching the sales reports and inventory trends, a technician can begin to know enough to assist the pharmacist in suggesting the most appropriate minimum and maximum inventory levels to be set in the inventory control software.

9.7 Pharmacy Informatics and Computer System Health

Name Exchange

Pharmacy informatics is also known as pharmaco-informatics.

As you have seen, computers, software, and automation play an essential role in the everyday practice of a pharmacy technician. Pharmacies are dependent upon computers and software to process prescriptions swiftly, accurately, and safely; run the cash registers and process credit; track inventory; purchase and receive deliveries; and run measurements to assess productivity and profitability. This is the realm of **pharmacy informatics**, and it encompasses the use of computer systems and software, online processing, and technology for the integration of pharmacy-related data, information, expertise, and automation.

Technicians who have a love for information technology have a great opportunity to combine their two loves into one by specializing in pharmacy informatics and helping pharmacies tailor their software to their specific needs.

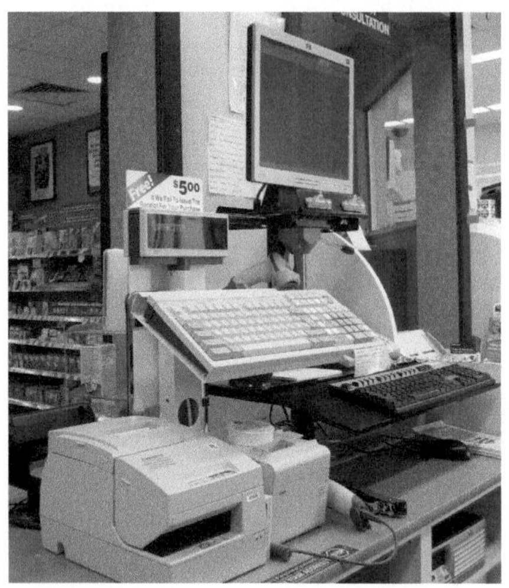

The workstation of the pharmacy technician often consists of a computer monitor, cash register, bar code, scanner, credit machine, telephone, and fax machine.

Productivity Reports

In addition to the many cash register, spreadsheet, inventory, and automation reports that the pharmacy informatics provide, **productivity reports** can also be generated. These reports compare staff time to prescriptions filled and other income-generating activities. They are formatted in different ways, such as by individual or group staff hours versus prescriptions generated or by individual or group hours versus sales income and reimbursements. Tracking productivity trends can be made visually clear with line and bar graphs.

Productivity reports need to be compared to safety reports. Do safety errors go up as productivity or swiftness of prescription filling goes up? Does customer satisfaction (i.e., waiting time) go up as productivity goes up? Community pharmacies do best when they emphasize safety and customer satisfaction while keeping productivity high. Experienced technicians can help establish and run needed reports, and also design customer satisfaction surveys and safety tracking mechanisms.

Concerns of Security and Stability of Information Systems

Though the move to digital systems makes the data sharing of the cash register, accounting, inventory, and pharmacy records easier and storage more stable, there are some concerns. Most of them revolve around data security. Software programs and online data must be guarded from viruses, data corruption, and hacking. Firewalls

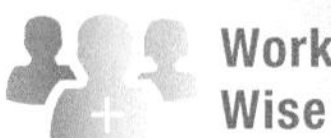

Some computer-savvy pharmacy technicians specialize as pharmacy informatic technicians. They help tailor software programs and maintain and repair the systems to fit the needs of the particular pharmacy in which they work.

from vendors of pharmacy software management systems minimize some of these risks. In recent years, databases of some PBMs and health insurance companies have been compromised by hackers. Technicians need to follow the pharmacy's procedures for protecting privacy and avoiding viruses.

Copies, or **backups**, of all data should be made by the main pharmacy computer(s) at regular intervals. A pharmacy can use remote storage, CDs, and other storage devices to back up its prescription records, usually on a daily basis. Some computer systems automatically collect and store prescription data daily with different storage options according to the pharmacy's **database management system (DBMS)**. For example, Computer-Rx offers two options to its community pharmacy: a nightly backup on an external hard drive that can be taken offsite for safekeeping in an emergency, or a backup system that immediately downloads the data to remote data centers in three different cities. Different pharmacies have different processes, based on their DBMS and their software vendor.

Electronic data storage and shared data information have offered great advantages in times of emergencies—as in fires, tornadoes, and floods—when paper records are often lost.

Computer Maintenance and Emergency Storage

Both the hardware and software of the pharmacy's computers, programs, and automated technology need to be cared for and maintained to stay high functioning. The equipment manuals for all the equipment must be followed to keep them running well.

Keeping the Pharmacy Software Up to Date

All of the pharmacy computer programs and automated technology must also undergo periodic software updates and upgrades. A **software update** brings all the information and programming of a currently installed program in line with the highest-functioning version available and the most current resource data. A **software upgrade** is a new edition of the software product with improved and enhanced capabilities. It is sold by the developer as a separate software product or an upgrade to a current version.

The pharmacy software services or vendors generally have programmed in regular updates and upgrades, or they will notify the pharmacy and technicians that the updates and upgrades are due. Online transmission of new data and programming can then be scheduled during off-hours (such as at night) or a nonpeak period. For regular maintenance and these program changes, the system usually has to be temporarily shut down.

Power and Data Backups for Emergencies

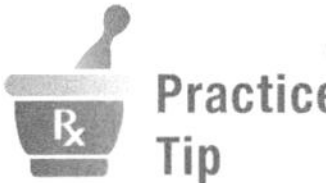

Pharmacies need to take time for data backup and to make contingency plans for natural disasters such as pandemics, tornadoes, floods, and fires.

In certain areas of the country, pharmacies may have backup generators for power outages to keep the lights on, computers going, cash registers operating, and refrigerators and freezers running. This is extremely important, as not only the prescription processing and billing depend on electricity, but the drug inventory depends on stable temperatures.

Many pharmacies in the areas affected by Hurricane Katrina sustained extreme losses due to the power outages and the hot weather that followed. Tracie Hoch, a commercial insurance underwriter, counseled in an emergency planning information brief, "You need a backup generator to not only secure your refrigerated products but also the stock on the shelf. During Hurricane Katrina, the stock on the shelf was condemned by the DEA because it was exposed to such high temperatures and high humidity for a number of days. Those pharmacies were a total loss...." (A change in temperature is not covered in most insurance policies.) Rallying to help, some pharmacies from unaffected areas sent pharmaceutical stock to help meet patient medication needs.

In most cases with a temporary interruption of power during a storm, prescription processing is halted until the power returns, and the pharmacy software system is able to be rebooted. Online insurance processing is also delayed until after internet access resumes. In emergencies, internet and cell phone transmissions can be down, intermittent, or slow, as happened in different areas of New York City right after 9/11. Because of the difficulties of accessing medical records during disasters, many state pharmacy boards allow pharmacists the discretion in an emergency to fill prescriptions based on patient bottles.

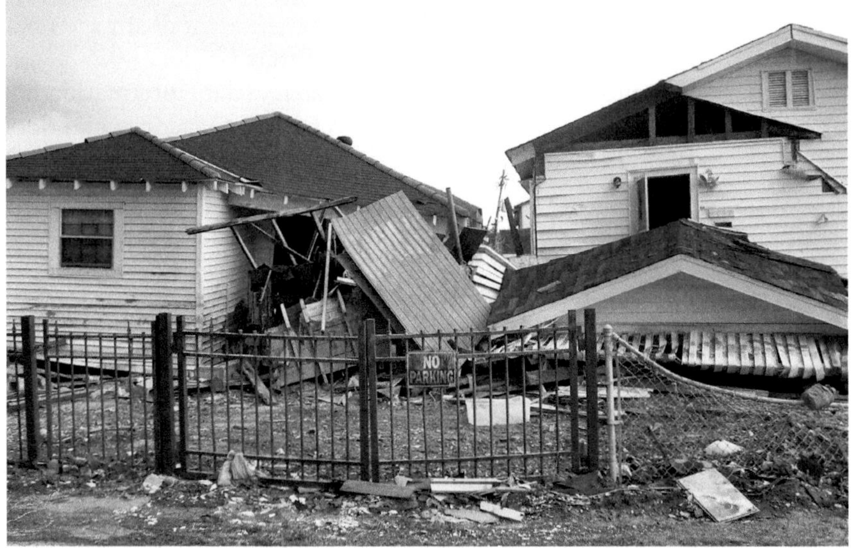

Many health records were lost in the flooding from Hurricane Katrina.

IN THE REAL WORLD

On Monday, August 29, 2005, Hurricane Katrina hit New Orleans, washing away stored patient records in hospitals, clinics, and pharmacies. Many healthcare providers, like their patients, had to flee the city, so patients were left with no medical records or even prescriber memories to guide them.

With the help of public and private organizations, the US government set up KatrinaHealth, a website to help pharmacies, prescribers, and patients access any medical record information available in other data systems or found paper records. Veterans were in the best position because the Veterans Health Administration had been storing records since the 1970s in their VistA electronic health record system. As the entire healthcare system moves to electronic health records and shared data that extends beyond a particular community or region, patient medical records can be reconstructed after an area emergency by drawing on these remote sources.

After Hurricane Katrina, some pharmacies found that the data backups made during the storm were no longer functional, some because of systematic glitches (no backup testing had occurred prior to the storm to see if the systems worked) and some because of computer storage water damage. Technology companies had to try to recover and reconstruct the missing information.

Jon Nolen, VP of information technology at Computer-Rx, told an *Elements* magazine reporter, "We understand the importance of data backup and what it can mean for a business following a disaster. Our company was devastated by the EF-5 tornado that traveled through the Oklahoma metro area in 1999." Disaster planning has become more a part of long-range vision in community and hospital pharmacies. (To read the full article in *Elements* "Preparing Your Business for a Natural Disaster," go to https://PharmPractice7e.ParadigmEducation.com/PBAHealth.)

9.8 Becoming the Business-Savvy Technician

Clearly, the work of the pharmacy technician is key not only to safe, efficient prescription processing and accurate insurance billing, but also to the pharmacy's profitability. To accomplish work successfully in this retail context, you will need to acquire many marketable skills, from excellent customer sales service to pharmacy software processing skills and automation operation to effective inventory management.

All of these are areas you can learn through studying in your educational program, training in labs, and practice. Program-arranged externships are a great way to get a start on the hands-on aspects of the job. Once hired, you can continually grow in your career through on-the-job training, everyday classes, and additional workshops and specialty certification courses. As you progress in knowledge and responsibilities, you can find opportunities to specialize. Pharmacy informatics, inventory, and business administration are areas you can consider. A technician who possesses these skills will be a major asset to the profitability of the pharmacy and will find progressive employment and advancement.

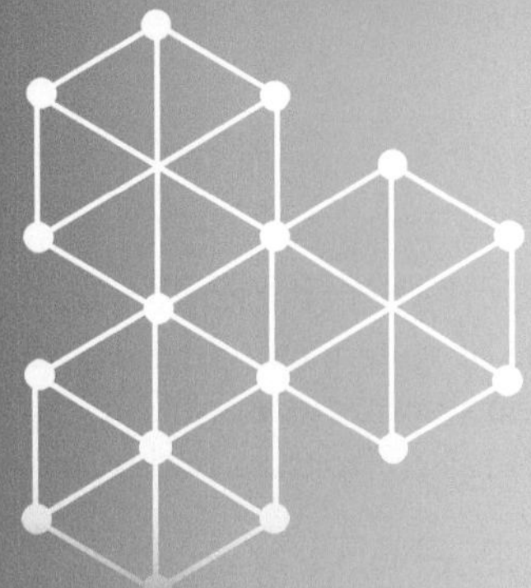

Review and Assessment

CHAPTER SUMMARY

- The technician has an important responsibility in assisting customers in locating needed OTC drugs and home health medical supplies and helping them interpret the labeling.
- Some OTC drugs—such as Schedule V cough syrups and decongestants containing pseudoephedrine—require specific procedures prior to sales.
- Holistic treatments focus on bringing the body back in balance as a path toward healing. Integrative medicines combine traditional medicine with non-traditional remedies.
- Dietary supplements (such as vitamins, minerals, herbals, and probiotics) do not have as extensive product labeling or testing as OTC drugs and are labeled with recommended "serving sizes" instead of doses.
- Vitamins, minerals, and herbals can have side effects and cause drug interactions.
- Dietary supplements labeled "USP Verified" have additional quality control assurances and can be recommended.
- The technician can assist patients with diabetes who need syringes, needles, test strips, glucometers, and related medical supplies.
- Patients with asthma or COPD may need a nebulizer, nebulizer solutions, a spacer, or a peak flow meter to treat or monitor their disease.
- The technician must be competent in all cash register management functions, including sales by cash (among them counting change), check, credit cards, debit cards, flex cards, and gift cards.
- The technician must become familiar with EMV-embedded chip credit card technology.
- Prescribed drugs and medical supplies are exempt from taxes by federal law. Other merchandise, including for health needs, can be taxed.
- State laws determine the rate of sales tax and what items can be taxed.
- A basic knowledge of both computer and mathematical skills is necessary for the technician to manage pharmacy business functions successfully.
- Adding the pharmacy markup to product prices and computing any discounts are often the responsibilities of the technician, who needs to understand how they are calculated and why.
- The technician's responsibilities in inventory management include the purchasing, receiving, and return of drugs for credit.

- Purchasing, receiving, counting inventory, and disposing of controlled substances all require specific legal documentation procedures.
- Checking expiration dates and returning unused drugs for credit to the wholesaler adds to the bottom line of the pharmacy.
- A technician is very important in handling any level of drug recall and the associated communication to patients and wholesalers.
- An experienced technician can assist the pharmacist in generating reports and setting periodic automatic replenishment (PAR) levels and minimum and maximum stock levels for each drug in the automated inventory control system.
- Computer software, hardware, and automation technology are essential and require ongoing maintenance and updating as well as sometimes individualized programming. Technicians can assist or specialize in pharmacy informatics.
- A technician can assist in running inventory, productivity, and safety reports as well as customer satisfaction surveys. · Pharmacies need to have plans for emergency backup systems for electricity, electronic storage, and internet service
- Pharmacies need to have plans for emergency backup systems for electricity, electronic storage, and internet service.

CHECK YOUR UNDERSTANDING

To ensure that you recall and understand the key chapter concepts, please read the question or statement and select the appropriate lettered option.

1. With OTC drugs the pharmacy technician is legally permitted to do all the following *with the exception of*
   a. making the sale.
   b. reviewing labeled directions.
   c. counseling.
   d. helping to locate the desired product.
2. The FDA discourages the use of which class of drugs for children under the age of 6 years old due to a high risk of adverse reactions?
   a. pain relievers
   b. fever reducers
   c. homeopathic medications
   d. cough and cold products
3. Which of the following is a restricted drug requiring special documentation?
   a. pseudoephedrine
   b. regular insulin
   c. probiotics
   d. dextromethorphan
4. For insurance to cover a nebulizer and medications, the pharmacy technician will need to submit
   a. ICD-10 diagnostic codes.
   b. NDC numbers of DME.
   c. the DEA number of the provider.
   d. a letter of justification from the provider.

5. Which of the following is not considered a dietary supplement?
   a. vitamin
   b. mineral
   c. OTC drug
   d. herbal

6. Which dietary supplement is used to treat insomnia in overnight shift workers?
   a. ginger
   b. ginkgo
   c. policosanol
   d. melatonin

MAKE CONNECTIONS

Take a moment to consider what you have learned in this chapter and respond thoughtfully to the following prompts. Note that some of these activities will require internet access.

1. As part of a team or a pair, create an informative, 15-minute PowerPoint presentation on the topic of diabetes, specifically the economics of diabetes. Use the internet to research the following questions, and be sure to address them in your presentation. Include your references in the presentation.
   a. What is the average annual medical cost for a patient with diabetes?
   b. What is the breakdown of that annual medical cost?
   c. How much do diabetic supplies cost per year?
   d. Why is it so important for the technician to provide customer-oriented services to this population?
2. Pharmacy technicians have a very important role in the inventory management and profit of a community pharmacy. Write a short essay (250–500 words) on these issues and the pharmacy technician role in inventory management. Identify five important financial measures that are necessary to operate a successful independent pharmacy operation. How does the average pharmacy compare to the top 25% of pharmacies? Discuss the significance of each of these financial measures and how they can improve your bottom line.

The online course includes additional review and assessment resources.

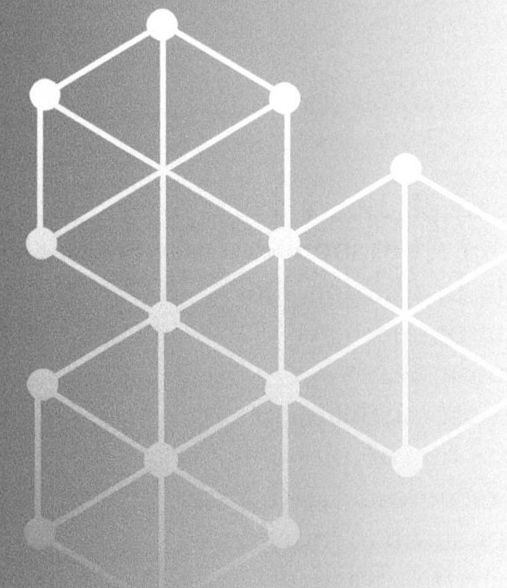

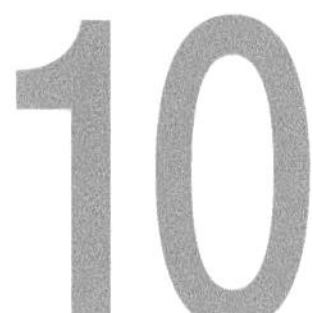

Extemporaneous, Nonsterile Compounding

Learning Objectives

1. Define the terms *compounding, extemporaneous, nonsterile, sterile,* and *anticipatory*, *compounding*.
2. Understand the distinction between a manufactured drug product and a compounded nonsterile preparation, and preparation and the purpose of Chapter <795>. (Section 10.1)
3. Understand the role and training requirements of pharmacy technicians in nonsterile compounding.
4. Explain the contemporary demands for nonsterile compounding and and the process for accreditation of specialty compounded pharmacies.
5. Describe the distinct purposes of the master formulation record and the compounding record.
6. Understand nonsterile compounding hand hygiene and garbing requirements.
7. Identify and describe the functions and limitations of the equipment used for the weighing, measuring, and compounding, and the proper techniques for using them.
8. Define the term *percentage of error* and its function.
9. Discuss the types of compounding ingredients and how to determine their quality and safety, and store them.
10. Define the various methods for the *comminution* and blending of ingredients.
11. Explain the differing techniques by which solutions, suspensions, ointments, creams, powders, suppositories, rapid dissolving tablets, troches, and capsules are prepared.
12. Understand the final compounding steps including calculating *beyond-use-dating*, labeling, offering patient education, and doing cleaning-up and equipment maintenance.

ASHP/ACPE Accreditation Standards
To view the *ASHP/ACPE Accreditation Standards* addressed in this chapter, refer to Appendix B.

Though most medications are manufactured in a drug production facility, the practice of compounding in the pharmacy is on the upswing. Today, approximately 40–120 million prescriptions are compounded in the United States each year, which is estimated to be 1%–3% of prescriptions dispensed (according to the International Academy of Compounding Pharmacists). General community and hospital pharmacies and their pharmacy personnel often do some simple compounding and even a little moderately complex compounding, but most complex nonsterile compounding occurs at dedicated pharmacies.

Nonsterile pharmaceutical compounding is both a necessary pharmacy skill and, on the complex end, a pharmacy specialty. It comes with a unique set of supplies, techniques, terminology, calculations, and decisions to be made. In addition, like other areas of pharmacy practice, nonsterile pharmaceutical compounding is governed by specific federal and state laws, regulations, and standards.

Because many high-volume chain pharmacies (and even most independent pharmacies) do not have the time, space, equipment, or expertise for complex compounding, specially trained community pharmacists and their technicians are increasingly being called upon to prepare a recipe or compound a preparation in individualized doses or strengths for human or veterinary use. To engage in this practice, pharmacy technicians must have advanced training and experience and devote the majority of their workday to performing precise calculations and mixing ingredients rather than dispensing prescriptions, billing insurance companies, or communicating with patients.

Even if you will not be doing this work intensely in the first years of being a technician, it is important to be able to do simple compounding in case you are called upon to do so. It is also helpful to have an understanding of what is involved to see if this may be a specialty you may someday want to pursue.

10.1 Types of Compounding

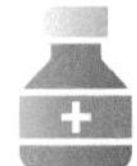

Pharm Fact

Simply following manufacturers' directions for reconstituting, flavoring, or diluting is not compounding. It is only considered compounding in the United States when preparations are made for products not available from manufacturers in the needed form, dosage, concentration, or other integral characteristic.

Compounding is, as they say, both an art and a skill. It is defined as the process in which a pharmacist or a technician uses bulk ingredients to prepare a prescribed medication that treats a specific patient's medical condition. It involves preparing, mixing, assembling, altering, packaging, and labeling a prescription according to a formulated recipe and prescription by a licensed prescriber who individualizes the appropriate quantity and dosage form for the patient. This can include steps of reconstituting, diluting, concentrating, flavoring, or changing a dosage form. However, if one is just reconstituting, diluting, or flavoring a manufactured medication according to the directions on the product package insert or labeling, this is not compounding. It is merely following product-specific dispensing directions.

For instance, mixing a powdered antibiotic according to the manufacturer's directions with a compatible diluent such as distilled water to make an oral suspension (or adding the recommended flavoring) is *not* considered compounding. But if you reconstitute a medication and then put it into a different dose or dosage formulation than the usual, or combine it with another medication in an individualized way, this *is* compounding.

Compounding is getting off the beaten path of dispensing the manufactured products to creating something more individualized that is not available on the market. In the most complex compounding, it is not just a skill but an art, where the pharmacist has to interpret the best way to individualize an established formula to fit the prescriber's unique instructions for the patient. The specially trained technician becomes an assistant in this artful application of tailored medication creation.

Sterile Compounding

Sterile compounding uses aseptic technique to prepare solutions free of microorganisms for parenteral products or ophthalmic preparations. Sterile compounding is performed in a cleanroom environment. These are found in hospitals and in home care infusion and nuclear pharmacies as well as in specialty compounding facilities.

Sterile compounding must be performed under strictly controlled environmental conditions to minimize the risk of contamination of the **compounded sterile preparations (CSPs)**. The guidelines for sterile compounding—including a clean-room environment, correct aseptic technique, and specialized equipment and training—are discussed in Chapters 12 and 13.

Nonsterile Compounding

Though not prepared in as controlled an environment as sterile compounding, **nonsterile compounding** follows particular guidelines to keep medications as contamination-free as possible within a sanitized compounding space in a community or compounding pharmacy. These guidelines are found in *United States Pharmacopeial Convention (USP)* General Chapter <795>. Since the drug formulations (such as capsules, tablets, ointments, creams, solutions, suspensions, powders, and suppositories) are not injected directly into a vein, aseptic technique and sterility are not required, but drug safety, stability, and integrity remain important concerns.

Put Down Roots

Extemporaneous comes from the Latin *ex tempore*, meaning "out of the time," or coming from the time. So it means compounding for an immediate need made for the occasion.

Current laws require that nonsterile compounding occurs only for medications, dosages, and forms that are *not commercially available*. When compounding occurs for a specific need of the moment for a particular patient, it is known as **extemporaneous compounding**. This is the majority of nonsterile compounding in a community pharmacy. Common compounding prescription requests include creating an oral suspension from crushed tablets or a topical ointment from a drug administered by a different route, or mixing two solutions for an ear drop. Medical specialists (especially dermatologists and gynecologists) and dentists often prefer to individualize their prescriptions for their patients. Physicians from hospice care for the terminally ill and pain management clinics often use the services of a compounding pharmacy to meet patients' specific pain needs.

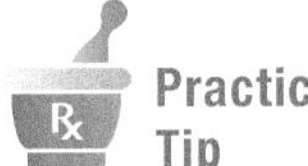

Practice Tip

Compounding uses more individualized instructions and calculations than the manufacturer's general directions.

Nonsterile compounding comes in three levels of complexity:

- Simple—reconstituting and recombining commercial products following USP monograph directions or peer-reviewed articles with specific quantities, common formularies, or a manufacturer's guidelines established and requiring no unknown calculations
- Moderate—requiring some special calculations
- Complex—requiring special calculations, decision making, training, procedures, equipment, and environment

To gain a better understanding of the circumstances in which nonsterile compounding is performed in the pharmacy setting, here are some possible scenarios:

- For a young, underweight child, a prescriber orders a medication dose smaller than any dose commercially available. For example, the prescription calls for 10 mg per dose of a medication available only in 30 mg unscored tablets. The technician (under pharmacist supervision) may pulverize the tablets and then mix the powder with an inactive powder to fill capsules containing the weight equivalent to 10 mg of the active medication.

Compounding, or the art of pharmacy, involves combining patient-specific medications.

- A medication typically available in a solid dosage form is prescribed in another dosage form—such as a liquid, suspension, or suppository—for administration to patients who cannot or will not swallow the solid form or are experiencing severe nausea. The tablets may need to be triturated using a mortar and pestle and then the powder added to a suitable suspending agent.
- A prescriber requests a commercially available dose or dosage form that is no longer available due to a drug shortage or back order, so it must be specially prepared.
- To ensure that a child will take an oral medication (currently in a tablet or capsule form) usually dosed for adults that has an unpleasant bitter taste, it must be prepared first in a child's dosage amount and then compounded in a syrup vehicle with a more palatable, flavor-masking base.
- A topical gel formulation must be prepared for a patient whose oral medication has had adverse effects on the stomach (such as causing ulcers).
- A patient has allergies to a commercial medication's preservatives, colorings, or other ingredients, so an alternative without the unwanted ingredients needs to be prepared.
- To reduce side effects, a postmenopausal woman may have the need for a hormone replacement therapy formulation besides the commercially available fixed-dose tablets. A compounded mixture of hormones in a cream or gel formulation can be individualized to relieve the patient's symptoms and minimize side effects.

Products compounded for veterinary use cannot be used in humans.

Many drugs used in humans can also be used to treat other animals in different dosages and forms. Veterinarians frequently require the compounding expertise of pharmacies to fulfill the unique medication requirements of the animals in their care, such as a thyroid medication for a cat or seizure medications for a dog.

That is why many community pharmacies receive a portion of their business from veterinary referrals. Nonsterile compounding allows medications to be catered to an animal's species and size. Technicians need to be aware of the rules of the American Veterinary Medical Association (AVMA), as spelled out in its "Guidelines for Veterinary

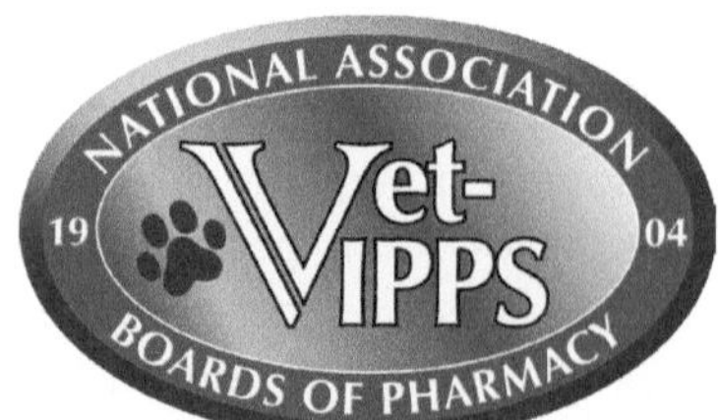

Online pharmacies that compound animal medications require verification in much the same way as pharmacies that compound human medication.

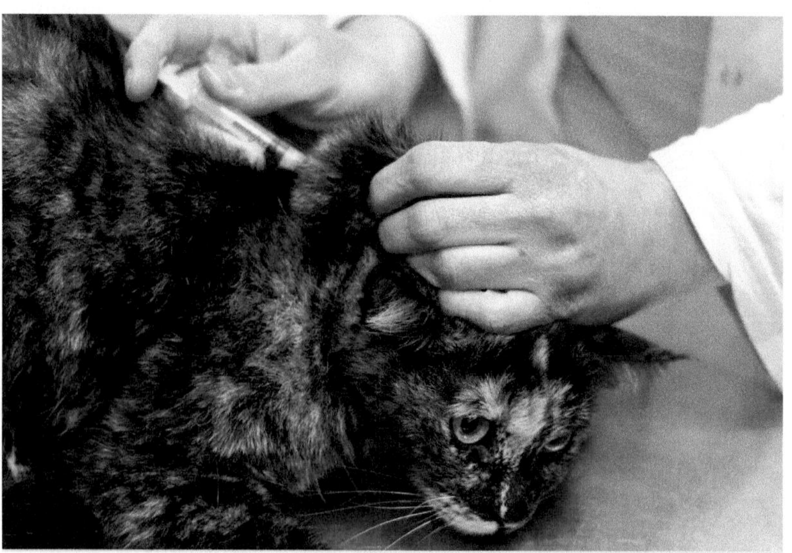

Compounding pharmacies often prepare a drug originally manufactured for humans in a special formulation for a pet.

Prescription Drugs" at https://PharmPractice7e.Paradigm Education.com/AVMA. The medications must be compounded from FDA-approved animal or human drugs. The AVMA assumes that the compounding pharmacy follows all *USP* Chapter <795> guidelines and is accredited. If the pharmacy is online, it should apply for the National Association of Boards of Pharmacy's Veterinary-Verified Internet Pharmacy Practice Sites accreditation.

10.2 Nonsterile Compounding Laws, Regulations, and Standards

According to the International Academy of Compounding Pharmacies, approximately 7,500 independent pharmacies offer *advanced compounding services*; fewer than half of these pharmacies compound sterile preparations. Both nonsterile and sterile compounding practices and facilities are regulated by federal and state laws and regulations, as well as by United States Pharmacopeial Convention (USP) guidelines and standards.

Food and Drug Administration Modernization Act of 1997

Before 1997, there were no specific federal or state laws governing the practices of pharmacy compounding; thus, the distinction between manufacturing and compounding was not defined. The Food and Drug Administration Modernization Act (FDAMA) of 1997—an amendment to the Federal Food, Drug, and Cosmetic (FD&C) Act—clarified the status of pharmacy compounding. This legislation allowed pharmacists to compound nonsterile medications for individual patients if these medications met established USP standards.

The amendment distinguishes compounding from manufacturing practices. The major provisions state that compounded products do not need to follow new drug approval processes and legislation as **manufactured drug products** do. In addition, compounding pharmacies *are not required to* follow all the specifics of **current good manufacturing practices (CGMPs)**, which are the main regulatory standards for the manufacturing of pharmaceuticals. Instead, they need to follow the compounding guidelines set out in *USP* Chapters <795>, <797> (rev. 2019), and the newly implemented <800> (2016).

Compounding pharmacies *do not* need to adhere to product labeling regarding directions for use or submit drug approval applications. The law assumes that public health concerns are minor when mass production is not involved. The exemptions are not meant to undermine the safety and effectiveness of compounded products; rather, they are based on the assumption that compounded products are typically used for a small group of patients with specific medical needs. With adherence to USP standards, the compounder can control quality if drug products are prepared in small quantities. The goal is to achieve a safe, stable, effective product that is **pharmaceutically elegant**, which means that it is aesthetically pleasing, both in appearance and application.

Medications are typically compounded only after the specific prescription is received at the pharmacy. However, pharmacies are allowed to prepare more than they need at that moment to have some on hand for refills or a similar need—a practice called **anticipatory compounding**. The excess quantity, however, must be limited to what will be reasonably used in a short time period and must be labeled with a lot

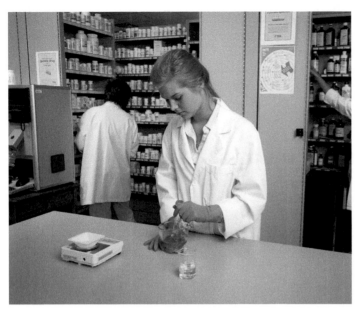

Many compounding pharmacies specialize in preparing and dispensing only nonsterile prescriptions.

number and a beyond-use date (discussed later in this chapter). For example, the original prescription may call for a quantity of 30 rapid-dissolving hormone tablets, but the mold to compound this dosage form has the capacity for 96 tablets. Therefore, 30 tablets are dispensed with the prescription, and the remaining 66 tablets are appropriately labeled and stored for this patient's refill or a future prescription.

Like retail pharmacies, compounding pharmacies must be licensed by both the federal government (including a license by the Drug Enforcement Administration if the pharmacy is compounding controlled substances) and the state government. If a facility specializes in compounding a prescription product in bulk for the projected needs of the market (nonextemporaneous compounding) and selling it to other pharmacies or healthcare professionals, the facility must apply for a manufacturing license as outlined by the Drug Quality and Security Act (DQSA) of 2013. The manufacturing license requires additional regulations, procedures, and quality-control checks.

Practice Tip

Compounding pharmacies are overseen by FDA, USP, Accreditation Commission for Health Care, and state standards.

If this compounding facility sells preparations to an out-of-state pharmacy or healthcare facility, it also is required to apply for a pharmacy license in the other state(s). The compounding disaster that prompted the DQSA was the 2012 outbreak of fungal meningitis from epidural injections of a contaminated cortisone injection solution. This product was prepared in a sterile compounding pharmacy that failed to follow guidelines, and the product was distributed to many states. The effects of this law upon compounding pharmacies were discussed in Chapter 2.

In addition, other federal and state regulations must be followed. If the compounding involves hazardous ingredients, the appropriate requirements of the Occupational Safety and Health Administration (OSHA) and the **National Institute for Occupational Safety and Health (NIOSH)** must also be followed (addressed in Chapter 13).

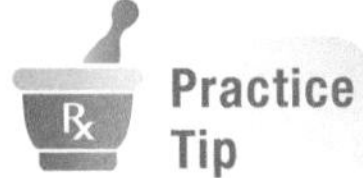

Practice Tip

State regulations on nonsterile compounding are often very similar but can be different, so they must be checked and followed.

State and Professional Oversight

As with community pharmacies, compounding pharmacies must be licensed by the state board of pharmacy, which oversees their activities. However, for situations in which significant violations of manufacturing practices are identified, the Food and Drug Administration (FDA) cooperates with state authorities for inspections and follow-up actions. Inspection and enforcement require time and expertise and thus vary considerably among the states. Additionally, compounding quality checks can be problematic in states where compliance is voluntary. Working with the state boards are several nationwide professional organizations, including the International Academy of Compounding Pharmacists (IACP), the American Pharmacists Association (APhA), the American Society of Health-System Pharmacists (ASHP), the National Community Pharmacists Association (NCPA), and, most significantly as already noted, the USP.

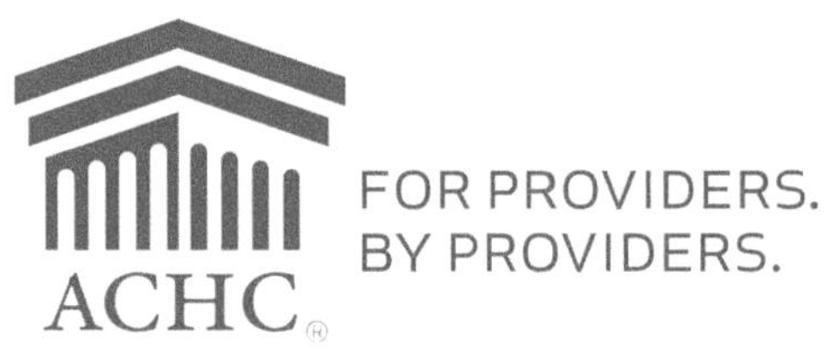

Compounding pharmacies can receive accreditation through the Pharmacy Compounding Accreditation Board (PCAB), a service of the Accreditation Commission for Health Care (ACHC).

Compounding pharmacies that go above and beyond the minimum regulation standards generally seek accreditation so that they can be recognized for the quality of their **compounded preparations**. The **Accreditation Commission for Health Care (ACHC)** specializes in accrediting facilities and pharmacies particularly oriented toward home health care, hospice care, alternative healthcare institutions, and medical supplies. The ACHC also administers the **Pharmacy Compounding Accreditation Board (PCAB)**, which offers a certification process for those pharmacies that comply with all national standards and the best industry practices in nonsterile and sterile compounding. Compounding pharmacies are allowed to advertise and market their compounding services, quality record, credentials of their personnel, and their certifications—*but not* the specific preparations they compound.

As part of maintaining accreditation, ACHS standards require that the facility have a **continuous quality improvement (CQI)** process to identify and resolve any problems in an ongoing way. It must do a monthly or quarterly spot check of each technician's work. A random product is selected and sent to an outside analytical lab for analysis of the exact measurements of the components and its sterile qualities. The product must be +/- 2% of the potency of the individual ingredients. If the analysis suggests that steps in a procedure were not followed or ingredients were not measured correctly, then the pharmacist must take, document, and date the corrective action, often requiring the technician to have additional training.

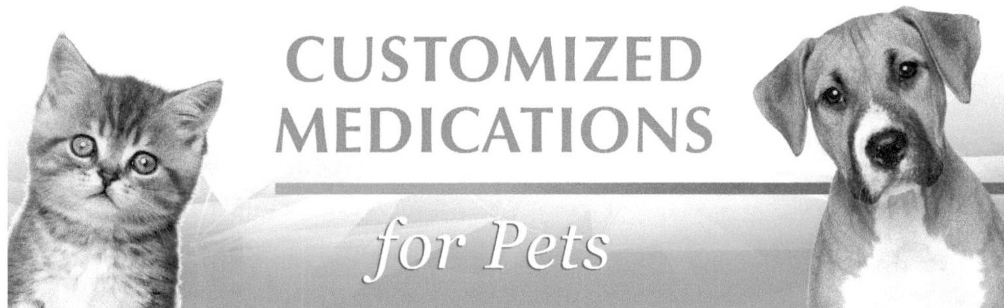

Customized compounding services may be offered at certain pharmacies for nonsterile and sterile prescription preparations for women, men, children, and pets.

USP Chapter <795> Standards

In lieu of current good manufacturing practices (CGMPs), the USP requires that a compounding pharmacy follow **good compounding practices (GCPs)**, as outlined in Table 10.1. The pharmacist and the pharmacy technician share the responsibility to ensure that all the GCPs are accomplished.

The *USP-NF* (a combination of the *United States Pharmacopeia* and *National Formulary*), the official global publication whose guidelines are a mainstay for pharmacists and pharmacy technicians, devotes a chapter to each type of compounding: *USP* Chapter <795> for nonsterile compounding, *USP* <797> for sterile compounding, and *USP* <800> (2016) for hazardous drugs. Although USP is not affiliated with any governmental agency, the FDA and state boards of pharmacies use and enforce these USP standards in the inspection of compounding pharmacies.

TABLE 10.1 USP Good Compounding Practices

Components of GCPs	Standards
Facility	A designated area with adequate space and a separate area for sterile compounding
Personnel	Staff members with education, training, and proficiency in this specialized area; compounders must wear protective clothing
Equipment	Appropriate design, size, and space of balances and measuring devices; equipment must be cleaned and calibrated
Ingredient selection	Only high-grade chemicals; ingredients are used and stored appropriately
Compounding process	Each step reviewed by the pharmacist, who makes a final check of the completed product
Packaging and storage	All ingredients and containers properly labeled
Controls	Quality control programs implemented by the pharmacist
Labeling of excess product	Labels showing quantity and lot number
Beyond-use dating	Stability (and sterility in some cases) of preparation reflected in beyond-use dating
Records and reports	Documents including Master Formulation Record, Compounding Record, and equipment maintenance, and logs and records of the ingredients
Patient counseling	Discussion with patient on safe administration and storage of the compounded preparation

In addition to the nonsterile compounding guidelines in *USP* <795>, compounding technicians need to utilize the guidelines in related *USP* Chapters:

- <1151> Pharmaceutical Dosage Forms
- <1160> Pharmaceutical Calculations in Prescription Compounding
- <1163> Quality Assurance in Pharmaceutical Compounding
- <1176> Prescription Balances and Volumetric Apparatus
- <1191> Stability Considerations in Dispensing Practice
- <1265> Written Prescription Drug Information Guidelines

10.3 The Role of the Technician in Nonsterile Compounding

The pharmacy technician often assists the pharmacist with the time-consuming and labor-intensive tasks:

- retrieving the recipe
- gathering all necessary ingredients and equipment
- calibrating the equipment if necessary
- weighing, measuring, mixing, and preparing products
- checking and ordering quality inventory ingredients
- calculating beyond-use dates

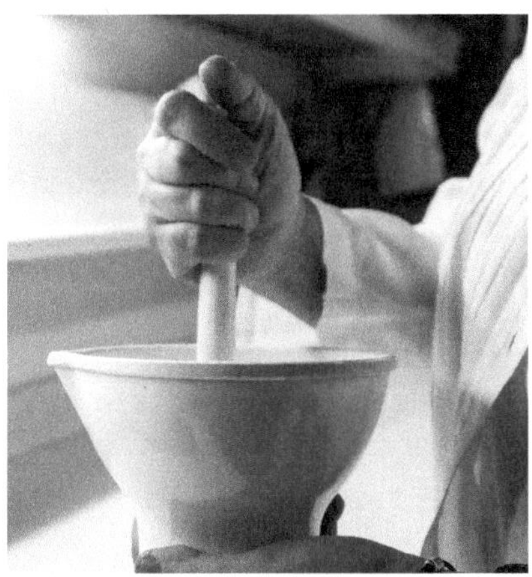

Technicians may prepare nonsterile compounds in either a community pharmacy or a compounding pharmacy, as long as a pharmacist is always present in the room.

- printing and affixing labels
- maintaining a clean work environment

Any compounding tasks undertaken by the technician must, in any case, be directly supervised in the same room and checked by the pharmacist. The equipment and techniques utilized are discussed later in this chapter.

Technicians who do simple and moderate compounding in community and hospital pharmacies should have successfully passed one of the general national pharmacy technician certification examinations (discussed in Chapter 1 and explained in more detail in Chapter 16) and have experience. Technicians must also have sufficiently studied and practiced calculations and compounding skills.

To work in a dedicated compounding pharmacy, both pharmacists and pharmacy technicians require special training. The technicians are encouraged to complete mini-certifications and laboratory training in nonsterile compounding. The knowledge and skills necessary to pass these specialty certification exams are presented as workshops and labs by the **Professional Compounding Centers of America (PCCA)**. It is now an international organization, uniting compounding pharmacists and technicians in the United States, Canada, Australia, and other countries of the world. Some academic pharmacy programs—like the one at the Austin Community College in Texas for pharmacy technicians and the one at the University of Florida Health in Gainesville for pharmacists—also offer special compounding courses.

To compound nonsterile drug products with hazardous substances, technicians must have additional training on the storage, handling, and disposal of these chemicals. Specialty training, experience, and certification must be documented, as it is generally necessary for employment and for the compounding pharmacy to attain or maintain accreditation with the ACHC. The training must be ongoing and reevaluated annually.

The required education credits and training for hazardous substances can be found from less traditional sources. Cardinal Health offers the ChemoPlus Chemotherapy Training and Certification Program for Compounding Hazardous Drugs. Critical Point, a training company, also offers a hazardous drug compounding program. The University of South Carolina's Kennedy Pharmacy Innovation Center offers seven hours of live continuing education credits in hazardous drug compounding.

10.4 The Nonsterile Compounding Process and Documentation

Nonsterile compounding is initiated by the receipt of a provider's prescription. The prescription is entered into the patient medication profile, which includes all the original prescription orders and the compounds dispensed to the patient. In compounding, however, the pharmacist seeks out or, in rare cases, develops an appropriate delineated formula of instructions, or a recipe, called the **Master Formulation Record**. Using this master formula, the technician and the pharmacist create an individualized version for the specific patient's batch that is generated, called the **Compounding Record**. This is followed (or modified with notes) and documented for tracking. It is important to understand in depth how these records are related and work.

As with any prescription, the Drug Utilization Review (DUR) must be run, and close attention must be paid to patient allergies and any interactions with other medications or medical conditions.

Master Formulation Record

Formulas for the master recipe can be found via USP or PCCA formularies, medical literature, research institutions, professional organizations, hospitals, physicians, and other compounding pharmacies. A Master Formulation Record can also be provided by a subscriber compounding software service, such as Compounder Lab and The Compounder Rx from the Professional Compounding Centers of America's PK Software. The recipes have to have been proven effective and safe, and they must provide all the active and inactive ingredients, quantities and/or proportions, directions for proper sequencing, mixing, and calculations. The pharmacist uses their best professional judgment to assess the safety and suitability of compounding the prescription as well as its intended use, especially on new orders for which a recipe must be found or created. Physicians are open to suggestions from the pharmacist to improve the quality or safety of the compounding prescriptions.

The chosen formula then becomes the source of the compounding pharmacy's Master Formulation Record, which will be stored in the pharmacy's computer database or as a hard copy on recipe-like cards stored in a file box for current and future use. Figure 10.1 is an example of a computerized Master Formulation Record from the PCCA. The Master Formulation Record must have an identifying number and list each prescribed drug's name, strength, and dosage form, and the ingredients and their quantities. In addition, this record contains the following useful information:

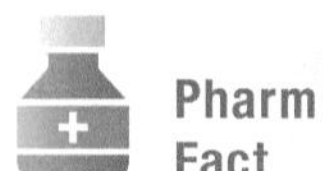

Community pharmacies usually use Master Formulation Records developed by specialized organizations or businesses such as the USP or PCCA.

- calculations needed to determine doses of active ingredients
- compatibility and stability information on ingredients and final compound
- equipment needed to prepare the preparation
- detailed mixing instructions, including sequencing, duration, and temperature
- required labeling information, including beyond-use dating
- packaging and storing requirements, including container used in dispensing
- quality control procedures/tests

When Master Formulation Records are updated or changed, the obsolete ones need to be deleted or thrown out to avoid confusion.

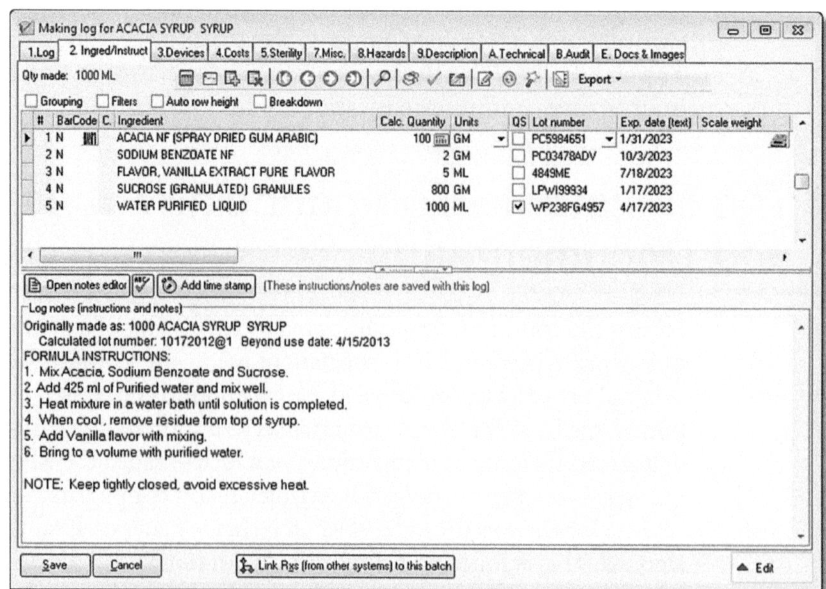

FIGURE 10.1
Computerized Master Control Record

This Master Formulation Record was created using PCCA's PK Software.

Compounding Record

A printed Compounding Record is generated for each patient's prescription, which is a unique batch of the master formula. Calculations for the amounts of individual ingredients for the specific prescription must be made initially by the pharmacist and be documented on the printout. The pharmacist also identifies on the record any special equipment the technician needs to use when compounding the preparation. This Compounding Record is then turned over to the pharmacy technician to initiate the preparation of the product.

The Compounding Record lists the following information:

- name of the compound, strength, and dosage
- Master Formulation Record reference number
- names and quantities of all ingredients, including source, lot numbers, and their individual expiration dates
- total quantity made
- name of the person who prepared the preparation, the one who performed the quality control procedures, and the one who approved the preparation
- date of compounding
- assigned control or Rx number
- assigned beyond-use dating
- duplicate label
- description of final preparation
- results of quality control procedures performed by the pharmacist
- documentation of any quality control problems or adverse reactions reported

The calculations are double-checked by the pharmacy technician in the compounding process and verified by the pharmacist after the preparation has been compounded.

For an example of a Compounding Record, see Figure 10.2, which shows the ingredients and directions for compounding a preparation called Magic Mouthwash.

FIGURE 10.2
Compounding Log

This record is for a commonly made formula of Magic Mouthwash.

Patient Name ____________ Date Prepared 12/2/202X

Rx # ____________ Master Control Record # ____________

Compounding Formula for Magic Mouthwash

Ingredient Name	Amount Needed	Manufacturer	NDC #	Lot #	Expiration Date	Prepared By	Checked By
Lidocaine 2% viscous	60 mL	Hi-Tech	50838-0775-04		12/10/202X		
Diphenhydramine 12.5 mg/mL	60 mL	Walgreens	00363-0379-34		07/12/202X		
Mylanta, generic	60 mL	Qualitest	00603-0712-57		03/12/202X		
Nystatin suspension	60 mL	Qualitest	00603-1481-58		09/11/202X		
Total quantity	240 mL						

Prepared by ____________

Approved by ____________

Date ____________

Directions ____________

Auxiliary Labeling: SHAKE WELL

This formula has many variations in different regions of the country and is commonly compounded in many community pharmacies. It is prepared by mixing together commercially available liquids or suspensions to make a new product. The technician should always list the source of the ingredients, the NDC number, and the product expiration date on the Compounding Record, especially if the manufacturer of any bulk ingredient has recently changed.

Safety Alert

Accuracy is crucial when compounding medications. In order to give yourself time to double-check your work, compounding should never be rushed.

The Compounding Process Steps

Table 10.2 summarizes the 14 steps required by *USP* <795> to compound a nonsterile preparation. These steps, or something similar, should appear in the **Policy and Procedure (P&P) Manual** for the community or compounding pharmacy. Each step is checked and initialed by the pharmacist and the pharmacy technician. If these steps are followed on each and every compounded prescription, the preparation's quality and effectiveness will be maximized while the risk of medication errors will be minimized. Following these steps also minimizes legal liability and ensures continuing accreditation status.

TABLE 10.2 Steps in the Compounding Process

1. The pharmacist does a Drug Utilization Review and judges the suitability of the prescription for safety and intended use.
2. The technician retrieves and reviews the Master Control Record in the computer.
3. The technician prints out a Compounding Record or log sheet for the technician to make the nonsterile preparation.
4. The technician performs all necessary mathematical calculations and identifies the necessary equipment for the technician; the pharmacist double-checks all calculations.
5. A medication container label is created by the computer software using information in the compounding log. The label includes the following:
   a. patient name
   b. physician name
   c. date of compounding
   d. name of preparation
   e. internal ID or lot number
   f. beyond-use date
   g. initials of compounding technician and pharmacist
   h. directions for use, including any special storage conditions
   i. any additional requirements of state or federal law
6. The pharmacy technician uses appropriate protective clothing and handwashing technique.
7. The technician gathers all necessary active and inactive ingredients as well as prepares and calibrates any necessary equipment.
8. The technician weighs and adds all ingredients for the preparation, initials each step, and adds documentation (such as source and NDC number) to the Compounding Record.
9. The technician stores the medication in a suitable container.
10. The technician affixes the medication label to the proper container.
11. The pharmacist reviews the Compounding Record (with the printout of the weights of all ingredients) and the medication container label and assesses appropriate physical characteristics of the preparation, such as any weight variations, adequacy of mixing, clarity, odor, color, consistency, and pH.
12. The pharmacist signs and dates the Compounding Record and/or prescription, files the records (computer entry and printed copy), and places the compounded preparation in a storage bin for patient pickup or mails the preparation to the patient.
13. The technician cleans all equipment thoroughly and promptly, reshelves all active and inactive ingredients, and properly labels and stores any excess preparation.
14. The pharmacist counsels the patient at the time of pickup.

10.5 Personnel Preparation for Nonsterile Compounding

Though nonsterile compounding does not require a sterile cleanroom, aseptic garb, equipment, and processes, it does require a dedicated facility area and its own special garb, equipment, and processes.

CDC Handwashing and Hand Hygiene

Before putting on the proper attire for nonsterile compounding, technicians should wash their hands thoroughly or perform hand hygiene. According to the Centers for Disease Control and Prevention (CDC), simple handwashing and hand hygiene are the single most important practices for minimizing touch contamination and reducing the transmission of infectious agents.

Handwashing with soap and water while rubbing can effectively remove dirt, stains, grease, harmful chemicals, and germs. Hand hygiene sometimes refers to the use of alcohol-based wipes, gels, foams, and rinses that disinfect. These hand sanitizers can reduce microbes but not all types of germs. So hand hygiene with alcohol-based products should be done after washing. The effectiveness of both handwashing and hand hygiene for infection control are affected by technique (see Table 10.3) as well as the presence of artificial fingernails and jewelry, which can harbor microorganisms.

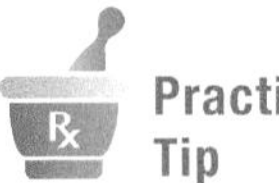

Practice Tip

The CDC states that handwashing with soap and water with vigorous rubbing is superior to alcohol-based hand wipes, lotions, or gels. However, if used, these should contain at least 60% alcohol.

TABLE 10.3 Handwashing and Hand Hygiene Guidelines

The handwashing and hand hygiene guidelines described here are appropriate for infection control procedures in a hospital setting. These procedures are followed by healthcare personnel in several departments, including pharmacy and nursing. *However, it should be noted that special, aseptic handwashing must be performed by personnel preparing sterile products, per* USP *<797> guidelines (as described in Chapter 12).*

Handwashing Technique

- First remove artificial fingernails and any hand and wrist jewelry, such as rings and bracelets.
- Wet hands first with water, apply an amount of product recommended by the manufacturer to hands, and rub hands together vigorously for at least 30 seconds, covering all surfaces of the hands and fingers, removing any debris from under nails. The rubbing time is needed to remove the temporary skin microorganisms effectively.
- Liquid, bar, or powdered forms of plain soap are acceptable when washing hands with a nonantimicrobial soap and water. When bar soap is used, small bars of soap and soap racks facilitating drainage should be used.
- Rinse hands with water and dry thoroughly with a disposable towel. Use the towel to turn off the faucet. Avoid using hot water; repeated exposure to hot water may increase the risk of skin irritation.
- Dry hands with single-use towels or air-dry them. Multiple-use cloth towels of the hanging or roll type are not recommended for use in healthcare settings because they can transfer infectious agents.

continues

TABLE 10.3 Handwashing and Hand Hygiene Guidelines—*Continued*

Hand Hygiene with Alcohol-Based Sanitizing Products
• Hand hygiene is defined as using special alcohol-based rinses, gels, or foams that do not require water. • When disinfecting hands with an alcohol-based hand rub, apply product to the palm of one hand and rub hands together, covering all surfaces of hands and fingers, until hands are dry. Follow the manufacturer's recommendations regarding the volume of product to use. • Hand hygiene is required even if gloves are used or changed.

Source: The Centers for Disease Control and Prevention (CDC), www.cdc.gov

Though many people use antimicrobial soaps, these can be very harsh on the skin. Scrubbing with a brush can also be harsh and encourages more flaking of skin cells, especially if you need to wash your hands numerous times a day. That is why the USP recommends that nonsterile compounders thoroughly wash their hands according to CDC recommendations, attending to the palms and webbing between fingers, but not use a scrub brush unless there is an unusual need for it.

In most community pharmacies or nonsterile compounding facilities, you will put on your compounding garb other than your gloves, wash your hands and sanitize them, and then finish your garbing by putting on your gloves.

After you have washed your hands, you do not want to contaminate them by touching the faucets. So use the sterile, clean, drying towel to turn off the water.

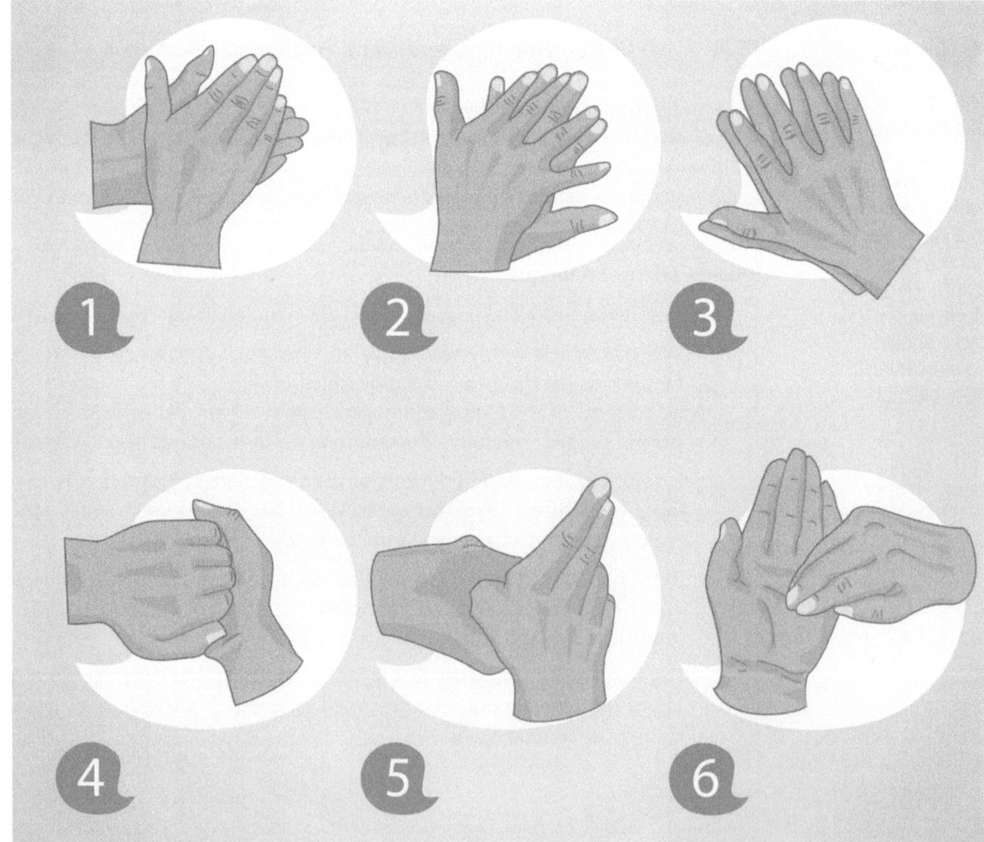

Proper handwashing is the first defense against catching or passing on harmful microorganisms that cause illness and infection. The steps above should be done vigorously and for a total of at least 30 seconds.

Proper Garb for Nonsterile Compounding

Performing simple compounding tasks in a community or hospital pharmacy is different from doing moderate or complex compounding in a special nonsterile compounding facility. For simple nonsterile compounding, you may need only clean clothing, a lab coat, gloves, and secured hair (as in a hairnet).

The specific requirements for nonsterile attire are provided by OSHA and in *USP* <795> as well as in each facility's P&P Manual. In a special compounding facility, the minimum requirements for nonsterile compounding garb include clean protective clothing, a hairnet, a long lab coat, shoe covers, and disposable gloves. Understandably, the garbing requirements for nonsterile compounding (excluding hazardous drugs) are less rigid than the attire for sterile compounding (discussed in Chapter 12). The nonsterile garb should not be worn outside the immediate compounding area.

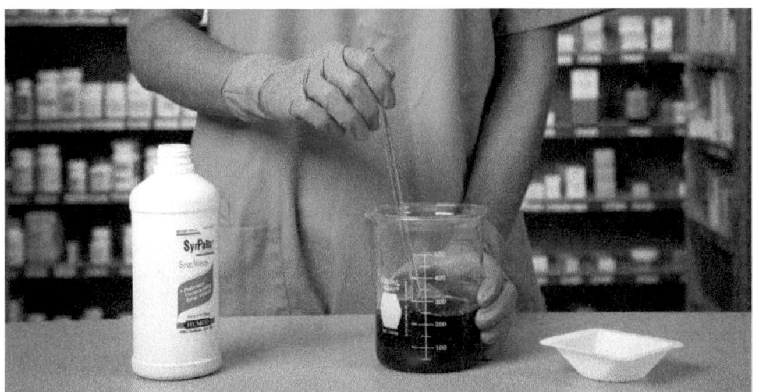

A pharmacy technician often wears scrubs or a lab coat, gloves, and a hairnet when preparing nonsterile products.

If hazardous chemicals are used, a special protective lab coat, eye goggles, respiratory mask and shield, hairnet, shoe covers, and double gloving with official chemotherapy gloves are all necessary. (For more on hazardous compounding, go to Chapter 13.)

10.6 Nonsterile Compounding Environment and Equipment

Before preparing a drug for compounding, gather the Master Formulation Record, Compounding Record, mixing directions, ingredients, measuring and mixing equipment, and packaging material. Adequate, uninterrupted time is also very important to minimize measurement or calculation errors. A nonsterile compounding area must have adequate space and storage as well as appropriate equipment that is properly maintained, calibrated, used, and cleaned. The space must meet high cleanliness and sanitation standards, have sufficient ventilation, and have counters that are free from potential contaminants. The compounding area itself should:

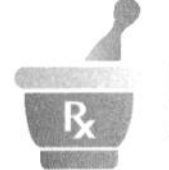

Practice Tip

It is important to have proper ventilation and lighting, hot and cold running water, and smooth counters with no cracks, as cracks can foster microbial growth or cross contamination.

- be free of dust-collecting overhangs, such as ceiling pipes and light fixtures;
- have an eyewash station in case of accidental contact with or exposure to a toxic chemical;
- have access to refrigeration and freezer equipment;
- have potable water for washing of hands and equipment;
- have purified water for compounding and rinsing of instruments;
- have a non-shedding work surface of sufficient space that is level, smooth, and free of cracks;
- have plumbing without defects, and with hot and cold running water; and
- have no food items stored or consumed in the staging area.

If coupled with a dispensing pharmacy, the nonsterile pharmacy must be physically separate. If the pharmacy also prepares sterile preparations, a separate cleanroom environment (see Chapter 12) and special equipment must be utilized. Hazardous compounding should also be kept separate (see Chapter 13).

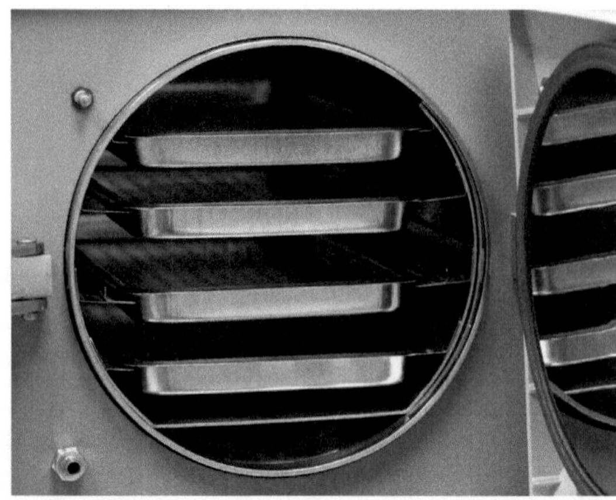

Heated autoclaves are often used in compounding pharmacies to sterilize metal instruments and glassware.

Staging Area

The work surface's **staging area**, or assembly space, should contain only the equipment and pharmaceutical ingredients needed for the compounding process. Clutter can cause confusion and potential errors. Equipment must be placed in areas where air currents will not interfere with or compromise the accuracy of the delicate electronic digital balance or scale. The ventilation system should be free of contaminants.

Within easy, organized reach should be the myriad of equipment elements used in a specialty compounding pharmacy for measuring, mixing, and molding. The large appliances needed within the space include a convection oven to create rapid-dissolving tablets, pellets, and suppositories; a microwave or hot plate to warm ingredients; and, for quality control, an incubator to test compounded preparations for bacteria. Also required is an **autoclave**—an intense heating appliance for chemical heat compounding processes. Additionally, it is used to sterilize instruments and measuring vessels and devices with steam heat and pressure. The process of **sterilization** kills the germs on the metal and glass surfaces.

Measuring and Compounding Vessels and Tools

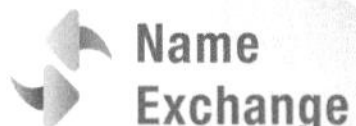

Name Exchange

The electronic digital balance and Class III prescription balance are also known as analytical balances because they measure very small weights.

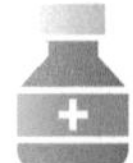

Pharm Fact

Glassine paper is a thin paper that has been coated with a nonabsorbent paraffin wax.

In establishing your staging area on the counter, you will need access to a variety of smaller equipment elements:

- mortar and pestle (glass and porcelain)
- electronic mortar and pestle
- ointment slab or parchment pad
- stainless steel and plastic spatulas (of various sizes)
- scoops and spoons
- beakers and Erlenmeyer flasks (those with flat bottoms, conical bodies, and slim necks)
- funnels and sieves
- ointment jars and tubes
- electronic digital balance
- graduated cylinders
- pipettes and droppers
- pipettes and droppers
- oral syringes
- glass stirring rods
- magnetic stirrer
- suppository molds (reusable or disposable)
- prescription vials, bottles, and containers
- pharmacy weights (metric, particularly)
- weighing papers (usually glassine)
- weighing boats (weighing canoes)
- disposable weight dishes
- ointment mill

With the exception of an electronic digital balance, electronic mortar and pestle, and ointment mill, these basic supplies are generally found in community pharmacies and are used for the occasional measuring of ingredients for a compounded nonsterile preparation. The precise devices, tools, and supplies for weighing and how to use them will be described in the weighing section of the compounding process.

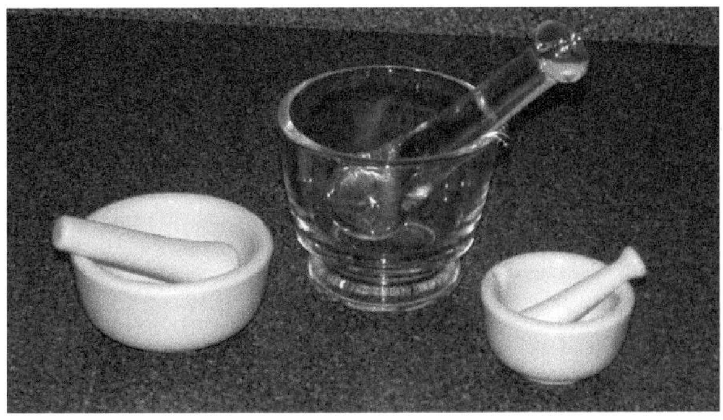

Glass and porcelain mortar and pestles are used to mix or grind substances: glass for liquids, stains, or oily substances; porcelain for particles, crystals, and powders.

Mortars and Pestles

The **mortar and pestle**, which come in matched sets made of glass or porcelain, are suited for hand grinding and pulverizing. You will select the appropriate one to use, based on the master formula. A coarse-grained porcelain mortar and pestle set is ideal for triturating (or pulverizing) crystals, granules, and powders; a glass mortar and pestle, with their smooth surfaces, are preferred for mixing liquids and semisolid dosage forms such as creams, ointments, and gels. A glass mortar and pestle also have the advantage of being nonporous and non-staining.

An electric mortar and pestle unit is often used in a high-volume compounding pharmacy to reduce particle size and to mix the pharmaceutical compound more thoroughly after the weighing and manual manipulation of ingredients with a spatula. An electric mortar and pestle can mix at a low rate (50 revolutions per minute, or RPMs) or a high rate (2,500 RPMs). This equipment can be calibrated to a specific product if necessary, but it generally produces a pharmaceutically elegant cream or ointment after three minutes of constant automated mixing.

Put Down Roots

A pharmaceutically elegant product is one that looks smooth and creamy and feels good on the skin, not too oily, watery, waxy, or gritty.

Ointment Mills

A three-roller ointment mill mixes and greatly reduces the particle size of ingredient powders used to compound a dermatological ointment or cream preparation. The result is a smoother, more pharmaceutically elegant end product for consumer use. The speed of the rolling or milling is easily controlled, and the rollers can be removed for easy cleaning after each preparation.

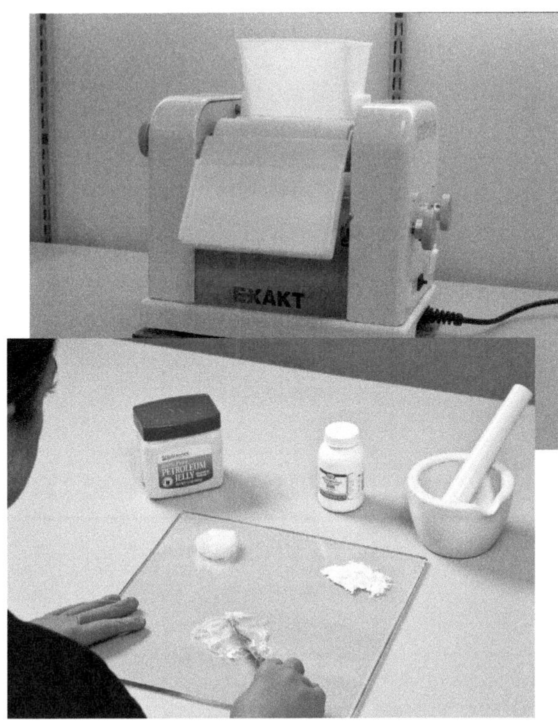

An ointment slab is used to prepare specialized prescriptions for creams and ointments.

Ointment Slabs and Pads

An **ointment slab**, also known as a compounding slab, is a plate made of ground glass that has a flat, hard, nonabsorbent surface ideal for mixing topical compounds. In lieu of a compounding or ointment slab, mixing may be performed on special disposable nonabsorbent parchment paper, which is discarded after the compounding operation has been completed.

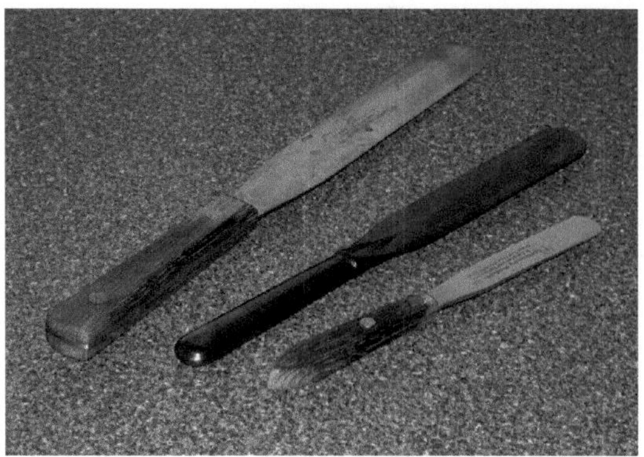

Spatulas are a common tool in a compounding pharmacy for combining ingredients on a slab.

Spatulas

A **spatula** is an instrument used for transferring solid pharmaceutical ingredients to and from weighing pans. This instrument is also utilized for various compounding tasks, such as preparing ointments and creams, loosening material from the surfaces of a mortar and pestle, and transferring the compounded preparation into its final container. Spatulas come in stainless steel, plastic, and hard rubber. Hard rubber spatulas are used when corrosive substances, such as iodine and mercuric salts, are handled. Spatulas must be thoroughly cleaned and sterilized before each use.

Beakers, Flasks, Funnels, and Sieves

Glass beakers and Erlenmeyer flasks (with flat bottoms and conical bodies sloping up into cylindrical necks as used in chemistry labs) are available in various sizes and are considered **nonvolumetric glassware**. This means that they are inappropriate for precise volume measurements. These beakers and flasks usually have only general markings and therefore can provide only approximate measurements of larger volumes of liquids (usually eight fluid ounces or more). So their role is to store, contain, and mix liquids. To transfer liquids from or to these containers, use plastic or glass funnels or sieves.

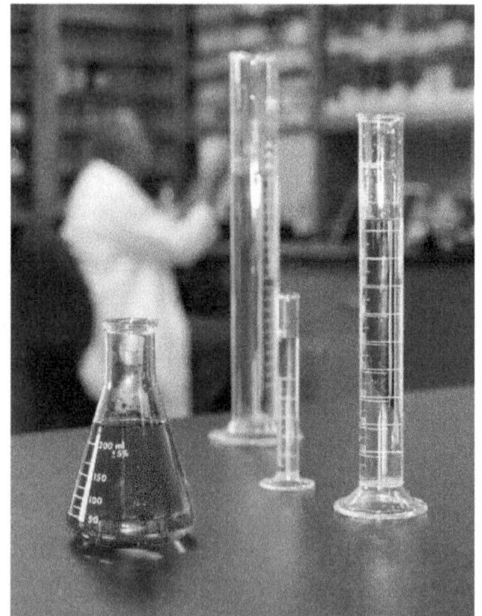

Simple compounding uses different measuring tools.

Molds and Presses

You use hot plates and microwaves to melt down powders or mix ingredients with various solvents for vaginal or rectal suppositories, pellets, and rapid-dissolving tablets or lozenges. The warm liquids are then poured into aluminum metal molds like candy molds to cool into shapes. The mold pans come in a variety of numbers and sizes of cavities in one pan (up to 100). Common ingredient doses are in the range of 1 g to 2.5 g. To compound an implantable urethral medication pellet, a pellet press is used.

10.7 Compounding Ingredients

To compound a safe and effective medication, start with quality ingredients, or **components**. The components needed for any preparation come in different types. An **active pharmaceutical ingredient** is any substance (or mixture of substances) in a compounded preparation that confers pharmacological activity. **Added substances** are ingredients that are necessary to compound a preparation but do not confer pharmacological activity. As explained in earlier chapters, added substances are

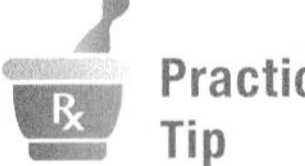

Practice Tip

As with dispensing manufactured oral solutions, flavorings for compounded oral solutions are important.

Practice Tip

A certificate of analysis provided by the American Chemical Society ensures that an ingredient is a high-grade, purified product.

sometimes called inactive ingredients, or **excipients**. One of the inactive ingredients (or a combination of them) is called the **vehicle** since it is the substance or solution that carries the active ingredients. Liquid, semisolid, or solid active ingredients can be dissolved or suspended in the vehicle solution.

Sources for Bulk Ingredients

The quality of the final product is in part determined by the quality of its ingredients. The pharmacist typically makes the decisions about what sources are used to purchase ingredients—both active and inactive. The decisions are based on cost, quality, and purity of product. Pharmacy personnel must secure a high-grade, purified product along with filing a certificate of analysis from the American Chemical Society. All chemicals or products should be properly labeled with their expiration dates. They should also have ranges of drug bioavailability in the ingredients (explained more in the percentage of error section to come.)

As *USP* <795> specifies, FDA-registered ingredient sources for *USP-National Formulary* (NF) pharmaceutical-grade (as opposed to cosmetic-chemical-grade) ingredients should be selected whenever available. Many large-volume compounding pharmacies use their membership with the PCCA as a primary source of ingredients because they have been certified after undergoing extensive research and scientific testing. The PCCA also provides a reputable source for new compounding recipes, as well as information and research on compatibility and stability of prepared or new compounds.

Often, the pharmacist must balance the higher cost of PCCA ingredients with other lower-cost sources that also provide certified *USP-NF*-grade ingredients. Pharmacists should have more than one source in case of a shortage, back order, or drug product recall. On request, any manufacturer of bulk ingredients will provide an analysis certificate for any of its ingredient products.

Accompanying each ingredient delivery will be a **Safety Data Sheet (SDS)**, formerly the Material Safety Data Sheet (MSDS). It is a document from the manufacturer on safe storage and handling that is required by OSHA for all bulk hazardous chemicals and drug substances. The SDS, as demonstrated in Table 10.4, includes information important for technicians and other pharmacy personnel to prevent an emergency or to address it if one occurs. These should be kept on hand in a pharmacy loose-leaf folder for quick reference and documentation.

Storage of Bulk Ingredients

Ingredients are commonly ordered by the technician two or three times per week, depending on the volume and inventory of the compounding pharmacy. The ingredients are received the next business day from one of several overnight mail services and are properly recorded and stored by the technician.

Bulk ingredients are typically stored in tight, light-resistant containers at room temperature. If you are unsure about temperature requirements, check product labeling or refer to the *USP-NF* compendia. You must always check expiration dates prior to mixing any ingredients. In addition, make sure that you have all the materials you will need for proper packaging and labeling of the end product.

TABLE 10.4 Safety Data Sheet Requirements

Components	Standards
Substance and Manufacturer	Product identifiers; manufacturer or distributor name, address, phone number; emergency phone number; recommended use; restrictions on use
Hazard(s)	Any hazards regarding the chemical and required label elements
Composition/Ingredients	Chemicals and any claims about them
First-Aid Measures	Important symptoms or effects from exposure (mild, acute, and delayed) and the required treatment
Fire-Fighting Measures	Hazards from fire and suitable extinguishing techniques and equipment
Accidental Release Measures	Emergency procedures, protective equipment, and proper methods of containment and cleanup
Handling and Storage	Precautions for safe handling and storage, including incompatibilities
Exposure Controls/Personal Protection	OSHA's permissible exposure limits (PELs); American Conference of Governmental Industrial Hygienists (ACGIH) Threshold Limit Values (TLVs); any other exposure limits used or recommended by the chemical manufacturer, importer, or employer; engineering controls; personal protective equipment (PPE)
Physical and Chemical Properties	Chemical characteristics
Stability and Reactivity	Chemical stability and possibility of hazardous reactions
Toxicological Information	Routes of exposure; related symptoms and acute and chronic effects; numerical measures of toxicity
Ecological Information*	Toxicity test on aquatics or terrestrials; persistence or degradation; bioaccumulation; potential to move from soil to groundwater, etc.
Disposal Considerations*	Appropriate disposal containers and processes, discouragement of sewage; precautions for landfill or incineration
Transportation Information*	United Nations (UN) number, guidance for transport and handlers, ecological hazards
Regulatory Information*	Any appropriate national, state, regional, or local safety, health, or environmental statutes
Other Information	Date of SDS preparation and updates, changes, other pertinent information

Source: OSHA website, 2015. *Indicates regulatory information not overseen by OSHA but included on form

Storage and Use of Controlled Substance Ingredients

If the compounding pharmacy receives prescriptions for hospice care or pain management patients, it may be necessary to compound controlled substances. Most vendors of bulk narcotic ingredients allow the online, identity-secure Controlled Substance Ordering System (CSOS). With this process, ingredients may be ordered and delivered for the preparation of the compounds the next business day.

As expected, the procedures and record keeping for Schedule II compounds are much more detailed and extensive, with these prescriptions filed separately. Each and every milligram of the narcotic ingredients must be accounted for on the compounding log and be deducted from the inventory. Some ingredients may need to be in locked storage. The pharmacist is held accountable for all controlled substance ingredient use and compounds. The pharmacy's procedural manual should outline the exact procedures to follow in order to meet state and federal regulations.

Storage and Use of Hazardous Ingredients

Hazardous chemicals must be stored separately in the drug inventory, with policies and practices in place for hazardous drug segregation and disposal. For example, protective clothing must be worn when such ingredients are received, and they must be labeled and stored separately from nonhazardous agents (even in refrigeration). The exact storage conditions and location of hazardous drugs are based on a risk assessment profile by NIOSH. This will be covered in Chapter 13.

10.8 Weighing, Measuring, and the Percentage of Error

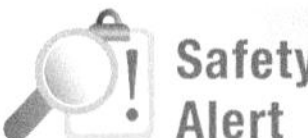

Pharmacy technicians should always work within the acceptable percentage of error range for their ingredients and equipment.

Knowing the proper techniques to measure and weigh ingredients is one of the most essential skills for a compounding technician. You must carefully and continually practice to feel confident in calculating and weighing products on various prescription balances. Any error in weighing or measuring ingredients could result in serious drug toxicity for the patient, and improper mixing or molding could result in a poor quality preparation and/or a product that is not pharmaceutically elegant.

Amount of Potential Error and Percentage of Error

The ideal for all measurements, of course, is no errors. However, there are ranges in the precision of the weighing and measuring instruments that can cause differences in the formulation recipes and compounded outcomes.

The amount of actual error is equal to the difference between the intended amount in the formula and the actual amount.

$$\text{actual amount measured} - \text{desired (prescribed) quantity} = \text{amount of error}$$

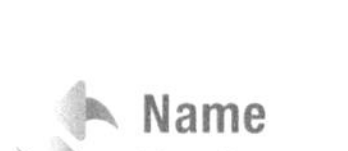

The sensitivity requirement is also known as the sensibility reciprocal, both abbreviated as SR. This is the basis of the +/- sensitivity range, or range of potential error.

Each different weighing or measuring device has a different potential range of error, or **sensitivity range**. It is the incremental unit that the device uses to measure, which is how much it can be off in measurement. For instance, a perfectly calibrated **Class III balance** measures in increments of 6 mg. This amount is the smallest amount of weight needed to move the measurement indicator one notch. So a weighed measurement can potentially be off by plus or minus 6 mg (+/− 6 mg), which is this device's sensitivity range, or range of potential error.

The **percentage of error** is the range of potential error in the weight or measurement, compared to the desired quantity. To calculate this, divide the sensitivity range by the desired (prescribed or formula) quantity, and multiply it by 100%.

$$\frac{\textit{sensitivity range}}{\textit{desired quantity}} \times 100 = \text{\% of error in product}$$

Or if you do not know the sensitivity range but you do know the amount of error, you can use the following formula:

$$\frac{\textit{error amount}}{\textit{desired quantity}} \times 100 = \text{\% of error in product}$$

The official USP guidance allows for a deviation range of plus or minus 5% in weighted measurements. Differences or errors within this range are not consequential in most cases. If the percentage of error is higher, then it is unacceptable.

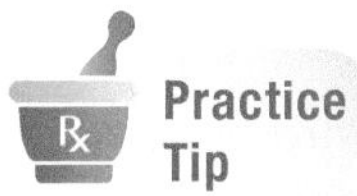

Practice Tip

Keep all the original ingredient containers and packages, as many pharmacists would like to double-check them to ensure that the right ingredients were used. Also be ready to show them the calculations used.

Example 1

The Master Formulation Record asked for 120 mg of a drug powder. Using a Class III balance, the amount was weighed. The amount was double-checked on a digital scale. It showed that the weighed amount was actually 100 mg. What are the amount of error and the percentage of error?

Step 1 Follow the amount of error equation to determine how over- or under-weight the measurement was.

100 mg − 120 mg = (−) 20 mg (The amount was 20 mg underweight.)

Step 2 Use the amount of error to determine the percentage of error that occurred.

$$\frac{(-)20 \text{ mg}}{120 \text{ mg}} \times 100 = -16.67\% \text{ (This is the percent of error.)}$$

If a scale is underweight by 16.67%, it may also be overweight by this much, meaning that this scale for 120 mg would have a +/−16.67% of error. This high percentage of error is unacceptable, as it is over the USP limit of +/− 5%. This scale should not be used for weighing.

The lower the ingredient quantity and the closer the measurement is to the sensitivity range, the higher the percentage of potential error. For instance, consider that you are trying to weigh out 90 mg of an ingredient on the Class III balance (which has a sensitivity range of 6%). To determine the percentage of error, you must divide the sensitivity range by the desired quantity and multiply by 100.

$$\frac{+/- 6 \text{ mg}}{90 \text{ mg}} = \times 100$$

$$+/- 6.7\%$$

This error range is above the +/− 5% allowed by USP standards, so this weighing device *should not be used* for this 90 mg ingredient.

Least Weighable Quantity per Scale

Most balances are marked with their degree of accuracy and their **least weighable quantity (LWQ)**. When any substance is weighed, the scale will appear to have measured correctly. However, weighing too small an amount for a specific scale (as in the above example) will result in an unacceptable margin of error.

To calculate an unmarked weighing device's LWQ to check for the 5% or less error percentage, divide the device's incremental unit by the highest allowed percentage of error and multiply it by 100.

$$\frac{\textit{scale's incremental unit}}{\textit{\% error}} \times 100 = \text{least weighable quantity}$$

$$\text{For the Class III balance: } \frac{6 \text{ mg}}{5\%} \times 100 = 120 \text{ mg}$$

(If you use the decimal form of the percentage of error as the denominator, there is no need to multiply by 100; you will get the incorrect answer if you do.)

For the Class III balance, you may not weigh ingredients for amounts lower than 120 mg (which is standard practice, so the calculation does not need to be done each time). That is another important reason for making a larger batch of a compound preparation—the percentage of error in measurement goes down.

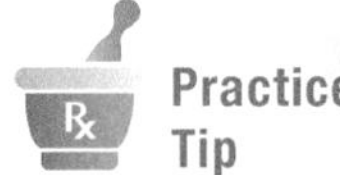

Practice Tip

To maintain an acceptable error of <5%, no less than 120 mg should be measured on a Class III balance.

Most compounded nonsterile preparations—tablets, capsules, ointments, creams, and gels—are prepared in larger quantities than the original prescription, especially if the prescription will be refilled. For example, instead of preparing 30 capsules of a medication each month, the Master Formulation Record or recipe may call for preparing a minimum quantity of 100 capsules. The reasons for this include both the lower percentage of error in measuring larger quantities of the ingredients and the lower costs in terms of staff time engaged in preparation.

Bioavailability Range

Each active ingredient will also have a bioavailability range written on its label along with the range of error. The **bioavailability range** is the percentage of how much of the substance is absorbed in this product form. For example, a new national brand of vitamins claims to have a bioavailability error range of +/− 9% of the full ingredient weight in its products. Therefore, in its stock of 1,000 mg of vitamin C, the range of error is 9% less and 9% more than the labeled amount of 1,000 mg, or 910–1,090 mg. Compounded nonsterile preparations, though, must have an error range of less than or equal to 5%. Most FDA-approved drugs must have a bioavailability in the range of +/− 5%.

10.9 The Processes of Weighing and Measuring

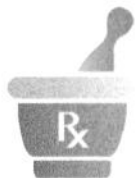

Practice Tip

A technician must be trained in weighing techniques and then checked in skill by a pharmacist or by another technician (as in tech-check-tech).

The art and skill of compounding relies greatly on knowing how to weigh and measure accurately with the different devices and vessels. Most active and inactive bulk ingredients for compounding come in powder form—either to be pressed into tablets, inserted into capsules, or added to liquids. To a layperson, a powder is any finely ground substance. To a technician or a pharmacist, however, powders range in textural size from extremely coarse to extremely fine, like sandpaper. The official powder sizes include very coarse (No. 8), coarse (No. 20), moderately coarse (No. 40), fine (No. 60), or very fine (No. 80). These are measured according to the amount of the powder that can pass through mechanical sieves of wire cloth of various dimensions (such as No. 8 sieve, No. 20 sieve).

Many types of balances and weights are used to measure powders. To operate any type of balance in a community or compounding pharmacy, you must become familiar with the calibration of weights of the device. The following balances are frequently seen in the pharmacy setting.

Using an Electronic Balance

An **electronic digital balance** uses a single pan and is easier to learn to use and more accurate than a Class III prescription balance or a counterbalance (to be described). However, electronic balances tend to be much more costly ($1,000 or more), so they are typically used in large-scale or dedicated pharmacy compounding labs and hospitals. Electronic balances do not need to use pharmacy weights. The sensitivity of an electronic balance is often in the range of +/− 1 mg to +/− 30 mg, depending on the volume capacity of the balance. The +/− 30 mg digital balance is used for heavier volumes of stock ingredients. Weighing bulk ingredients is more efficient and accurate, compared with the two-pan balances.

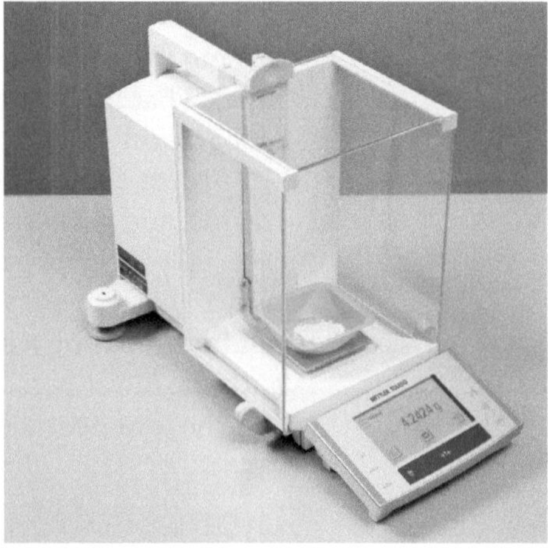

A digital electronic balance is very accurate with a capacity of 100 g or more and a sensitivity as low as +/− 2 mg.

An electronic balance should be placed on a secure, level, non-vibrating surface, at waist height. It must be perfectly level—both side to side and front to back. Leveling is often the most time-consuming process for beginners. The levelness should be checked often throughout the day if the balance is heavily used. Place the balance in a well-lit area free from air current drafts, dust, corrosive vapors, or high humidity, which might affect the ingredients or the weight measurements. In fact, electronic balances are usually enclosed on three or four sides to minimize any air current impacts during the weighing process.

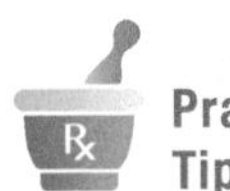

Practice Tip

Never place anything to weigh on an unlocked balance of any kind, since this can result in a sudden, forceful drop of the pan.

Turn on the electronic balance 30 minutes prior to use, and then calibrate it. You must document the calibration process each day. Lock the balance. Place a **weighing paper** (or **weighing boat**) on the scale to hold the powder, protect the balance from damage, and avoid contact between the pharmaceutical ingredient and the metal tray. The weight of this paper (or any weighing container) is called the **tare weight**. It must be subtracted from the total during the measuring process, or the final ingredient weight will be short by that much. To do this, place the paper on the scale and press the "tare" key of the balance to set the weight to zero. Typically, glassine paper is used.

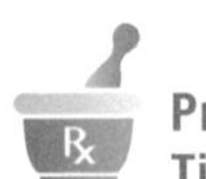

Practice Tip

Avoid spilling materials onto the balance itself. In the event of a spill, place the balance in a locked position to wipe it up. Then recalibrate the balance. Also, always lock the balance when moving it and recalibrate it afterwards.

The procedure for measuring an ingredient with an electronic digital balance is outlined in Table 10.5. Be sure that all panel doors, side doors, and top doors are closed to reduce air movements and resistance.

Many electronic balances produce a hard-copy printout of the weights of the individual ingredients measured; some advanced balances have bar code scanning of the drug's NDC to add to the printout for accurate tracking. This printout is then attached to the Compounding Record for the pharmacist's final check of the compounded preparation. This is especially important for nonelectric scales that do not provide a tracking printout.

Safety Alert

Use a digital electronic scale when preparing a compound in which very small ingredients will be weighed (such as a compound for a premature baby, infant, or young child).

TABLE 10.5 Steps for Using an Electronic Digital Balance

1. Place the weighing paper (or plastic weighing boat) on the balance and calibrate to the zero point, including the weight of the weighing paper or boat.
2. Using a spatula, place a small amount of the chemical or drug to be measured (from the Compounding Record) onto the paper on the pan.
3. Once a nearly precise amount of material has been transferred to the pan, a very small adjustment upward can be made by placing an additional small amount of material on the spatula, holding the spatula over the paper, and lightly tapping the spatula with the forefinger to knock granules of the substance onto the pan until the weight is correct; this is done with the balance unlocked to weigh the adjustments. Lock the balance and remove sufficient powder if above desired weight.
4. Read the final digital weight measurement.
5. Lock the balance before removing the measured substance.
6. Collect the printout to assemble with the final compounded product for the pharmacist's check.

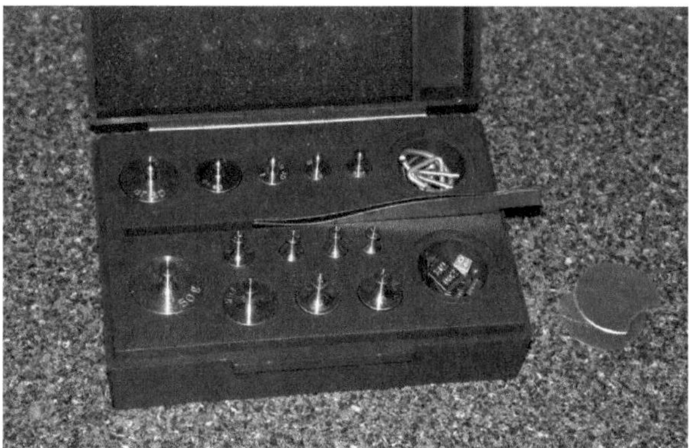
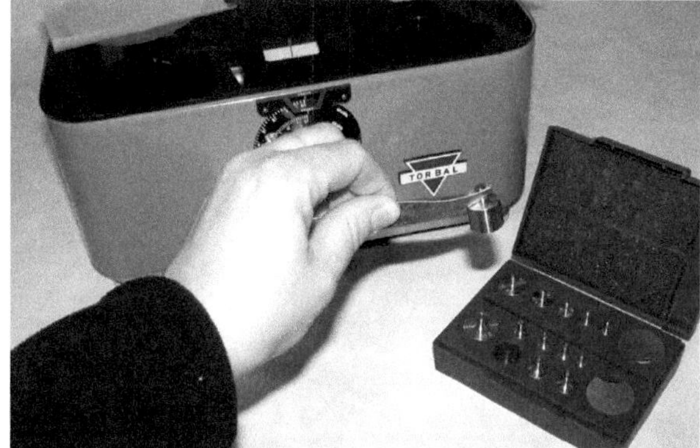

This set of pharmacy weights has metric weights in the front and apothecary weights in the back. Weights should be transferred using forceps, never touched with bare skin. They should always be placed on weighing papers or containers of some kind.

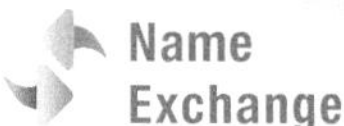
Name Exchange

Two-pan balances are also referred to as "torsion" balances.

Using Two-Pan Balances

If a digital electronic balance or scale is not available, two types of two-pan balances are used to weigh ingredients in nonsterile compounding: a **Class III prescription balance** (with two mechanical balancing pans) for compounding small amounts, and a larger counterbalance for bulk ingredients (to be explained below). Place the appropriate number of **pharmaceutical weights** totaling the desired amount in the right pan and the ingredient to be measured in the left pan until the two pans balance exactly evenly. The weights come in full gram and fractional gram amounts. A set of gram weights usually includes 1, 2, 3, 10, 20, 50, and 100 g and are generally made of polished brass. The weights may be coated with a noncorrosive material such as nickel or chromium. Fractional gram weights come in amounts of 10, 20, 50, 100, 200, and 500 mg. They are made of aluminum and are usually flat, with one raised edge to facilitate being picked up.

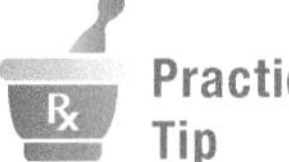
Practice Tip

Always use forceps or cloth when transferring weights.

Weight sets usually contain both metric and apothecary weights, though the metric weights are the standard in pharmacy. (For information about the metric and apothecary measurement systems, see Chapter 6.) To grasp and transfer weights, use a pair of forceps or a cloth, not your fingers. Over time, the moisture and oil from hands would change the fixed quantity of the weights and introduce a potential source of error in measuring small ingredient amounts, such as for pediatric patients. A pair of **forceps** is a tweezer-like instrument used for grasping and holding small, light objects. You typically use a cloth to handle the larger weights. When weights are not in use, store them in their containers to avoid dust and humidity so they maintain their stated values.

Place weighing papers on both pans to hold the ingredients and to put a barrier between the ingredient and the metal. The paper on each balance pan should be of exactly the same size and weight, and the edges of the paper on the pan may be folded upward to hold the ingredient to be weighed. Weigh the paper prior to adding each ingredient to be measured, and discard the paper after each ingredient is measured to prevent contamination. To weigh larger quantities of chemicals, use plastic weighing boats. The boats should also be weighed before beginning the measuring process.

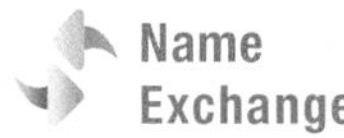
Name Exchange

A Class III prescription balance was formerly known as a Class A prescription balance, so now you will find it referred to by either name.

Class III Prescription Balances

Mechanical scales are still in use. Class I and II two-pan balances are for high-precision laboratories. The Class III prescription balance, formerly known as a Class A prescription balance, has been and continues to be a common fixture in many pharmacies. The Class III prescription balance is sufficiently accurate for infrequent, non-rushed compounding within its balance capacity in a community pharmacy. Since the balance has a sensitivity requirement in the range of +/- 6 mg, it can be used to weigh mid-range prescription amounts. It has internal weights that measure amounts from 120 mg to 1 g. For amounts larger than 1 g, there are the external pans on the balance. Depending on the model, the balance can measure quantities from 120 mg (0.12 g) to 15 g or 120 mg (0.12 g) up to 120 g. When the weight of the ingredients in the left pan exactly balances the pharmaceutical weights in the right pan, the dial registers the weight.

The correct technique for weighing ingredients with a Class III prescription balance is demonstrated in Figure 10.3. The balance must first be checked to be level front to back and side to side and then calibrated. Set the internal weights to zero and place the weighing papers or boats on both sides. **Arrest**, or lock, the pans in place before adding or subtracting any materials to the pans. Then add the desired number of weights to the right pan and gradually add ingredients to the left until even.

Lock the final weighing balance in place so that it can be checked by the pharmacist. Variations in technique could easily result in a small but serious error, resulting in a subtherapeutic (below correct dosage) or a toxic overdose of medication. Weighing the exact amount prescribed is essential because, once mixed, the ingredient amount cannot be easily checked. A pharmacist must inspect the weight measurements of all ingredients you have weighed on any nonelectronic balance.

FIGURE 10.3 Weighing with a Class III Prescription Balance

(a) After the scale is level and locked, transfer weights with forceps to the right pan and ingredients to the left. (b) Make final measurement and check with the cover down.

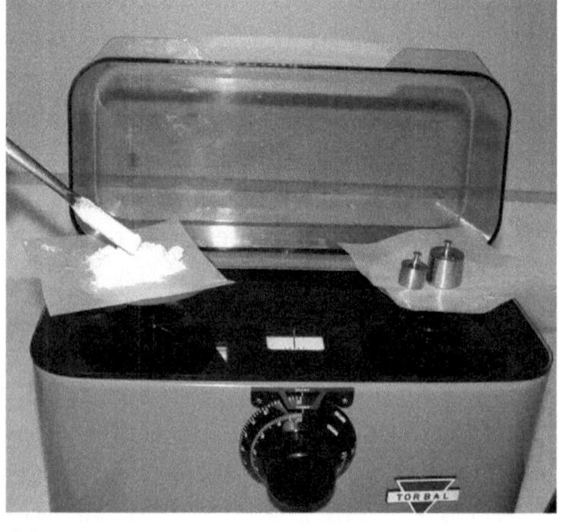

(a)

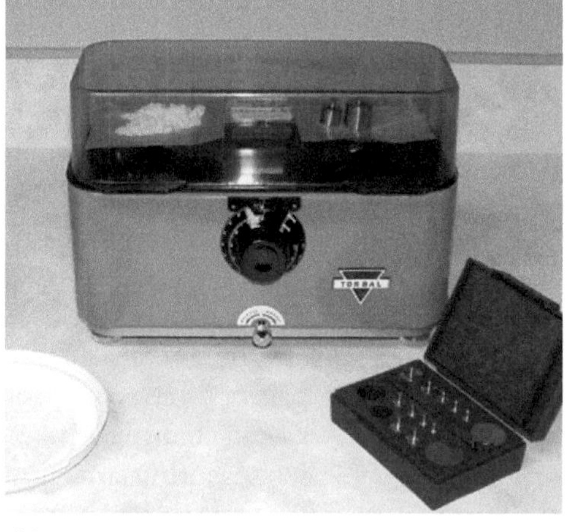

(b)

Practice Tip

Never choose a large container for measuring a liquid that will fill less than 20% of the container's capacity. Select a container that is very close to the amount being measured while being a little more than sufficient to hold all the volume.

Bulk Ingredient Counterbalance

Like a Class III prescription balance, a **bulk counterbalance** also contains two pans, but this device is used for weighing larger amounts, from 100 g up to about 5 kg. It has a sensitivity range of +/-100 mg. Because of its lesser sensitivity, a counterbalance is not used in compounding but for measuring bulk products, such as Epsom salts. Use a weighing boat to hold the larger quantities.

Measuring Processes for Liquids

Liquid volumes are often much easier to measure than solid ingredients. To perform **volumetric measurement**, you can choose from a wide variety of glassware that is designed to measure—not mix—liquids. These containers include graduated cylinders, pipettes, oral syringes, and droppers.

A general rule of thumb is to always select the device that yields the most accurate volume, which is the smallest possible cylinder of sufficient volume. It will offer the most precision and accuracy. In no case should you measure a liquid volume in a container that is more than 80% larger in capacity. For example, 10 mL of a liquid should not be measured in a graduated cylinder exceeding 50 mL in capacity. The closer the total capacity of the container is to the volume to be measured, the more accurate the measurement will be.

Practice Tip

Always add ingredients into the center of a container to avoid liquids adhering to the sides.

Using Graduated Cylinders

A **graduated cylinder** is a glass or polypropylene flask used for measuring liquids. The flasks come in two varieties: conical and cylindrical. Conical graduates have wide bases and narrow tops, tapering from the bottom to the top. These are used for larger, more general amounts because they are less accurate in the bottom levels where the diameter increases. They range in size from 10 mL to 4,000 mL. Cylindrical graduates are more accurate and have the shape of a uniform column. They vary in size from 5 mL to more than 1,000 mL. Select a container that will become at least half full during measurement or the smallest device that can hold the required volume and display the **meniscus**.

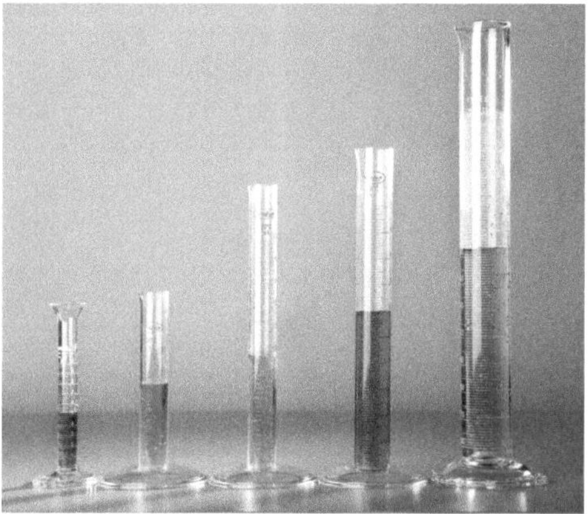

Choosing the appropriate-sized graduated cylinder is important to accurately measure liquids.

When measuring liquid volumes in a graduated cylinder, be sure that the cylinder is on a flat surface before following the procedure outlined in Table 10.6. Always view it at eye level to see that the liquid's meniscus aligns with the desired measurement line. As the illustration shows, the liquid level in the graduated cylinder is concave in appearance, with slightly higher edges, and the meniscus is the half-moon-shaped dip in the center surface of a liquid (see Figure 10.4). The accurate volume measure is level with the bottom of the meniscus.

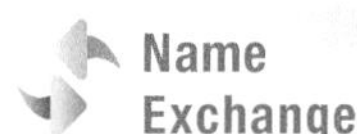

Name Exchange

Pharmacy technicians need to remember that milliliters (abbreviated as mL) and cubic centimeters (abbreviated as cc) are equivalent and interchangeable terms of liquid measurement though the cc measurement is being phased out for safety reasons.

FIGURE 10.4 Meniscus

Take measurements at eye level, lining up the bottom of the concave dip of the meniscus with the measurement line of the vessel.

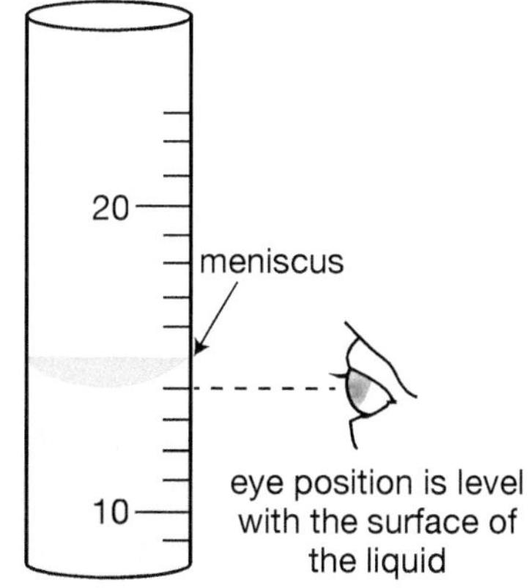

Viscous liquids, such as syrups, propylene glycol, mineral oil, and glycerin, move slowly and particularly adhere to the edges of the container. For this reason, always add new liquid ingredients into the center of the container and avoid moving the container. Wait as the liquid settles in after adding the substance. It may take as long as 60 seconds before an accurate measurement of the meniscus can take place.

TABLE 10.6 Steps for Measuring Liquid Volumes

1. Choose a graduated cylinder with a capacity that equals or very slightly exceeds the total volume of the liquid to be measured. Doing so reduces the percentage of error in the measurement.
2. Note that the narrower the column of liquid measured, the less substantial any reading error will be. Thus, for very small volume measurements, a pipette dropper or an oral syringe is preferable to a cylindrical graduate, and, for larger measurements, a cylindrical graduate is preferable to a conical graduate.
3. Pour the liquid to be measured slowly into the center of the graduated cylinder, watching the level of the liquid in the container as you do so.
4. Wait for any liquid clinging to the sides of the graduated cylinder to settle before taking a measurement.
5. Read the level of the liquid at eye level, and read the measure at the bottom of the meniscus (refer back to Figure 10.4).
6. When pouring the liquid out of the graduated cylinder, allow ample time for all of the liquid to drain. Depending on the viscosity of the liquid, more or less of it clings to the sides of the container. For a particularly viscous liquid, you may need to use a spatula and/or make some compensation or adjustment to the measurement for this clinging amount of liquid.

Using Pipettes and Droppers

A **pipette** is a long, thin, calibrated hollow glass tube (similar to a glass straw). The types of pipettes include a one-volume-only transfer pipette (for a specific volume of liquid, such as 10 mL); a calibrated pipette (usually with inner plungers or suction mechanisms, for measuring precise, multiple volumes of liquid); and a micropipette (for measuring a very small volume of liquid).

To measure and transfer small volumes of liquid, pipettes are often used. To use a pipette, attach a pipette filler or a rubber bulb to the end. Cautiously press and release the bulb to suction the liquid up the pipette. The use of this attachment is particularly important when drawing up a hazardous substance such as an acid.

On March 20, 1944, Private First Class Johnnie Mae Welton used standard laboratory practices with pipettes for doing a test in a military blood lab. Using the mouth for suction with a pipette is now considered an unsafe practice. Pipette droppers are now used instead.

When measuring liquids with a graduated cylinder, pipette, dropper, or oral syringe, always use the smallest size that can contain the volume to be measured. Doing so minimizes your percentage of error in measurement.

Pipette **droppers** have a suction bulb on one end that allows for calibrated drop measurements of liquids. They're available in both glass and plastic and are often used to transfer small volumes of liquid, such as medication dosages for infants. The glass pipettes can be cleaned and reused, whereas the one-piece, bulb-ended plastic droppers are disposable.

Each liquid in a pipette delivers a different drop volume based on the different density, weight, and viscosity of the liquid. That is why, to use it for measurement purposes, one must first **calibrate** the dropper, or fill it with the appropriate liquid, and count how many drops it takes to make a certain volume. A standard way to measure a dropper is to count the amount of water drops it takes to fill a dry 10 mL cylinder. Once you know that, you can divide the drop amount by 10 to find out how many drops are required for a 1 mL measurement and round off the number of drops. For pediatric doses, you always round the drops down.

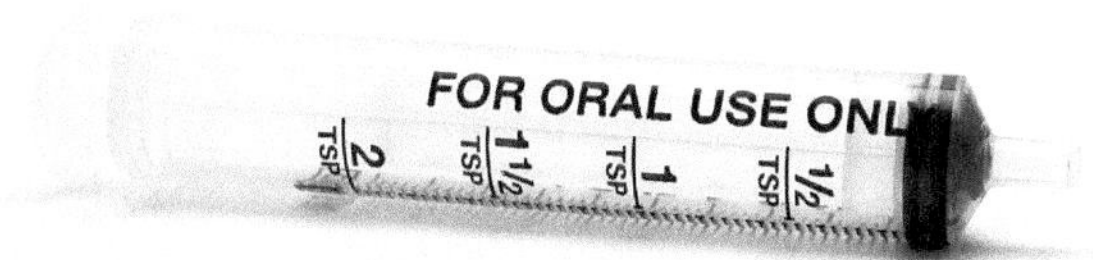

Be sure to thoroughly clean syringes between uses to avoid contamination.

Using Oral Syringes

Oral syringes (or hypodermic syringes without a needle) may also be used to measure small or large quantities of liquids. Pull the plunger back to create suction to pull in the liquid. Tap out all bubbles and add more liquid as needed. Place the syringe vertically on a counter with the tip up. Line up the bottom of the rubber plunger tip (not the top) with the measurement lines on the syringe. Oral syringes are more accurate than a graduated cylinder, especially when measuring thick, viscous liquids.

10.10 Techniques for Ingredient Preparation and Blending

After you have accurately weighed or measured out the individual ingredients, you must use the best technique to mix the active and inactive ingredients for a tablet, capsule, cream, ointment, gel, suppository, or other dosage formulation. The mixing directions should include the sequencing of the addition of ingredients and any dilutions needed. These directions should be included in the Master Formulation Record or suggested by the compounding pharmacist; you may also be using automated equipment. Some of the mixing methods are described below.

Comminution is the act of reducing a substance of one particle size to a smaller one through various methods. The exact procedure utilized will depend on recommendations contained in the Master Formulation Record and the type of nonsterile compound being prepared.

Blending is the act of combining two substances. It is not one technique but includes many different ones, applying what is needed in the recipe. The techniques include spatulation, sifting, tumbling, and the use of the geometric dilution method (which will be described). They are often mixed with the comminution techniques of trituration, levigation, and pulverization. With repetition and experience, the technician can become more proficient in knowing when and how to use these techniques individually, together, and in succession for the preparation of high-quality, pharmaceutically elegant compounded preparations.

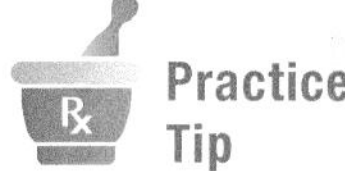

In trituration or pulverization, use swift rotations with minimal pressure. Too much pressure can result in damage to the mortar and pestle.

Trituration

The process of rubbing, grinding, or pulverizing a substance to create finer particles is called **trituration**. Using minimal pressure on the ingredients in a mortar, you rotate the pestle rapidly to rub and grind the ingredients into a powder. It can also be used to combine different substances to get a standardized blended powder. To gain a better understanding of trituration in the compounding process, refer to Figure 10.5.

Trituration is also used when a potent or hazardous drug is mixed with a diluent powder. At first, equal amounts of the potent drug and the diluent are triturated with a mortar and pestle. When these are thoroughly mixed, more of the diluent is added, equal to the amount already in the mortar. This process is continued until all of the diluent is incorporated into the compound.

FIGURE 10.5 Preparing a Solution for Sparky the Dog

(a) A pharmacy receives a prescription from a veterinarian to compound a preparation for Sparky the dog. This illustration shows the compounding log for this prescription.
(b) To prepare this medication, the pharmacist carefully weighs the product (potassium bromide).
(c) Next, the product is placed in a mortar to be triturated and combined with the beef flavoring.
(d) The ingredients are mixed, but more trituration is needed to get the particles to a more even texture.
(e) The pharmacist uses a wall-mounted source of distilled water (also used to reconstitute antibiotic powders) to add to the veterinary mixture.
(f) The mixed and triturated ingredients are put into an amber bottle, using a glass funnel. Then, the bottle is shaken well and labeled.

04-Feb-X1 Ron Holly — 3659.69 62
RX NO. 6600008 — AQ COST 13.05
PATIENT LLOYD, SPARKY K-9 01/01/202X 12Yrs — $ PROFIT 2.04
3000 MAPLE RD, FORT WAYNE, IN — Tax
(219) 555-1234 — Discount
09/03/XX ALLERGY NOT KNOWN—NO MED INFO — New total 15.09
DOCTOR [Notes]
Prescription:
Product — Patient: — 15.09
Disp — Prescriber:
Product: 48 G KBR QS TO 240 ML W/ H_20 +
Disp Qty — Product: 1 TEASPOONFUL BEEF FLAVOR POWDER
G 134 — Std PC KT: — KT
Give 1 — KT
Days 60 — Total O/R
Refills Auth Remain Total # — Copay O/R
DAW 0 First 02/04/X1 Comply — P Code O/R KT
Drug Exp 02/04/X2 Last 02/04/X1 [1] Status
Rx Exp 02/03/X2 Labels 01 166 002 #RX/OR Y
Written 02/04/X1 Auth by TECH
Exit Enter: Select

(a)

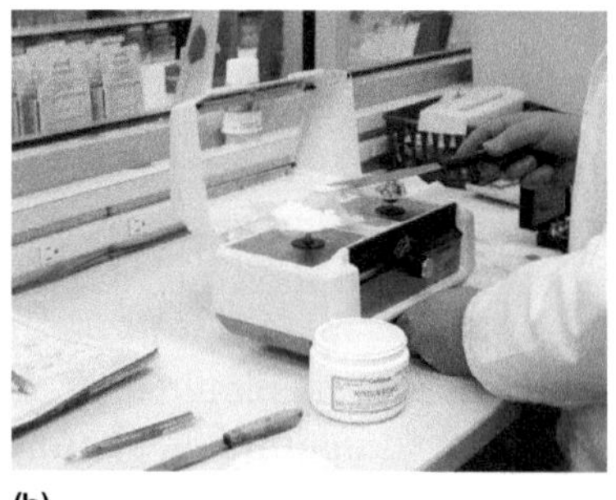

(b)

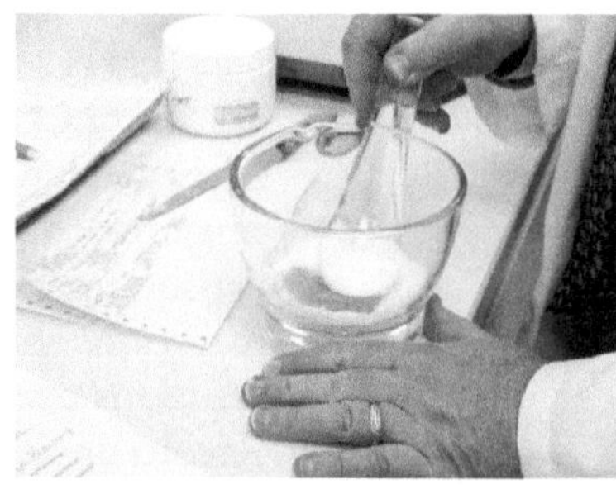

(c)

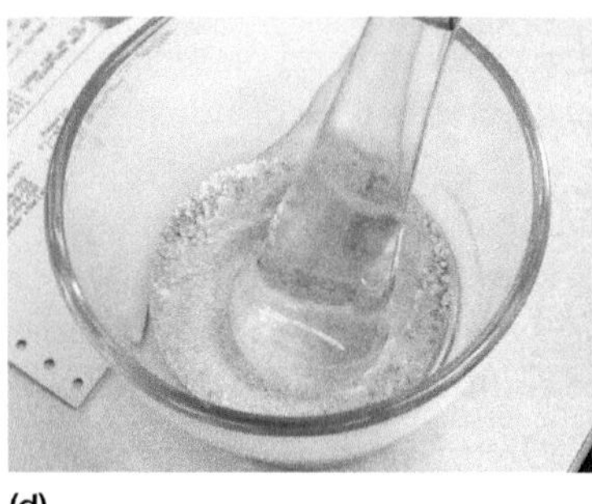

(d)

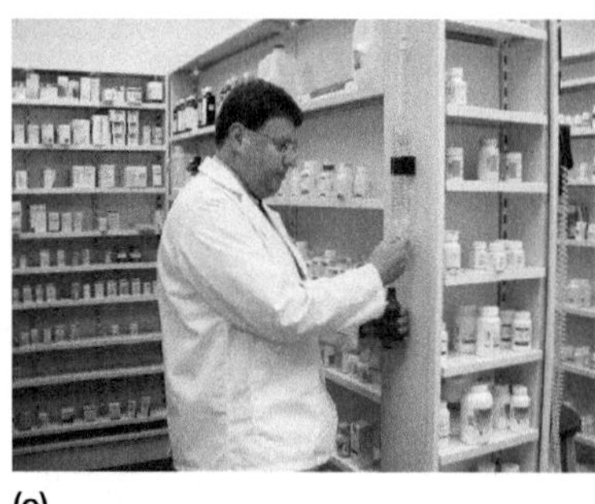

(e)

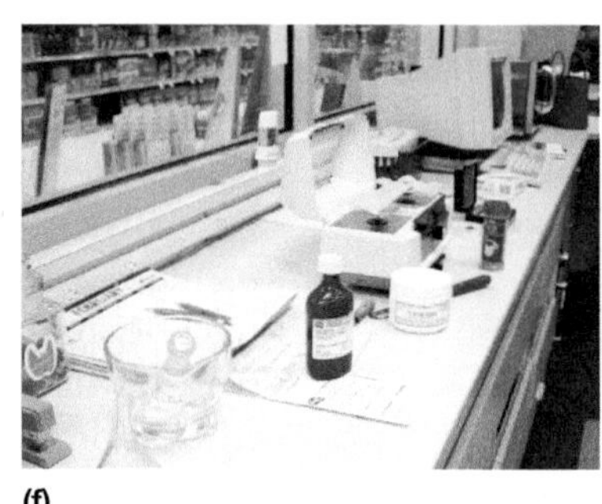

(f)

Sifting

In nonsterile compounding, **sifting** is a process not unlike sifting flour in baking. This process blends or combines powders using a wire mesh sieve. Select the mesh size based on the particle size needed. Pour the powders through the sieve, and use a rubber spatula to force the powder through the sieve and onto the glassine paper.

Tumbling

In the **tumbling** technique, you place the powders being combined into a container such as a resealable plastic bag or a glass bottle and "tumble" or rotate the container to mix the ingredients well. An inert coloring agent may be added to one or both of the substances to detect an adequate mixing of the ingredients. This technique is frequently used when combining hazardous substances.

Spatulation

The process of combining and mixing substances by means of a spatula, generally on an ointment slab or tile, is called **spatulation**. This technique is effective when mixing fine-particle powders. It is often used in the preparation of creams and ointments.

Pulverization by Intervention

In nonsterile compounding, **pulverization by intervention** is the process of reducing the size of particles of a solid with the aid of an additional ingredient in which the substance is soluble. A volatile solvent such as camphor, alcohol, iodine, or ether is often used for this process. The solvent is added in small amounts per mixing directions on the Master Formulation Record, then the mixture is triturated. The solvent is permitted to evaporate so that it does not become part of the final product.

Levigation

The **levigation** technique is typically used to further reduce the particle size of a solid during the preparation of an ointment. A levigating agent–such as castor oil, glycerin, propylene glycol, or mineral oil–is slowly added to the large particles of the dry ingredients in a glass mortar or on an ointment slab to wet (not dissolve) the insoluble chemicals. The resulting paste is triturated with a pestle or metal spatula and then added to an ointment base. The amount of levigating agent added depends on the desired consistency and is included in the Master Formulation Record. One example of levigation is adding glycerin to reduce the particle size of bismuth subnitrate.

Heating and Dissolving

When mixing a solid that is not easily dissolvable, you can gently melt the ingredient in a hot water bath or on a special low temperature hot plate (or at times in a microwave) and stir. Heating generally makes the solid dissolve faster and more uniformly with less precipitation, preventing the solute from clinging together in particles of unacceptably large size.

10.11 Compounding Specific Delivery Forms

In nonsterile compounding, different dosage forms require different compounding approaches to fit their unique qualities. (For learning more about the process of alligation to calculate the correct amounts of ingredients for combining manufactured drug products into a new product, refer back to Chapter 6.)

Powders

In earlier times, the pharmacist commonly prepared prescription medicines simply in the form of **powders**. The pharmacist measured, mixed, and divided the powders into separate units and placed them on pieces of paper to be dispensed. These pieces of paper were then folded and given to the patient. This dispensing method is all but obsolete in current compounding pharmacy practice. Some over-the-counter (OTC) medicines still come in powders, often in bulk packaging or individualized foil packets. In traditional Chinese medicine practice, fresh herbs are still prepared in wrapped paper packets and sold in herb shops.

Powders dispensed in bulk amounts have the disadvantage of inaccurate dosing. For example, Metamucil is a bulk powder used as an OTC fiber supplement in which the "approximate" dose may be one teaspoonful added to a glass of water or juice. For prescription drugs, the dose must be more exact.

Tablets

A tablet may be compounded with dry powdered ingredients in a traditional compression formulation using a single-punch tablet press to blend active and inactive ingredients (or excipients) into one solid form. You weigh the powders and place them in the die of a tablet press and then lower the handle to compress the ingredients. However, compression tablets are rarely compounded in most pharmacies, as this process requires expensive equipment, expertise, and labor-intensive preparation. It is often easier to triturate or pulverize ingredients and use them in the compounding of a capsule or suspension formulation.

Rapid-dissolving tablets (RDTs) are a unique tablet formulation that can be more easily prepared in a specialty compounding pharmacy. In addition to the active ingredient, a base, a sweetener, and flavoring agents are used for taste because these tablets dissolve on the tongue within 30 seconds. There are binders as well, such as gelatin, dextran, alginate, and maltodextrin. After the active and inactive ingredients are mixed, they are placed in a special Teflon mold (using a rubber spatula only, no metal) and then baked in a convection oven for a specified period. After cooling, the compound is then packaged and labeled in a blister pack for consumer use. (Some RDTs are formulated through freeze-drying.) Hormones such as estrogen, testosterone, and thyroid hormone may be prepared as RDTs. Since hormones are generally considered hazardous substances, they are typically compounded under a special contained hood to minimize airborne contamination (as will be explained in Chapter 13).

FIGURE 10.6 **Types of Hard-Shell Capsules**

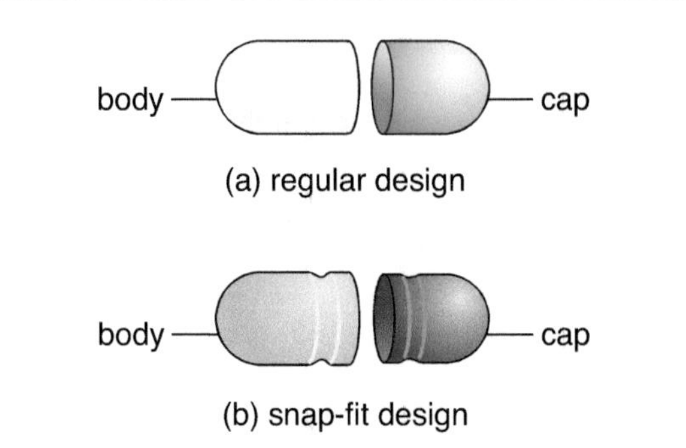

FIGURE 10.7 **Hard-Shell Capsule Sizes**

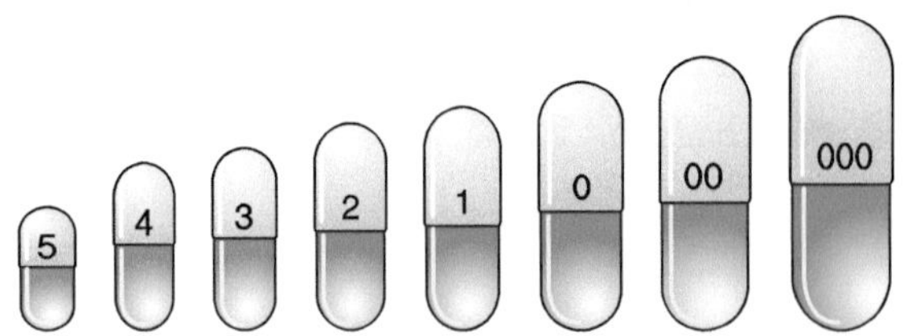

Capsules

In a capsule, the enclosed pharmaceutical contents may be a powder, granule, or liquid. The hard shells of capsules are made of gelatin, sugar, and water and consist of two parts: (1) the body, which is the longer and narrower part; and (2) the cap, which is shorter and fits over the body. In some cases, capsules have an interlocking design (marketed as Snap-Fit®), with grooves on the cap and the body that fit into one another to ensure proper closure (see Figure 10.6). Hard-shell capsules come in standard sizes indicated by the numbers 5, 4, 3, 2, 1, 0, 00, 000 (from smallest to largest). The largest capsule, size 000, can contain about 1,000 mg of medication; the smallest, size 5, contains about 100 mg (see Figure 10.7).

Capsules are often compounded to provide unusual dosage forms, such as those containing less of an active ingredient than is readily available in commercial tablets or capsules.

For example, in order to create an oral capsule in a pediatric dose that is not commercially available, the pharmacist may have you pulverize, or triturate, commercially available tablets, mix the resultant powder with a diluent powder, and use that powder mixture to fill capsules. This diluent powder provides bulk and stability to the capsule.

Most hard-shell capsules are meant to be swallowed whole; however, some capsules are intended to be opened so that their contents can be sprinkled on food or in drink. Therefore, patients should be advised as to which administration method should be used with their medications. They should also be warned that opening and ingesting the contents of certain capsules can adversely affect the controlled-release properties of certain medications and may upset the stomach.

When filling capsules, two methods are most common, the one-by-one punch method and the capsule machine.

Punch Method

To use the **punch method**, count the number of capsules to be filled. Then place the powder on a clean surface of paper, porcelain, or glass and, with a spatula, form into a cake approximately one-quarter to one-third the height of the capsule body. Punch the capsule into the cake repeatedly until the capsule is full. Then place the cap snugly over the body. To fill the capsule body with granules, pour them from the paper into the body before capping it. Check the doses by weighing the filled capsules.

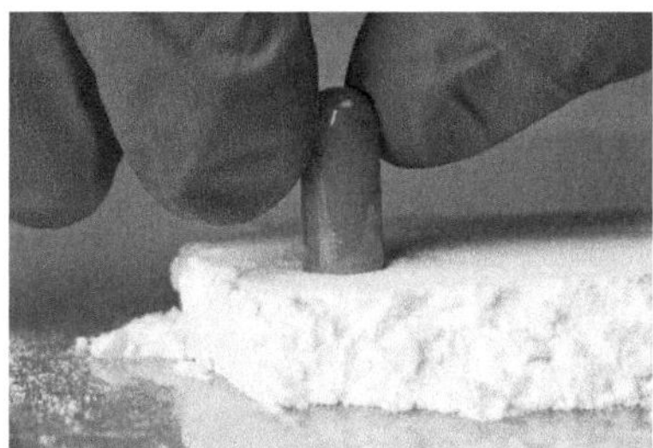
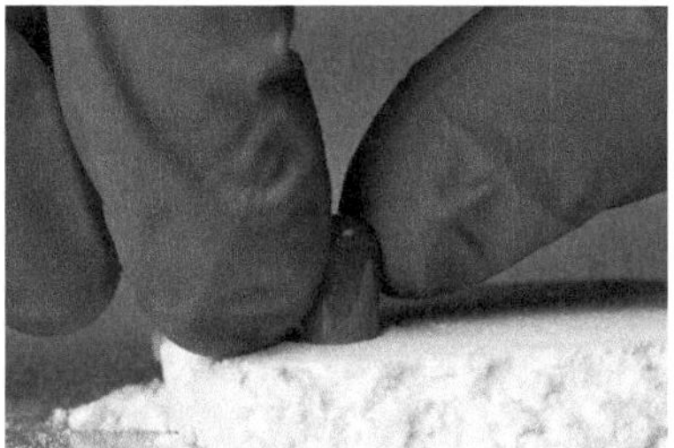
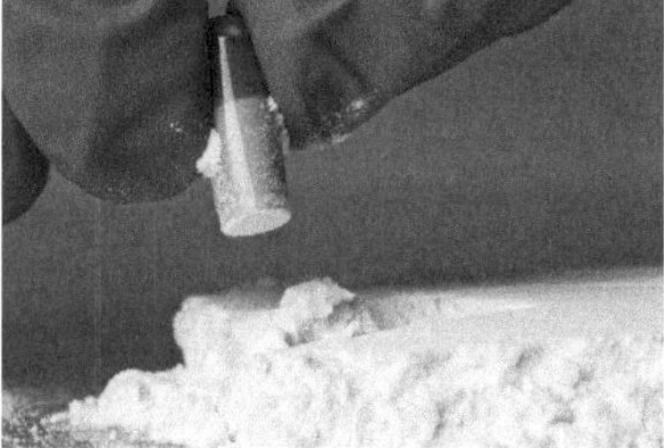

In the punch method, the body of the capsule is filled by "punching" it into a pile of dry power. Weigh the filled capsule to verify the dose.

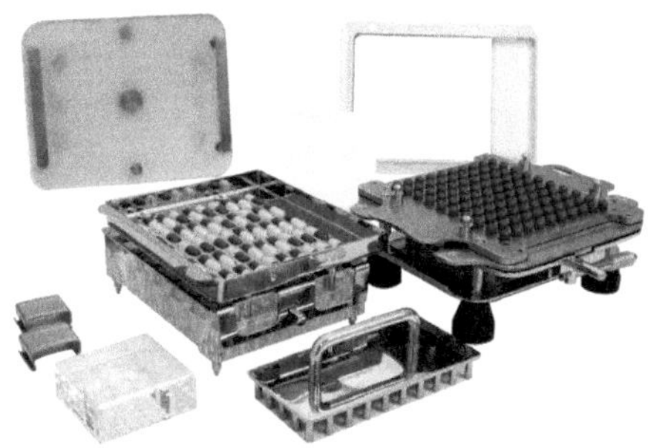

A capsule-filling machine is used in most compounding pharmacies.

Capsule Machine

A capsule machine with multiple metal or plastic plates may be used to replace the one-at-a-time punch-and-fill method. A capsule machine can make 100 capsules within a short period. The capsule bodies are poured into the slotted trays and shaken until they fill the slots and are arranged properly to receive ingredients. The drug ingredients are then poured over and smoothed into the capsules. The tray with the caps is placed over and pressed down to seal the filled bodies. To see a demonstration of one model, go to https://PharmPractice7e.ParadigmEducation.com/CapsuleFiller.

Example 2

Nystatin powder has a strength of 100,000 units/g. How many grams of nystatin would you use in each capsule if the final preparation is supposed to be 1,500,000 units per capsule?

Step 1 Convert 100,000 units/g to units/milligram using dimensional analysis.

$$\frac{1{,}500{,}000 \text{ units}}{1 \text{ capsule}} \times \frac{1 \text{ gram}}{100{,}000 \text{ units}} = 15 \text{ g per capsule}$$

Step 2 Determine the number of milligrams needed in each capsule using the dimensional analysis ratio and proportion method. You can then convert that to grams.

$$15{,}000 \text{ mg} \times 1 \text{ g}/1{,}000 \text{ mg} = 15 \text{ g}$$

This problem could also be solved using the ratio and proportion method. (For review of metric conversions and more examples of the ratio-proportion method, please refer back to Chapter 6 on pharmaceutical calculations.)

Troches

The small circular or oval lozenges that are designed to dissolve in the mouth (or within the vagina in some cases) rather than be swallowed are called **troches**. Because the ingredients are partially or fully absorbed through the mucous membranes, the powders for troches are often measured and mixed in cleanrooms under compounding hood fans to avoid contamination. The oral troches commonly include a base such as polyethylene glycol, suspending agents, sweeteners, and flavorings for taste. In compounding, the active medication in the powder form is slowly added to a base (and other agents as specified in the Master Formulation Record) over heat, thoroughly stirred and dissolved, and then poured into a troche mold and allowed to cool. The procedures for compounding troches are demonstrated at the following web link: https://PharmPractice7e.ParadigmEducation.com/Troches.

Troches are well-absorbed because the lining of the mouth (and vagina) is thin and rich in blood supply. An example of a prescription-only troche formulation is the antifungal drug clotrimazole; however, troches are also used to deliver bioidentical hormones and pain-relieving medications. Medicated lollipops can also be compounded with special molds, ingredients, and equipment.

Solutions

A solution is a liquid dosage form in which the powdered active ingredients, or **solute**, are dissolved in a liquid vehicle, the **solvent**. Solutions are prepared by dissolving the solute in the liquid solvent or by combining or diluting existing solutions.

Solutions may be aqueous (made with water), alcoholic, or hydroalcoholic. Hydroalcoholic solutions contain both water and alcohol, which may be necessary to dissolve some solutes. Colorings or flavoring agents may be added to solutions for appearance or improved palatability (taste); for example, a syrup—known as Simple Syrup NF—can be made by combining 85 g of sucrose with 100 mL of purified water.

Otic solutions are a commonly requested preparation in a compounding pharmacy. An example of a recipe or Master Formulation Record for an otic solution to remove ear wax is shown in Figure 10.8.

FIGURE 10.8
Master Control Record for Otic Solution Compound

Compound Title

urea and hydrogen peroxide otic solution

Compound Ingredients

carbamide peroxide .... 6.6 g

glycerin, as much as necessary to total .... 100 mL

Compounding Procedure

Dissolve the carbamide peroxide in sufficient glycerin to volume; then package and label. A beyond-use date of up to six months can be used for this preparation.

When mixing two or more liquids that are incompatible or insoluble, you can reduce or avoid a precipitation of solutes and make the end solution more stable if you dilute each solute ingredient with a portion of the solvent and stir or blend this diluted solute before adding it to the full solvent.

Regardless of their apparent stability, all suspensions should be dispensed with an auxiliary label stating "Shake Well."

Suspensions

In a suspension, as opposed to a solution, the active ingredient is not dissolved but rather is dispersed throughout the liquid vehicle. An obvious problem with suspensions is the tendency of the active ingredient to settle. The point (and rate) at which the suspending agent is added in the mixing procedure can be crucial. Therefore, you must always remember to add the ingredients in the proper order according to the recipe contained in the Master Formulation Record.

Ingredients can be judged according to their **suspendibility**, or ability to become and remain suspended in a liquid rather than dissolving into it or clumping up into **agglomerations** (lumps or globs).

To avoid settling of the insoluble drug, vigorously triturate the tablets into a powder and then add the suspending agent. Such suspending agents include tragacanth, acacia, and carboxymethylcellulose (CMC). Still, the auxiliary medication label "Shake Well" should always be affixed to a suspension container.

Flavoring agents may sometimes be incompatible with the active ingredient because of pH or acid/base balance. That is why many vendors provide flavoring vehicles that have been proven to be safe and effective in children for compounded preparations as well as commercially available reconstituted antibiotic suspensions.

Many pediatric suspensions that are commercially unavailable can be prepared in the pharmacy from adult tablets or capsules. A good example is compounding a pediatric suspension of captopril for patients under age six. The drug is available only in 12.5 mg, 25 mg, 50 mg, and 100 mg oral tablets. The pediatric dose is approximately 0.2 mg/kg. For a child weighing 10 kg (22 lb.), the dose is 2 mg. Tablets must be crushed, and suitable suspending and flavoring agents must be identified for stability and palatability.

Another example is calculating a dose for the cardiovascular drug carvedilol (Coreg) for a child. See the example below for a step-by-step explanation of the calculation and compounding processes.

Example 3

The pharmacy receives the following.

℞ **60 mL of a suspension of carvedilol (Coreg) at a concen tration of 5.5 mg/mL**

Carvedilol (Coreg) is not available commercially as a suspension but only as tablets in strengths of 3.125 mg, 6.25 mg, 12.5 mg, and 25 mg. How would you compound this prescription for the pediatric patient?

Step 1 Determine how many milligrams of carvedilol (Coreg) are needed using the ratio and proportion method.

$$\frac{y \text{ mg}}{60 \text{ mL}} = \frac{5.5 \text{ mg}}{1 \text{ mL}}$$

$$y \text{ mg} = 60 \text{ mg} \times 5.5 \text{ mg}$$

$$y \text{ mg} = 330 \text{ mg}$$

Step 2 Determine the tablet sizes and number of each that must be crushed or ground up with a mortar and pestle to equal approximately 330 mg.

$$\begin{aligned} 12 \text{ tablets} \times 25 \text{ mg/tablet} &= 300 \text{ mg} + \\ 2 \text{ tablets} \times 12.5 \text{ mg/tablet} &= 25 \text{ mg} + \\ 1 \text{ tablet} \times 6.25 \text{ mg/tablet} &= \underline{6.25 \text{ mg}} \\ & \quad 331.25 \text{ mg} \end{aligned}$$

After crushing the 15 tablets of different strengths, add a suspending agent until a volume of 60 mL is reached. Then add a small amount (usually one-half to one dropperful) of a flavoring agent and agitate vigorously. Beyond-use dating for nonsterile compounded suspensions for children is generally a maximum of 14 days (reviewed later in this chapter). Place a prescription label with prescriber directions and two added auxiliary labels: "Shake Well" and "Refrigerate." Present to the pharmacist for verification.

℞ **Put Down Roots**

In pharmacy, *occlusiveness* means the characteristic of holding moisture and resisting absorption. *Emolliency* refers to the characteristic of softening and soothing.

Ointments, Creams, and Lotions

The vast majority of nonsterile compounding is preparing individualized topical products, mostly hormonal medications. Ointments, creams, and lotions are semisolid dosage forms that are meant for application to the skin. The dry ingredients need to be triturated into a fine powder before being slowly added to the ointment or cream base. This is necessary to avoid a gritty, nonuniform appearance of the preparation.

IN THE REAL WORLD

A community pharmacist used clonidine powder (provided in containers labeled by weight in grams) to prepare a prescribed suspension for administration to a five-year-old boy for attention deficit disorder. The prescribed doses for clonidine in pediatrics range from 25 mcg (0.025 mg) to 125 mcg (0.125 mg). Clonidine has several medical indications, but in high doses, it can lower the blood pressure to unsafe levels, especially for children. There was a mix-up during the conversions among grams, milligrams, and micrograms, and the concentration of the suspensions dispensed was 1,000 times greater than intended. The boy began to hyperventilate and was admitted to the hospital, where he was saved. Careful conversions and compounding are essential to preventing medication errors.

To create a pharmaceutically elegant product, add the powder in small amounts, and constantly work the mixture in the ointment or cream base with the spatula on a compounding slab. A cream or lotion is best prepared using glass equipment. The edge of the spatula should press against the slab to provide a shearing force, which allows for a smoother preparation. An electric mortar and pestle or an automated ointment mill can be used if available to maximize the mixing of ingredients and to improve the appearance of the final preparation.

Ointments

Since an ointment is a water-in-oil (w/o) emulsion, it is greasy and not water washable. The properties of the various ointment bases such as lanolin, petrolatum, and Aquaphor vary in their degree of occlusiveness, emolliency, water washability, and water absorption. An **occlusive** ointment base has the ability to hold moisture in the skin and is best used when additional hydration is needed, such as for a patient with dry skin. An **emollient** base has the ability to soften skin, such as with bath oils.

White petrolatum is an example of a lipophilic (fat-soluble) base with high occlusive and emollient properties. Most ointment bases are commercially available from a wholesaler or pharmacy compounding vendor and are best prepared using water-repellent plastic equipment.

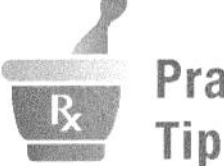

Practice Tip

The abbreviation *qs* means "a quantity sufficient up to the necessary amount," which means to fit the dosage and days' supply for the duration of the prescription.

Creams

A cream is an oil-in-water (o/w) emulsion that is nonocclusive, nongreasy, and water washable. Water washability and absorption relate to cosmetic appearance as in vanishing creams. Polyethylene glycol is an example of a water-soluble base.

Lotions

A lotion is a liquid suspension or an oil-in-water emulsion used topically on areas of the body such as the skin or the scalp where a lubricating effect is desirable. Calamine for poison ivy is an example of a commercially available skin lotion.

Compounding Ointments, Creams, Gels, and Lotions

When compounding these products, you often have to add powdered active ingredients to ointment, cream, gel, and lotion bases. This requires calculations, measuring, manipulations of the powders to make them fine and able to disperse in the base (as in pulverizing or levigation), and then adding them gradually into the base. You can then use the spatula with the ointment slab or mill to combine them into a smooth elegant product.

Example 4

℞ **3 ounces of an analgesic gel containing 10% ketoprofen, 10% gabapentin, and 3% lidocaine.**

Describe the process for compounding this prescription. Include a calculation for the amount of gel base needed to compound the product.

Step 1 Convert 3 ounces to grams.

$$1 \text{ ounce} = 30 \text{ g}, \quad \text{thus } 3 \text{ oz} \times \frac{30 \text{ g}}{1 \text{ oz}} = 90 \text{ g}$$

Step 2 Determine how many grams of each bulk ingredient are needed to make the correct active ingredient percentages in the final product.

$$\textbf{ketoprofen: } \frac{90\text{g} \times 3 \text{ g ketoprofen}}{100 \text{ g}} = 9 \text{ g}$$

$$\textbf{gabapentin: } \frac{90 \text{ g} \times 3 \text{ g gabapentin}}{100 \text{ g}} = 9\text{g}$$

$$\textbf{lidocaine: } \frac{90 \text{ g} \times 3 \text{ g lidocaine}}{100 \text{ g}} = 2.7 \text{ g}$$

Step 3 Weigh out these amounts of each medication.

Step 4 Add their weights together: 9 g + 9 g + 2.7 g = 20.7 g

Step 5 Subtract 20.7 g from the final product amount of 90 g to know how much gel base to add.

$$90\text{g} - 20.7 = 69.3 \text{ g of gel base}$$

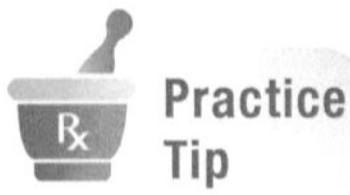

Practice Tip

To review conversion of measurements and percentages, please refer to Chapter 6.

Step 6 Mix each of these weighed powders with a sufficient amount of propylene glycol as a levigating agent to wet and smooth the powders (per the Master Formulation Record), and then gradually add them one by one to the gel base to make 90 g of the final gel product.

Practice Tip

The alligation method (alternate) is used for calculating the amounts of two drug products of differing percentages of active drug to create the proper amount of a middle percent of concentration. (It is nicknamed "Tic-Tac-Toe Math" and is covered in Chapter 6.)

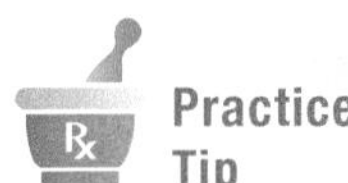

Practice Tip

Remember that prepackaged topical treatments come in the number of grams to 100 units (w/w), such that 1% hydrocortisone cream is 1 g/100 g cream.

Dermatologic therapies may call for a prescriptive strength that does not exist in commercial products. So you will have to take an existing commercial product of a more potent strength and one with a weaker strength, and combine them in different amounts to come to the prescribed strength in between. To do this, you will need to use the alligation alternate method, and the pharmacist will need to double-check the calculations before you do the compounding. To review and practice alligation calculation, go to percent in Chapter 6.

Example 5

How much 2% Nitro-Bid ointment is required to make 100 g of a 0.4% ointment?

Step 1 Determine the amount of Nitro-Bid needed to make 100 g of 0.4% Nitro-Bid ointment.

$$\frac{0.4 \text{ g of Nitro-Bid}}{100 \not{\text{g}} \text{ of } 0.4\% \text{ ointment}} \times \frac{100 \not{\text{g}} \text{ of } 0.4\% \text{ ointment}}{1} = 0.4 \text{ g of Nitro-Bid}$$

Step 2 Determine how much 2% Nitro-Bid ointment is needed to obtain 0.4 g Nitro-Bid.

$$\frac{0.4 \not{\text{g}} \text{ of Nitro-Bid}}{1} \times \frac{100 \text{ g of } 2\% \text{ Nitro-Bid ointment}}{2 \not{\text{g}} \text{ of Nitro-Bid}} = \begin{matrix} 20 \text{ g of } 2\% \\ \text{Nitro-Bid} \\ \text{ointment} \end{matrix}$$

This means that 20 g of 2% Nitro-Bid ointment is needed to make 100 g of 0.4% ointment.

Step 3 You can also solve this problem using the dimensional analysis one-step method.

$$\frac{0.4 \cancel{\text{g of Nitro-Bid}}}{100 \text{ g of } 0.4\% \text{ ointment}} \times \frac{100 \cancel{\text{g of } 0.4\% \text{ ointment}}}{1} \times \frac{100 \text{ g of } 2\% \text{ Nitro-Bid ointment}}{2 \cancel{\text{g of Nitro-Bid}}} = 20 \text{ g of } 2\% \text{ Nitro-Bid ointment}$$

Geometric Dilution Method for Combining If you are mixing two or more ingredients into the ointment or cream base, it is best to add them a little at a time sequentially using the **geometric dilution method** mentioned earlier. Place the most potent ingredient (often the ingredient that occurs in the smallest amount) into the mortar first. Then add an equal amount of diluent (least potent) and mix well. Repeat the process if a second active ingredient needs to be blended. Continue in this manner by adding, each time, an amount equal to the amount in the mortar until successively larger amounts of all the ingredients have been added.

FIGURE 10.9 **Master Formulation Record for a Topical Pain-Relief Gel**

Compound Title	
ketoprofen 10% and ibuprofen 2.5% in pluronic lecithin organogel	
Compound Ingredients	
ketoprofen	10 g
ibuprofen	2.5 g
lecithin:isopropyl palmitate 1:1 solution	22 mL
Pluronic F127 20% gel qs to total	100 mL
Compounding Procedure	
Mix the ketoprofen and ibuprofen powders with propylene glycol to form a smooth paste. Incorporate the lecithin:isopropyl palmitate solution and mix well. Add sufficient Pluronic F127 gel to volume and mix using high-shearing action until uniform. Package and label.	

Any small amounts of leftover diluent should then be added and mixed well. It is similar to the process of diluent trituration of powders. This method of gradual integration is time-consuming but creates a smooth dispersion of the drug(s) in the cream or ointment base, which allows for more drug stability and a more pharmaceutically elegant end preparation. (Other combining calculations are found in Chapter 6.)

Example 6

A prescription is received to prepare a compound for three ingredients in a ratio of 1:1:6 = 80 g. How much of each of the three ingredients will be needed?

Step 1 Find the number of total parts by adding all the elements of the ratio together.

$1+1+6 = 8$ parts. Then divide the total weight by total ratio parts.

$$80 \text{ g} \div 8 \text{ parts} = 10 \text{ g per part}$$

Step 2 Multiply each ingredient ratio by the weight for one part to find the ingredient ratios.

$$\begin{aligned} A &= 10 \text{ g} \\ B &= 10 \text{ g} \\ \underline{C} &\underline{= 60 \text{ g}} \\ &\ \ 80 \text{ g} \end{aligned}$$

The total amount of the preparation equals 80 g with ingredient C (the diluent) added at six times the amount of the two active ingredients A and B.

Here is the method you use to gradually combine them (if appropriate to the master formula directions):

1. Add C10 g to the A10 g.
2. Add C10 g to the B10 g.
3. Mix the combined C20 g with C-A 20 g mixture.

4. Add and mix the C20 g to the combined C-B 20 g mixture.
5. Then add and mix the C-A 40 g and C-B 40 g together.

Compounding Hormone Formulations Gynecologists in particular are requesting more compounded formulations to individualize the hormone treatments for their patients. **Hormone replacement therapy (HRT)** consists of a combination of estrogen, progestin, and androgen (male hormone) to relieve specific postmenopausal symptoms. **Estrogen replacement therapy (ERT)** consists of hormones and is sometimes used in postmenopausal women and premenopausal women who have had complete hysterectomies. Many commercially available hormones are available in a fixed-dose, oral synthetic formulation as well as sprays and transdermal patches.

Many women prefer creams, lotions, and ointments to tablets. With that in mind, more specialists are prescribing compounded topical preparations of bioidentical hormones that attempt to match each woman's individual medical needs based on the different levels of varied hormones present or missing in her blood or saliva. (Men are also being prescribed these specially compounded hormone formulations to treat male hormone deficiencies.)

Table 10.7 lists the most common abbreviations for the various estrogen hormones contained in a compound prescription. The dose is often based on symptoms, clinical observations, and laboratory analyses of serum, saliva, or urine levels. During hormone therapy treatment, a woman maintains a symptom diary so that the dose can be fine-tuned if necessary. A compounded cream or gel formulation may release the active ingredients more slowly and provide more long-lasting relief (fewer peaks and valleys) than a commercially available oral preparation. Because the various hormones in a topical formulation do not have to be eliminated through the liver like an oral tablet, it may be safer to use, although the long-term effects are unknown. Even with topical hormone compounds, the risk versus benefit must be assessed by the physician on an annual basis.

TABLE 10.7 Abbreviations on Bioidentical Hormone Compound Prescriptions

Bioidentical Hormone	Abbreviation	Percentage
estrone	E1	100%
estradiol	E2	100%
estriol	E3	100%
biestrogen	E3/E2	80%/20%
triestrogen	E3/E2/E1	80%/10%/10%

Practice Tip

In some cases, the mold must be properly calibrated and/or lightly lubricated to avoid difficulty removing the compounded products.

Suppositories

Since suppositories are solid dosage forms that are inserted into the body's orifices, generally the rectum or the vagina (less commonly, the urethra), they are composed of one or more active ingredients placed into one of a variety of water-soluble bases (such as glycerinated gelatin and polyethylene glycol) or oleaginous bases (such as cocoa butter and hydrogenated vegetable oil). These dosage forms melt or dissolve when exposed to body heat and fluids. Compounding high-quality suppositories typically requires the skills of a highly experienced pharmacy technician or a pharmacist.

Suppositories are produced by molding and by compression. The preparation of suppositories involves melting the base material, adding the active ingredient(s), and pouring the resultant liquid into a mold. (When using an aluminum metal mold, a light coating of lubricant such as mineral oil or glycerin must be applied prior to filling the mold.) Let each mold cavity slowly fill, ensuring that no air bubbles are entrapped. To prevent layering in the suppositories, do not stop the pouring process until all the cavities have been filled. Once filled, allow the contents of the mold to congeal or solidify at room temperature. When dispensing the suppositories, advise patients to refrigerate the medication to minimize premature melting of the active ingredients.

To view a demonstration on the technique of making suppositories, go to https://PharmPractice7e.ParadigmEducation.com/Suppositories.

10.12 Medication Containers and Beyond-Use Dating

To contain and store compounded preparations, there are various sizes of prescription bottles, capsule vials, suppository boxes, ointment jars, and special delivery units. It is important that you select the appropriate container to extend the integrity and stability of the product as much as possible. Packaging standards for the most common compounds are provided by USP in the *Pharmacists' Pharmacopeia* (see Table 10.8). Specialized packaging is needed for certain compounds. For example, rapid-dissolving tablets may need individualized blister packaging similar to many unit dose products in the hospital pharmacy.

TABLE 10.8 Compounding References

To stay up to date in the compounding field, refer to standard reference works on the subject, such as the following:

- USP's United States Pharmacopeia and National Formulary (USP-NF)
- Professional Compounding Centers of America (PCCA) web resources
- International Academy of Compounding Pharmacists (IACP)
- Remington: The Science and Practice of Pharmacy

UV-Protective Containers

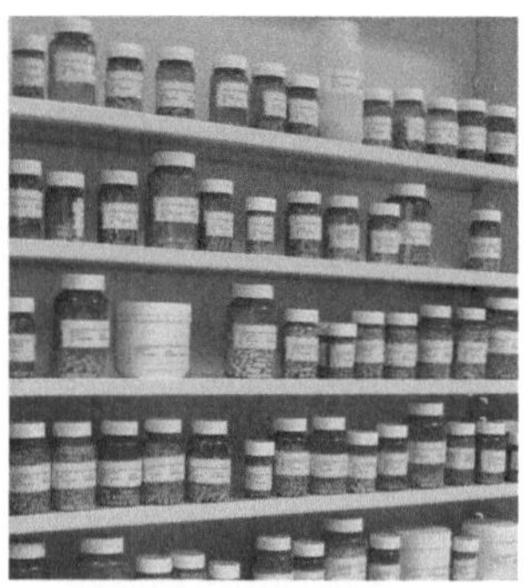

Most compounded tablets and capsules for future dispensing require special storage. Amber, light-protected vials are commonly used to protect the compounded products from UV light.

Most tablets, capsules, and liquids need to be stored in amber-colored vials or bottles or other ultraviolet (UV) light-protected packaging to prevent premature degradation of the products. Ointments and creams may be placed in white ointment jars of various sizes. Suppositories and pellets may be dispensed in cardboard packages. For precision in dosing, cream or gel hormone formulations are often dispensed to consumers in a needle-less (oral-style) syringe with the dosage calibrated in milliliters. These syringes can also come in amber plastic for protection against UV light.

Another accurate delivery method for topical creams is the easy-to-use Topi-CLICK. Well-accepted by physicians and patients, the patented, metered-dose applicator delivers a small measured squirt of a topical treatment of gel or cream. The unit is made of UV-blocking plastic and can hold up to 35 mL. Depending on the dose, the Topi-CLICK applicator may provide one to three months of medication. To operate, patients twist the base a quarter turn (one click) to move the plunger, thus delivering a given amount (0.25 mL per click) of medication in a topical base. The patient simply rubs the top of the container over the skin and then rubs it in. If applied to the inside of one arm or wrist, the patient can use the inside of the other arm or wrist to rub it in. (The patient needs to continually rotate the placement of the medication to avoid creating rashes or skin reactions from using the same patch of skin over and over.) Depending on blood levels, the patient dose may be one or more clicks per day. For patients on more than one hormone, the units are color coded to limit errors.

For less convenient skin regions, Topi-CLICK provides an applicator pad to rub in the cream so that the patient does not use their hands (since the hands are great absorbers and can remove some of the medication from the intended area). Using one's hands can also increase the chances of others accidentally being exposed to someone else's prescription when holding or shaking hands.

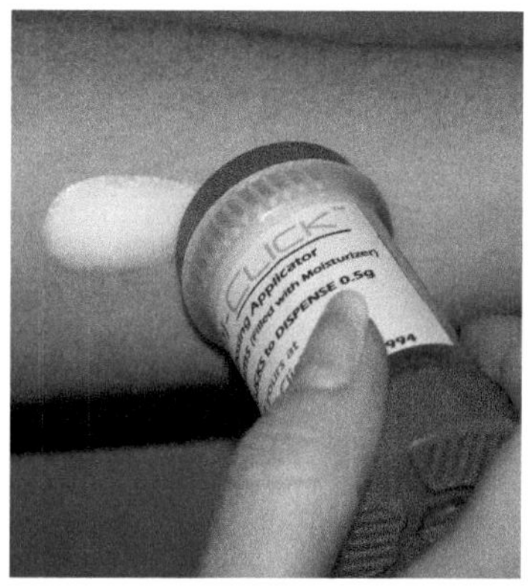

Topi-CLICK is a patented delivery system to dose hormone creams and gels accurately.

Stability Criteria and Beyond-Use Dating

Before a compound is mixed and formed, its stability needs to be assessed according to the expiration dates of its ingredients, and, from this, a **beyond-use date (BUD)** needs to be calculated. The BUD is the last date of recommended use. (The labels often say "discard after this date.") This assessment and calculation are performed by the technician or pharmacy software and double-checked by the pharmacist. **Stability** is defined as the extent to which a product retains the same properties and characteristics that it possessed at the time of preparation. Stability considers assessments of the physical properties (appearance, taste, uniformity, dissolution, and suspendibility) and chemical properties (potency). Some allowable variation (typically +/- 2%), however, is to be expected and accepted.

Calculating Beyond-Use Dating

Compounded preparations are meant for immediate use by the patient or a limited storage time. Because of this, the beyond-use dating of the preparation is by its nature very conservative and short-termed, beginning *at the time of compounding and not at the time of dispensing.* Therefore, compounded medications should be prepared as close to the time of dispensing to the patient as possible. Numerous considerations come into play:

- nature of the drug and how it degrades
- presence or lack of preservatives
- dosage form and components
- potential for microbial proliferation in the preparation
- packaging container

- prescribed length of therapy
- any scientific data

USP <795> provides guidelines for calculating beyond-use dating. For example, *a refrigerated aqueous solution or suspension always has a beyond-use date of 14 days (or less) with proper storage,* especially for pediatric solutions and suspensions. Semisolid formulations containing water are labeled with a 30-day beyond-use date or duration of therapy, whichever date is earlier.

Solids, such as tablets and capsules, and nonaqueous solutions have a beyond-use date of six months or less, depending on the ingredients of the compound. Determining the beyond-use date for a prescription having two or more active or inactive ingredients with varying expiration dates is a bit trickier, requiring calculation. If a manufactured or bulk drug is used, the beyond-use date is determined by taking 25% of the remaining expiration date of the drug stock or six months, whichever date is earlier. If dates differ among ingredients, the earliest expiration date is always used.

If the two ingredients both have long expiration dates, such as a year, the six-months clause ends up being applied. *This means that no compounded drug product should ever have a BUD beyond six months.* Examples 7–9 demonstrate the calculation of beyond-use dating for two nonsterile preparations.

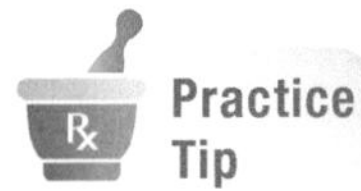

Compounds with water in them have deadlines of 14 days (liquid) and 30 days (semisolid) or less. A pediatric suspension must always have a BUD of 14 days (or less).

Example 7

A low-dose pediatric capsule of a blood pressure medication is combined with a suspending agent on March 30, 2023, with the following drug sources and expiration dates. What should the beyond-use date be?

Drug	Drug Source	Expiration Date
Lisinopril	Manufacturer	July 2023
Suspending agent	Bulk chemical	October 2024

The earliest expiration date is July 2023. March 30 to July 30 is 4 months, so 4 months $\times$ 0.25 = 1 month from date of compounding. However, because this is a pediatric suspension, it should be only 14 days.

Example 8

A pain compound is formulated with two different pain medications on June 1, 2023, with the following drug sources and expiration dates . What should the beyond-use date be?

Drug	Drug Source	Expiration Date
Ibuprofen	Bulk chemical	June 2025
Ketoprofen	Bulk chemical	August 2026

The labeled BUD should be December 1, 2023, or six months after compounding. The earliest expiration date of the bulk chemical is for ibuprofen, but 25% of the remaining expiration date (in two years) would be greater than six months. The more conservative BUD is used. The six-month expiration date should be used for this prescription, and any additional product (anticipatory compounding) should be stored for future prescriptions or refills.

Example 9

A bioidentical cream is formulated with two different hormones on June 15, 2025, with the following drug sources and expiration dates. What should the beyond-use date be?

Drug	Drug Source	Expiration Date
Hormone A	Bulk chemical	December 2026
Hormone B	Bulk chemical	October 2027

The earliest expiration date is December 2026. June 15, 2025, to December 15, 2026, is 18 months. So, 18 months $\times$ 0.25 = 4.5, or 4 ½ months from date of compounding. The beyond-use date is October 31, 2025.

10.13 Labeling, Final Check, Dispensing, and Cleanup

With the product compounded, it must be properly labeled and checked by the pharmacist before being dispensed to the patient with educational materials and counseling. Then reimbursement must be obtained and the product tracking information be documented for quality control. Tools and equipment must be cleaned and maintained.

Labeling

After the compounding operation, the preparation must be labeled with a medication container label containing all information for the consumer as required by the governing laws and regulations of the state and federal government. As noted earlier in Table 10.2, it should include the following:

- patient name
- physician name
- date of compounding
- name of preparation
- internal ID or lot number
- beyond-use date
- initials of compounding technician and pharmacist
- directions for use, including any special storage conditions

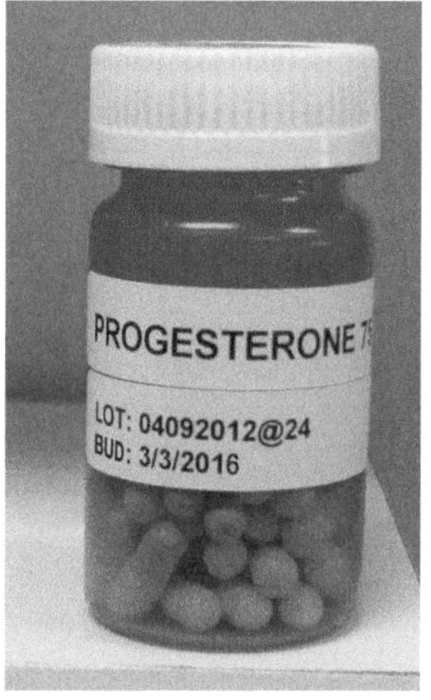

Excess nonsterile compounds must be labeled with the drug name, lot number, and beyond-use dating, and stored properly.

- any additional requirements of state or federal law

The original sig, or directions from the prescriber, must be prominently displayed on the label for patient attention, along with any auxiliary colored labels as special reminders about warnings and storage. If commercial products are used, then the brand or generic drug names should be listed on the medication container label. Do not use abbreviations of the active drug ingredients, because they need to be immediately obvious to the patient and any medical personnel in the rare event that the drug must be identified in an emergency. If Topi-CLICK is used, the medication container label can be directly affixed to the sides of the plastic container.

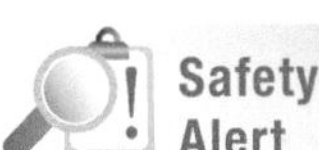

Counseling by the pharmacist is very important, because many extemporaneous compounds are unique to the patient, and there may not be much prepared information to print out for the patient regarding the completed compound.

The excess compounded product must be stored in the appropriate temperature conditions and stock container and labeled with drug, dose, lot number, beyond-use dating, and sometimes the initials of the pharmacist and the compounding technician. The stock medication must be checked for expiration dates and potential disposal monthly or as specified in the pharmacy's P&P Manual.

Final Check by the Pharmacist

The pharmacist is legally responsible for checking the final product, including ensuring that the correct Master Formulation Record was used, that mathematical calculations were accurate on the Compounding Record, and that weighing of amounts or printouts on all weighed ingredients were verified. The medication container label must also be checked. A careful record of the compounding operation—including ingredients and amounts of ingredients used, the preparer of the compound, and the name of the supervising pharmacist—should be kept.

Finally, the pharmacist checks the pharmaceutical elegance by performing a physical inspection of the preparation. The pharmacist uses their knowledge and experience to review the adequacy of mixing, odor, color, consistency, and pH (acid or base balance) if necessary. The pharmacist initials the Compounding Record and the label and then places the product under proper storage conditions for future pickup or mailing to the patient.

After the product is prepared by the technician and checked by the pharmacist, a printed copy of the Compounding Record is filed with the original prescription for later retrieval. Easy retrievability is important if there is a drug recall of any ingredients in the compounded prescription or if an adverse effect occurs in the patient. In addition to printed copies of the formula and the prescription, most records are stored on a CD, flash drive, passport, internet cloud, or an on-site computer or that of an off-site vendor. Storage of the compounded products must also be considered. Some compounded preparations require freezing or refrigeration, and pharmacy technicians must monitor and document their temperatures as well as room temperatures on a daily basis in order to maintain the stability of the stored prescriptions and anticipatory compounds.

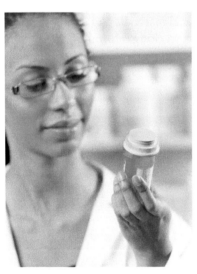

As with any prescription, the pharmacist must provide a final check of the medication and label before dispensing to the patient.

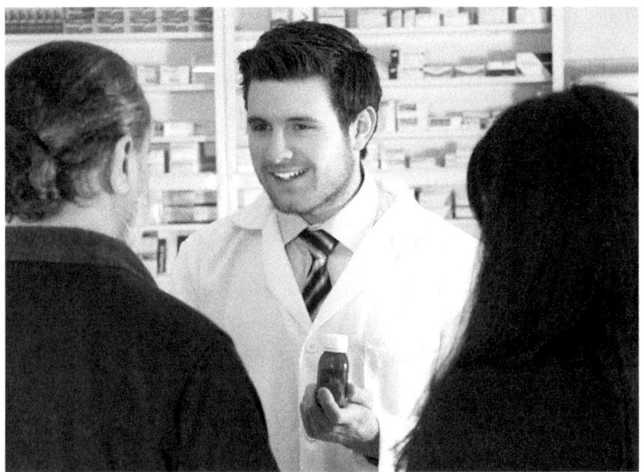

Counseling by the pharmacist on proper use, storage, and beyond-use dating is important on any compounded preparation.

Dispensing and Patient Counseling

Once the compound has been approved, you need to inform the patient that their prescription is ready and has been individually prepared and compounded pursuant to a prescription. The patient should be counseled by the pharmacist on the proper use, storage, handling, and beyond-use dating requirements. A written medication information printout should accompany the prescription.

As with all prescriptions, you must offer pharmacist counseling to all patients. They must be made aware of all the ingredients contained in the compounded prescription and their expected therapeutic and potential adverse effects. The pharmacist in particular must be sure that the patient understands how to take the medication, especially if an unusual delivery system is used. For example, how does the dosage compare to the milliliters (mL) or cubic centimeters (cc) on a syringe or to the clicks on a Topi-CLICK? How is this delivery device primed, or how often does it need to be primed? The pharmacist should demonstrate how the medication should be applied—for example, placed on one arm and rubbed in by the other arm for 15 to 20 seconds.

Reimbursement

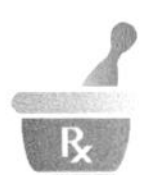

Practice Tip

It is best practice to secure partial or full payment prior to executing the actual compound. If the patient finds the cost unaffordable *after* the technician has prepared the compound, then time, money, and inventory have been wasted.

Insurance generally does not cover compounded preparation costs. This lack of coverage is a major reason for the growth of specialized compounding pharmacies. Since independent pharmacies have been financially struggling because of the low reimbursements from insurance, many have moved into specialized compounding. The patient cost for a compounded medication is based on the time and experience of the pharmacist and the technician rather than on the specific ingredient costs, which are often relatively minimal except with newer specialty drugs. Most compounded prescriptions take a minimum of 30 to 60 minutes to prepare.

Though patients generally pay out of pocket for compounded preparations, sometimes if they complete the proper online or paper forms, they may be reimbursed by their insurance at a later date. You can provide the patient with all necessary information regarding the compounded preparation on a universal claim form (UCF) so that the patient can pursue this option, submitting the necessary documentation to the insurance company for personal reimbursement. The information the patients need includes the NDC number and the cost of each ingredient, as well as the time necessary to prepare. Reimbursement success for a compounded medication tends to be greater if the patient, rather than the pharmacy, submits the claim, billing a third-party insurer.

Patient Follow-Up, Tracking, and Quality Control

Compounding pharmacies often want to track the success of their products and the patients' health out of concern for them, for quality control, and for continued accreditation. *USP* <1163> outlines a holistic approach to quality control for compounding pharmacies that takes a robust look at each stage of compounding to ensure best practices and feedback when things go wrong. *USP* <1163> also offers quality assurance testing methods to ensure that the best possible product has been compounded before it is dispensed.

The need for these types of quality control features are part of the continuous quality improvement required by the Professional Compounding Centers of America. The PCCA markets a user-friendly software package for dedicated compounding pharmacies to accomplish quality assurance and improvement called The Compounder Rx. This software offers a sophisticated database for compounding prescriptions quickly, efficiently, and safely. The software logs all ingredients in the Compounding Record and is integrated with measuring scales and bar code readers for easier pharmacist verification. The Compounder Rx also tracks the prescriptions (including lot numbers), patients, and prescribers. It generates labels, allows for mandated patient counseling, and provides documentation for a quality assurance tool for accreditation. A screen shot of The Compounder Rx can be viewed in Figure 10.11.

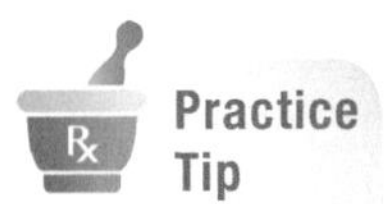

Chemical *ignitability* refers to the potential for sparking and causing flames when meeting air, water, other chemicals, or environmental triggers.

Corrosivity is the potential to damage or destroy other substances through an intense acidic, base, or other chemical composition.

Reactivity is the potential to cause chemical reactions when encountering other chemicals, molecules, or substances.

Cleanup and Maintenance

Cleaning up and maintaining tools and equipment are essential technician tasks in compounding. Once each product has been compounded, the equipment and work area must be thoroughly cleaned, and ingredients should be returned to their proper storage areas. Even the balances must be cleaned after each use, with documented daily calibration. As stated earlier, the prescription balance, when not in use or in transit, should be placed in the locked position and covered, with weights (if used) placed back in their original container.

You must pay special attention to the correct cleaning and disinfecting procedures to minimize any cross-contamination and potential allergic reactions. An ingredient that has beneficial effects on one patient can cause a deadly adverse reaction in an allergic patient from even trace amounts left on a mortar or measuring device. In addition, many active pharmaceuticals and bulk ingredients used in compounding are considered hazardous chemicals. This designation is not only for

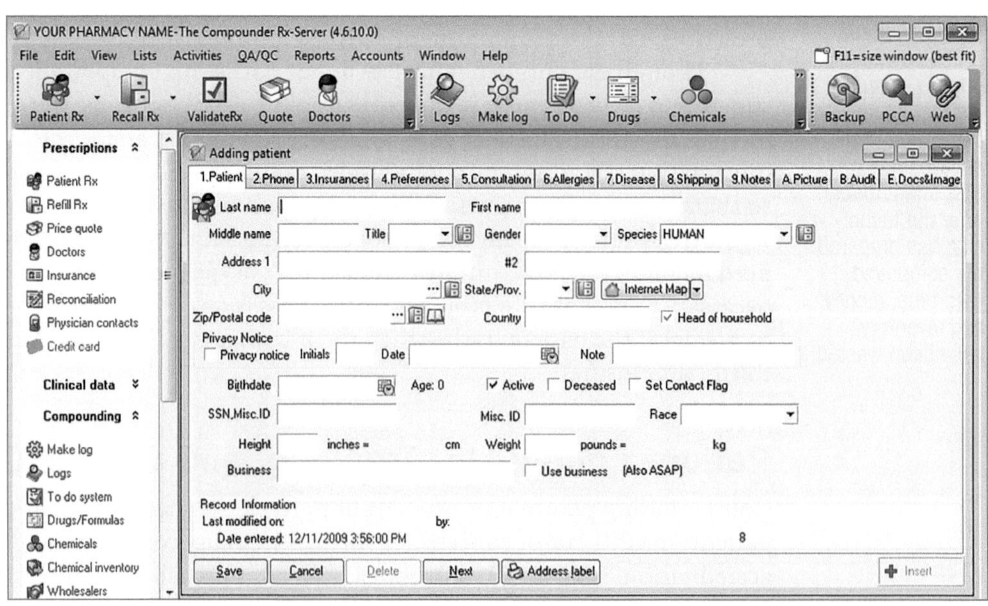

FIGURE 10.11 Screenshot of The Compounder Rx

This is a sample of a compounding software program designed to help compounding pharmacies manage quality control, prescription tracking, and patient monitoring.

toxicity, but also for higher than usual levels of chemical ignitability, corrosivity, and reactivity to other compounds.

In the compounding and cleaning up of hazardous substances, you must wear the required protective clothing. (More discussion on this is in Chapter 13.) A sodium hypochlorite 2% solution is recommended for the cleaning, decontamination, and disinfecting. This should be followed by a solution of sodium thiosulfate 10% or a similar neutralizing agent (to make the chlorine in the disinfecting solution chemically neutral or harmless), as outlined in the facility's P&P Manual. You must discard any expired or unusable product containing a hazardous chemical in a sealed container in the designated biohazard container (not the wastebasket), again according to the written policies and procedures. The pharmacist must then verify and sign off on the contents, and an outside vendor will take the receipt and the contents and discard the hazardous materials properly in a medical waste incinerator or by other means per state and federal regulations.

10.14 Progressing in the Field of Nonsterile Compounding

With this overview of nonsterile compounding and some hands-on practice in a lab class and in an externship, you will have a firm base of knowledge for preparing for the certification exam. You can grow on this specialty path through targeted compounding classes and workshops, and learning from the compounding pharmacists with whom you work.

Keeping Up to Date with Resources

Part of the challenge of compounding and pharmacy in general is keeping up with the field. The USP offers online the *USP-NF*, which serves as the primary guide for pharmacy personnel involved in both sterile and nonsterile compounding. Its collected materials include approved monographs for more than 120 compounded preparations, in addition to all the necessary guidelines and standards for the safe preparation, packaging, and storing of many compounded prescriptions mentioned earlier.

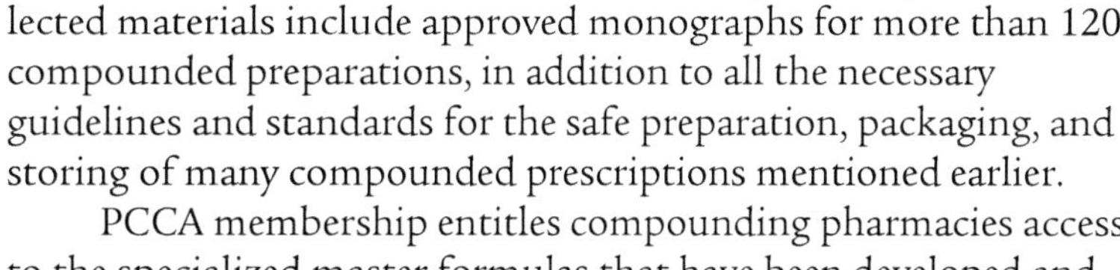

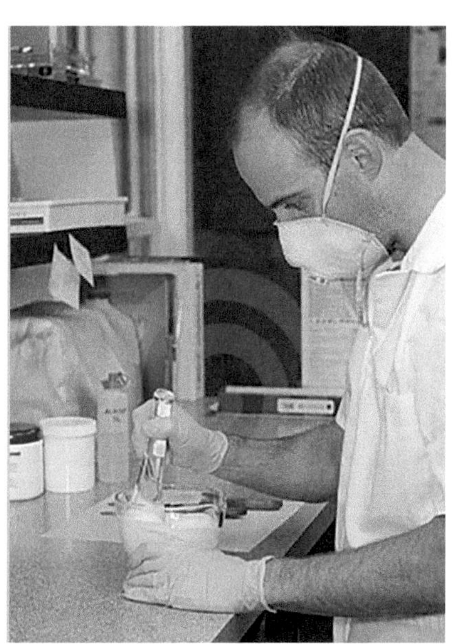

This pharmacy technician is using a mortar and pestle to compound a prescription.

PCCA membership entitles compounding pharmacies access to the specialized master formulas that have been developed and proven safe and effective over the years. In addition, the PCCA holds national and regional educational and training seminars in sterile and nonsterile compounding for both pharmacists and pharmacy technicians. The PCCA is also a source of pharmacy software, as well as marketing, business, and clinical consultations.

The International Academy of Compounding Pharmacists (IACP) is a political action group; membership is open to both pharmacists and pharmacy technicians. The group's mission is to promote and advance personalized medication solutions for patients. In addition, the organization keeps compounding pharmacy personnel alert to legislative challenges that have an impact on their profession. For example, the FDA has suggested in the recent past that all compounded preparations should be considered new drugs and thus be subject to undergoing a new drug application (NDA) process similar to the requirements for pharmaceutical manufacturers. If such legislation were passed, compounding pharmacies—the embodiment of a long-standing tradition that lies at the heart of pharmacy practice—would cease to exist. Keeping attuned to changes in the pharmaceutical industry is essential to fulfilling the responsibilities of practicing safe and effective patient care.

The latest print and online edition of *Remington: The Science and Practice of Pharmacy* has been a mainstay of information for pharmacists for more than 100 years; it is continually updated. It is considered a comprehensive pharmacy resource and can provide helpful background knowledge for technicians as well, especially if you would like to go further in the field in any specialty or perhaps someday become a pharmacist.

Another helpful local source of information for the compounding community pharmacist and technician is a local or area hospital pharmacy, especially a pediatric hospital pharmacy, where a pharmacist may have a needed recipe or formula and has experience compounding and flavoring formulations for neonates, infants, and pediatric patients.

Accepting the Compounding Challenge

As a pharmacy technician working in a community or hospital pharmacy, you will occasionally be asked to prepare a nonsterile compound according to a prescription or medication order. However, as you can see, working in a full-time dedicated compounding pharmacy is anything but an introductory skill. One cannot underestimate the importance of experience and practicing skill in calculating, weighing, mixing, and measuring of various ingredients. Being able to follow a detailed compounding process to prepare a safe, effective medication for patients of all ages is also significant. Providing easy-to-understand patient education materials and in-person directions, accurate beyond-use dates, and proper storage conditions for each product is also key so that patients can use the medication appropriately. Each prescription must meet all state and federal regulations and the *USP* Chapters <795> and <800> (2016) standards for enforcement and accreditation.

The environment in an extemporaneous nonsterile compounding pharmacy is radically different from a typical community pharmacy—you use sophisticated equipment in a segregated area without interruption from walk-in patients, telephone calls, or insurance processing. Advanced training and certification in this specialty area of pharmacy are required, but you are rewarded with higher pay and benefits. Another benefit similar to that of the work of a pharmacy technician in general is that your work will always be varied and continue to change as drugs and their master formulas and delivery methods change.

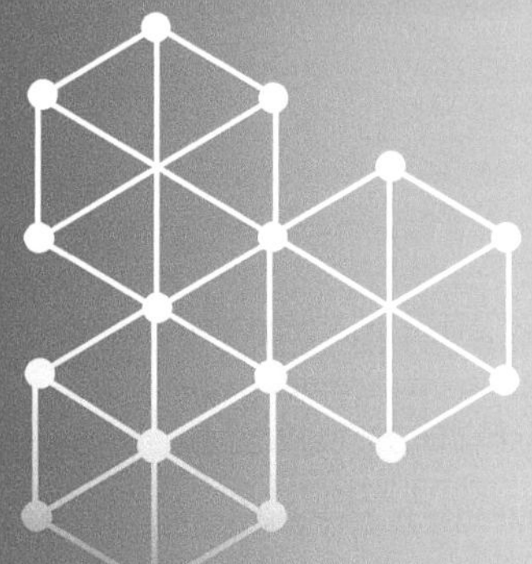

Review and Assessment

CHAPTER SUMMARY

- Nonsterile compounding is used to prepare medications in strengths, combinations, or dosage formulations that are not commercially available.
- Pharmacy technicians generally need national certification and additional training to practice in a dedicated nonsterile compounding pharmacy.
- The FDA Modernization Act differentiated manufacturing from compounding.
- Compounding pharmacies must follow standards set in *USP* Chapters <795> and <800> (2016) as well as other *USP* standards and state and federal regulations.
- Product quality for bulk ingredients is important in compounding a high-quality product.
- A Safety Data Sheet is required to be on file for all bulk ingredients stored in the pharmacy.
- Many specialty compounding pharmacies seek national accreditation for marketing and reimbursement, though they can only advertise their services, track record of quality, and credentials of their personnel, not their specific products.
- Minimum proper attire includes a long lab coat, shoe covers, hairnet, and disposable gloves.
- Compounding hazardous preparations requires additional personal protective equipment, such as a special coat, double gloving, a respiratory mask, a face shield, shoe and hair covers, and goggles.
- The Master Formulation Record documents the correct ingredients, equipment, and technique (like a recipe) that must be used to prepare a quality preparation of a specific type.
- The Compounding Record documents the ingredients and steps taken in the specific preparation process for each patient's prescription.
- The technician must carefully follow each step in the compounding process as outlined in the Master Formulation Record and USP standards.
- Instruments for weighing and measuring extemporaneous compounds commonly include a digital scale or an analytical two-pan balance, pharmaceutical weights, forceps, spatulas, weighing papers, a compounding or ointment slab, parchment paper, mortar and pestle, graduated cylinders, and pipettes, among others.
- Mortars and pestles are available in glass and porcelain varieties.

- Graduated cylinders come in various sizes of both conical and cylindrical shapes, the latter being smaller in volume and consistent in shape. They are therefore more accurate for measuring.
- The volume of a liquid must be measured by the level of the center of the meniscus.
- Proper technique and use of correct measuring devices are crucial when weighing and measuring pharmaceutical ingredients.
- The calculations and measurements for individual ingredients must be double-checked by the pharmacist.
- Compounding hazardous drugs must be accomplished in a separate room with specialized equipment.
- Several techniques are used for the comminution and blending of ingredients, including trituration, pulverization, spatulation, sifting, tumbling, levigation, alligation, and the geometric dilution method.
- Geometric dilution is utilized when mixing two or more ingredients of different strengths or concentrations with a diluent, such as a solute, cream, or ointment base.
- The compounding of lozenges or troches often requires heating the solution and pouring it into molds to form their shapes as the liquid cools.
- Hormone creams and ointments are the most common nonsterile compounded preparations, and they often require mixing the ingredients on a slab with a spatula or in an ointment mill.
- Topi-CLICK is a unique patented drug delivery system to more accurately and safely administer bioidentical hormones.
- Beyond-use dating is the assignment of an end date for recommended use of a compounded preparation that meets USP guidelines or is supported by independent scientific research.
- The completion of the compounding process includes selecting the most appropriate medication container, calculating beyond-use dating, affixing a label, keeping accurate prescription records, cleaning up, and maintaining equipment.
- The pharmacist is legally responsible for the final check of the compounded prescription (including all calculations, measurements, and labeling) and for counseling the patient.
- Proper storage of ingredients and finished and excess product is important, especially for hazardous drugs.
- Nonsterile compounding is an art to be learned under the tutelage of an experienced pharmacist, with additional learning to come from training workshops and programs, professional organizations, and compounding resources.

CHECK YOUR UNDERSTANDING

Take a moment to review what you have learned in this chapter and answer the following questions.

1. Pharmacies are allowed to compound more product than what is needed at that moment to have some on hand for refills or a similar need; this practice is called
   a. anticipatory compounding.
   b. extemporaneous compounding.
   c. sterile compounding.
   d. manufacturing.
2. A pharmacy involved in nonsterile compounding is required to follow good compounding practices as required by
   a. *USP* Chapter <795>.
   b. *USP* Chapter <797> (rev. 2019).
   c. the Food, Drug, and Cosmetic Act.
   d. the Orphan Drug Act.
3. Mini-certifications and laboratory training in nonsterile compounding for both pharmacists and technicians are provided by the
   a. PCCA.
   b. PCAB.
   c. FDA.
   d. USP.
4. The certification process for compounding pharmacies that comply with all national standards and the best industry practices in nonsterile and sterile compounding is administered by the
   a. USP.
   b. FDA.
   c. PCCA.
   d. ACHC.
5. The master formulation record contains
   a. the original prescription.
   b. the recipe with all the ingredients and mixing directions.
   c. the beyond-use dating of all active and inactive bulk ingredients.
   d. the cost of the final compounded preparation.
6. When preparing a nonsterile compound, pharmacy personnel should wash their hands with soap and water
   a. before donning a sterile gown, shoe covers, a hair cover, and a face mask.
   b. after the preparation of each compound.
   c. before donning disposable gloves.
   d. if hazardous ingredients will be utilized.

MAKE CONNECTIONS

Take a moment to consider what you have learned in this chapter and respond thoughtfully to the following prompts. Note that some of these activities will require internet access.

1. Use the internet to research Magic Mouthwash, and address the following in a short essay (approximately 300 words):
   a. What are the indications for this compound?
   b. What information needs to be documented in the compounding record?
   c. What are common patient instructions?
   d. List all of the ingredients you can find in the various formulations of Magic Mouthwash.
2. Research the background on the establishment of the Pharmacy Compounding Accreditation Board (PCAB) and the advantages it offers to prescribers, pharmacists, and customers. Write a short essay (approximately 300 words) that addresses the following:
   a. What is and is not permissible to use in marketing of services?
   b. Find (and visit if possible) an accredited compounding pharmacy in your geographical area, and make a report on your findings; what are the accreditation dates and services offered?

 The online course includes additional review and assessment resources.

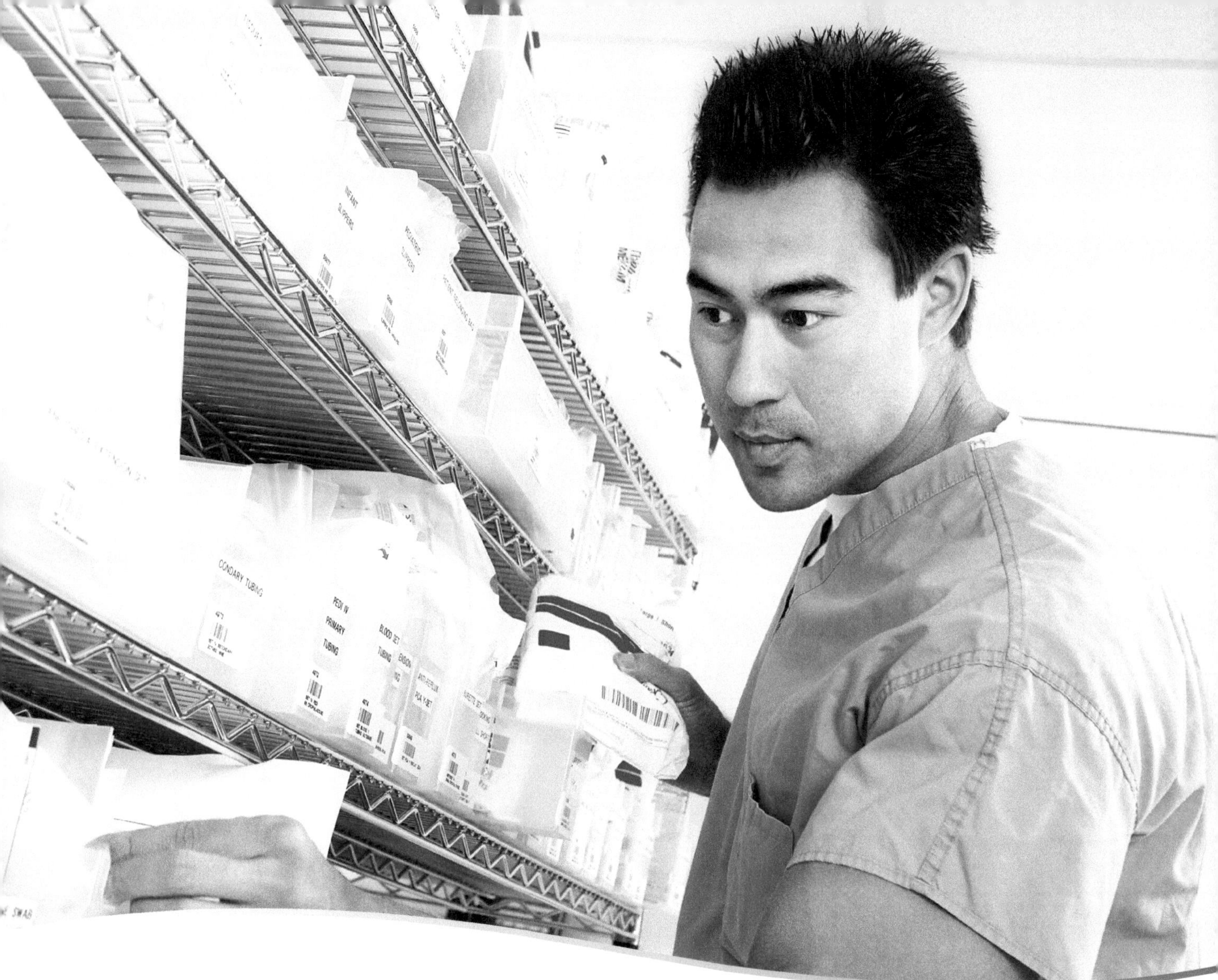

UNIT 4 Institutional Pharmacy Practice

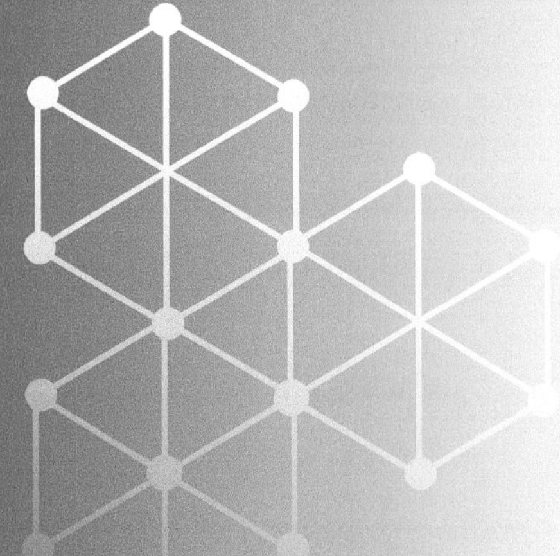

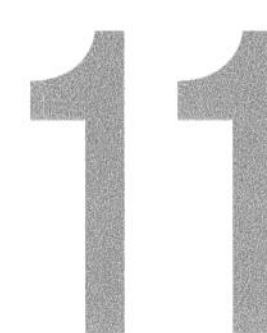

Hospital Pharmacy Dispensing

Learning Objectives

1. Describe the functions of a hospital and its organizational framework. (Section 11.1)
2. Define the roles and functions of the Pharmacy and Therapeutics Committee (especially on the hospital formulary) and the Institutional Review Board (on investigational drug studies). (Section 11.1)
3. Explain the functions of the pharmacy department within the hospital structure and the roles and responsibilities of the director of pharmacy, the pharmacist, and the pharmacy technician. (Section 11.2)
4. Identify the training and certifications required for a technician to work in a hospital pharmacy. (Section 11.2)
5. Paraphrase the role of the interoperability of hospital management software, different types of electronic health records, medication orders, and automated technology. (Section 11.3)
6. Discuss the functions and benefits of CPOE, AMDS, BPOC, and eMARs. (Section 11.3)
7. Describe the different dispensing systems for medication orders, such as unit dose carts, robotic filling and dispensing equipment, automated dispensing cabinets, and specialty cleanroom services. (Section 11.4)
8. Explain the proper procedure for preparing, labeling, and repackaging unit dose medications. (Section 11.4)
9. Describe the ordering, receipt, and documentation of controlled medications, including the advantage of utilizing an automated dispensing storage unit. (Section 11.4)
10. Understand inventory management of pharmaceuticals, including drug bidding, ordering, receiving, and storage processes. (Section 11.5)
11. Describe other institutional pharmacy practice settings that serve the aging population. (Section 11.6)
12. Explain the major role of the Joint Commission in establishing accreditation standards for hospitals. (Section 11.7)
13. Identify the importance and types of various measurements of productivity in the pharmacy department. (Section 11.8)

ASHP/ACPE Accreditation Standards

To view the *ASHP/ACPE Accreditation Standards* addressed in this chapter, refer to Appendix B.

As compared to community pharmacy practice, hospital practice has different organizational structures and medication filling/distribution systems. In addition, the services and policies of a large urban hospital pharmacy will vary from an academic university hospital, a veterans hospital, or a 50-bed rural hospital. Yet they all share many important commonalities.

If you wish to work in hospital practice, you generally must be certified and often must have specialized education, experience, and/or training in areas such as medication reconciliation, unit dose medications, repackaging, floor stock, narcotic inventory, or intravenous (IV) and chemotherapy medication preparation. Even more than in the community pharmacy, hospitals rely on computer software, technology, and automation in medication ordering, filling, distribution, inventory control, and bedside drug administration. Therefore, pharmacy technicians must be familiar with all these advanced technologies that have made a significant impact on reducing medication errors.

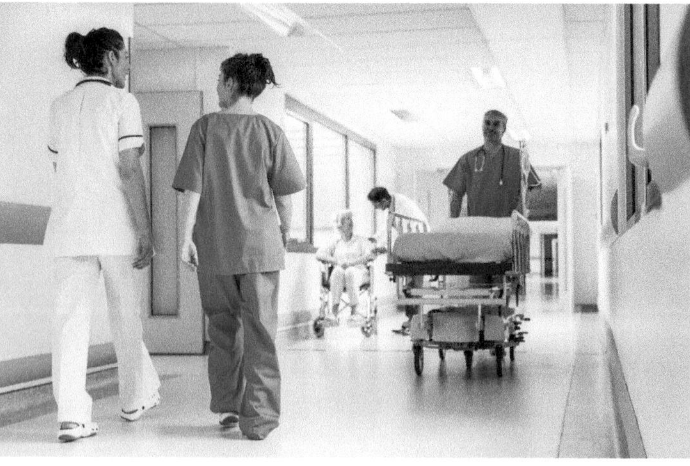
Working in a hospital pharmacy environment presents unique challenges, compared to working in a community pharmacy.

This chapter provides an overview of hospital pharmacy practice, including regulatory controls and standards, and it outlines the roles and responsibilities of pharmacy technicians in providing safe, effective patient care. It also highlights the importance of hospital care teams and accreditation.

11.1 Hospital Organization and Functions

A hospital is a facility that provides many different kinds of medical care, including emergency, trauma, surgical, medical, and public health services, so the facility's pharmacy services must also be varied to support these functions.

TABLE 11.1 Functions of a Hospital

The major functions of a hospital include:

- diagnosis and testing (laboratory, x-ray, and so on)
- treatment and therapy, including surgical intervention
- emergency services for individuals and the community
- patient processing (including admissions, record keeping, billing, and planning for post-discharge patient care and discharge education)
- promotion of public health and wellness through educational programs, such as smoking cessation, weight loss, and peer support
- preventive health initiatives, such as mammography, colonoscopy, blood pressure readings, and cholesterol screenings
- training of healthcare professionals, including medical residents and interns, nurses, and pharmacy students
- conducting research studies that add to the sum of medical knowledge

Organizational Framework

Not all hospitals provide the same depth and breadth of services. Since hospitals perform numerous major functions, as outlined in Table 11.1, they are generally categorized by a set of defining characteristics:

- bed capacity
- type of service (general or specialized) and targeted patient population (such as children's hospital versus VA facility)
- affiliation (university or teaching hospital versus private or nonteaching hospital versus HMO facility)
- urban versus rural and the size of the population being served
- ownership (state-owned versus community-owned, government versus nongovernment)
- financial status (for-profit versus not-for-profit)

Quite often, hospitals establish an organizational structure that mimics a corporate framework. With the many recent changes in healthcare regulations and reimbursements, many hospitals in a specific area or servicing a particular type of patient have merged into one corporation to improve efficiencies in communications, inventory control, and billing to insurance. A president, or chief executive officer (CEO), runs the hospital and reports to the hospital's board of directors or that of a larger healthcare system. The CEO guides the overall direction and long-range planning of the hospital and—depending on bed size and scope of services—may supervise several vice presidents and directors who preside over various departments in the hospital.

TABLE 11.2 Common Hospital Departments and Acronyms or Abbreviations

Department	Acronym or Abbreviation
Ambulatory Patient Care	APC
Heart Catheterization Laboratory	Cath Lab
Coronary Care Unit	CCU
Endoscopy	Endo
Emergency Room/Department	ER/ED
Intensive Care Unit/Medical ICU	ICU/MICU
Labor and Delivery	L&D
Neonatal Intensive Care Unit	NICU
Operating Room	OR
Pediatrics	Peds
Post-Anesthesia Care Unit/Recovery Room	PACU
Surgical Intensive Care Unit	SICU
Transitional Care Unit	TCU
Radiology	X-ray

For example, a vice president of patient care typically oversees such departments as the laboratory, medical records, rehabilitation, respiratory care, social services, and pharmacy. Other vice presidents may oversee medicine, nursing, and finance departments. In larger hospitals, a chief operating officer (COO) usually supervises hospital operations and directs the departmental vice presidents. The pharmacy department interacts with all departments.

A hospital also requires committees of cross-department specialists to ensure the sharing of information and expertise for the best policies and solutions. The main committees relating to pharmacy include the Pharmacy and Therapeutics Committee, the Institutional Review Board, and the Infection Control Committee (to be discussed in Chapter 12).

Pharmacy and Therapeutics Committee

The **Pharmacy and Therapeutics (P&T) Committee** oversees the policies for all drug-related hospital issues. It handles numerous key tasks:

- reviewing, approving, and revising the hospital's drug formulary
- maintaining the drug use policies of the hospital
- reviewing studies on the appropriate use of drugs within the hospital
- monitoring medication error reports (including computerized adverse drug event monitoring reports)
- reviewing investigational drugs after the Institutional Review Board has approved them for onsite clinical studies

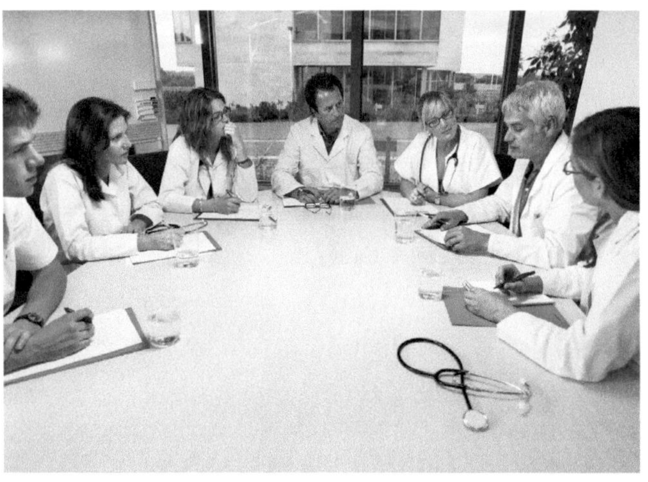

The Pharmacy and Therapeutics Committee meets monthly to discuss drug formulary recommendations and review medication error reports and safety recommendations.

The P&T Committee is composed of several members of the medical staff as well as representatives from the hospital, nursing, and pharmacy administration. The director of pharmacy and a drug-information pharmacist often represent the pharmacy department. The director of pharmacy often acts as the committee secretary, recording and disseminating each meeting's minutes. The drug-information pharmacist researches and makes objective, data-based drug formulary recommendations. In some hospitals, a pharmacy technician, called the procurement technician, is also part of the committee, representing the technicians and assisting the drug-information pharmacist in drug data collection.

Drug Formulary

Most P&Ts adopt a **drug formulary**, or a list of approved drugs for the institution, based on the committee's recommendations about the best drugs to provide the most effective medications that can fit insurance reimbursements and hospital budgets. (Drug formularies do not exist in the community pharmacy setting with the exception of some HMO pharmacies, such as Kaiser Permanente.) It is important for technicians to get to know their specific hospital formulary well.

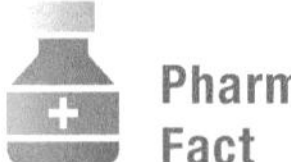

The technician who works with the P&T Committee on the drug formulary data collection and medications selection is often called the "procurement pharmacy technician."

If medical staff members want the P&T Committee to consider adding a new drug to the hospital's drug formulary, they must submit an extensive medication application form to the committee. The drug-information pharmacist then reviews the application's information and completes an independent search of the medical literature. The cost, advantages, and disadvantages of the new drug are then compared with an existing formulary drug, and these findings are presented to the entire committee for its consideration.

At times, formulary approval of a particular high-cost or unusual drug may be restricted to an approved use for a specific department. For example, a new, high-cost antibiotic with limited indications and high resistance patterns may be restricted to use by members of the infectious disease service department. A prescriber outside of this department could not write a prescription for this new antibiotic, and the pharmacy could not fill this medication order without the approval and signature of an appropriate infectious disease prescriber.

If a hospital prescriber writes a medication order for a **nonformulary drug**—one *not* on the approved hospital list—they will probably need to justify the patient necessity for it to a member of the P&T Committee. In a teaching hospital, a medical resident usually needs to get approval from the supervising physician first to order a nonformulary drug.

Medication Error Reports

The P&T Committee also reviews all medication error reports that have been forwarded to the pharmacy department from medical, nursing, or even pharmacy teams and units. The pharmacy's drug-information center researches, collates (a technician may assist in this information gathering), and analyzes these medication error reports. The adverse drug events are easily tabulated through the pharmacy software and electronic health records if the events have been reported and input properly in the system. When the committee reviews a medication error report, the focus is not to assign blame but to identify and correct any systematic problem to prevent similar errors from occurring. To receive hospital accreditation—approval of service quality—by the Joint Commission, each hospital needs to demonstrate stringent, accurate medication error reporting, resolution processes, and improvement achievements. (The Joint Commission and its standards will be described in detail at the end of the chapter.)

The Institutional Review Board

Some hospital physicians engage in pharmaceutical research studies with university or government researchers or manufacturers to test new medications and treatments. However, any clinical investigational drug research must first be approved by both the P&T Committee and the hospital's **Institutional Review Board (IRB)**. The IRB—also known as the Human Use Committee—typically meets monthly to review the proposed use of **investigational drugs** (not yet approved by the FDA or approved for a new indication) for hospital clinical studies or innovative surgical or therapeutic procedures. The IRB seeks to provide appropriate safeguards for the patients. It consists of representatives from the departments of medicine, pharmacy, nursing, and hospital administration as well as a consumer member.

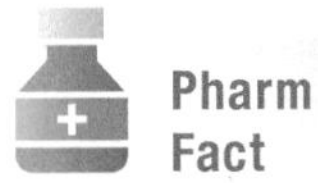

Pharm Fact

A technician on an investigational drug study may manage the study's drug inventory, distribute the drug in the hospital, assist with clinical study protocols and documentation of the trials, perform training or educational functions, and/or prepare the drug products.

The key investigator submits an application outlining the goals of the study and the participating patient population, including the number of subjects, their ages, and their healthcare status (such as patient or healthy volunteer). Both the IRB and the investigator must meet federal and state regulations that apply to clinical research investigational studies.

The IRB protects the patient by ensuring both adequate knowledge of the risks of the study and confidentiality of the personal medical information. The investigator must submit to each patient participant an **informed consent form**, or a document describing clearly (in layperson terms) the study, risks, potential benefits, reimbursement (if any), and follow-up responsibilities and procedures in the case of an adverse event. To participate in the study, the patients must read and sign the consent form to indicate their knowledge and approval. Special protective procedures exist for potentially vulnerable populations such as newborns, children, women of childbearing age, older adults, and those with mental health problems. A drug-information (or clinical) pharmacist is commonly responsible for educating nurses and monitoring investigational drug use within the hospital.

The investigational data collected may be collated and sent outside the hospital to a government agency or private sponsor; or it may be analyzed to be published in a medical or scientific journal. However, the individual patient's identity and medical data must remain protected. Most commonly, patients are assigned an ID number as a study subject (separate from their hospital number) to maintain anonymity.

If an adverse reaction occurs during the study, it must be reported immediately by the nurse or the pharmacist to the primary physician investigator. Depending on the severity of the reaction, the Adverse Drug Reactions (ADR) may need to be reported to the IRB so that it can evaluate whether or not the study should continue.

11.2 The Hospital Pharmacy Department

Depending on the hospital size and specialization, hospital pharmacies provide a number of wide-ranging pharmaceutical products and services. The services fall into four categories: administrative (overseeing of the drug formulary, budget, inventory, and information); distribution (filling and delivering medications); clinical (consulting with and on patients); and educational (training pharmacists, technicians, patients, and the public).

However, how these services are provided and to what depth and range vary considerably. Some of the variations among hospital pharmacies include the following:

- the specialty services being offered and how they are offered
  - ~ satellite or small pharmacies located within specific patient care units
  - ~ clinical pharmacists making rounds with physicians and monitoring patients

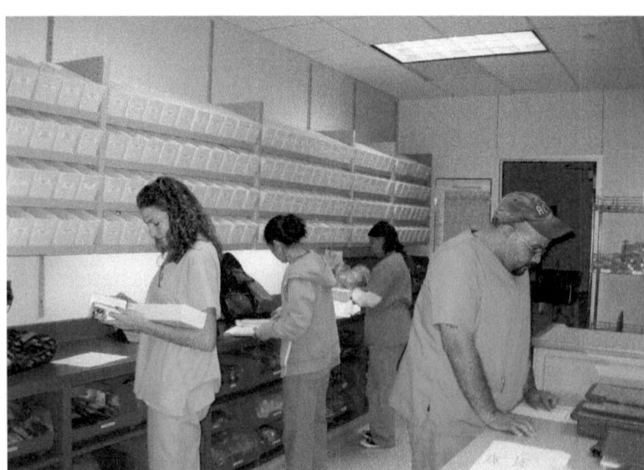

Hospital pharmacy technicians often work at multiple workstations.

- ~ consultation services for pharmacokinetics and individual patient dosing
  - ~ pharmacy personnel staffing of a drug-information center
  - ~ discharge pharmacy service versus outsourcing to a retail pharmacy
- the medication distribution systems
  - ~ medication delivery with unit dose cart exchange versus an automated floor stock system
  - ~ frequency of unit dose cart exchanges (more than once daily, daily, or less often)
  - ~ use of an automated or robotic dispensing system
  - ~ centralized versus decentralized narcotic inventory control system
  - ~ presence of an IV admixture program, including preparation of hazardous agents
  - ~ in-house total parenteral nutrition (TPN) or nutrition service versus offsite preparation or outsourcing
- the service availability (24 hours a day, 7 days a week, or less)
- the pharmaceutical inventory processes, including those for the processing of bids, contracts, and purchase orders
- the pharmacy protocol in providing medications and supplies in emergency codes
- the instructional support for pharmacy residents and students
- the procedures and measurements for safety, quality control, and productivity

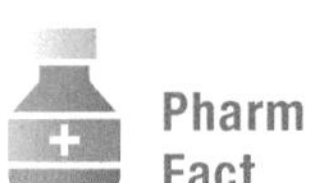

Pharm Fact

Hospitals have now incorporated scanning systems with bar code recognition for repackaging medications to reduce medication errors. Technicians have to place bar codes on medications that do not have them to work with the scanning system.

Several of these variations, including the range and processes of medication distribution systems and pharmaceutical inventory, are discussed later in this chapter.

Location and Structure

In a traditional hospital setting, the pharmacy department occupies a centralized location that is readily accessible to the emergency room/department and to the patient care units and surgical suites (or to the elevators leading to them). The pharmacy also needs to be in close proximity to a central storage area for bulk items such as boxes of IV solutions.

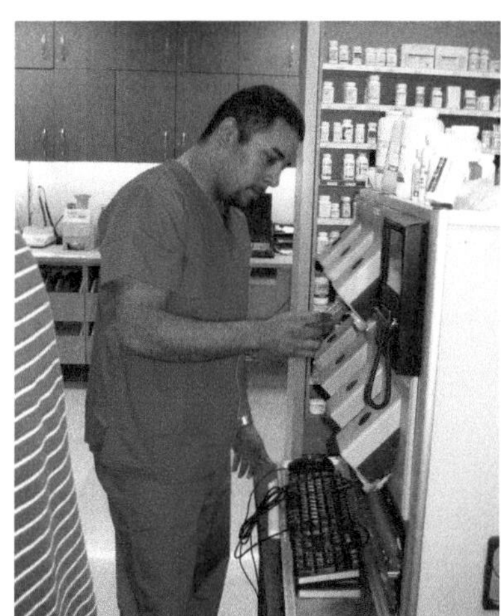

Both small and large automation units are incorporated in hospital pharmacies to improve efficiency in carrying out the many diverse pharmacy responsibilities and to reduce medication errors.

The interior layout of the pharmacy typically has several designated areas for different tasks: filling medication orders for individual patients, filling the medication carts, repackaging medications, and storing narcotics and investigational drugs, among other functions. The preparation of sterile and hazardous products occurs separately in a cleanroom or a hazardous compounding area.

Aside from the typical pharmacy equipment, hospital pharmacies usually have a unit dose cart for each care unit as well as repackaging equipment. Many large hospitals have incorporated robotic automation equipment for selecting and repackaging medications to improve efficiency and reduce medication errors. The cleanroom and the hazardous substance preparation areas have additional, large equipment for aseptic, sterile, and protective compounding (addressed in Chapters 12 and 13).

Director of Pharmacy

The hospital pharmacy staff is typically composed of a director of pharmacy, additional associate or assistant directors of pharmacy (for larger hospitals), pharmacists, and pharmacy technicians. Appointed by the CEO and hospital administrators, the **director of pharmacy**, also known as the pharmacist in charge (PIC), oversees the day-to-day and strategic operations of the department, such as managing the pharmacy budget; handling the staffing (hiring, evaluating, and firing of personnel); developing a strategic vision (long-term planning); complying with all federal and state regulations and laws; and establishing department policies and procedures with the P&T Committee to conform to the hospital's overall policies and accreditation standards.

The director of pharmacy usually reports to a vice president of professional or patient care services (or similar title) and works closely with the director of nursing and the chief of staff in medicine to provide high-quality patient care.

Determining Pharmacy Services and Budget

The director determines the scope and level of pharmacy services based on available resources. The hospital's overall annual budget determines the amount allocated to the pharmacy department for its budget, and the hospital's budget is affected by patient census and government and insurance rates of reimbursements. Thus the pharmacy budget varies from year to year according to that of the hospital as a whole.

The director is responsible for projecting pharmacy needs and allocating funds for pharmaceuticals, staff, supplies, vendors, software, automation, and other needs. This annual projected budget is then submitted to the hospital administration for approval. The director is also in charge of implementing and monitoring the pharmacy budget that finally gets approved.

A vast majority of the budget must go to the purchase of pharmaceuticals. Drug budgets, in particular, can be difficult to predict, especially one to two years in advance. Newer, more expensive drugs or biotechnology advances are always coming into the marketplace, replacing lower-cost medical therapies and approaches. An example might be that a new transplant service is being implemented in the hospital that requires the use of new, expensive immunosuppressive drugs. Consequently, this will require a juggling of the current drug budget to free up the funds for these drugs or to find new sources for these budgetary funds. The director continually assesses the budgetary impacts of new drugs and hospital services.

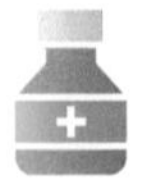

Pharm Fact

The ASHP Practice Advancement Initiative is being put in place most actively in hospitals, where pharmacists are taking more and more responsibility for patient health outcomes related to medications. The ASHP works to support this movement with resources, research, and case studies.

The high costs of implementing state-of-the-art pharmacy software and automation technologies must also be calculated into the department budget, considering costs versus potential benefits, but these expenditures are more predictable and easier to plan.

Determining Staffing and Resources

The pharmacy's general budget and the amount allocated for drugs affect how much can be used for onsite staffing. Per day shift, a large city hospital may staff ten or more each of pharmacists and pharmacy technicians, with fewer on evening and night shifts. In addition, larger hospitals usually have pharmacy students, interns, and postgraduate residents.

In small, rural hospitals, there are fewer full-time pharmacists and technicians. Part-time pharmacists can make up the entire pharmacy staff, using "on-call" pharmacists for after-hours needs. No matter the size of the staff, the overall roles and responsibilities of the hospital pharmacy personnel remain the same.

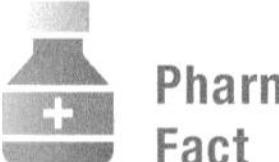

Pharm Fact

Hospitals plan staffing based on their state requirements. Some hospitals can staff two technicians per one pharmacist or three to one, depending on their state regulations and whether or not the technicians are certified.

Staffing decisions are based on the pharmacy's dispensing rates and the projected bed occupancy numbers for the next year (or a select time period as well as hours of operation) and scope of services. Support personnel may include administrative support staff, part-time professional staff, and pharmacy students, interns, and residents. The hospital's human resources department generally advertises for personnel positions and screens candidates. However, the director of pharmacy makes the final decision when pharmacy staff members are hired.

Though staffing needs are generally more predictable than drug budgets, they can also fluctuate in unplanned ways. For instance, if there is a local epidemic, this quickly escalates hospital use by the community, resulting in the need for more staff. Staffing decisions are also affected by space restrictions. Because of space and staff budget limitations, the director may outsource some medication preparation, distribution, or pharmacist clinical services. For example, a smaller hospital pharmacy may contract with an infusion pharmacy outside the hospital to formulate and deliver nutrition or hazardous drug products to the hospital. A hospital may also lease space to a local community pharmacy to provide outpatient pharmacy services within the hospital's lobby or public space.

Overseeing the Policy and Procedure Manual

For a hospital to retain accreditation, each pharmacy department must have and follow an official **Policy and Procedure (P&P) Manual**. It outlines the mission of the department, its organizational components, and all the many policies and procedures for department operations with step-by-step instructions for both pharmacists and technicians. The director must see that the P&P Manual is implemented correctly and consistently and updated appropriately and frequently. The policies and procedures are drafted to fit all state and federal laws. The director of pharmacy may ask a technician to be involved in helping update the P&P Manual items directly related to pharmacy technicians. If you fail to follow the rules and processes of the P&P Manual, it may result in the termination of your employment.

Hospital Pharmacists

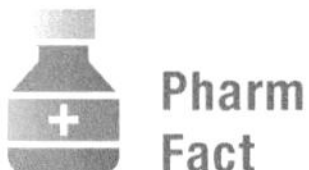

Pharm Fact

A code blue emergency team usually consists of a physician who is the team leader, a critical care/ ICU RN who leads until the physician arrives, a unit RN, a pharmacist, and a respiratory therapist. An emergency department technician may also be part of the team.

A large traditional or university hospital's onsite pharmacy department is typically staffed 24 hours a day, 7 days a week with pharmacists and technicians. Hospital pharmacists oversee the accurate and safe dispensing of the medication orders. They also spend time advising hospital prescribers and nurses, and in clinical work consulting with patients and the healthcare teams for medication therapy management. The pharmacists who work in a hospital must have an extensive knowledge of the specific hospital formulary medications to provide thorough, expert drug consultations to the medical and nursing staff. For this reason, the pharmacists have a great responsibility to keep up to date on drugs moving through FDA approvals into the market, including high-potency injectable drugs and high-cost biotechnology drugs that are rarely, if ever, dispensed in a community pharmacy.

In addition, the lead code blue pharmacist must have the skills to prepare (and document) emergency medications that are needed in code blue emergency critical care situations. Hospital pharmacists typically wear name tags with their white lab coats so that they are easily recognizable for consultation in the hospital.

Major Pharmacist Responsibilities

The responsibilities of a hospital pharmacist include the following:

- review medication histories of all newly admitted patients
- verify medical drug orders in the computer
- check medication orders against patient medical history and medication reconciliation alerts
- visit patients and provide patient care services as part of a healthcare team (when assigned to a team)
- verify medication cart fills, repackaging, and the preparation of sterile products
- closely monitor controlled drug usage on each patient care unit
- order and receive Schedule II controlled drugs
- provide necessary drug information to prescribers and nurses
- monitor automated robotic systems in the pharmacy and narcotic floor stock on patient care units
- assist in cardiopulmonary resuscitation (CPR) codes by providing lifesaving drugs
- dispense investigational drugs and complete the necessary documentation
- provide medication education for patients soon to be discharged from the hospital
- investigate medication error reports
- provide quality control and productivity measurements within the department
- represent the pharmacy department on select hospital committees as needed

Practice Tip

Many medical scientists are finding that different age groups, especially those of children, have different metabolism rates and organ effects. Some pediatric practices call for calculating dosages through additional formulas. That is why pediatric drug therapy is becoming a specialty for pharmacists and technicians.

Specializing Pharmacists

Many larger hospital pharmacies also have specialty-trained clinical pharmacists in internal medicine, emergency medicine, oncolocy, organ transplant, pediatrics, neonatal care, intensive care, surgery, nutrition, and pharmacokinetics. These specialists serve on healthcare teams that make daily rounds to visit or consult on patients. They may assist prescribers in ordering TPN solutions or offer recommendations in dosing high-risk medications. These clinical pharmacists work closely with the medical and nursing staff to resolve medication issues and improve the quality and safety of patient care. Some pharmacists specialize in compounding sterile products or chemotherapy and other hazardous drug compounding.

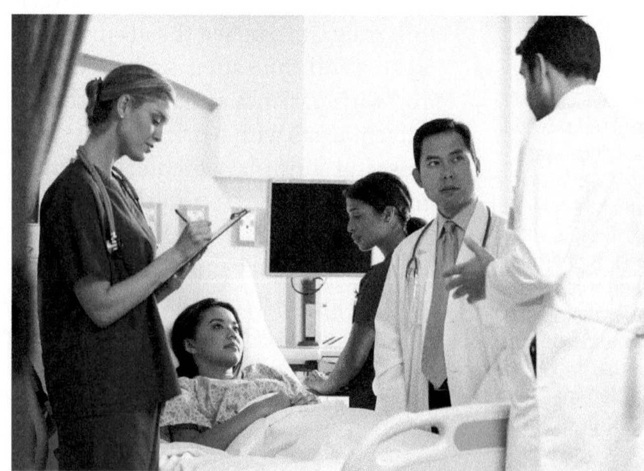

Hospital pharmacists are called in to consult on patient drug therapies as part of a healthcare team. The pharmacists' clinical tasks can include visiting with patients and consulting with nursing teams and all the involved prescribers and specialists.

Hospital Pharmacy Technicians

The pharmacy technicians support the pharmacists (and the nurses) in preparing, packaging, and delivering the drugs to each nursing unit by filling the unit dose carts, stocking the automated central pharmacy and floor dispensing units, monitoring inventory and controlled substances in both the pharmacy and the nursing units, stocking the emergency crash cart, and, if trained, preparing sterile products. The drug types they dispense in the hospital are radically different from those used in the community pharmacy. Hospital drugs are generally more potent and targeted, and many are administered via the IV route of administration. Patients are often maintained on various IV fluids (with or without medications), IV nutrition solutions, and chemotherapy infusions.

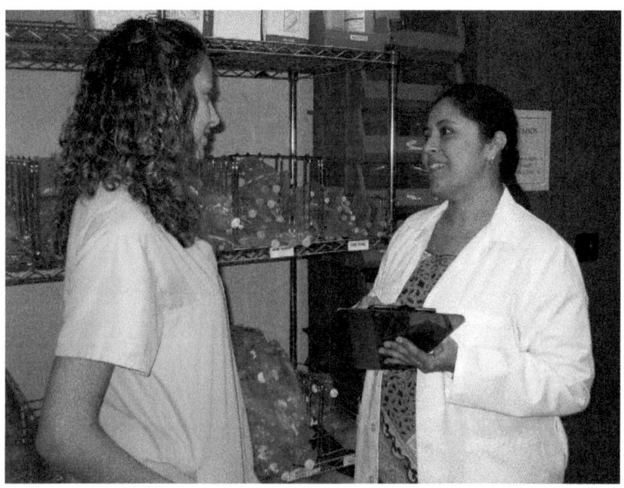
The hospital pharmacy technician wears a particular colored scrub to be distinguished from the lab-coated pharmacists.

Work Environment

A hospital pharmacy setting is a more controlled work environment than a community pharmacy. Instead of handling patients at the counter, drive-through window, and on the phone, hospital pharmacy technicians have minimal interactions with the patients and the public. They communicate mainly with physicians, nurses, and other staff members via computer or phone. Most communications and medication orders are transmitted through the hospital software network.

Unlike in a community pharmacy, the pharmacy technician does not process insurance for each medication dispensed to a patient. The hospital's billing department prepares and submits all the charges for each patient at discharge. The charges not being assumed by Medicare, Medicaid, Tricare, or private insurance (unless it is an HMO facility, where there will be no other insurers involved) are billed to the patient. The costs per dosage unit are far higher than at a community pharmacy because, instead of the community pharmacy's small dispensing fee, the hospital adds a markup per drug to cover a portion of the overhead costs (including for pharmacy and nursing) for 24/7 care, which are substantial.

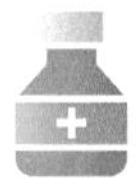
Pharm Fact

Because pharmacy technicians handle controlled substances, most healthcare facilities require technicians to wear security photo ID badges along with all the rest of the healthcare workers.

The pharmacy technicians typically wear name tags and scrubs or lab coats in a designated color to differentiate themselves from the pharmacists. This protocol for attire has been implemented by many hospitals in response to a need to quickly identify hospital personnel in the event of an emergency. Wearing pharmacy-designated uniform colors also helps identify pharmacy technicians who frequently deliver medications to patient care units.

In addition, all pharmacy personnel must follow the same hygiene and infection control procedures used by the rest of the healthcare staff for personnel and patient safety (addressed in Chapter 12, Infection Control, Aseptic Technique, and Cleanroom Facilities). For technicians who serve in the hospital cleanroom, additional processes and garbing elements are required for aseptic technique (also covered in the next chapter).

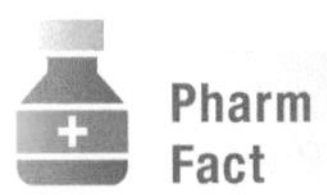

The University of Wisconsin Hospital and Clinics, Cedars-Sinai Medical Center (Los Angeles), and Long Beach Memorial Medical Center have all implemented tech-check-tech (TCT) programs and recorded a > 99.8% accuracy rate for trained and certified technicians filling unit dose delivery carts. This rate is comparable to pharmacists' rates.

Technician Training and Orientation

Because of the complex environment of a hospital pharmacy department, the learning curve for technicians may be three months or longer to develop the necessary skills. Many large, urban hospitals will hire only certified technicians who have graduated from an American Society of Health-System Pharmacists (ASHP)-accredited training program who bring with them hospital experience. All technicians must pass criminal background checks (like other pharmacy personnel) due to access to potent narcotic drugs. To keep up with new drug and policy changes, the department requires frequent all-staff informational sessions with mandatory annual retraining.

To maintain flexibility in scheduling, each technician generally goes through training to perform all major department functions. They rotate through these functions during their orientation and training. However, most pharmacy technicians do not rotate through the cleanroom or hazardous compounding area without specialized training.

Technician Advancement and Specializations

Though the technicians rotate in the general pharmacy, they often end up specializing in one area, such as medication reconciliation, unit dose filling, managing robotics, maintaining floor stock, managing inventory control, staff training, or sterile compounding. In larger hospitals, there are often different grade levels among the pharmacy technicians, allowing technicians to advance in responsibilities and pay depending on their skills and experience.

For example, in some hospital pharmacies, a senior pharmacy technician may be given additional administrative responsibilities, such as supervising other technicians in their daily responsibilities. This is the **tech-check-tech (TCT)** function, where a senior technician checks another technician's work. This adds another layer of safety verification to the process of medication ordering. State boards of pharmacy have authorized TCT programs in at least nine states.

To encourage the technician staff to continually develop their capabilities, many large hospital corporations have developed their own formalized certification programs, especially in the areas of sterile and hazardous drug compounding. Since the medications and supplies needed on a surgery nursing unit will be much different from those on a pediatric one, a pharmacy technician may become specifically trained and assigned to a decentralized specialty satellite unit. For example, a certified technician with time and experience can become a valuable resource in a specialty nursing unit.

11.3 Electronic Hospital Records and Medication Orders

Taking advantage of the digital age, hospitals now utilize hospital management software systems that collect patient data and communicate between medical departments, billing, and finance, and with external healthcare providers. These overall management systems need to interface well with each department's specific software, technology, and records, such as that in the pharmacy department. Some common hospital management software systems include Cerner, Epic, Net Health Systems, Pro Med, and eHospital Systems. This capacity for **interoperability**—interactive communication and operation between internal record programs, software and hardware systems, and external information sources—is one of the greatest advantages of a system based on **electronic health records (EHRs)**.

Some of the key forms of EHRs pertinent to the pharmacy include intake records and patient medical/medication histories, bar code point-of-care scanning information, electronic medical charts, medication orders, and electronic medication administration records. The EHR software provides the following benefits to members of the healthcare team:

- immediate access to a patient's medical record and hospital medication profile
- streamlined workflow processes
- improved documentation
- enhanced coordination of patient care
- clear communication with other healthcare personnel
- data collection and trend tracking information to measure safety to meet hospital accreditation standards

Intake Records

Upon admission to the hospital, the patient or guardian must be interviewed about the patient's medical and medication history to assemble an accurate **intake record**. The record also includes key personal, insurance, and billing information and the doctor's admitting diagnosis. Collecting this information is often done by an admitting staff person or a nurse who inputs the information into the hospital computer system.

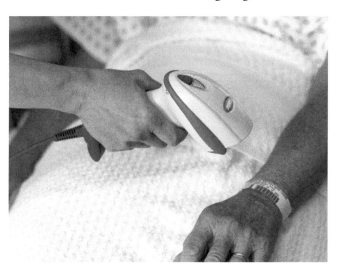

A patient's wristband with its bar code helps the healthcare team follow a specific patient's care plan and keep the patient's EHR up to date with each medication administration and procedure.

Patient Wrist Bands

To follow a patient through the hospital system and keep the EHR complete, all patients receive a wristband that has their name, birth date, and a bar code at intake to the general hospital or emergency department. As nurses in the care units enter a shift, it is common practice for them to introduce themselves and ask the patient for name and date of birth (if it is possible for the patient to respond). The nurse then verifies the patient's identity by scanning the bar code on the wristband prior to each medication administration.

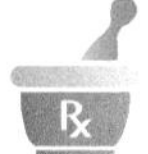

Practice Tip

When discussing medication history with a patient, keep your voice low to avoid being overheard to protect the patient's privacy per HIPAA regulations.

Medication Histories

As with the community pharmacy, accurately documenting the medication history of new patients is often time-consuming and frustrating. It can be especially problematic for an admitting nurse who is not as knowledgeable about brand and generic drug names and indications. Problems arise with patient memory, confusion, and understanding of questions; limited access to patient records; time constraints; and language or cultural problems. More and more hospitals are working with Surescripts and its record locator and exchange service to access more of a patient's medical history and medication records from external physicians and pharmacists, even if out of state.

Patients may also bring in **home medications (home meds)** or those medications prescribed to them prior to admittance. These labeled and unlabeled bottles of medications from home must be identified and added to the medication history. If patients know they are taking a medication but the bottles are not available, the admitting staff person needs to call the community pharmacy or the prescriber to get the drug, dose, and schedule. That is why some hospitals are assigning experienced and specially trained pharmacy technicians to identify the home meds and assist in assembling the medication information in the initial admitting process.

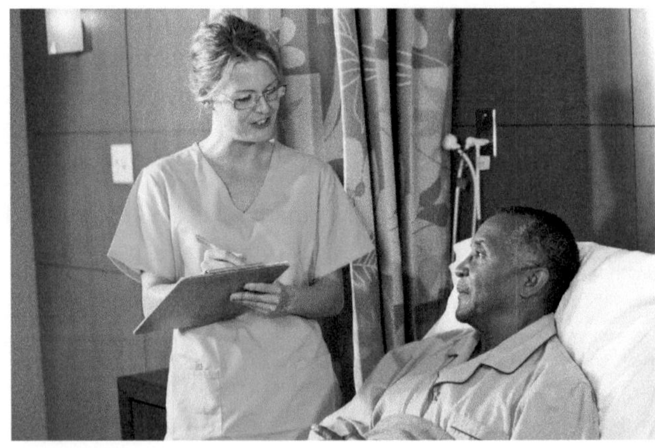

This pharmacy technician is interviewing a patient about his medication and allergy history.

As in a community pharmacy or doctor's office, the patient (or guardian) will need to be shown a privacy protection statement and sign it, as is necessitated by HIPAA regulations.

IN THE REAL WORLD

At North Memorial Hospital in Tucson, Arizona, a number of experienced technicians and pharmacy interns were selected for specialized training in obtaining patient medication histories and seeking additional intake information when information was missing or medication problems surfaced. They would contact the patient as well as the patient's family, healthcare providers, and community pharmacy. The technicians and interns had a dedicated work space and had been drilled in common critical medications that should not be stopped during a hospital stay, proper medication dosages, and dangerous drug interactions.

Over the two years of the pilot project, the new medication reconciliation process found over 1,240 patients needed continuation of at least one critical medication (particularly thyroid drugs, anticonvulsants, and antidepressants) that would otherwise have been missed. The recommendations of the technicians and interns alerted the pharmacists, who made suggestions to the prescribers for modifications in the drug therapies. For example, over two months in 2010, the pharmacists made 178 interventions for 132 patients. The prescribing physicians accepted 102 (57%) of these recommendations, showing the value of these technician- and intern-prompted alerts. After the study was over, North Memorial continued and expanded the program. Better outcomes resulted, and nursing, physician, and pharmacist staff time was freed up for other tasks.

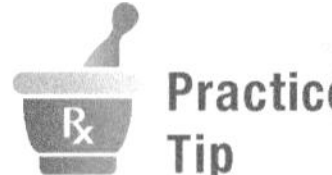

Practice Tip

All information collected using automation must be used in a way that protects patient privacy, according to HIPAA.

Admitting Orders

After intake, the nurse electronically transmits the **admitting order** to the pharmacy department. An admitting order is a request for specific medications and medical procedures (see Figure 11.1) that was written in the emergency department or in a patient's room by the physician who met with the patient and is admitting them. This order may contain a suspected diagnosis and requests for lab tests or radiology examinations; nursing staff instructions; dietary requirements; as well as medication orders with the allergy and medication history.

A pharmacist, pharmacy resident, or pharmacy intern then must review the compiled medication history and home medication drug list to ensure that no critical medications have been discontinued or missed and that there are no problematic allergies or interactions. If not involved earlier, a specially trained pharmacy technician may be assigned to check the medication and allergy history and home medication list for completeness and accuracy, doing follow-up calls and even visiting the patient to ask questions to fill in any incomplete information.

Once the medication history information is complete and accurate and the admitting medication orders are submitted, a drug utilization review (DUR) will be run, and the software will highlight allergy and drug interaction problems as it does in the community pharmacy. The pharmacist will assess any medication-related issues and provide the admitting physician with recommendations or counsel about the admission medication order.

FIGURE 11.1 Admitting Order

Whether a written or digital admission order, these are common required informational elements.

DATE	HOUR	PHYSICIAN'S ORDERS
9-1-202X		Admit to: Dr. Chung
		Diagnosis:
		1. lower abdominal pain with history of diverticulitis
		2. asthma
		3. chronic back pain
		4. anxiety
		Condition: fair
		Vitals: per routine
		Labs: chem 12, electrolytes, ABG
		X-ray: lungs
		Allergies: codeine, Floxin, Biaxin, PCN, Ceclor, doxycycline
		Diet: clear liquids, low salt, 1800 kcal/day
		IVFs: NS @ 125 mL per hour
		Meds: Phenergan 25 mg IV q6 h prn nausea/vomiting
		Levaquin 500 mg IV daily
		Levsin 0.125 mg po tid
		zolpidem 10 mg po hs prn sleep
		carisoprodol 350 mg po tid prn muscle spasm
		Advair 250/50 1 puff bid
		montelukast 10 mg po daily
		Lorcet 10/325 po bid
		famotidine 40 mg po bid
		albuterol 0.083% 1 unit via nebulizer q6 h prn
		Nasonex 2 sprays in each nostril daily
		sertraline 100 mg 2 tabs po daily

IN THE REAL WORLD

In 2011 in Joplin, Missouri, St. John Hospital (known today as Mercy Hospital Joplin) converted its medical records from paper to EHRs with digital storage. Three weeks after completion, a tornado with 200-mph winds ripped through Joplin, destroying the hospital and throwing its paperwork to the sky. Because of the transition to an EHR system, the hospital was able to recover its patient records after electricity was restored. Questions remain about how to handle access to records when electricity or internet access has not yet been restored. Hospitals and hospital pharmacies have to do various kinds of emergency disaster planning to handle the contingencies of many different types of threats and hazards from tornadoes, floods, hurricanes, and fires–to acts of terrorism, shooters, and infectious diseases.

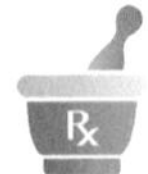

Practice Tip

Nurses cannot dispense home medications unless a hospital prescriber writes a medication order allowing this. Then the medication needs to be brought to the hospital pharmacy for a label and bar code to allow the nurse to scan before administration.

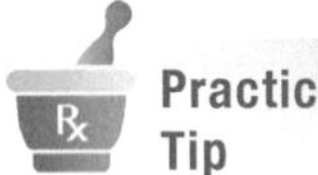

Practice Tip

All pharmacy personnel are trained to identify random medications and unlabeled drugs brought in by patients.

The medications patients brought from home or which were prescribed before arriving at the hospital may not be on the hospital's approved drug formulary. Even so, the physician may decide that it is in the patient's best health interest to continue these nonformulary drugs, and, to do so, the physician will write "continue home meds" on the admission order.

If approved by the pharmacist, the home meds may be sent to the pharmacy to be distributed through the hospital unit dose delivery system or, depending on hospital policy, may be kept at the patient's bedside for self-administration. To do this, the patient's physician must write an order for "Bedside medications," which alerts the pharmacy personnel and the nursing staff to allow the administration. At discharge, the patient brings along any remaining "at bedside" medications.

Electronic Medical Charts

In the hospital rooms of the past, at the patient's bedside was a **medical chart**–handwritten charted notes on observations and vital signs at different times, medication administrations, physician diagnoses and recommendations, and other documentation held together on a clipboard. But now, the medical chart is digitally transportable and interactive, holding all this information plus the full EHR along with the medication history and list. For example, McKesson has a ProMedica Electronic Charting System (iCare), and Epic has the EpicCare Inpatient Clinical System. Both of these allow electronic communication to all departments in the hospital and include the patient's personal identifying demographics, daily physician and specialist notes, nursing assessments, medication and lab orders, tests, dietary necessities, problem list, and, eventually, discharge summary.

As the nurse and provider continually add notations to the digital medical chart, the patient's real-time bedside information is shared with everyone on the patient's hospital healthcare team, including the pharmacist. For pharmacists, these charts provide easy access to current patient care information to provide better medication therapy management. For instance, the pharmacist may call up lab results to monitor the patient's drug blood levels for efficacy or toxicity before allowing a medication refill or dosage change.

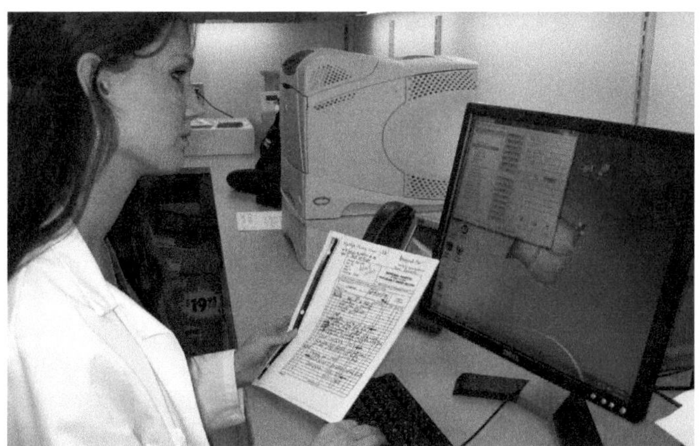

St. John's Hospital (known today as Mercy Hospital Joplin) in Missouri was able to recover its EHRs after the devastating tornado on May 22, 2011.

Medication Orders

As with the admission medication order, any request by the physician for drugs for a patient comes to the hospital pharmacy as a **medication order** (an official hospital prescribed drug request). A medical order often includes much more information than a community pharmacy prescription: the individual patient's diagnosis, allergies, diet, activity level, vital signs, requested radiology images and laboratory tests, and medications (both routine scheduled and oral drugs as well as parenteral medications and IV fluids), among other pertinent information.

Types of Medical Orders

Besides the initial admitting order, there are several other kinds of medication orders:

Daily Order After the physician checks on the patient each day, a **daily order** is placed for any new medications that have not been requested through the admitting (or home med continuation) order. The daily order may also modify those earlier orders, such as providing a change in dose or schedule based on how the patient is responding.

Continuation Order If the physician checks on the patient the next day or later in the week and wants to continue the same daily drug regime, they submit a **continuation order**. Most hospitals have a policy that the physician must review, approve, and electronically resubmit (or rewrite) all daily medication orders at least weekly to decide whether or not a continuation order is the best therapy. Continuation orders of antibiotics for patients fighting an aggressive infection are often checked and renewed on a more frequent than weekly basis, or per hospital policy, to prevent unnecessary use. Continuation orders are also sent to the pharmacy for patients who transfer from one unit of the hospital to another (e.g., from surgery to medicine).

Standing Order A **standing order** is a standard medication order for each patient who receives a common treatment or surgery in which the same set of medications and treatments applies. For instance, there will be a standing medication order for every patient who goes through a typical appendectomy without complications. The physician simply pulls up the screen with the appropriate standing order in that hospital for the appendectomy (or any surgery or specific treatment) and modifies it as needed to fit the patient before transmitting the standing order to the hospital pharmacy. Postoperative (postop) orders written after surgeries are also common examples of standing orders.

Stat Order A **stat order** is an emergency order typically sent electronically or telephoned to the pharmacy. These orders must receive priority attention and be immediately input, digitally verified, and filled without delay. After final pharmacist verification, the pharmacist or technician delivers the medication in person as soon as possible for the nurse to administer.

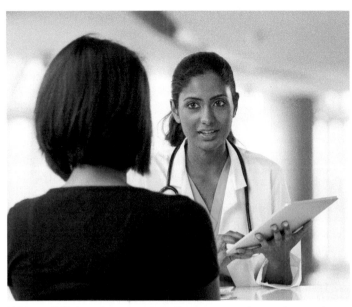

With an EHR-based system, prescribers, nurses, pharmacists, and other hospital healthcare specialists can access patient medical records and send medical orders electronically via computerized prescriber order entry (CPOE) to the pharmacy from their handheld devices or unit/room computers.

Discharge Order A **discharge order** is an order that provides take-home instructions for a patient who is leaving the hospital. This order includes all prescribed medications and dosages. Prescriptions are commonly written for a seven-day or one-month period until the patient's follow-up visit with the primary care physician or specialist.

In receiving and filling these medication orders and working with the patients' EHRs, it is important to remember that you must be on guard to protect the patient's privacy. That means no discussion of patient information with others for unauthorized reasons or with unauthorized persons, or where others can hear (such as in the dining room or elevator); no discussion of confidential information outside the hospital and no removal of files; no leaving up on the screen any information that is private or allowing staff without legitimate reasons or authority to look over someone's shoulder at a screen, medication list, or order. These are just some of the provisions of the HIPAA legislation that is part of the practice in handling medication histories and orders. These are laid out in the hospital pharmacy's P&P Manual.

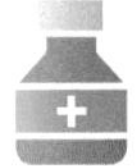

Pharm Fact

By 2018, 65% of hospitals already adopted CPOE (at a minimum 85% of medication orders) according to the Leapfrog Hospital 2018 Survey. Government financial incentives have accelerated the adoption process.

Portable Computerized Prescriber Order Entry

Most hospital medical orders are electronically sent to the pharmacy via a **computerized prescriber order entry (CPOE)** from the physician's mobile device or hospital room computer. The CPOE software can even allow hospital prescribers who are off-shift to order medications from their home or private office. CPOEs reduce ordering and transcription medication errors from the misinterpretation of a prescriber's handwriting (the number one preventable error). CPOEs have also simplified the posting of patient hospital charges and inventory ordering.

Hospital adoption of CPOEs, however, has been delayed in some facilities due to high costs for initial implementation and maintenance, insufficient time and costs for training staff, resistance by prescribers to embrace change, and the complexities of converting existing department-specific software to hospital-wide software.

Pharmacy Input of Handwritten Orders

Not all orders are delivered to the pharmacy via electronic transmission, especially in hospitals that have not completed full implementation of an EHR system. Handwritten orders may be delivered to the pharmacy via personal delivery, fax, phone order, or a pneumatic tube (like at the bank) from the prescriber or nursing unit. However, these handwritten hospital orders must then be entered by a pharmacist into the hospital/pharmacy software or by a technician who will have it verified by the pharmacist.

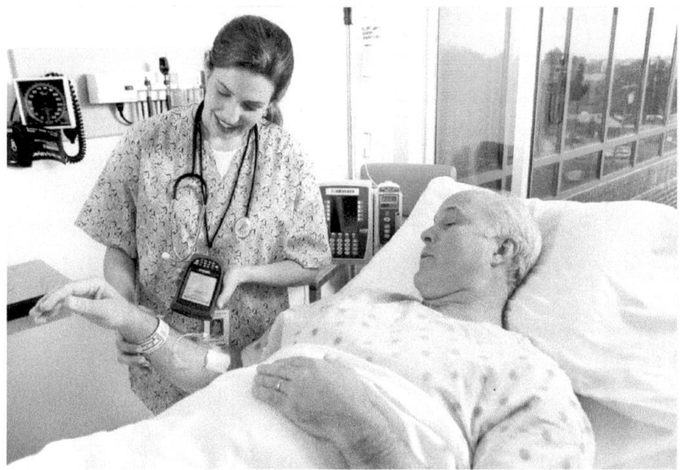

Using BPOC technology, the nurse can verify that the right drug at the right dose and by the right route gets to the right patient at the right time.

Electronic Medication Administration Records

The electronic tracking of drug therapies continues through the hospital software system. Once the pharmacy delivers a medication for administration, the nurse scans the patient's bar-coded wristband and accesses the patient's EHR from a computer or a notebook in the patient's room or on a mobile cart. The nurse verifies the medication order and compares the scanned bar code to the scanned bar code on the medication label and EHR. Using this **bar code point-of-care (BPOC)** scanning reduces the potential for medication errors because of the software's embedded safeguards.

The scanning process enters an **electronic medication administration record (eMAR)** into the patient's EHR medical chart. The eMAR system automatically records and documents the name of the drug, dose, route of administration, administration time, and start and stop date, plus any special instructions for the nursing staff. This BPOC scanning and eMAR documentation must occur for all medication orders, including oral and IV drugs. Because of BPOC technology, medication reconciliation can occur once more at the bedside, sending any safety alerts to the nurse before the medication is administered (see Figure 11.2).

FIGURE 11.2 Printout of an Electronic Medication Administration Record (eMAR)

SCHEDULE II DRUG ADMINISTRATION FORM				
Drug Demerol	**Strength** 100 mg	**Quantity** 25	**Form** ☐ Tablet ☐ Capsule ☑ Injection ☐ Liquid	**Control Number** A 3735
Issued By Andy Saul		**To Station** CCU		**Date Issued** 10/10/202X
Received By (Nurse in Charge) David Anderson				**Date Received** 10/10/202X

Date	Time	Patient Name	Room No.	Medication	Dosage Given	Dosage Wasted	Physician	Administered By	BAL
10/11/202X	0550	Martelli	CCU	Demerol	100 mg		Schnars	Lynch	24
10/12/202X	1245	Singh	CCU	Demerol	100 mg		Fields	Bond	23
10/14/202X	1625	Kappel	CCU	Demerol	90 mg	10 mg	Serrao	Richards	22
10/15/202X	1130	Gehrig	CCU	Demerol	75 mg	25 mg	Aicher	Fibich	21

RECORD OF WASTE AND SPOILAGE					
Dose No	**Date**	**Amount**	**Explain Wastage**	**Signature #1**	**Signature #1**
	10/15/202X	25 mg	defective syringe	Updegraff	Anderson

11.4 Filling and Delivery of Medication Orders

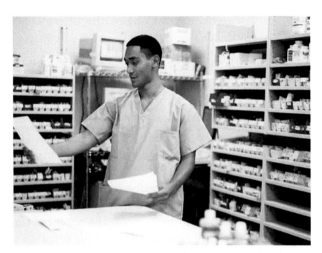

The pharmacy technician receives the printout of the medication order list to begin the process of filling it.

Prior to the electronically tracked administration, the medication order must be properly filled in the pharmacy. The software reconciles the medication orders with the patient's diagnosis and treatment and guidelines from the software's database of medical and pharmacy literature on "best practices," such as clinical guidelines, hospital protocols, and dosing guidelines for different patient populations.

As in community pharmacy prescriptions, the software also reconciles the medication order with the patient's personal medication history, allergies, and other drugs being administered. The program looks for duplicate drugs, incorrect doses, and laboratory test results that may have an impact on the choice of drug or dose.

For pharmacists, the EHR system provides easy access to clinical information contained in the patient medical record and provides better medication therapy management. If an issue is flagged by the medical software, the order will not be filled until the pharmacist can review it, or the physician is notified and the issue resolved.

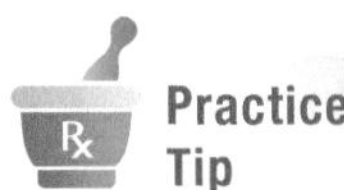

Practice Tip

When technicians are handling patient information and working with EHRs, they must follow strict hospital protocols to protect patient privacy per federal HIPAA law.

After the medication order has been checked and verified by the pharmacist, a medication label is generated, and the order can then be filled by the pharmacy technician (or the robot) using bar codes, verified again by the pharmacist, and sent to the patient care unit for administration by the nurse.

Medication orders in a hospital are dispensed to patients through one of the following distribution systems: dispensing carts (unit dose and emergency carts), robotic filling and dispensing, automated floor stock, or an IV admixture service. Pharmacy technicians are actively involved in all of these pharmacy methods of delivery to the nurses for administration.

The Unit Drug Packaging System

Unlike a 30-day or 90-day supply of medication dispensed in the community pharmacy, technicians in a hospital pharmacy typically prepare enough single-unit medications for only 24 to 72 hours (depending on the size and scope of the hospital pharmacy). A **unit dose** is a drug amount prepackaged for a single administration. Most common oral medications—such as tablets, capsules, and some liquids—are commercially available in a unit dose formulation.

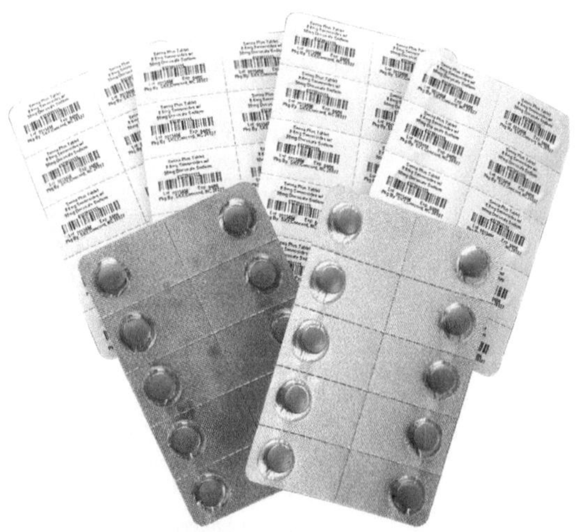

With prepackaged individual dose units, the manufacturer puts a bar code on the label for scanning and an expiration date and lot number for tracking in case of a drug recall.

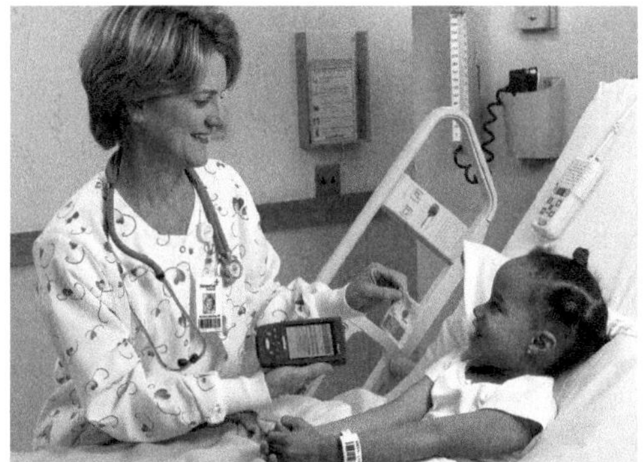

Bar code scanning and automation technologies help reduce errors by ensuring the right drug and dose are delivered to the right patient.

Costs and Benefits of the Unit Dose System

The cost of one dose of medication is proportionately higher in a hospital than one dose from a retail pharmacy. That is because this cost usually includes a portion of the staff time of the pharmacy and nursing personnel and the other hospital overhead as well as the unit dose packaging. Consequently, a dose of Tylenol in the hospital may cost $5 or more per tablet.

However, traditionally the unit dose drug distribution system has offered several benefits for patients, healthcare personnel, and hospitals that offset the higher packaging costs and more labor-intensive activity involved in utilizing this system:

Streamlined Work Flow Process With the drug formulation already prepared, packaged, and labeled, nurses on the patient care unit can administer the medication to the patient more efficiently, thus saving nursing staff time for other patient care responsibilities.

Decreased Medication Errors The bar code on the unit dose package label offers another medication safety check. If a medication does not scan correctly to match the patient's wristband (BPOC), then the wrong medication (or wrong dose) has been sent, and the error is detected before patient administration.

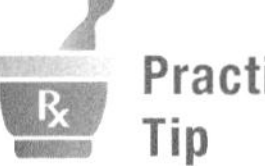

Practice Tip

Only unopened unit doses can be returned to stock. For ease of reuse, the unit doses are labeled with the name of the drug, its strength, and the expiration date.

Increased Medication Security A unit dose system is locked at all times for added security when not in use by the nurse administering medications. The administration of each dose for each patient must be documented by the initials of the nurse in the eMAR.

Reduced Medication Waste In the unit dose system, unused medication whose packaging has not been compromised and bears a valid expiration date can be returned to inventory in the original, unopened package and reissued.

Increased Cost-Effectiveness for Hospital and Patient A unit dose system provides an easier method for the hospital accounting department to maintain patients' accounts (including charges and credits), as each medication dose that is administered is billed to the patient's account.

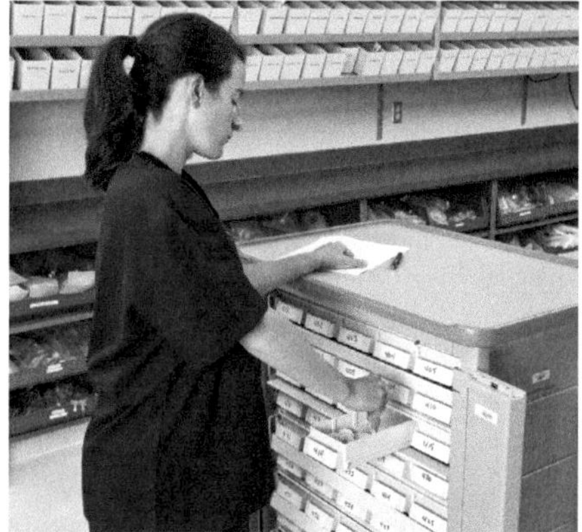

A unit dose cart has individually labeled drawers that contain medications for patients assigned to a room in a designated nursing area.

Design of the Unit Dose Delivery Cart

The unit doses are delivered with a mobile cart—a small rolling cabinet that contains a number of small removable cassette drawers. There are different kinds, such as the daily dose unit cart, which gets delivered on a regular schedule to the nursing units, and the emergency crash cart, which holds all the most needed crisis drugs for ready use. The hospital pharmacy is responsible for stocking as many unit dose carts as there are nursing units, plus the emergency crash carts, drug boxes, and any other mobile carts.

In a **unit dose cart**, each drawer houses the daily medications for a specific patient on the nursing unit. Typically, the cart has two sets of drawers: one set for delivery to the patient care unit and a replacement to be filled by the pharmacy while the cart is on the nursing unit. These drawers are filled and

Practice Tip

Necessary medical supplies such as insulin vials and pens, inhalers, and other multiple-use items have to be delivered to the patients and charged to their accounts.

maintained by the pharmacy technicians. Each cassette drawer is labeled with the patient's name and room number until discharge from the hospital or transfer to another care unit. Each drawer contains a sufficient quantity of the patient's medications for a 24- to 72-hour span (per hospital policy), though smaller hospitals may exchange patient drawers less frequently. The drawers in the unit dose carts are typically exchanged after the scheduled morning dose administrations and then returned to the nursing station to be locked for security until the next administration time later in the day.

Filling the Daily Unit Dose Cart

The pharmacy software collates the medication orders of every patient in a nursing unit to generate a complete medication order list, or **cart fill list**. Each morning, it is printed out by the pharmacy technician (see Figure 11.3) prior to cart filling.

More than one technician is commonly involved in cart filling at the same time. **Pick stations**, as they are called, store frequently used unit dose medications arranged in small, stacked storage bins that are readily available. Each technician has a designated pick station for cart filling. Multiple pick stations in a larger hospital pharmacy allow more efficient patient drawer filling for more technicians.

As a technician, you will read the list description of each medication order and its signa codes to determine the type and number of unit doses required for the patient's dosage schedule (see Figure 11.4). For example, if a prescriber orders *Zofran 4 mg po every six hours prn*, this translates to 4 milligrams of Zofran, in oral form, to be taken every six hours as needed. With these **signa code directions**, or sigs, a maximum of four doses is designated for any 24-hour period. If the unit dose cart is exchanged every 72 hours, then 12 doses of Zofran would be needed.

Each hospital has a standard schedule for dose administrations in regular staggered hours, such as every 4, 6, 8, or 12 hours. For example, if a patient is prescribed *penicillin VK 500 mg po every six hours*, the doses should be administered at 0600, 1200, 1800, and 0000 according to the military (24-hour) clock. These times would be 6 a.m., noon, 6 p.m., and midnight. (For more on the conversion from the 12-hour to 24-hour clock, see Chapter 6.)

As with the community pharmacy, it is important to memorize the sigs. For common dosage sigs for scheduled dosages, see Table 11.3. The "q"s for "every" are crossed out in many of the acronyms to indicate that they should no longer be in use in US hospitals because the Joint Commission (JC) and the Institute for Safe Medication Practices (ISMP) have put them on their lists of "Do Not Use" or "Error Prone" abbreviations. In many cases, the word "every" should be fully written out, but you may see the q still used. (For additional common sigs, see the Common Prescription Abbreviations Table in Chapter 7.)

FIGURE 11.3 Cart Fill List

℞

Amina Ali	**Room 532**			
#06051957				
cyclobenzaprine 10 mg PO				
Q12 H	**0800**	**2000**		
ibuprofen 800 mg PO				
Q6 H	**0000**	**0600**	**1200**	**1800**
diphenhydramine 25 mg PO				
HS	**2200**			
Irma Elmore	**Room 638**			
#12121926				
trazodone 100 mg PO				
Q HS	**2200**			
sertraline 100 mg PO				
QAM	**0900**			
Patrice Anderson	**Room 714**			
#11121956				
amoxicillin/clavulanate 875 mg PO				
TID	**0800**	**1400**	**2200**	
diphenhydramine 25 mg PO 10 mg				
Q6 H	**0000**	**0600**	**1200**	**1800**

TABLE 11.3 Hospital Dosage Timing Signa Codes

Acronym	Timing of Dosage	Acronym	Timing of Dosage
q	every	*~~q~~wk*	every week
~~q~~h	every hour	*q__h*	every [#] hours
~~q~~am	every morning	*bid*	twice a day
~~q~~pm	every evening	*tid*	3 times a day
~~q~~hs	every night at bedtime	*qid*	4 times a day
~~q~~d	every day	*x_d*	times [#] days
~~q~~od	every other day	*prn*	as needed

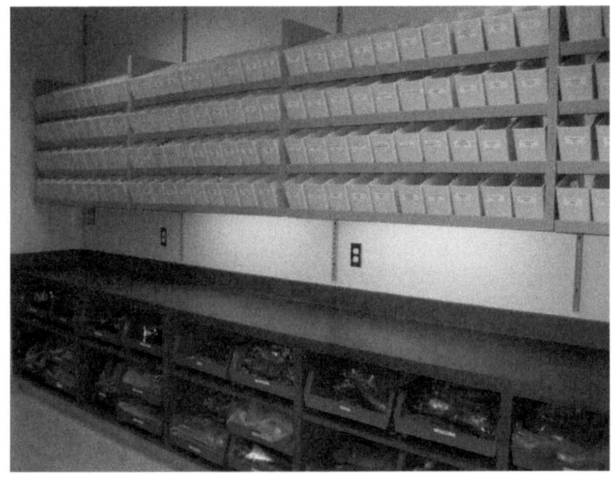

Each of these two pick stations, red and blue, contains the common oral unit doses that are needed to fill the individual drawers of a unit dose cart.

After you select each medication out of the pick station, select the correct dose, dosage form, and amount of unit doses needed. The quantity of unit doses to place in the drawer will depend on the dosing frequency and the hospital policy on frequency of unit dose cart exchanges (i.e., every 12, 24, or 72 hours or once weekly). Each **unit dose product label** includes the following information:

- generic or brand name of the drug
- dosage and special instructions
- strength of the drug
- manufacturer's name, lot number, and expiration date
- bar code of the product

Safety Alert

Remember that *po* means orally or "by the mouth" whereas *npo* indicates that nothing should be given orally, so infusions, patches, suppositories, or other means of delivery will be needed.

Verify the information to make sure that it matches the cart list and what you collected. Place the medication in the unit dose drawer that is labeled with the patient name and room number. If the patient is receiving other medications, add those unit doses to the same drawer. Before delivery, the pharmacist in charge must do a final check. (If there is a tech-check-tech supervisor, this check would occur before the pharmacist's final approval.)

Unlike formulary drugs, Schedule II, III, and IV substances are not dispensed in a unit dose cart per hospital policy. Instead, they are obtained from the locked, secure automated medication delivery system on each nursing floor, where the administration of each dose for each patient is documented by the nurse, which will be addressed later in this chapter. This restriction and security minimize illegal drug diversion.

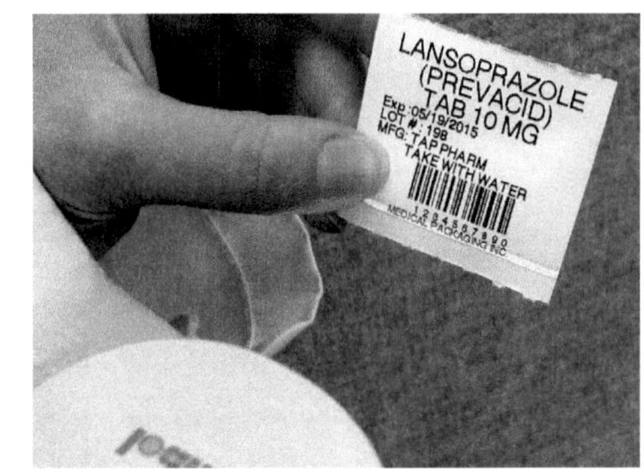

Commercially available unit dose labels contain the drug, dose, and bar code.

Robotic Filling

Many medium- to large-size hospital pharmacies now use a centralized, automated **robotic dispensing system** to more efficiently and accurately fill unit dose orders. This automated medication

FIGURE 11.4
Medication Order Printout

Patient Name	Order	Room #
Jessica Shirley	labetalol 200 mg IV every 8h	825
	phenergan 25 mg IV every 6h prn nausea	
	D5½NS 20 mEq KCl at 50 mL/h	
	NPO after 12PM	
Bobbie King	gentamicin 20 mg IV every 8h	432
	baby powder	
	ASA gr v po every 6h	
Roscoe Mack	Nitrostat SL prn chest pain	503
	Capoten 25 mg po STAT, then bid	
Megan Mills	10,000 units heparin IV STAT	407
	gentamicin 60 mg IVPB tid	
	Bentyl 10 mg po tid prn stomach cramping	
Shannon Bell	continue Rocephin 1 g IV every 24h	335
	continue Zithromax IV 500 mg every 24h	

filling and dispensing system, which is housed in the pharmacy department, is also integrated with hospital and pharmacy software. Larger models can store more than 1,000 (or 90%) of the most frequently prescribed medications, and, in some systems, they may even send the dosages directly to the nursing floors through pneumatic tubes. Similar to a vending machine, this type of dispensing system can hold most of a hospital's drug inventory of selected drugs for three days and can accommodate most dosage forms—tablets, capsules, prepackaged unit dose liquids, patches—even those items requiring refrigeration. It does not handle cleanroom IV infusions and injections.

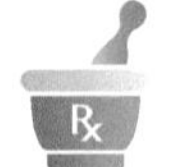

Practice Tip

Some hospital pharmacies have a technician supervisor check (tech-check-tech) the steps in a prepared medication order prior to the pharmacist as an added safety verification step.

For security reasons, there are no controlled substances stored in the robot. Robotic dispensing is sometimes done offsite due to space requirements, and the facility that houses this technology is often centrally located to serve several area corporate hospitals, much like a mail-order warehouse.

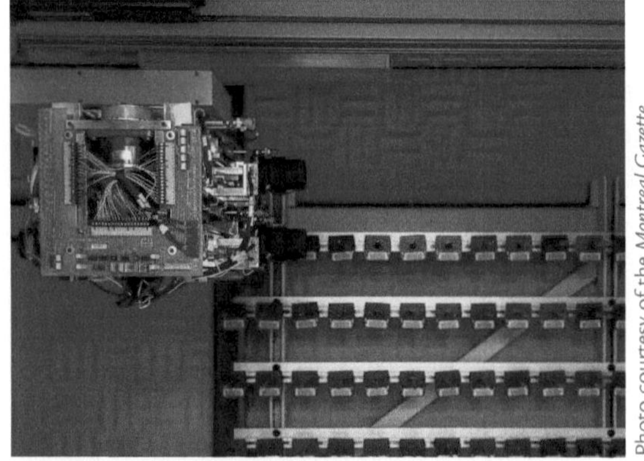

Photo courtesy of the *Montreal Gazette*.

This ROBOT-Rx was installed in 2015 in the new Montreal Children's Hospital.

Operation of the Robot

After a medication order is digitally entered into the system and checked by the pharmacist, the robot takes over. Using bar code technology, the robot can pick, count, package, label, store, and dispense the unit dose medication. (The automated robotic dispensing system can also be used to repackage a high volume of drugs if needed and programmed to do so.) The robotic arm uses suction and pneumatic tubes to pull the correct bar-coded medication and transfer it to a collection area, where it is packaged into an envelope or dispensed onto a tray for the technician to insert into the proper drawer of a unit dose cart or dispensed directly to the nursing floor. In addition, the robot can process drug returns, credits, inventory reordering, and record keeping. A designated technician has the responsibility of restocking the robot's pick station with replacement inventory.

To utilize a robotic system, a hospital or warehouse pharmacy has to process a high-enough volume of medications to justify the cost and the amount of space it takes up.

Benefits of Robotic Filling and Dispensing Systems

There are many advantages to using automation for dispensing medications in the hospital setting, including the following:

Decreased Medication Errors For instance, when used in combination with CPOE and BPOC technologies, ROBOT-Rx (Omnicell) automation has resulted in an accuracy rate of 99.9%. The human rate is about 97.2% with an error rate of 2.8% (according to the company's statistics). One-third of medium- and large-size hospital pharmacies currently use ROBOT-Rx automation for medication dispensing, and half of these hospitals have also adopted BPOC technology.

Reduced Pharmacy Workload Dispensing requires more than 10 discrete steps from physician order entry to nurse administration of the drug at the patient's bedside. Robotic dispensing has been estimated to reduce the workload of pharmacists by 90% and the workload of pharmacy technicians by 72%, allowing them to redirect their energy to other needed areas.

Increased Long-Term Cost Savings The high short-term costs associated with purchasing and installing the robotic dispensing system (which amount to approximately $750,000 to $1 million) are substantial. For smaller hospitals, these costs are prohibitive. Cost savings may be realized in staff efficiencies, improved productivity, and fewer medication errors, resulting in fewer litigation and settlement costs. As costs decrease in the future, such automation will likely become the standard of care within the hospital pharmacy community.

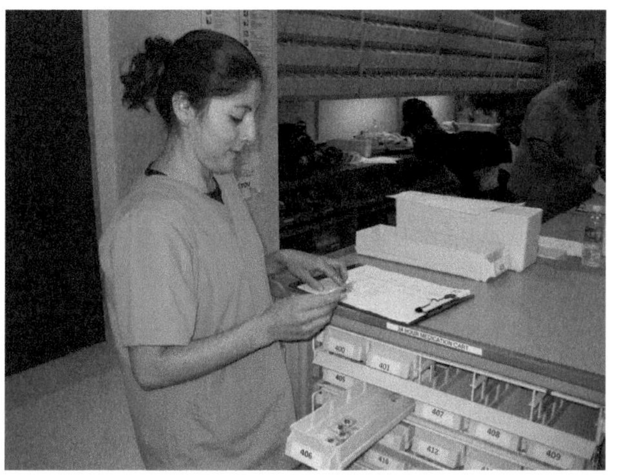

Pharmacy technicians are responsible for filling the daily unit dose carts with packaged medications for each patient's individual drawer.

Processing the Returned Unit Dose Cart

When the unit dose cart is returned to the pharmacy, the pharmacy technician empties all patient cassette drawers and reconciles any returned medications. Unit dose medications may not have been administered for a variety of reasons. The patient may have been undergoing a procedure such as an x-ray at the scheduled medication time; or was told not to take oral medications before surgery per physician's order (NPO, or nothing by mouth); or may have become nauseated so that an oral medication was changed to an injectable or a suppository dosage form. These notes are commonly recorded in the EHR.

Though the dose may have been intentionally skipped, it may also have been missed accidentally and not administered. Some pharmacy departments use the *medications remaining* as a quality assurance tool—they may prompt an investigation into why a medication was missed. The pharmacy technician plays a crucial role in bringing missed doses of drugs, such as antibiotics, or a pattern of several missed doses to the pharmacist's attention. The technician may be asked to visit the nursing unit and conduct an investigation as to why the medication dose was not administered to the patient.

Labeling and Documentation of Repackaged Unit Dose Medications

Not all drugs are commercially available in unit dose packaging, so the pharmacy technician often needs to repackage medications from bulk containers into unit doses and give them a bar-coded label. A **medication special** is a single dose preparation that is repackaged for a particular patient and checked by the pharmacist. The process of creating patient-specific unit doses from stock drugs is labor intensive and often the responsibility of a designated pharmacy technician.

To hand package solid oral medications in unit doses, you will generally use heat-sealed bags, adhesive-sealed bottles, blister packs, and heat-sealed strip packages. For oral liquids, you will measure the medication into plastic or glass cups, heat-sealable aluminum cups, and plastic syringes labeled "For Oral Use Only." Whatever packaging is used, it needs to provide an airtight and light-resistant delivery system to ensure the drug's physical stability.

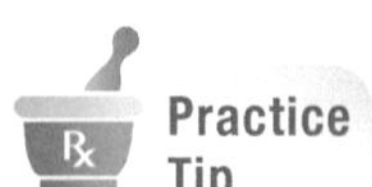

Expiration dates and lot numbers must be included on all repackaged medications. When a drug is repackaged, the expiration date changes from the stock expiration date.

All repackaged unit doses are placed in an envelope or a plastic bag and labeled with the patient's name, the drug name and dose, the medication administration time, lot number, expiration date, and an identifying bar code. As a final check, scan the bar code of the computer-generated unit dose label and/or envelope before the medication order is placed in the unit dose drawer.

After repackaging, you must legally document the essential information about the repackaged medications in a digital **repackaging control log** (or handwritten repackaging logbook, though this is now less common). (See Figure 11.5.) This information must include your initials as the repackaging technician as well as the initials of the pharmacist who checked the medication.

Any home meds that are to be delivered in the daily dose carts also need to be repackaged as unit doses, affixed with a bar-coded label, and portioned out in correct scheduled doses for the cart fill. At discharge, any remaining stock of the home meds will be returned to the patient.

Large hospital pharmacies use a variety of time- and cost-saving devices to assist technicians in medication preparation and repackaging, such as automated pill counting machines and high-speed packaging and dispensing machines for oral

FIGURE 11.5 **Repackaging Control Log Information**

This information must be entered and filed in the computer or logbook to document and track repackaging.

Repackaging Control Log Department of Pharmaceutical Services							
						Initials	
Date Repackaged	Pharmacy Lot Number	Drug Name, Strength, and Dosage Form	Manufacturer and Lot Number	Expiration Date	Quantity Packaged	Prep. By	Approved By

medications (for example, PACMED by McKesson). Such automation can improve efficiency by reducing cart fill times, lowering inventory costs, and improving patient safety. Such automation can also interface with robotic systems, which will be explained, to produce additional efficiencies and safety in hospital pharmacy operations.

Processing Missing Orders

If an order is received in the pharmacy department after the unit dose cart has already been delivered to the nursing floor, an individual medical order will have to be filled and delivered to the nursing unit. You will need to calculate the sufficient amount of the unit dosage needed for the patient until the next cart exchange (and have it checked by the pharmacist). For example, if an order is received at 1300 (1 p.m.) for *Zyrtec 300 mg every 8 h* (0600, 1400, 2200) and the next cart exchange is at 0800 (8 a.m.) the next morning, then three doses need to be delivered for the administrations at 1400 (2 p.m.), 2200 (10 p.m.) and 0600 (6 a.m.).

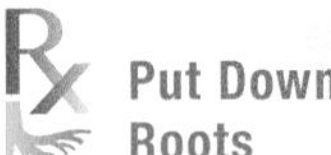

Put Down Roots

Code blue is thought to have come from a code of procedures to assist someone turning blue from lack of oxygen.

Stocking Emergency Drug Crash Cart and Drug Box

Another significant drug cart that technicians are responsible for stocking is the **crash cart**—a mobile cart that holds necessary drugs for an emergency code, such as a **code blue** calling for immediate resuscitation of a patient in respiratory failure or cardiac arrest. The pharmacist verifies the select drugs necessary for restocking the depleted cart, and the technician fills the crash cart with these drugs and checks the expiration dates of all the remaining medications to replace them if they are near expiring. The technician then presents the cart to the pharmacist for review and verification. This cart (or carts) may be housed in the pharmacy, on a nursing unit, or in the emergency department. Pharmacy technicians may also be responsible for restocking the paramedics' emergency drug box after an ambulance run. The crash cart or emergency drug box is sealed after the pharmacist's final check until it is needed.

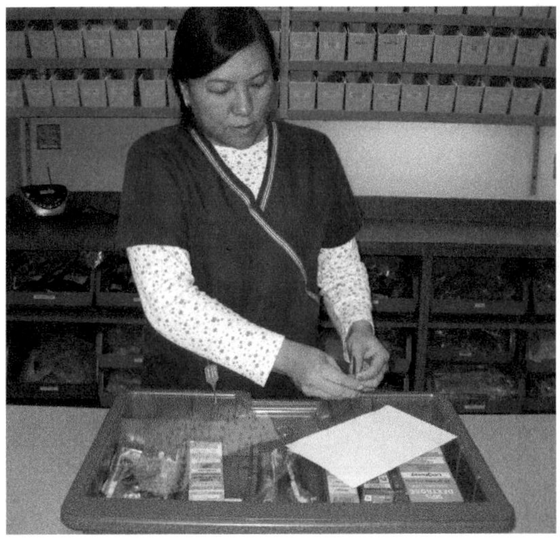

The pharmacy technician checks missing stock and expiration dates to restock the emergency drugs for the hospital crash cart.

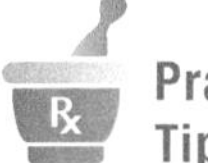

Practice Tip

Technicians are responsible for finding out which patient received a crash cart medication to have that patient's account billed.

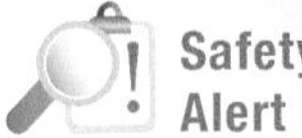

Safety Alert

Robotic and automated dispensing equipment is only as safe and accurate as the pharmacy technicians who fill it, the pharmacists who verify the fills, and the nurses who administer the medications.

Stocking Floor Stock Automated Dispensing Cabinets

Not all medications are delivered through unit dose carts. **Floor stock** is a secured inventory of frequently prescribed drugs and IV solutions that are stored on the patient care unit. Historically, floor stock was limited to commonly selected drugs used on a *prn*, or as needed, basis and it included mainly over-the-counter medications. Ointments, creams, antacids, ear drops, and eye drops—considered bulk items—were all commonly supplied as floor stock and placed at the patient's bedside upon a physician's order.

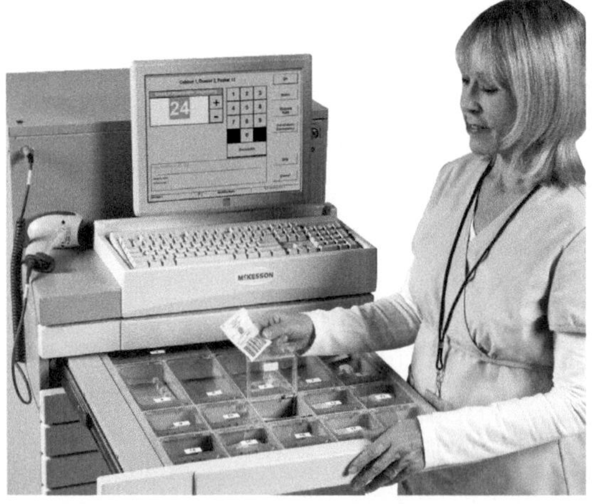
This automated delivery system dispenses stock drug items to the nurse on the patient care unit.

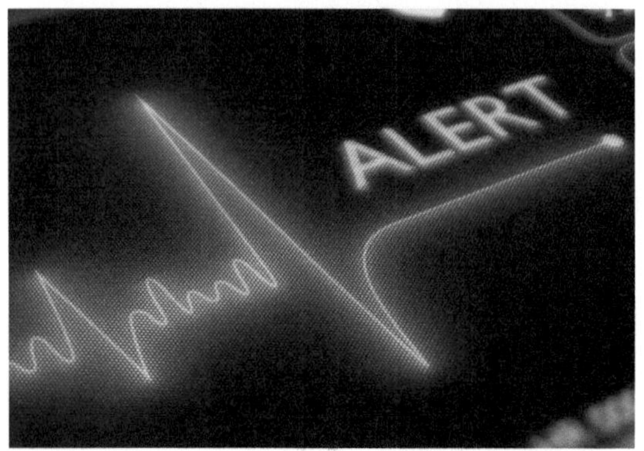

Integrating automated robots, AMDS, CPOE, BPOC, and eMAR has reduced many types of hospital medication errors.

Almost all US hospitals now place floor stock (plus other commonly used Rx medications) in a high-technology **automated dispensing cabinet (ADC)**. An ADC is a mechanized locked cabinet with several drawers for medications, which is specifically designed for each nursing unit to dispense unit doses, similar to a vending machine. Some drawers of the cabinet may be refrigerated; other drawers contain oral and injectable narcotics with a higher level of security and documentation required. These cabinets work with **automated medication dispensing system (AMDS)** software that is integrated into the hospital's patient management system to increase efficiency, safety, and security.

The pharmacist must initially approve all new medication orders that are to be filled in the ADC. The nurse then logs onto the computer located on the dispensing cabinet and uses touch screen technology to match a patient's specific medication order with the floor stock stored in the ADC. The AMDS software highlights the status of each medication order, indicates the exact location of the prescribed medication in the storage cabinet, and then records the time and initials of the nurse who retrieves and administers the medication. (There is a specific labeled compartment for each medication in the ADC.) Each dose of each drug is documented in the AMDS and registers on the computerized screen. The drug bar codes from the ADC and the patient wristband are scanned for a match before each drug administration.

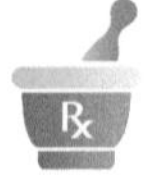
Practice Tip

Bar code scanning of each drug before restocking it in the automated dispensing machine reduces restocking and potential medication errors.

Automated Dispensing Cabinets Restocking

A technician is responsible for restocking the ADCs on different floors with common medications on those units. The AMDS provides automated reorders of inventory levels to be sent to the pharmacy. For each drug in the ADC on each nursing unit, the **PAR level**, or the minimum stock level to spur a reorder (with the maximum reorder amount), is set by the pharmacy department. (PAR stands for periodic automatic replenishment). These automated systems optimize inventory control by minimizing costs and out-of-stock items.

Throughout the day, the nursing units also send reports, sometimes called "out-of-stock reports," to the hospital pharmacy requesting that selected drug inventory be replaced. Before a technician refills the automated dispensing cabinet, a pharmacist checks all of the medications to be sent up to the floor by request or procedure. Double-checking as you fill the cabinet or the robotic dispensing unit shelves is essential. If a technician absentmindedly places Fiorinal where Fioricet should be, the wrong medication could be dispensed. That is why you need to scan the bar code of the drug and label before restocking the ADCs (or a robot in the central pharmacy). This scanning will prevent a restocking error. You also need to check all the medication expiration dates and adjust inventory levels as needed.

IN THE REAL WORLD

One technician recalls, "There have been several medication errors that I have encountered while filling medications in the Pyxis machine. I was filling the Bupropion XL spot when I found that another technician had filled it with Bupropion SR instead, and the pharmacist had verified it." Other errors she caught were hydroxyzine filled instead of hydralazine and Plavix instead of Paxil. "As pharmacy technicians," she added, "we always have to be the second eye of the pharmacist and always double-check all of the medications even if the pharmacist has verified them."

Since ADCs are locked, narcotics are now commonly included in the floor stock inventory of each patient care unit in the hospital, though type and quantity will vary by unit. Depending on hospital policy, the exchange of narcotics from the pharmacy technician (or the pharmacist) to the floor ADC and a nursing staff member requires documentation, including the names of both parties, the name and quantity of each dose of narcotics being delivered, and the date and time of delivery. A careful audit trail must exist from the manufacturer to the pharmacy to the patient in order to account for each dose of each Schedule II drug to comply with strict regulations established by the DEA.

Though medications are stored on the nursing units, the Joint Commission holds the pharmacy department accountable for monitoring the safety, security, and inventory of the AMDS.

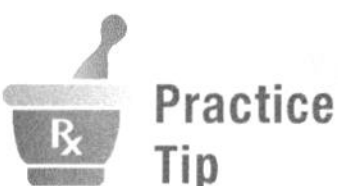

Practice Tip

Each hospital has its own mix of automated equipment and storage/dispensing units that technicians must know how to fill and run.

Automated Dispensing Cabinet and Automated Medication Dispensing System Advantages

The nursing floor ADC run by the AMDS offers several advantages for patients, healthcare personnel, and the hospital. These benefits offset the high equipment cost that is initially involved in implementing this type of drug distribution system. The use of AMDS reduces the incidence of medication errors. In one study, the Pyxis AMDS reduced medication errors by 82%. This streamlined process also saved time and allowed nursing personnel to administer medications in a timelier manner and spend more time providing patient care. With nursing floor ADCs, pharmacy technicians can spend more time on refilling, repackaging, and sterile compounding duties. By having the most frequently needed medications on each nursing unit, there are fewer telephone calls and interruptions of daily activities in the central pharmacy.

The ADCs offer great security advantages too because they can be set up for various security levels, such as *prn* medications, frequently used drugs, and controlled substances. The system can be programmed with different security and process parameters set for pharmacists, pharmacy technicians, nurses, and nursing supervisors. The AMDS documents each step of the medication dispensing and administration process, tracking all medications by type of drug, dose, patient, and caregiver. It also captures all charges for dispensed medications. The security and accountability incorporated in the AMDS provides a strong deterrent to illegal drug diversion and medication theft of controlled substances.

Robotic dispensing and automated cabinets are just the beginnings of the automated solutions. There are large and small varieties of automated storage and filling units (including specialized narcotic stations), carousels, packaging, and bar code labeling equipment. As a technician, you will have to learn well the specific handling of all automated equipment.

Cleanroom Services

Many medication orders that cannot be filled in unit dose carts or general floor stock must be individually prepared in sterile controlled environments with aseptic technique for administration into the patients' veins through IVs and injections. These drugs include, among many different kinds, infection-fighting antibiotics, hazardous drugs, and **total parenteral nutrition (TPN)**, also known as intravenous feeding. TPN is a specially formulated IV solution that provides for the entire nutritional needs of a patient who cannot or will not eat solid food. It may contain more than 20 ingredients, including amino acids, carbohydrates, fats, sugars, vitamins, electrolytes, and minerals. Recipients of TPN include patients of all ages, among them premature infants and newborns. A TPN service team usually is composed of a physician, a nurse, a nutritionist, and a pharmacist—all of whom have specialty training and/or certifications. This team sees all TPN patients each day, writes medication orders, and monitors patient progress.

Unlike other parenteral medications, TPN is usually administered directly into a large vein (often the vena cava), so it is extremely important that the solution be sterile. The solution may be hanging at room temperature for up to 24 hours or longer, and it is essential that it be contaminant free so that nothing microbial grows within that time.

Preparing TPN and all parenteral sterile solutions is called an **intravenous (IV) admixture service** or infusion service (also known as an IV additive service). Technicians in the general hospital pharmacy are not preparing or handling these solutions, as this is left to the specially trained technicians and pharmacists in the hospital cleanroom and hazardous compounding areas (the processes of which will be described in more depth in Chapters 12 and 13). However, certain common infusions and injection solutions can be made by automated sterile compounding systems, such as RIVA (Robotic IV Automation) and Intellifill IV. These are installed in the hospital cleanrooms to help the technicians compound more parenteral products.

Smaller hospitals may elect to outsource their TPN preparations to a larger hospital pharmacy or an offsite infusion pharmacy. In this situation, the physician order for TPN is received by the hospital pharmacy, reviewed and verified by the hospital pharmacist, and then forwarded to the outsourced pharmacy. The offsite pharmacy is then responsible for the preparation, expiration dating, verification, labeling, and transport of the final product to the hospital. The director of the hospital pharmacy must be assured that the offsite pharmacy meets all state and federal laws and regulations as well as adhering to the standards set by the USP and the Joint Commission (which will be described in greater detail later on).

11.5 Inventory Management

Inventory control is an important task for the hospital pharmacy technician. Since up to 70% or more of the department budget is spent on pharmaceuticals, the efficient turnover and accurate tracking of inventory are extremely important responsibilities. Many hospital pharmacies have assigned inventory management to a senior pharmacy technician. This individual (with the assistance of the drug-information pharmacist) assumes the position of the pharmaceutical buyer and is responsible for helping to prepare contracts and bids, ordering the medications, and receiving shipments of these ordered items. These technician duties are performed under pharmacist supervision.

Information technology greatly assists the technician in meeting and adjusting drug inventory. In addition to pharmaceuticals, the budget often includes IV solutions, bulk ingredients, administration sets, and pumps, as well as various other medical supplies. Pharmacy storage space is often limited, so managing to have sufficient inventory without shortages is essential to providing good patient care. For this reason, hospital pharmacy personnel usually perform a physical inventory of their drugs annually.

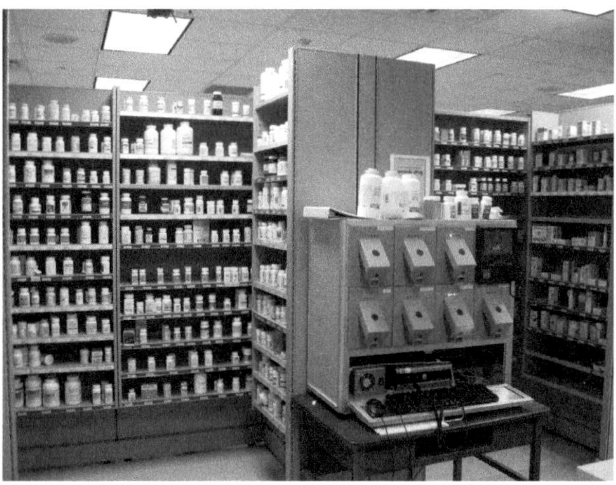

Drug inventory comprises a majority of the hospital pharmacy budget and must be carefully monitored and tracked.

Bidding Pharmaceuticals and Purchasing Contracts

The pharmacy department must ensure that its patients receive the highest-quality pharmaceuticals at the lowest cost. Most hospital pharmacies order their pharmaceuticals from a prime vendor wholesaler (such as McKesson or Cardinal Health) and their IV solutions, ingredients, tubing, administration sets, and pumps directly from a specialty pharmaceutical compounding manufacturer. Software from the hospital pharmacy and the wholesaler makes inventory management more accurate and less costly.

Many large hospitals use an annual or biennial competitive, confidential, sealed-bid process for selecting the prime vendor wholesalers and manufacturers of drugs and IV solutions. The inventory-control technician is often responsible for collecting the information necessary for the drug-bidding process. For example, the technician may be asked to estimate the annual total hospital units for the antibiotic Zosyn in its many dose formulations or to estimate the number of cases of dextrose 5% in water (D_5W) IV solutions for the next year. The technician with the pharmacists and the director must arrive at accurate estimates of the units needed of each of the many thousands of formulary drugs for the next calendar or fiscal year.

Most hospital pharmacies accept bids with a one year "lock in" of medication costs. Changing manufacturers of generic medications (or switching from brand name drugs to generics) too often may cause confusion for the pharmacist, nurse, and physician because the color, shape, or packaging may differ from that of the previously stocked medication. If the hospital operates an outpatient community pharmacy, many states require a separate bidding process and physical inventory.

Contracts with the IV compounder and supplies manufacturer are generally made for a longer period (typically five years). Switching IV solutions and IV administration sets requires massive re-education of nursing personnel, and completing this task on a yearly basis would be neither feasible nor cost-effective. Plus, constant fluctuation in IV solutions and equipment increases the risk of medication administration errors.

Ordering the Pharmaceuticals

Once bids and purchasing contracts are finalized, an important responsibility of the inventory control technician is ordering from these drug vendors. However, there are two situations in which special ordering may be required. Each situation is described below.

Nonformulary Drugs

Occasionally, a nonformulary drug must be purchased from a different wholesaler (or community pharmacy) if prescribed and approved for a specific use. Depending on hospital policy, the patient receiving the medication may be charged by the hospital for the bulk purchase (for example, a quantity of 100 tablets or capsules). The nonformulary drug is then repackaged by a technician into a unit dose formulation with a bar code for scanning by a nurse. If charged to the patient, any remaining medication is returned to the patient at discharge.

Drugs Borrowed from Other Facilities

At times, a hospital pharmacy may need to borrow a medication from another hospital or a community pharmacy. The P&P Manual will outline the process, and the borrowed drug must be returned when the next shipment is received from the wholesaler. Once the restitution has occurred, each facility's inventory is settled at the month's end. Of course, if controlled substances are borrowed, even more careful documentation with more signatures is required so that substantial proof is evident in case of an audit.

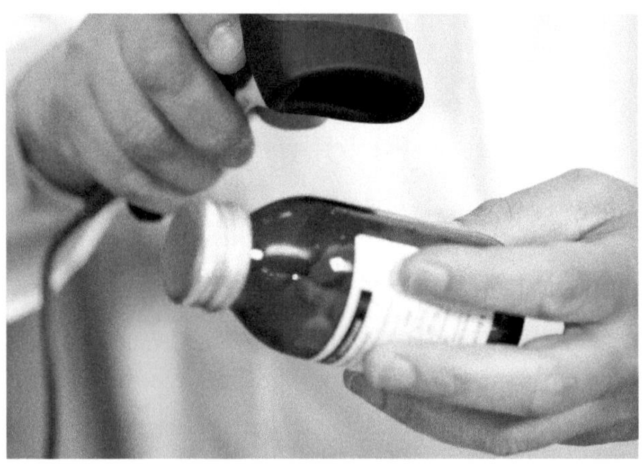

The pharmacists and pharmacy technicians use a handheld bar code scanner to track inventory usage in the pharmacy.

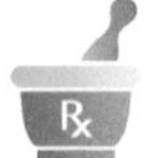

Practice Tip

Pharmacy and nursing refrigerators and freezers are designated solely for medication storage. No food or beverages can be stored alongside the medications.

Receiving and Storing Drug Inventory

Once the regularly ordered drugs are received, the technician must check each drug in the order against the wholesaler's or manufacturer's invoice. The order must be reviewed for potentially damaged or expired goods. Unusable goods must be refused.

If items are missing from the invoice, the technician alerts the pharmacist in charge of inventory. The wholesaler may not have been able to acquire the requested medication due to an FDA or manufacturer drug recall or a drug shortage. If the drug cannot be received in a timely manner, the pharmacist may need to notify the prescriber and help to find an alternative drug. Shortages for needed chemotherapy drugs and even IV fluids are not an uncommon problem. The inventory technician should also check special order deliveries (medications not routinely stocked) on a daily basis in case a patient is waiting for a newly received medication.

Whereas the inventory control technician is the one primarily responsible for purchasing and ordering medications, all pharmacy technicians assist in receiving, storing, and restocking the ordered items once they are verified by the invoice. Boxes of various IV solutions must be stored in a warehouse; they must be removed from boxes and wiped down before being placed in a designated area outside the IV cleanroom.

The technicians store the medications on their designated shelves, in the refrigerator, or in the freezer. The storage guidelines for each pharmaceutical can be found in the attached product package inserts or by consulting pharmaceutical references, such as the American Hospital Formulary Service Drug Information. Prior to storing the drugs, temperatures (in degrees Celsius) in the pharmacy and nursing refrigerator, freezer, and automated units should be documented per the hospital policy.

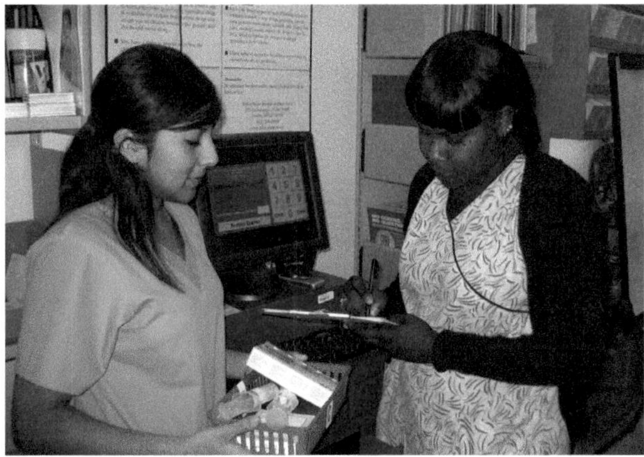

The pharmacy technician is responsible for delivering narcotics and any other controlled substances to each nursing unit floor stock. Each time the inventory must be checked and signed off by the nursing supervisor.

Special Handling of Certain Pharmaceuticals

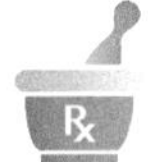

Practice Tip

All unused, returned, damaged, or missing narcotics and other controlled substances must be recorded on a special DEA Form 106 signed by the pharmacist. An investigation will be conducted to make sure the missing drugs weren't stolen.

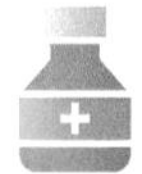

Pharm Fact

Hospitals that use automated narcotics storage reduce the time spent reconciling controlled substance inventory by more than 90%.

Two types of pharmaceuticals require special consideration in inventory control: narcotics and investigational drugs.

Narcotics

The Controlled Substances Act (CSA) defines the proper processes for ordering inventory, filing, and record keeping for controlled substances. As in the community pharmacy, the purchase of Schedule II controlled substances must be authorized by a pharmacist and executed using the online or paper Drug Enforcement Administration DEA Form 222. Vendors also have DEA-approved online **Controlled Substance Ordering Systems (CSOS)**. Unlike the receipt of other pharmaceuticals, the pharmacist must personally check in Schedule II substances, completing the DEA 222 receipt forms, and signing and filing the invoices. The pharmacist must check each Schedule II drug, dose, quantity, and NDC number.

Multiple checks and balances exist for the secure storage and accountability of narcotics in the pharmacy as well as on the nursing units. As in the community pharmacy, all Schedule II controlled substances in a hospital pharmacy must be secured in a locked cabinet or safe. The pharmacist must conduct a physical inventory of Schedule II substances a minimum of every two years per DEA regulations. Any destruction of Schedule II drugs in the pharmacy or on the nursing unit must be witnessed and documented in the pharmacy department records. Returns of Schedule II drugs (due to theft, loss, or damage) are rare and must be recorded on a special DEA Form 106 signed by the pharmacist. Nurses must also maintain a **Schedule II drug administration record** on each unit to account for each dose of each Schedule II narcotic administered to a patient.

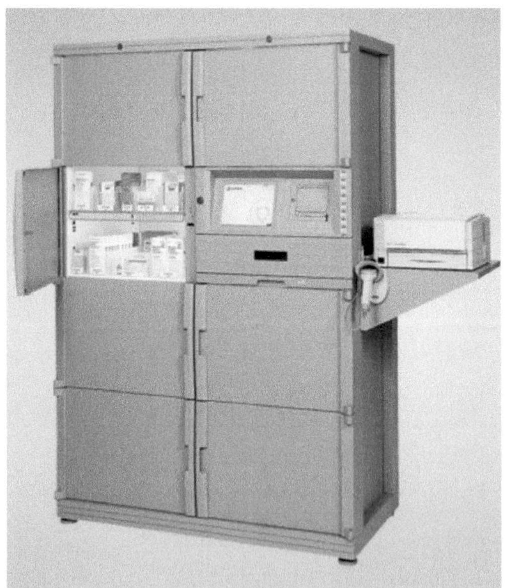

The Pyxis C^{II}Safe is an example of an automated narcotic software system and vault that is used to store and track controlled substances in the central pharmacy.

Since pharmacy technicians deliver controlled substances to nursing units, they are also responsible for reporting any unusual increases in inventory or discrepancies of nursing unit narcotics to the pharmacist. The pharmacist must immediately resolve any discrepancies with the nurse supervisor.

NarcStation and Pyxis C^{II}Safe are specialized AMDS units that may be used in the centralized pharmacy. They provide compatible software tracking systems using state-of-the-art bar code technology to maintain the record keeping, reporting, and transaction date for all controlled substances from the wholesaler to the patient. These systems also provide separate reporting for Schedule II, III, and IV drugs to meet DEA, state, and federal requirements. The software is compatible with many hospital systems and automatically reorders needed Schedule II drugs with an electronic sign-off for the DEA Form 222. Bar coding technology is used for receipt.

Automated dispensing systems offer perpetual inventory record keeping that continually updates the balance of remaining doses of each drug.

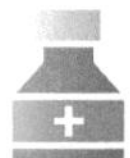

Pharm Fact

An AMDS provides real-time reports and immediate access to information that identifies trends in controlled substance usage on each patient care unit.

Investigational Drugs

Pharmacy technicians also have the responsibility of storing investigational drugs under proper conditions (locked, refrigerated) and maintaining them separate from other hospital drug inventory. Investigational drugs require special ordering (directly from the manufacturer), handling, and record keeping procedures by the pharmacy technician. They may be received directly from the manufacturer or from a research department within the hospital.

Like controlled substances, investigational drugs must be maintained in a secure and separate area of the pharmacy, often a locked cabinet. They cannot be accessed without a valid written medication order received from the primary physician investigator. In most of these research studies, the drug is *not labeled with a name or strength*, but instead, the technician labels them with a drug study code, lot number, and expiration date. At the study's conclusion, the technician in charge of storage returns all unused drug amounts, information, and data to the primary investigator.

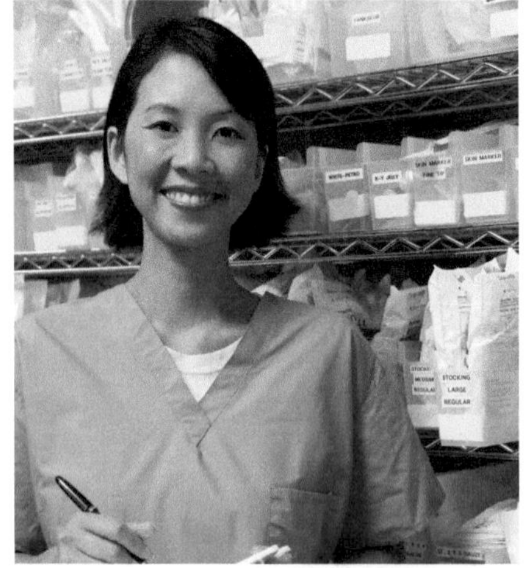

Technicians need to rotate the stock and keep track of any low or missing stock.

Performing Ongoing Inventory Responsibilities

Besides correct storing of the inventory and documenting point of use, technicians have other hospital inventory responsibilities.

Rotating Inventory

As in the community pharmacy, shelf stock must be rotated so that the most recent inventory is not used first. Once a month, all technicians need to inspect all of the stock in the pharmacy and on the nursing units for expired drugs, including opened multidose vials of sterile water and normal saline in the pharmacy or on the nursing units. Automation may alert the technician to the lot numbers of drugs that will soon be out of date. Inventory turnover is rapid, and expired drugs rarely are found. Documentation for checking expired drugs in the pharmacy and nursing units is required for hospital accreditation.

Checking for Drug Recalls

Any medications recalled by the FDA or a manufacturer must be immediately pulled from the inventory shelves, unit dose carts, crash carts, automated filling and dispensing cabinets, and robots. A recall notice may come from the wholesaler or from a letter sent from the drug manufacturer to the director of pharmacy. The technician must compare the lot number of the drug in the recall notice with the inventory. Then, typically, the technician fills out, signs, and returns a form to the wholesaler indicating drug, strength, amount, and lot number to receive credit. A copy is kept in the pharmacy department records. (Drug recalls are also addressed in Chapter 2 on the laws involved and Chapter 14 on medication safety. It is important to know the many aspects of drug recalls, as they are likely part of the knowledge needed for certification exams.)

11.6 Other Institutional Pharmacy Practice Settings

If serving a large enough patient population, skilled nursing facilities (SNFs), home healthcare agencies, long-term care facilities (LTCFs), and health maintenance organizations (HMOs) often have their own institutional in-house pharmacies with pharmacist and pharmacy technician staffing. These institutional pharmacies are run more like a hospital pharmacy than a community pharmacy. The HMOs often have both a community pharmacy and a hospital pharmacy among their facilities.

It is estimated that, by 2025, more than 20 percent of the country's population will be over 65 years old. With the aging population, many retirement communities offer different levels of residential and nursing care on the same campus. These levels may include independent living, assisted living, SNFs, and LTCFs with memory care programs. Residents can transition to various levels of medical and nursing care as they age or progress in an illness. A variety of pharmacy services need to be available to serve these patients. Still, most of the medications are prepared off the premises and delivered to the institution.

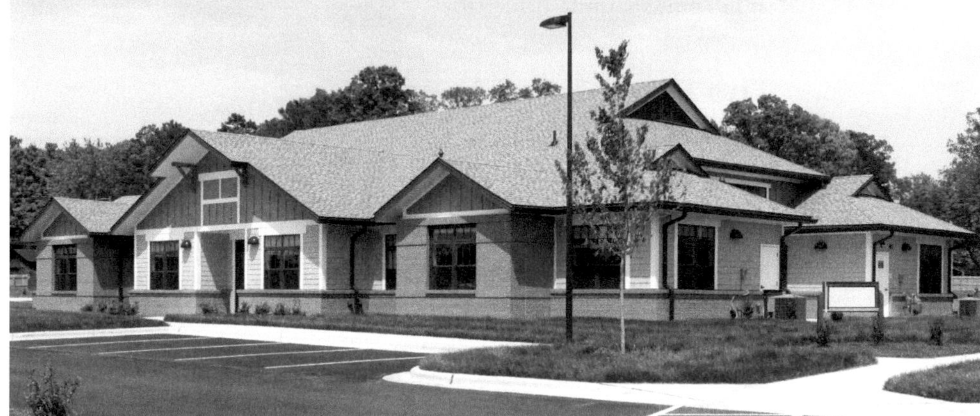

Most assisted living homes contract with a community pharmacy. However, if it runs a large enough complex, an assisted living company may have its own pharmacy.

The other popular option to care for the nation's aging population is home health care, where nursing and pharmaceutical services are delivered to the patient's residence. These services, though, are not only for the aging. A patient of any age may be discharged from a hospital (or skilled nursing facility) and still need nursing care for rehabilitation, chronic disease, intravenous fluids and nutrition solutions, chemotherapy, antibiotic or pain infusions, or specialty high-cost drugs.

A **home infusion pharmacy** is a specialty pharmacy set up particularly to serve home healthcare dispensing. Many of the drugs are prepared in a cleanroom environment by certified pharmacy technicians and verified by the pharmacist, similar to a hospital cleanroom. The major difference between a hospital and an infusion pharmacy is that a technician is preparing a batch of sterile preparations for up to a week or longer in the home infusion pharmacy rather than for an emergency need or a 24-hour supply. ASHP recommends that a pharmacy technician working in either of these sterile compounding environments graduate from an accredited pharmacy technician training program and be certified by the Pharmacy Technician Certification Board (PTCB), as well as receiving specialized training in sterile compounding.

The home infusion pharmacies generally have contracts with many small home healthcare companies, and they need to abide by the Joint Commission and USP compounding standards as well the ASHP guidelines on home infusion pharmacy services, which are posted on the ASHP website. To access them, visit https://PharmPractice7e.ParadigmEducation.com/ASHPInfusion.

11.7 The Joint Commission for High Standards of Care

Hospitals and other healthcare institutions must all comply with state and federal regulations and standards, and each pharmacy department within them must also abide by all state pharmacy board regulations and oversight. In addition, every US hospital (and many other healthcare institutions) seeks initial accreditation and reaccreditation by the Joint Commission to receive reimbursement from Medicare, Medicaid, and private insurance companies. To receive accreditation, every hospital department, including the pharmacy, must follow and document standards for high-quality care and patient safety. That is one reason why contracted compounding pharmacies must follow Joint Commission standards, and the pharmacy technicians in hospitals should be certified.

The Process of Accreditation

The **Joint Commission** accredits more than 19,000 hospitals, home healthcare systems, and skilled and long-term care facilities. If a hospital meets the standards and is approved, accreditation or reaccreditation lasts for three years.

The Joint Commission acts as a patient and healthcare advocate, making sure that the facility is following the appropriate standards and procedures. The organization sets evidence-based standards of care developed in consultation with healthcare experts, providers, and researchers. Hospitals and their pharmacies must submit documentation that they have met these standards. All departments, including the pharmacy, must submit an up-to-date online P&P Manual following the criteria required by the Joint Commission. They also must offer annual documentation of technician training on the manual and drug updates.

The Joint Commission's standards for the hospital pharmacy include best practices for reconciling a patient's profile upon admission to the hospital, processes to improve the safety of medication use and drug infusion pumps, and to reduce medication errors and the risk of hospital-acquired infections, among others. These standards address a number of significant patient safety issues, including the implementation of patient safety programs, the response to adverse events when they occur, and the prevention of accidental harm.

The emphasis of the Joint Commission is on addressing safety issues that are significant not only for patient care, but also for hospital financial viability. Medicare no longer reimburses hospitals for the additional cost of treating preventable medication errors, injuries, and infections. Medicare also no longer reimburses for preventable readmissions to the hospital within 30 days of discharge.

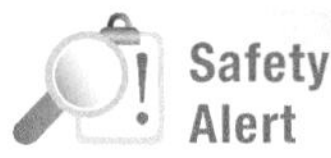

Approximately 50% of the Joint Commission standards relate directly to safety.

The Onsite Joint Commission Survey

After the application with documentation is fully submitted, the Joint Commission visits the site without warning and evaluates a hospital's performance in each specific area of care, as compared against the defined standards. The Commission awards accreditation status if the facility meets or exceeds those standards. The facility inspection is sometimes referred to as a *survey*. It requires extensive, multiday, onsite visits by a surveying team composed of healthcare professionals who are extensively trained, certified, and educated in quality-related performance evaluation. When the survey team arrives unannounced to conduct its evaluation, it is not done to seek problems and be punitive, but to assure patients that the hospital is at all times living up to the required standards or instituting improvements to be in compliance.

The survey team evaluates the facility's performance data, reviews the P&P Manual for compliance with quality and safety standards, and often interviews hospital personnel. For example, the survey team may discover that a hospital pharmacy recently implemented multiple personnel cuts for budgetary reasons, and some data suggest that it may be leading to a compromise in the care quality or safety level. The survey team will interview personnel to find out if they believe this is the case and what they recommend. The Joint Commission survey team, having noticed any problematic areas, has the authority to require prompt corrective action by hospital administration.

If the Joint Commission finds enough evidence that inappropriate antibiotic use by hospital prescribers may be leading to an increase in surgical site infections, resistance patterns within the hospital, and healthcare costs, the Commission might then request that a plan be put in place to address the situation, such as establishing hospital-wide criteria that must be met for prescribing antibiotics with the pharmacist in charge, flagging any use patterns that do not match these criteria, and providing counsel about alternative therapies. The hospital and its pharmacy would then have a set time period to demonstrate that an improvement strategy has been determined and implemented.

The survey team generally provides a summary report to the administrative staff and employees. In addition, the Joint Commission offers education and guidance to improve the facility's overall performance. The final accreditation report of each healthcare facility is available on the Joint Commission's website for public review by any consumer or healthcare professional.

Quality Assurance and Quality Control

Both the USP and the Joint Commission require each hospital and other healthcare facilities to have written policies and procedures for quality standards, training, and documentation of implementing all practices. These are required for hospital accreditation, which is required for insurance reimbursement. Site inspections that include the sterile and hazardous compounding facilities are essential to initial and maintained accreditation. Also required are quality monitoring and improvement procedures.

Quality assurance (QA) is a system of procedures, activities, and oversight that ensures that operational and quality standards are consistently met. **Quality control (QC)** involves the sampling, testing, and documentation of results that, taken together, ensure that specifications have been met. Where quality assurance is about how a process is performed or how a product is created, quality control is more about the inspections used to manage quality.

Setting National Quality of Care Standards

The Joint Commission not only sets individual facility improvement goals but also sets National Quality Improvement Goals for raising patient care quality across the country for select at-risk patient populations. Hospitals must then report on key indicators of care quality for these specific populations, such as those for heart attack, heart failure, community-acquired pneumonia, and surgical infection rates. The survey team often requests a number of medical charts to randomly review for compliance with the National Quality Improvement Goals. For example, in assessing the hospital performance for the care of heart attack patients, several medication-related factors may be evaluated, measured, and compared with those at other hospitals accredited by the Joint Commission. The clinical pharmacists are commonly the ones responsible for measuring progress in the following areas (and they may ask technicians to help gather the data):

- use of aspirin, prescribed on arrival and at discharge because it decreases the risk of recurrent blood clots and improves survival
- use of certain heart drugs, called beta blockers, within the first 24 hours and at discharge to minimize damage to the heart
- timely use of thrombolytic or clot-buster therapy within 30 minutes of arrival to the hospital or emergency room to reduce heart muscle damage
- use of certain heart drugs, called *angiotensin-converting enzyme (ACE) inhibitors* or *angiotensin receptor blockers (ARBs)*, at discharge if the patient has a diagnosis of heart failure

Comparative analysis is performed at a national and state level by the Joint Commission and is also made available to employers and patients at its website.

11.8 Pharmacy Department Productivity Measurement Processes and Tools

Traditionally, the productivity of the hospital pharmacy department has been measured by the number of medication orders processed, various labor or drug cost ratios, labor hours invested, or a hospital census. Error rate assessments, error-to-medication order ratios, and trend tracking have also been included, and all these productivity measurements have been made easier by the new patient management software systems.

These measurements, however, do not reflect the impact of pharmacy personnel on improving patient outcomes and lowering the cost of patient care. Hospital pharmacy departments are increasingly utilizing other benchmarks contained in EHRs and other pharmacy software to better measure productivity, such as the following:

- the number of medication orders entered, verified, discontinued

- patient profiles reviewed
- progress notes written by clinical pharmacists
- adverse drug reaction reports investigated or even prevented
- participation in CPR codes
- involvement in hospital formulary control committees
- pharmacist dosing of medications (such as certain antibiotics and anticoagulants)
- pharmacist adjustment of medication doses based on patient-specific parameters (such as kidney function)

The American Society of Health-System Pharmacists (ASHP) has established benchmarks to measure the total department impact on the safe, effective, and efficient use of drugs through the hospital pharmacy services and pharmacist consultations with prescribers and patients. Hospitals can use these benchmarks and their software programs to track these and other productivity and safety impacts to find ways to build efficiencies and identify areas leading to wasted time or medication errors. Technicians are often asked to be part of the data gathering and processing.

The number of staffed pharmacy technicians and the ratio of technicians to pharmacists have a direct impact not only on labor costs, but also on the hospital's goal to improve patient outcomes and lower hospital costs and potential liability.

11.9 Being a Hospital Pharmacy Technician

Whether working in a small rural hospital or a large university teaching hospital in a metropolitan area, you as a technician will be exposed to unit dose, repackaging, institutional automation, inventory control, and perhaps even sterile or hazardous IV compounding (which will be covered in the following chapters). Being a technician in a hospital requires more training and experience than in a community pharmacy. This can be gained only by completing an ASHP-accredited program and becoming PTCB certified.

As a hospital pharmacy technician, you will generally receive a higher hourly wage to compensate for your additional training, experience, certification, and working fewer traditional hours. Having weekend and night shifts is normal since most hospital pharmacies are open 7 days a week—and many are open 24 hours per day. If you work in larger hospitals, you will likely gain a breadth of experience and elect to specialize in one of many different areas, such as unit dose filling, tech-check-tech, automation management and filling, investigational drugs, or inventory. You may even decide to get additional training to become certified to do sterile and/or hazardous compounding. For these reasons, the opportunities for advancement are often greater within a larger institutional system than in a community pharmacy. There are compelling reasons to choose to work in a hospital or other healthcare institution. There will always be something new happening and challenges to take on.

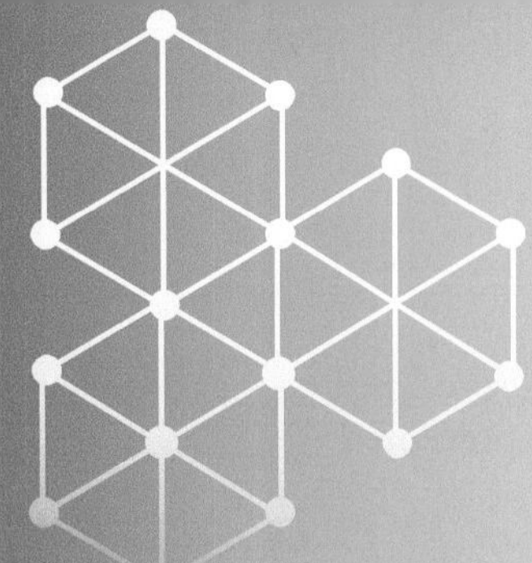

Review and Assessment

CHAPTER SUMMARY

- The hospital is a complex organization of many different departments that interact to provide quality patient care. It is helpful to know department acronyms as they appear on patient medical orders.
- Hospitals are often run like corporations with CEOs and boards of directors.
- The Pharmacy and Therapeutics Committee is primarily responsible for making the final decision on the medications included in the hospital's drug formulary.
- The Institutional Review Board, also known as the Human Use Committee, oversees the consideration and approval of investigational drug studies on patient populations within the hospital.
- The director of pharmacy is in charge of the department budget and budgetary allotments for the drugs within the formulary, staffing decisions, and the implementation of the Policy and Procedure Manual, as well as other operational decisions.
- Responsibilities for the pharmacy technician in the hospital vary considerably from working in a community pharmacy, with less patient interaction, no insurance billing, more emphasis on single-dose packaging and repackaging, sterile compounding, dispensing formulary medications to nurses for administration, automated dispensing, and managing drug inventory.
- Technicians need to understand the value and use of electronic health records (EHRs), computer prescriber order entry (CPOE), bar code scanners and bar code point-of-care (BPOC) patient wristbands, robotic filling, automatic dispensing cabinets (ADCs), and automated medication dispensing system (AMDS) software to enhance productivity and minimize errors to improve safety.
- A hospital prescription is called a medication order—it is written as an admitting, stat, daily, continuation, standing, or discharge order.
- A unit dose drug distribution system saves money and also reduces the chance of medication errors.
- A cart fill list is used by the technician to fill the unit dose cart or the emergency crash cart with 24- to 72-hour allotments (or longer) of patient medication.
- The pharmacy technician is often responsible for repackaging drugs into single-unit doses when they are not commercially available in unit dose packaging.
- Most hospitals today have extensive automated floor stock dispensing systems at the different nursing stations; these systems consist of frequently needed unit dose drugs as well as narcotics and IV solutions.

- The pharmacy technician assists in ordering, purchasing, and receiving the hospital medications—both formulary and nonformulary drugs.
- The ordering, receipt, and storage of narcotics and investigational drugs require specific procedures to be in compliance with federal laws and hospital policies.
- Pharmacy productivity can be measured in many different ways, including patient medication records reviewed, medication orders filled, and consultations done.
- Hospitals strive for Joint Commission accreditation to improve quality and safety and receive reimbursements from government and private insurance programs.

CHECK YOUR UNDERSTANDING

Take a moment to review what you have learned in this chapter and answer the following questions.

1. Patient confidentiality for participation in investigational drug studies is a function of the
   a. P&T Committee.
   b. Infection Control Committee.
   c. Institutional Review Board (IRB).
   d. Joint Commission.
2. Investigation of medication error reports is a function of the
   a. P&T Committee.
   b. Infection Control Committee.
   c. Institutional Review Board (IRB).
   d. Joint Commission.
3. Which of the following is not a key responsibility expected of the director of pharmacy?
   a. hiring, evaluating, and firing of personnel
   b. managing the pharmacy budget
   c. establishing the hospital's drug formulary
   d. assuring that the P&P Manual is appropriately updated
4. Which of the following is not a requirement to start working as an IV technician?
   a. criminal background check
   b. community pharmacy experience
   c. graduating from an ASHP-accredited training program
   d. passing the PTCB certification exam
5. Interoperability is the greatest advantage of a(n)
   a. electronic health record.
   b. drug inventory management system.
   c. robotic dispensing system.
   d. automated medication dispensing system.
6. Medication errors can be greatly reduced by use of all of the following technologies except
   a. robotic dispensing systems.
   b. computerized prescriber order entry.
   c. bar code scanning technology at the patient's bedside.
   d. computer-generated daily cart fill list.

MAKE CONNECTIONS

Take a moment to consider what you have learned in this chapter and respond thoughtfully to the following prompts. Note that some of these activities will require internet access.

1. Technology is heavily used in the hospital, especially in the pharmacy to minimize medication errors. Write a short essay in which you analyze the various ways technology can help reduce errors. Compare and contrast at least three advantages and disadvantages of a robotic dispensing system.
2. There are major differences in the role and responsibilities of pharmacy technicians working in a hospital versus community pharmacy. Write a short essay in which you compare and contrast these roles and responsibilities. Be sure to address the following:
    - participation in CPR codes
    - How do responsibilities differ?
    - How does the work environment differ?
    - How do type of drugs/route of administration differ?
    - How do qualifications differ?

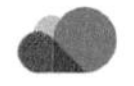 The online course includes additional review and assessment resources.

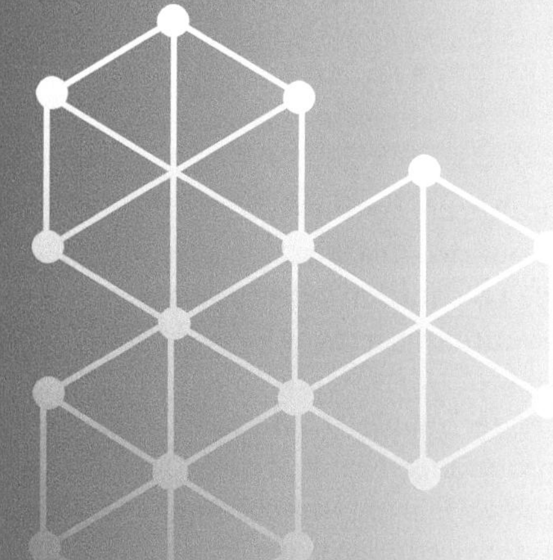

12 Infection Control, Aseptic Technique, and Cleanroom Facilities

Learning Objectives

1. Explain the role of pathogenic organisms in causing disease and distinguish between bacteria, viruses, fungi, and protozoa. (Section 12.1)
2. Discuss the dangers of antimicrobial resistance, superbugs, and healthcare-associated infections. (Section 12.1)
3. Identify common modes of contamination and the preventive measures. (Section 12.2)
4. Explain the role of CDC guidelines (including the universal precautions), the Infection Control Committee, and *USP* Chapter <797>. (Section 12.3)
5. Discuss the advantages and disadvantages of various forms of sterilization. (Section 12.4)
6. State the preparatory processes that must be completed prior to assembling compounded sterile preparations (CSPs). (Section 12.5)
7. Describe the different types of sterile products. (Section 12.5)
8. State the training requirements of becoming a sterile compounding technician. (Section 12.5)
9. Paraphrase the layout of a cleanroom and its ISO air environment standards, and the different levels of air quality controls, including primary and secondary engineering controls. (Section 12.6)
10. Describe methods of aseptic technique, including garbing and washing. (Section 12.7)
11. Describe basic cleanroom quality assurance and control procedures. (Section 12.7)
12. Identify the role and function of equipment used in sterile compounding, including syringes, needles, intravenous sets (and their components), and filters. (Section 12.8)

ASHP/ACPE Accreditation Standards
To view the *ASHP/ACPE Accreditation Standards* addressed in this chapter, refer to Appendix B.

For pharmacy technicians working in the hospital setting, a good understanding of infection control procedures is critical. Patients with severe diseases often have compromised immune systems and are more susceptible to serious, and sometimes life-threatening, infections. In addition, microorganisms have a greater ability to adapt and become resistant to potent antibiotics in a hospital setting. In light of these facts, it is important for you to understand how infection spreads and how hospitals can employ special infection control practices to limit the possibility of contamination. Any breach in protocol increases the risk for serious infections for patients and healthcare workers.

Many drugs ordered for patients in hospitals and other healthcare settings are administered directly into veins, so they must be specially compounded in a strictly controlled environment that is as germ-free as possible. Though a technician (and pharmacist) needs special training to work in one of these compounding areas, it is essential that every pharmacy technician understands an overview of *USP* Chapter <797> and the goals, key concepts, cleanroom layout, and aseptic technique, in addition to the intravenous (IV) supplies and equipment for sterile compounding. Many of the concepts and supplies also apply in sterile hazardous compounding. Having this context will prepare you to understand the overview of the processes and procedures of sterile and hazardous compounding addressed in the next chapter.

12.1 Types of Microorganisms

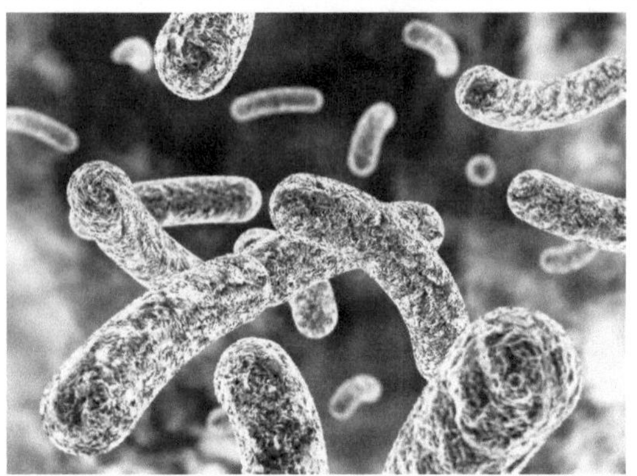

In 1873, using the first microscope (which he made himself), Anton van Leeuwenhoek first saw moving shapes like these bacteria, and understood that they were independent organisms living within humans.

As explained in an earlier chapter, 17th century European scientists discovered the existence of **microorganisms** that cause infection, launching the field of microbiology, or the study of microorganisms. Understanding how these microbes function is key to infection control because harmful microorganisms, especially bacteria, are everywhere. Microorganisms are mainly single-celled living organisms that are classified according by type—bacterium, virus, fungus, or protozoan—as well as by effect: pathogenic versus nonpathogenic.

Bacteria

A **bacterium** is a type of small, single-celled microorganism. Bacteria exist in three main forms as categorized by the shapes viewed under the microscope (see Figure 12.1): spherical (such as cocci), rod-shaped (such as bacilli), and spiral-shaped (such as spirochetes). Bacteria are responsible for causing a wide variety of illnesses, such as food poisoning, strep throat, ear infections, rheu- matic fever, meningitis, pneumonia, tuberculosis, and conjunctivitis. Normal human skin is colonized by several kinds of bacteria, some of which are potentially harmful, or **pathogenic**, and others that are beneficial or neutral, or **nonpathogenic**. Bacteria are easily passed off to others by touching, coughing, sneezing, brushing hair, kissing, and exchanging fluids.

FIGURE 12.1 Characteristic Bacterial Shapes

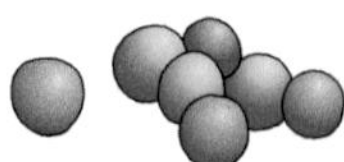

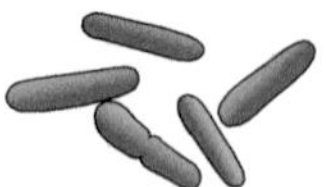

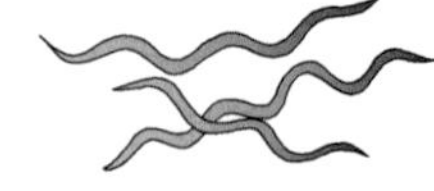

Viruses

A **virus** is a microorganism that consists of genetic material enclosed by a casing of protein. Viruses need a living host in which to reproduce, and after replicating, these organisms cause a wide variety of illnesses and diseases, including influenza (flu), colds, polio, mumps, measles, chicken pox, shingles, hepatitis, and human immunodeficiency virus (HIV). They are passed on in similar ways to bacteria and other parasites. For instance, the pandemic-causing Zika virus is transmitted mainly via the mosquito.

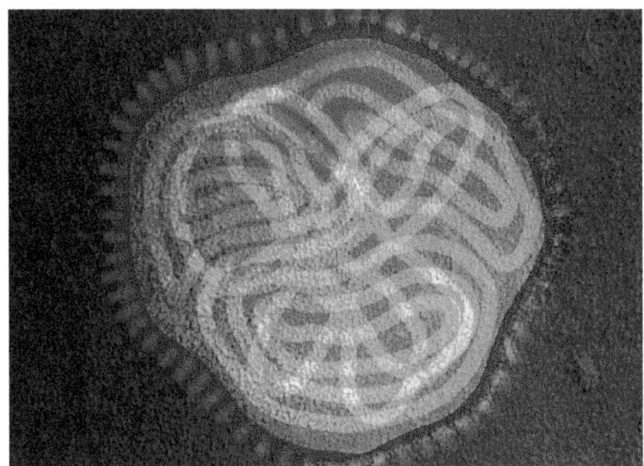

A virus is much smaller than a bacterium and can be viewed only with an electron microscope, as seen here. The virus does not have all of the components of a cell and requires a living host to replicate itself.

Fungi

A **fungus** lives on organisms by feeding on living or dead organic material. Fungi reproduce slowly by means of spores. Spores are microscopic reproductive bodies that travel through the air and can develop into molds, mildews, mushrooms, or yeasts. Some molds are the source of antibiotics, such as penicillin. Other fungi cause skin conditions such as athlete's foot and ringworm or vaginal yeast infections. In more serious cases, systemic fungal infections can form in the lungs and other areas deep within the body, which can be potentially life-threatening. The air and surfaces of objects have fungus living on them, emitting fungal spores into the air for dispersal.

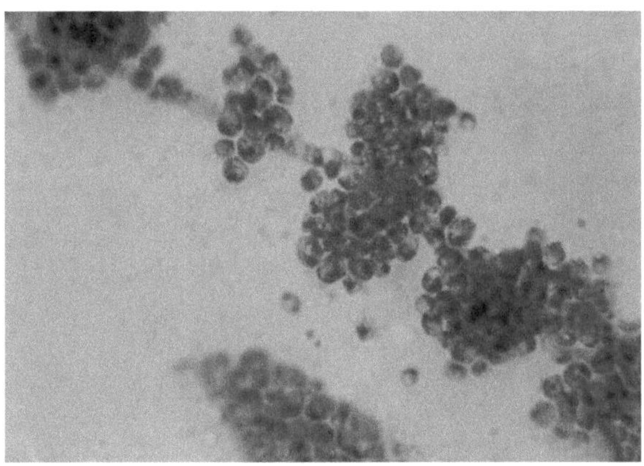

This photomicrograph of the fungus *Candida albicans* indicates its multicellular structure.

Protozoa

A **protozoan** is a microscopic organism made up of a single cell or a group of identical single cells. Protozoa live in water or as parasites inside other creatures. Examples of protozoa include paramecia and amoebas. Amoebic dysentery, malaria, and sleeping sickness are examples of illnesses caused by protozoa.

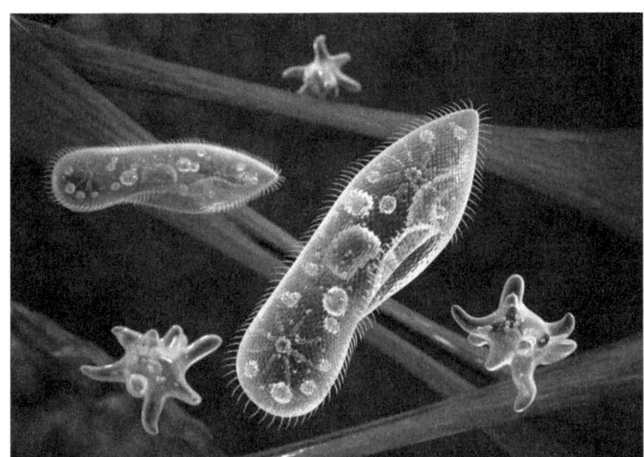

Paramecia and amoebae are protozoa commonly found in freshwater lakes.

Effects of Microorganisms

As mentioned earlier, microorganisms can be either nonpathogenic (harmless or beneficial) or pathogenic (harmful).

Nonpathogenic Microorganisms

The majority of microorganisms are nonpathogenic, meaning they are not dangerous, and besides not being harmful, many actually perform essential functions, such as keeping pathogenic populations down or helping the body break down various food substances. Outside the body, they can create by-products that are used to formulate medicines, ferment wine, fix nitrogen in the soil, and other important functions. For example, yogurt consists of "good" bacteria that can reestablish the positive bacteria typically found in the gastrointestinal (GI) tract after a course of antibiotics that kills them. The beneficial bacteria can also reduce the incidence of diarrhea and yeast infections from antibiotics.

Pathogenic Microorganisms

Pathogenic microorganisms, as noted, have led to widespread illness and disease throughout the world. Some of these microorganisms have been the catalysts of **epidemics** (regional contagious disease outbreaks) and **pandemics** (worldwide contagious disease outbreaks, such as the Spanish flu in 1918). Public health diseases and ongoing epidemics kill thousands of people annually in different locations in the world by different local organisms (such as Ebola, tuberculosis, swine flu, bubonic plague, yellow fever, malaria, cholera, and others).

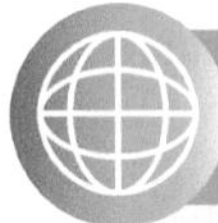

IN THE REAL WORLD

Throughout history, many pandemics have killed millions of people. The HIV/AIDS pandemic is well known and feared, especially now in countries in sub-Saharan Africa, such as South Africa, where 13.1% of people live with the disease (according to a 2018 South African report). Some other notable pandemics include:

- **Zika**–a virus that is passed by certain mosquito species. It has been active in Africa and Asia from the 1940s on, but since 2007 it has been rapidly spreading in South, Central, and North America and the Caribbean, causing neurological damage in those infected and a high risk of birth defects in the children of women infected while pregnant.
- **Ebola**–a virus that causes victims to essentially bleed to death internally. The latest major outbreak of the virus ravaged West Africa and killed over 8,000 people.
- **Spanish flu**–or influenza, a disease caused by the H1N1 virus. This 1918 pandemic was spread around the world after World War I and killed approximately 50 million people worldwide, including an estimated 675,000 people in the United States. It has been called the worst pandemic in human history.
- **Cholera**–an illness caused by bacteria that is spread through contaminated food or water. There have been seven pandemics of cholera since the 19th century, killing millions of individuals on five continents.
- **Polio**–a pandemic in the first half of the 20th century. It has killed or crippled millions, and continues to do so at a slower rate.
- **Bubonic plague**–a disease caused by bacteria and spread by the fleas of diseased black rats. This pandemic killed 25 million people throughout Europe and Asia during the 14th century.
- **Smallpox**–caused by strains of a virus. It was a virulent killer for centuries, responsible for the deaths of more than 300 million people in the 20th century alone.

Though these organisms (other than smallpox) continue to wreak havoc in many people's lives in various places in the world, the presence of vaccinations and/or other public health efforts have prevented them from causing the regional and worldwide harm they once did. Scientists are working to contain and prevent the spread and damage of the Zika virus. However, as microorganisms build up resistance to antimicrobials, there is fear of their resurgence to create epidemics and pandemics again.

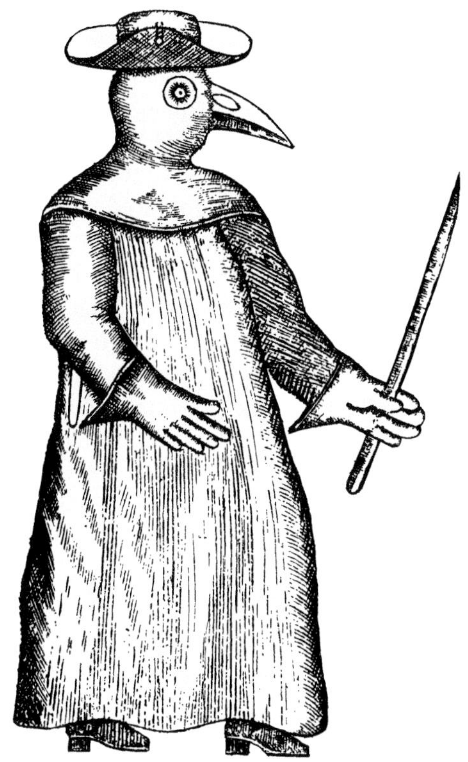

During the bubonic plague of the 14th century, doctors worked in full-body garb to protect themselves from the disease. This was an early hazmat suit, so to speak. The beak of the mask held pungent herbs to purify the "bad air," and included a full-length heavy robe covered in wax, leather breeches, and leather gloves and boots.

Antimicrobial Resistance

Many antimicrobial medications—the antibiotics, antivirals, and antifungals—are effective in killing or neutralizing pathogenic microorganisms in humans. However, microorganisms adapt rapidly and can become resistant to both some sterility techniques and medications. A medication can kill the majority of a **colony**, or community of microorganisms, so that the disease symptoms decline or go away. However, a remnant of the microorganism colony may remain that was either immune or only weakened by the medication. These remaining microorganisms can reproduce a new strain that is resistant to the medication.

This growth in microbial resistance is even more likely to occur when patients do not complete their prescribed therapy regimens of antibiotics and antivirals, stopping when disease symptoms go away. Also, the overprescribing of antibiotics by providers for unnecessary reasons (like prescribing an antibiotic for a viral illness) or incorrect administration by patients can result in ever more virulent microorganisms. In particular, noncompliance with HIV therapy is leading to rapid viral resistance.

Microbial Resistance and Superbugs

Antibiotic-resistant bacteria have led to the rise of **superbugs**, microorganisms that are immune or highly resistant to conventional antibiotic therapies. These superbugs are a growing worldwide healthcare concern both inside and outside of the hospital. One in five urinary tract infections, is resistant to most sulfa drugs. Antibiotic- resistant strains of tuberculosis kill 65,000 people each year worldwide. Many strains of salmonella, a common cause of food poisoning, are resistant. Many sexually transmitted infections, such as gonorrhea, are increasingly difficult to treat because of their resistance. Hospitals, which are centers for both disease and health, are places where the most virulent diseases can meet the most vulnerable individuals if strict infection control techniques are not applied.

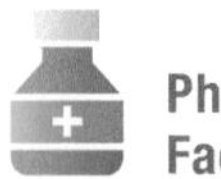

Pharm Fact

There is a MRSA that is acquired in healthcare facilities and one that is acquired in the community. The HAI form of MRSA tends to be more virulent and deadly.

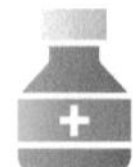

Pharm Fact

The deaths of Muhammed Ali and Patty Duke (Astin) from sepsis in 2016 made people more aware of the behind-the-scenes health issue it can cause.

Healthcare-associated infections (HAIs) are infections that patients contract while receiving care at a medical facility. They are an ongoing threat in all hospitals, requiring intense attention. HAIs result in extended, higher drug doses and multiple drug therapies, costly hospitalizations, and sometimes death. Common organisms causing HAIs include the **methicillin-resistant Staphylococcus aureus (MRSA)** bacteria that can cause serious bloodstream infections. MRSA is often passed by contaminated hands. *Clostridium difficile (C. difficile)* is a resistant bacterium that can cause potentially serious diarrhea in patients on certain antibiotic therapies; the antibiotics have killed the good bacteria in their digestive systems that generally keep *C. difficile* populations too low to cause harm. Particularly susceptible to these HAIs are patients who have compromised immune systems or open wounds, scratches, or devices that need frequent cleaning and changing, such as urinary catheters, ventilators, or intravenous catheters.

HAIs, and any infection, can trigger **sepsis**, often referred to as "blood poisoning." Sepsis arises when an infection is so threatening to the body that the immune system goes into overdrive. It begins to attack the body's own blood vessels and organs, causing inflammation, leaky vessels, organ failure, and septic shock. Infections such as pneumonia, urinary tract infections from catheters, meningitis, a burst appendix, or even an untreated cut that becomes radically infected can lead to sepsis. According to the CDC, sepsis is more common than a heart attack and claims more lives than cancer, killing more than 258,000 US citizens each year. Yet swift recognition and finding the right antibiotic therapy and offering organ support can save lives.

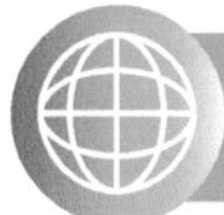

IN THE REAL WORLD

According to the CDC, one out of every 25 patients hospitalized develops 5% of the cases. The CDC estimates that 2.25 million patients per year acquire a new infection while being hospitalized, which adds an additional cost of over $10 billion per year; 37,000 deaths per year are due to HAIs.

In 2015, at Ronald Reagan UCLA Medical Center, more than 100 patients were exposed to the carbapenem-resistant Enterobacteriaceae (CRE) during specialized endoscopy procedures. CRE has become known as the "nightmare" bacteria because of its resistance to antibiotics. At least seven people were infected, and two died. UCLA is just one of many hospitals to have an outbreak of an HAI. In fact, a hospital in Kentucky had an outbreak of CRE that involved 23 patients between 2016 and 2017. These cases further highlight the challenges hospitals face with the growing risk of drug-resistant superbugs. Adherence to recommended infection control guidelines significantly decreases the transmission of infectious agents.

12.2 Sources of Contamination

Microbes cannot cause an infectious disease unless they are transmitted to humans and enter their bodies. This can occur through inhaling, ingesting, touching mucosal linings, contact with piercings or open sores, or injection. Unfortunately, these transmission processes are easily accomplished without knowing it through various avenues, including touch, air, and water. One must be keenly aware of the modes of microorganism transmission in order to understand how to control infection and to avoid contamination during hospital work and the preparation of compounded sterile drug products.

Touch

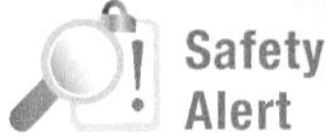

Nonsterile touch is the most common and dangerous source of contamination, especially when performing sterile compounding— even when wearing gloves.

Besides living on our skin, millions of bacteria live in our hair and under our nails. Therefore, properly washing hands and fingernails is essential in all hospital work. Following the strict recommended procedures before handling and preparing sterile materials is also essential. Touching is the most common method of contamination and the easiest to prevent. In addition to frequent handwashing, the use of disposable gloves can minimize touch contamination, which is why they are commonly used by healthcare personnel.

Air

Microorganisms inhabit the air by floating, resting on dust particles, and inhabiting moisture droplets. For this reason, sterile compounded products need to be prepared in a designated area where these possible contaminants are minimized to as low a level as possible. Special equipment within these areas controls airflow and filter contamination, as will be discussed later in this chapter.

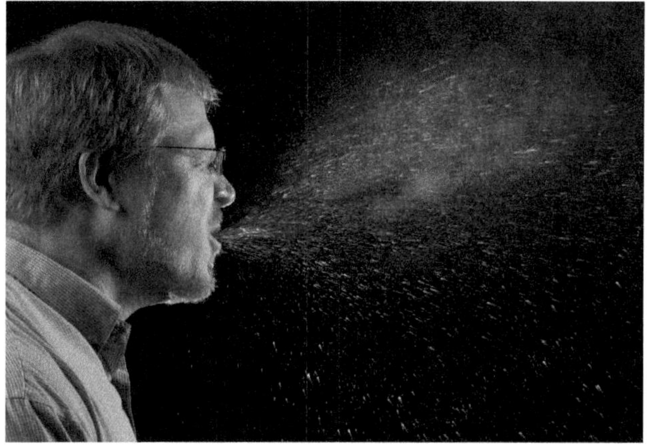

Sneezing causes air contamination up to seven feet by emitting thousands of microorganisms in tiny water particles.

Water

Moisture droplets in the air, especially after a sneeze or cough, often contain harmful microbes. Even tap water is not completely free of microorganisms. Exposure to droplets of tap water or other sources of moisture can contaminate sterile compounds, which is why distilled, sterile water is used in various pharmacy cleaning and compounding procedures. Any pharmacy technician assigned to prepare sterile products who has a common cold should notify his or her pharmacist supervisor for a temporary change in work functions. Sterile compounding personnel use special techniques and garb to reduce or eliminate potential moisture contamination.

12.3 Hospital Infection Prevention

Infection control is the responsibility of all healthcare workers. It involves two aspects—stopping transmission of disease agents (prevention) and killing germs that exist on instruments and surfaces and in facilities (destruction). Healthcare facilities must continually do both.

Patients and employees are only safe from infectious processes when everyone working in the hospital follows good infection control techniques. Guidelines and recommendations to prevent infections are developed at the national, state, and facility level.

The Centers for Disease Control and Prevention

At the national level, the **Centers for Disease Control and Prevention (CDC)** set guidelines for hospitals and healthcare workers. State departments of health also set policies and procedures to prevent and address state public health issues and disease outbreaks. The CDC recommends that healthcare workers receive an annual flu shot (usually free of charge), and the CDC developed the **universal precautions for preventing transmission of blood-borne infections** for all healthcare workers who have any potential contact with any blood or bodily fluids (mucous, urine, semen, lymphatic fluid, excrement, and sebum). These precautions work to protect healthcare workers and patients from HIV, tuberculosis, hepatitis B and C, MRSA, and many other HAIs.

Generally, technicians in hospital pharmacies or sterile compounding facilities do not have potential contact with blood or other bodily fluids, but they need to be cautious to cover any open wound and follow the universal precautions and infection-control procedures of the department. Pharmacists who provide direct patient care and administer vaccines at healthcare fairs do encounter situations where they have potential contact; in these situations, they apply the prevention and disposal precautions shown in Table 12.1.

TABLE 12.1 Universal Precautions for Prevention of Blood-Borne Infection Transmission

- Universal precautions apply to all individuals within the hospital.
- Universal precautions apply to all contact or potential contact with blood, other bodily fluids, or body substances.
- Disposable gloves must be worn when contact with blood or other bodily fluids is anticipated or possible.
- Hands must be washed thoroughly after removing gloves.
- Blood-soaked or contaminated materials (such as gloves, towels, or bandages) must be disposed of in a wastebasket lined with a plastic bag.
- Properly trained custodial personnel must be called if cleanup or removal of contaminated waste is necessary.
- Contaminated materials (such as needles, syringes, swabs, and catheters) must be placed in red plastic containers labeled for disposal of biohazardous materials. Proper institutional procedures generally involve incineration.
- A first-aid kit must be kept on hand in any area in which contact with blood or other bodily fluids is possible. The kit should contain, at minimum, the following items:

continues

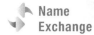

Name Exchange

Another term for healthcare-associated infections (or healthcare acquired infections) is nosocomial. The Greek term nosokomos refers to someone who tends the sick, so a nosocomial infection comes from someone working to heal those who are ill.

TABLE 12.1 Universal Precautions for Prevention of Blood-Borne Infection Transmission—*Continued*

- adhesive bandages for covering small wounds
- alcohol
- antiseptic or disinfectant
- bottle of bleach, which is diluted at the time of use to create a solution containing 1 part bleach to 10 parts water, for use in cleaning up blood spills
- box of disposable gloves
- disposable towels
- medical adhesive tape
- plastic bag or container for contaminated waste disposal
- sterile gauze for covering large wounds

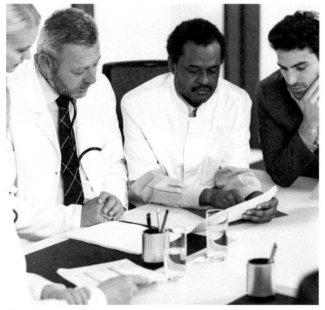

The Infection Control Committee (ICC) develops procedures with the hospital to prevent or address HAI outbreaks as well as other infection-fighting issues.

The Infection Control Committee

Each hospital's Infection Control Committee is responsible for following CDC guidelines by developing hospital-specific policies and procedures. The **Infection Control Committee (ICC)** is generally composed of physicians, nursing staff, infection control practitioners, quality assurance personnel, and risk management personnel, as well as representatives from microbiology, surgery, central sterilization, and environmental services. A pharmacist with an interest and expertise in antibiotics is also a member of the team. The goal of this interdisciplinary team is to bring together individuals with expertise in different areas of health care to oversee the infection control procedures and training of all healthcare workers, track hospital infection rates, monitor trends in antimicrobial medication use, and address any specific threats and ongoing problems.

The CDC recommends that the hospital's ICC documents the incidence of HAIs and the use of antibiotics, and periodically checks to assess the adherence of staff members to hand-hygiene guidelines. The committee is also responsible for educating hospital personnel on the importance of receiving all necessary vaccines. Lastly, the committee plays a major role in ensuring that the hospital maintains compliance with the Joint Commission accreditation standards regarding all infection control procedures.

Tracking and Addressing Healthcare-Associated Infections

To reduce the possibilities of occurrences of HAIs, also known as "nosocomial infections," the ICC works to identify and fix any gaps or problems in procedures or training. When outbreaks occur, the committee is responsible for investigating to determine the infective source(s). They then recommend implementation of changes in protocols and new education measures and materials to correct the deficiency. For instance, the committee may evaluate whether new sanitizing chemicals or sterilization processes should be used in the surgical operating rooms. If resistance of particular microorganisms to a specific antibiotic is increasing, then the committee may review whether the antibiotic is being ordered or administered inappropriately. The hospital ICC might also recommend that all employees are properly vaccinated and that certain healthcare workers receive TB skin tests to ensure that they have not contracted the disease or are not carriers.

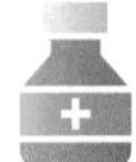

Pharm Fact

Severe adverse effects from vaccines are rare (less than 1 in 100,000 administrations, according to the CDC).

Implementing Healthcare Worker Vaccinations

The most common vaccines recommended in the hospital are the annual flu vaccine and for specific personnel, a series of vaccines against hepatitis B given over a six-month period. The hepatitis B virus is transmitted by exposure to blood and body fluids; it can cause acute and chronic infections of the liver.

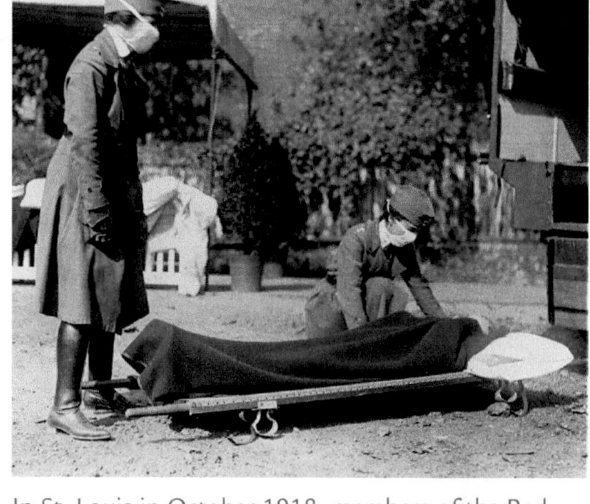

In St. Louis in October 1918, members of the Red Cross Motor Corps, all wearing masks against the further spread of the Spanish influenza epidemic, carry a patient on a stretcher into their ambulance. Spurred to prevent a recurrence of the devastation of the 1918 flu pandemic, scientists work on annual flu vaccines.

The best time to get a flu vaccination is in September or October each year in North America because the immune system can take a few weeks to respond fully to the vaccine before the usual winter flu season starts. The benefits to the healthcare workers are that the flu shot usually keeps those individuals, their family members, and hospitalized patients safe from the flu strain that it was formulated to address, reducing the number of sick days.

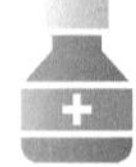

Pharm Fact

In most years, when the most circulating seasonal influenza viruses are similar to the one in the vaccine, the flu vaccine is 60% to 70% effective. It is not 100% effective because the most current injectable flu vaccine is developed based on last year's virus (it takes a year for development).

Many individuals, especially those who are young and healthy, feel as though a flu shot is unnecessary; yet research has shown that the flu virus can be carried by asymptomatic healthy individuals and passed on to hospital patients with whom they have contact. Since many of these patients, especially older adults and young infants, have compromised or weakened immune systems, exposure to the flu virus can be deadly.

There are a few restrictions for obtaining a flu vaccine. Personnel with minor illnesses, such as a cold, can be vaccinated, but those who have an acute feverish illness need to wait at least 24 hours after the fever has subsided before getting the vaccine. Women who are pregnant can be vaccinated, but individuals who are hypersensitive to eggs should not receive the flu vaccine as the virus is incubated in eggs.

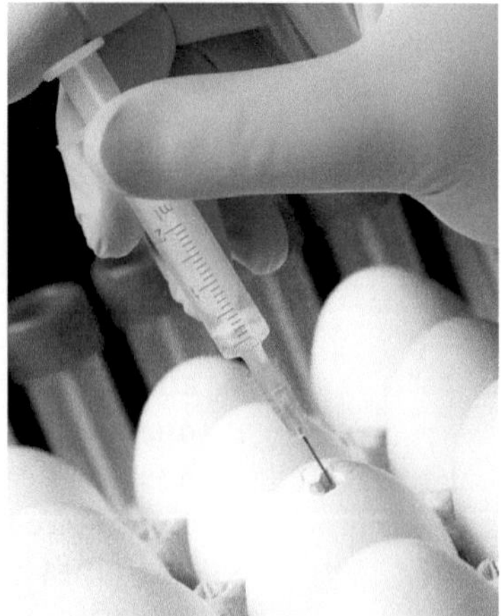

Vaccine developers use chicken embryos. These embryos incubate a form of the virus that is processed into a vaccine. Because of the egg connection, those with egg allergies need to receive a different flu vaccination formulation.

Safety Alert

All pharmacy personnel should receive an annual flu vaccine to protect both themselves and their patients and families from contracting this virus.

IN THE REAL WORLD

The flu virus mutates or changes every year, and scientists never know how virulent or contagious it will be. Occasionally, a virulent pathogenic influenza virus appears like the 1918 flu. The 1918 Spanish flu pandemic killed far more people than World War I—675,000 US citizens and servicemen died, which was 10 times the number of US soldiers killed in the war. In case of any epidemic or pandemic flu outbreak, all healthcare workers need to be fully vaccinated to protect themselves and care for the sick.

Despite these compelling reasons, 2018 CDC studies showed that only 78% of all healthcare workers received an annual flu shot, leaving approximately one out of four healthcare workers (and their patients) vulnerable. In October 2018, the CDC reported that only 37.1% of people age 18 and older in the United States received a flu vaccine, leaving most persons without the protection afforded by flu vaccination.

Contrary to popular myth, individuals cannot get the flu from most vaccines because these inoculations generally contain an inactivated (killed) virus. There is, however, a live **attenuated virus** (a weakened form) present in the nasal flu vaccine marketed as FluMist. This product is indicated for healthy children and adults from ages 2 to 49 who do not want a shot. Pharmacy personnel should be aware that some studies report that the use of the intranasal antiviral drugs may not be as protective as the injectable vaccine. In fact, the CDC recommended against the use of FluMist vaccine for the 2016–2017 flu season. However, FluMist was included in the recommended vaccine list for the 2018–2019 season.

The Advisory Committee on Immunization Practices (ACIP) has expressed concern over the use of the live, attenuated nasal flu vaccine for healthcare workers who care for patients in protective environments, such as intensive care or cancer care units. However, no documented transmission of this vaccine to patients has been reported. Most healthcare facilities allow healthy personnel up to age 49 who work in any setting to use the nasal flu vaccine, except those who care for severely immunocompromised patients.

12.4 Sterilization to Eliminate Microorganisms

All areas of the hospital or healthcare facility, including the general pharmacy, are responsible for cleanliness and infection-control procedures. The hospital aims for clean and sterile tools and sterile or aseptic surfaces, equipment, and intravenous fluids and medications. **Sterile** is the absence of *any* microorganisms while **asepsis** is the absence of any destructive or harmful pathogens.

Aseptic technique is the set of special procedures used to ensure that harmful germs are not passed on or introduced onto surfaces and equipment, into the air, or into the compounded drug preparations. A person can never be "sterile" or completely free of germs. In everyday life, we wash our hands before we eat and after using the bathroom, cover our mouths and noses when we cough or sneeze, and avoid eating from each other's plates or drinking from others' cups when anyone is sick. These are all examples of simple everyday acts of infection control. We clean wounds with disinfectants and antibiotics before putting on bandages. These acts are a mix of preventive, aseptic, and sterile practices.

In the hospital, these methods become stricter and part of everyday routine. For example, rigid aseptic procedures are followed in the surgical, special care, and sterile compounding areas, and hospital instruments are either disposable or sterilized. **Sterilization** is the process that destroys all microorganisms or eliminates the conditions they need to live on surfaces, in liquids, and in the air. When an object (such as a medical instrument) is sterilized, the microbial life forms present are destroyed.

Many types of sterilization exist—dry and moist heat, distillation, mechanical, chemical, and ultraviolet—and a mix of all of these techniques is used in large hospitals. In some large university hospitals, the hospital pharmacy runs the central supply department that provides sterile supplies and sterilizes the surgical instruments. Consequently, pharmacy technicians particularly have to be familiar with sterilization methods and their clinical applications.

Heat Sterilization

Using heat to kill microorganisms is a an effective, economical, and easily controlled method of sterilization. It comes in two forms: dry heat and moist heat sterilization.

Dry Heat Sterilization

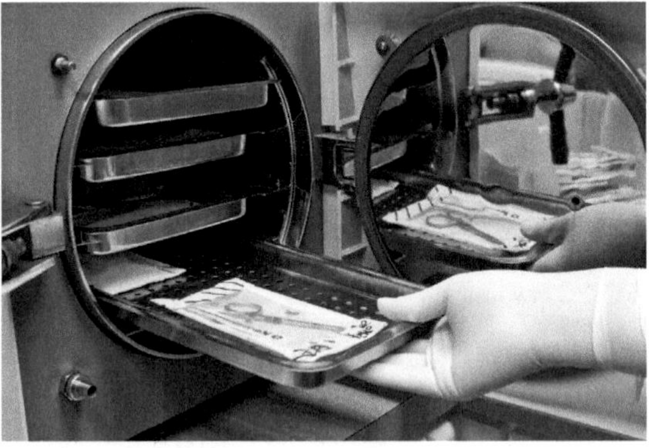

An autoclave generates heat and pressure to sterilize. Most known organisms are killed in about 15 minutes.

A traditional method of sterilization by dry heat is baking, which destroys microorganisms at intense temperatures. The higher the temperature, the shorter the time. Dry heat radiates off an object or organism first before penetrating, so higher temperatures and longer times are necessary for dry heat sterilization than for moist heat sterilization (to be explained next). For sterilization, a dry temperature of at least 170°C (338°F) must be maintained for a sufficient time, such as nearly two hours. For instance, hospitals bake blankets this way to sterilize them. Obviously, higher temperatures can also destroy the integrity of the tool, substance, or vehicle holding the microorganisms if it burns, boils, or melts. Therefore, one has to choose the right temperature and process. Facilities often use flame incineration for the disposal of contaminated objects.

Moist Heat Sterilization

Another traditional method for killing microbes is the moist heat sterilization method of boiling or steaming. Boiling kills many parasites, bacteria, viruses, and fungi in about 10 minutes, but more time is required to kill other microorganisms, such as bacterial and fungal spores and hepatitis viruses. If a water supply is of questionable quality, it should be boiled for a half hour before drinking. Automatic dishwashers loosely borrow concepts of both moist and dry heat sterilization during their hot water and drying cycles.

To sterilize instruments, the hospital and compounding facility use an **auto-clave**, a device that generates steam heat and pressure simultaneously (as mentioned in Chapter 10). When moist heat of 121°C (270°F) under pressure of 15 psi (pounds per square inch) is applied to instruments, solutions, or powders, most known organisms—including spores and viruses—are killed in about 15 minutes. At home, pressure cookers use the concept of heat and pressure to cook (and sterilize) vegetables. Moist heat is usually able to permeate into the microorganisms' cells. However, hospitals are using moist and dry heat sterilization less frequently due to space requirements, equipment expense, and personnel training issues.

Distillation—Heat with Condensation

When a liquid like water is boiled to kill microorganisms, chemical contaminants like mercury, lead, or arsenic remain. However, if the water is boiled and the steam gas vapor is sent through tubes to condense into distilled water, the chemical contaminants are removed. That is why distilled water, which is water in its purest liquid form, is the water that is boiled once more (for a sufficient time to kill any microbes that traveled with the vapor) to be used in sterile compounding. **Distillation** is an important decontamination process for liquids that can be boiled without changing their desired qualities.

Mechanical Sterilization—Filtration

For liquids and gases that would be radically changed by distillation or heat sterilization, one can use the mechanical sterilization method of **filtration**, which is the funneling of a liquid or gas through a screen-like material with pores small enough to block microorganisms. This method is used for heat-sensitive materials such as a culture medium (needed for growing colonies of bacteria or other microorganisms), enzymes, vaccines, and antibiotic solutions. Filtration can also be used to sterilize drinking water.

Filter pore sizes must be 0.22 **micrometer** (or **micron**) for bacteria and 0.01 micrometer for viruses and some large proteins. (A micrometer is 0.001 mm, or a millionth of a meter—for perspective, there are 25,400 micrometers to an inch.) Pharmaceutical manufacturing plants use both of these filters; hospitals and infusion facilities for home health care commonly use the 0.22 micron filters. Inserting a micrometer in-line filter in the lines of IV administration sets has been shown to reduce the incidence of infusion-related inflammation of the veins, as will be explained later in the chapter.

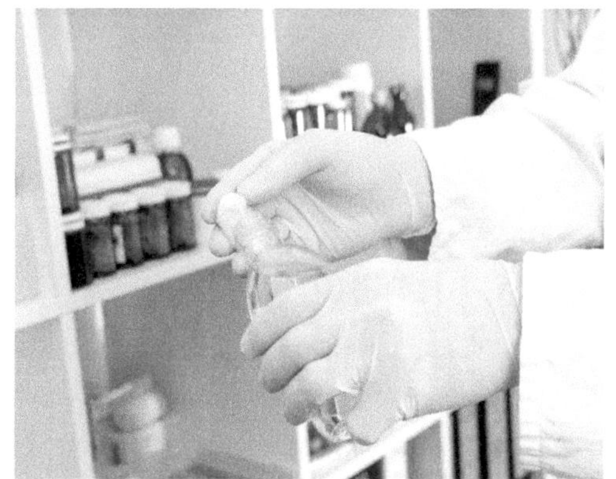
In hospitals, many different disinfecting agents are selected for use, depending on whether they are used to clean tools, injuries, or hands. Chlorhexidine gluconate is an antiseptic germicidal agent used for aseptic handwashing in sterile compounding.

Chemical Sterilization

On surfaces that cannot be heated, hospitals use chemical sterilization with chemical gases, sprays, liquids, or wipes. As explained in Chapter 3, the English surgeon Joseph Lister first applied this technique during surgeries in the 19th century using a mild carbolic acid solution to prevent infection. Some forms of chemical disinfecting are still used to prevent pre- and postoperative infections. Few chemicals produce complete sterility, but many reduce microbial numbers to safe levels. Any chemical applied to an object (or the body) for sterilization purposes is known as a **disinfectant**. Iodine, isopropyl alcohol (IPA), and chlorinated bleach are common topical or surface disinfectants. The disinfecting solution of choice to clean equipment in surgical and sterile compounding areas is sterile 70% IPA solution.

Gas Chemical Sterilization

Gas sterilization uses chemicals in their gaseous, or vapor forms, for disinfecting. Gas sterilization requires special equipment and aeration after application. Sealed equipment can automatically spray the gas ethylene oxide to sterilize objects that are too difficult or large to wipe down or that could be destroyed by heat. Ethylene oxide is highly flammable and is used only in large institutions and manufacturing facilities that have adequate equipment and ventilation to handle the gas. Many prepackaged IV fluids, IV administration sets, and bandages are manufactured in facilities that apply this type of sterilization. Ethylene oxide leaves a slight, harmless residue that can be detected as an odor.

Ultraviolet Sterilization

Light is also used for sterilization. Light rays come in different lengths, intensities of energy, and colored hues, all of which are on a spectrum and some of which our eyes are not able to detect and distinguish. The smaller the wavelength of rays, the more radiation of energy there is. Ultraviolet light is on the shorter spectrum, and it is more dangerous because of this. That is why we wear sunscreen to protect our skin from the sun's ultraviolet rays, which are damaging to skin cells.

Ultraviolet (UV) radiation is the focused energy of these UV rays. UV radiation is damaging to living organisms, causing deterioration of cellular processes. That is why people for centuries have hung out their laundry and diapers in the sun to disinfect them. UV radiation can be used to sterilize air, gases, and surfaces. However, UV radiation does not permeate deeply, so only those elements directly touched by the UV rays are actually sterilized. Also, UV radiation is harmful to human eyes and skin, which is why you must avoid direct contact with the UV sterilization processes. That is why UV lights are turned on to sterilize rooms in evenings or off hours when personnel are not present.

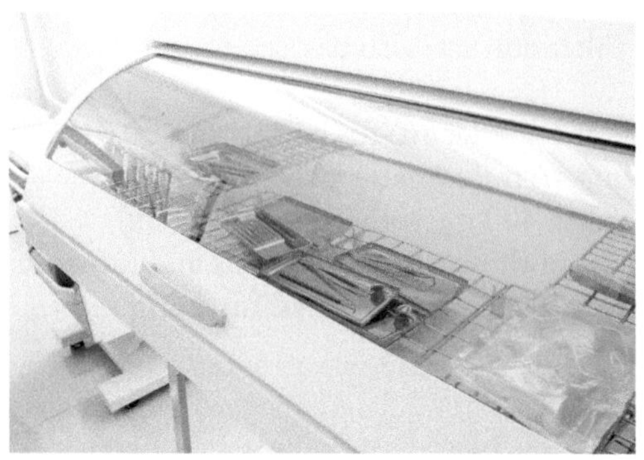

Sterilization boxes are used to sterilize surgical instruments.

12.5 The Need for Sterile Compounding of Drug Products

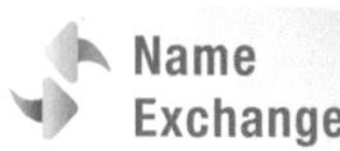

IV solutions are also known as IV "infusions" and "admixtures."

Many drug products also need to be sterile. Since many medications are for parenteral administration–administered into a vein, muscle, organ, skin, or under the skin–the bacteria or other contaminants in a nonsterile compound could enter into the the patient's body and cause a serious infection, leading to illness and possibly death. Patients often depend for survival upon swift administration of individualized sterile drug products, called **compounded sterile preparations (CSPs)**. A CSP is a medication compounded in a sterile cleanroom environment with sterile instruments and equipment using aseptic technique. These include the following kinds of CSPs:

- **Large-volume parenteral (LVP) preparations**—IV solutions of more than 250 mL that may contain medications, nutrients, or electrolytes
- **Small-volume parenteral (SVP) preparations**—IV solutions of generally 25 to 250 mL, typically administered as an IV piggyback (infusing into the LVP)
- **Parenteral nutrition (PN)**—specialized LVP solutions that provide nutrition and nutrient requirements to patients who require a long-term alternative to oral and digestive feeding (both supplemental and total parenteral nutrition)
- **Syringe injections**—smaller volume sterile solutions administered via a syringe; IV push, intramuscular (IM), subcutaneous (subq), intradermal (ID), and **intrathecal** (into protective membrane around the spinal cord)
- **Noninjected CSPs**—miscellaneous sterile solutions that include ophthalmic drops and ointments, aqueous nasal and bronchial inhalations, baths and soaks for live organs, irrigations for wounds and body cavities, tissue implants, and medical imaging diagnostics dyes and tracers
- **Sterile hazardous drugs (HD)**—toxic drugs that are injected into the body, including biological agents; many HDs are chemotherapy medications aimed at killing cancerous cells and destructive tumors
- **Sterile nuclear drug products**—radioactive compounded drugs (such as irradiated iodine) that diagnose and treat various diseases, primarily administered by the IV route

USP Chapter <797> Sterile Compounding Standards

To ensure the safest CSPs, the *USP* publishes a set of sterile compounding standards in ***USP* Chapter <797>** on the preparation of sterile products in the most suitable environment using properly trained personnel and personal protective equipment (PPE), or the proper garb and gear. It outlines how CSPs must be compounded using proper aseptic technique in specially designed and designated rooms that utilize specially filtered air and have specially designed workbenches within which the CSPs are prepared. CSPs are classified into Categories 1 and 2, each with different guidelines for determining their beyond-use date (BUD). The BUD is the date *and* time after which the CSP may not be used. It is determined by many factors, including the date and time it was compounded, the nature of the product, and the environment in which it was compounded.

USP <797> is frequently revised to reflect new science and information as it becomes available. Once the revised chapter is made available, it is important for all sterile compounding personnel to read it, ask questions as necessary to gain understanding, and then follow all of the standards set forth in the chapter. Until the revised *USP* <797> is confirmed, it is important to read and follow the guidelines presently in place. To read the standards, go to https://PharmPractice7e.ParadigmEducation.com/SterilePrep.

Based on the current *USP* <797> standards, all sterile compounding facilities are required to establish written **standard operating procedures (SOPs)** that integrate the guidelines in *USP* <797> to bring consistency of sterility, accuracy, and quality. The SOPs work to ensure that the entire sterile compounding operation is well designed, functions properly, and yields CSPs that are safe for administration to patients. The SOPs are contained in the pharmacy department's policy and procedure manual.

Practice Tip

Pharmacy technicians who prepare sterile products are referred to as sterile compounding technicians, IV technicians, or IV admixture technicians.

All sterile compounding technicians should be so well trained in these SOPs that they can immediately recognize and report any potential problems, deviations, or errors associated with preparing a CSP (related to equipment, facilities, materials, personnel, compounding process, or testing) that might result in contamination or negatively affect the quality of the CSP.

Sterile Compounding Personnel Credentials and Training

To work in a growing number of sterile compounding facilities and hospitals, you must be a nationally certified pharmacy technician and also obtain additional training for sterile compounding. Most sterile compounding personnel are either required to, or elect to, complete an accredited course in sterile compounding and aseptic technique. Education and training facilities that provide this type of education are generally accredited by the Accreditation Council on Pharmacy Education (ACPE). Training for sterile compounding personnel should include didactic components, such as reading, viewing training videos, classroom instruction, and home-study assignments. It should also include an experiential, hands-on component conducted in the laboratory or simulation environment. Upon completion of your didactic and experiential training, you will undergo written examination and skills process validation procedures. *USP* <797> sets out the standards for training sterile compounding personnel. The requirements of *USP* <797> are far more stringent than for nonsterile compounding *USP* <795> (discussed in Chapter 10).

The *USP* <797> standards apply to all sterile compounding settings, including hospital compounding pharmacies and nuclear, home health, or infusion pharmacies. When a pharmacy outsources, or sends out, its prescription or medication orders for the preparation of CSPs, the pharmacy must be assured that the outsource facility is meeting all *USP* <797> requirements to ensure safe, sterile products for administration to their patients.

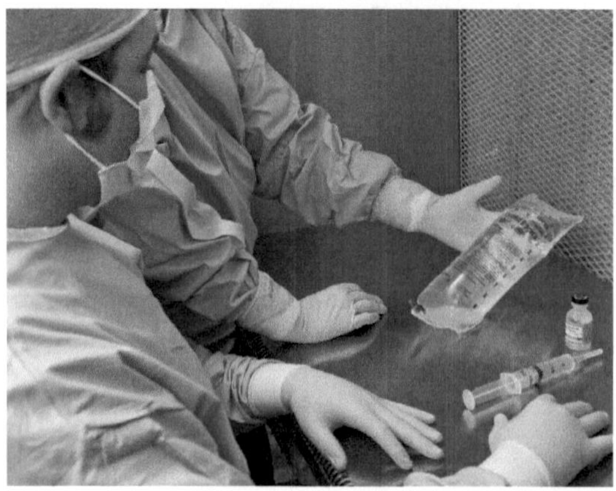

Technicians preparing IVs, injections, and other CSPs must be carefully trained to follow aseptic technique.

Besides classes and lab training, it is important for aspiring IV technicians to read, understand, and regularly refer to the most recent *USP* <797> requirements. The competencies that sterile compounding technicians must exhibit are specified in the current version of *USP* <797>. Sterile compounding personnel must pass written tests and skills assessments at least annually, in addition to completing gloved fingertip sampling and media fill testing twice a year, to provide the evidence needed to meet *USP* guidelines and Joint Commission accreditation standards.

In addition to knowing well all of the *USP* <797> guidelines, sterile compounding personnel will utilize some of the same processes as are required in nonsterile compounding (explained in Chapter 10). For example, you must work with a master formulation record, do accurate, exacting calculations and measurements, and compile a compounding record. Some of the *USP* <797> requirements include being able to demonstrate competency in the following (see Table 12.2):

- properly and accurately doing calculations and measurements and following formula directions in precise sequential order
- undergoing training and testing in principles and practices of aseptic technique
- performing aseptic hand washing and donning appropriate sterile compounding garb
- working in a cleanroom environment that meets the *USP* <797> standards for air quality
- disinfecting supplies, equipment, and work surfaces
- properly using special equipment and the varied workbench equipment
- monitoring environmental quality specifications of airflow, ingredients, and supplies
- identifying contamination risk levels and checking beyond-use dating of CSPs

In addition to understanding all of the *USP* <797> guidelines, sterile compoundingpersonnel will utilize some of the same processes as are required in nonsterilecompounding (explained in Chapter 10). For example, you must work with a Master Formulation Record; do accurate, exacting calculations and measurements; and compile a Compounding Record. Some of the *USP* <797> requirements include beingable to demonstrate competency in the skills listed in Table 12.2.

TABLE 12.2 Sterile Compounding Skills Proficiencies

- Undergoing training and testing in principles and practices of aseptic technique
- Performing aseptic handwashing and donning appropriate sterile compounding garb
- Working in a cleanroom environment that meets the *USP* <797> standards for air quality
- Cleaning and disinfecting supplies, equipment, and work surfaces
- Aseptic manipulation
- Proper cleanroom behavior
- Properly and accurately doing calculations and measurements and following formula directions in precise sequential order
- Use of equipment and tools
- Properly using special equipment and the varied workbench equipment
- Understanding the HEPA-filtered unidirectional airflow within the rooms and equipment
- Understanding the potential impact of personnel activities, such as moving materials into and out of the compounding area
- Documentation of the compounding process (e.g., Master Formulation and Compounding Records)
- Methods of sterilization
- Monitoring environmental quality specifications of airflow, ingredients, and supplies
- Identifying contamination risk levels and checking beyond-use dating of CSPs

You must also know and apply the relevant standards for related skills and knowledge contained in the following *USP* chapters:

- <1151> Pharmaceutical Dosage Forms
- <1160> Pharmaceutical Calculations in Prescription Compounding
- <1163> Quality Assurance in Pharmaceutical Compounding
- <1176> Prescription Balances and Volumetric Apparatus
- <1191> Stability Considerations in Dispensing Practice
- <1265> Written Prescription Drug Information Guidelines

The hospital pharmacy also has its own quality assurance program to ensure that prescription errors do not occur and that high quality CSPs are consistently prepared. Such a program tracks and documents personnel qualifications; drug selection and handling; design, operation, cleanliness, and maintenance of building, facilities, and equipment; compounding processes and aseptic technique; and final CSPs and dispensing processes. The role and duty of each pharmacist and technician involved in the sterile compounding process are carefully delineated in the quality assurance program and the SOPs. The Occupational Health and Safety Administration (OSHA) and your state board of pharmacy also have regulations that must be followed.

The greatest risk of CSP contamination are from failure to follow established procedures and failure to adhere to quality standards. A written training program for each sterile compounding area must be in place to list the requirements and frequency for training as well as processes to evaluate performance.

The hospital pharmacy also has its own quality assurance program to ensure that prescription errors do not occur and that high quality CSPs are consistently prepared. Such a program tracks and documents personnel qualifications; drug selection and handling; design, operation, cleanliness, and maintenance of building, facilities, and equipment; compounding processes and aseptic technique; and final CSPs and dispensing processes. The role and duty of each pharmacist and technician involved in the sterile compounding process are carefully delineated in the quality assurance program and the SOPs. The Occupational Health and Safety Administration (OSHA) and your state board of pharmacy also have regulations that must be followed.

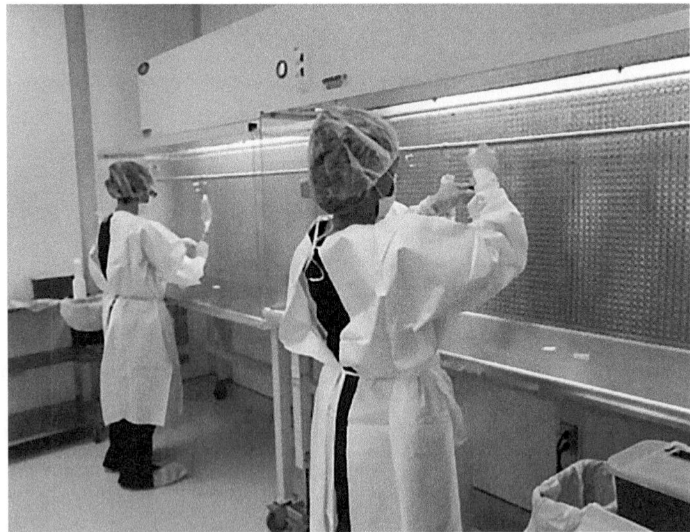

Students at the new, state-of-the-art compounding laboratory at Lipscomb University in Nashville, TN, are learning aseptic technique in sterile compounding.

12.6 The Cleanroom

According to *USP* <797>, CSPs need to be compounded in a **cleanroom**, which has highly controlled air quality to ensure an environment as germ free as possible with no dust and low levels of particulates in the air to avoid contamination. The standard compounding cleanroom is separated into two separate rooms: a preparatory anteroom and a buffer room that provides space for the sterile compounding equipment (which will be described in depth later in the chapter).

Globally, air quality is measured by the fractional number (in micrometers) of particles (contaminants) that can be found per cubic meter (m3) of air. This classification system is from the **International Organization for Standardization (ISO)**. Particles in the air are counted with a light scattering device that tallies the particles of different sizes in a cubic meter of compressed air. The lower the fractional number of particles, the lower the ISO class number and the better the air quality. Sterile compounding needs to be done at ISO Class 5 or less as opposed to typical indoor room air, which is a Class 9 environment (see Table 12.3). The anteroom must have Class 8 or better air, the buffer room must have Class 7, and the **direct compounding area (DCA)**, which is inside an engineered compounding workbench, must have Class 5.

TABLE 12.3 ISO Clean Air Classes by Airborne Particulate Amounts

Class	≥ 0.5 μm/m3*	Cleanroom Compounding Area
ISO 1	0.0029	
ISO 2	0.029	
ISO 3	0.29	
ISO 4	2.9	
ISO 5	29	direct compounding area (DCA)
ISO 6	290	
ISO 7	2,900	buffer room
ISO 8	29,000	anteroom
ISO 9	290,000	room air

* The maximum number of particles of different size ranges per cubic meter of compressed air. The cleanest air is the lowest class number while the dirtiest air is the highest. Cleanroom air for sterile compounding needs to be Class 5 or cleaner, while indoor room air is usually Class 9.

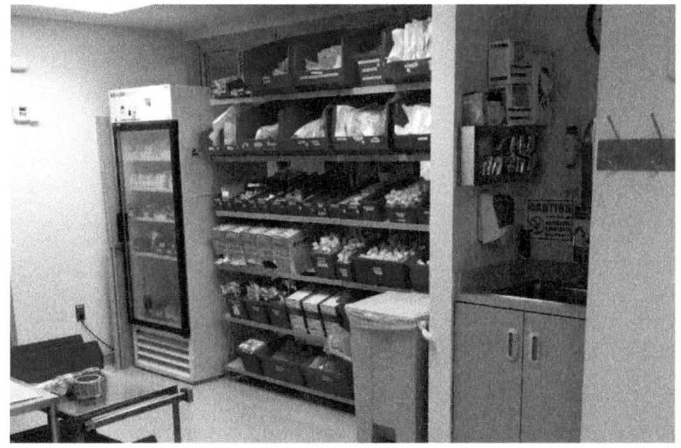
The anteroom serves as a supply preparation area and washing area, and as preparation for the buffer room.

Anteroom

The **anteroom** is the preparatory room that comes before the buffer room. Prior to entering this room, the compounding technicians remove their outerwear and put on light scrubs. Once inside, they collect and prepare their ingredients and supplies, wash, and put on their compounding garb. As noted, the anteroom must be maintained at nothing less clean than an ISO Class 8 environment, so the air quality level needs to be periodically checked.

Only necessary supplies, furniture, and equipment (such as a stainless steel table, supply transport carts, and the refrigeration and freezer units for the ingredients needing cold storage and completed CSPs) are allowed in the anteroom. It also holds pens, calculators, cleaning supplies, and nonrefrigerated CSP ingredients and packaged supplies. Many state standards require a "touch-free" sink and a "touch-free" non-wood door between the anteroom and the cleanroom.

The Buffer Room

The inner room to which the anteroom leads is known as the **buffer room** (it is technically the actual "cleanroom," which is sometimes called the "IV room"). The buffer room is able to maintain the required cleaner air standard (ISO Class 7) than the anteroom because it is separated physically from the heavy foot traffic of the main hospital and pharmacy by the anteroom.

Only properly trained and garbed pharmacy personnel have access to the buffer room. The design elements include heat-sealed floors and smooth, nonporous walls and ceiling tiles that are easily cleaned. It contains only the items absolutely necessary for sterile compounding, including the stainless steel counters and workstations. The temperature and humidity of this room are maintained at specific levels to inhibit the potential for bacterial growth.

Practice Tip

Garbing and degarbing should never occur at the same time in the same place.

Within the buffer room are the **primary engineering controls (PECs)**, which are the ventilated workbenches that have the DCAs within them. As cited, each DCA *must have* ISO Class 5 air quality. The ISO Class 5 environment is maintained within the PEC by its **high-efficiency particulate airflow (HEPA) filter** system that forces sterile, unidirectional air across the work surface of the DCA. The HEPA filters are 99% efficient in removing particles as small as 0.3 micrometers (microns) in size. The different kinds of sterile compounding PECs will be described later in the chapter.

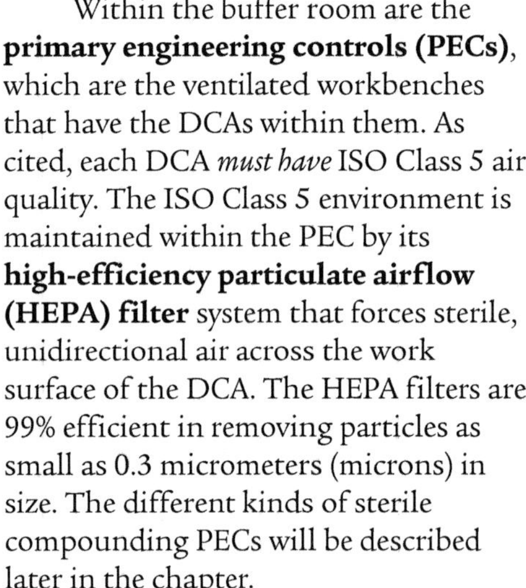

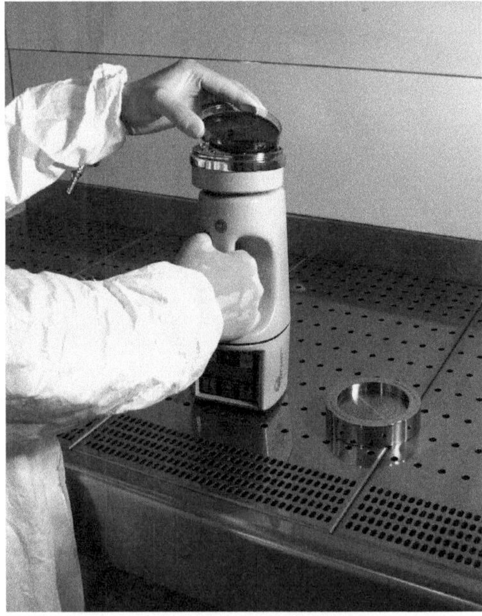

The SAS Air Sampler (which comes in different styles) is used to measure the air quality of the laminar flow workstation, buffer room, and anteroom.

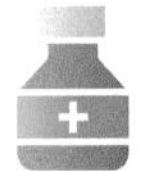

Pharm Fact

The HEPA filter removes particles that are 0.3 microns in size, which is about 300 times smaller than the average diameter of human hair.

Safety Alert

The technician should keep in mind that the greatest risk of contamination in a sterile compounding area comes from human error or touch contamination, despite the presence of equipment, filters and engineering controls.

Secondary Engineering Controls

The **secondary engineering controls (SECs)** for air quality are the ventilation and HEPA systems built into the cleanroom area's heating, ventilation, and air conditioning (HVAC) systems. The SECs are calibrated to maintain the ISO Class 7 air quality in the buffer room as a whole and ISO Class 8 or better in the anteroom. **Positive pressure** is created when air is forced through the HEPA-filtered HVAC system into rooms of the sealed cleanroom. Positive pressure is required for a sterile compounding area to help keep contaminants from entering the cleanroom. The **unidirectional airflow** sweeps particles away from the room where CSPs are being compounded toward the lower-pressure anteroom and then outward toward the lowest-pressure outer area (see Figure 12.2).

As new air is HEPA-filtered and cycled into the room by the HVAC system, it replaces the old air in the room. The air replacement is called an **air exchange**. The rooms must have a *USP*-specified amount of air exchanges per hour. This is another way the air quality is maintained.

FIGURE 12.2 Sterile Cleanroom Facility Layout

Compounding technicians enter the anteroom (ISO Class 8) and, after preparation, enter the buffer room (ISO Class 7) to work in the DCAs (ISO Class 5) of the PECs. Notice that the airflow goes in the opposite direction, carrying air and any contaminants out of the high positive pressure buffer room through the lower pressure anteroom and to the outer area.

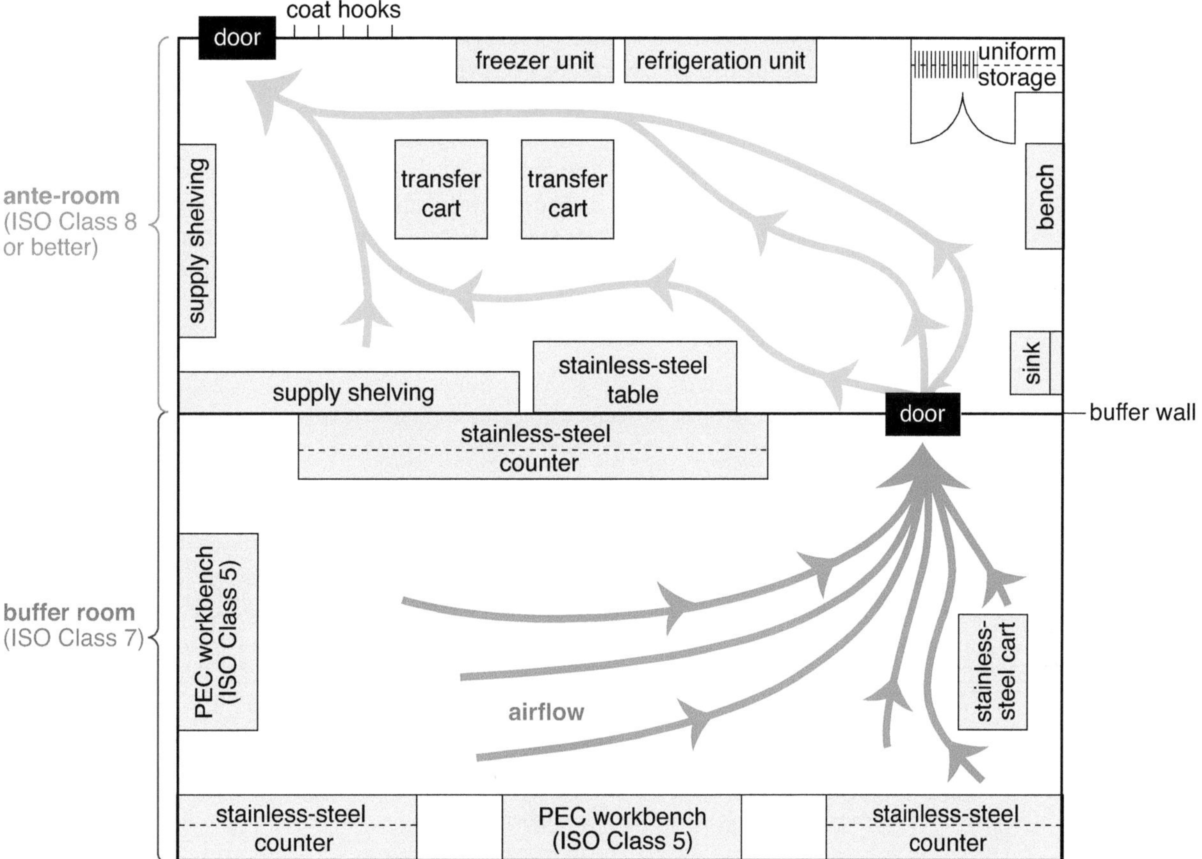

Cleanroom Facilities without a Separate Anteroom and Buffer Room

Some hospital and inpatient care facilities may not have the space for a full anteroom and a buffer room with all the filtered ventilation systems for their sterile cleanroom compounding. Though it is not ideal, some establish a semi-enclosed **segregated compounding area (SCA)** away from the outer doors, windows, traffic, sink, and garbing areas. Some hospitals also are erecting small enclosed, ventilated, modular HEPA-filtered cleanroom compounding areas within larger rooms. Hospitals using SCAs and modular cleanrooms have to follow the *USP* <797> guidelines that fit those types of spaces.

12.7 Aseptic Technique

Despite the engineering controls, the sterile compounding area will not remain clean if sterile compounding personnel introduce contaminants into the environment from their skin, hair, jewelry, and clothing. One of the primary focuses of aseptic technique is to prevent carrying microorganisms and other contaminants into the workspace and CSPs.

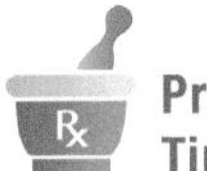

Practice Tip

Prior to entering the anteroom, compounding technicians remove all cosmetics, jewelry, outer garb, and anything else they have with them. They can store these items in lockers and put on light scrubs.

Aseptic Preparation

Before even coming to work in sterile compounding, a technician has to prepare. Sterile compounding personnel must not wear jewelry, cosmetics, perfume, artificial nails, or nail polish. These substances can flake and compromise the aseptic environment. No earbuds, headsets, devices, or cell phones are allowed in the cleanroom. If you have jewelry that cannot be removed, it must be covered.

Individuals who have certain medical conditions that increase the risk of contamination during the compounding process are also banned from the sterile compounding area. These conditions include communicable diseases, respiratory colds or infections, weeping sores, oozing tattoos, rashes, and sunburn. Food and beverages are not permitted in either the anteroom or the cleanroom, and you must not chew gum or engage in horseplay in these areas. Street clothes should be removed and clean scrubs donned right before entering the anteroom.

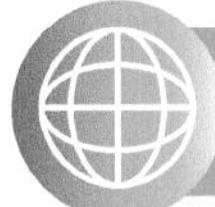

IN THE REAL WORLD

In the fall of 2015, Duke Raleigh Hospital was undergoing renovations but it needed to keep the hospital open. So it chose to take advantage of the new mobile cleanroom created by Germfree Labs that was completely suited to *USP* Chapter <797> standards at the time. Duke Raleigh was the first US hospital to use a mobile unit. The unit is a combined hospital pharmacy, cleanroom (with anteroom and buffer room with laminar flow workstations), and a hazardous compounding room (with Class II biological safety cabinets) in a specially designed semi-trailer facility. This unit allowed Duke Raleigh Hospital to have uninterrupted service during its renovations.

The possibilities, though, for this transportable cleanroom and hazardous compounding station go beyond hospital renovations. The mobile cleanroom offers great hope for hospitals and facilities in disaster-hit areas where the pharmacy has been damaged. It also offers hope for rural areas and even hospitals in developing countries that cannot afford a full cleanroom facility.

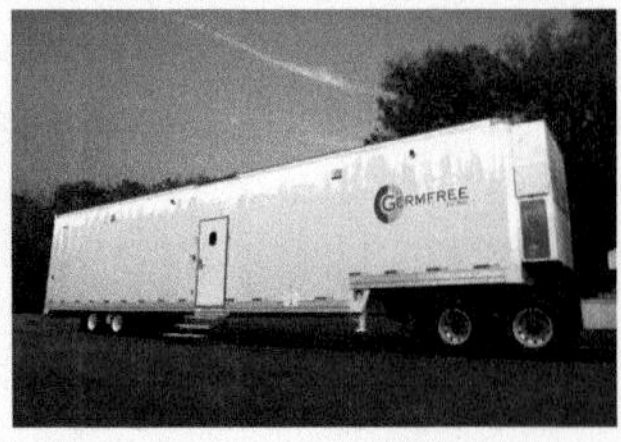

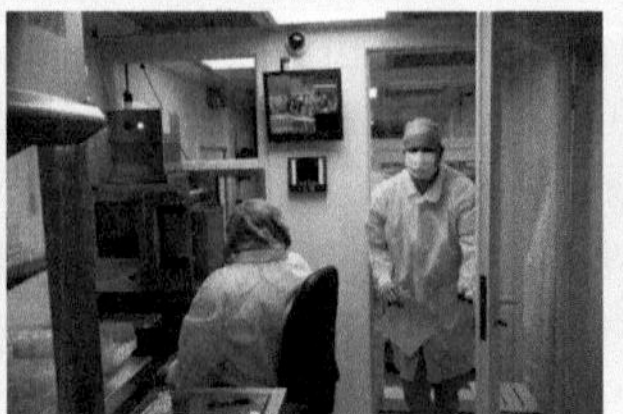

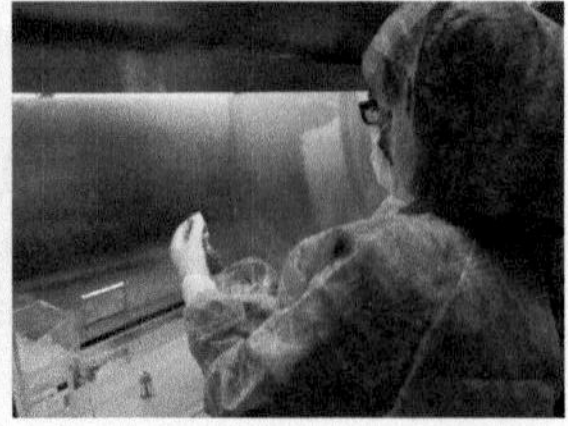

Many key duties have to be fulfilled in the anteroom before garbing, such as gathering supplies and finishing any calculations on dilutions. The technician places the pharmacist-approved label, compounding directions, and calculations along with the medication order (if needed) in a clear plastic bag and wipes it down with sterile 70% isopropyl alcohol (IPA) so the bag can come into the cleanroom. The PEC cleaning supplies, compounding ingredients, and supplies are also wiped down and placed in a sanitized, nonporous molded plastic or stainless steel bin on a stainless steel cart for transport into the buffer room. Then the technician is ready to garb.

Safety Alert

The order for putting on sterile compounding personal protective equipment (PPE) is dependent on the placement of the sink and facility specific standard operating procedures (SOPs).

Aseptic Garbing and Washing

The garbing process for sterile compounding personnel follows a strict sequence. You put on the protective garb in a specific order: first shoe covers, hair cover, and face mask. Then comes handwashing and arm scrubbing. The sterile gowns (with sleeves) and gloves must be the cleanest items, so they are put on last; the gown goes on in the anteroom, and the gloves are donned in the buffer room.

Safety Alert

Sterile compounding personnel who prepare CSPs are required to perform aseptic handwashing, a more rigorous handwashing practice than the general guidelines dictated by the CDC.

Aseptic Handwashing and Hygiene

Aseptic handwashing is a more vigorous and thorough washing than the CDC handwashing guidelines. The aim of aseptic handwashing is not only to reduce the number of resident and transient flora to a minimum but also to inhibit their regrowth for as long as possible—not just on the hands but also on the wrists and forearms. It means performing specific hand-washing procedures with unscented soap (plain or antimicrobial) and water followed by an alcohol-based sanitizer as will be explained below.

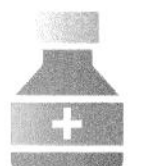

Pharm Fact

Skin cells are naturally shed at the rate of 30,000 to 40,000 every hour and a million cells per day, and with them come multitudes of microorganisms. Thousands of bacteria live on a square centimeter of skin, which is why washing, scrubbing, and garbing are so important!

Hand and Forearm Washing

The most ideal sink situations are those with a touchless faucet controlled by a foot pedal or electronic sensor. Proper handwashing includes first removing any debris under the fingernails with a nail pick, sponge, and cleaner under warm running water. Then, using unscented soap and water, rub your hands together vigorously, cleaning each finger individually and the webbing between each finger for 30 seconds at a minimum.

Clean the back of each hand by starting at the wrist, moving up the forearm to the elbow in a circular motion (see Figure 12.3). Rinsing should be done in the same order, working from the fingers down the forearms with the hands always pointed upward to allow the water to wash toward the elbows and off. The aseptic hand-washing technique radically affects how effective the process will be in terms of infection control, so it must be understood and done properly as practiced in a lab.

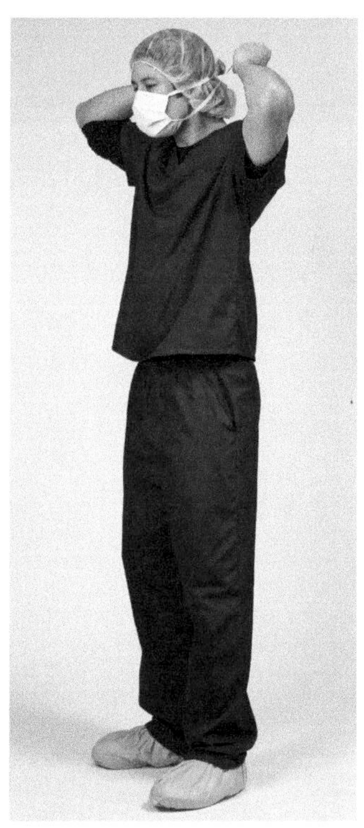

The pharmacy technician demonstrates putting on the face mask before handwashing, scrubbing the arms, and adding the gown.

The cleansing sequence should end with drying your hands on a lint-free disposable towel until they are completely dry. After donning a low lint gown, then apply an alcohol-based hand wipe, gel, or spray (where the liquid evaporates) for sanitizing hygiene. This entire hand-washing process must be completed multiple times during a shift in the sterile compounding area, including:

- upon entering the sterile compounding area,
- after a major contamination,
- after touch contamination, such as scratching your face,
- after eating, sneezing, coughing, or using the restroom, and
- after every 30 minutes during batch CSP procedures.

FIGURE 12.3 Proper Aseptic Forearm Washing

This technician is completing the forearm scrubbing and rinsing sequence.

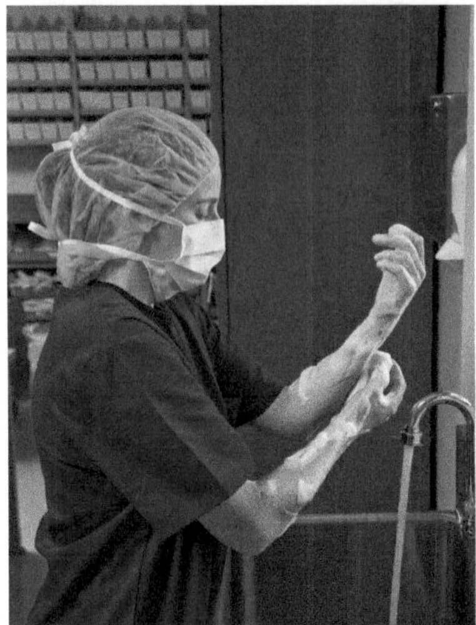

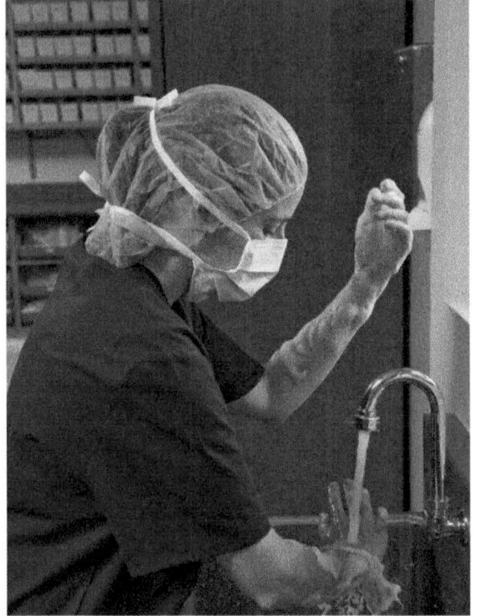

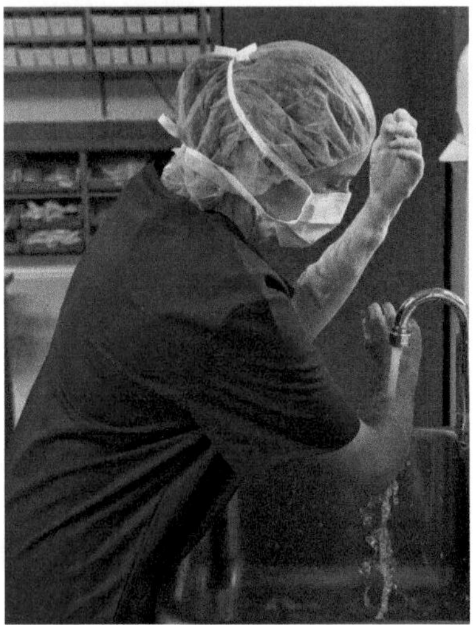

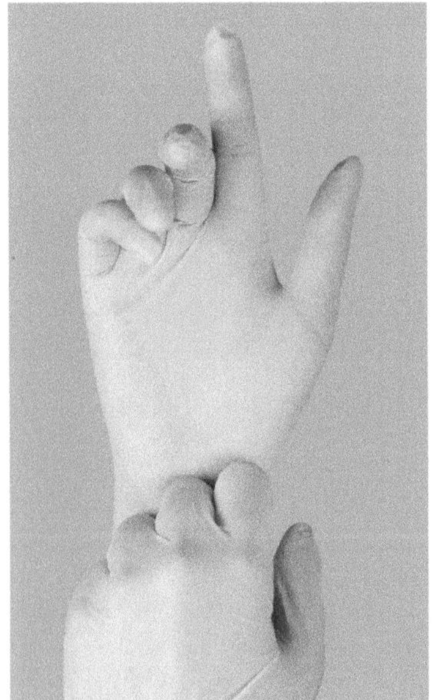

Gloving by the pharmacy technician provides an extra safeguard to touch contamination, but gloves too can become contaminated.

Sterile Gowning and Gloving

After the handwashing and hygiene, the last two procedures are gowning and gloving. With clean hands, open the sterile gown package (which has been wiped down), and put it on, one arm at a time. Be sure the gown does not touch the floor or any surfaces. Secure it in the back. Once gowned, sanitize your hands with sterile 70% IPA, and now you may safely enter the buffer room with the supply cart to be gloved.

Gloving To finish the hand hygiene and disinfect the hands from using the cart and doors, the technician applies a long-lasting antimicrobial alcohol-based rub again and lets it dry before donning the sterile gloves. The gloves should be powder-free and compatible with alcohol disinfectants. The gloves are labeled "left" and "right." The outer area of the gloves should never be touched. Grasping the inside of the cuff, the first glove should be pulled over the hand and the cuff of the gown so that no skin shows. Then the second glove should be put on in a similar way. Gloves must be worn at all times inside the cleanroom, especially while preparing CSPs.

The gloves need to be sanitized and inspected regularly during a shift for tears or punctures, and if they are found, the gloves must be

Safety Alert

Pharmacy personnel should not use petroleum-based ointments, creams, or lotions before donning sterile gloves, as these products may decrease the integrity of the sterile gloves.

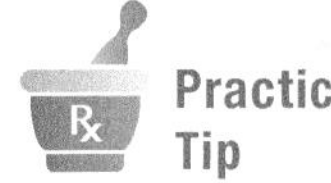
Practice Tip

If a technician leaves the sterile compounding area (to use the restroom, to go to lunch or breaks, and such), then the entire garbing and hand-washing process must be repeated.

replaced with a new pair. In addition, every time a glove touches a nonsterile surface or object while you are working in the cleanroom or DCA, the glove must be sanitized with sterile 70% IPA spray. Gloves should also never be washed or reused. Discard them after leaving the cleanroom.

Quality Assurance and Quality Control

Within the cleanroom facility, hospital quality assurance and quality control programs are implemented. Site inspections of the sterile compounding areas are required to initiate and maintain accreditation. Also required are quality monitoring and improvement procedures.

Aseptic Technique Testing

Prior to working in the buffer room, each technician who is training in sterile compounding procedures must successfully pass a competency evaluation and a **fingertip sampling** three separate times. To do this, immediately after gloving, the technician places gloved fingers on a petri dish medium (agar) for growing cultures, and the dish is monitored to see if any microorganisms grow over the next few days. If they do, that means the glove was contaminated and the aseptic procedure was not done properly.

Compounded Sterile Preparation Testing

In addition to the fingertip testing of sterile compounding personnel, the quality control (QC) program in a sterile compounding area involves a sampling of the CSPs and drug products by the pharmacist before their release to the nurse and administration to the patient. Periodically, products will be sent for **sterility testing**—an established laboratory procedure for detecting viable microbial contamination in a sample or preparation. **Release testing** involves the final visual check of the CSP by the pharmacist for particulates, foreign matter, or discoloration against a lit background. If detected, the CSP is immediately discarded.

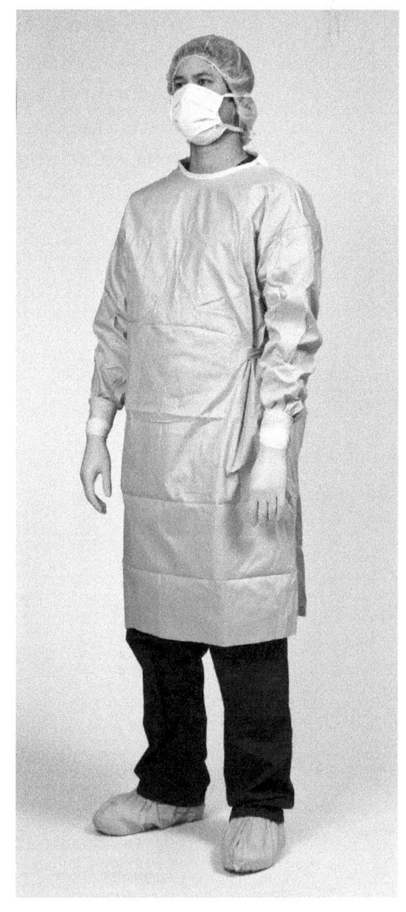
The full protective clothing of a technician helps keep CSPs sterile. After a shift, the aseptic garb must come off in the anteroom and be discarded properly in the reverse order of donning it.62

Ongoing Technician Testing

Sterile compounding technicians are observed by their pharmacist supervisors and given periodic aseptic testing. The testing frequency is dependent upon the risk level of the CSPs, facility SOPs, and *USP* <797> guidelines. A technician's CSPs also receive periodic spot testings. The technique of all sterile compounding personnel must also be re-evaluated at a minimum of every six months. With such training, certifications, and experience, technicians are rewarded in higher salary for their higher-level, CSP-related responsibilities.

Degarbing

Upon completion of the CSP(s), the technician will return to the anteroom for the pharmacist check (if not done in the buffer room). If no one is in the process of garbing, the technician can properly discard the used garb. (If someone is preparing to enter the cleanroom, she or he must wait to degarb until the new compounder has entered the buffer room.) Unless otherwise instructed, the technician removes the PPE in the opposite order as putting it on: gloves, gown, face mask, hair cover, and shoe covers.

12.8 Sterile Compounding Supplies and Their Care

There are a variety of commonly used supplies that sterile compounding personnel work with. These include IV solutions, ampules and vials, syringes and needles, IV administration sets, medication cassettes, and personal pain pumps. Since ampules and vials have special ways to open and use them, they will be described in the next chapter on the processes of sterile compounding.

Solution Bottles and Bags

Sterile compounding facilities often use sterile water or manufactured mixtures of 5% dextrose in water, 0.9% normal saline, and other solutions as a medication base or diluent. Technicians choose the proper base in the correct bottle or IV bag based on the medical order, and once in the DCA, they use the right-sized syringe and needle sets to inject the drugs, diluents, or nutritional substances into these bases. (Ways these solutions are used will be explained in more depth in Chapter 13.)

Syringes and Needles

To withdraw solutions from sterile containers or inject solutions into sterile containers, a needle-and-syringe unit is necessary. Technicians use this syringe transferal process to reconstitute a powdered medication, dilute an existing medication, withdraw fluid from a vial or ampule, or transport fluid from one container to another.

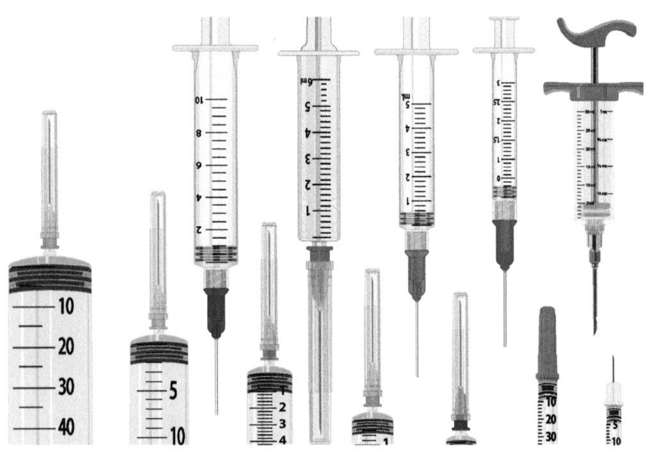

Various sizes of syringes used in sterile compounding range in volume from 60 mL (left) to 1 mL (right), with different incremental measuring units to calibrate them.

Syringes

Syringes are made of plastic or glass. Most sterile compounding syringes are made of sterile plastic components that are disposable. Glass syringes are expensive, and since they are rarely reused, they are only selected when a drug is incompatible with plastic or when certain chemotherapy products are prepared. (In rare compounding scenarios, glass syringes may be cleaned and sterilized in an autoclave for reuse.)

The main components of a syringe include the syringe tip, the barrel containing the calibration marks, and the rubber-tipped piston plunger (see Figure 12.4). Because the piston plunger, the inner plunger shaft, and the syringe tip must always remain sterile, they must never be touched, not even with a sterile glove.

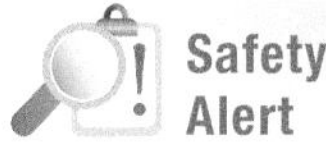

Always be careful to touch only the barrel and top of a syringe and never the piston plunger, inner plunger shaft, or syringe tip, even with a gloved hand. If they are touched, they need to be thrown away.

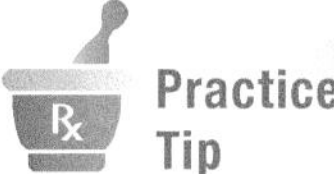

Always measure the amount of liquid in the syringe by aligning the shoulder of the plunger with the desired calibration mark on the syring barrel.

Syringe Selection and Measurement Various sizes of syringes deliver significantly different volumes. During the sterile compounding process, choose the smallest syringe possible to hold the desired volume while being at least three-quarters full. A syringe is considered accurate to half of the smallest calibration mark (usually mL or cc) indicated on its barrel.

To get an accurate measurement reading, you need to know the total volume and the number of marks between labeled measurement units. For example, the 10 labeled calibration marks on a 1 mL syringe indicate that each mark is equivalent to $^{1}/_{10}$ of 1 mL (0.1, 0.2, 0.3, . . .). The small lines in between measure an equal proportion of that $^{1}/_{10}$ unit. On a 50 mL syringe, each labeled calibration equals 10 mL, with each small line marking 1 mL. It is important to study syringes to learn their individualized calibration measurements.

To measure the volume of solution drawn into a syringe, air bubbles must first be tapped out. The volume is measured not where the rubber plunger tip lines up to a calibration line, but where the measurement edge of the rubber piston lines up to a calibration (see Figure 12.4).

FIGURE 12.4 **Syringe Components**

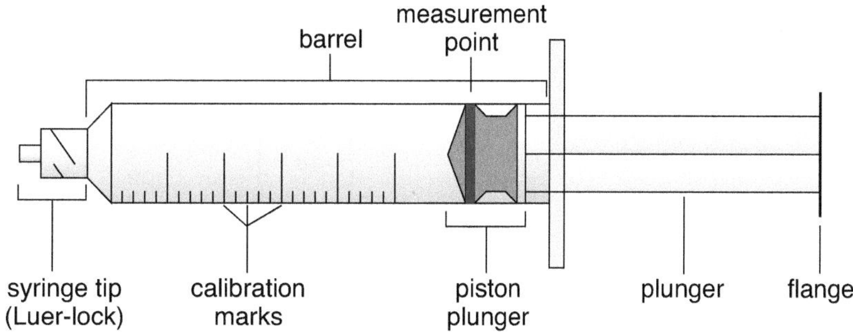

Only touch the shield of the needle. Never touch any of the metal—shaft, heel, bevel, or tip—or the needle is contaminated and must be thrown away in the sharps container. Besides, the needle is obviously sharp and could pierce your glove and skin.

Needles

Sterile compounding needles are made of stainless steel or aluminum and are individually wrapped to maintain their sterility. A needle consists of several parts: the needle hub, lumen, shaft, heel, bevel, and tip (see Figure 12.5). A needle has a hard plastic cap that covers the shaft and tip until the needle is ready to be used. Even with gloves, this cap is the only place that can be touched. Accidentally touching any part of the needle itself leads to contamination and requires the disposal of the needle in a **sharps container** (secure needle disposal bin).

FIGURE 12.5 **Needle Components**

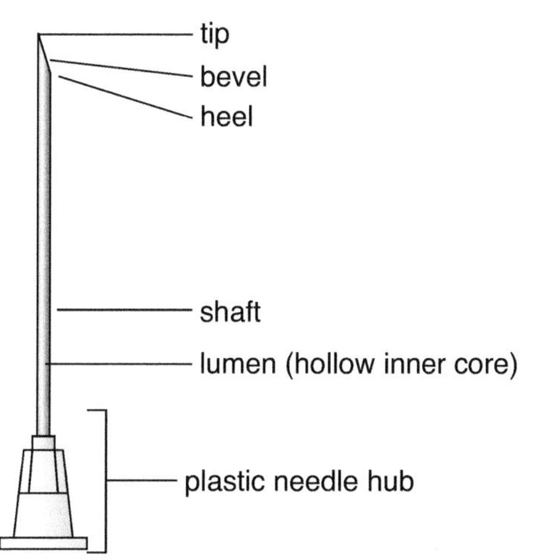

A needle's size is determined by its length and gauge. The needle's gauge refers to the diameter of the shaft's hollow inner core and opening, or lumen. There is an inverse relationship between the gauge number and the size of the lumen. For example, a 16-gauge needle has a wider diameter than a 25-gauge needle. The smaller gauge numbers (with thicker lumens) are appropriate for thicker, more viscous liquids, and the higher gauges (thinner lumens) are used for injecting less dense solutions.

In sterile compounding, 1-inch and 1.5-inch long needles are commonly used, and they have needle gauges ranging from 16 (wider) to 25 (narrower) as shown in Figure 12.6a.

The **critical sites** of a needle and/or syringe are the parts that include fluid pathway surfaces or openings (see Figure 12.6b). These sites must never be touched.

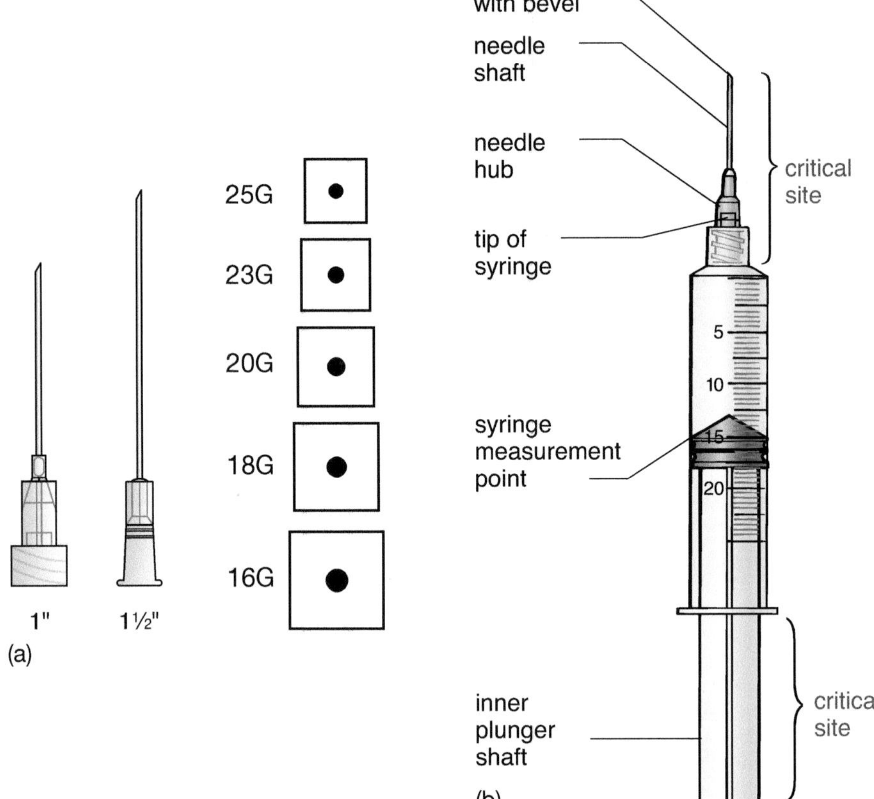

FIGURE 12.6 Common Needle Lengths and Gauges in Sterile Compounding and Critical Areas of a Needle and Syringe

(a) Needle lengths and gauges
(b) Critical sites

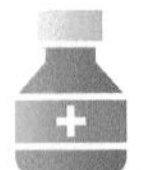

Pharm Fact

IV sets do not have expiration dates, but they do contain the following legend: "Federal law restricts this device to sale by or on the order of a physician."

Administration Sets and Their Components

Sterile compounding personnel sometimes use IV administration sets to prepare CSPs. An **IV administration set** is a sterile, disposable device of many linked components that is used to deliver the IV fluids. These fluids flow from the bag through the tubing and other components through an **injection port** with a needle into the patient's vein. Often called "IV tubing" or an "IV set," the assembled unit comes in a sterile, sealed package.

Sterile compounding personnel may use IV administration sets to:

- transfer fluids between containers while working in a PEC
- prime IV sets to prepare hazardous drug CSPs for patient administration

Regardless of the manufacturer, IV administration sets have certain basic components (see Figure 12.7), which will be described in more depth:

- a universal spike adapter (commonly called a "tubing spike" or "spike"), which pierces the stopper port on the IV solution bag

- a drip chamber, which allows healthcare personnel to view and count the drops of IV fluid before the solution flows down the tubing
- flexible tubing, which delivers the fluid
- a roller clamp, which adjusts the flow rate of the IV fluid from the source container into the receiving container or patient
- injection ports, to infuse fluids with primary IV
- in-line filters, to remove contaminants from the tubing
- a needle adapter set, which attaches a needle or a catheter to the patient and the IV tubing set

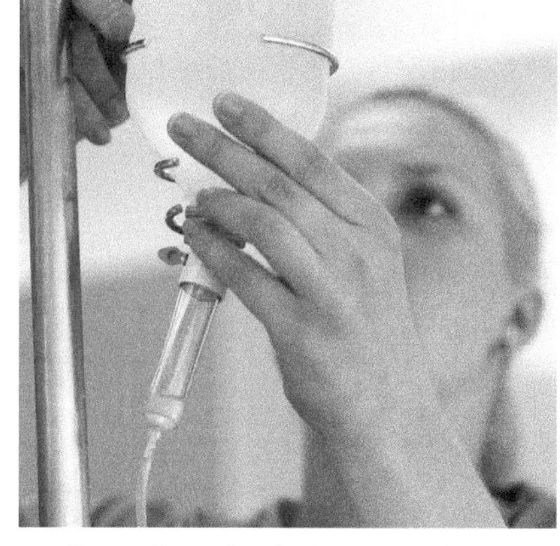

Sterile medicated solutions are often delivered to a patient via an IV administration set.

- Sterile medicated solutions are often delivered to a patient via an IV administration set.

Universal Spike Adapter

The sharp, plastic bag **spike adapter** is used to pierce the IV bag's tubing port to attach the drip chamber and tubing. Some IV sets have an air vent with a bacterial filter cover positioned below the spike. This vent allows air to enter the bottle or bag as fluid flows out of it.

FIGURE 12.7 Sterile IV Solution and Administration Set

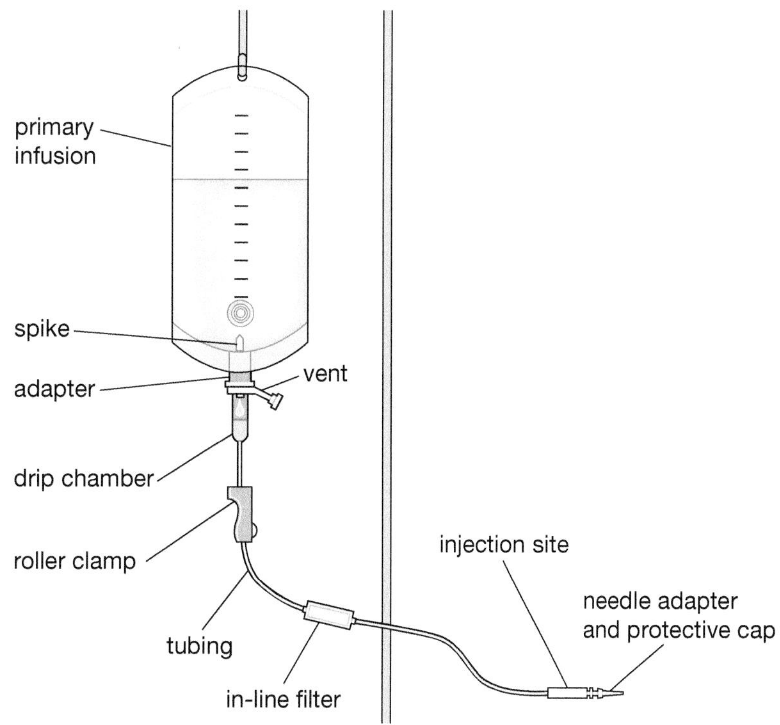

Safety Alert

If possible, do not use PVC IV sets for nitroglycerin, amiodarone, most biotechnology drugs, and fat emulsions due to the absorption of the drug by the plastic. PVC and DEHP-free IV bags and sets are also specifically recommended for pregnant women, neonates, children, ongoing IV patients, and other high-risk populations.

Drip Chamber

Sitting below the spike is the transparent, hollow drip chamber. The **drip chamber** allows any air bubbles to rise to the top of the IV fluid, thus preventing the air bubbles from entering the tubing and, subsequently, the patient. The drip chamber also allows the attending nurse to set the medication flow or infusion rate by counting the drops and then making adjustments to the pump, clamps, tubing, or height of the bag.

IV Tubing Types and Sizes

IV sets deliver either a primary IV solution or a secondary one. The secondary medication has a smaller bag with less volume. This medication is often more concentrated, and it needs to be diluted by the primary solution, so the **secondary tubing** is inserted into the **primary tubing** line to merge the liquids, which is called "piggybacking." The nurse hangs the **IV piggyback (IVPB)**—another name for the secondary IV—higher than the first IV bag to allow the additional gravitational force to push the secondary IV solution into the primary line to the patient (see Figure 12.8).

IV Tubing Length The majority of the IV set is made of clear, flexible plastic tubing. The length of IV tubing in the sets varies, with extensions ranging from 6 to 120 inches. The length of tubing is dependent on the patient's needs, the number of IV lines, and the procedure being performed. Longer tubing is used for primary IV lines in most hospital settings. Shorter tubing lengths are used for the IV piggyback secondary lines and in surgical settings where many people are working around a patient in a small space.

FIGURE 12.8 **Primary Versus Secondary IV Lines**

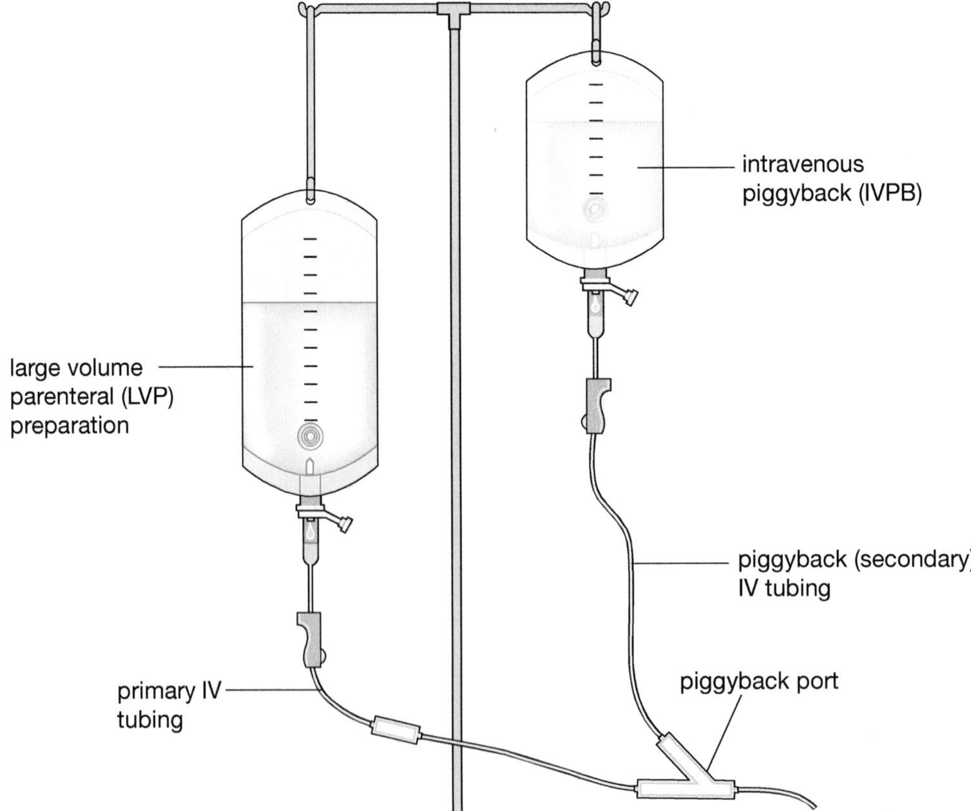

Practice Tip

Because so much of nitroglycerin is absorbed by PVC containers and IV sets, nitroglycerin is best compounded into a glass IV bottle and infused through a non-absorbing IV line. The same is true for vitamin A acetate, warfarin, methohexital, terbutaline, lorazepam, and insulin.

IV Tubing Diameter Size—Drop and Drip Factors The diameter size of the tubing selected is determined by the prescribed number of drops per mL the tubing needs to deliver. This calibration is referred to as the tubing's **drop factor**, with larger diameter tubing delivering larger, fewer drops per mL, and smaller diameter tubing delivering smaller, more numerous drops (gtts) per mL. You will need to know this drop factor to determine how many bags will be needed for 24 hours or the next resupply. The equations to do these calculations will be addressed in Chapter 13.

The most common IV set sizes for adults are **macrodrip tubing sets** that deliver 10, 15, 20 drops per milliliter—(10 gtts/mL, 15 gtts/mL, 20 gtts/mL as shown in Figure 12.9. IV tubing sets that provide smaller drops like 60 gtts/mL are used for pediatric patients and for particular IV medications requiring tight control. The smaller diameter tubing sets are called **microdrip tubing sets** (also known as minidrip sets).

FIGURE 12.9
Microdrip and Macrodrip Drop Sets

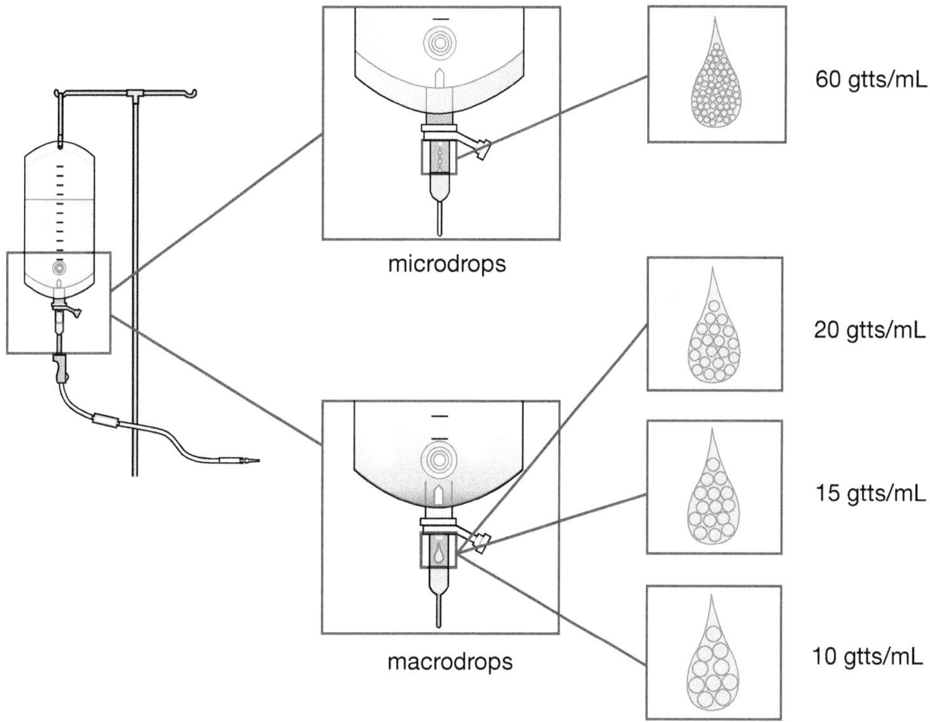

IN THE REAL WORLD

When PVC tubing is manufactured or incinerated, dioxins, chloride, and other toxic compounds are produced and/or emitted, and a portion of these substances is usually released into air, water, or soil. Both chloride and dioxin are known toxins that affect organs and bodily systems and are carcinogenic. They can bioaccumulate in one's body and the bodies of wildlife.

Because of these health and environmental issues, there is a medical move to go PVC-free. Europe is phasing out PVCs. Kaiser Permanente, one of the largest healthcare providers in the United States, and Dignity Health, the eighth largest healthcare system in the nation, are among those that have gone 100% PVC- and DEHP-free in their IV materials. Non-PVC IV tubing is available from most pharmaceutical manufacturers.

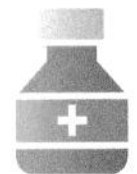

Pharm Fact

B. Braun Medical and Hospira are just two of the manufacturers of non-PVC bags and tubing. Non-PVC alternatives are 30 times less toxic when disposed of by incineration and are significantly lighter, resulting in reductions in landfill costs.

IV Tubing Plastic and Health Issues Some blood bags, IV solution bags, and IV tubing are made of a type of plastic known as PVC (polyvinyl chloride). Many common drugs, though, are partially absorbed by the PVC plastic tubing and/or IV bag. For example, when nitroglycerin is in a PVC IV bag and administration set, 70% of the drug is absorbed after 24 hours. This absorption reduces the amount of drug delivered intravenously to a patient.

Besides drug absorption issues, there are concerns about PVC chemicals leaching into the CSP solution and being absorbed by the patient. In addition, disposal of PVC causes environmental issues, and the chemical compound Di(2-ethylhexyl) phthlate (DEHP) often used to make the PVC tubing flexible creates other health issues. For these reasons, hospitals are moving toward non-PVC IV bags and tubing.

Roller Clamp

The **roller clamp** contains a small roller that can move freely along the length of the tubing between the spike adapter and the needle adapter to manually regulate and adjust the solution flow rate. When the clamp is rolled up toward the universal spike adapter, the clamp loosens, increasing fluid flow and drip rate. When the clamp is rolled down toward the needle adapter, the clamp tightens, resulting in a reduced flow of fluid. The roller clamp is always closed when an IV solution is being attached to the tubing. There is also an **auxiliary clamp**, or slide clamp, that is used to completely stop the IV solution from flowing when needed.

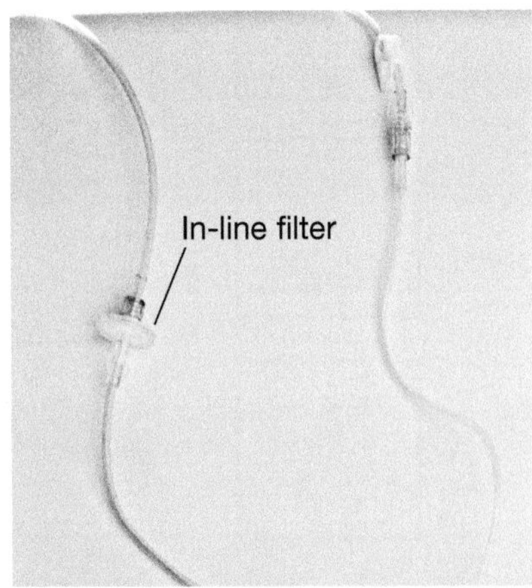

In-line filters vary in size and can minimize the risk of phlebitis or infection.

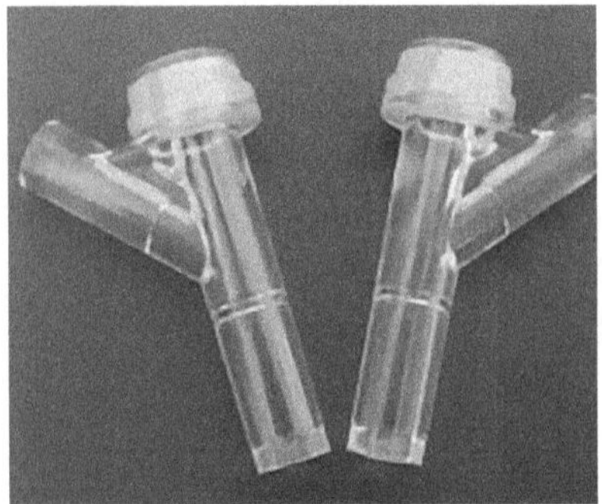

This Y-site injection port allows a secondary IV or injection to be added to the main IV line.

In-line Filters

In-line filters are included in many IV administration sets. An in-line filter is a device used to remove contaminants flowing through the tubing, such as glass particles, fibers, and tiny bits of rubber that may have inadvertently entered the CSP during the sterile compounding procedures. The filters are built into the tubing or added to it and are classified by the size or nature of the particles they remove.

A 0.45 micron filter provides a final filtration of the fluid before it enters the patient, but it is not a sterilizing filter. Final filtration protects the patient against air bubbles, particulate matter, bacteria, and **phlebitis**. Phlebitis is vein inflammation caused by undissolved drug particles, plastic particulate matter from IV tubing, or infectious agents.

Manufactured IV solutions without drugs generally have very low particle counts and do not require filtration. However, when compounded drugs are added to these manufactured solutions, the particle count increases. A total parenteral nutrition (TPN) solution with multiple additives often requires an in-line filter.

Filters do not remove viruses as viruses are too small to be caught by the filter. However, a 0.22 micron filter is optimal for blocking bacteria. These filters, however, are so fine that they slow down infusion rates and can get clogged. IV solutions that contain a fat emulsion must utilize a larger micron size filter.

Injection Ports

A self-sealing injection port is needed to allow IV fluids or medications to be infused along with the primary IV into the patient's vein through the tubing. The Y-site injection port (see Figure 12.10) provides a site for inserting the piggyback and IV push medications, reducing the pain of a new injection site for the patient.

FIGURE 12.10
Example of Y-site Injection Ports

These ports are used to administer various medications with the same primary IV set. A syringe can be injected into the port nearest the patient's vein and a secondary tubing port can be connected to the line closer up the line to the drip chamber of the primary solution.

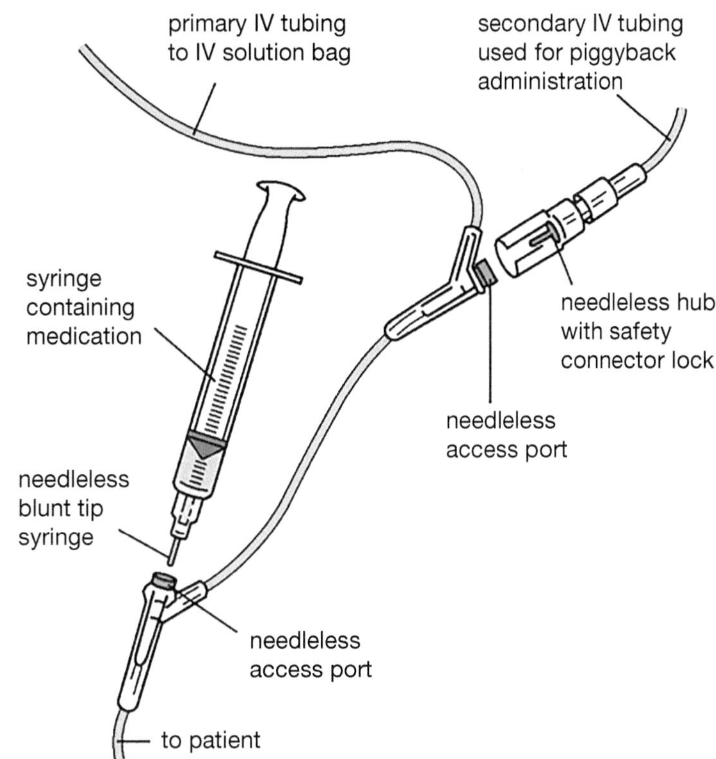

Catheter Set

A catheter set is located at the patient end of the IV set. The tubing delivers medication through the implanted needle in the patient's vein. When an IV solution set is changed, the old tubing is removed from the catheter connection port and the new IV tubing is attached. This saves the pain and effort of repuncturing the patient each time.

Medication Reservoir Cassettes and Personal Pain Pumps

A new approach to sterile drug delivery is through devices that allow greater power to the patient in managing the rate of administration, especially in terms of pain medications. This delivery method is called **patient-controlled analgesia (PCA)**—or patient-controlled sedation (PCS). Personal infusion pumps can administer sterile intravenous admixtures that come stored in medication reservoir cassettes, such as those for the CADD-Prizm PCS II.

Experienced sterile compounding technicians will receive medication orders to prepare epidural and morphine cassettes. (Some drug manufacturers offer premixed sterile drug solutions in medication cassettes.)

These CADD medication cassette reservoirs and the ON-Q* Fixed Flow Pump are examples of new carriers for sterile compounded medications.

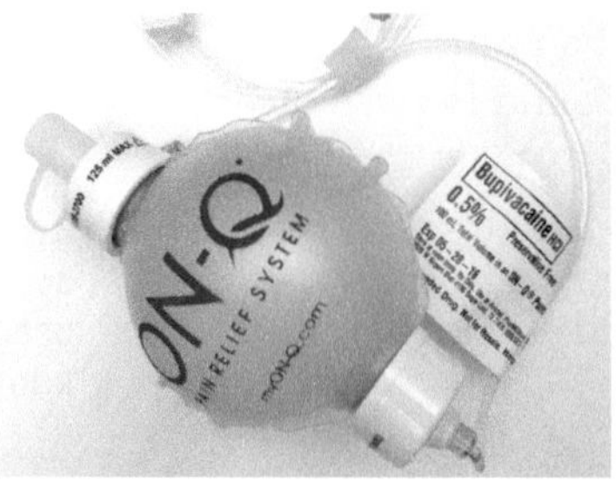

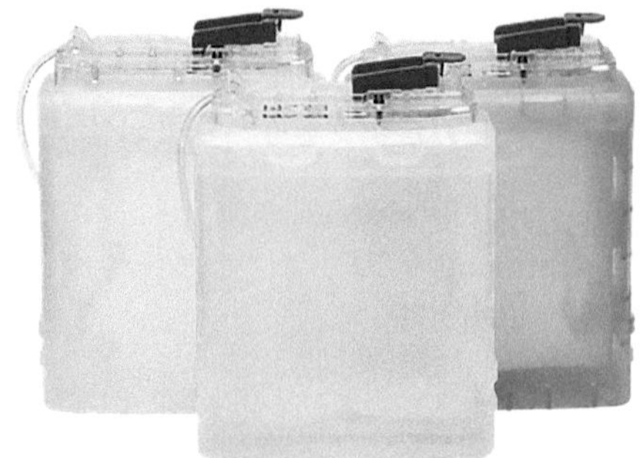

Another new sterile delivery device is a small, solution-filled sterile plastic ball attached to a sterile catheter line that is sewn into a surgery site. The ball, such as the ON-Q* Fixed Flow Rate Pump, slowly deflates, administering the pain medication as the patient heals. Sterile compounding technicians fill these balls with the medications ordered for patients' specific needs.

12.9 Types of Primary Engineering Controls

A variety of different primary engineering controls are used in sterile compounding. The type of PEC that is used in a sterile compounding facility is dependent upon the environment in which the PEC is placed (i.e., ISO Class 7 or ISO Class 8), and the number and type of CSPs being prepared within the PEC. The two most frequently used PEC types in sterile compounding are the horizontal laminar airflow workbench and the compounding aseptic isolator (CAI). Hazardous drugs are compounded in different types of PECs that will be discussed in the next chapter.

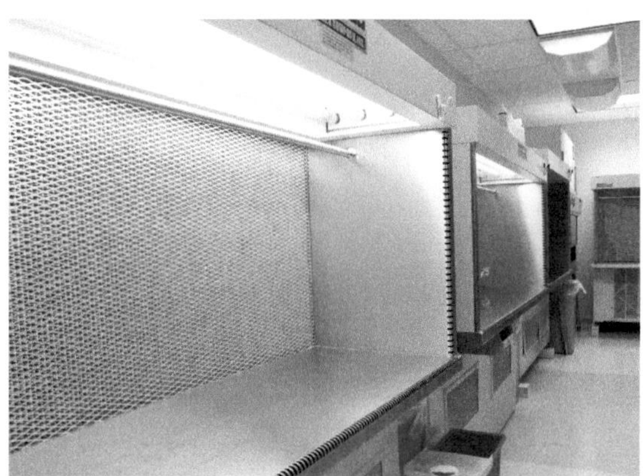

More than one horizontal laminar airflow workbench may be needed in a hospital cleanroom to handle all the IVs and other CSPs needed.

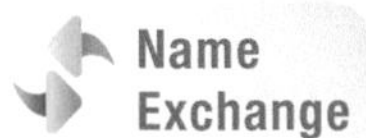

Name Exchange

The H-LAFW is also known as the horizontal airflow workbench, horizontal clean bench, horizontal laminar hood, or some combination of these titles. Laminar workbenches are a type of primary engineering control (PEC) and are commonly called "hoods."

Horizontal Airflow Workbench

The **horizontal laminar airflow workbench (H-LAFW)**, sometimes referred to as the "hood" or "cabinet," is a three-sided surgical steel framework with a stainless steel work counter, an open back, and an interior illuminated by overhead lights. The components of the hood work in tandem to maintain a controlled air environment through continuous HEPA filtration. The constant movement of filtered air prevents contaminants from entering and tainting the sterile compounding process. The blower, or fan, is sealed within the rear of the cabinet. The blower draws the room air through the prefilter and then pushes it through the HEPA filter and grilled vent across the nonporous work surface and DCA (see Figure 12.11). Technicians can feel the air blowing on them as they work. The DCA is in front of them near the grilled vent.

FIGURE 12.11 Side Cross Section of Horizontal Laminar Airflow Workbench

In an H-LAFW, the room air is drawn into the cabinet through the prefilter and then blown up and through the HEPA filter, and fanned horizontally across the DCA toward the worker to help prevent CSP contamination during compounding procedures.

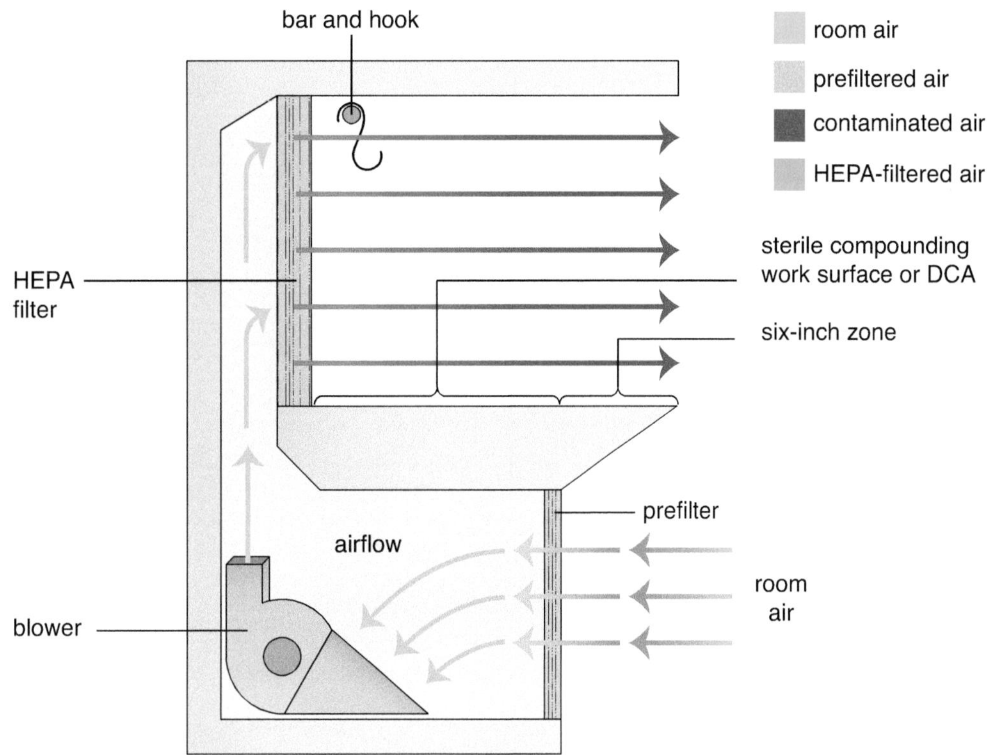

The prefilter is located in the front under the counter; it prevents large particles of dust, hair, and other debris in the buffer room air from entering the hood. The HEPA filter is located behind the back wall grill; it traps 99.97% of microbial contaminants, viruses, fungi, bacteria, and other pollutants that are 0.3 micrometers or larger.

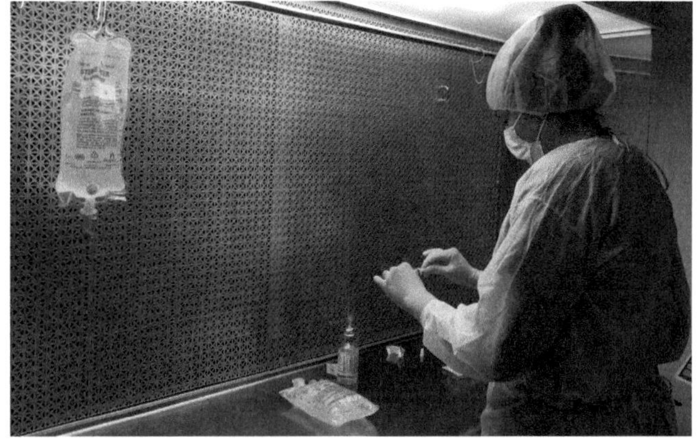

Technicians need to ensure that their hands are in the inner DCA, in a space where there is direct, uninterrupted airflow of filtered air, without blockage or shadowing.

Safety Alert

Sterile compounding personnel should avoid coughing and talking while working in the H-LAFW to avoid the risk of contaminating the environment during sterile product preparation.

When working at an H-LAFW, you must work at least six inches inside the semi-enclosed space to avoid compounding where the filtered air and room air mix at the counter's edge. The DCA is the space closest to the system's HEPA filter wall, the spot that receives an uninterrupted flow of sterile air during the compounding process.

Wherever the air is blocked or interrupted from having unidirectional airflow, a **turbulence of air is** created. Turbulence occurs where the PEC airflow meets the buffer room air, behind the supplies, and wherever the body of the person compounding is moving or blocking the air. A **zone of turbulence** is created between the DCA and the compounding technician in the act of compounding (see Figure 12.12). That is why technicians have to be very careful not to let their hands or supplies be closer to the air vent than the CSP or they will shadow, or block, the CSP from the cleansing airflow. To avoid any **shadowing**, supplies always go to the outer edges of the counter (another zone of turbulence) on either side of the technician, lined up in the order they will be used.

FIGURE 12.12
Overview of Horizontal Laminar Airflow Workbench

The technician preparing CSPs must work within the direct compounding area to maximize the protective filtered airflow of the H-LAFW.

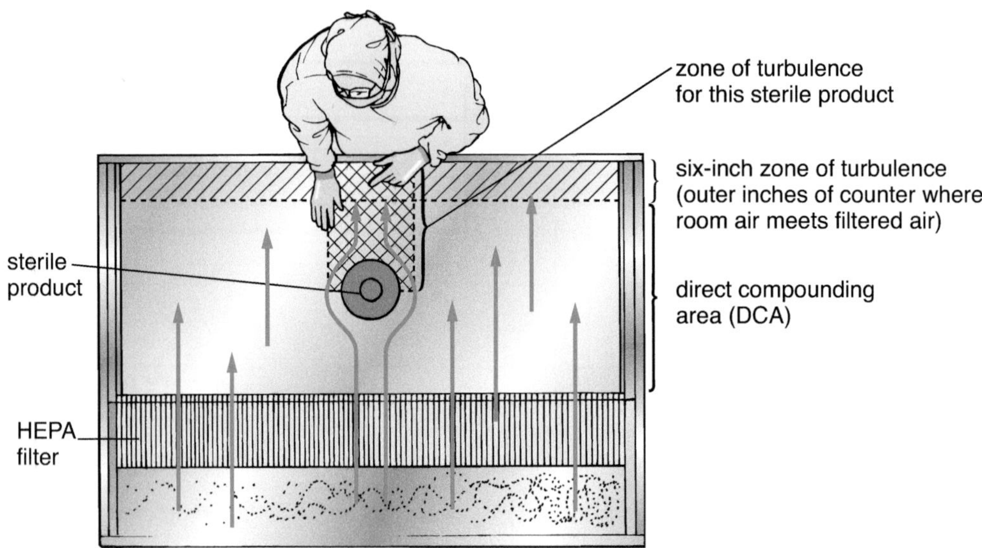

In cleaning, never allow fluid to come into contact with the grill. These actions may cause irreparable damage to the HEPA filter.

Aseptic Isolators

The **compounding aseptic isolators (CAI)** style PEC offers even more of a physical and aerodynamic barrier through an enclosing box shield around the DCA to protect the product, person, and environment. No breathing, coughing, or sneezing can affect the compound. As in all the other PECs, the DCA is maintained at ISO Class 5 air quality by the HEPA-filtered ventilation system in the unit. The shield has heavy-duty gloves projecting through it. The gloves provide the ability to work in the DCA without any exposure of the CSP to the buffer room air. CSP supplies and ingredients are moved inside the DCA via a transfer port (an enclosed movable chamber that is not fully sealed).

In a CAI, the airflow is from a top vent flowing downward, so the zone of turbulence is different from an H-LAFW. The technician must be careful not to block the airflow down to the CSP by putting fingers or tools above it.

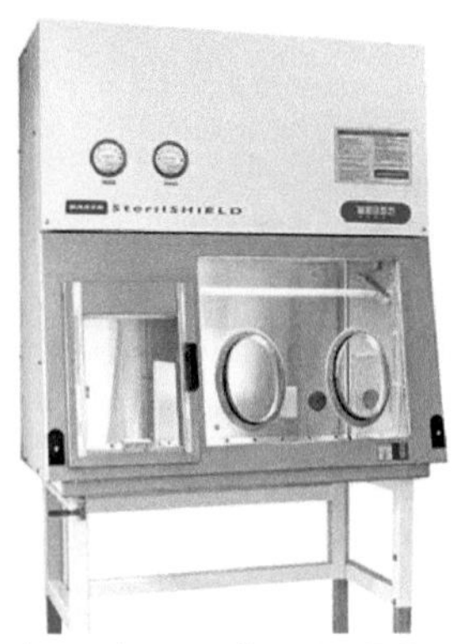

The Baker Steril-SHIELD® Barrier Isolator is just one example of a compounding aseptic isolator (CAI) for sterile cleanroom compounding. It offers a slanted shield with a top hinge to open for loading and unloading of tools and ingredients and for cleaning.

Cleaning and Maintenance of the Primary Engineering Controls

Technicians are responsible for maintaining the overall cleanliness of the PECs and the sterile compounding environment, following a routine cleaning schedule of these areas, as outlined in Table 12.4. The equipment must be cleaned before a shift, after spills, and at proper intervals prescribed by *USP* <797>, with each cleaning documented. Technicians must be properly garbed and use lint-free, aseptic hood-cleaning wipes, sterile water, and sterile 70% isopropyl a lcohol (IPA), and the PECs must be running during the cleaning.

TABLE 12.4 Cleaning in the Sterile Compounding Area

Site	Frequency
H-LAFW main work surface	At the beginning of each shift and before each batch, with the DCA cleaned every 30 minutes during continuous compounding periods, after spills, and when surface contamination is known or suspected
Counters and easily cleanable work surfaces	Daily
Floors	Daily
Walls	Monthly
Ceilings	Monthly
Storage shelving	Monthly

Cleaning the Horizontal Hood

The entire H-LAFW, including the protective sides, needs to be cleaned first with sterile water and then with the sterile 70% IPA for disinfecting. The cleaning follows a particular sequence, starting with wiping the hood's hang bar and hooks (if present), followed by the hood's ceiling, both sides of the hood, and, finally, the work surface. A separate wipe is used for each section.

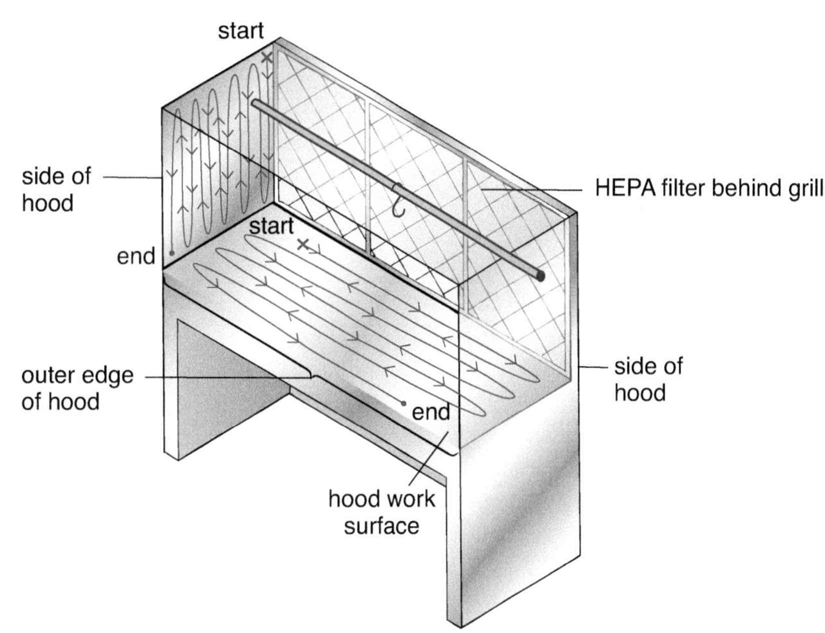

FIGURE 12.13 Procedures for Cleaning the H-LAFW

The cleaning of the horizontal H-LAFW is important in maintaining a sterile DCA and compounding work environment.

Each section also requires its own cleaning motion. The top (ceiling) is cleaned in a singular motion using minimally overlapping, side-to-side strokes, and the sides must have minimally overlapping, down-and-up strokes. The work surface comes last and is done similarly to the ceiling (see Figure 12.13). The back wall, where the grill covers the HEPA filter may be wiped lightly or it may not be cleaned to avoid harming the HEPA filter, depending upon the facility's SOPs and the hood manufacturer's specific instructions for grill cleaning.

Prefilter and HEPA Filter Maintenance

Sterile compounding personnel must replace all PEC prefilters every 30 days and document this process on a checklist located in the anteroom. The HEPA filter must be recertified every six months (usually by the manufacturer) or whenever the PEC is moved. This action must also be documented by sterile compounding technicians. If a PEC is turned off for installation, repair, maintenance, or relocation, then it should be recertified before being used again according to *USP* <797>. If you become a compounding technician, you will need to learn the requirements for each piece of equipment you use.

12.10 Keeping the Purpose of Aseptic Technique and Infection Control in Mind

In working against HAIs, fighting microbial contamination and infection must be a primary job of all healthcare workers and every hospital pharmacy technician, whether working in the general pharmacy or in the sterile compounding area. The work of the Infection Control Committee, the Joint Commission, and the *USP* all are aimed at providing standards and procedures to keep patients safe. The requirements of *USP* <797> for sterile compounding, aseptic technique, air quality and airflow in the cleanroom and PECs, and quality testing are designed to achieve these safety goals.

Understanding the reasons for the strict precautions and for the established protocols can help provide the lifesaving medications needed by patients. This background will also help you understand some of the processes involved in sterile and hazardous compounding that are presented in Chapter 13.

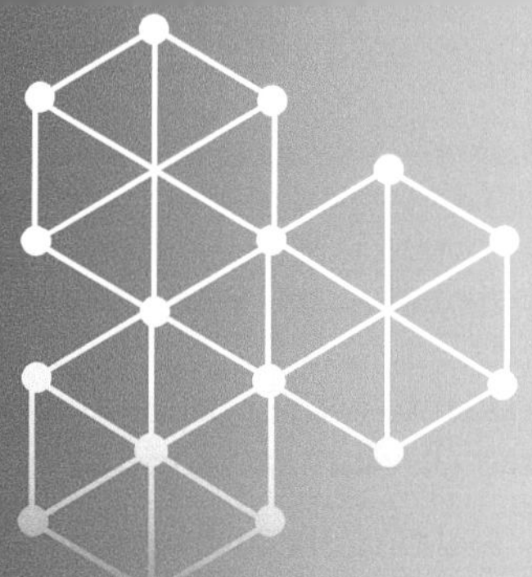

Review and Assessment

CHAPTER SUMMARY

- Bacteria, viruses, fungi, and protozoa are examples of microorganisms that can be harmful, or pathogenic.
- Pathogenic bacteria can mutate and become resistant to antibiotics.
- Common sources of contamination are touch, air, and water.
- The Center for Disease Control and Prevention (CDC) publishes guidelines to minimize the transmission of infectious disease, and the Infection Control
- Committee establishes and implements policies within the hospital.
- The major role of the Infection Control Committee (ICC) is the prevention of health-associated infections (HAIs), or healthcare-associated infections.
- Every healthcare worker, including an IV pharmacy technician, should have up-to-date immunizations.
- Various types of sterilization are available to kill microorganisms on medical instruments, devices, and surfaces, including heat (dry and moist), distillation, filtration, chemical (including gas), and ultraviolet light.
- *USP* Chapter <797> provides guidelines for sterile compounding.
- Sterile compounded products include small and large volume IV medications (including parenteral nutrition—peripheral and total): IV, IM, subq, and ID injections; miscellaneous noninjectable CSPs, sterile hazardous drugs (HDs), and nuclear drug products.
- Compounding sterile drugs requires a separate compounding area that includes an anteroom, buffer room, and primary engineering control units with direct compounding areas (DCAs).
- Each cleanroom area has a specific ISO air standard requirement: Class 8 for the anteroom, Class 7 for the buffer room, and Class 5 for a DCA.
- Sterile (nonhazardous) compounding requires positive pressure to push contaminants out of the buffer room.
- Numerous other *USP* chapters are significant for sterile compounding, including *USP* Chapters <1151>, <1160>, <1163>, <1176>, <1191>, and <1265>.
- The pharmacy technician needs specialized training before working in a sterile compounding environment.
- To minimize the risk of contamination, sterile compounding personnel must become trained in aseptic technique. Aseptic technique encompasses handwashing and hygiene, garbing, and disinfecting of supplies and PECs, among other steps, done in a special order.
- Proper aseptic practices, including aseptic handwashing and hygiene, are the most important ways to minimize touch contamination, especially in an IV compounding room.

- A pharmacy technician must become familiar with various syringes and needles as well as the components of each IV administration set, including the universal spike adapter, drip chamber, roll clamp, flexible tubing, and in-line filter.
- An in-line filter in the IV administration set for select medications helps to protect the patient against phlebitis.
- Primary engineering controls (PECs) come in various kinds of HEPA filtering systems, with horizontal airflow hoods generally used for sterile compounding.
- A zone of turbulence occurs wherever the filtered air meets resistance or blockage, so care must be taken to avoid placing fingers or tools between air vents and the CSP.
- The pharmacy technician must become familiar with the proper cleaning and maintenance of the H-LAFWs, including changing the prefilters.

CHECK YOUR UNDERSTANDING

Take a moment to review what you have learned in this chapter and answer the following questions.

1. HIV is caused by a
   a. bacterium.
   b. fungus.
   c. protozoan.
   d. virus.
2. The most common source of contamination is
   a. touch.
   b. air.
   c. water.
   d. dust.
3. The CDC recommends that all healthcare workers receive which vaccine?
   a. hepatitis A
   b. shingles
   c. influenza
   d. HIV
4. The CDC's Universal Precautions deal with infections by disease-causing microorganisms found in
   a. tap water and other liquid sources.
   b. blood and other bodily fluids.
   c. immediate-use medication vials.
   d. TPN solutions.
5. A major role of the Infection Control Committee is to
   a. approve antibiotics for the hospital formulary.
   b. purchase antibiotics.
   c. approve investigational studies of antibiotics.
   d. track hospital infection rates.
6. What type of sterilization uses an autoclave?
   a. heat sterilization
   b. chemical sterilization
   c. gas sterilization
   d. mechanical sterilization

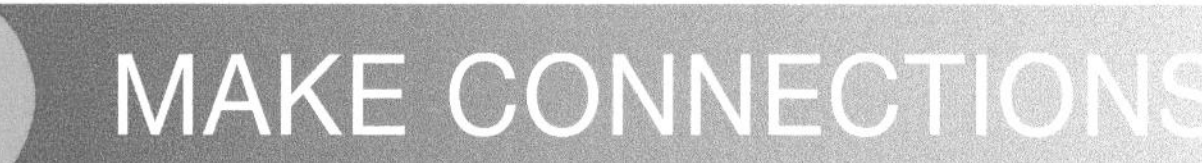

MAKE CONNECTIONS

1. Healthcare-associated infections (HAIs), also known as nosocomial infections, can occur in any setting but are especially prevalent in a hospital. Research and prepare a slide presentation on CDC HAIs recommendations. Be sure to include a references slide and address the following:
   - How does the CDC define HAIs?
   - Include types of infections and discuss MRSA infections.
   - What is the top CDC recommendation for prevention of HAIs that impact pharmacy technicians?
   - How effective are recent efforts to reduce these types of infections with common organisms?
2. To understand how to control infection, one must be keenly aware of the modes of microorganism transmission to avoid contamination during hospital work and the preparation of compounded sterile drug products. Write a short essay in which you outline the common sources of contamination and how an IV compounding technician can prevent and/or minimize each. When should the DCA surface be cleaned?

The online course includes additional review and assessment resources.

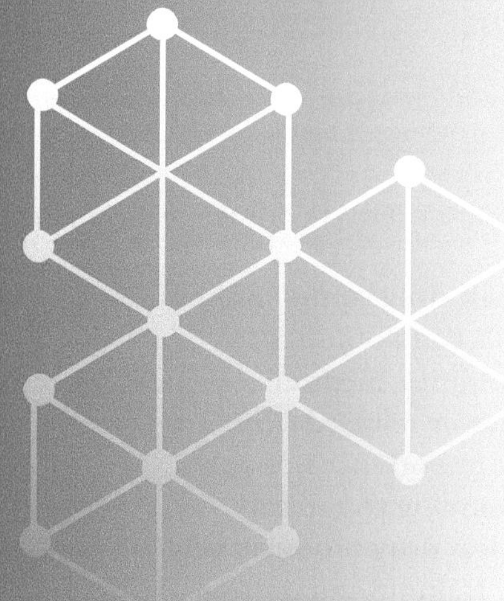

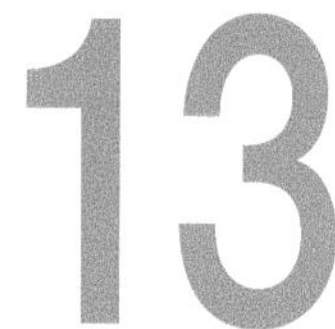

Sterile and Hazardous Compounding

Learning Objectives

1. Explain why an intravenous (IV) medication must have compatible characteristics to blood plasma in terms of pH value, osmotic pressure, and tonicity and have chemical compatibility with other medications. (Section 13.1)
2. Describe the sterile compounding process, which follows *USP* Chapter <797>. (Section 13.2)
3. Identify parts of a CSP medication order and label and the types of IV solutions. (Section 13.2)
4. State the functions of the Master Formulation Record and the Compounding Record. (Section 13.2)
5. Describe handle overfill concerns and calculate the infusion rates and 24-hour supply quantities for IV solutions. (Section 13.3)
6. Explain general principles in sterile and hazardous compounding with vials, ampules, and automated sterile compounding equipment. (Section 13.4)
7. Paraphrase the handling of premade parenteral products, including vial-and-bag systems and frozen intravenous sterile solutions. (Sections 13.5, 13.6, 13.7)
8. Define a hazardous drug and the categories of risks of exposure and the different levels of primary engineering controls for compounding them, according to *USP* Chapter <800>. (Section 13.8)
9. Describe the importance of a medical surveillance program for those preparing hazardous compounded sterile and nonsterile products. (Section 13.8)
10. Discuss the key techniques for receiving, storing, handling, delivering, and disposing of hazardous drugs and ingredients, and the function and the contents of a spill kit. (Section 13.8)
11. Define personal protective equipment and primary engineering controls for preparing hazardous drugs. (Section 13.8)
12. Understand the role of the USP's evolving standards in nuclear pharmaceutical compounding. (Section 13.9)

ASHP/ACPE Accreditation Standards
To view the *ASHP/ACPE Accreditation Standards* addressed in this chapter, refer to Appendix B.

In the hospital pharmacy, sterile and hazardous compounded drug products are used on a regular basis. Therefore, having an overview of the nature of the compounded sterile preparations (i) and the compounding processes entailed in their preparation is useful.

This chapter describes the required chemical properties of CSPs and the most common parenteral solutions. Some of the processes that will be explored include calculations of overfill and infusion rates, adding medications into solutions with vials and ampules, and operating automated compounding devices.

The advantages of commercially available vial-and-bag systems and frozen IV solutions for specific drugs and situations will also be considered.

Hazardous drug compounding shares many aspects of sterile drug compounding because many hazardous preparations must be sterile. Hazardous compounding, however, requires additional training, equipment, supplies, procedures, medical surveillance, and cleanup regulations, which are covered in the newly released ***USP* Chapter <800>**. These guidelines for hazardous drugs stress the importance not only of protecting the patients but of protecting yourself as a compounding technician from the toxicity of hazardous drugs. The compounding of nuclear drug products falls under the extremely hazardous category and requires even more training and protection. With the overview in this chapter, you will have a better understanding of some of the fields of specialization that you could choose from within the institutional setting.

13.1 The Nature of Compounded Sterile Products

Safety Alert

It is essential that the base solution selected is compatible with the medication chosen. The measurements must be calculated correctly in order to maintain the capability between the diluent and the solute and between the CSP and the patient's blood.

CSPs are often called "admixtures" because they are made by starting with a base solution that is compatible with human blood and adding medications and other ingredients to it. The body is primarily an aqueous or water-containing entity, so most CSPs and parenteral solutions consist of ingredients added to a sterile-water medium, a **normal saline (NS)** solution (0.9% sodium chloride with sterile water), or a base dextrose solution (sugar and sterile water mixture as in D5W). You, as a sterile compounding technician, will then add ingredients that include medications, electrolytes, vitamins, and nutrients. **Electrolyte solutions** contain micronutrients that carry important electrical energy for cellular function.

To assimilate properly into the patient's blood supply, CSPs must be sterile while having chemical properties or characteristics that do not damage blood cells or vessels or alter the blood's own chemical makeup. In other words, the CSPs must be compatible with blood in order to be safely administered. If they are not, they may cause a patient to have an adverse reaction. Sterile compounding technicians need a basic knowledge of these chemical properties to understand why the concentrations and measurements to compound a CSP must be followed so precisely—they have to be formulated to address these key necessities of the human body.

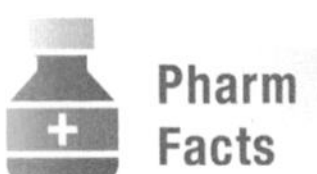

Pharm Facts

Sodium chloride (0.9%) was originally called "indifferent fluid" because it had properties similar to human blood and did not cause visible cell rupture. It is now referred to as normal saline and is isotonic.

The chemical properties that must be matched to human blood include pH value, osmotic pressure, tonicity, and compatibility. Each of these concepts requires some explanation. As a sterile compounding technician, you will not be making these determinations, but each compounding pharmacist, manufacturer of IV ingredients, and Master Formulation Record considers these characteristics in the "recipes" for the parenteral solutions.

pH Value

The degree of acidity (acid) or alkalinity (base) of a solution is known as its **pH value**. Common household acids are vinegar and citrus juices. Bases include baking soda. All substances are on the spectrum from acid to base. Too intense an acid or a base can cause irritation or damage to the body, which is why it hurts if you get orange or lemon juice or baking soda in a cut.

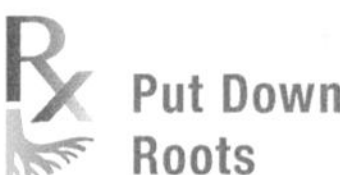
Put Down Roots

Osmosis comes from the Greek word *ōsmos*, which means "impulsion" or "push."

Most high-school chemistry classes teach pH value by using litmus paper to test various solutions on a rating range of 0 to 14, with 0 as the most acidic. If the litmus paper turns pink when dipped, the solution is acidic—with a pH value less than 7.0. With a dark pink, lemon juice has a rating of 2.2; common white vinegar has 2.4; tomatoes, 4.5; and milk, 6.6.

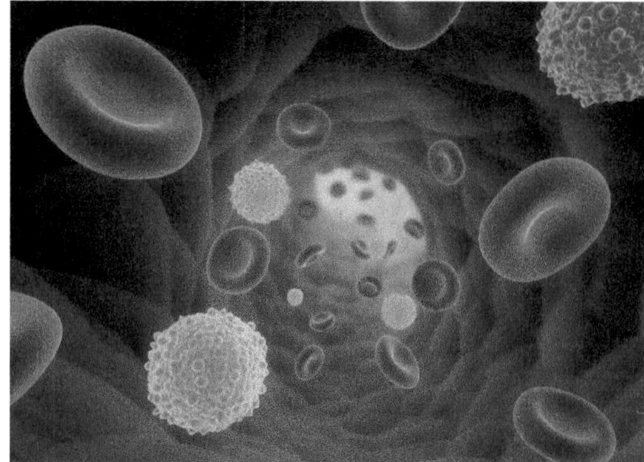
Blood plasma has a pH value of 7.4 and an osmolarity near 285 mOsm/L. Most IV solutions have similar osmolarity so as not to damage red blood cells.

If the litmus paper turns blue when dipped, then the solution is alkaline—with a pH value of more than 7.0. Baking soda (sodium bicarbonate) has a rating of 8.3; milk of magnesia has 10.5; ammonia, 11.0; and lye, 13, which turns litmus paper a very dark blue.

Blood plasma is near the very middle with a pH of 7.4; therefore, it is slightly alkaline. IV solutions with a pH near neutral (or near 7.0) are less likely to affect the natural pH of the blood.

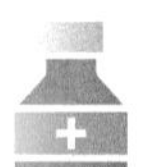
Pharm Facts

In laboratories, the osmotic pressure of solutions is measured on various kinds of osmometers. One type of osmotic measurement uses osmoles per liter (Osm/L) or milliosmoles per liter (mOsm/L).

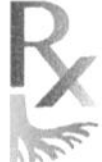
Put Down Roots

The Greek word *isos*, means "equal to" or "the same as," and *iso-osmotic* means equal to the osmotic pressure of blood plasma, which is considered the universal normal for all human solutions. *Isotonic* comes from the additional Greek word tonos, which means "tone" or "level."

Osmotic Pressure

Another key factor in parenteral solutions is managing osmosis. **Osmosis** is the natural flow of molecules in a solution through semi-permeable cellular or organ walls to equalize the concentrations of minerals on both sides. Proper **osmotic pressure** is needed to maintain a state of balanced movement across cellular membranes so as not to burst any membranes from undue pressure. Solutions cannot be too concentrated with solutes (dissolved ingredients) because the pressure to move those solutes through the cellular walls too fast will burst the walls.

Generally speaking, an IV solution must be **iso-osmotic**, meaning that the solution should have the same number of particles in solution per unit volume producing the same osmotic pressure as blood plasma, or blood fluid. IV solutions with too high a concentration of solute particles can cause blockages, so these solutions need to be diluted or administered to larger veins. These highly concentrated solutions can also be administered in a small volume parenteral (SVP) solution via an IV piggyback line that flows into a large volume parenteral (LVP) primary line of sterile normal saline or medication.

Complicated chemical equations are used to calculate different measurements of a solution's osmotic characteristics. **Osmolarity** refers to the concentration of all molecules—those that cross the cellular membranes and those that do not—in a volume of fluid. Osmolarity is measured in milliosmoles per liter (mOsm/L). The osmolarity of blood plasma, for instance, is approximately 275–300 mOsm/L. The osmolarity of a solution affects whether water flows out of a cell or into a cell to equalize osmotic pressure, or remains equal in the osmotic exchanges of water and solutes.

Tonicity

Blood has to have a certain level of water content to be healthy, as do organs and individual cells. Low water levels indicate problems, such as dehydration or high glucose levels associated with uncontrolled diabetes.

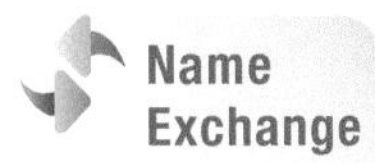

Maintenance solutions typically refer to fluids used for maintenance therapy. Maintenance therapy replaces the ongoing losses of water and electrolytes under normal physiologic conditions via urine, sweat, respiration, and stool.

Tonicity is the directional flow pattern of water in cells based on concentrations and osmotic pressure within their environments. The tonicity of a solution determines whether it catalyzes an inward flow, an outward flow, or a balanced molecule exchange between the inside and outside of a cellular wall. A solution's tonicity is classified as isotonic, hypotonic, or hypertonic (see Figure 13.1 and Table 13.1).

Isotonic Solution

An **isotonic solution** has a similar concentration of solute particles to blood plasma, prompting an exchange of water molecules through the semi-permeable cell walls with equal flow moving inward and out. There is no net loss or gain of water or electrolytes in the cells. An isotonic solution that has a similar pH to blood will flow even more easily through the system without damage. Examples of isotonic solutions are NS (0.9% sodium chloride) and lactated Ringer's solution (a parenteral nutritional solution). At times, a pharmacist may need to check and adjust the tonicity of parenteral preparations to ensure that they are isotonic or nearly isotonic.

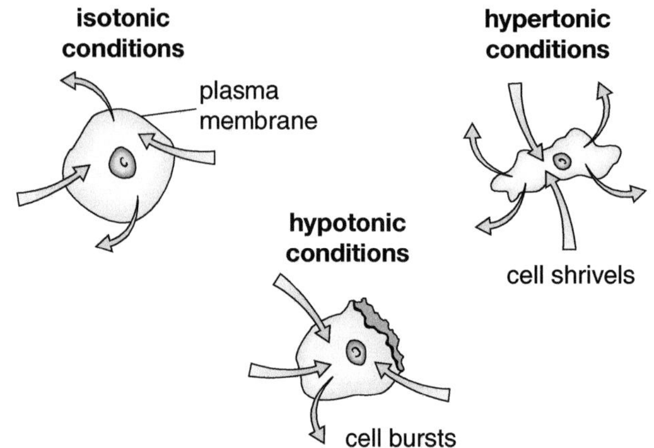

FIGURE 13.1 Tonic Conditions in Cells

When a cell is bathed in an isotonic solution, the amount of water entering and leaving is the same. In hypotonic solutions, more water enters a cell and may result in a cell rupture. In hypertonic solutions, more water leaves a cell and may result in cell shriveling and dehydration.

TABLE 13.1 **Common Parenteral Solutions and Tonicity**

Tonicity	Solution	Osmolarity per Liter
Isotonic solutions	Dextrose 2.5% in 0.45% NaCl ($D_{2.5}W$ in ½ NS)	280 mOsm/1000 mL
	Dextrose 5% in sterile water (D_5W)	300 mOsm/1000 mL
	0.9% NaCl (normal saline [NS])	310 mOsm/1000 mL
	Lactated Ringer's solution (LR)	275 mOsm/1000 mL
Hypertonic solutions	Dextrose 5% in 0.45% NaCl (D_5W in ½ NS)	405 mOsm/1000 mL
	Dextrose 5% in 0.9% NaCl (D_5W in NS)	560 mOsm/1000 mL
	Dextrose 10% in sterile water ($D_{10}W$)	600 mOsm/1000 mL
	3%, 5%, 14.6%, and 23.4% NaCl concentrates	Varies
Hypotonic (hydrating) solutions	0.45% NaCl (½ NS)	155 mOsm/1000 mL
	Dextrose 2.5% in sterile water ($D_{2.5}W$)	140 mOsm/1000 mL

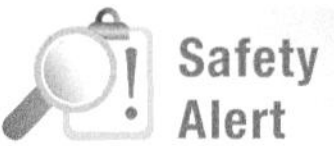

Safety Alert

Patient recipients of hypotonic and hypertonic solutions must be closely monitored for potential risks, as these types of solutions are short-term therapies to quickly rebalance a system. Hypotonic solutions can cause a potentially life-threatening electrolyte imbalance. Hypertonic solutions can cause collapse of cells and veins.

Hypotonic Solution

A **hypotonic solution** has fewer solute particles than blood plasma and cells so water is drawn into the cells to equalize the differing concentration, causing the cells to swell. The directional flow of molecules is *into* the cell. This is important for individuals who are dehydrated, such as those with diabetic ketoacidosis or those who are low on minerals. The flow should be inward to replenish the depleted cells. An example of a hypotonic solution is 0.45% sodium chloride (sometimes called $^1/_2$ NS).

Hypertonic Solution A **hypertonic solution** has more solute particles than the blood plasma and cells themselves, so water is drawn *out* of the cells, which causes them to shrivel. This can be helpful to reduce swelling in cells or to draw toxic elements out of the cells. On the rare occasions when hypertonic solutions must be administered to patients, these infusions must be done cautiously and gradually by an experienced nurse or a physician, or the infusions can cause congestive heart failure. Examples of hypertonic solutions are TPN solutions, 20%–50% dextrose in water (D20W to D50W), and 3%–5% sodium chloride (3% saline to 5% saline). Hypertonic solutions often require a slower infusion rate or administration via a larger vein to prevent phlebitis (inflammation of the veins).

Chemical Compatibility

Finally, each compounded sterile IV solution must have chemical compatibility with the blood, with other medicated solutions in the body, and among its own ingredients. **Chemical compatibility** is the ability of two or more base components (or additives within a solution) to combine without resulting in significant physical or chemical reactions to the components or the encountered solutions. For example, fat emulsions are incompatible with electrolyte solutions. Trissel's *Stability of Compounded Formulations* is an excellent reference for checking IV drug incompatibilities. The book also provides stability and storage information in monographs on many compounded drug formulations.

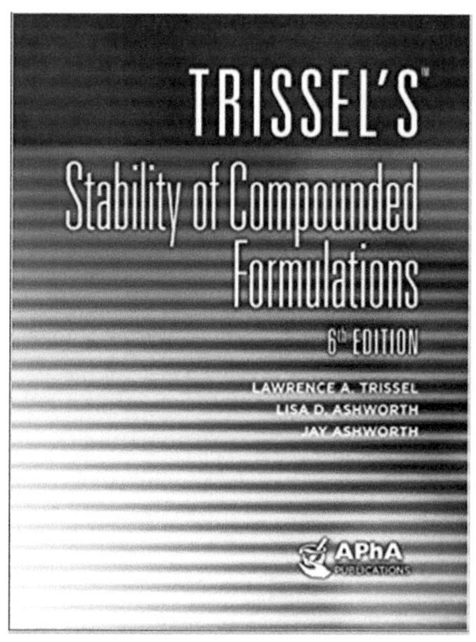

Practice Tip

Product package inserts also provide information on the properties of each medication and directions on how to mix and use it to create and maintain compatibilities.

13.2 Overview of the Sterile Compounding Process and Components

As noted, there are many steps in the sterile compounding process, many of which are complicated. The process begins with the medication order, which generates a drug utilization review and a label with all its components. The process ends with verification by the pharmacist and delivery for nurse administration. It is helpful to get a sense of the full sweep of the steps and components before exploring each more closely. Table 13.2 provides a summary.

TABLE 13.2 Overview of Steps in Sterile Compounding

This is a general outline of process steps for sterile compounding in a two-room cleanroom area. Each facility is slightly different, based on its layout and standard operating procedures. It is essential to take a sterile compounding course with practice labs to get a real sense of the detailed steps involved. *USP* Chapter <797> is the ultimate source for all sterile compounding guidelines.

1. In the main hospital pharmacy, receive medication orders and labels, run drug utilization review, and the pharmacist will do the initial calculations from the Master Formulation Record.
2. Receive pharmacy verifications, do any remaining calculations, and initiate a compounding or log record (may be done in the pharmacy or the anteroom, depending on area procedures; outerwear must be removed before entering the anteroom).
3. Wipe down supplies, and follow aseptic techniques for garbing and handwashing.
4. Collect compounding supplies, ingredients, and primary engineering control (PEC) cleaning materials, and transport them into the buffer room on a disinfected cart.
5. In the buffer room, disinfect hands and don sterile gloves.
6. Clean the PEC per manufacturing directions and *USP* <797>.
7. Compound the CSPs in the PEC according to *USP* <797>; processes often include withdrawing medications from vials or ampules and then injecting them into IV base solutions or containers.
8. Complete a quality check of each CSP by comparing the label and the medication order and doing a visual check.
9. The pharmacist will verify the final CSP, label, and ingredients in the buffer room or the anteroom before applying the label and any auxiliary labels.
10. The CSP will be delivered to the nursing unit for administration.

The Medication Orders and Sterile Compounding Considerations

Medication orders for CSPs are delivered to the hospital pharmacy from the physician via handheld devices, computers, faxes, pneumatic tubes (like in banks), or hand delivery (see samples in Figure 13.2). Once the hospital pharmacy receives the CSP order, a pharmacist (or in certain facilities, a senior technician) enters the order into the pharmacy's computer system. However, many hospitals utilize computerized physician order entry (CPOE) and the prescriber may have already entered the order into the computer system. Either way, the entered order prompts software to run a Drug Utilization Review (DUR). The DUR will check the order against the patient's medical history and medication profile to alert the technician of any allergies, cross-sensitivities, drug-drug or drug-food interactions, duplicate therapies, or contraindications.

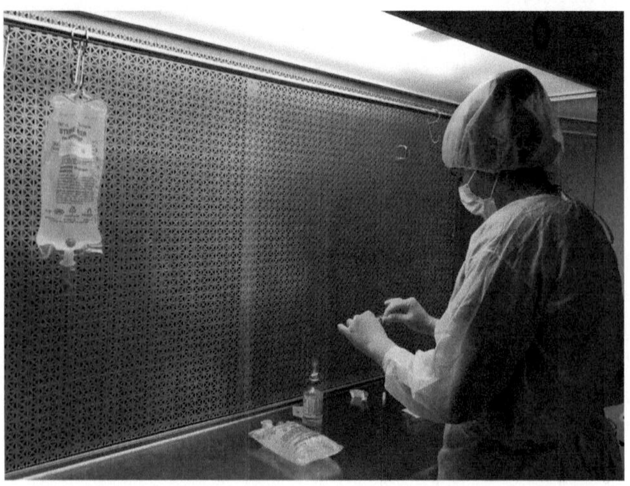

Sterile compounding requires special training and equipment.

The pharmacist resolves all computer-generated warnings and either modifies the order with the physician or approves it, and the sterile compounding labels are generated. Rather than just issuing a single label for the medication order, a separate label is issued for each individualized dose to be compounded. These are provided to the sterile compounding technician in the pharmacy.

FIGURE 13.2
Common Physician's Orders for Parenteral Solutions

These are medication orders with sterile compounding sigs and abbreviations. To translate, see Table 13.3.

℞ cefoxitin 1 g IV every 6 h over 24 hours

℞ nafcillin 1 g IV every 4 h

℞ penicillin 2 million units IV every 4 h

℞ add 100 units Humulin R regular insulin to 500 mL NS @ 20 mL/hour (label ℞ concentration 0.2 units/mL)

℞ begin magnesium sulfate 5 g in 500 mL NS to run over 5 hours × 1 dose only

℞ change IV fluids to 0.45 NS with 20 mEq KCl @ 125 mL/hour

In addition to the patient-specific medication orders, the sterile compounding technician is also generally responsible for preparing all of the ongoing CSPs needed for a day. This is called the daily IV run, or the **batch**—a 24-hour supply of every CSP for each patient in a unit, wing, or the hospital. (A "batch" can also mean the preparation of specified amounts of CSPs for storage and future use.) Labels are generated for each dosage in the batch.

Since parenteral solutions are the core products ordered in sterile compounding, you must become familiar with the different kinds, the common ways of compounding them, and the abbreviations for terms used for parenteral solutions (see Table 13.3).

Three basic forms of parenteral IV solutions may be ordered; the large volume parenteral, small volume parenteral, and parenteral nutrition solutions. The large and small volume parenterals are the most commonly ordered. There are key distinguishing features that affect how each parenteral is compounded and administered.

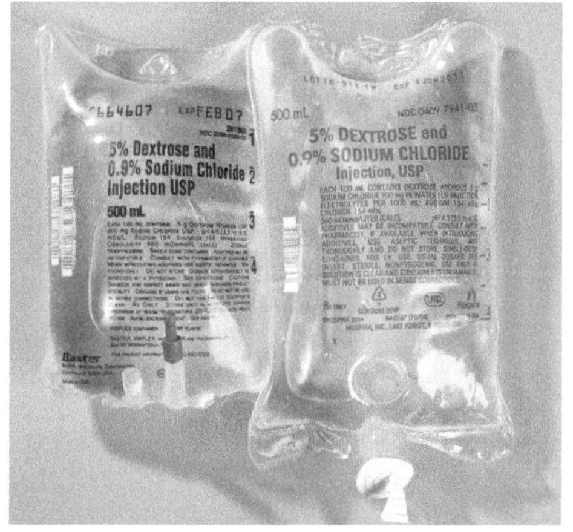

Dextrose 5% in normal saline (0.9%) is a common 500 mL large-volume parenteral IV (as is the 1 L [1,000 mL size]).

Large-Volume Parenteral (LVP) Solutions

These solutions, which are administered through primary IV bags and tubing sets, replenish fluids and provide drugs, electrolytes, and nutrients to patients. **Large-volume parenteral (LVP) solutions** are generally administered over a prolonged period that ranges from 8 to 24 hours, so they are available in 250 mL, 500 mL, and 1,000 mL IV bag sizes. Since electrolytes carry important electrical energy for cellular function, an LVP usually contains one or more electrolytes that have been added to the IV solution. Potassium chloride is the most common electrolyte, but other salts of potassium, as well as magnesium or calcium, can be added based on the requirements of the individual patient. Other common additives to LVPs include trace elements, vitamins, andminerals. (See Figure 13.3 for a sample of an LVP label.)

FIGURE 13.3
Large-Volume Parenteral Solution Label

****Large-Volume Parenteral****

Memorial Hospital

Pt. Name: Van Ingen, Will **Room:** Neuro ICU
Pt. ID#: 8873662 **Rx#:** 74521

Potassium Chloride 30 mEq
Lactated Ringer's 1000 mL
Rate: 40 mL/hr

Date Prepared _____ Time prepared _____
RPh _____ BUD/Expiration Date _____
Tech _____ BUD/Expiration Time _____

Keep refrigerated – warm to room temperature before use.

TABLE 13.3 Commonly Used IV Products and Abbreviations

Component		Abbreviation
Fluids	2.5% dextrose in water	$D_{2.5}W$
	5% dextrose in water	D_5W
	5% dextrose and lactated Ringer's solution	D_5RL or D_5LR
	10% dextrose in water	$D_{10}W$
	5% dextrose and 0.9% sodium chloride	D_5NS
	2.5% dextrose and 0.45% sodium chloride	$D_{2.5}$ ½NS
	5% dextrose and 0.45% sodium chloride	D_5 ½NS
	0.9% sodium chloride; normal saline	NS
	0.45% sodium chloride	½NS
	Lactated Ringer's solution	RL or LR
	Sterile water for injection	SW for injection or SWFI
	Bacteriostatic water for injection	BW for injection or BWFI
	Sterile water for irrigation	SW for irrigation
	Normal saline for irrigation	NS for irrigation
Electrolytes	Potassium chloride	KCl
	Potassium phosphate	K phos or KPO_4
	Potassium acetate	K acet
	Sodium phosphate	Na phos or $NaPO_4$
	Sodium chloride	NaCl

continues

Practice Tip

Depending upon the patient, medications may also be added to an LVP, such as insulin or famotidine (Pepcid).

TABLE 13.3 Commonly Used IV Products and Abbreviations–*Continued*

Component		Abbreviation
Additives	Multivitamin for injection	MVI
	Trace elements (combinations of essential trace elements such as chromium, manganese, and copper)	TE
	Zinc (a trace element)	Zn
	Selenium (a trace element)	Se

One common LVP solution that contains a specific mixture of electrolytes—called **lactated Ringer's solution (LR)**—is used often for fluid restoration after blood loss from injury, surgery, or burns. LR is a mixture that includes sodium chloride, sodium lactate, potassium chloride, and calcium chloride. It may be used alone or in combination with a dextrose solution. Other types of medications that may be administered by LVP include nutritional solutions and many chemotherapy drugs, both of which will be explained in more depth later in the chapter.

Small-Volume Parenteral (SVP) Solutions

Because this IV solution has less volume and contains a concentrated prescribed medication, it is either administered directly to the patient by being syringed into the port of the primary IV line or "piggybacked" into the IV tubing of an LVP using a secondary IV line (as described and diagrammed in Chapter 12).

The majority of **small-volume parenteral (SVP) solutions** prepared by sterile compounding personnel are IV piggybacks (IVPBs). They are comprised of medication injected into a minibag (such as 25, 50, 100, or 150 mL) of a base solution like sterile NS or D5W. The solution volume needed is dependent upon the drug's dose and solubility, according to the manufacturer's recommendations or Master Formulation Record. (See Figure 13.4 for a sample SVP label.)

An SVP is typically administered intermittently over a short period ranging from 10 minutes to an hour (sometimes longer), based on the physician's or manufacturer's recommendations. Since the IVPB line is connected to a port in the primary IV line, this secondary line can be turned on and off for the required periods of intermittent drug administrations. To obtain a more gradual release over an extended time, some medications may be mixed in the LVP to obtain a more dilute concentration, thus avoiding possible phlebitis and patient discomfort.

Parenteral Nutrition Solutions

These IV solutions are specialty LVPs. Parenteral nutrition (PN) is a means of supplying needed nourishment to patients who cannot or will not take in sufficient (or any) food or water through their mouths or port in the GI system. Parenteral nutrition can be **peripheral parenteral nutrition (PPN)** or **total parenteral nutrition (TPN)**. PPN provides partial nutritional support for shorter-term hospital stays; TPN provides complete and sustaining nutritional support for patients who are unconscious or who cannot receive food, water, or medication by mouth (designated on the medical order as *npo*). This inability to take nutrition by the mouth can be the result of surgery, infection, or inflammation in the GI tract. TPN administration is generally for extended stays in the hospital (or sometimes even at home with home health care).

FIGURE 13.4
Small-Volume Parenteral Solution Label

****IV Piggyback****

Memorial Hospital

Pt. Name: Ogard, Christopher **Room:** 560
Pt. ID#: 898372 **Rx#:** 03127

Ampicillin 500 mg
Sodium Chloride 0.9% (NS) 50 mL
Rate: over 20 min

Date prepared ______ Time prepared ______ Administration time ______
RPh ______ BUD/Expiration Date ______
Tech ______ BUD/Expiration Time ______

Keep refrigerated – warm to room temperature before use.

Sterile Compounding Label Components

The medication label provides patient identification information, such as the patient's name and ID number (or bar code), and the patient's hospital room or unit number. In addition, the sterile compounding labels must also contain very specific information about the product, dose, dosing interval or infusion rate, storage requirements, beyond-use date (or expiration date if premanufactured), and initials of preparers.

Often the label includes directions. The label and formatting will differ among hospital pharmacies and software vendors, but labels generally include information contained in Table 13.4.

TABLE 13.4 Sterile Compounded Labeling Requirements

Each compounded product must have affixed upon it a label that encompasses most or all of the following information:

- medication order number
- name and identification (ID) number (or bar code) of the patient for whom the medication is prescribed
- name, concentration, and amount of base solution (such as *D_5W 500 mL*)
- brand or generic name and amount (or concentration) of each drug or additive in the compound (such as *potassium chloride 20 mEq*)
- infusion rate (such as *100 mL/hr* or *infuse over 20 min*), dosing interval, and/or administration time
- form and route of administration (such as *for intravenous administration*)
- beyond-use date (or manufacturer's expiration date)
- storage requirements (such as *keep refrigerated* or *protect from light*)
- auxiliary labels or special instructions (such as *shake well before administering; warm to room temperature before administering;* or *for wound irrigation only*)
- any device-specific instructions (such as *MINI-BAG Plus must be activated and mixed prior to administering*)
- preparer's and pharmacist's initials
- address and contact information of the infusion pharmacy or compounder if the CSP is to be sent outside of the facility in which it was compounded

Note: Consult the hospital pharmacy's policies and procedures manual for an institution's specific labeling requirements.

Solution, Drug, and Additive Information

Each CSP requires a base solution and additives, and the label must mention both. For the base solutions, you need the name, concentration, and amount. For instance, the base solution listed as 0.9% NS 1 L (1,000 mL) indicates the concentration (0.9%, or 900 mg of saline per 100 mL of fluid), the type of solution (NS), and the amount (1L or 1,000 mL).

The label must also list each additive and the amount of each. A compounded product may have more than one additive. For example, a TPN solution may have as many as fifteen or more additives, including electrolytes, minerals, vitamins, and trace elements (and occasionally antacids).

Administration Directions for Infusion Rates, Intervals, and Times

The medication administration time or **infusion rate** (the rate in mL/hour that it takes for the IV bag to be fully infused in the patient) may be indicated by the medication order written by the physician, or it may be determined by consulting the manufacturer's package insert. If the medication's administration is not ordered by the physician and the package insert is unavailable, the pharmacist may find this information by consulting one of the pharmacy reference manuals, such as the *Handbook on Injectable Drugs* (available in print or digital online format).

For CSPs, the most common medication timing information for LVPs is noted as the infusion rate (see Figure 13.3 earlier). The physician usually orders an infusion rate for an LVP in milliliters per hour, such as *125 mL per hour*. At this rate, one liter (1,000 mL) of the LVP will run for approximately eight hours.

Occasionally, the physician will order an IV infusion rate based on the amount of drug per hour. For instance, the infusion rate of heparin is often ordered in *units* per hour, such as *1,000 units per hour*. Once the administration time or infusion rate has been calculated, the pharmacy is then responsible for ensuring this information is added to the label. (The calculations of infusion rates comes later in this chapter.)

In general, only IV piggyback (IVPB) and IV push (drug injection directly into a vein via syringe) medications require a specific administration time as in Figures 13.4 and 13.5. For instance, cefazolin 1 g IVPB may be administered at a specific time using an IV pump. A phenytoin sodium (Dilantin) 500 mg IV push is administered by a nurse or physician who slowly injects over a 10-minute period the solution into the patient's IV line at specified 6-hour intervals. The administration time varies widely between different types of medications and the route of administration or dosage of the drug.

FIGURE 13.5
Syringe Label

****Syringe****

Pt. Name: Decoteau, Kaya **Room:** ICU-7
ID#: S114971441 **Rx#:** 17725909

Ceftriaxone 250 mg/2 mL 1% Lidocaine Hydrochloride

For IM administration only

Preparation Day/Time ______________________
Administration Day/Time ______________________
Expiration Day/Time ________ Tech ______ RPh ______

The label may also indicate that the entire solution needs to be administered (to address potential overfill issues, which will be described later in this chapter).

Storage Requirements

Storage requirements (such as *refrigerate, keep frozen—thaw immediately prior to administration, do not refrigerate*, or *protect from light*) must also be included on the label, per the medication order, Master Formulation Record, or manufacturer's instructions. The storage conditions of the CSP will often dictate the beyond-use dating along with *USP* Chapter <797> guidelines. Typically, sterile compounds stored in a refrigerator or freezer have a longer beyond-use date than those stored at room temperature. Many IV medications must be refrigerated (or even frozen) to maintain their ability to provide the full effects for therapy. Once a CSP is thawed, it cannot be refrozen. Other IV solutions must be covered with an amber-colored bag to protect the drug from exposure to light. An example of a light-sensitive agent is an IV infusion of the antifungal drug amphotericin B.

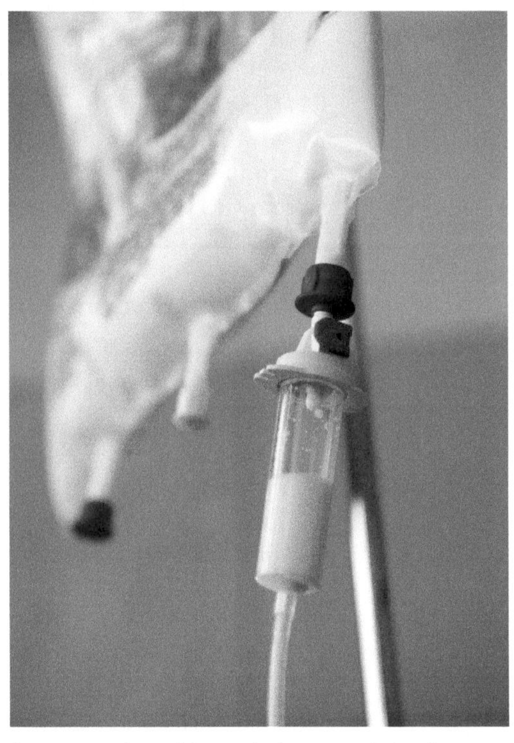

A parenteral nutrition solution containing fatty acids (Liposyn) gives the IV a white color. The solution should be refrigerated for storage.

Beyond-Use Dating

For each manufactured IV solution, the label bears an expiration date, which is based on the product's stability under the designated storage conditions. However, once a technician in a sterile compounding facility adds a medication like penicillin to a manufactured stock IV bag, that IV bag is now a CSP, and it requires a calculated beyond-use date (BUD) based on *USP* <797> guidelines, which is far shorter than the manufacturer's expiration date. The BUD is the date *and time* after which the CSP may not be used as determined from the day and time the sterile compound was prepared and how it was stored. The drug's stability, or its ability to maintain integrity in its compounded form, is affected by the number of ingredients as well as the storage conditions.

Usually the label software automatically generates the BUD, but when using the Master Formulation Record, the BUD will need to be determined by the technician and checked by the pharmacist. For most CSPs, the beyond-use dating is counted in hours rather than in days and months. The possibility of microbes multiplying within a CSP increases over time as the physical and chemical stability and integrity of the product decrease. **Preservatives**, or ingredients to extend integrity, are not in single dose vials. The determination of BUDs is complicated, and one must refer to the *USP* Chapter <797>. The guidelines consider the environment where the compound was made, the starting ingredients, and the storage conditions of the CSP. It will be important to always read and follow the most current *USP* Chapter <797> guidelines.

Auxiliary Labels

In addition to the compounding label, the pharmacist can recommend that auxiliary labels be added to call the nursing staff's attention to unique conditions of the CSP, such as an unusual administration route (like an epidural or via a central catheter); proper storage conditions; special IV tubing; a change in administration procedure or dosage concentration; or a coupling with commercially available products. Special high-alert medications like heparin and cancer drugs *require* such stickers to minimize any chance of a medication administration error. Table 13.5 presents some examples of the many auxiliary labels available.

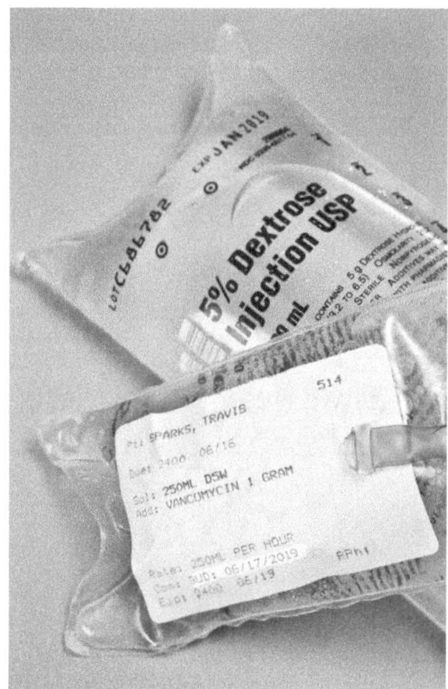

Remember, expiration dates are used for manufactured products while BUDs are used for CSPs, according to USP guidelines.

Accountability on Label

Every CSP label must also identify the compounding personnel with their initials in the provided blanks to allow traceability and accountability.

The blank headings vary widely among institutions. In some facilities, the label may provide separate blanks, one preceded by *prep by*, *preparer*, or *tech*, and the other blank preceded by *checked by* or *RPh*. Some labels simply have blank spaces where both the technician and pharmacist must sign their names.

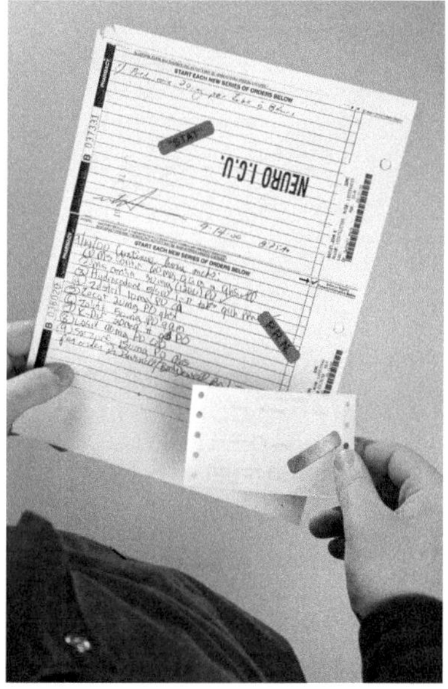
The IV technician is comparing the CSP label to the medication order to verify accuracy.

Master Formulation Record

Some pharmacy labeling programs provide sterile compounding instructions directly on the label. For instance, the label might contain instructions that direct the IV technician to draw up 5 mL of a 1.36 mEq/mL concentration of calcium chloride 10% solution in order to provide a 6.8 mEq dose of the medication. (See Chapter 6 on calculating milliequivalents.)

However, per the guidelines in *USP* Chapter <797>, a **Master Formulation Record** (or control record) must be followed when the labels do not provide compounding instructions and also when CSPs are prepared *in a batch for multiple patients*. This information is contained in the pharmacy software. As in nonsterile compounding, the Master Formulation Record is like a tested and approved recipe that lists the ingredients, specific procedures, equipment to be used, and testing required for each specific kind of CSP (see Table 13.6).

TABLE 13.5 Auxiliary Labels Commonly Used in Sterile Compounding

Auxiliary Labels with Blanks for Required Information

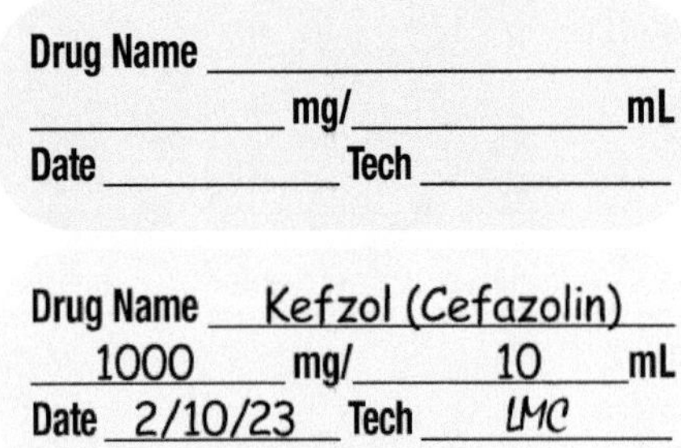

These labels are for powdered drug vials: one label is blank and one is completed by the sterile compounding technician, who attaches the label to the powdered drug vial upon dilution; in addition to recording the drug name, the final drug concentration, and the date and time of dilution, the technician diluting the powdered drug records their initials.

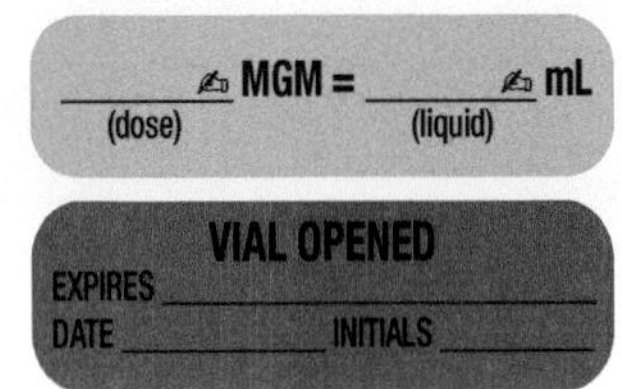

Some facilities use two auxiliary labels to provide information similar to that provided on the larger labels above.

Preprinted Auxiliary Labels

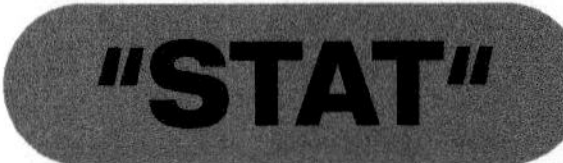

This label indicates that a CSP should be delivered to the nursing unit and administered to the patient immediately.

P.R.N.

This label indicates that the medication is to be used as needed.

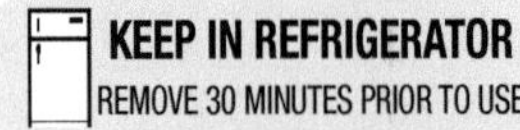

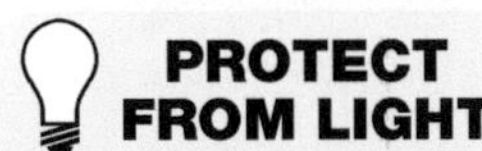

Storage labels highlight how the CSP must be treated to maintain integrity, potency, and stability.

INSULIN

This warning label reminds nurses that they do not need to give additional insulin to the patient because it is included in the CSP delivered.

CAUTION
High Concentration

This label warns that special cautionary procedures should be applied because of a dangerously high concentration (most often used on bulk potassium chloride bottles).

KCL ADDED

This label alerts handlers that this CSP contains potassium chloride, a potentially dangerous drug.

FOR IRRIGATION ONLY

This label cautions that a CSP is to be administered only for irrigation of a wound, dressing, tube, etc.

Note: This table presents but a small sample of some of the most frequently used CSP auxiliary labels. Many other auxiliary labels are used in sterile compounding.

TABLE 13.6 Sterile Master Formulation Record Components

A Master Formulation Record must include at least the following information:

- Name, strength or activity, and dosage form of the CSP
- Identities and amounts of all ingredients
- Type and size of container-closure system(s)
- Complete instructions for preparing the CSP, including equipment, supplies, a description of the compounding steps, and any special precautions
- Physical description of the final CSP
- BUD and storage requirements
- Reference source to support the stability of the CSP
- Quality control (QC) procedures (e.g., pH testing, filter integrity testing)
- Other information as needed to describe the compounding process and ensure repeatability (e.g., adjusting pH and tonicity, sterilization method (e.g., steam, dry heat, irradiation, or filter)

The Compounding Record

For sterile products that are assembled according to manufacturer's direction, such as standard reconstitution of powders for injectable medications, no Compounding Record is required. However, for every compounded product using a Master Formulation Record, a **Compounding Record**, or log, must be established by the technician on the computer for each patient, as in nonsterile compounding. This record documents the ingredients, calculations, and compounding process, allowing for traceability. It is critical that the record also describes in detail any deviations from the label directions or Master Formulation Record and any compounding problems or errors experienced. Each Compounding Record must be reviewed and approved with the pharmacist's signature or initials and the date before the CSP is released. See Table 13.7 for recommended components of the sterile Compounding Record.

TABLE 13.7 Sterile Compounding Record Components

Compounding Records must include at least the following information:

- Name, strength or activity, and dosage form of the CSP
- Date and time of preparation of the CSP
- Assigned internal identification number (e.g., prescription, order, or lot number)
- A method to identify the individuals involved in the compounding process and verifying the final CSP
- Name of each component
- Vendor, lot number, and expiration date for each component for CSPs prepared for more than 1 patient and for CSPs prepared from nonsterile ingredient(s)
- Weight or volume of each component
- Strength or activity of each component
- Total quantity compounded
- Assigned BUD and storage requirements
- Results of QC procedures (e.g., visual inspection, filter integrity testing, pH testing)

If applicable, the Compounding Record must also include:

- Master Formulation Record reference for the CSP
- Calculations made to determine and verify quantities and/or concentrations of components

13.3 Calculations

Safety Alert

The IV technician is referring to a medication label to perform calculations.

Though the label or Master Formulation Record may provide most or all of the calculations for compounding, there may be times when mathematics is required. Many pharmacy software programs automatically print the needed calculations for measurements and dosages of the drugs (the amounts needed to be drawn up or added) on the CSP labels.

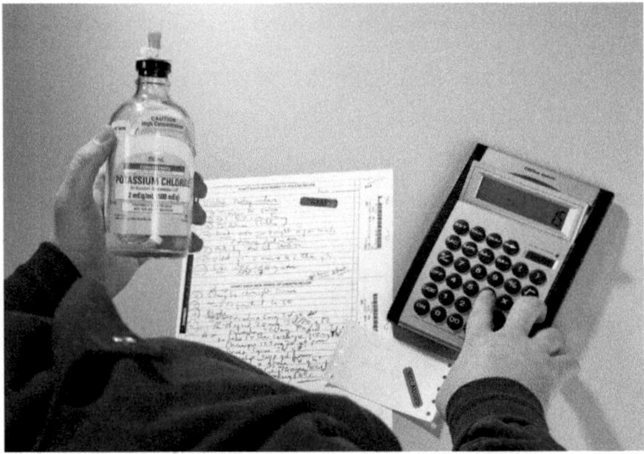

The IV technician must always double-check the medication order, labels, and calculations, documenting them all in the Compounding Record

However, inside the anteroom, the technician may need to compare the concentration of the dose ordered with the concentration of stock drug on hand and perform calculations to determine the desired volume of each ingredient to add to the LVP or SVP. The IV flow rates are also typically provided on the physician's medication order. The technician then uses the ordered IV flow rate to calculate the days' supply for IVs and IVPBs, and the pharmacist verifies the accuracy of the technician's calculations as a double check. Hospital pharmacy technicians may also serve on cardiopulmonary resuscitation (CPR) or code teams that need to calculate dosages and drip rates for heart medications, prepare IV infusions and tubing, and attach IV sets.

For certain TPN preparations, neonatal (newborn) IVs, and chemotherapy IVs, the process is reversed. For these products, the pharmacist typically performs the first set of calculations, which are then verified by another pharmacist. The pharmacy technician then provides the "third-line check" of these calculations.

Common Compounding Calculations

As was demonstrated in Chapter 6 on calculations, numerous calculations may need to be done for different CSPs. The first calculations needed are often ones of measurement conversions, so it is essential to memorize the equivalents and metric conversions provided in Chapter 6. You will also need to know conversions from standard time (clock time) to military time since drug administration times in hospitals and other institutions are generally based on military time. Knowing how to translate temperatures in Fahrenheit to Celsius and back is essential for refrigerator and freezer storage conditions. (These conversions are also explained in Chapter 6.)

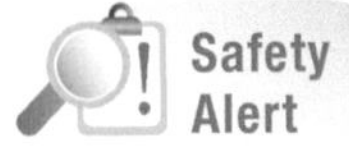

Safety Alert

Never rely solely on the directions on the CSP label or pharmacist's calculations, or on your own. Always do the calculations and compare them to ensure accuracy.

Numerous other calculations are needed, and certain scenarios favor specific formulas and methods for the greatest accuracy. (But you will also have favored methods, based on what you know best.)

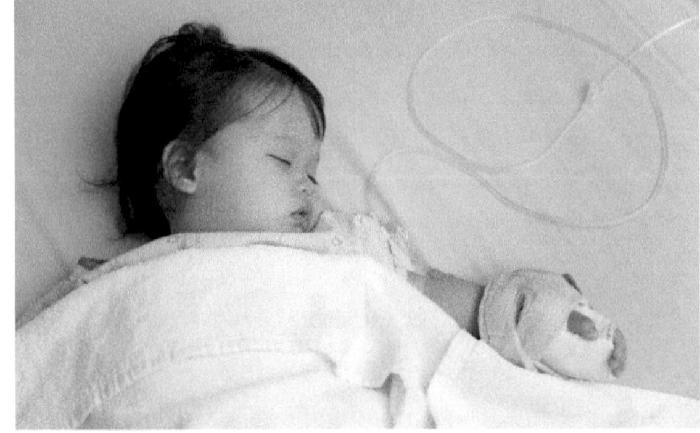

Checking and double-checking conversion measurements and IV calculations for children is especially important.

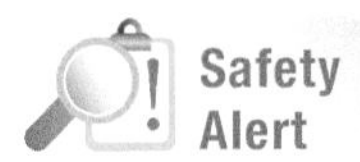

The metric system is typically used in the hospital setting. For this reason, all equations involving nonmetric measurements must be converted into metric (typically in the first step).

- **When a measurement is missing in an equation involving equal ratios, proportions, or fractions,** the *rate and proportion calculation method* may be best.
- **For multi-stepped problems using conversions**, *dimensional analysis* is usually favored.
- **For calculating concentrations based on the body surface area**, use the proper *equal ratios and proportion formula.*
- **For addressing dilutions of powders and solutions**, a combination of the ratio and proportion method and dimensional analysis can be used.
- **For mixing two different concentrations of the same drug**, use the *alligation method* to find the amounts needed of each these solutions.
- **For working with milliequivalents for electrolytes and other solutes**, there are specialized formulas.

These are not the only calculations needed. In addition, one must know how to handle overfill concerns and calculate drip rates, drop rates, and infusion rates to determine 24-hour IV supply needs. Descriptions of these calculations are to follow.

Since there are often various ways to calculate the same answer, the best method to use is the one you are most comfortable with using the information provided to you by the medication order, the CSP label, and the medication label.

Overfill Concerns in Admixtures and Dilutions

Although manufactured bags or bottles of medicated solutions are labeled to contain a set number of mL (e.g., 25, 50, 100, 250, 500, or 1,000 mL), the actual volume is greater because the containers include overfill. **Overfill** is the amount of solution that manufacturers add to make up for the loss of water due to evaporation through plastic. This loss is somewhat dependent on conditions during transport and storage and the ratio of fluid volume to the surface area. The larger the base solution of the IV bag, the greater the potential loss, so the more the manufacturers add overfill to compensate.

Manufacturers are not consistent in their addition of overfill amounts, and they do not always label the overfill percentages they use. (See Table 13.8 for an example of overfill amounts.) Some overwrap their non-PVC (a type of plastic) IV solutions to reduce evaporation. These wraps should stay on until right before compounding or administration.

TABLE 13.8 Examples of Overfill in IV Bags

- 100 mL bags contain 7 mL overfill (7% overfill)
- 250 mL bags contain 25 mL overfill (10% overfill)
- 500 mL bags contain 30 mL overfill (6% overfill)
- 1000 mL bags contain 50 mL overfill (5% overfill)

The amount of overfill varies with the manufacturer.

Overfill Effects on IV Compounding Processes

There are four major ways to create admixtures for IV infusions, each affected by overfill rates to differing degrees:

Practice Tip

IV solutions that are in non-PVC plastic may be more permeable to air and tend to evaporate, so manufacturers often place an outside wrap on them. You should leave the outer wrap on until going into the buffer room to discourage evaporation.

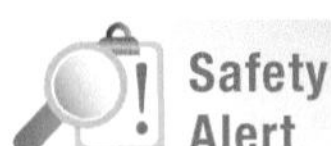

Safety Alert

An epidural pain medication must always be exact, with no overfill, so the base solution and the medication must be drawn into new syringes and then injected into a sterile medication reservoir cassette.

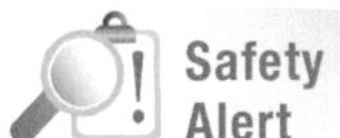

Safety Alert

The only sure way to know a dosage is if the mixture is compounding into a new sterile container, and the label accurately indicates the percentage of drug solute to solvent, with no overfill to address.

Small-Volume Medication Addition for a Simple Admixture In this, you add the medication to the manufacturer's base solution. But before doing so, you may need to reconstitute a powdered medication or dilute a concentrated medication by adding a diluent. These substances increase an IV's volume. Generally, the SVP IV solution is meant to be infused to a patient until the bag is empty over a short period of time (such as 30 minutes)—as with antibiotics in an IV piggyback. In this situation, there is no need to compensate for overfill because the entire contents will be used and the full dosage will be received. However, the label should list the total amount of the drug and the total estimated amount of solution (including the estimated overfill). The label must also indicate that the CSP is meant for a single dose for a single short-term administration, and the IV tubing should be flushed to ensure that the whole dose is administered.

For example, you may receive a medication order for 20 mL of a drug solute in 100 mL of D5W to be administered over 30 minutes. To prepare the drug, you must add the 20 mL. The estimated overfill of the base solution bag is 7 mL, so the total volume in the SVP is equal to 127 mL. The IV label must read "Infuse entire contents for full dose."

Volume Withdrawal and Medication Addition Another process is used when adding a large amount of medication to an LVP that is meant to be continuously administered until another IV filled with the same drug follows. Before adding the medication to the IV, a similar volume to that of the drug additive has to be removed first. For example, if you need to add 150 mL of a drug to 1,000 mL of a D5W solution, you must first withdraw 150 mL of the base solution before adding the medication. As with a simple admixture, the label should indicate the total drug amount and the estimated total volume of the solution, which would be the original 1,000 mL plus the overfill of the original base solution.

Larger Volume Withdrawal and Medication Addition When a large-volume of an intensely concentrated dose is required, such as with a cancer chemotherapy drug, you may need to remove both the volume (diluent) of the medication to be added plus the estimated amount of the manufacturer's overfill. That way, when the medication is added to the solution that remains, it will hold the prescribed dosage with no extra overfill solution to dilute it. However, if the overfill amount is not known but is just estimated, then it will still not be a precise dosage. Yet it will be far closer than if the overfill amount was never estimated for some accommodation of the volume. (See overfill calculation Example 1.)

New Container with Solute and Solvent For medications that need to be the most precise, as in chemotherapy, sterile compounding technicians need to work with accurate medication amounts and add them as well as the diluents and base solvent into a new sterile container. This can be done manually or in an automated compounding machine (as with TPN solutions). Using a new container means that there will be no overfill to calculate or estimate.

Overfill Policies

Each hospital and home infusion pharmacy will have written protocols for dealing with overfill calculations when using base solutions that have overfill. Small and large parenteral solutions are the majority of sterile compounded solutions, and normally the overfill amount does not appreciably affect the amount of IV fluids or drug dosages administered. In the case of IV neonatal drugs or cancer chemotherapy drugs that come in premixed solutions that must be reconstituted with a diluent before being transferred into a small or large volume parenteral solution, the combination of

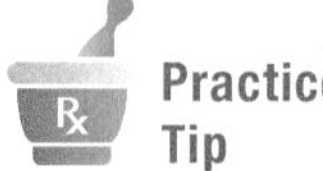
Practice Tip

At the time of compounding sterile preparation, the volume of the actual overfill in manufactured products can only be estimated even if labeled because it is impossible to know how much solution has evaporated by the time of use.

the overfill in the IV bag plus the diluent can cause an overdilution of the prescribed dose, especially if the entire contents of the IV solution are not administered. A diluted or less than prescribed dose of a critical drug may adversely affect the disease outcome.

Many pharmacies implement a 10% overfill rule for most medications where overfill issues are encountered. If the total calculated final volume to be administered equals 10% or less additional fluid, it is not necessary to withdraw any of the base solution.

For example, a medication order is received for a doxorubicin 90 mg solution to be added to a 1,000 mL (1 L) NS, with the compounded IV to be infused over six hours. Doxorubicin is available as a 2 mg/mL solution concentration; therefore, a 90 mg dose requires 45 mL of doxourbicin solution to be used.

If the manufacturer offers IV products with overfill amounts like those in Table 13.8, one liter of NS will contain approximately 50 mL of overfill. So 1,000 mL + 45 mL (of the diluent) + 50 mL (of overfill) = 1095 mL. Ten percent of 1,000 is 100, so an overfill of an additional 10% would total 1,100 mL. Because 1,095 is under the limit of 10% more, no adjustment in the volume of the base solution (NS) would be needed, according to the 10% rule of hospital policy.

When the total calculated final volume to be administered equals more than an additional 10%, it is necessary to withdraw a volume of the base solution equal to the overfill volume plus the diluent of the drug.

Using the same example, if the 90 mg solution (45 mL) was to be added to 500 mL NS instead of 1,000 mL NS, then the final volume would have been 500 mL + 45 mL (volume of doxorubicin) + 30 mL (overfill) for a total of 575 mL. Since this volume is greater than the limit of 10% more of 500 mL (550 mL), the protocol states that 75 mL (45 mL + 30 mL) NS should be withdrawn before adding the medication solution of 90 mg and 45 mL results in a final (and labeled) concentration of 90 mg of doxorubicin in 500 mL NS.

Example 1

A medication order says: Mitomycin 40 mg (0.5 mg/1 mL sterile water dilution), added to 1000 mL NS, infused over 6 hours. If the institution utilizes the 10% overfill rule, will this CSP result in an overfill that needs an adjustment of the base solution? Assume the manufacturer uses overfill according to Table 13.8.

Step 1 Mitomycin 40 mg is available as a dry powder that recommends a concentration of 0.5 mg/mL. The amount of sterile water diluent to be added must be determined.

First, convert $\frac{0.5 \text{ mg}}{1 \text{ mL}}$ from a decimal: $\frac{10}{10} \times \frac{0.5 \text{ mg}}{1 \text{ mL}} = \frac{5 \text{ mg}}{10 \text{ mL}}$

Next, use the ratio and proportion method to calculate the volume of mitomyin required for a 40 mg dose.

$$\frac{5 \not{\text{mg}}}{10 \text{ mL}} = \frac{40 \not{\text{mg}}}{y \text{ mL}};\ 5\,y = 400 \text{ mL};\ y \text{ mL} = \frac{400 \text{ mL}}{5} = 80 \text{ mL}$$

IN THE REAL WORLD

In August 2013, it came to light that more than 1,000 patients in some Ontario and New Brunswick hospitals received less than their required doses of their chemotherapy drugs because of confusion over the IV admixtures of cyclophosphamide and gemcitabine supplied by the compounding pharmacy. The problematic understanding arose between what the supplier contract requested and what was delivered, a problem increased by poor product labeling. The hospital pharmacy compounding personnel thought that the supplied IVs were concentrated forms of a multi-dose medication that required dilution while the manufacturer was providing single doses with overfill.

Because of this error, the cancer patients who received the compounded multi-doses were estimated to have received doses diluted between 3% and 20% from their medication orders. Family members of those who died of cancer may wonder whether their loved ones would still be alive if they had received their full-strength, medically ordered doses of the chemotherapy drugs.

Step 2 One liter (1,000 mL) of NS will contain approximately 50 mL NS of overfill if the manufacturer's proportion of overfill is similar to Table 13.8. Estimate the amount of overfill plus diluent.

1,000 mL + 50 mL (overfill) + 80 mL (diluent) = 1,130 mL

The final volume of the IV solution is equal to 1,130 mL, which is more than 10% of a liter (or 1,100 mL). Therefore an adjustment in the volume of the base solution (NS) *is needed.*

Step 3 The hospital protocol states then that 130 mL (the amount of the overfill plus diluent) should be withdrawn from the 1,000 mL NS IV bag before injecting the medicated solution.

Determining the Days' Supply with IV Administration Flow Rates

To determine the correct number of IV bags needed for a 24-hour period and the time when a new IV bag will be needed, technicians at times must calculate the IV administration flow rates based on the size of the IV tubing and on the prescribed infusion rates. These calculations typically address the following questions that affect each other:

- What is the infusion rate in mL/hour?
- What is the size of the tubing and the drip rate (in gtts/min)?
- How long will this bag last?
- How much fluid has the patient received?
- What time will the next bag be needed?
- How many bags will be needed for the patient in a 24-hour period?

To answer these questions, you need to know the total volume of the ordered parenteral solution and either the prescribed infusion rate in milliliters per hour (mL/hr) *or* the number of hours over which the solution is to be infused. This information can be found in the physician's medication order or in the Master Formulation Record directions. You then perform a series of IV flow rate calculations using either multiplication or division.

In the most simple sense, the infusion rate (R) is the volume divided by the time it takes (*Volume/Time*), and the time can be expressed in hours or minutes (and seconds if desired). The volume is expressed in mL.

$$\frac{\text{Volume}}{\text{Time}} = \text{Rate (mL/hrs or min)}$$

To answer the question, *"What is the infusion rate in mL/hr?"* you must divide the IV volume in mL by the number of hours (hr) over which the CSP is to be administered (see Example 2, which follows):

$$\frac{\text{total mL}}{\text{total hours}} = \frac{y\text{ mL}}{1\text{hr}}$$

To answer the question, *"How long will this IV bag last (or take to administer)?"* you must divide the total mL by the infusion rate (mL/hr) to determine the hours per IV bag (see Example 3):

$$\frac{\text{Volume (mL)}}{\text{Rate (mL/hr)}} = \text{Time (hrs or min per bag) or } z; \quad z \text{ is how long until 1 bag is empty}$$

To answer the question, *"What time will the next bag be needed?"* you must add this length of time in hours (z) to the standard military time of the last administration of the infusion (see Example 4).

To answer the question, *"How many bags will be needed for the patient in a 24-hour period?"* you must divide 24 (the number of hours till resupply) by the number of hours calculated (z) that each bag will take to be infused (see Example 5). It is important to practice calculating examples of each equation.

Example 2

A physician orders

℞ **4,000 mL of D_5NS to be administered over 24 hours**

What is the infusion rate in milliliters per hour?

Step 1 Begin by identifying the numbers to insert into the equation.

Volume/Time = Rate

$$\frac{4{,}000\text{ mL}}{24\text{ hr}} = 166.67\text{ mL/hr, rounded to 167 mL/hr}$$

The answer rounded up is the infusion rate: 167 mL/hr.

Step 2 Any hourly infusion rate can be converted into milliliters per minute by multiplying the answer by the conversion rate of 1 hour to 60 minutes.

$$\frac{167\text{ mL}}{1\text{ hr}} \times \frac{1\text{ hr}}{60\text{ min}} = \frac{167\text{ mL}}{60\text{ min}} = 2.7833\text{mL/min rounded to } 2.8\text{ mL/min}$$

Example 3

A physician orders

> ℞ **500 mg of cefazolin in 50 mL of D_5W to be administered as a secondary IV at 100 mL/hr**

How long will it take to administer this medication, or how long will it last?

$$z\text{ hr} = \frac{50\text{ mL}}{100\text{ mL/hr}} \text{ or } 50\text{ mL} \times \frac{1\text{ hr}}{100\text{ mL}} = \frac{5\text{ hr}}{10} = \frac{1\text{ hr}}{2} = 0.5\text{ hr or half hour}$$

$z = {}^1/_2$ hour. The IV bag will take a half hour or 30 minutes to administer.

Example 4

A physician orders

> ℞ **20 mEq of medication in 1,000 mL of D_5W to be administered at 125 mL/hr**

If the first bag is hung at 10:00 a.m., when will the next bag be needed?

Step 1 Apply the formula: $\frac{V\text{ (mL)}}{R\text{ (mL/hr)}} = \text{Time (hrs)}: \frac{1{,}000\text{ mL}}{125\text{ mL/hr}} = T$

$$\text{or } 1{,}000\text{ mL} \times \frac{1\text{ hr}}{125\text{ mL}} = \frac{1{,}000\text{ hrs}}{125} = 8\text{ hrs}$$

One 1,000 mL bag will last 8 hours.

Step 2 Add the 8 hours to the last administration time of 10 a.m.

$$10\text{ a.m.} = \left\{ \begin{array}{r} 1000 \\ +800 \\ \hline 1800 \end{array} \right.$$

So 1000 military time plus 8 hours equals 1800 military time or 6:00 p.m.

Example 5

A 1-liter LVP is running at 150 mL/hr. How many IV bags will be needed in a 24-hour period?

Step 1 Begin by converting 1 L to 1,000 mL, and then identifying the amounts to insert into the equation:

$$\frac{V\,(\text{mL})}{R\,(\text{mL/hr})} = T\,(\text{hrs})$$

$$\frac{1{,}00\cancel{0}\ \cancel{\text{mL}}}{15\cancel{0}\ \cancel{\text{mL}}/\text{hr}} = T\,(\text{hrs}) = 6.67 \text{ hrs per bag}$$

Step 2 Divide the 24 hours of the day's supply by the hours per bag:

$$\frac{24\ \cancel{\text{hr}}}{6.67\ \cancel{\text{hr}}/\text{bag}} = 3.6 \text{ bags for a 24-hour period}$$

So 3.6 bags will be needed, rounded to 4 full bags for a day's supply.

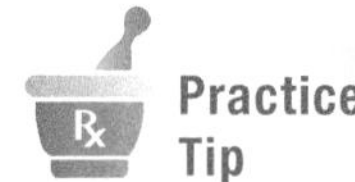

Practice Tip

If a calculation yields that a number of bags expressed by a decimal are needed, then an additional full bag is made. Fractional bags are never made.

Calculating Infusion Rates in Drops per mL and Drops per Minute

Sometimes it is important to know an even more precise calculation than the infusion rate to figure out how much medication a patient is receiving per drop and per minute. As described in an earlier chapter, the types of IV tubing selected have an influence on the infusion rates because they have a different **drop factor**, or drops per milliliter.

Macrodrip IV tubing may deliver either 10, 15, or 20 drops per milliliter. (Macro tubing comes in different diameters from manufacturers, resulting in some variance in drop factors.) In contrast, microdrip IV tubing delivers 60 drops per milliliter, so the drops are far smaller than the ones with macrodrip tubing. Macro tubing is generally used when more than 50 mL per hour needs to be administered, while microtubing is used when fewer milliliters per hour are needed, such as in intensive care, pediatrics, or neonatology, when counting drops is important.

Most simple IV sets, if hung properly, use gravity to force the solution through the IV set to the patient, much like a water tower works to deliver tap water to city residents. However, many hospitals use an IV infusion pump or controller, which automatically adjusts the volume and administration rate of the infusion to fit the desired rate. The infusion pump is often integrated into the electronic medical record (EMR) and bar code point-of-care (BPOC) technologies to improve the accuracy of the IV administration and reduce medication errors.

Put Down Roots

The Latin word for "drops" is *guttae*, which is then abbreviated as *gtts.*

Nursing personnel simply program the prescribed rate into the electronic infusion pump at the patient's bedside. The rate can be digitally adjusted, causing the pump's internal clamp to slow or quicken the rate at which the fluid flows through tubing routed through a chamber in the pump. Pumps can be set to give IV fluids in milliliters per hour or drops per minute.

To determine the rate in drops per minute, when the total volume and infusion time are known, the following formula is used (see Example 6):

$$\frac{\text{Volume (mL)}}{\text{Time (min)}} \times \text{Drop factor (gtt/mL)} = \text{Rate of drops per minute (gtt/min)}$$

Practice Tip

Always round down drips and minutes in drip rate solutions, especially for pediatric and neonatal patients.

Dimensional analysis may also be used to solve this type of equation. Since you cannot administer partial drops, it is common practice to round down answers with partial drops or minutes. For example, if the calculated answer is 20.6 gtts/min, it would typically be rounded down to 20 gtts/min.

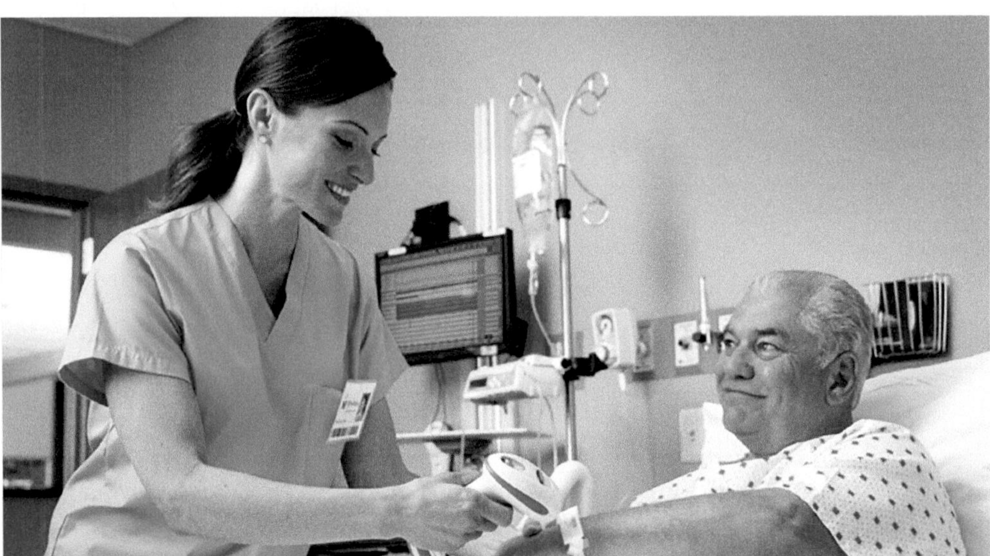

An example of an IV set integrated with an infusion pump and bar code software records is the B. Braun Synchronized Intelligence Infusion Platform.

Example 6

An IV solution has a total volume of 250 mL and is being administered over 60 minutes using macrodrip tubing with a drop factor of 15 gtts/mL. What is the rate in drops per minute?

Step 1 Recall the drip rate formula previously given.

Identify the values to insert into the drip rate formula.

volume = 250 mL

time = 60 min

drop factor = 15 gtts/mL

Step 2 Insert the values into the drip rate formula.

Step 3 Round down the answer to 62 gtts/min.

Example 7

An IV of D5W with 20,000 units of heparin is being administered at a rate of 40 mL/hr using macrodrip tubing with a drop factor of 20 gtts/mL. How many drops per minute is that?

Step 1 Use the drip rate formula previously given.

$$\frac{\text{Volume (mL)}}{\text{Time (min)}} \times \text{Drop factor (gtt/mL)} = \text{Rate of drops per minute (gtt/min)}$$

Begin by identifying the amounts to insert into the formula.

IV flow rate = 40 mL/hr
drop factor = 20 gtts/mL

Step 2 Insert the values from the problem statement into the formula to determine the drops per minute rate. First convert 1 hour to 60 minutes.

$$\frac{40 \cancel{\text{mL}}}{60 \text{ min}} \times \frac{20 \text{ gtt}}{1 \cancel{\text{mL}}} = 13.3 \text{ gtt/min}$$

$$80 \div 6 = 13.33 \text{ gtts/min}$$

The rate is 13 drops per minute (as rounded down to the nearest whole number).

This problem can also be solved using the following dimensional analysis:

$$\frac{20 \text{ gtt}}{1 \cancel{\text{mL}}} \times \frac{40 \cancel{\text{mL}}}{1 \cancel{\text{hr}}} \times \frac{1 \cancel{\text{hr}}}{60 \text{ min}} = 13.33 \text{ gtt/min, rounded down to } 13 \text{ gtt/min}$$

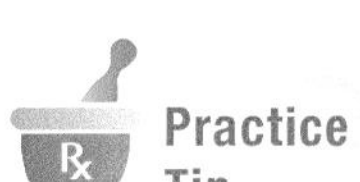

To set up a problem logically, first identify the type of units needed for the final answer. Then list all the pertinent information, especially conversion rates, and their units. You can keep canceling out unneeded units, circling the ones that are needed.

Drop Rate Calculations for Medication Infusion Amounts Occasionally, pharmacy personnel can use drop factor calculations to determine the precise amount of a drug that will be infused per minute. These types of problems are sometimes referred to as IV drip rate calculations and can be solved by using dimensional analysis.

Example 8

The prescriber has ordered a dopamine drip of an IV 800 mg in 250 mL of D5W. The IV will be administered at 10 mL/hr through microdrip tubing with a drop factor of 60 gtts/mL. How many milligrams of dopamine are in each drop? How many milligrams are received by the patient each minute?

Step 1 First determine the mg of dopamine per drop of the infusion using dimensional analysis.

$$\frac{800 \text{ mg}}{250 \cancel{\text{mL}}} \times \frac{1 \cancel{\text{mL}}}{60 \text{ gtt}} = 0.053 \text{ mg/gtt}$$

The patient will receive 0.053 mg of dopamine per drop.

Step 2 Now calculate the mg of dopamine per minute of the infusion using dimensional analysis.

$$\frac{800\ \text{mg}}{250\ \cancel{\text{mL}}} \times \frac{10\ \cancel{\text{mL}}}{\cancel{\text{hr}}} \times \frac{1\ \cancel{\text{hr}}}{60\ \text{min}} = 0.53\ \text{mg/min}$$

The patient will receive 0.53 mg of dopamine per minute.

13.4 The Processes of Adding Ingredients to Base Solutions

With completed calculations and labels per IV dose in hand, the technician needs to have the pharmacist compare them to the medication order to verify their accuracy before preparing the CSPs. A large portion of sterile compounding entails injecting the proper measurements of medications from vials and ampules into the prepackaged IV bag solutions. You have to work to master these skills, since withdrawing medications from vials and ampules with syringes and injecting them into IV bags or other containers requires complex manipulations. Aseptic technique must be followed, which requires training and practice. The following section gives an overview of the major steps in sterile compounding.

In compounding, stay free from interruptions to keep mentally focused on following proper aseptic technique. Any breach in technique may lead to product contamination and medication errors.

Sterile Compounding with Ingredients in Vials

A **vial** is a sealed glass or plastic sterile container with a rubber seal and hard plastic cap. Vials contain sterile diluents or medications in either a liquid or powdered form and are commonly available in sizes ranging from 1 mL to 100 mL (for batch CSPs). Vials come as **single-dose vials (SDVs)**, which *do not contain preservatives*, and **multiple-dose vials (MDVs)**, which do contain preservatives. (Insulin often comes in MDVs.)

The vial label contains the stock drug's concentration and the manufacturer's directions for reconstitution or use (see Figure 13.6). Before using the vial contents, the expiration and in-use dates need to be checked.

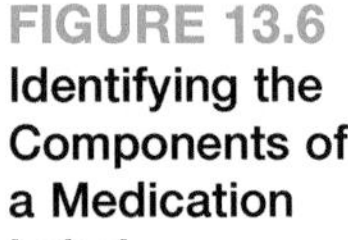

FIGURE 13.6
Identifying the Components of a Medication Label

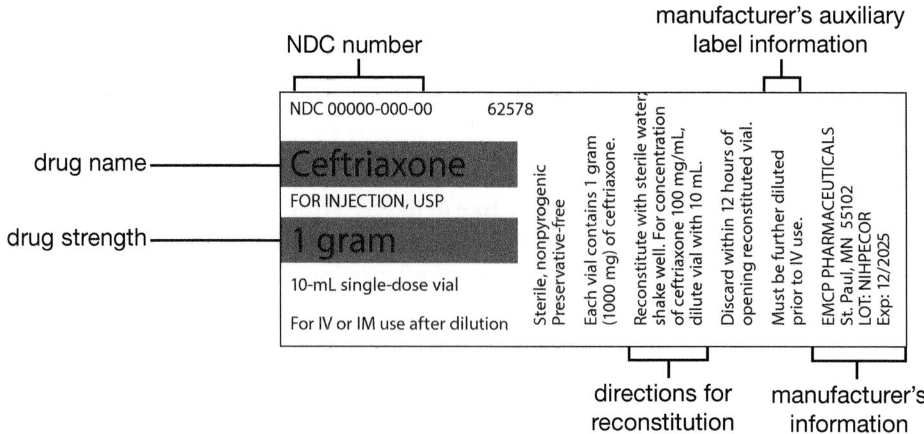

The absence of a preservative in an SDV makes this container an ideal medium for microbial growth, so the contents change to must be used within 12 hours of opening in the direct compounding area (DCA) and then be discarded. The contents of an MDV, on the other hand, are considered stable (with a preservative) for up to 28 days from its initial opening unless otherwise specified by the manufacturer. Once an MDV is opened, mark the beyond-use date and time on the MDV to ensure that the vial is stored under appropriate conditions (usually refrigeration) and to alert other pharmacy personnel of the opening and the medication's change from an expiration to BUD.

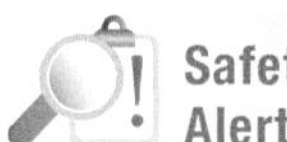

It is important to know if a patient is allergic to latex. If so, a vial with a latex-free rubber top is needed or special tools to remove the contents from the vial.

Withdrawing Fluid from a Vial

During sterile compounding in the DCA, all processes must be aseptically performed according to strict procedures dictated by the *USP* Chapter <797> and the facility's standard operating procedures. The processes are complicated and must be practiced in a training lab. The vial's flip-top plastic cap must be opened to expose the rubber top and wiped with a sterile 70% isopropyl alcohol (IPA) swab. Once the appropriate needle unit has been aseptically unwrapped and uncapped, the needle's bevel must be carefully placed on the vial's rubber top, with the bevel pointing up toward the ceiling at a 45-degree angle (see Figure 13.7). The needle tip should then be pressed to pierce and penetrate the rubber closure at this angle and then be straightened to 90 degrees and pushed down so the bevel heel will enter the closure at the same point as the tip.

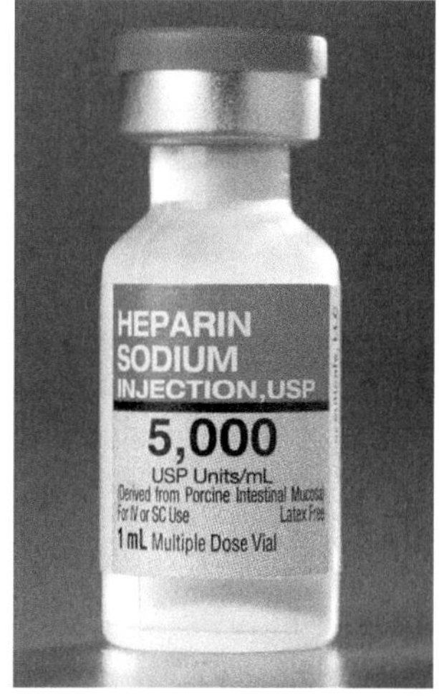

This sealed, sterile, multi-dose vial contains several doses of medication stabilized with a preservative.

FIGURE 13.7
Correct Needle Insertion into a Vial

Note the slight bend of the needle during the insertion.

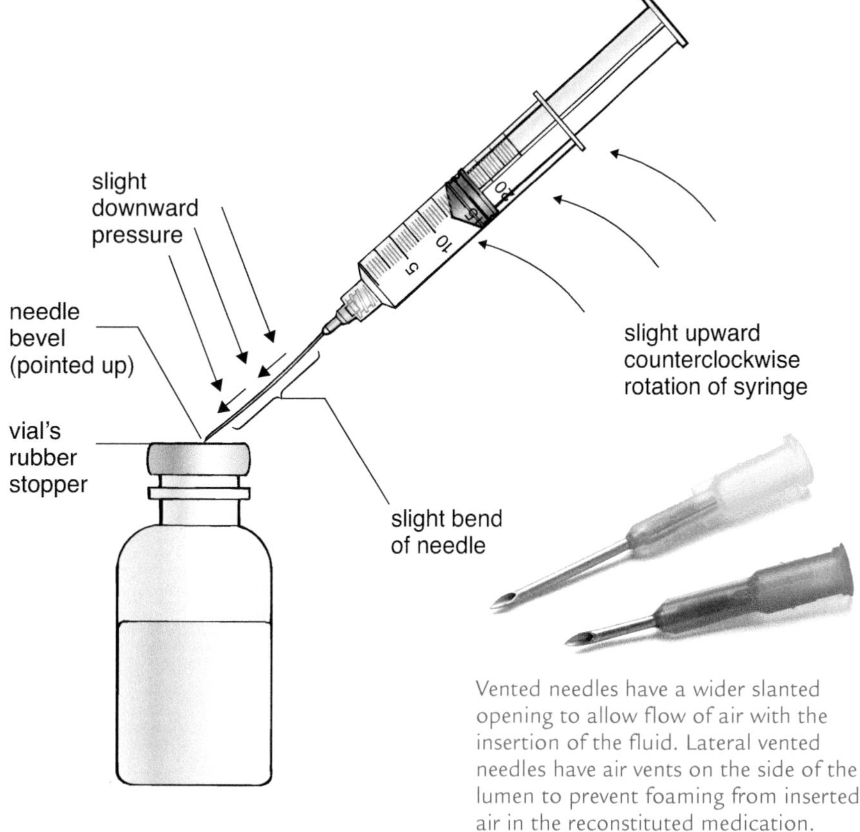

Vented needles have a wider slanted opening to allow flow of air with the insertion of the fluid. Lateral vented needles have air vents on the side of the lumen to prevent foaming from inserted air in the reconstituted medication.

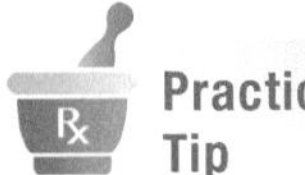
Practice Tip

During sterile compounding in the DCA, you must always hold the vial and syringe so that the airflow to the critical area—which includes the syringe tip, needle, and the vial's rubber top—remains unobstructed.

This technique prevents **coring**, or the inadvertent introduction of a small piece of the rubber top into the solution. If coring does occur, you must discard the contaminated vial and needle-and-syringe unit and repeat the process with new supplies. Because a vial is a closed-system container, the air cannot freely flow in or out, so you must use a milking technique. For milking, use a syringe to insert a small amount of air into the vial that is equal to, or slightly less than, the volume of liquid needing to be withdrawn. Then draw up some solution into the syringe. This insertion and withdrawal process is done a little at a time in alternating steps, easing sufficient fluid into the syringe. (If the vial contains powdered medications, a **vented needle** is used to add the diluent. The vented needle, with its hole in the lumen, allows the fluid to be injected into the powder while simultaneously venting the positive pressure that has built up within the vial without milking. Vented needles are used when inserting a solution into a vial containing a powered medication for reconstitution.)

Once the fluid measurement seems to be reached, the sides will have to be tapped to make the bubbles rise and be released so that only fluid is in the syringe. More fluid may be needed. When the correct amount of fluid is precisely measured, it may be injected into an IV or IVPB bag, or into an IV port for an IV push, or into another vial with powder for reconstitution.

Safety Alert

Check the product package insert that accompanies each stock drug to verify which diluent and what volume should be added to the medication vial to make the correct concentration of a sterile medication.

Reconstituting Powdered Medication in a Vial Many antibiotics for parenteral solutions, such as cefazolin, are available as a lyophilized, or freeze-dried, powder. This allows the medication to have an extended expiration date and shelf-life, but it also means the powder has to be reunited with a fluid. Use a syringe (with vented needle) of the correct diluent, such as sterile water or normal saline, to perform this reconstitution. After injecting the diluent into the powder vial, the vial will need to be gently swirled or mixed according to manufacturers instructions to dissolve the powdered medication and turn it back into a liquid medication for parenteral administration.

Safety Alert

The special procedures of safe aseptic needle changing and vial swabbing must be learned through training to avoid contaminating the needle, fluid, or medication, or pricking yourself with the needle or putting a hole in the glove and your skin.

Inserting the Vial's Contents into Compounded Sterile Products

The reconstituted liquid medication must be withdrawn by syringe to be added to an IV bag or used for an IV push or intramuscular (IM) administration. Once the correct dosage volume has been measured in the syringe (as explained earlier), its needle should be recapped. This can be done by the **scoop method**, which involves placing the needle tip into the inside of the cap and scooping it up before putting pressure on the cap to secure it. The capped syringe, IV bag, and vial should be laid out in the DCA for the pharmacist (and/or supervising technician) to check the drug name and concentration, the base solution type and volume, and the volume in the syringe against the label and medication order.

After this verification, the vial top or the IV injection port (if for an IV) must be swabbed with 70% IPA in the DCA. Then using proper aseptic technique, the needle must be inserted into the port and the medication injected into the base solution. The final CSP will be checked again before being approved and sent to the nursing floor.

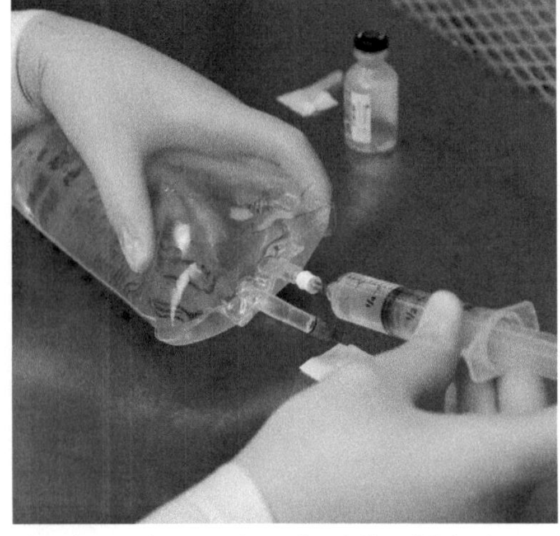
This shows the injection of a vial's additive into an IV bag.

If you are preparing a syringe for nurse administration and you have withdrawn the reconstituted medication into the proper syringe, remove the needle and dispose of it in a sharps container. Then, cap the syringe with a sterile cap before labeling the syringe, having it checked and verified, and sending it to the nursing unit.

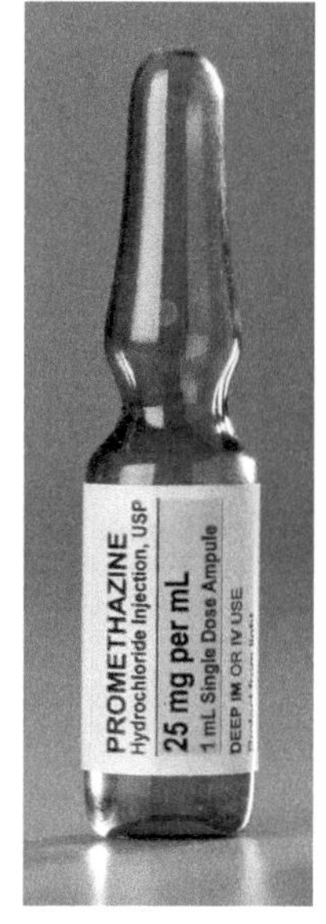

An ampule, with a neck ring for proper opening, contains no preservatives or ways to reseal the container, so any unused medication must be discarded.

Preparing Ampule-Based Compounded Sterile Preparations

In addition to using medications from vials, you may also need to use medications stored in ampules. An **ampule** is a small, hermetically sealed sterile container. Made of thin glass, an ampule stores a single dose of sterile medication in either a liquid (most common) or powdered form. You need to be aware that ampules *contain no preservatives* and some drugs are available *only* as a solution in an ampule because these drugs are incompatible with the rubber top or any plastic sealing components of vials.

Opening an Ampule

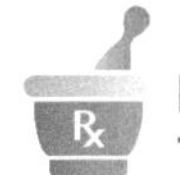

Practice Tip

All medications contained in ampules are considered single-dose only.

One must be familiar with the parts of an ampule to understand the directions on how to open this specialized container. An ampule has a head, an elongated neck, a shoulder, and a body (see Figure 13.8). Because it is a completely whole glass container without an opening, it is typically designed with a break ring. A **break ring** is a scored, or weakened, ring around the glass neck that marks the site where a technician will break it to access the ampule's contents. Therefore, the process of opening an ampule has some inherent risks, including getting injured when breaking the glass, contaminating the medication with glass shards, and damaging and/or contaminating the hood with broken glass. You should be aware of these risks and should have sufficient training and practice in this skill before compounding CSPs.

Before breaking an ampule, hold it upright and gently tap or swirl the container to clear the medication contents from the head and neck of the ampule. The neck must be wiped with 70% IPA swab to remove any microorganisms. Some technicians wrap a sterile 70% IPA swab around the neck of the ampule before breaking it. (Alcohol-soaked gauze may not be used, per *USP* <797>.) Grasp the ampule body in your nondominant hand with thumb and fingers below the ampule neck. Position your other hand holding the top of the ampule with your thumbs on each side of the break ring, away from the critical site. Holding the ampule toward the side of the DCA away from the HEPA filter but still within first air, exert a gentle but firm pressure on the break ring by pushing both thumbs forward to snap the ampule's neck cleanly towards the side wall of the hood (see Figure 13.9).

FIGURE 13.8
Critical Site of an Ampule

Pharmacy technicians must not contaminate the critical site of an ampule through touch contamination or incorrect handling or positioning of the ampule within the hood.

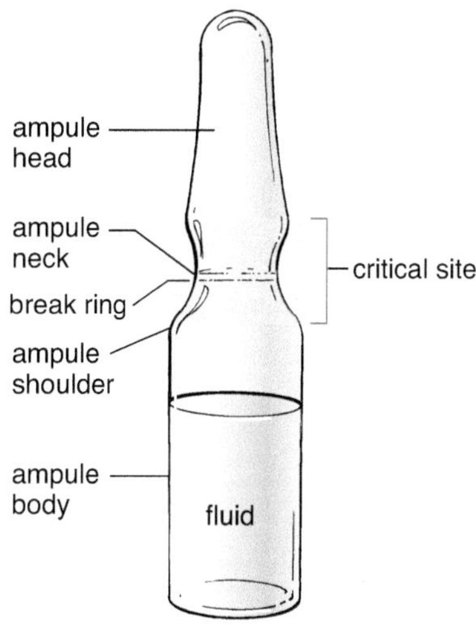

FIGURE 13.9
Opening an Ampule

With vial upright, gently tap the head to bring the medication down to the body. Swab the neck, and, if needed, use the swab to grip the ampule (though this is not the preferred method). If not, simply grasp it firmly. Then snap the neck away from you toward the inner side wall of the PEC but still within first air.

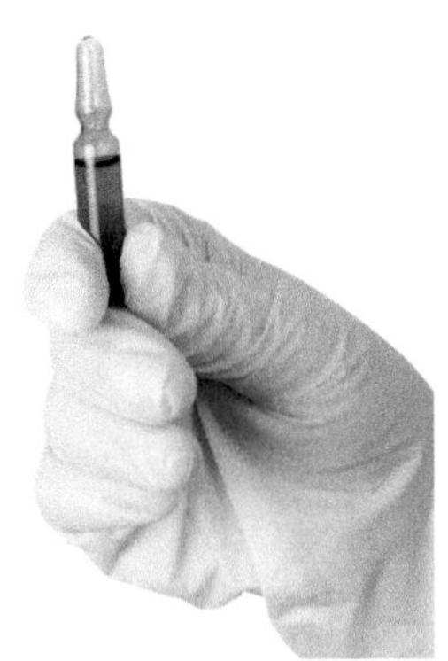

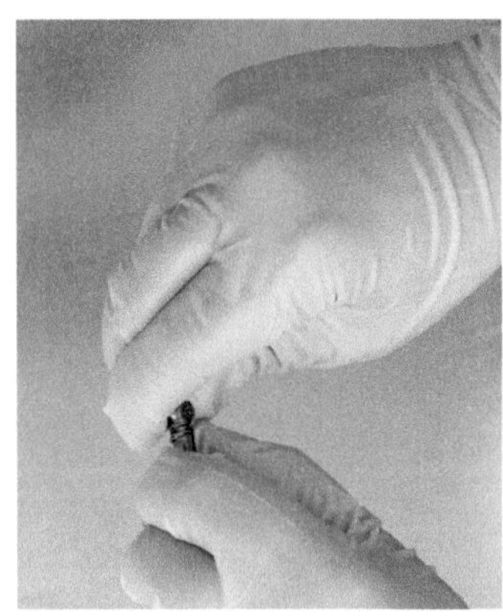

Withdrawing Medication from an Ampule

Because you must break glass to access the medication, a **filter needle** or a **filter straw** must be used to withdraw the medication according to *USP* <797>. The needle or straw must have a 5-micron (or finer) filter within its core to catch any microscopic glass shards to prevent them from entering the CSP. The filter needle or filter straw should be attached to the syringe just like a regular needle.

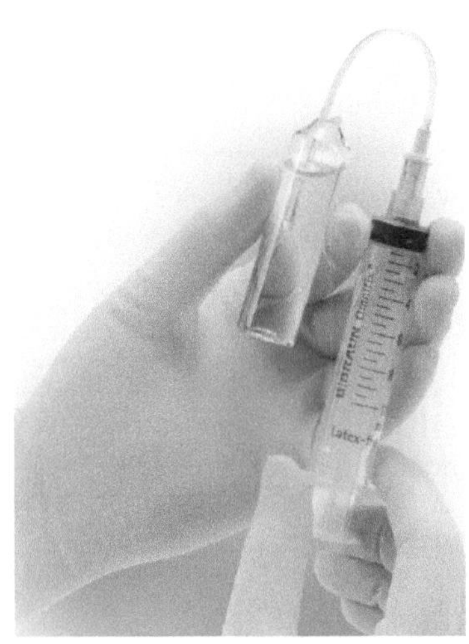

A filter straw can be used instead of a filter needle for withdrawing medication from an ampule. To see how to use one, watch the "Using the Filter Straw" video at https://PharmPractice7e.ParadigmEducation.com/FilterStraw.

To withdraw the medication, the ampule must be held upright in first air, and the filter needle bevel (pointing down) or the tip of a filter straw needs to be placed into the liquid surface to withdraw the liquid. Filter needles are for one-directional use only, meaning that the needle may be used only to withdraw fluid from an ampule *or* inject fluid into an IV or IVPB. The same needle may *not* be used to both withdraw from and inject into a container. When the ampule is nearly emptied, the technician should tilt the ampule slightly to allow easier access to the remainder of medication.

Before injecting the contents of a syringe into an IV, change to a regular needle in first air of filtered air to avoid introducing glass or particles into the IV admixture. If a regular needle is used to withdraw the drug from the ampule, then the needle must be replaced with a filter device before the drug is pushed out of the syringe and into an IV or IVPB solution. Small glass fragment contamination has to be prevented, because it can lead to systemic side effects such as phlebitis (irritation of the veins), especially in pediatric and neonatal patients.

When the pharmacist verifies the dose in the DCA by checking the drug name and concentration against the medication order and compounding label, the base solution type and volume, and the syringe volume, the pharmacist will also verify that you used a filter needle or straw to prevent the transfer of glass particles into the CSP.

Preparing Parenteral Nutrition Solutions

Since parenteral nutrition formulas are a mix of pharmaceutical and dietary elements, many hospitals have special parenteral nutrition teams comprised of specialized physicians, nurses, dietitians, and pharmacists who work together to design individualized patient medication orders and administration rates for these vulnerable patients. They monitor their progress to change the formula according to health progressions or declines. There are some general principles to know for preparing these CSPs.

IN THE REAL WORLD

Numerous studies have been done about glass-related injuries resulting from medications made from glass ampules, including pain from phlebitis, organ inflammation, pain at the infusion site, and other issues. In a 1992 survey of postmortem studies of newborns who died after receiving medicated IVs from glass ampules without filter needles or straws, scientists found glass particles in the babies' lungs. The glass particles caused pulmonary granulomas and hypertension in 5% of the late infants. The glass particles have also been known to cause immune system suppression and other harmful and sometimes fatal problems in newborns, children, and adults. Even so, filtered needles and inline filters in IV tubing are not consistently used with glass-ampule-based medications.

The USP, ASHP, and Infusion Nurses Society all recommend blunted filter needles when preparing medications from glass ampules. An analysis of the many studies on the dangers of nonfiltered medications from glass ampules can be found in the 2014 doctor of nursing thesis by Debran L. Harmon of the University of Northern Florida. This article can be seen at https://PharmPractice7e.ParadigmEducation.com/FilterNeedle.

Peripheral Parenteral Nutrition Components

PPN supplies only a portion of the patient's daily nutritional requirements via a **peripheral IV line**, or a line to a vein in an arm or leg rather than in the chest. PPN is recommended for short-term use (less than 10 to 14 days). It decreases the risk of infection and is easier to use compared to TPN. PPN is often used after a surgery before a patient is ready for full meals. The solutions are simpler to compound than TPNs as PPNs have fewer ingredients. A PPN can be provided by a carbohydrate solution, such as D5W, or a fat emulsion.

Examples of commercially available **parenteral intravenous fat emulsions (IVFEs)** used for nutritional support are Intralipid 20% and Liposyn II/III (10%–20%). They are administered to patients who need more calories than can be supplied by maintenance carbohydrate solutions like dextrose solutions. Neither of these solutions contains important building blocks for protein, such as amino acids, which are important to maintain a good immune system.

Total Parenteral Nutrition Components

In contrast, TPN supplies all of the patient's daily nutritional requirements including proteins, amino acids, and electrolytes via a catheter to a central vein (usually in the chest cavity). TPNs are recommended for longer-term use, generally defined as more than 14 days. TPNs are more expensive and have more potential complications, so they require more sterile compounding expertise than a PPN. TPN IVs are generally infused slowly over 24 hours in the hospital (and sometimes in home health care); hence the need for large volume IV bags holding 2,000 mL or more of solution.

Although there are guidelines for typical adult, pediatric, and neonatal daily requirements, the components of a patient's TPN are tailored to each patient, based on laboratory findings and clinical responses, and are often changed daily based on the patient's vital signs and bodily responses. The healthcare team uses specialized computer order forms or sheets with a list of all common ingredients to check off. Figure 13.10 is an example of a paper TPN medication order for an adult patient, though most TPN medication orders are now done electronically.

A typical TPN solution contains many additives including the following:

- sterile water for hydration
- dextrose for calories and energy (carbohydrates)
- amino acids for protein synthesis
- additives such as electrolytes, vitamins, minerals, and trace elements for chemical processes
- fatty acids for chemical processes and energy (fatty acids may be infused separately from the TPN solution)
- sometimes medication such as insulin to control blood sugar

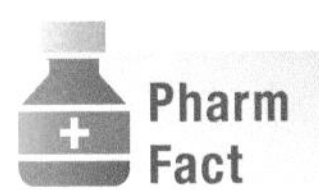

Pharm Fact

To avoid any kind of inflammaion or infection, the nurse must also cleanse the catheter site, flush the catheter, and check the catheter site regularly during TPN administration.

2 in-1 Versus 3-in-1 TPN Solutions A TPN **2-in-1 solution** contains a formulation of dextrose and amino acids with the lipid emulsion administered via piggyback in a separate bag. A total parenteral nutrition solution that contains the third component (fatty acid emulsion) in the same IV bag/bottle becomes a 3-in-1 solution. The major disadvantage of the **3-in-1 solution** is that the macronutrients can change the pH of the solution and cause precipitation of some of the ingredients, which may be undetectable due to the presence of the opaque fat emulsion.

Once the IV fat emulsion (rather than solution) has been added to the IV, the 1 in-1 solution can be difficult to keep stable. These 3-in-1 preparations often have an oily surface since the fatty emulsion, which is an oil, does not blend with the water. Because of this, the 3-in-1 TPNs often lead to some vein irritation and potential infection issues.

In addition, with all the additives in the 3-in-1 TPN solution, there is some risk of physical incompatibilities and a greater risk of medication and calculation errors, especially for pediatric and neonatal patients. Some prescribers prefer to administer an IV with a carbohydrate solution like dextrose along with a premixed fat emulsion piggyback or a peripheral line IV instead of a single 3-in-1 TPN IV solution for the patient's total nutritional needs.

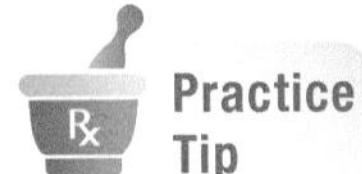

Practice Tip

TPN solutions must be administered via an IV set with an in-line filter into the subclavian vein.

Administering TPNs Administration of a TPN solution requires the insertion of a **central venous catheter (CVC)**, also called a *central line*. Central lines are often inserted into the subclavian vein of the chest near the clavicle. The larger vein accommodates the hypertonic concentration of all the ingredients and the large amount of fluid (usually 2,000 mL per day) that must be diluted in the bloodstream. TPN solutions are most commonly administered continuously via an infusion pump.

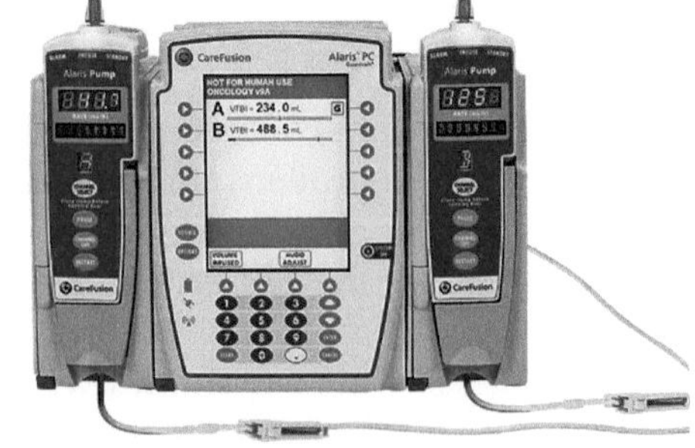

Many medications are administered using an infusion pump at the patient's bedside; the pump accurately controls the rate of IV delivery.

FIGURE 13.10 Sample of a TPN Medication Order

Memorial Hospital Pharmacy

Pt. Name: Sarah Mansfield **Pt. ID#:** 66734
Room: TCU-07 **Rx#:** 126981

Physician Orders

TOTAL PARENTERAL NUTRITION (TPN) ADULT

Primary Diagnosis: Multiple Trauma – post MVA **Ht:** 181 cm Dosing Wt: 80 kg

DOB: 2/11/80 **Allergies:** NKDA

Instructions: This form must be completed for a new order or continuation of PN and faxed to the pharmacy by 2 p.m. to receive same-day preparation. TPN administration begins at 6 p.m. daily.

Administration Route: ☒ CVC or PICC *Note: Proper tip placement of the CVC or PICC must be confirmed prior to PN infusion.*
❑ Peripheral IV (PIV) (*Final PN Osmolarity ≤ _________ mOsm/L*)

Monitoring: Daily weights; strict input & output; bedside glucose monitoring every 8 hours
☒ Na, K, Cl, CO_2, Glucose, BUN, Scr, Mg, PO_4 every Day
☒ T. Billi, Alk Phos, AST, ALT, Albumin, Triglycerides, Calcium every Week

Base Solution: *Total parenteral nutrition **MUST** be administered through a dedicated infusion port and filtered with a 1.2-micron in-line filter at all times. Discard any unused volume after 24 hours.*
Select one

❑ **PERIPHERAL 2-in-1**	☒ **CENTRAL 2-in-1**	❑ **CENTRAL 3-in-1**
Dextrose _______ g	Dextrose 15%	Dextrose _______ g
Amino Acids (*Brand*_______) _______ g	Amino Acids (*Brand* Aminosyn) 3.5%	Amino Acids (*Brand*_______) _______ g
For patients with PIV and established glucose tolerance; provides _____ kcal; maximum rate not to exceed _____ mL/hour.	*For patients with CVC or PICC and established glucose tolerance; provides _____ kcal; maximum rate not to exceed _____ mL/hour.*	Fat Emulsion (*Brand*_______) _______ g
		For patients with CVC or PICC and established glucose/fat emulsion tolerance; provides _____ kcal; maximum rate not to exceed _____ mL/hour.
		Use of additional fat emulsion not required with 3-in-1 base solution.

RATE & VOLUME: 40 mL/hour for 24 hours = 960 mL/day
Must specify

or CYCLIC INFUSION: ______ mL/hour for ______ hours, then ______ mL/hour for ______ hours = ______ mL/day

Fat Emulsion (Brand 0) – via PIV or CVC with 2-in-1 base solutions (select caloric density & volume)

❑ 10% ❑ 20% Infuse at ____ mL/hour over ____ hours. Frequency ____

❑ 250 mL ❑ 500 mL *(Note: Infusions < 4 or > 12 hours not recommended)* *Discard any unused volume after 12 hours.*

Additives: (per liter)		**Normal Dosages**
Sodium Chloride	40 mEq	*1–2 mEq sodium/kg/day*
as Acetate	_____ mEq	*pH or CO_2 dependent*
as Phosphate	_____ mmol of PO_4	*Consider if hyperkalemic*
Potassium Chloride	20 mEq	*1–2 mEq potassium/kg/day*
as Acetate	_____ mEq	*pH or CO_2 dependent*
as Phosphate	12 mmol of PO_4	*20–40 mmol/day(1 mmol Phos = 1.5 mEq K)*
Calcium Gluconate	10 mEq	*5–15 mEq/day*
Magnesium **Sulfate**	_____ mEq	*8–24 mEq/day*
Adult **Multivitamins**	10 mL/day	*Contains vitamin K 160 mcg*
Adult **Trace Elements**	5 mL/day	*Zn __ mg, Cu __ mg, Mn __ mg, Cr __ mcg, Se __ mcg (with normal hepatic function)*
H_2 Antagonist	_____ mg	*____ mg/day with normal renal function*
Other:		

Additives: (per liter)
Regular Insulin 60 units
Recommended if hyperglycemic; start with 1 unit for every 10 g of dextrose.

Pharmacy Use Only: Ca/PO_4
Limit Checked MKing, RPh
(Note: Some brands of amino acids contain phosphate.)

Physician's Signature Kumar Singh, MD Pager Number: 6-5411 Date/time: 8/14/2021

Orders transcribed by: RMcManus Date/time: 8/14/21 11:30 am Orders verified by: MKing, RPh Date/time: 8/14/21 2:45 pm

IN THE REAL WORLD

Children's Hospital, a 350-bed facility in Salt Lake City, Utah, developed in-house software to electronically order TPN solutions. The prescriber initiates the order and the software does all the calculations, including patient weight and dosage, checking for any incompatibilities. If an error is detected, the software provides the user with real-time solutions. After seven years and more than 84,000 TPN orders, there were 230 errors (a lower rate than with pharmacy personnel doing the calculations of each additive). Most of the TPN errors that did occur happened during administration; all transcription errors were eliminated because of the automated software!

The IV tubing for TPNs includes a special 0.22-micron in-line filter to screen out contaminants and maintain sterility. This in-line filter and tubing must be changed every 24 hours (or per hospital policy) or with each new TPN bag (or bottle) to minimize bacterial contamination and infection. So new filters and IV sets must be sent along with the TPNs at the daily resupply rounds.

Automated Compounding Devices for Parenteral Solutions

In small hospital pharmacies, the pharmacy technician may have to perform manual sterile compounding to prepare the TPN solutions. In this time-consuming process, the technician prepares the base solution, draws up each of the various additives into separate syringes, and then injects the additives into the base solution per the prescriber's order. Compounding the many additives of a TPN is especially time-consuming.

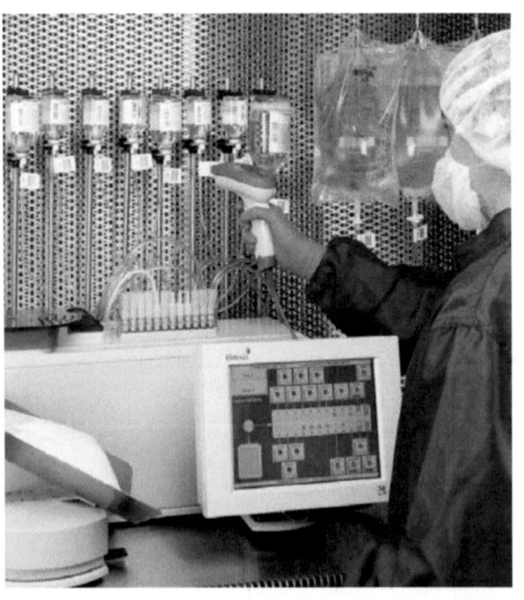

A sterile compounding technician uses an Exacta-Mix 2400 from Baxter, which is an automated compounding device that allows up to 24 ingredients to be inserted in TPN bags, producing a sterile 3 L bag in about four minutes.

In large hospitals and in many infusion compounding pharmacies for home care, an **automated compounding device (ACD)** is generally used. The ACD generally comes with 12 to 24 fluid ports within it that each have sterile containers of the commonly needed nutritional additives for the TPN bags. The ACD uses a pumping system calibrated with metric measurements of volume or gravity to fill the bags with the correct elements. The technician who oversees the ACD must measure each compounded bag to check that it is of the desired volume or weight. The ACD must also be checked for accuracy and correct calibration each day, both of which must be documented.

The technicians must be trained in the proper aseptic technique and ACD-filling and maintenance procedures to work with an ACD, according to the manufacturer guidelines and standards and procedures set by the USP and the American Society of Health-System Pharmacists (ASHP). If used and maintained properly, ACDs have had a better safety record than pharmacy compounding personnel.

IN THE REAL WORLD

Using an automated compounder is not an answer for all safety questions. As reported by the Institute for Safe Medication Practices, a physician ordered a TPN for a premature infant. The physician prescribed a total of 14.7 mEq of sodium chloride and 982 mg of calcium in the infant's TPN. The order was faxed to the pharmacy after midnight, at which time a pharmacy technician made an error entering the order into the automated compounder software. Apparently, the technician accidentally entered the prescribed dose of calcium ("982" mg) into the mEq field for sodium. The technician then prepared the TPN with a total of 982 mEq of sodium, using an automated IV compounder. The technician affixed the automated printed label to the TPN, which showed the erroneous sodium content.

Unfortunately, the error was not detected when the pharmacist checked the final product. The original order was not checked against the automated printed label, and a different label that listed the originally prescribed amount (sodium content as 14.7 mEq) was applied directly over the label produced by the automated compounder. Thus, the nurse who eventually started administration of the TPN solution was unable to detect the error.

It is very sad to say that a few hours after the TPN was started, routine lab studies showed that the infant's sodium level was abnormally high. The infant's physician assumed the study results were inaccurate and asked for the lab test to be redone. This was never accomplished before the infant experienced a cardiac arrest and died. So this reminds all to check, double-check, and triple-check the orders and labels and calculations even with ACDs.

13.5 Completing Compounded Sterile Preparation for Storage and Delivery

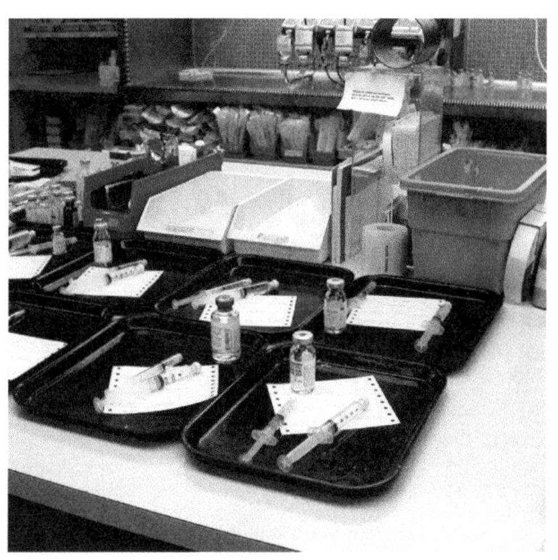

Medications compounded by the technician must await approval by the pharmacist along with all the syringes, vials, and ampules used.

After the various types of CSPs are prepared and labeled, but before they are transferred for short-term storage or immediate delivery, they must be inspected once more by the technician and pharmacist and assigned a BUD on the label (if not preprinted), with a sign-off from both the preparer and pharmacist. As noted, the *USP* Chapter <797> guidelines specify procedures for dating, labeling, storage, handling, packaging, and transporting of CSPs in the hospital or infusion pharmacy. Improper procedures could adversely affect the sterility or stability of the CSP.

The Final Physical Inspection and Verification

The technician checks to make sure there are no precipitates, incompatibilities, or leaks in any of the IVs, then lays out all the CSP and all the components used in the compounding for the pharmacist's approval. The pharmacist's final CSP inspection will include checking for accuracy in the proper selection and quantities of ingredients, technique for aseptic mixing and sterilization, packaging, and labeling or reviewing photos that have been taken with dedicated cameras in the clean room that have been used to capture the volumes and medication drawn up and added to the final container.

Physical appearance of the CSP is a key element for inspection. As explained, often more than one drug must be added to an LVP IV solution. Once those medications are reconstituted with sterile water (or normal saline) and then mixed with the others in the base solution, there is always the possibility of a physical incompatibility or particulate contamination. If one medication is an acidic salt like potassium chloride and the other an alkaline salt like sodium bicarbonate, a solid precipitate such as sodium chloride (salt) may form when the two are mixed together in the LVP. To avoid any solid precipitates, all final CSPs are inspected by the pharmacist and technician against a white or black background to confirm that precipitates (and particulate matter) are not present. If there is concern about a potential physical drug incompatibility, Trissel's *Stability of Compounded Formulations* should be consulted.

If any particulate matter is identified, then the CSP is discarded to prevent the introduction of any particles in the solution into a vein that could cause an obstruction in a vein or blood vessel. The use of SVPs that contain medication minimizes the risk of physical incompatibility since the medications are not in prolonged contact with the additives or drugs in the LVP base solution.

Storage of Compounded Sterile Preparations

Once approved and labeled, the CSPs are either delivered or are placed in short-term storage until delivery. The storage conditions vary according to the preprinted label instructions. The pharmacy technician is often responsible for monitoring and documenting the conditions under which CSPs are stored—at room temperature, or in the refrigerator or freezer. Each controlled temperature area must be checked daily and recorded in a temperature log. If a CSP has been exposed to temperatures that exceed the acceptable range (such as greater than 4 hours at 40 degrees), it must be discarded.

Practice Tip

General rule of thumb for all CSPs in terms of sterility or integrity is, "When in doubt, throw it out!"

Inspecting, Packaging and Handling

If not immediately delivered, the CSP must be reinspected by the pharmacist before delivery for any defects, such as precipitation, cloudiness, or leakage, that may have developed during storage. The closure of the container must also be inspected for integrity. With any noted defect, the CSP must be discarded.

How you package the CSPs for delivery can determine how well they maintain their physical integrity, sterility, and stability from this point on. The transport packaging must protect CSPs from damage, leakage, contamination, degradation, and particle adhesion while simultaneously protecting transport personnel from harm if hazardous compounds are present. Tamper-evident closures and seals on CSP

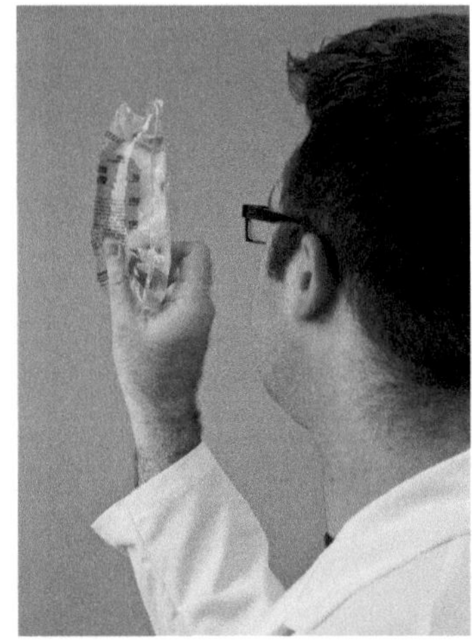

If a CSP has been stored before delivery, the pharmacist must reinspect it for its physical properties to see that it has maintained its integrity.

ports can provide an additional measure of security. If the CSP is sensitive to light, light-resistant materials must be used. In some cases, the CSP should be packaged in a special container (e.g., a cooler) to protect it from temperature fluctuations.

At times, you must also select the best transport mode to deliver the properly packed CSPs to arrive in an unshaken, undamaged, sterile, and stable condition. The exterior packaging must be clearly labeled with the specific patient information and delivery handling instructions along with the storage and administration counsel and any necessary highlighted warnings.

Priming and Administration of the IVs

After the CSPs are compounded and approved, a technician often delivers them to the nursing unit. Just prior to administration, the nurse will check that the CSP is still sealed and has its packaging and labeling intact. Then the nurse will hang the IV bags one at a time, keeping all ports and needles sterile. Priming is needed for both the primary and secondary tubing. Sometimes the technician does the priming, depending on the CSP, especially if it is a chemotherapy drug.

Bedside Priming

Priming is the action of letting fluid run through the system before administration, tapping at all the connections to dislodge bubbles to be sure that all of the air is out of both lines prior to attaching to the patient. The amount of fluid needed to prime the tubing depends on its length—up to 18 mL for longer primary sets, down to 3 mL for the shorter secondary extensions. Sometimes technicians do this priming just before delivery. See the presentation on priming the IV line at https://PharmPractice7e.ParadigmEducation.com/PrimingIV.

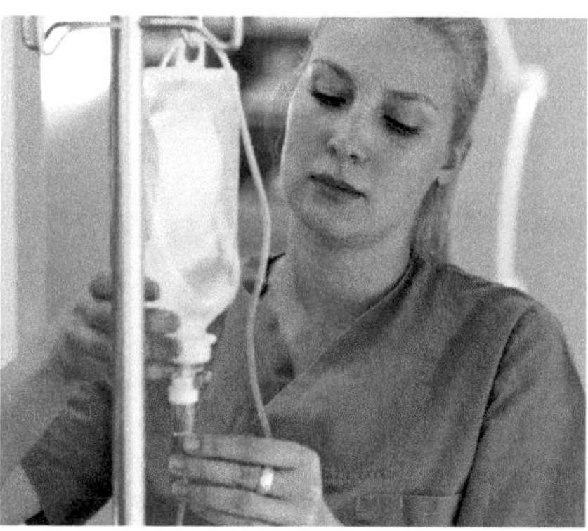

Before administering the IV, the nurse will prime the tubing (if not preprimed) to clear the lines of air bubbles and to check and calibrate the drip rate.

13.6 Premade IV Solutions Not Requiring Sterile Compounding

For some parenteral administrations, premade IV solutions are available. Recent innovative IV technologies from commercial pharmaceutical manufacturers, such as vial-and-bag products and frozen antibiotics, offer many advantages over cleanroom CSPs. They minimize measurement and compounding errors.

Vial-and-Bag Systems

A **vial-and-bag system** provides a single vial of powdered medication attached with an adapter to a specified IV bag solution that acts as the diluent. After scanning the product's bar code, the nurse uses aseptic technique to break the seal of the attached powder vial, releasing the medication into the IVPB bag. This action "activates" the medication, which, once fully dissolved, is administered in short order to the patient via the secondary line tubing.

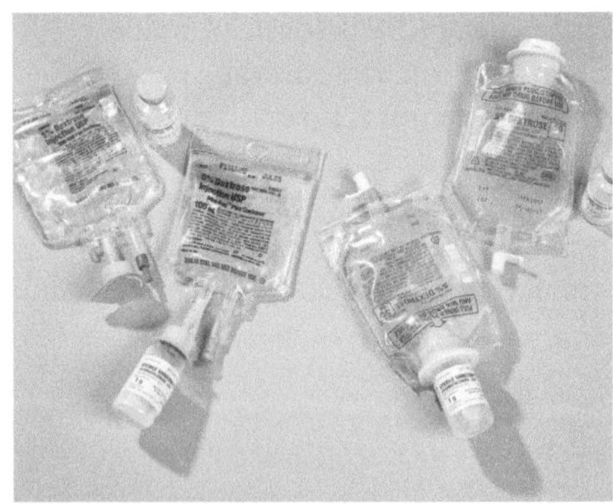

A vial-and-bag IV system is assembled by the technician but activated by the nurse at the patient's bedside.

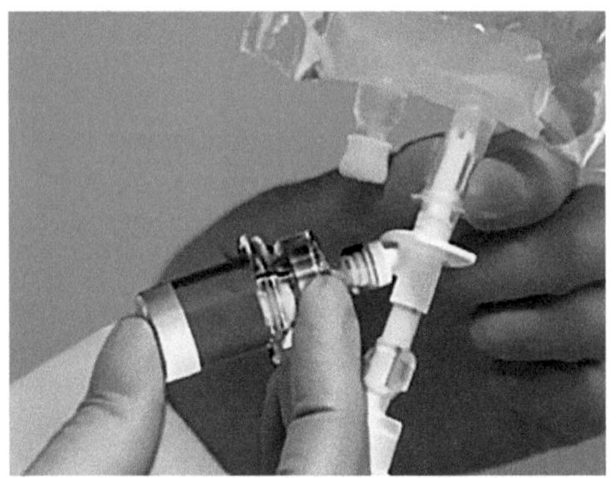

The technician assembles the vial-and-bag system in a cleanroom DCA, preparing the IV for the nurse to activate at the patient's bedside when it is time to administer it. With different systems, there are various ways to insert the vial contents into the bag.

Though the technician does not compound the vial-and-bag product, it must be assembled (linking the vial and the bag with the connector device. Docking and activation of proprietary bag and vial systems (e.g., addEASE, ADD-Vantage, Mini Bag Plus) in accordance with the manufacturer's labeling for immediate administration to an individual patient is not considered compounding and may be performed outside of an International Organization for Standardization (ISO) 5 environment. Docking of the proprietary bag and vial systems for future activation and administration is considered compounding and must be performed in accordance with this chapter, with the exception of 14. Establishing Beyond-Use Dates. Beyond-use dates (BUDs) for proprietary bag and vial systems must not be longer than those specified in the manufacturer's labeling.

Vial-and-bag systems are marketed under many trade names, such as ADD-Vantage (Pfizer) and Mini-Bag Plus (Baxter Healthcare) and addEASE (B. Braun Medical). Each vial-and-bag system differs somewhat in design, but the concept is similar. The vial of drug—which has not been reconstituted—is coupled (with or without an adapter) with an appropriate volume of IV solution. Minibags are usually available in 50 mL, 100 mL, and 250 mL sizes with many diluent options (D_5W, D_5NS, NS, lactated Ringer's, and so on). However, only select products are available in vial-and-bag systems—mostly in-demand antibiotics.

CSPs are a time-consuming and labor-intensive process. Though initially more costly, vial-and-bag systems offer a variety of benefits for healthcare personnel. In addition to fewer returns to the pharmacy and less wastage, other advantages are improved safety, efficiency, and cost-effectiveness.

Safety

Preparation errors are minimized with vial-and-bag systems because doses are standardized. Enhanced labeling and bar coding of both the vial medication and IV solution are provided so the nurse knows exactly what is in the IV solution. The closed-system sterile packaging also minimizes the risk of contamination. Finally, these devices do not use needles, thus preventing the possibility of inadvertent needle sticks by the pharmacist, technician, or nurse.

Efficiency

Vial-and-bag systems are efficient because doses are premeasured for rapid reconstitution and easy assembly by the nurse. There is no need for freezing, thawing, or refrigeration of the solution in the pharmacy or nursing unit because the product is immediately administered to the patient.

Cost-Effectiveness

With the vial-and-bag system, there are no additional personnel or supply costs incurred—such as for syringes, needles, gauze, and so on. With fewer plastic syringes and other supplies used, less waste is produced for disposal. There is also less wastage when an order is changed. The expiration dates of these non-activated manufacturer products far exceed the beyond-use dating of a compounded product required by *USP* Chapter <797> so they last longer. These advantages may well outweigh the additional cost per unit.

Frozen IV Solutions

Manufactured frozen IV solutions are premixed products and, consequently, are also not considered CSPs. Most frozen IV products are antibiotic solutions for SVPs. Like the vial-and-bag IV solutions, the frozen IV solutions are also more costly than compounding standard IV solutions and additives. However, hospital pharmacies purchase these frozen products for a number of the same reasons that they purchase the vial-and-bag systems—the longer expiration dates, reduced risk of microbial contamination, and less labor-intensive preparation for pharmacy personnel. The reconstituted vials of antibiotics in CSP solutions have much shorter half-lives than the frozen solutions and thus there is potentially more wastage in CSPs. These benefits partially offset the higher acquisition cost and the additional freezer space needed for the frozen IVs.

Until a medication order is received, premixed IV products are kept in the hospital pharmacy freezer. When a frozen IV is ordered, it is thawed at room temperature or in the refrigerator (if there is sufficient time). The use of a warming bath or microwave to expedite the thawing process ("forced thaw") is *not* recommended. Manufacturers' recommendations for thawing vary among products, so personnel must be sure to check each product's label or package insert.

After thawing, the technician prepares a patient-specific label that includes the manufacturer's expiration date. Again, the expiration date varies with the drug and storage conditions. For example, a frozen Ancef antibiotic solution has an expiration date of 48 hours at room temperature or 30 days if stored in the refrigerator. A Zosyn antibiotic solution has an expiration date of 24 hours at room temperature or 14 days if stored in the refrigerator. Once thawed, these frozen preparations cannot be refrozen.

After preparing the label, affix it to the bag for pharmacist review and, once approved, send the medication to the nursing unit for administration.

13.7 Handling CSP and Manufacturer Product Returns

What if an IV or other CSP is returned from the nursing unit unopened and unused? The patient may have been discharged, transferred to another hospital, or died, or the physician may have changed the medication order. The decision as to whether to reuse any CSP or commercially available product is influenced by the nursing unit's storage conditions, the hospital's policies and procedures, and *USP* Chapter <797> directives. An unopened CSP can be returned for a short period of time to pharmacy storage, relabeled, and redispensed *only* when the pharmacist or technician is certain that it was stored by the nursing unit in compliance with instructions and remained sterile and chemically stable per *USP* <797>. Is there any doubt that it was refrigerated properly and protected from light as the instructions dictated? Is there evidence of compromises in package integrity? If so, the CSP must be discarded.

In the case of a proprietary vial-and-bag system that has not been "activated," the vial-and-bag system may be returned to the pharmacy for reuse and relabeling.

Depending on the manufacturer's recommendations, once the product has been removed from the exterior sterile packaging, there is a 14- to 30-day shelf life for future use. The manufacturer's product package insert should be consulted for precise expiration dating. Activated doses returned to the pharmacy, however, *must be discarded.*

If a premade, frozen IVPB is stored for a short time at room temperature, the pharmacist must determine in accordance with manufacturer recommendations and hospital policies whether it can be relabeled and used soon after with a shorter expiration date. If the turnaround is quick enough that it can be used for another patient, then a new patient-specific label may be generated with an updated beyond-use date.

13.8 Hazardous Sterile Compounding

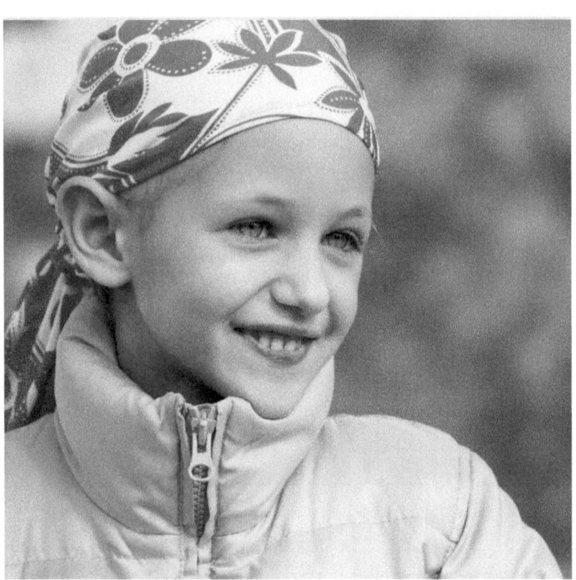

Many cancer treatment drugs are very toxic. Patients often lose their hair, but it will grow back after treatments are completed.

A subcategory of sterile compounding is hazardous compounding. Cancer-fighting, or **antineoplastic**, drug therapies generally apply toxic agents to kill or inhibit the cancer cells, which are faster-growing than normal healthy cells. However, these are not the only hazardous agents. Destructive compounds also include antivirals, hormones, dangerous biological agents, and radiation treatments (nuclear pharmacy). Any drug that is known to have a risk of at least one of the following six criteria is considered a **hazardous drug (HD)**:

- carcinogenicity (causes cancer)
- teratogenicity (causes development damage/problems)
- reproductive toxicity (causes reproductive damage/problems)
- organ toxicity (causes organ damage/problems)
- genotoxicity (causes genetic damage)
- new drugs that mimic hazardous drugs in structure or toxicity

Put Down Roots

The term *carcinoma*, meaning "cancerous tumor," originated from the Greek words *carcinos*, meaning, "cancer," and *onkos*, meaning "mass."

Many pharmacy technicians, especially those working in a hospital setting, occasionally handle hazardous agents, especially in compounding nonsterile and sterile medications. Others specialize in hazardous or nuclear compounding.

Clearly, *there is no acceptable level of exposure to HDs*. Recent scientific studies have shown that even those handling the toxic agents in receiving and delivery of ingredients and final products experience far more exposure than was previously known. The CDC has a special center for hazardous substances: the **National Institute for Occupational Safety and Health (NIOSH)**. The CDC and OSHA have published the *NIOSH Alert: Preventing Occupational Exposures to Antineoplastic and Other Hazardous Drugs in Health Care Settings*, and the ASHP has established its own new HD guidelines. The *USP* Chapter <800>, which was finalized in 2016, had to be fully implemented by institutions doing hazardous compounding before December 1, 2019.

USP <800> outlines requirements for receipt, storage, mixing, preparing, compounding, dispensing, and administration of hazardous drugs to protect the patient, healthcare personnel, and environment. This chapter can offer only an overview. For more information about *USP* <800>, go to **https://PharmPractice7e.ParadigmEducation.com/USP800FAQ**.

FIGURE 13.11
Safety Data Sheet

Safety Data Sheets (SDSs) on each toxic agent with colorful pictographs about the danger level and response must be available to employees, according to OSHA rules, *USP* <800> (2016), and the Globally Harmonized System (GHS) of classification and labeling of chemicals.

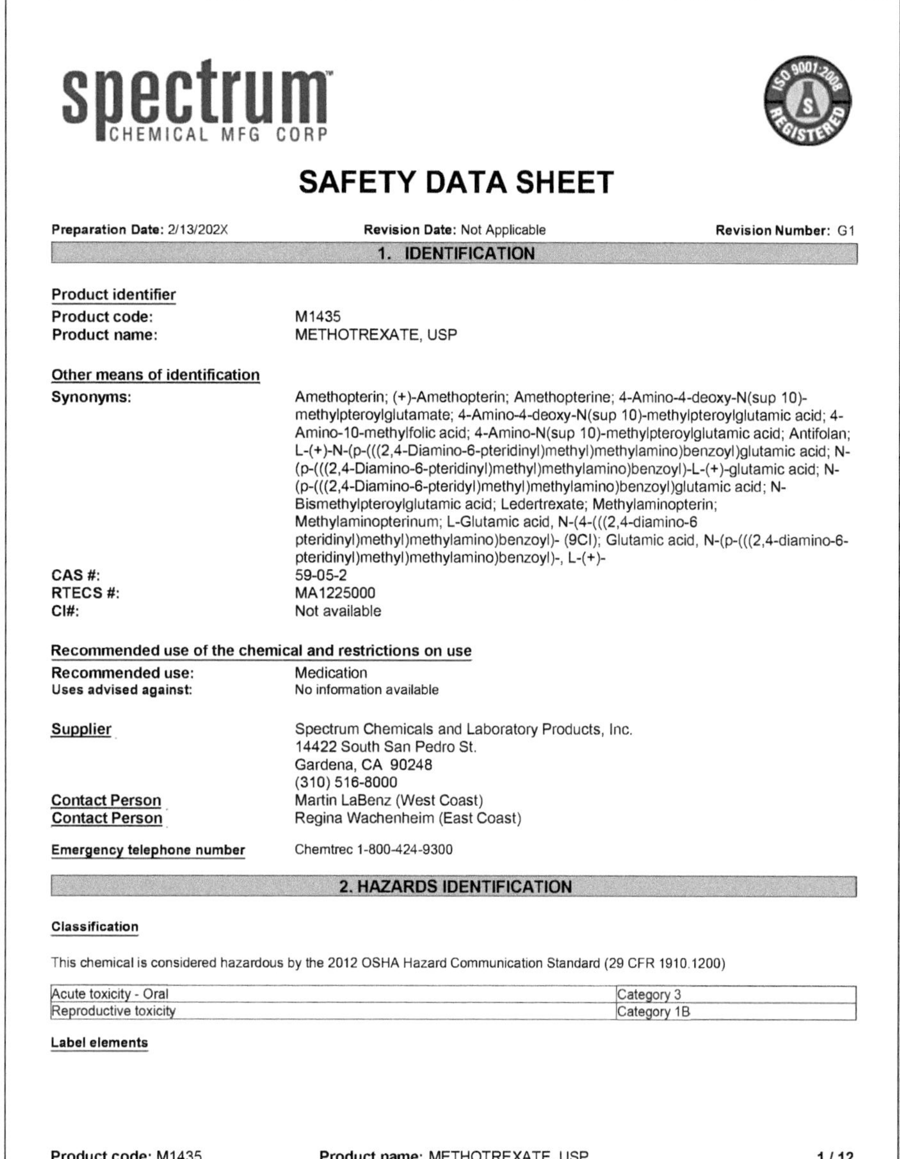

spectrum™ CHEMICAL MFG CORP

SAFETY DATA SHEET

Preparation Date: 2/13/202X | **Revision Date:** Not Applicable | **Revision Number:** G1

1. IDENTIFICATION

Product identifier

Product code: M1435
Product name: METHOTREXATE, USP

Other means of identification

Synonyms: Amethopterin; (+)-Amethopterin; Amethopterine; 4-Amino-4-deoxy-N(sup 10)-methylpteroylglutamate; 4-Amino-4-deoxy-N(sup 10)-methylpteroylglutamic acid; 4-Amino-10-methylfolic acid; 4-Amino-N(sup 10)-methylpteroylglutamic acid; Antifolan; L-(+)-N-(p-(((2,4-Diamino-6-pteridinyl)methyl)methylamino)benzoyl)glutamic acid; N-(p-(((2,4-Diamino-6-pteridinyl)methyl)methylamino)benzoyl)-L-(+)-glutamic acid; N-(p-(((2,4-Diamino-6-pteridyl)methyl)methylamino)benzoyl)glutamic acid; N-Bismethylpteroylglutamic acid; Ledertrexate; Methylaminopterin; Methylaminopterinum; L-Glutamic acid, N-(4-(((2,4-diamino-6 pteridinyl)methyl)methylamino)benzoyl)- (9CI); Glutamic acid, N-(p-(((2,4-diamino-6-pteridinyl)methyl)methylamino)benzoyl)-, L-(+)-
CAS #: 59-05-2
RTECS #: MA1225000
CI#: Not available

Recommended use of the chemical and restrictions on use

Recommended use: Medication
Uses advised against: No information available

Supplier
Spectrum Chemicals and Laboratory Products, Inc.
14422 South San Pedro St.
Gardena, CA 90248
(310) 516-8000

Contact Person Martin LaBenz (West Coast)
Contact Person Regina Wachenheim (East Coast)

Emergency telephone number Chemtrec 1-800-424-9300

2. HAZARDS IDENTIFICATION

Classification

This chemical is considered hazardous by the 2012 OSHA Hazard Communication Standard (29 CFR 1910.1200)

Acute toxicity - Oral	Category 3
Reproductive toxicity	Category 1B

Label elements

Product code: M1435 | **Product name:** METHOTREXATE, USP | **1 / 12**

According to *USP* <800>, personnel in a hospital or compounding facility who come into *any level of contact* with HDs require specialized equipment, training, protective equipment, and procedures for the handling, preparation, and disposal of these substances. Hospitals are required to develop written policies and procedures for each aspect of HD use to be in compliance with the USP and the Joint Commission, as well as state and federal regulations.

Safety Data Sheets (SDSs) for each hazardous agent or investigational drug must be readily accessible so that employees can see what they are handling and what should be done in the case of an accidental exposure or spill (see Figure 13.11). For an extended explanation, see Chapter 10.

Risks of Exposure

NIOSH categorizes risk for exposure to hazardous agents through four routes: (1) trauma, (2) inhalation, (3) ingestion, and (4) direct skin contact. The routes are illustrated by the following examples:

- **Trauma or injury:** A technician uses a syringe to add a drug to an IV bag and accidentally gets pricked with the needle or receives a cut from a broken container of the hazardous drug.
- **Inhalation of the hazardous substance:** A technician drops and breaks a bottle containing a volatile substance or uses poor manipulation technique with a vial, thereby releasing a fine mist and inadvertently inhaling the toxic substance.
- **Ingestion:** A technician gets minute powder particles on lips when crushing an oral tablet or even cleaning a counting tray and unconsciously licks lips.
- **Direct skin contact:** A technician accidentally spills a medication when pouring it from a large container into a smaller container or flask, and a drop splashes their skin. Direct contact with many cancer drugs can cause immediate reactions, such as the following:
  - Doxorubicin can cause tissue death and sloughing if introduced into a skin abrasion.
  - Nitrogen mustards can cause damage to the eyes, mucous membranes, and skin.

Within the hospital pharmacy, many activities have potential to result in HD exposures through the various routes without care and protection (as seen in Table 13.9).

TABLE 13.9 Routes of Exposure to Hazardous Agents

- Receiving and unpacking HD orders
- Counting individual oral doses and tablets from bulk containers
- Crushing tablets or opening capsules to make oral liquid
- Pouring oral or topical liquids from one container to another
- Mixing topical dosage forms
- Weighing or mixing components
- Constituting or reconstituting powdered or lyophilized (freeze-dried) HDs
- Withdrawing or diluting injectable HDs from parenteral containers
- Expelling air from syringes filled with HDs
- Expelling HDs from a syringe
- Coming into contact with HD residue present on drug container exteriors, work surfaces, floors, and final drug preparations (e.g., bottles, bags, cassettes, and syringes)
- Inhaling HD residue or vapors
- Handling contaminated waste generated at any step in the preparation or dispensing
- Deactivating, decontaminating, cleaning, and disinfecting areas contaminated or suspected of being contaminated with HDs
- Undergoing maintenance activities for contaminated equipment and devices
- Spilling substances, cleaning up a spill, and disposing of cleanup materials

The use of unprotected, incorrect technique in HD compounding not only poses contamination risks for the patient but also jeopardizes the and the area and people around them due to cross contamination.

With exposure to HDs, workers can suffer acute, chronic, and long-term health consequences if proper precautions, procedures, and training do not take place. The acute responses include skin rashes or allergic reactions. In women and men of reproductive age, chronic exposure can result in infertility, miscarriages, or neonates with low birth weight or congenital malformations. Long-term chronic exposure for all workers includes a higher risk for certain cancers, including skin and bladder cancers and leukemia.

Medical Surveillance

To prevent the serious health issues that can be caused by exposure to HDs, a medical surveillance program by the hospital or compounding facility should be implemented according to *USP* <800> guidelines. The goal of **medical surveillance** is to collect and interpret data on HD workers to detect any changes in their health status due to potential exposure. The surveillance is meant to identify the earliest reversible biologic effects in every worker so that exposure can be identified, eliminated, or reduced before the employee sustains irreversible damage.

The program consists of an initial baseline of health (including reproductive history); exposure assessment; monitoring of health through regular physical examinations, laboratory tests, and questionnaires; response plans when there is evidence of HD toxicity; and an exit physical exam on termination of employment. If exposure-related health changes occur, it should prompt immediate re-evaluation of primary preventive measures (e.g., administrative and engineering controls, PPE, and others). In this manner, medical surveillance acts as a check on the effectiveness of controls already in use.

Any person of reproductive age who routinely works with hazardous agents must confirm in writing an understanding of the the reproductive risks of handling hazardous drugs. A pharmacy technician who is pregnant, breast-feeding, or trying to conceive should notify their supervisor so that so that they can discuss if they want to be reassigned to a different department position, take extra precautions, or have different work responsibilities, so as to minimize contact with any hazardous substances.

Personnel Training

Specialized training to avoid exposure is essential for all HD employees. (Sterile hazardous compounding technicians need training in both specialties.) The US Occupational Safety and Health Administration, or OSHA, requires each hospital or pharmacy to establish a **hazardous communication standard (HCS)** outlining the policies, procedures, and practices to ensure worker safety in all aspects of the manipulation and distribution of these drugs and chemicals for all workers.

The HD training must be documented, and each technician must be assessed for competency prior to any HD compounding and then reassessed at least every 12 months. The training must include at least the following:

- Overview of entity's list of HDs and their risks
- Review of the entity's SOPs related to handling of HDs
- Proper use of PPE
- Proper use of equipment and devices (e.g., engineering controls)
- Response to known or suspected HD exposure

- Spill management
- Proper disposal of HDs and trace-contaminated materials

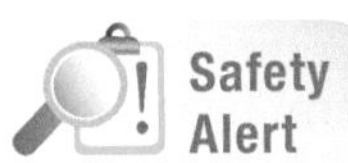

If you deal with HDs in any capacity—even if not compounding—PPE must be worn!

The hospital or facility must designate a pharmacist to be the compounding supervisor responsible for personnel competency and developing and implementing appropriate HD procedures in compliance with *USP* Chapter <800> as well as applicable federal and state laws, regulations, and standards.

Protective Clothing

According to *USP* Chapter <800>, personal protective equipment (PPE)–specialized clothing and gear–must be worn when working with hazardous agents. These guidelines are similar to the ones discussed in Chapter 12 for preparing CSPs, but HD compounding has additional requirements. The PPE must meet the NIOSH standards and include (among other potential equipment) the following:

- a non-permeable chemo rated gown
- hair cover and two pairs of shoe covers
- eye protection (goggles and shields)
- two pairs of chemo rated gloves; the top must be sterile when compounding

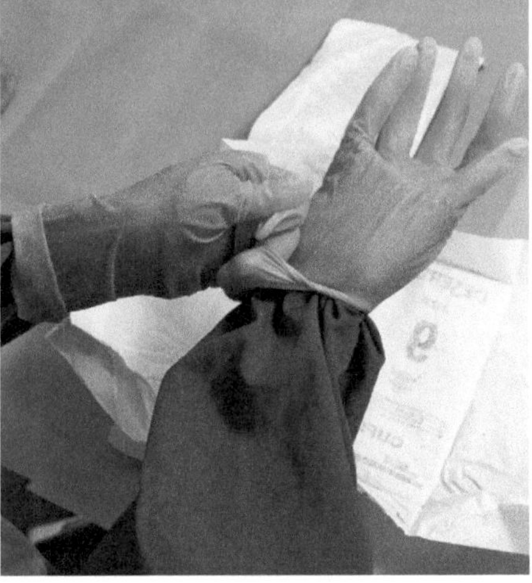

When working with hazardous drug agents, pharmacy technicians must use additional precautions, such as double chemotherapy gloves.

The goggles and face shields are designed to guard compounders' eyes and faces, as well as breathing passages and lungs, and must particularly be NIOSH approved. The gown must be disposable, lint-free, and impervious to liquids and solids, with a closed front and long stretchy cuffed sleeves to close off airflow. (Cloth laboratory coats, surgical scrubs, or isolation gowns are not appropriate when handling HDs because they permit the permeation of HDs and can hold spilled drugs against the skin and increase exposure. Chemotherapy gowns must be changed according to manufacturer recommendations or every 2–3 hours if no recommendation exists for the chemo-rated gown.)

Simply wearing sterile compounding gloves is not sufficient for hazardous compounding. Two layers of non-permeable **chemotherapy gloves** that are powder-free and tested by the ASTM (an international standards testing organization) are required. **Double gloving** should be done after proper hand hygiene per CDC guidelines, as described in Chapter 12. The outer gloves should be changed every 30 minutes or whenever torn or punctured, and must be sterile if sterile compounding.

The hazardous compounding PPE should be worn by a pharmacy technician when handling HDs and performing any of these functions:

- receiving intact supplies (remote from the compounding area)
- receiving broken or potentially broken supplies
- transporting intact supplies or compounded HDs
- receiving intact supplies in the compounding area
- stocking and inventory control of the compounding area

- nonsterile compounding
- sterile compounding
- collecting and disposing of compounding waste
- routine cleaning
- managing spills

Safety Alert

If a technician is working with hazardous drugs, additional protection such as a second pair of sterile gloves (known as double gloving) is required. A new gown must be worn if you have a spill or splash.

Before leaving the hazardous drug preparation area, *all disposable protective garb* must be discarded as trace chemotherapy waste in a specially marked container. No gloves, masks, and so on, can be reused (even after a short break), and no contaminated protective clothing can be worn outside the hazardous compounding area.

Secondary Engineering Controls to Contain Hazardous Agents

Hazardous substances and sterile hazardous substances must be compounded away from sterile products in a **containment secondary engineering control (C-SEC)** area with an exterior venting system. This way the trace hazardous substances do not flow into other CSP compounding areas and the hospital or the rest of the compounding facility.

As explained in Chapter 12, sterile compounding requires a cleanroom facility with two rooms with ISO air quality standards of Class 8 in the anteroom and Class 7 in the buffer room. To achieve these ISO standards, secondary engineering controls with high-efficiency particulate air (HEPA) filters are integrated into the heating, ventilation, and air conditioning systems (HVAC) of the rooms to create unidirectional airflow and air exchanges. For nonhazardous sterile compounding, filtered air is *pumped into* the buffer room to create positive air pressure and to have it flow out of the cleanroom areas, taking contaminants with it.

Hazardous compounding airflow, however, goes in the reverse pattern of that in the sterile compounding cleanroom. Hazardous compounding areas must provide **negative pressure**, with the ventilation system *suctioning away* the air around the compounder and hazardous product into a filtered exhaust system to keep the toxins away from the compounder and the buffer room.

There are two acceptable basic configurations for the C-SEC. In order to get full dating in *USP* <797> the C-SEC must be an ISO 7 negative pressure buffer room with appropriate air changes per hour (ACPH) with ISO 7 anteroom. An alternate option is a segregated compounding area with appropriate ACPH, but may only dispense CSPs with a 12 hours beyond-use date. Both room configurations still require the use of a negative pressure primary engineering control and both C-SECs must follow *USP* <800> standards.

For both sterile and nonsterile HD compounding, a sink must be available outside the buffer area for handwashing as well as for emergency access to water but at least one meter away from the entrance to the negative pressure area. An eyewash station within the contained HD compounding area is necessary for removal of hazardous substances from the eyes and skin.

Primary Engineering Controls to Contain Hazardous Agents

Per *USP* Chapter <800> standards, all HD compounding must be done in **containment primary engineering controls (C-PECs)**, which provide some level of shielding, enclosed isolation of the DCA, or sealed isolation to contain the HD substances and protect the compounding personnel. These C-PECs must still provide ISO Class 5 air quality in the DCA through the use of a ventilation system with HEPA filtering of the circulating air, air exchanges, and some level of exhausting of the circulated air. The C-PECs, however, have **vertical airflow**, or downward moving air, instead of the horizontal airflow that occurs in nonhazardous sterile compounding. (See Figure 13.12, which shows how vertical airflow works in one of the types of C-PECs.) The vertical airflow keeps the contaminants from blowing at the person doing the compounding. C-PECs come in various classifications, according to the level of toxicity of the agents compounded within them and the needed protection level to keep the compounder safe from exposure.

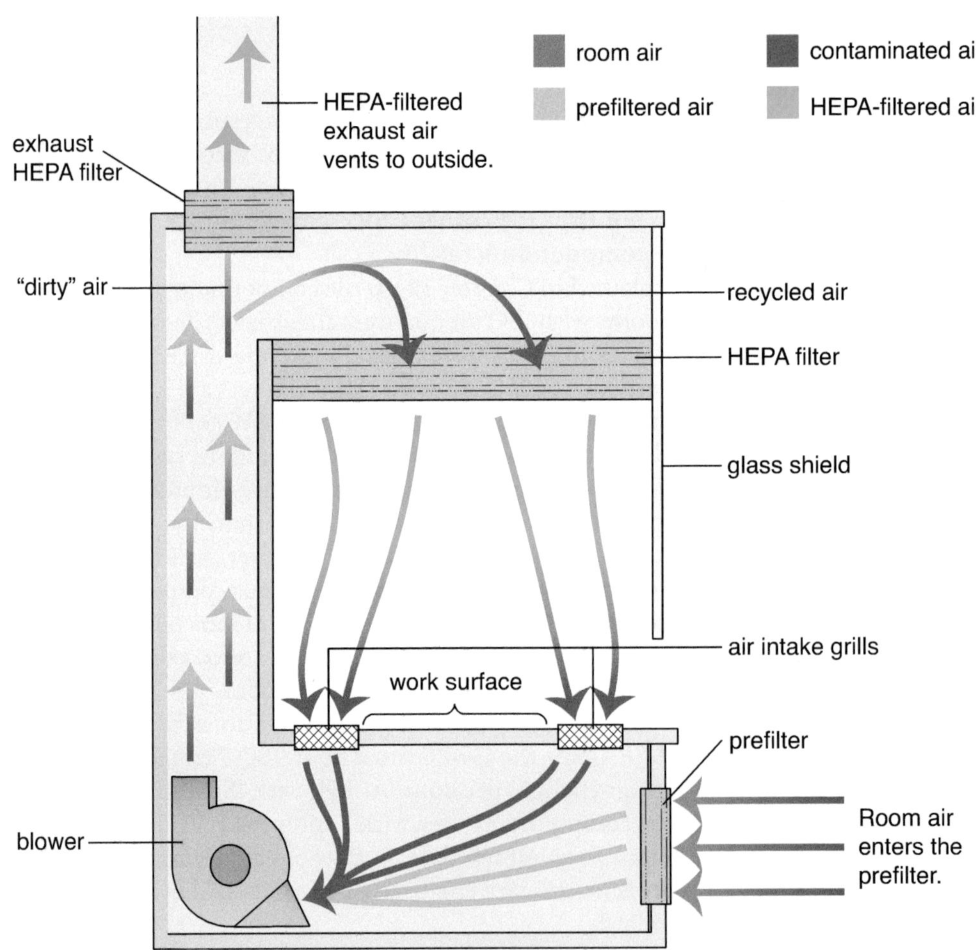

FIGURE 13.12 Side Cutaway of a Class II Biological Safety Cabinet

In a C-PEC with vertical airflow, the room air enters a prefilter and is forced upward through the HEPA filter, then a portion is blown down vertically from the hood onto the DCA to the work surface, where it is sucked back into air intake grills, drawing the air away from the compounder and the outer room. The rest of the air is exhausted through another HEPA filter to an outside space or exterior ventilation system.

Levels of Hazardous Drug Risk and Contained Primary Engineering Controls

NIOSH publishes a list of HDs based on groups of risk. This list is updated every two years and includes a review of existing HDs as well as the addition of newly approved drugs. The NIOSH groups of risk include the following.

- Group 1: Antineoplastic drugs. Many of these drugs may also pose a reproductive risk for susceptible populations.

- Group 2: Non-antineoplastic drugs that meet one or more of the NIOSH criteria for an HD. Some of these drugs may also pose a reproductive risk for susceptible populations.
- Group 3: Drugs that primarily pose a reproductive risk to men and women who are actively trying to conceive and women who are pregnant or breastfeeding (some of these drugs may be present in breast milk).

TABLE 13.10 General Types of Containment Primary Engineering Controls for Sterile Hazardous Compounding

Each unit has vertical HEPA-filtered airflow, air exchanges, and some level of HEPA-exhausted air, according to *USP* Chapter <800> (2016) standards.

Containment Primary Engineering Controls

Class II biological safety cabinets—provide a containment barrier through a partial or full shield for hazardous compounding protection in various levels

- **Class II-A biological safety cabinets** (including the vertical laminar airflow workbench): partially shielded units with downward filtered airflow onto the DCA, with little exterior venting and high amounts of recirculated air
- **Class II-B biological safety cabinets:** similar units (with barriers and vertical airflow) though with exterior filtered venting and little to no recirculating air

Compounding aseptic isolators—an enclosed PEC with an ingredient transfer station or interchange zone

- **Compounding aseptic containment isolator (CACI):** used to provide worker protection from exposure to undesirable levels of airborne drugs throughout the compounding and material transfer processes and to provide an aseptic environment with unidirectional airflow for compounding sterile preparations.

Sealed sterile compounding isolators—units with completely sealed DCAs and transfer chamber systems with self-cleaning/gas sterilizing

- **Class III biological safety cabinet:** sealed unit for high-risk hazardous compounding, vented, and filtered to outdoors with no recirculating air
- **Radiopharmacy isolator:** a lead-shielded, sealed unit designed specifically for compounding radioactive diagnostic and therapeutic agents

Types of Containment Primary Engineering Controls

Various levels of HEPA-filtered C-PECs are designed to protect the workers and the environment from toxic exposure to the HDs in the aforementioned NIOSH risk groups. Hazardous C-PECs include the many levels of **biological safety cabinets (BSCs)**, the **compounding aseptic containment isolator (CACI)**, and the radio pharmacy isolator used in nuclear pharmacy. These BSCs come in different Class levels of protection and safety to align with the risk level of the substances: Class I, Class II, and Class III. A Class I BSC protects personnel and the environment but does not protect the product/preparation and is not appropriate for sterile compounding. Class II BSCs for compounding come in different levels of filtered venting and recirculated air. Class III is a sealed isolator offering the most protection for the most hazardous compounds.

Table 13.10 shows an overview of the general types of C-PECs. Manufacturers produce variations of the different PEC types, creating hybrid models as they work to continually improve their equipment offerings and keep up with the new *USP* <800> guidelines. Each HD compounding facility has to train its staff on the ins and outs of its own specific equipment, but there are some standard principles to learn.

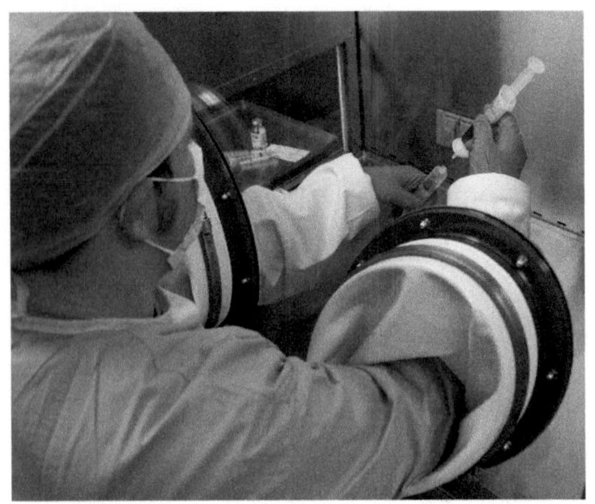

A technician prepares hazardous drugs in a CACI.

Class II Biological Safety Cabinets Class II BSCs are subdivided into even more categories of Class II-A2, B1, and B2 with increased containment at each level. Some C-PECs that are in the Class II-A categories are also known as vertical laminar airflow workbenches (V-LAFWs). Because the airflow is moving downward from the ceiling vent onto the DCA rather than from the back wall, the zone of turbulence is in a different place. The compounding technician must be careful not to block the airflow to the CSP in the DCA.

Class II-A2, B1, and B2 have less recirculated air and more filtered venting to the outside of the cleanroom environment for cleaner air exchanges. The Class II-B cabinets also have a lower shield for additional protection, some extending to the counter like a hinged door.

Since the filtered airflow flows down onto the DCA, the key zone of turbulence has changed from a horizontal LAFW. So, the zone exists below any action or supplies. Technicians have to be very careful that they do not put their hands or tools above the CSP in the DCA. They do not want to block air flowing down on the CSP or compounding actions in any way.

Compounding Aseptic Isolators (CAI) The CAI creates a positive pressure clean air controlled environment. Whereas the compounding aseptic containment isolator (CACI) creates a negative pressure clean air controlled environment. Both CAIs and CACIs are types of PECs known as RABS or Restricted Access Barrier Systems. RABS are treated no differently than other primary engineering controls and all personal protective equipment is required when compounding in a RAB. Beyond-use dating is determined by the environments the PEC is placed in and not they type of PEC it is compound in. The CACI, like the compounding aseptic isolators, is an enclosed PEC, with an ingredient transfer station or interchange zone and ingredient transfer stations. As in all the other PECs, the DCA is maintained at ISO Class 5 air quality by the HEPA-filtered ventilation system in the unit. The CACI has heavy-duty NIOSH-approved gloves projecting through it. The hazardous CSP supplies and ingredients are moved inside the DCA via a transfer port (an enclosed movable chamber that is not fully sealed). The RABS shield must be opened to conduct a full deep clean and decontamination. This includes cleaning under the work tray. Daily cleaning and decontamination is more difficult and requires special tools to reach all surfaces of the RAB.

Placing a biological safety cabinet Class II-B in a separate negative-pressure room decreases the risk of employee exposure to dangerous contaminants, which is why it is required.

Class III Biological Safety Cabinets The Class III BSC is like the compounding aseptic isolator in having a completely sealed DCA and sealed supply transfer chamber and a self-cleaning gas and vacuum system, so the unit is not opened by the technician. However, the BSC Class III has vertical airflow and complete filtered external venting with no recirculated air, and some units have robotic arms instead of a DCA for extra protection.

Nuclear Compounding Isolators The radiopharmacy isolators are also completely sealed, though they have lead or tungsten shielding (including leaded glass) to protect the compounding personnel from nuclear exposure. Many of these isolators have computer screens to view the compounding for even greater protection.

Supplemental Engineering Controls for Hazardous Compounding

In hazardous sterile compounding, slightly different processes are used for working with vials and ampules than in general sterile compounding, and a few additional protective supplies should be used: a chemotherapy compounding mat, closed-system transfer devices, and chemotherapy **engineering controls**. A supplemental engineering control is an adjunct control (e.g., CSTD) that may be used concurrently with primary and secondary engineering controls. Supplemental engineering controls offer additional levels of protection and may facilitate enhanced occupational protection, especially when handling HDs outside of primary and secondary engineering controls such as for nursing during adminstration.

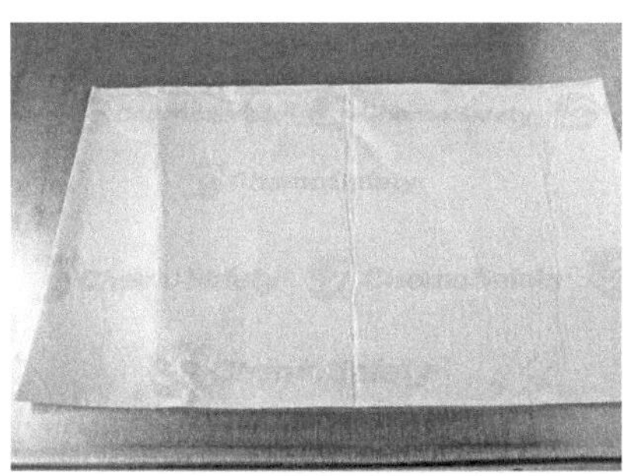

A chemotherapy compounding mat is placed on the work surface before each session to catch toxic contaminants.

Chemotherapy Compounding Mat

A **chemotherapy compounding** covering for the counter that has o of absorbent material to soak up po spills within the DCA. The other side of the mat is made of a low-permeability material that prevents fluid from seeping through to the work surface. Before beginning each HD compounding session, the mat is laid on the counter, and afterwards the mat is discarded as contaminated waste in a designated container.

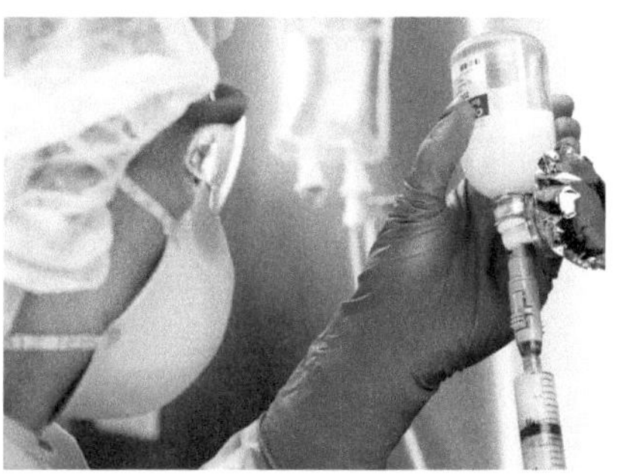

This CSTD (the blue plastic piece connecting the syringe to the bottle) around the vial to the needle-and-syringe site offers the compounder additional protection from vapors within a BSC or CACI.

Closed-System Transfer Devices

Supplemental engineering controls are needed to reduce trace hazardous substance exposure during the transfer of toxic agents from one container to the next in compounding. For this purpose there are commercially available **closed-system transfer devices (or CSTDs)**. These are hand-manipulated devices that attach to transfer sites of HDs between containers, such as syringes to vials. CSTDs come in different forms and styles. They use double membranes to provide tightly sealed and dry connections that allow the safe withdrawal of fluid from a vial into a syringe and the safe injection of fluid from a syringe into an IVPB or LVP. The closed system also circumvents pressurization issues with vials, thus preventing the escape of toxic vapors. CSTDs should be used as a supplemental control for compounding inside a BSC or CACI when the HD dosage form allows, and must be used for administration when the dosage form allows.

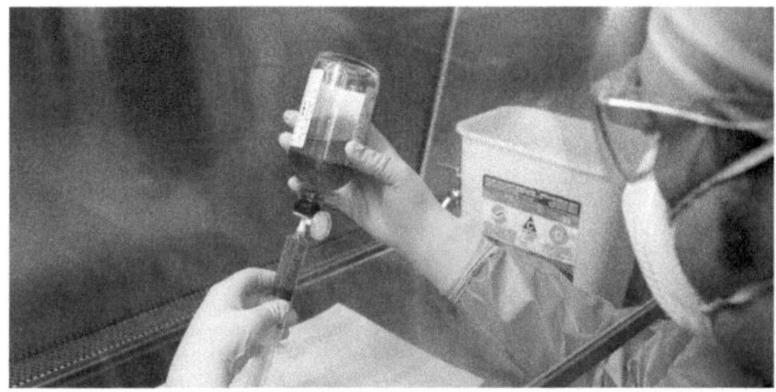

A Class II biological safety cabinet is commonly used to prepare hazardous cancer drugs in the hospital or the infusion pharmacy HD compounding area.

Compounding with Hazardous Agents

When a pharmacy technician is required to prepare a hazardous CSP from a vial medication, a CSTD should be used. If possible, it is recommended to use an injection solution rather than a powder for the active pharmaceutical ingredients.

Occasionally, a pharmacy technician will need to prepare a hazardous CSP from an ampule with an HD. This is done in a similar manner to the general sterile compounding procedures. Some examples of common toxic chemotherapy drugs can be seen in Table 13.11.

TABLE 13.11 Samples of Common Chemotherapy Drugs

Generic	Brand	Indication
abiraterone	Zytiga	Prostate cancer
bevacizumab	Avastin	Colon, lung, renal, ovarian, and brain cancers
bortezomib	Velcade	Multiple myeloma, mantle cell lymphoma
chlorambucil	Leukeran	Chronic lymphocytic leukemia
cyclophosphamide	Cytoxan, Neosar, Endoxan, Procytox, Revimmune, Cycloblastin	Lymphomas, brain cancer, leukemia, prostate cancer
etoposide	etoposide	Lung cancer, testicular cancer
gemcitabine	Gemzar	Pancreatic, lung, bladder, breast, and ovarian cancers, soft tissue sarcoma
imatinib	Gleevec	Leukemia and other cancers of blood cells, gastrointestinal stromal tumors
irinotecan	Camptosar, Onivyde (lipsome injection)	Metastatic colon or rectal cancer
lenalidomide	Revlimid	multiple myeloma
mercaptopurine	Purinethol	Some types of leukemia
methotrexate	Trexall, Folex	Breast, bladder, bone, lung, head and neck, ovarian, cervical, and testicular cancers and others
pembrolizumab	Keytruda	non-small cell lung cancer, classical Hodgkin lymphoma, melanoma, gastric and cervical cancer
rituximab	Rituxan	Leukemias and lymphomas, rheumatoid arthritis
oxaliplatin	Eloxatin	Colon or rectal cancer
trastuzumab	Herceptin	Breast cancer

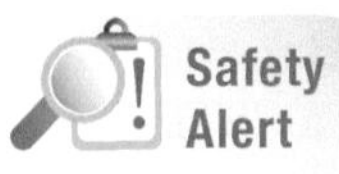

With HD vials, do not inject a volume of air equal to or greater than the volume of drug to be withdrawn.

Dispensing Hazardous Oral Drugs

Hazardous oral drugs may be handled in community, home health care, long-term care, and hospital pharmacy settings. HDs that are in sealed unit-dose or unit-of-use dose packaging and do not need modification do not require workers to wear any additional protection unless there are manufacturer cautions or compromises in the packaging.

During routine handling of hazardous tablets and capsules, workers should wear one pair of HD gloves of sufficient quality and thickness, a gown, or any PPE dictated by facility SOPs, according to the faculties' assessment of risk. Counting and pouring these drugs (such as methotrexate) should be done carefully, and contaminated equipment like counting trays should be immediately cleaned with detergent and/or a decontaminating agent and rinsed after each use. HD tablet and capsule forms of hazardous materials should not be placed in automated counting or packaging machines. When hospital pharmacy technicians repackage a hazardous oral agent into unit-dose bubble packaging, they must wear personal protective equipment. Manipulation of any HDs (such as crushing tablets or opening capsules) should be performed carefully within a C-PEC using appropriate PPE.

Handling Hazardous Drug Stock and Products

Even when receiving, stocking, inventorying, and disposing of HDs, pharmacy technicians must wear double gloves and often other forms of PPE, per hospital and OSHA policies. A **spill kit** must be readily accessible in the receiving area. A spill kit is a container of supplies, warning signage, and related materials used to contain an HD spill. Its contents and use will be discussed in more detail in the cleaning and disposal of HDs section later in this chapter.

Damaged packages should be inspected in a segregated, isolated area that is negative, neutral, or normal pressure. The receipt of broken vials of HDs should be treated as a hazardous agents spill, and reported to the compounding pharmacist supervisor.

Cleanup should follow established written procedures, as discussed later in this chapter.

Transporting Hazardous Compounded Sterile Products

Personnel who transport HDs to the compounding area, storage, and nursing units also must be trained and their competency documented. HD handling requires safeguards, particularly to minimize the potential for breakage or spill exposure. Technicians should be well versed in how to respond to exposure, breakages, and spills, and should know how to use a spill kit.

Within the hospital, the HDs must be transported in closed protective containers. If the final delivery is outside the hospital, infusion, or compounding pharmacy, the technician must select packing containers and protective materials to maintain physical integrity, stability, and sterility (if needed) of the HDs during transit. All CSPs must be delivered to the nursing unit (or home) in a sealable plastic bag to prevent damage, leakage, contamination, or degradation; this becomes especially important with hazardous CSPs.

Storage

Hazardous drugs should be delivered directly to the storage area upon delivery and immediately inventoried. During this process, the HDs should be separated from other medications to prevent contamination and exposure as well as to reduce the potential error of pulling a look-alike container from an adjacent shelf or bin.

Storage areas, including drug cartons, shelves, bins, counters, and trays, should carry appropriate, brightly colored warning labels ("Caution: Hazardous Agents") and be designed to maximize product recognition and minimize breakage. For example, storage shelves should have a barrier at the front; carts should have rims; and HDs should be stored at eye level or lower. Ideal storage is in a room with frequent air exchanges and negative air pressure to dilute or remove potential airborne contaminants.

Hazardous drugs requiring refrigeration should be stored separately from other drugs in bins that prevent breakage and that would adequately contain the leakage if it should occur. This dedicated HD refrigerator must be located in the designated HD storage area or in the HD buffer area. Access to storage areas and work areas for hazardous materials should be limited to specified trained personnel. A list of hazardous drugs should be compiled and posted in appropriate locations throughout the workplace.

Labeling

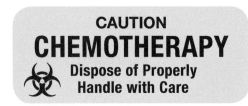

All CSPs containing hazardous agents must be properly labeled. The labels must contain the patient's name and room number, the solution name a volume, the drug name(s) and dosage, CSP administration information, and storage requirements. Hazardous agents also require additional labeling that clearly identifies the CSP as a hazardous agent.

All CSPs that contain HDs need to be assigned appropriate beyond-use dates. If the HD CSP is prepared and sent off-site, then the medication must be insulated and stored at the appropriate temperature during transit.

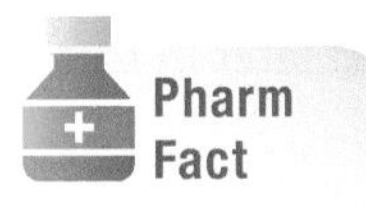

Technicians prime the IV tubing before they inject the HD into the bag.

Administration of Hazardous Products and Compounded Sterile Products

Besides being clearly labeled as hazardous, all HD CSPs should be primed according to institutional guidelines and *USP* Chapter <800>. Syringes filled with hazardous agents should *never be filled more than* $^3/_4$ *full* because overly full syringes have a greater potential for the syringe plunger to become separated from the barrel. If the medication is to be dispensed from the syringe, then the HD solution should be cleared from the needle and hub, and the needle should be replaced with a locking syringe cap. The exterior surface of the prepared syringe should be cleaned with a lint-free wipe saturated with sterile 70% IPA and then labeled. If the HD medication is to be added to an IV bag, special care should be used to prevent a puncture of the bag.

Priming an IV Administration Set

As opposed to general CSPs, HD IV administration sets should always be primed in the DCA of the biological safety cabinet to avoid endangering the nurse or patient at the bedside. To prime the IV administration set before adding the HD, the technician should insert the spike of the administration set into the CSP's tubing port as would have been done by the bedside. This action allows fluid to run from the CSP through the tubing, thus priming the tubing. As with the other CSPs, the chamber, connections, and ports must be tapped to remove air bubbles. The exterior surface of the administration set and the entire bag should then be wiped with sterile 70% IPA and labeled.

Administration

Depending on the specific type of CSP, the nurse may administer the hazardous CSP through the primed IV administration set or a drug-specific closed-system transfer device at the bedside.

To administer the hazardous medication, the nurse must also wear a shield (if there is a risk of splashing), chemotherapy gloves, and a chemo gown, like the HD compounding technician. Typically, two nurses check the medication dose and labeling before administering it to the patient. This precautionary measure minimizes the risk of drug administration errors. An incorrect HD dose, especially in a pediatric patient, could prove deadly.

Once the administration of the medication is completed, the nurse disposes of the HD protective garb in a designated hazardous waste container. As with any other medication, the nurse must do the proper documentation.

Cleaning and Decontamination

A technician should never use bare hands to handle hazardous fluids or glass shards. Broken glass should be placed in an appropriate, puncture-proof container.

In general, the standard HD personal protective equipment, including eye and face protection and ASTM chemotherapy gloves, should always be worn for cleaning, disinfecting, decontaminating the C-PECs and CACIs, and deactivating HDs in the compounding area, using appropriate products. Chemical **deactivation** of an HD should be done with 2% sodium hypochlorite or other appropriate agent. Alcohol is not an effective deactivating or HD cleaning agent.

Decontamination is the inactivation, neutralization, or removal of HD residue from surfaces. This is done with a low-lint wipe, which is then contained and discarded as contaminated waste. HD contamination in a BSC or CACI may be reduced by wiping down HD containers before introducing them, as studies show the outside of the vials have trace contamination on them when they arrive in the pharmacy. The BSC or CACI should also be decontaminated at least daily or any time a spill occurs.

Since the HEPA filter is located in the ceiling of the hood in a vertical airflow C-PEC, the pattern of the cleaning strokes and order is different from the horizontal hood. Clean the HEPA filter cover, being careful not to get the HEPA filter wet, then the back wall of the hood, the bar, sides, and the front facing. The main work surface will be the last surface cleaned as it is the dirtiest surface. Use linear, overlapping strokes, following the direction of airflow starting at the top and moving horizontally to the bottom. Use a decontaminating agent, a cleaning agent and then a disinfecting agent like sterile 70% IPA. Keep in mind that some decontaminating agents will require the surface to be wiped twice. The procedures for working with and cleaning PECs that encased hazardous drugs are even more rigorous and are outlined in manufacturer specifications. Though the CACI is enclosed while in use, it also must be opened at least monthly to clean under the work tray and clean with a sporicidal agent. Personnel should also wear respiratory protection whenever they clean under the work tray of the BSC or CACI.

BSCs and CACIs used for compounding HDs need to be disinfected at the beginning of the workday, between batches of compounding medications, at the beginning of each subsequent shift, routinely during compounding, and after any time the units have been powered off. The area under the work tray should be cleaned at least monthly to reduce the contamination level in the BSCs and CACIs, *USP* <800> also requires that the hood is decontaminated between the compounding of different HD's.

Cleaning a Hazardous Spill

Spills must be contained and cleaned immediately by trained workers. Only trained workers with appropriate PPE should manage an HD spill, and they must post warning signs to restrict access to the spill area. The goal is to ensure that the staff, patients, and visitors are not exposed and that the healthcare environment (both inside and outside the medical facility) is not contaminated.

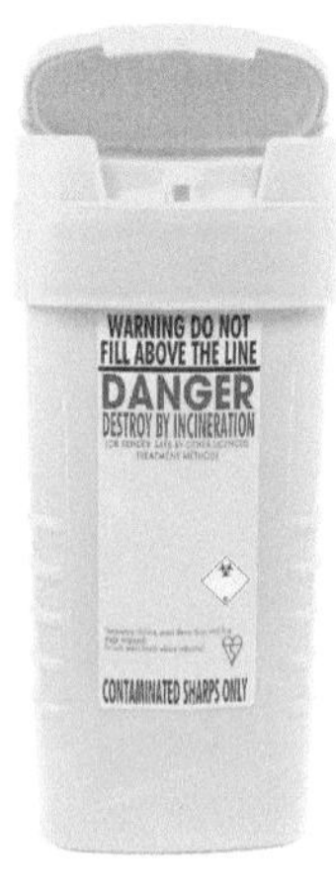

Some sharps can be placed in sealed containers and in a sharps disposal container in a C-SEC, *if* approved by facility policies. Other HD waste must go in specific hazardous waste disposal containers.

When cleaning spills, the trained personnel must wear proper attire–including a gown, double gloves, goggles, and a mask or a NIOSH-certified respirator.

HD spill kits that contain all of the materials needed must be readily available in all areas where HDs are routinely handled. Spill kits contain materials to control, clean up, and decontaminate spills of up to 1,000 mL (see Table 13.12).

TABLE 13.12 Typical Contents of a Spill Kit

Appendix I—Recommended contents of HD spill kit

1. Sufficient supplies to absorb a spill of about 1,000 mL (volume of 1 IV bag or bottle).
2. Appropriate PPE to protect the worker during cleanup, including 2 pairs of disposable gloves (1 outer pair of heavy utility gloves and 1 pair of inner gloves tested to ASTM D6978).
3. Disposable HD-resistant gown or coverall tested against HD permeability.
4. Disposable HD-resistant shoe covers.
5. Chemical splash goggles.
6. Protective face shield to be used with goggles (for full range of splash protection).
7. NIOSH-approved disposable respirator.
8. Absorbent, plastic-backed sheets or spill pads.
9. Disposable toweling.
10. At least 2 sealable, thick plastic hazardous waste disposal bags (prelabeled with an appropriate warning label).
11. One disposable scoop for collecting glass fragments.
12. One puncture-resistant container for glass fragments.
13. An approved cartridge respirator for use with contents of spill

In cleanup, technicians first start by absorbing up the bulk of the spill with a large absorbent mat. They start from the edge and work inward, using absorbent sheets, spill pads, or pillows for the liquids, and damp cloths or towels for solids. Then they should use spill pads and water to rinse the area, and detergent to remove residue. The spill area should be wiped down with a detergent solution at least three times to ensure that the hazardous agent has been removed from the spill area.

Spills within the BSC or CACI require additional cleaning steps. The drain trough should be thoroughly cleaned and the cabinet decontaminated according to manufacturer specifications. All contaminated materials from a spill should be sealed in hazardous waste containers and placed in leak-resistant containers. The spill, cleanup, and any personnel exposure must be documented.

Disposal of Hazardous Agents and Supplies

When disposing of all HD waste (including unused and unusable HDs) from the C-SECs, BSCs, CACIs, and spills, technicians must comply with all applicable federal, state, local, and facility regulations. They must be aware of the hospital's proper procedures for the disposal of contaminated drugs, supplies, and clothing. Direct spill waste must be placed in hazardous waste containers. Supplies that held the HDs–such as vials, ampules, IV bags, needles, straws, and syringes–contain **trace hazardous waste**, which is why they must be treated as hazardous waste. Similarly, so must all items used in the handling, compounding, dispensing, administration, or disposal of HDs–such as gowns, gloves, goggles, and wipes. The worker should remove contaminated garments and gloves and dispose of them in specially designated hazardous or chemotherapy waste containers. No protective clothing should be taken outside the area where the exposure occurred.

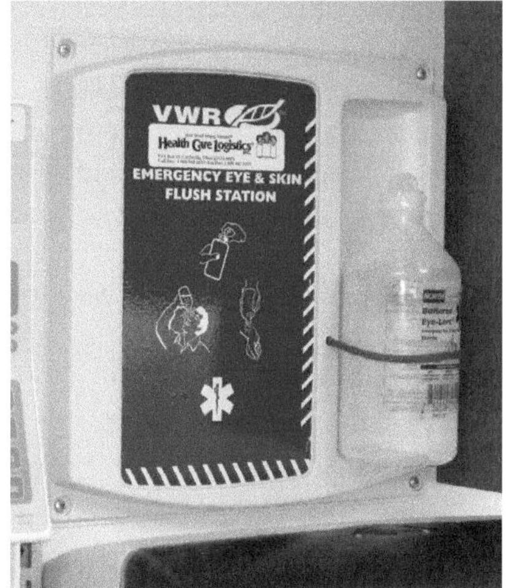

A sink and an eyewash station must be located near to the HD compounding area.

Workers who have direct exposure to HDs during sterile compounding or are contaminated during the spill or spill cleanup, require immediate treatment. Written policies should delineate exact procedures to follow. Every hazardous substance has its Safety Data Sheet filed within the pharmacy department, as explained earlier, outlining specific recommendations on how to treat various exposures.

If the skin is exposed, the worker should use water to flush the affected area immediately and then thoroughly cleanse the area with soap and water. If the substance comes in contact with the eyes, the worker should flush the eyes with large amounts of water or use an eye-flush kit. Workers must also wash their hands thoroughly and be sent or escorted to the emergency room. The accidental exposure should be reported to the supervisor, who should notify other staff members to avoid the spread of contamination. An incident report documenting the spill, exposure, and cleanup must be completed. Follow-up medical surveillance of the exposed worker is required in *USP* Chapter <800>.

Hazardous Drug Containment Quality Control

To ensure containment of HDs, procedures for **containment quality control**, such as environmental wipe sampling, should be performed routinely (such as initially as a benchmark and at least every six months, or more often as needed, to verify containment in the C-SEC room) to detect uncontained HD traces. This sampling should include surface wipe sampling of the working area of C-PECs; countertops where finished preparations are placed; areas adjacent to BSCs and CACIs, including the floor directly under the working area; and patient administration areas.

13.9 Radioactive Pharmaceuticals

A specific kind of hazardous compounding occurs in a **nuclear pharmacy**, which prepares radioactive materials to diagnose and treat specific diseases. Nuclear medicine records radiation emitting from elements injected into the body, rather than from external elements like x-rays **Radiopharmaceuticals** are irradiated HDs.

Unlike a hazardous chemical CSP, these preparations are not prepared in a hospital pharmacy. They are most commonly prepared off-site in a nuclear pharmacy by specially trained and certified nuclear pharmacists and pharmacy technicians. One nuclear pharmacy may serve nuclear medicine departments in several hospitals, with the radioactive drugs carefully transported to

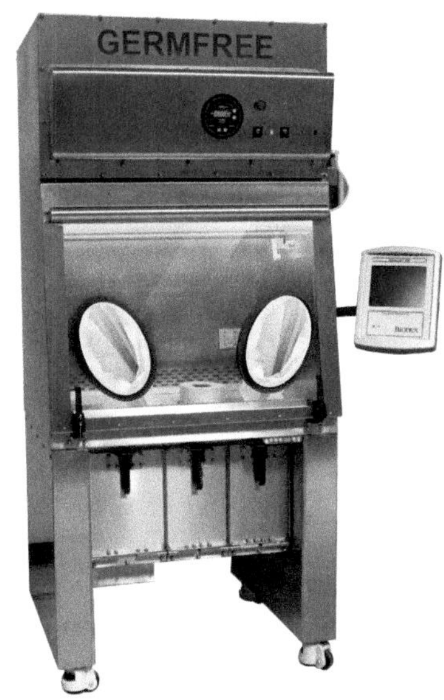

A compounding nuclear pharmacist or technician must be behind sealed lead protective casing with leaded glass shielding or have a computer screen for viewing the DCA.

their sites. A nuclear pharmacy is similar to a compounding pharmacy in that it utilizes extensive, sophisticated equipment with no direct interaction with patients.

A **nuclear pharmacy technician (NPT)** prepares the radioactive pharmaceuticals. Working knowledge of these nuclear drugs and their risks and benefits is essential, as these technicians often advise medical providers regarding their toxic nature and their dangers. The NPT's major tasks are to compound and dispense radiopharmaceuticals under direct supervision of the pharmacist; prepare and maintain compliance documentation of preparing and shipping products; and select, prepare, and stock medications and supplies.

The worker protection and medical surveillance programs for the nuclear pharmacy workers are even stricter than those for chemical hazardous drugs. Everyone working in a nuclear pharmacy, including the pharmacy technicians, must wear a radiation badge to detect exposure to radiation. Radiation exposure is kept to a minimum by the use of specifically designed equipment, syringes, gloves, and other devices. The radiopharmacy compounders must use leaded or tungsten glass syringe shields, transfer devices, and containers in the radiopharmacy isolator.

USP Chapter <821> Standards on Nuclear Medications

As with chemical HDs, the USP has articulated standards on radioactive medicine and pharmaceuticals. Chapter <821> *Identification and Assay of Radionuclides.* However, a need for change arose when the the **positron emission tomography (PET)** scan was developed. It is an imaging test that uses a radioactive drug as a tracer to help reveal the function of tissues and organs. Because of the short half-life of the radionuclide and the mode of production, PET drug products have unique storage, shipping, and handling concerns. *USP* Chapter <823> sets forth requirements for PET drug production, including control of components, materials, and supplies; verification of procedures; stability testing and expiration dating; quality control; and sterilization and sterility assurance. A full description of this chapter is beyond the scope of this text.

In 2018, the USP proposed a new General Chapter <825> tailored to the specific needs of sterile and nonsterile radiopharmaceutical preparations. *USP* Chapter <825> was written by an expert panel to provide clear standards that focus on the unique patient and provider needs of radiopharmaceuticals.

Training and Job Possibilities for Nuclear Pharmacy

To work in a nuclear pharmacy, a pharmacist must undergo 200 hours of classroom training and another 700 hours of experience under the observation of a qualified instructor. The nuclear pharmacy technician training program is intensive as well, though not quite as rigorous and time-consuming. These training programs are offered by the American Pharmacy Association (APhA).

There are fewer than 2,000 NPTs practicing in the United States. There is a shortage of certified technicians in this niche area of pharmacy, so it is a growing field, with salaries up to $55,000 per year with experience and credentials.

13.10 Challenges and Rewards of Sterile and Hazardous Compounding

As you have seen, extensive knowledge and practice are needed for both sterile and hazardous compounding. The importance of training, experience, and certification for compounding sterile products (CSPs), hazardous drugs (HDs), and radioactive products is quite clear. Knowing well the appropriate *USP* chapters is crucial as these guidelines are the standards for the industry.

In the previous chapter, you learned the importance of aseptic technique and use of sophisticated equipment in a cleanroom environment. In this chapter, the chemical properties of the various intravenous parenteral solutions, correct compounding processes for various IV solutions, and the techniques of withdrawing medications from vials and ampules were introduced. These can be put into practice with additional aseptic compounding steps in your labs or at the hospital during your experiential training. You now can understand the efficiencies of automated compounding devices (ACDs), vial-and-bag systems, and premanufactured frozen IV solutions.

The primary goal in compounding a sterile nonhazardous CSP is to *protect the patient* against contamination that may lead to a hospital-acquired infection, whereas the primary goal of the hazardous CSP requirements is to also *protect the worker* against health risks due to unnecessary exposure. You now have a clearer sense of what this hazardous compounding field entails as well as the even more specialized career path of the nuclear pharmacy technician.

You may be intimidated by all the requirements expected of a sterile compounding technician preparing CSPs, hazardous drugs, or radioactive drug products.

However, if you are among those who are willing to take on these challenges and training and gain the necessary experience, a promising career with commensurate higher salary and benefits may await you.

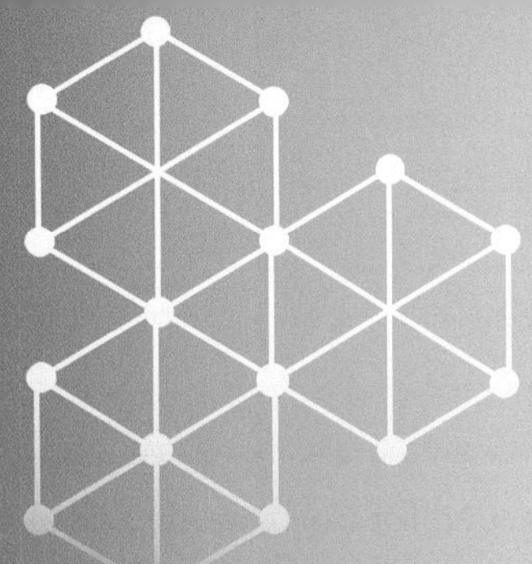

Review and Assessment

CHAPTER SUMMARY

- Compounded sterile preparations (CSPs) have many chemical properties, including pH value, osmotic pressure, tonicity, and stability, which must be compatible with blood and understood by the sterile compounding technician.
- Medication orders delivered to the hospital pharmacy start the CSP process, followed by a DUR for medication and allergy alerts before sending the order and generated label to the compounding cleanroom.
- Many types and volumes of base IV solutions, such as dextrose in water, normal saline (NS), and dextrose in NS, may be used in the compounding of parenteral medications.
- Peripheral parenteral nutrition (PPN) IV solutions are for short-term, partial replenishment and nutrition. They are administered in a peripheral vein, typically in the arm or the wrist.
- Total parenteral nutrition (TPN) IV solutions are more complex, being used for long-term nourishment and therapy, with medication including electrolytes, minerals, and nutrients, such as lipids, amino acids, sugars, and vitamins.
- TPN is administered through a major vein (usually in the chest cavity). It can be administered in a 2-in-1 bag plus IV piggyback, or in a 3-in-1 solution bag.
- Parenteral solutions may be administered via llarge-volume parenteral (LVP) infusions, small-volume parenteral (SVP) infusions, or IV push.
- Master Formulation and Compounding Records are required for individualized compounded orders and batch prepa- rations of CSPs.
- Labeling components of CSPs include both detailed medication and administration information.
- The assignment of BUDs for sterile products depends on the environment the CSP was prepared in, sterility of starting ingredients, and storage conditions determined by *USP* <797>.
- A CSP has more restrictive beyond-use dating than a manufactured sterile product or a nonsterile preparation because there are added products and more chances for microorganism growth and instability.
- Medications that need to be reconstituted from vials or withdrawn from ampules before adding them to the IV solution require special aseptic techniques and specialized equipment.
- To reconstitute powered medications in vials, you will need to use the milking technique of fluid introduction into a vial.

- After working with solutions in glass ampules, filtered needles or straws must be used to prevent the presence of glass particulates in the IV solutions.
- Specially premixed IV solutions, which include vial-and-bag systems and frozen IV solutions, need to be assembled or prepared for use in a DCA even though they will have product expirations dates instead of BUDs.
- All parenteral medications must be properly labeled, checked, and physically inspected by the pharmacist before being sent to the nursing unit.
- Unused and returned manufactured parenteral products and CSPs can be used if the beyond-use dating has not been exceeded and if proper storage conditions on the nursing unit can be verified.
- *USP* Chapter <800> handles guidelines for hazardous compounding
- Hazardous drug compounding, according to *USP* <800>, requires special training, personal protective equipment (PPE), techniques, supplies, and equipment to guard against HD exposure of employees—especially women who are pregnant, breast-feeding, or trying to conceive.
- *USP* <800> recommends baseline and periodic medical surveillance of all personnel working with hazardous drugs.
- Hazardous compounding also requires a contained area of negative pressure, air exchanges, ISO Class 7 air quality, and external filtered venting to keep the hazardous substances from contaminating other areas (according to the *USP* <800> standards).
- The primary engineering controls for hazardous compounding require a measure of toxic substance containment, so the contained primary engineering controls are used (C-PECs).
- Hazardous substances are grouped into different categories. There are ECs for compounding built with differing levels of containment and protection to accommodate them: biological safety cabinets in levels of Class II-A1, II-A2, II-B1, II-B2, CACI, and BSC Class III isolators. (Class II-A1 is no longer considered suitable for HD compounding.)
- Accidental spills or exposures require immediate treatment, cleanup, reporting to the supervisor, and completion of an incident report. Cleanup, decontamination, and disposal of hazardous drugs and supplies must be done with PPE, following strict protocols.
- Preparing radioactive pharmaceuticals is a specialty area of practice available to nuclear pharmacy technicians, requiring intensive course training and practice as well as additional protective equipment and gear.

CHECK YOUR UNDERSTANDING

To ensure that you recall and understand the key chapter concepts, please read the question or statement and select the appropriate lettered option.

1. The pH of blood is considered to be slightly
   a. acidic.
   b. alkaline.
   c. neutral.
   d. hypotonic.

2. Chemical incompatibility data on two or more medications added to an IV solution is best found in
   a. U.S. Pharmacopoeia.
   b. Prescribers' Digital Reference (PDR).
   c. Facts and Comparisons.
   d. Trissel's Stability of Compounded Formulations.

3. Which of the following is not a role expected of the IV compounding technician?
   a. Prepare a 24-hour supply of every CSP for each patient in the hospital.
   b. Wipe down IV bags prior to entering buffer area.
   c. Resolve computer-generated warnings on DUR.
   d. Complete a quality check of each CSP by doing a visual check.

4. An example of an isotonic solution that is often used after blood loss in surgery is
   a. lactated Ringers (LR).
   b. dextrose 50%.
   c. sodium chloride (NaCl) 3%.
   d. 0.45% normal saline (NS).

5. An IV order is received for 0.9% Normal Saline at an infusion rate of 125 mL/hour. How many 1-L bottles must be prepared for use over the next 24 hours?
   a. 2 1-L bottles
   b. 3 1-L bottles
   c. 5 1-L bottles
   d. 6 1-L bottles

6. A Master Formulation Record must be followed
   a. when CSPs are prepared in a batch for multiple patients.
   b. for every CSP prepared by the IV compounding technician.
   c. for standard reconstitution of powdered injectable medications.
   d. when documenting calculations for a CSP for an individual patient.

MAKE CONNECTIONS

Take a moment to consider what you have learned in this chapter and respond thoughtfully to the following prompts. Note that some of these activities will require internet access.

1. Using the internet, research and explore the complex topic of overfills in the making of compounded sterile preparations (CSPs). Write a short essay that summarizes your research. Be sure to include a description of two different practitioner-based methods for making CSPs, and demonstrate your understanding of the 10% rule.
2. While the protection of patients from microbial contamination is important with sterile CSPs, the protection of all personnel involved is a priority in the preparation and administration of hazardous drugs (HDs). Use the internet to research and review the CDC National Institute for Occupational Safety and Health (NIOSH) Alert on "Preventing Occupational Exposures to Antineoplastic and Other Drugs in Health Care Settings". Write a 250-word report on the safe handling of hazardous drugs, and focus on the potential adverse effects to health care workers involving genotoxicity, reproductive health, and cancer. List at least 10 NIOSH recommendations for the safe preparation of CSPs by a pharmacy technician in order to minimize exposure to HDs.

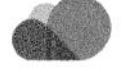 The online course includes additional review and assessment resources.

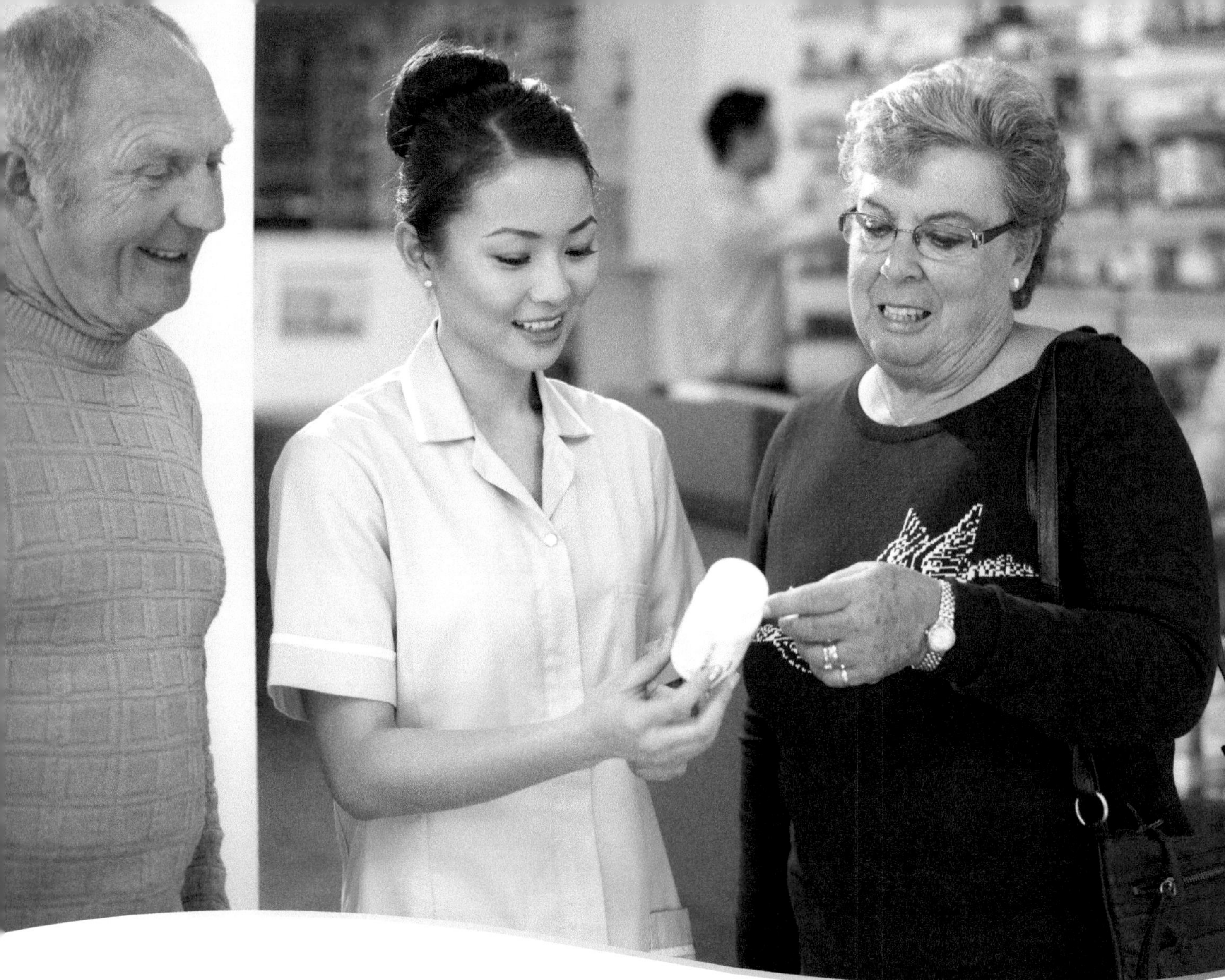

UNIT 5 Professionalism in the Pharmacy

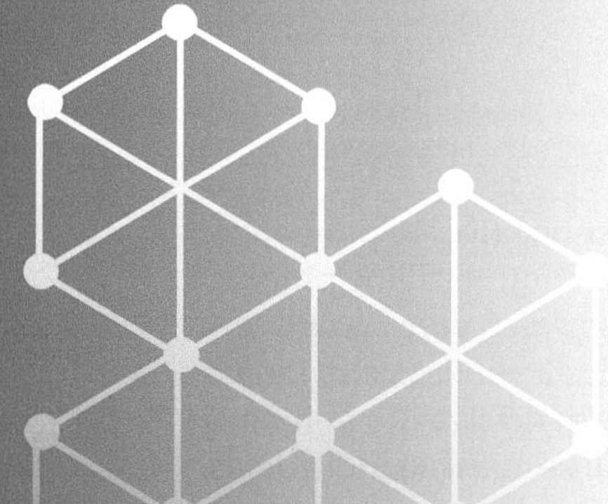

14 Medication Safety

Learning Objectives

1 Describe patient medication rights, the extent of preventable medication errors, and the effects of errors on patient safety and health-care costs. (Section 14.1)

2 Identify specific categories of medication errors, their causes, and how to avoid them. (Section 14.2)

3 Describe the various potential errors per each step of the dispensing process. (Section 14.3)

4 List tools to assist in preventing medication errors, including the use of automation and package design. (Section 14.4)

5 State why errors are unreported and what can be done to insure proper reporting. (Section 14.5)

6 Identify the common programs available for reporting medication errors. (Section 14.5)

7 Define FDA safety strategies to prevent adverse effects in high-risk drugs, including Medication Guide and REMS programs. (Section 14.6)

8 Differentiate the terms *drug tolerance*, *psychological and physical dependence*, and *addiction*. (Section 14.7)

9 Explain why prescription drug abuse is a public safety issue. (Section 14.8)

10 Describe ways to detect drug seekers and forged prescriptions for controlled drugs. (Section 14.8)

11 Identify and resolve drug abuse issues among coworkers. (Section 14.8)

12 Outline appropriate behavior during a robbery using the acronym REACT. (Section 14.8)

ASHP/ACPE Accreditation Standards
To view the *ASHP/ACPE Accreditation Standards* addressed in this chapter, refer to Appendix B.

With the increasing number of drugs dispensed and utilized in community and hospital pharmacies, there are also increasing medication errors and other issues. It takes a team effort to identify, address, and prevent medication errors as they involve prescribers, pharmacy personnel, and the nursing staff. This chapter examines the types and causes of medication errors, the strategies that pharmacies can implement to prevent or minimize these errors, and the automation technologies and drug safety monitoring systems that are making a positive impact. Several government and professional programs offer safety-promoting resources. With greater understanding and resources, you

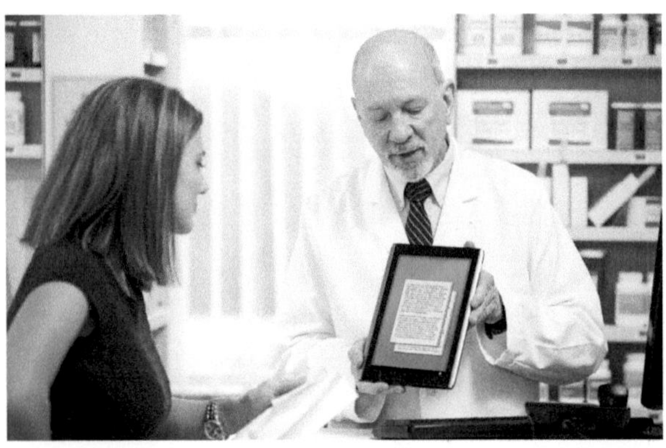

The profession of pharmacy exists to protect the safety of patients from medication errors and adverse effects of drugs. Technological innovations assist the pharmacist and technician in fulfilling this responsibility.

can establish personal best practices to promote safety throughout the prescription-filling process.

Medication safety, however, goes beyond the dispensing process to include public health safety. This means preventing birth defects from pharmaceuticals, as well as substance abuse in individuals, in pharmacy staff, and within communities. It also means working to avoid drug thefts and being ready to protect oneself during a robbery. The common goal of all of these safety initiatives is to protect the well-being of patients, personnel, and the community at large. As a pharmacy technician, you can play a crucial role in all of these safety arenas. By doing so, healthcare costs decrease, and quality of life improves for all.

14.1 Medication "Rights" and Preventable Errors

Working in health care means making a commitment to "first do no harm." This means that healthcare workers must put safety first. As a result, no acceptable medication error rate exists, and each step in the task of filling medication orders should be reviewed with a 100% error-free goal in mind.

The Seven Prescription Rights That Patients Expect

Prescribers and pharmacy personnel are responsible for ensuring the "seven Rs," or seven rights for the patients who trust in you (see Figure 14.1). In other words, you must work as part of a team to ensure that the medication each patient receives is for the right drug, at the right strength, in the right route formulation, for the right dosage time and supply, with the right documentation (including for insurance), for the right person, and accompanied by the right patient education.

In some ways, these rights may seem obvious, but, as you will see, errors can easily happen where the medication dispensed can be of the wrong kind; at the wrong strength; in the wrong formulation route; for the wrong dosage timing and days' supply; with wrong or missing profile, insurance, or hospital documentation; given to the wrong person; and given without the proper patient and administration education materials.

The Scope of Medication Errors

Medication errors are one of the most common types of medical errors. The National Coordinating Council for Medication Error Reporting and Prevention (NCC MERP) defines a **medication error** as "any preventable event that may cause or lead to inappropriate medication use or patient harm while the medication is in the control of the healthcare professional, patient, or consumer."

A medication error often results in an **adverse drug reaction (ADR)**, which is an appreciably harmful or negative consequence to a patient from taking a particular drug. It may be a short-term acute reaction, long-term injury, or even death.

FIGURE 14.1 Patient Rights in Prescription Drug Dispensing

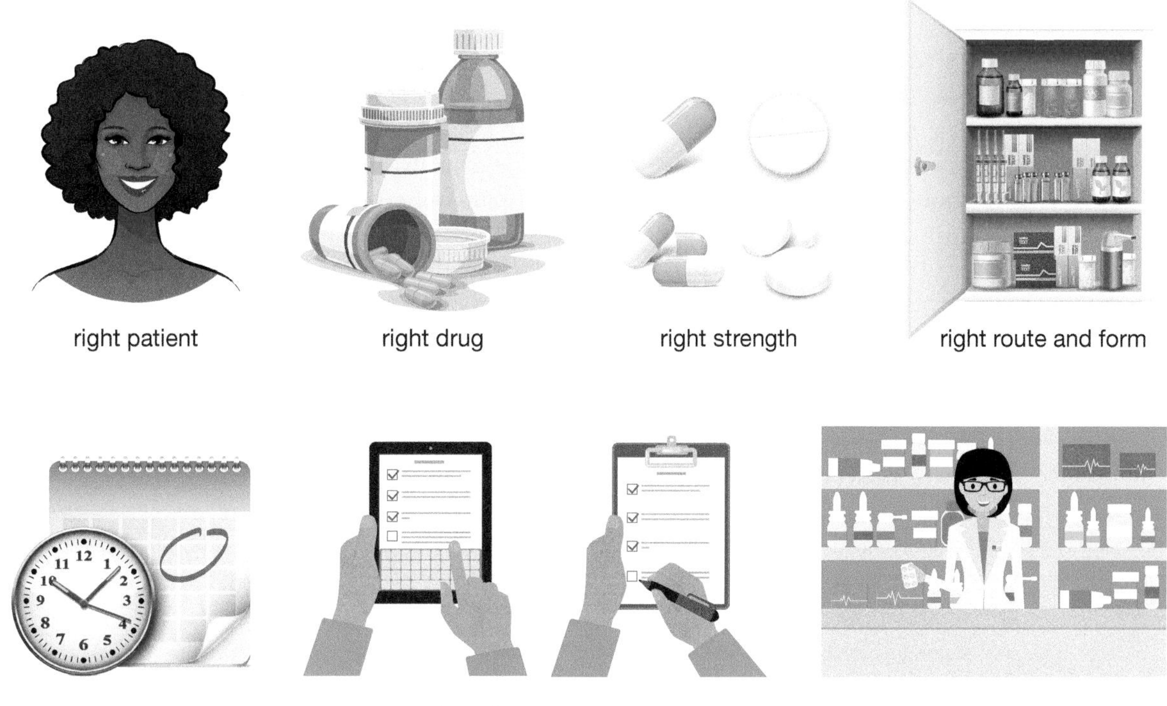

Medication errors are difficult to track because there are no national laws requiring the reporting of pharmacy personnel errors. Based on research, the Institute of Medicine (IOM) estimated in 2006 that more than 1.5 million medication errors cause harm in the United States every year, with deaths at about 7,000 annually. The study estimated that drug errors cause an estimated 800,000 preventable injuries in nursing homes, 400,000 in hospitals, and 500,000 among Medicare patients treated in outpatient clinics each year. Then a 2009 observational study of 50 community pharmacies found that 1.7% of prescriptions filled (4 out of 250) had an error, and an estimated 65% of these errors resulted in negative impacts on the patients' health. Since then, no new extensive studies have been published, but a great deal of effort has been put into reducing errors by tracking where they are arising and by looking for solutions.

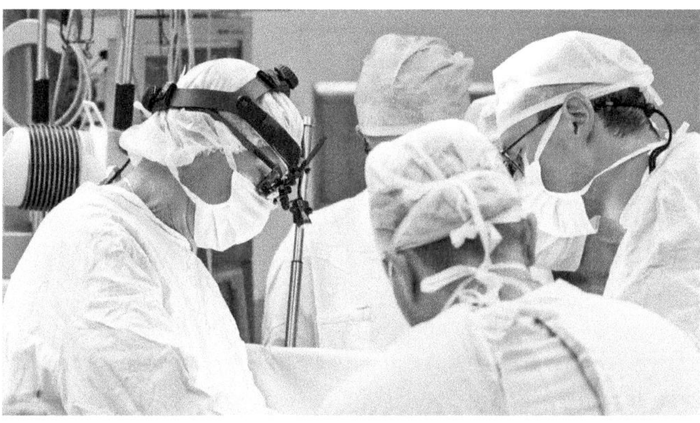

In a single operation, numerous medications are often administered to help the patient. With many different people involved, there are opportunities for miscommunication and missing some protocols, leading to medication errors.

Medication Error Reporting Rate

In 2012, the Institute for Safe Medication Practices (ISMP) and the American Pharmacists Association (APhA) surveyed members, and 700 pharmacists from various settings responded—44% admitted making errors, and, of these, 37% admitted that they *did not report the errors they made*. That shows how underreported prescriptive errors are and how necessary it is for an effective check-and-balance system.

IN THE REAL WORLD

The October 2015 issue of *Anesthesiology* published an eight-month study that uncovered medication errors in almost half of all surgeries at the Harvard-affiliated Massachusetts General Hospital (MGH). Since MGH had been a leader in patient safety initiatives, especially in the operating room, this study was particularly shocking. The patients were tracked before, during, and immediately after surgery.

Out of 275 surgeries, 3,671 medication administrations were observed, with 153 medication errors discovered and 91 adverse drug events recorded. They found problems in 1 out of 20 administrations (5%). Errors arose at each stage from everyone involved, including the pharmacy department personnel. Common errors were mistakes in dosage, labeling, documentation, and neglect of proper responses to vital signs that indicated problems. Of these, 80% of the errors were considered preventable, and more than 60% of the errors caused serious effects.

Because MGH has been very proactive in safety initiatives (and continues to be so as evidenced by its willingness to be part of this study), it is estimated that the error rates at other hospitals are similar if not higher. Faced with this study information, MGH and hospitals at large are redoubling efforts to address medication errors and find the gaps in communication and procedural systems.

Cost Impact of Medication Errors

Since medication errors are underreported, it is very difficult to assess the damage. Lives are lost, and patients are disabled or lose valuable time from work or school. A 2007 study estimated that the direct and indirect costs to the healthcare system for preventable medication errors occurring inside the hospital or institutional setting were $4.2 billion and outside were $16.4 billion. These costs are primarily caused by additional hospitalizations (millions of extra days), admissions to long-term care, physician visits, and emergency room visits. Lost time at work and lost productivity must be accounted for in addition to the bereavement when individuals die.

14.2 Root-Cause Analysis of Medication Errors

To prevent medication errors, one has to identify clearly what the error was, where it took place, and, through closer examination, what specifically caused it (i.e., the *why*). Medication errors are caused by numerous factors within the different systems of any pharmacy, from the organizational systems to the technical tools to the specific human decisions. In the 1940s, the US military developed a process of root-cause analysis that was called the **Failure Mode Effects Analysis (FMEA)**. This analysis breaks larger processes down into levels and tasks to find the root causes of failures (problems) and the rate or probability of failure occurrences, the consequences, and ways to fix the failures. Healthcare facilities are now using modifications of this form of analysis and others for quality control and safety initiatives.

Root-cause analysis is a systematic approach to identifying the deep causes of why something happened to prevent a recurrence. Administrators use facility data on error trends to figure out gaps in policies and procedures as well as technological problems. Pharmacy directors can apply root-cause analysis within their departments for investigating common errors, and technicians can use it to examine their own practice. Numerous failures can occur at once, contributing to each other and magnifying the possibilities and quantity of errors, so prevention strategies have to address all three levels of systems and processes.

- An **organizational failure** occurs because of a deficiency in organizational rules, leadership, culture, policies, or procedures. Examples of this type of failure include pressure for production and cutting corners over safety concerns; inadequate staffing, training, or breaks per workload; out-of-date or poor rules or procedures for preparing or admixing parenteral medicines, such as chemotherapy drugs; poor maintenance schedule of automated devices; and poor facility organization and cramped spaces.
- A **technical failure** results from equipment problems. Examples of this type of failure include a virus in the pharmacy software throwing off the information or losing patient information; a bar coding scanner that misreads the code and scrambles the numbers; and incorrect preparation of a total parenteral solution (TPN) due to a calibration error of the automated compounding device (ACD) in the hospital pharmacy.
- A **human failure** occurs at an individual action level. Examples include a technician pulling a medication bottle from the shelf based on memory without cross-referencing the bottle label with the prescription/medical order or without scanning the National Drug Code (NDC) bar code; anyone skipping an aseptic technique step; a pharmacist approving a medication without addressing the Drug Utilization Review (DUR) alerts or carefully checking a technician's calculations or medication selection; a patient not paying attention to the label, not adhering to prescribed drug therapy, or quitting therapy early.

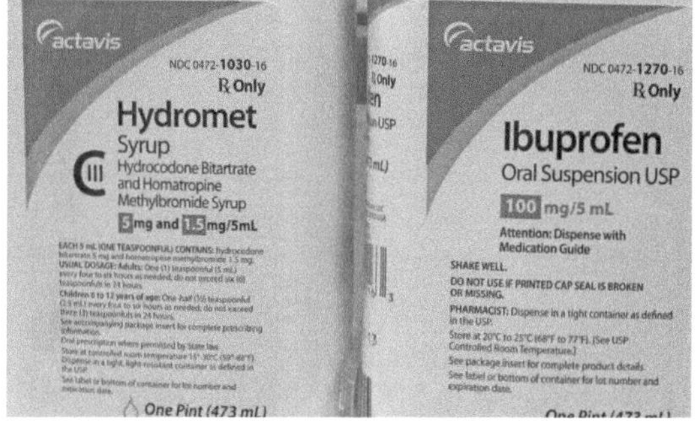

Identical label designs are a source of confusion and a cause for error when filling a prescription, especially if a technician uses memory instead of checking and double-checking the NDC number when selecting a medication.

Addressing Organizational and Technological Failures

Some issues must be addressed by the community or hospital pharmacy, not by the individual personnel.

A Safety-Oriented Work Environment

A pharmacy's physical setting can make a major contribution to fostering disorientation or enabling attention. Adequate space and clean, well-lit conditions are just some of the basic requirements for a well-working pharmacy in addition to adequate staffing. Work shifts of 12 hours or longer (or even more than 8 hours) by pharmacy staff, physicians, and residents-in-training can correlate with a higher incidence of medication errors. Table 14.1 outlines the best practices for a pharmacy work environment that promotes safety and reduces errors.

TABLE 14.1 Workplace Ergonomic Practices to Promote Safety

- Maintain a clean, organized, and well-lit work area.
- Provide adequate storage areas with clear drug labels on the shelves.
- Provide adequate computer applications and hardware.
- Automate and use bar code technology for all fill procedures for safety checking.

A Safety-Oriented Culture

Pharmacists are responsible for adequate on-site technician training, oversight, verification of prescription stages, patient education and counseling, and prescriber discussions about resolving prescription or medication order issues.

Within the pharmacy, a safety-promoting work culture is key. Pharmacists need to create a professional, nonpunitive environment where technicians are encouraged to take responsibility, ask questions, query prescriptions and DUR alert flags, and suggest contacting prescribers. It must be clear that safety is more important than who is at fault, time goals, or productivity measurements. To continually keep the mind fresh, break times must not only be encouraged, but enforced. Time-flow management principles must be indoctrinated to avoid interruptions and distraction errors at key points of the prescription filling process.

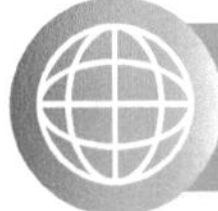

IN THE REAL WORLD

Pharmacy understaffing of both technicians and pharmacists is a significant cause of medication errors in all settings, but especially in large-scale chain and independent pharmacies. Though staffing levels have been minimized, the number of prescriptions and vaccine administrations have increased and clinical responsibilities have been added. At the same time there has been an emphasis on working faster to increase productivity and customer satisfaction.

In 2014 and 2015, NBC's I-Teams in Washington DC and New York City investigated claims of mounting prescription errors in the chain pharmacies of CVS and Walmart. Joe Zorek, a pharmacist for CVS for 30 years, filed a whistle-blower lawsuit against his company. "I was concerned we were going to kill someone." Another CVS whistle-blower explained that the errors were numerous. "I would say there's at least one a day if not more." Both blamed the pressure put on the pharmacists and technicians to hurry and reach time and productivity quotas.

At the time, then executive director of the National Association of Boards of Pharmacy, Dr. Carmine Catizone, confirmed the concerns: "We've heard the complaints about the large chains and how they're morphing or how they resemble fast food restaurants." Some large chains have been refusing to monitor errors effectively and turn over their error reports. In 2015, the executive vice president of the Institute for Safe Medication Practices, Allen Vaida, told the New York I-Team that an estimated 30 to 50 million prescriptions annually have some type of error.

Technicians usually do not make organizational policies nor are they responsible for purchasing automation tools. But technicians can contribute by offering suggestions to the pharmacists or pharmacy administration and through organizational suggestion structures when appropriate. You can also learn how to use, maintain, and calibrate automation, alerting the pharmacists when there are breakdowns or issues.

Accountable Care Organizations A voluntary movement for quality improvement, safety, and cost reduction is the accountable care organization (ACO) movement. ACOs are formal groups of physicians, pharmacists, and other providers, hospitals, and healthcare facilities that join together in a coordinated way to seek out measurable improvements in patient health outcomes. They study reports and trends about medical errors and expenditures to set and achieve specific goals to improve services and delivery while reducing costs. The healthcare ACO providers and facilities share both the business risks and the savings of the healthcare improvement efforts. The aim is to reward healthcare professionals for good health outcomes and the quality of healthcare decisions, services, and products rather than the quantity.

Medicare is encouraging and leading the formation of ACO groups and facilities. ACO organizations can market this positive approach as a benefit to patients and insurance companies. For more information on Medicare ACOs, visit the page devoted to ACOs at the Centers for Medicare and Medicaid Services website at https://PharmPractice7e.ParadigmEducation.com/FeeForService.

Safety-Oriented Technology and Utilization

Properly selecting, implementing, utilizing, and maintaining pharmacy technology and automation are key to the safe filling, dispensing, compounding, and administering of medications (such as the use of bar code scanning for drug verification). Pharmacists can encourage the prescribers they work with to use e-prescribing software and employ common terminology in their prescription and medication orders, avoiding any abbreviations that have proven confusing and unsafe (as determined by the ISMP). Technicians contribute to this effort by getting to know the ins and outs of each element of pharmacy software and automation equipment and following procedures without skipping steps.

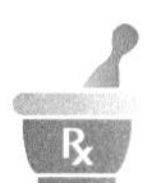

Practice Tip

Instead of asking "Do you have any drug allergies or health conditions?" it can be more effective to ask: "Can you think of any changes you have had in your drug allergies or health conditions? Have you started taking any new medications, dietary supplements, or herbal products since you have last seen us or that you may not have mentioned before?"

Addressing Psychosocial Causes of Human Errors

The level of errors where technicians and pharmacists have a great deal of influence is that of individual human errors. One may ask, if all personnel have been taught the correct procedures, why are they not always done? The answer lies in seven social and psychological reasons, including incomplete information error, incorrect assumption error, selection error, capture error, rushed error, distraction error, and fear error. These are helpful to be aware of to work against them in practice.

- An **incomplete information error** occurs when a full medication profile is not available because the patient was not asked sufficient or proper questions about their medications, supplements, and allergies; the answers were somehow not recorded in the profile; or the patient withheld information deliberately or by accident of memory. For instance, consider a patient who is allergic to penicillin receiving a penicillin-related antibiotic. It is crucial to strive for complete medication profiles in order to avoid these errors.

- An **incorrect assumption error** occurs when an essential piece of information is assumed to be true without verification; therefore, a wrong decision is made. An example of an assumption error is misreading a poorly written abbreviation, drug name, or direction on a prescription. Double-checking missing or questionable information is the only cure.

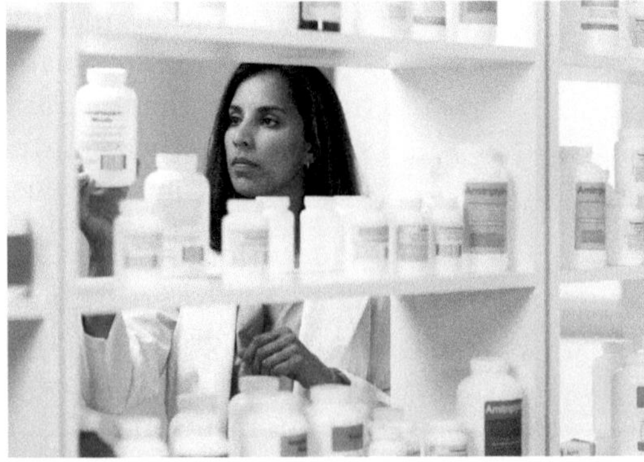
Technicians and pharmacists must be careful to double-check the desired NDC number on the prescription and on the stock medication and not go by memory of the package or usual dosage strength.

- A **selection error** occurs when two or more options seem to exist (or do exist), and the wrong option is chosen. The most common error in dispensing and administration is drug misidentification. An example of a selection error is mistakenly grabbing off the shelf a look-alike or sound-alike drug instead of the prescribed drug or choosing an immediate-release formulation instead of an extended-release drug. Similar manufacturer labels can also lead to a mistaken medication selection. Double-checking information and using the NDC bar code scanner can help eliminate these problems.
- A **capture error** is an error of inattentiveness and habit. It occurs when a more practiced behavior automatically takes the place of a less familiar one because of a failure to notice or capture the differences in the situation. For example, the usual prescription for alprazolam is 1 mg, but an elderly woman of low weight receives a prescription for 0.25 mg. Rather than attending to this difference, you simply fill it as if it were the norm, thus preparing the medication at four times the prescribed dose! (You assume it is up to the pharmacist or tech-check-tech supervisor to notice and correct the error.) The opposite can happen also. Suddenly a prescription comes in for a far higher dose than the usual range, which can be a danger signal that a prescriber has made a mistake. Instead of querying the pharmacist and prescriber, you just follow habit and fill the prescription. A mistake was made, but the pharmacist also approves the prescription without question, and the patient gets a medication that can cause harm.

  In both cases, the remedy for a capture error is to remind yourself with each and every prescription to focus on the details. Taking a new breath with each prescription can be a way to remind yourself to also refresh your mind with each new prescription.

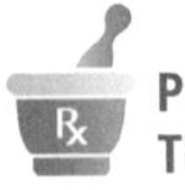
Practice Tip

At the end of any step, take five seconds to look over what you have done to ensure that no mistakes have been made, like proofing a paper.

- A **rushed error** is an error that is becoming increasingly common—an error made because of the pressure to meet corporate or self-imposed time constraints, resulting in cut corners and unnoticed danger alerts. The interior monologue is, "If I take the time to check this, I will be late and not meet the production quotas or customer satisfaction surveys," or "More waiting will make this patient even angrier." Elements that would have been carefully checked with more time are left unchecked, and errors go unnoticed. To address this, slow down rather than speed up when feeling this inner pressure, take a breath to clear your head, and remind yourself that patient safety always overrides speed, and you are not productive if you are harming the patient, which in the end also harms the pharmacy, your job, and your career.

Practice Tip

Not only can a cell phone create distractions, but it can also create opportunities for inadvertently compromising patients' privacy.

- A **distraction error** occurs when a technician or pharmacist is interrupted in the middle of a filling process and forgets a portion of key information or train of thought. An example is being interrupted in a metric measurement calculation by a patient query, a customer call, or a text on a cell phone. When you return to the calculation, the wrong decimal place that was going to be corrected is missed; or you dispense the wrong number of tablets (e.g., because the correct number was not double-checked at the conclusion of the phone call) or inadvertently override an alert due to the distraction.

  Determining when and where in the prescription-filling process it is safe to answer a customer call or query or be diverted for another work task is essential. For instance, when you are completing a medication-related task, what are the points in the process when stopping and answering the pharmacy telephone is not appropriate? When is it appropriate and necessary? The pharmacist and training personnel can help determine this. Knowing when to allow interruptions and when not to do so is vitally important in developing individual safety practices—and having the confidence to adhere to such practices during the pressure of a workday is key. You must also put your cell phone away from your body (along with other personal belongings or devices) and not check it except at breaks.

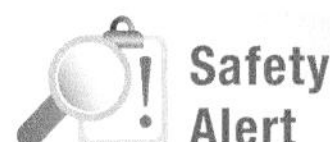

Safety Alert

Each person who participates in the filling process has the opportunity to catch and correct a medication error. Maintaining focused attention when filling prescriptions is important to avoid errors.

- A **fear error** occurs when a technician fears the consequences of speaking up and asking a technician colleague, a pharmacist, or a prescriber to assist or double-check a prescription element. As a technician, you usually are the one to enter a prescription, talk at length to the patient about their medication and allergy profile, submit the prescription for medication reconciliation and insurance claims, and fill it. As such, you "own" a substantial portion of the prescription-filling process and can many times spot errors. However, the fear of bothering, embarrassing, or angering someone can mistakenly become more important than patient safety.

  A lack of confidence in one's own knowledge may also make someone reluctant to speak up and say, "Can we check this?" The only way around these fears is to face them and know that if you choose this career, you must choose daily to be brave enough to speak the truth when you see it and to question those things that need questioning. Remind yourself that these courageous choices matter very much to the patients as you have their lives and health in your hands with each prescription.

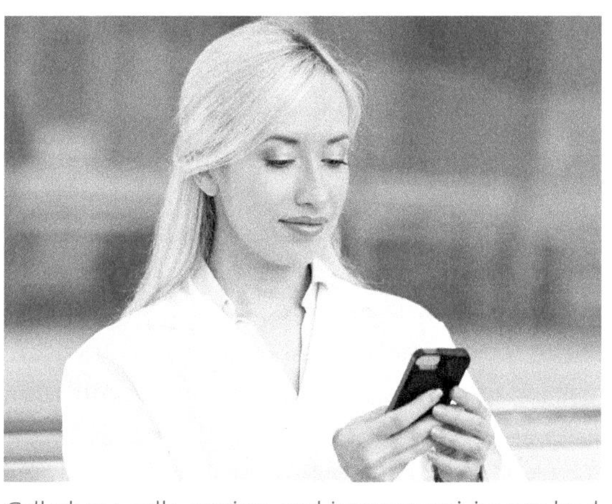

Cell phone calls, texting, and internet activity can lead to distractions, causing medication errors.

For a sense of how some of these errors work in everyday life, consider the case of Emily Jerry (described in Chapter 2), the two-year-old who died because of a medication error. Numerous psychosocial factors were involved. The uncertified technician was distracted on her cell phone making plans for her upcoming wedding. Though she *did* have the courage to admit that she might have made a mistake, the pharmacist (who lost his license) did not take the time to recalculate. The pharmacy was understaffed, and the pharmacist felt rushed. He was found guilty of involuntary manslaughter and sentenced to five years in prison and a maximum fine of $10,000. This case resulted in the passage of Emily's Law in Ohio, which establishes standards for qualified pharmacy technicians.

IN THE REAL WORLD

While entering new prescriptions, a technician named Thuy noticed an unusually high dose and nonstandard dosing regimen for the antipsychotic quetiapine (Seroquel)—300 mg in the morning, 450 mg in the evening. Thuy pointed out to the pharmacist that the dose seemed high and that it was odd that the morning and the evening doses were not the same. The pharmacist looked into it—this patient had not had Seroquel before, so this dose was too high to be an appropriate starting dose, and it was odd to start a patient with different morning and evening doses. The pharmacist called the patient's nursing home and learned that the wrong patient's name had been written on the order! So the technician's simple question spared the patient from receiving a high dose of a powerful antipsychotic medication that wasn't intended for them.

Step-by-Step Task Analysis of Prescription Filling

Human errors with medications occur most frequently at two crucial points in the process: prescription filling and administration. Knowing this can aid in the identification and prevention of future problems. Technicians and pharmacists use root-cause analysis to examine their own work flow to determine potential for errors and prevention steps to avoid them.

Incorrect drug identification is the most common error in dispensing or administration.

Prescription-Filling Errors

In most pharmacy programs, technicians are taught to check each prescription against the original prescription and medication information sheet at least four times:

1. during the computer order entry and printing of the label
2. when the medication is taken from the shelf
3. when the NDC number/bar code scan is verified
4. during the counting of the dosage to fill the prescription

Pharmacists check the medication profile and prescription entry at the beginning of the dispensing process; then they check the medication, label, and patient education material at the end. They also answer questions or verify elements during the filling process if needed for calculations or by technician request. Technicians and pharmacists are fully responsible for these specific technical errors in the filling process:

- A **wrong drug error**, occurs when the incorrect drug is substituted for the one prescribed; when the wrong drug has been prescribed by accident for the medical indication, and the prescriber is not alerted to adjust the prescription; when the wrong ingredients are mixed during drug compounding; or when the wrong medication label is applied and given to the wrong patient.
- An **adverse drug error**, occurs when the prescribed drug initiates an allergy or an adverse drug interaction because a flag is missed or the medication profile was incomplete.
- A **wrong amount error** (or wrong dosage error), occurs when a dose is either above or below the correct amount by more than 5% ; or when the wrong supply of medication is provided.

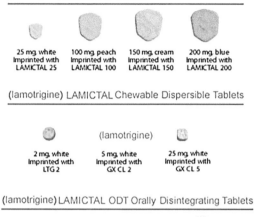

(lamotrigine) LAMICTAL Tablets

25 mg, white Imprinted with LAMICTAL 25

100 mg, peach Imprinted with LAMICTAL 100

150 mg, cream Imprinted with LAMICTAL 150

200 mg, blue Imprinted with LAMICTAL 200

(lamotrigine) LAMICTAL Chewable Dispersible Tablets

(lamotrigine)

2 mg, white Imprinted with LTG 2

5 mg, white Imprinted with GX CL 2

25 mg, white Imprinted with GX CL 5

(lamotrigine) LAMICTAL ODT Orally Disintegrating Tablets

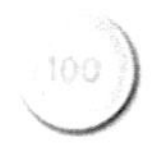

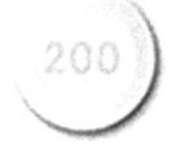

25 mg, white Imprinted with 25

50 mg, white Imprinted with 50

100 mg, white Imprinted with 100

200 mg, white Imprinted with 200

Lamictal 25 mg comes in many dosage formulations, including Lamictal XR (not shown), which can cause errors by inattentive pharmacy staff or unaware prescribers.

- A **mislabeling error**, occurs when a medication has incorrect information on it leading to incorrect usage; or when the wrong patient receives the medication
- A **wrong formulation error**, occurs when the dose formulation provided does not fit the physician's order. Examples include a drug given by mouth for a drug ordered as an intramuscular (IM) injection; a transdermal patch instead of a tablet; a drug prescribed for IM instead of subcutaneous administration; or an immediate-release drug dispensed instead of a controlled- or extended-release drug. How does this happen? Consider that the brand name drug Lamictal is available as an immediate-release, extended-release, chewable dispersible, and oral disintegrating tablet!
- A **documentation error**, occurs when essential information is missing or not properly noted, such as a prescription, an allergy, a patient request, or other information in the medication profile; or when insurance or billing claims are not properly processed.
- A **medication education error**, occurs when the proper medication education materials and counsel are not passed on to the patient or medication administrator.
- A **contaminated product error**, occurs when aseptic technique is not followed properly in compounding and the drug is no longer sterile, causing a microorganism infection.

Patient or Caregiver Drug Administration Errors

Many errors occur beyond the pharmacy walls at the point of administration. In the community pharmacy, the medications pass through the hands of the patient or guardian, so the technician and pharmacist must provide adequate education in the forms of medication label, information sheets, and pharmacist counseling about proper administration. In the hospital setting, the administering hands are those of the nurse (utilizing bar code technology at the bedside), so nurses, too, must be educated by the pharmacy staff. Without this education, the following errors are common:

- A **wrong time error** occurs when a drug is given 30 minutes or more before or after it was ordered to be administered, up to the time of the next dose. This is a common error in short-staffed hospitals and nursing homes and in patient homes.
- An **extra dose error** occurs when a patient receives more doses than were prescribed.
- An **omission error** occurs when a prescribed dose is due but not administered.

14.3 Step-by-Step Overview of Filling and Administration Education

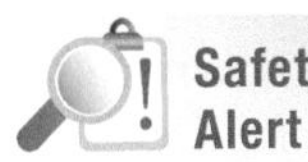

If information is missing from a prescription or medication order, a pharmacy technician must obtain that information from the prescriber. The technician should never make conjectures regarding the missing content.

The only way to stop medication errors is to review the steps in the filling process and key points where errors can be prevented. Figure 14.2 provides an overview of a typical step-by-step prescription-filling process for community and hospital pharmacy practice settings, medication. As the steps are briefly described, it is helpful to think of each as entailing three factors:

- information that needs to be obtained or checked
- resources that can be used to verify information
- potential medication errors that would result from a failure to obtain or check the information using the appropriate resources

FIGURE 14.2 Prescription-Filling Process

Each step in the prescription-filling process is an opportunity to do things correctly or make an error. At each step, there is also a chance to catch and correct any previous errors and to make a positive difference in someone's life.

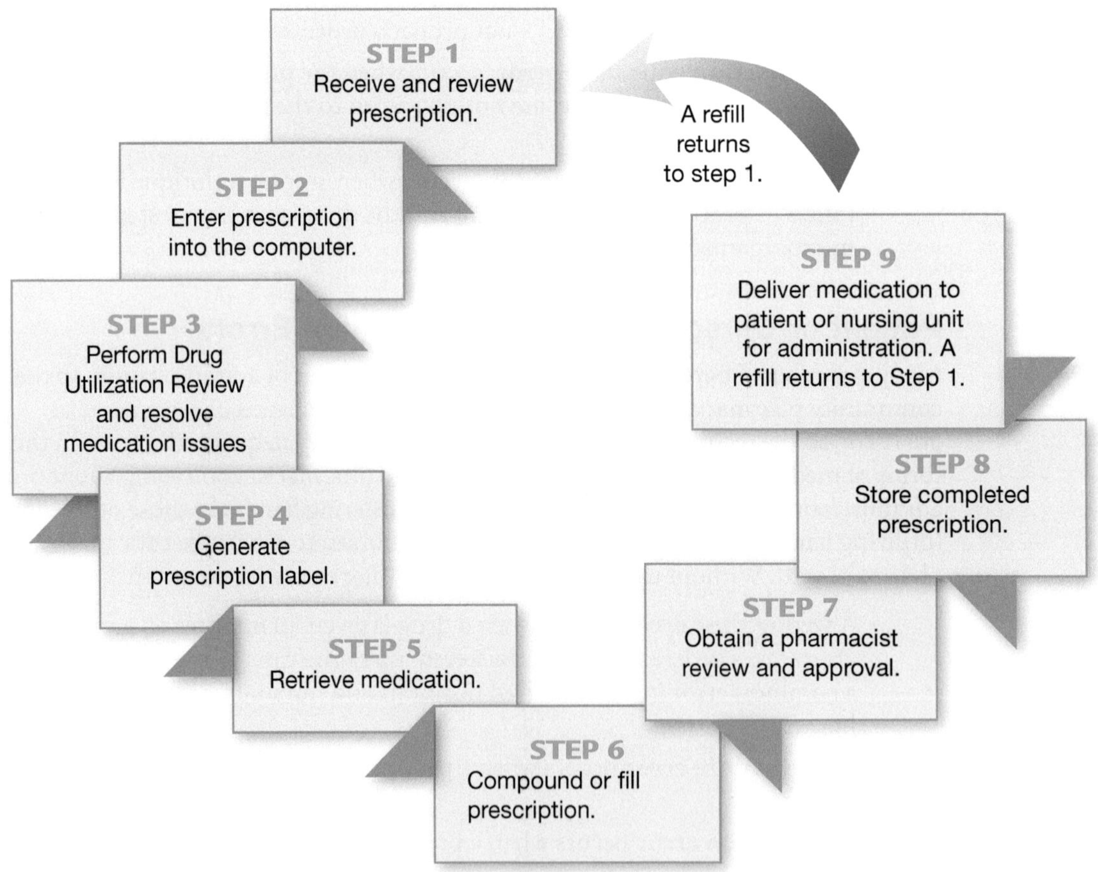

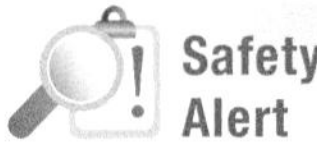

A prescriber's signature is required for an electronic or written prescription to be valid.

Step 1: Receive and Review Prescription

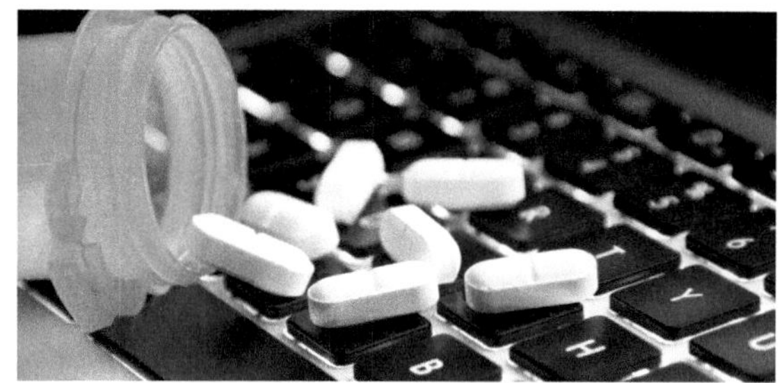

In at least 1.7% of all prescriptions dispensed in a retail pharmacy, some type of medication error occurs. Medication errors are generally not reported.

In receiving a prescription or medical order, an initial check of all key pieces of information is vital. Table 14.2 lists the data needed and the resources to avoid potential errors. A thorough review by the pharmacy technician and the pharmacist substantially reduces the chances that an unidentified error will continue throughout the filling process. Verify the legitimacy of the prescription or medical order first and then the individual components of the prescriber, patient, and prescription information. Any unclear information must be clarified.

TABLE 14.2 Step 1: Receive and Review Prescription

Information to Check	Resources to Verify Information	Potential Errors Resulting from Failure to Check/Verify Information
Legibility: Are there any typos or seeming errors in the e-Rx that are confusing? In a handwritten Rx, can the prescription be read clearly?	Physician, patient, independent reviewer, such as a pharmacist or a nurse	Prescription misread
Prescriber information: Is the prescription valid? Did the prescriber sign the prescription?	Physician, pharmacist, nurse	Out-of-date (i.e., invalid) prescription filled; fraudulent prescription filled; patient receives medication intended for another patient
For controlled substances, is the prescriber's Drug Enforcement Administration (DEA) number listed?		
Are the prescriber's name, address, and phone number printed on the prescription?		
Patient information: Is all necessary information included?	Physician, patient, immediate family member, patient profile, pharmacist, nurse	Incorrect patient selected; contraindicated drug dispensed
Is this prescription for this patient?		
Are the patient's name, date of birth, address, phone number, and allergies provided?		
Does the information match the profile?		
Medication information: Is all necessary information included?	Patient, physician, family member, patient profile	Wrong medication dispensed; wrong form or formulation dispensed; wrong dose dispensed; patient administers incorrectly; out-of-date (i.e., invalid) prescription filled
Are drug name, dose, dosage form, route of administration, refills, directions for use, and dosing schedule included?		
Is the prescription dated?		

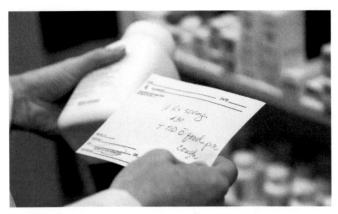
In a community pharmacy, handwritten prescriptions still come in that are incomplete. If you are unable to seek out the complete information, do not fill the prescription.

Verbal Order Precautions

A common cause of error in prescriptions over the phone or in person is sound-alike drugs; if the caller or prescriber did not spell out the name of the drug and the pharmacist (or the technician, in some states) is unclear about the correct name, the order should be spelled or clarified. If the nurse calls it in, the caller is encouraged to read back the order to minimize errors. Any verbal prescription order should include all of the information necessary to verify the credibility and legality of the prescriber, including the National Provider Identifier (NPI), DEA, or license number, depending on what is needed.

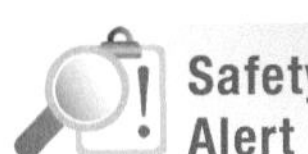
Safety Alert

C-III, -IV, and -V prescriptions should not be filled after six months; non-controlled medications should not be filled after one year from date of prescribing.

There are many occasions when a nurse will leave a voicemail for a new prescription. In some states, the technician is allowed to transcribe the prescription. In one case, a technician misheard "Pamelor" (an antidepressant) for "Tambocor" (an anti-arrhythmic); the error was not discovered for one month. Fortunately, the patient experienced no adverse outcomes. This error might have been prevented by reviewing the profile and calling the nurse back for clarification.

Abbreviation and Signa Code Errors

Prescribing errors include the use of nonstandard abbreviations, confusing look-alike and sound-alike drug names, poor handwriting, and "as directed" instructions. An "as directed" instruction does not allow a pharmacist to verify normal recommended dose scheduling or to reinforce the correct dosing regimen to patients. Though errors on sound-alike drugs are less common with e-Rxs, the "sig" could be inappropriate due to incorrect selection in the drop-down menu, or the refill field may be missing.

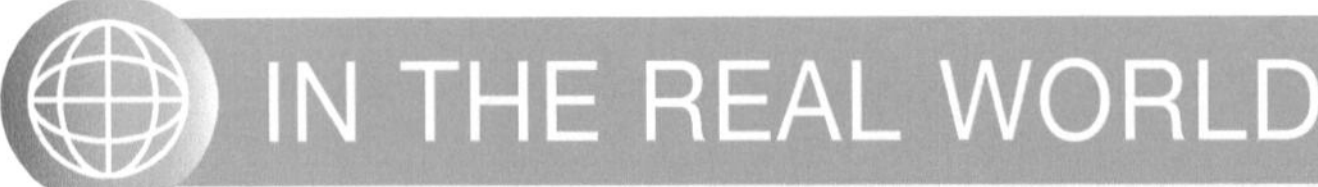

IN THE REAL WORLD

The very potent drug methotrexate is most often prescribed for arthritis in a specified oral dose of "q wk" or *once weekly*. An unsuspecting technician entered the dose as 28 mg *once daily* rather than once weekly. This damaging error was not caught by the pharmacist, and the patient continued taking the incorrect dose at seven times the prescribed dose, which was toxic to the bone marrow, until the damage was finally noticed by the prescriber!

In contrast, while entering an order for pregabalin (Lyrica), a drug used to treat neuropathic pain, an attentive technician named Nelya noticed that the directions on the order were not standard—1 to 2 tablets at bedtime "prn" (as needed). She called the pharmacist over to alert him: "I've never seen an 'as-needed' order for pregabalin before." The pharmacist agreed—and in the drug's labeling there is no such dosing. The pharmacist called the doctor's office, and the prescriber modified the directions. The patient was spared the additional dosing, which would not have been more effective at treating her pain and might have caused additional side effects.

The Joint Commission has assembled a list of problematic abbreviations to avoid (see Table 14.3), and if any of them occur on the prescription, make sure that they are verified and replaced with the appropriate substitution so that no errors result. Many of these potential "abbreviation errors" have been discussed previously, but they are listed here for reinforcement.

TABLE 14.3 The Joint Commission's Official "Do Not Use" Abbreviation List[1]

Do Not Use	Potential Problem	Use Instead
U, u (unit)	Mistaken for "0" (zero), the number "4" (four), or "cc"	Write "unit"
IU international unit	Mistaken for "IV" (intravenous) or the number "10" (ten)	Write "international unit"
Q.D., QD, q.d., qd (daily)	Mistaken for each other	Write "daily"
Q.O.D., QOD, q.o.d, qod (every other day)	Period after the Q mistaken for "I" and the "O" mistaken for "I"	Write "every other day"
Trailing zero (X.0 mg)*	Decimal point missed	Write X mg
Lack of leading zero (.X mg)	Decimal point missed	Write 0.X mg
MS	Can mean morphine sulfate or magnesium sulfate	Write "morphine sulfate"
MSO^4 and $MgSO^4$	Confused for one another	Write "magnesium sulfate"

[1] Applies to all orders and all medication-related documentation that is handwritten (including free-text computer entry) or on preprinted forms.
*Exception: A "trailing zero" may be used only where required to demonstrate the level of precision of the value being reported, such as for laboratory results, imaging studies that report size of lesions, or catheter/tube sizes. It may not be used in medication orders or other medication-related documentation.

Step 2: Enter Prescription into the Computer

In the community pharmacy setting, the pharmacy technician often enters the prescriptions into the computer database, whereas in the hospital it is the pharmacist or the prescriber who usually enters the medication order. As each piece of information is entered, the prescription should be compared with choices from the computer menu. Check the brand and generic drug options and their spellings to determine whether the information on the prescription and in the computer match. Special attention should be paid to dosages, formulations, concentrations, and the increments of measure. Prescriptions that contain unapproved, error-causing abbreviations must be reviewed carefully with a pharmacist or confirmed with the prescriber.

Once entered, each data element should be checked again before the entry process is finalized. In many pharmacies, the original prescription is scanned so that the pharmacist can check the technician's entry on the screen during the verification process. Table 14.4 lists the information needed and the resources used to avoid potential errors in the second step of the prescription-filling process.

TABLE 14.4 Step 2: Enter Prescription into the Computer

Information to Check	Resources to Verify Information	Potential Errors Resulting from Failure to Check/Verify Information
Are data choices from the computer menu and those on the prescription the same?	Cross-check brand/generic names for identical spelling.	Look-alike or sound-alike drug selection error made
Does the spelling on the prescription match the drug selection options?		
Do the increments of measure on the drug selection options match those on the prescription (e.g., gram versus milligram versus microgram)?	Cross-check measure prescribed with drug choices listed.	Patient given incorrect dose
For the dose selected, do available strengths or concentrations match?	Cross-check dose written with available strengths or concentrations on selection menu; cross-check dose or concentrations that use decimals or leading or trailing zeros.	Patient given incorrect dose
Does the dose or concentration have leading or trailing zeros?		
Does it require a decimal?		
Do available forms match the route selected?	Match route to formulation choices (e.g., injection route corresponds to intravenous [IV] or intramuscular [IM] drug; oral route corresponds to capsule, tablet, liquid, or lozenge).	Inappropriate form or formulation selected

Be sure to look for DAW status on prescriptions but especially for thyroid medications. If a new prescription is received, check the patient's profile for past history to see what generic or brand name was dispensed, and then verify if correct.

Brand Versus Generic

A common pharmacy dilemma is when a prescribed brand-name cough and cold remedy is not carried by the pharmacy, is no longer available, or is not covered by insurance. Most software will list a generic equivalent. However, if the recommended generic equivalent is not in stock, caution should be used before offering another generic equivalent. Other options would contain different ingredients, which could change their bioequivalency. The technician or the pharmacist then needs to contact the prescriber to discuss a therapeutically equivalent product with similar but not identical ingredients.

Another common problem arises when a brand name drug, such as Synthroid, is prescribed as a "*dispense as written*" (DAW, or do not substitute). If the technician does not enter the correct DAW code, the computer may default to the less expensive generic drug levothyroxine, and the wrong drug will be dispensed if not detected in the pharmacist check.

Dosage Form and Formulation Mix-Up Dangers

Does the dosage form or formulation match the route of administration? Be aware that certain concentrations or formulations of a medication are often associated with a particular administration route. For example, methylprednisolone acetate (Depo-Medrol) and methylprednisolone (Solu-Medrol) are both injectable and have similar dosages, depending on the clinical situation. However, Depo-Medrol is for IM administration only and is a cloudy suspension when reconstituted. Solu-Medrol is for IV administration and is a clear solution. A serious and potentially fatal medication error could occur if a suspension were inadvertently administered by the IV route, as the suspension could cause damage to veins.

Another mix-up may occur with morphine sulfate. Morphine sulfate is available in a concentrated liquid formulation (20 mg/mL) and a less concentrated liquid (4 mg/mL and 2 mg/mL). Entering or selecting the wrong concentration would result in a fivefold to tenfold error and cause serious respiratory depression in the patient. Other examples include ointments versus creams in topical products or solutions versus suspensions in ophthalmic and otic medications. In some cases, substituting a capsule for a tablet or vice versa is permissible. If you're unsure, always check with the pharmacist.

Related Drugs with Different Dosages and Sigs

If a related drug is entered instead of the correct one, the mistake can be more easily missed by both technician and pharmacist. Certain Schedule II pain medications are a particular source of potential error. For instance, OxyContin is the extended-release formulation, and oxycodone IR is the immediate-release formulation. Because of their different functions and metabolizing rates, these drugs should be prescribed differently. OxyContin is commonly dosed every 8 to 12 hours, whereas oxycodone is dosed every 4 to 6 hours. To make things worse, the two drugs are often prescribed together. Entering the right drug(s) into the computer profile with the right dosage directions is extremely important!

Teaspoons Versus Milliliters

Mix-ups occasionally occur with the teaspoonful and milliliter dosage amounts. A prescriber may either inadvertently write the wrong instructions, or the technician might enter an incorrect measurement form for the dosage into the computer. For example, a prescription may be written for 3.5 mL of an antibiotic, but the order is entered as 3.5 teaspoonfuls (or 17.5 mL). If the pharmacist misses the error, the pediatric patient would receive five times the recommended dose. Therefore, it is recommended to always use milliliters for computer entry and labeling to minimize errors.

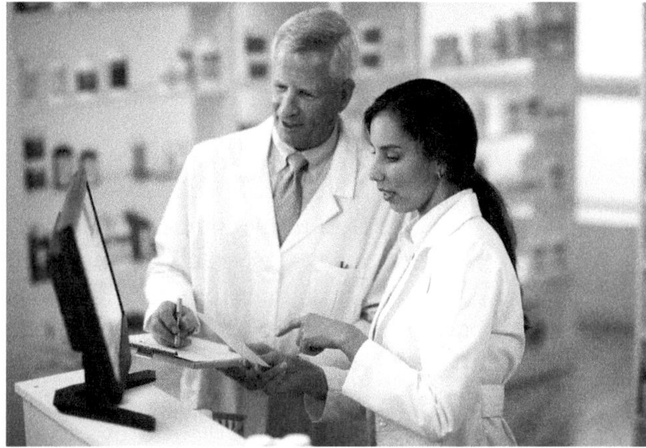

For each prescription, the technician has to stay attentive and focused while entering patient medication profile and prescription information into the computer and checking the DUR and insurance prompts, working against screen and alert fatigue.

Step 3: Perform Drug Utilization Review and Resolve Medication Issues

While working through DUR and insurance processes, multiple prompts and alerts will pop up on the screen about repetitive drug therapies, dosing ranges, existing allergies, contraindications in pregnancy or in women of childbearing potential, and problematic interactions with other medications (see Table 14.5). Beware of **alert fatigue**. This is when the technician and/or the pharmacist start to have a relaxed attitude toward the screen alerts. One has to find ways to stay alert, engaged, and focused with each new prescription and screen prompt.

TABLE 14.5 Step 3: Drug Utilization Reviews and Resolving Medication Issues

Information to Check	Resources to Verify Information	Potential Errors Resulting from Failure to Check/Verify Information
Drug screening: Does the prescribed medication interact with other conditions or medications listed on the profile?	Patient, physician, family member, patient profile, interaction screening program, electronic messages from insurance provider, drug information resources (e.g., books, call centers, package inserts, patient information handouts)	Contraindicated drug dispensed; drug-drug or drug-disease interaction occurs
Pediatric dosing: Are the prescribed dose and frequency of dosing in a pediatric patient consistent with manufacturer recommendations and pharmacy references?	Original prescription, physician, package inserts, electronic database, reference texts, pharmacist experience	Serious overdose (or underdose) leading to side effects, adverse reactions, or treatment failure
Geriatric dosing: Are the prescribed dose and frequency of dosing in a geriatric patient consistent with manufacturer recommendations and pharmacy references?	Original prescription, physician, package inserts, electronic database, reference texts, pharmacist experience	Serious overdose leading to side effects or adverse reactions
Pregnant (or potentially pregnant) and nursing women dosing: Is the prescribed drug indicated in pregnant women or women of childbearing potential? Does the drug pass into the breast milk?	Physician, package inserts, electronic database, reference texts, questions to patient, pharmacist experience	Congenital birth defects, side effects in breast-feeding infants

The risk of medication errors and harmful drug interactions obviously increases with the number of medications, pharmacies, and prescribers that an individual patient uses, especially among elderly patients. For example, if a patient is on many drugs from many prescribers and specialists and suddenly is prescribed clarithromycin (Biaxin) to fight an infection, it may interfere with and increase the risk of toxicity of other drugs, such as blood thinners, antiseizure medications, or cholesterol-fighting drugs. Certain high-risk drugs such as warfarin and the arthritis drug methotrexate can interact with many drugs and always require careful review by the technician and the pharmacist. Even at normal therapeutic doses, the interactions of drug accumulations can lead to serious adverse reactions or even death.

IN THE REAL WORLD

While inputting a refill request, Marina discovered a problem in the pattern of a previously entered order for the tapering drug therapy (decreased gradually before stopping) of the corticosteroid prednisone. Prednisone may be tapered so that patients do not experience withdrawal symptoms such as severe fatigue, weakness, body aches, and joint pain. The taper sequence had been entered this way:

> *50 mg daily × 7 days, 40 mg daily × 7 days, 30 mg daily × 7 days, 10 mg daily × 7 days, 5 mg daily x 7 days, 1 mg daily × 7 days, then stop.*

Marina tacked a sticky note to the prescription label printout: "Looks like the 20 mg dose was missed" and handed it to the pharmacist. The pharmacist checked the original prescription, found that the taper sequence had indeed been entered incorrectly, and fixed it.

Allergy-Related Alerts

The computer software generally flags allergies, but it is often the pharmacy technician who sorts through the questions and brings the problematic ones to the attention of the pharmacist for professional judgment. For example, if the patient is allergic to codeine, can they tolerate hydrocodone, a similar narcotic? Similarly, if a child is allergic to penicillin, there is a chance of cross-sensitivity with other antibiotics.

Problems arise if the patient or the caregiver has not told the technician, pharmacist, or prescriber about any allergies, so technicians need to remember to ask the patient, probing for any allergies that may have been missed. Also, how is the allergy manifested? Is the patient's allergy a gastrointestinal upset, rash, shortness of breath, or another symptom? This information is key for the pharmacist to make a correct decision.

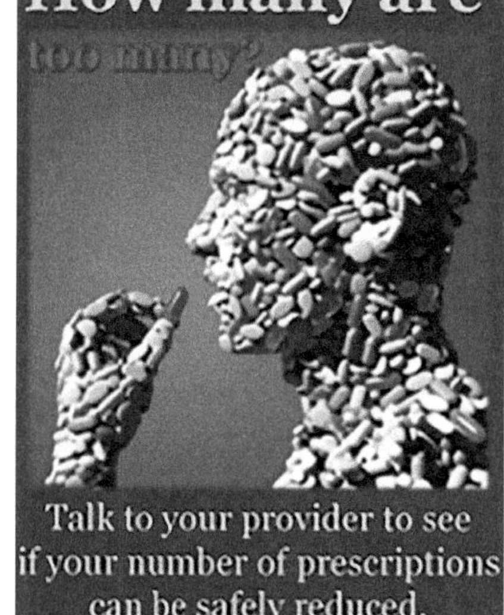

The more drugs and supplements one takes, the more likely the errors and adverse drug reactions. A 2013 Mayo Clinic study found that more than 50% of US citizens are taking at least two prescriptions while 20% are on five or more, and these numbers are rising. Many patients are also taking diet supplements, including herbal drugs, which also interact with prescription drugs. So all the more caution is needed in attending to DURs.

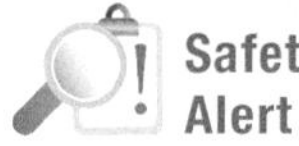
Safety Alert

The patient profile must always be checked for existing allergies or possible drug interactions prior to dispensing medications.

Interactions and Duplication Alerts

The computer software also flags duplicate therapy that may lead to serious adverse reactions. For example, a patient may be taking both ibuprofen and etodolac, which are similar anti-inflammatory and pain medications that, if taken together for a long period, can lead to a gastric bleed or ulcer. Another example may be a patient prescribed one cholesterol drug from a heart specialist and another one by the primary care physician.

Identifying these duplications saves money and reduces the risk of serious side effects or adverse reactions. The pharmacist must decide whether to counsel the patient or contact the prescribing physician before approving the filling of this prescription.

Special Considerations for Vulnerable Populations

As noted many times, special considerations must be paid to the prescription dosages for pediatric patients, especially those younger than age two. The prescriber must make the dosages appropriate for neonates (newborns), especially those born prematurely, and these must be triple-checked during input.

Also, if a woman is pregnant (or of childbearing potential), a more careful review of her prescriptions must always be done by the technician and the pharmacist to avoid any potential harm to a developing fetus. Finally, patients of low weight or older adult patients may require a lower dose of medication. Seniors often have age-related declines in liver and kidney functions and other body changes. In many cases, a drug may be contraindicated, or the dosage may need to be decreased from the average adult rate by 25% to 50% or more.

Physiological Causes of Medication Errors Every person is genetically unique, and the speed at which a body can process a medication varies tremendously from person to person. For instance, a patient may lack an enzyme that helps remove or eliminate medications from the body, thus leading to serious harm from what would normally be a safe medication at the prescribed dosage. A patient's reduced kidney function can also cause medication difficulties since the kidneys play an important role in excretion—the process by which drugs are removed from the bloodstream. Many patient populations have decreased kidney function because of age or disease.

Elderly patients, newborns, and premature babies have diminished kidney function, as well as patients with chronic renal failure, high blood pressure, diabetes, or alcohol abuse. If a medication dose is not lowered in consideration of these conditions, the drug can accumulate to toxic levels, causing an adverse reaction. Consequently, kidney function is one of many factors for the pharmacist to consider before approving and verifying a prescription. In the hospital, the pharmacist has access to pertinent laboratory results, such as kidney function. In the near future, community pharmacists may have access to the patient's lab results.

Patients are not always aware of the need to report their conditions, or they forget them. You can assist the pharmacist by being assertive and persuasive in drawing information out of patients for creating and updating medical condition notes and medication profiles in the computer database.

Narrow Therapeutic Index Drugs

There are certain medications where small differences in dose or blood concentration may lead to adverse reactions or therapeutic failures. These medications are said to be **narrow therapeutic index drugs**. For these drugs, there is a small difference between a therapeutic dose and a toxic dose.

Certain antibiotics (such as aminoglycosides), antiseizure agents (such as carbamazepine, phenytoin, and phenobarbital), and cardiac medications (such as digoxin, digitoxin, flecainide, and warfarin) are considered to have a narrow therapeutic index. It is common practice to carefully monitor patients who are taking a narrow therapeutic index drug. This often means laboratory testing of drug levels in the blood. Doses can be adjusted based on drug levels; if the drug level is too low, the dose may be increased. If the drug level is too high, the dose may be decreased.

Medication error rates are higher with narrow therapeutic index drugs. Furthermore, negative consequences of errors are amplified with these drugs. For example, if the blood levels of the injectable antibiotic gentamcin are too high, it can cause kidney damage and irreversible hearing loss. If too little of the blood thinner warfarin is used, a patient could suffer from a stroke or pulmonary embolism. As a technician, it is your job to familiarize yourself with narrow therapeutic index drugs so that you can keep your patients safe.

Step 4: Generate Prescription Label

After generating the label, cross-check it with the original prescription to make sure that a typing error or inherent program malfunction did not alter the information and that it is for the proper patient. Table 14.6 offers an overview to avoid potential errors in the fourth step.

TABLE 14.6 Step 4: Generate Prescription Label

Information to Check	Resources to Verify Information	Potential Errors Resulting from Failure to Check/Verify Information
Has the patient information been cross-checked?	Compare label generated with original prescription.	Wrong patient, medication, or dose selected
Are the label and original prescription identical?	Compare label generated with original prescription.	Wrong patient, medication, or dose selected
Are the leading or trailing zeros and unapproved abbreviations correct?	Check with pharmacist or prescriber.	Incorrect dose selected
Do all the data elements match those of the original prescription (e.g., prescriber information, patient information, medication information)?	Use additional information generated on label reference for verification (e.g., brand/generic names; NDC number; manufacturer's name; patient's address, phone number[s], date of birth).	Inappropriate form or formulation selected

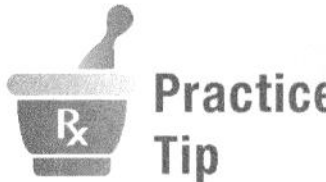
Practice Tip

Trazodone and tramadol are similar-sounding generic drugs with two distinct indications. Trazodone is an antidepressant while tramadol is an analgesic. Selecting one of these medications without checking the NDC number could have serious consequences.

Step 5: Retrieve Medication

The most common error is a selection error. Look-alike labels, brand or generic names, and medication shapes or colors can all contribute to medication errors. For instance, in one infamous case, *Troppi v. Scarf*, a pharmacist accidentally dispensed Nardil, an antidepressant, instead of Norinyl, a contraceptive. The woman who received the incorrect drug gave birth to a child, and the Michigan Court of Appeals held the pharmacist liable not only for the medical expenses incurred in the woman's pregnancy, but also for the costs of raising the child.

Sometimes manufacturers deliberately use look-alike and sound-alike labeling to attract customers. The manufacturer of Maalox was attempting to increase its market share by a **product line extension**—using a brand name to sell various combinations of active ingredients with different indications—leading to consumer selection errors. At the request of the FDA, the manufacturer voluntarily recalled its confusing products, changed the product names, provided educational programs for healthcare professionals and consumers, and added safety monitoring and a reporting program for its products.

Generics of both Fioricet and Fiorinal are dispensed as white tablets. An NDC bar code scan ensures that the correct medication is dispensed. If generic Fiorinal is dispensed in error to a patient with an aspirin allergy, a serious reaction can occur.

National Drug Code Matchups and Bar Code Scanning

To avoid an incorrect selection from the storage shelf, match the NDC numbers, drug names, and other information available on manufacturers' labels or patient information handouts, scanning the bar codes to lead you to the right choice. The reason that NDC numbers serve as such an effective cross-check is because each numeral in the NDC number combination is specific to a particular drug and a specific strength, dosage form, and packaging for it. For example, bupropion 150 mg SR will have a different NDC than bupropion 150 mg XL. The SR formulation is commonly dosed twice daily while the XL formulation is dosed once daily. Table 14.7 offers a safety overview of Step 5.

TABLE 14.7 Step 5: Retrieve Medication

Information to Check	Resources to Verify Information	Potential Errors Resulting from Failure to Check/Verify Information
Has the available information on the manufacturer's label been used to verify the medication selection?	Original prescription, shelf- or bin-labeling systems, manufacturers' names, NDC numbers, brand names and generic names, pictographic medication verification references or computer programs	Medication selection error made
Does the brand or generic name on the label match the product container?		
Do the dose strength and form on the label match those indicated on the product container?	Original prescription, shelf- or bin-labeling systems, manufacturers' names, NDC numbers, brand names and generic names, pictographic medication verification references or computer programs	Incorrect dose, form, or formulation selected
Do the NDC numbers and manufacturers' names match those listed on the label?	Bin-labeling systems, NDC numbers, pictographic medication verification references or computer programs	Incorrect dose, form, or formulation selected

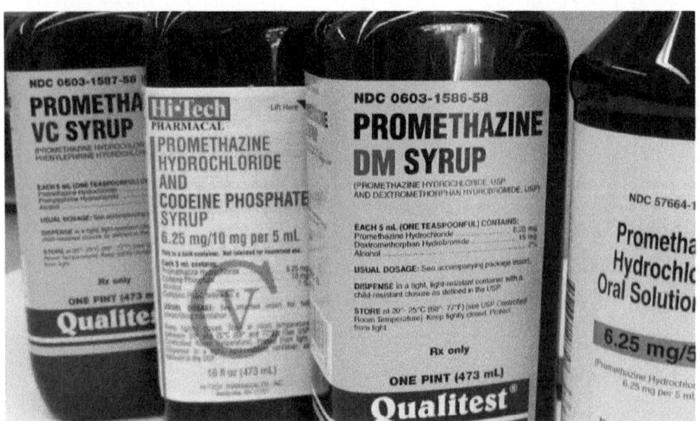

Medications with near-identical names and similar manufacturer packaging can lead to the wrong selection; always check the NDC number or scan the bar code.

Shelving Order and Medication Image Double-Checks

To prevent similarly labeled drugs or doses from being mixed up, drugs will often be shelved in a nonalphabetic or illogical order, so that the technician or pharmacist is less likely to select the wrong stock bottle with a similar name next to the right one. Some pharmacies use a shelf-labeling system to organize inventory and possess a computer-based tablet identification program. You can visually verify the medication selected by the NDC number and name with the picture called up by the bar code scan.

Take steps to minimize interruptions during the prescription-filling process. When necessary (such as when completing calculations), do not allow interruptions at all.

Step 6: Compound or Fill Prescription

Calculation and substitution errors are frequent sources of pharmacy-related medication errors in all practice settings as explained in Chapter 6. Do not allow interruptions, distractions, or multitasking during calculations. You should write out your calculations and have a second person check the answers. If you must stop before the calculations process is complete, be sure to start over from the beginning when you return. Table 14.8 presents safety tips for the sixth step.

Technology presents its own unique potentials for safety checks and for errors. All equipment must be maintained, cleaned, and calibrated on a regular basis. In most circumstances, technology failures are the result of user error, but inherent technology malfunctions and program glitches do occur, so safety monitoring must be standard. Good practices include consistent, timed checks of the technology's accuracy (e.g., computers, scales, robots, infusion pumps, automated dispensers, and compounders).

Proper safety checks are not limited to sophisticated equipment. The act of cleaning the counting trays and spatulas on a regular basis is an important part of medication safety. Consider the potential for serious harm to a patient if the residue or dust from an allergy-causing medication from one patient contaminated another patient's prescription. For example, penicillin- or sulfa-containing medications should preferably be counted on dedicated counting trays because of the high prevalence of penicillin and sulfa allergies. The counting tray must be cleaned with isopropyl alcohol after any of these drugs are dispensed. If you are dispensing oral hazardous substances, such as methotrexate, then the counting tray must also be carefully cleaned to prevent contamination.

TABLE 14.8 Step 6: Compound or Fill Prescription

Information to Check	Resources to Verify Information	Potential Errors Resulting from Failure to Check/Verify Information
Have the amount to be dispensed and the increment of measure (e.g., gram, milligram, microgram) been reviewed?	Amount dispensed (count twice), original prescription	Incorrect quantity or incorrect dose dispensed
Does the prescription require a calculation or measurement conversion?	Write out the calculation and conversions; ask another person to review the calculation.	Incorrect dose dispensed
If you are using equipment, has it been calibrated recently?	Equipment (check calibration), pharmacist, patient information handout, package insert	Incorrect dose dispensed
Does the medication dispensed require warning or caution labels?	Pharmacist, patient information handout, package insert	Administration error made by patient

Step 7: Obtain a Pharmacist Review and Approval

Though the pharmacist is legally responsible for every prescription or medication order filled, it is not practical for pharmacists to verify each step. Instead, the pharmacist verifies the initial computer entry and the original prescription/medication order, and the quality and integrity of the end product. You are responsible for laying out all the information in a logical order for the pharmacist to check, including the medication's stock bottle, calculations, labeled medication container, and original prescription. The same verification process is needed for a compounded sterile or nonsterile preparation. Table 14.9 offers safety counsel for the seventh step.

TABLE 14.9 Step 7: Obtain a Pharmacist Review and Approval

Information to Check	Resources to Verify Information	Potential Errors Resulting from Failure to Check/ Verify Information
Did the pharmacist review the prepared medication?	Original prescription, stock medication bottle or vial, calculations	Invalid or out-of-date prescription filled
Can the pharmacist verify the validity of the prescription using the finished product and the information you provide?	Original prescription	
Can the pharmacist verify the patient information using the finished product and the information you provide?	Original prescription, patient profile, patient, physician, or nurse	Wrong patient given medication
Can the pharmacist verify the correctness of the prepared prescription based on the medication information provided?	Physical appearance of prepared medication, calculations and conversions of technician, original manufacturer's container, pictographic medication verification programs, package insert	Medication selection error made; incorrect dose, form, or formulation selected; incorrect medication administered

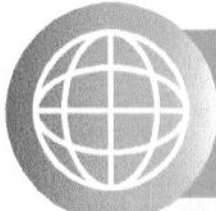

IN THE REAL WORLD

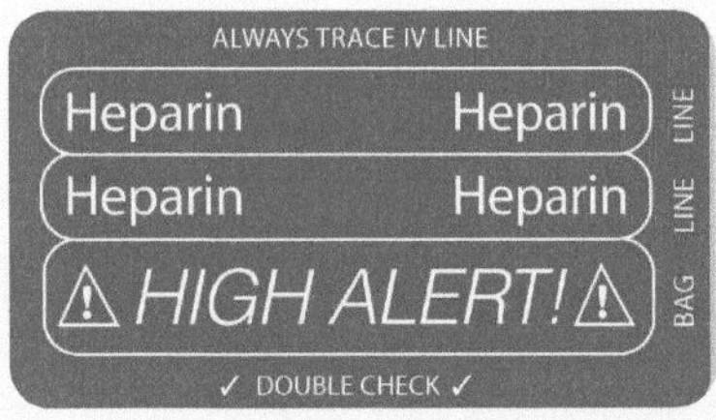

In the hospital setting, heparin is available in vials of concentrations from 10 units per mL to 10,000 units per mL. The lower concentrations are used to flush, clear, or maintain flow in an IV or dialysis line whereas the higher concentrations are used as adult blood thinners. Unfortunately, several serious medication errors, including death, have occurred when technicians and nurses have inadvertently selected the wrong heparin vial for patient recipients.

The FDA supported a USP proposal to revise the labels of Heparin Lock Flush Solution and Heparin Sodium Injection. The USP recommended that manufacturers clearly state the total drug strength by name and label call-out. Hospitals have also developed and implemented policies specifically for heparin administration. These policies include additional computer alerts, a a cross-check system between nurses, limited availability of certain concentrations on the nursing units, and colorful labeling to minimize heparin dosing errors.

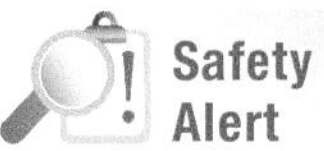

Safety Alert

The pharmacist must always check the technician's work before a prescription is dispensed, though a tech-check-tech supervisor can do a first check.

Checking Other Technicians' Work

A useful awareness exercise in considering what resources are needed for the pharmacist is to practice checking a colleague's work. After trading a finished prescription or medication order with another technician, consider the following questions: Can you retrace the steps taken to fill the prescription or medication order? Can you validate all of the key pieces of information? Undertaking this exercise on a regular basis helps highlight bad habits or shortcuts that may open the door for medication errors. This is also practice for someday becoming a tech-check-tech supervisor.

Auxiliary Labels and Medication Guides

Patient and nurse education is obviously key to appropriate administration. Several auxiliary caution and warning labels may be applied for each prescription and need to be checked by the pharmacist. They need to be prioritized, on the container, however, so that the most important warning is seen first. For example, if an antibiotic that interferes with birth control and makes a patient sensitive to sunburn is being administered to a woman on birth control, it may be important to make the birth control interference most prominent with the sun warning next (unless the patient also has a history of skin cancer). Before the technician affixes the auxiliary labels to the prescription vial, they should ask the pharmacist which ones to prioritize.

Similarly, **Medication Guides** with boxed warnings should not just be stuffed into the patient's prescription bag but should be stapled to the top of the bag so that they are in view. Common drugs that require an FDA-mandated Medication Guide are listed in Table 14.10. For more information, go to https://PharmPractice7e.ParadigmEducation.com/FDA-Common.

Step 8: Store Completed Prescription

Simple measures—such as establishing well-organized and clearly labeled storage, backup database, and temperature-controlled systems—can help keep a patient's medications together and separate from those of other patients while being properly stored.

Well-Organized Storage Systems

Orderly storage decreases the chances that patients will receive someone else's prescriptions or not receive their own because they were given to another patient. Off-site backup data storage systems are necessary in the event of natural disasters or fires.

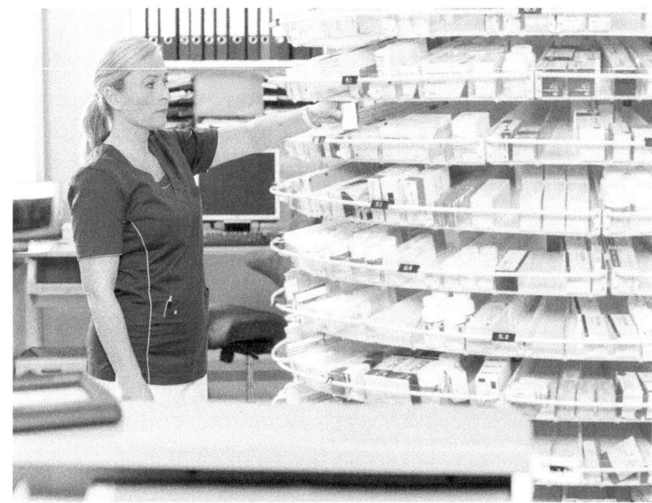

Having stock shelves that are well lit and neatly and systematically organized makes it easier and swifter to find the correct medications.

TABLE 14.10 Examples of Drugs Requiring a Medication Guide

Drug	Concerns Associated with Use
ADHD drugs (such as Adderall XR, Ritalin)	May cause heart-related problems (sudden death, stroke and heart attack in adults, increased blood pressure and pulse); mental health problems (thought problems, bipolar illness, aggressive behavior); circulation problems
Amiodarone (Cordarone)	May cause lung problems; may cause liver problems; may worsen heart problems
Antidepressants (SSNRI such as fluoxetine, sertraline, paroxetine, citalopram, escitalopram)	May be associated with an increase in suicidal thoughts and actions (especially in children, adolescents, and young adults)
Ciprofloxacin (Cipro)	May cause tendon rupture; may cause nerve damage; may cause seizures
Isotretinoin (Accutane)	Causes birth defects and miscarriage in pregnancy; may cause serious mental health problems
NSAIDs (such as celecoxib, diclofenac, ibuprofen, ketorolac, naproxen, sulindac)	May increase the risk of heart attack or stroke that can lead to death; may increase the risk of bleeding and ulcers
Transmucosal immediate-release fentanyl (TIRF)	May increase the risk of overdose and death; only for use in patients with pain severe enough to require around-the-clock, longterm treatment with an opioid; patients must already be using a regular opioid medication upon initiation
Warfarin (Coumadin)	May cause bleeding; may interact with other medications and supplements
Rivaroxaban (Xarelto)	May increase the risk of bleeding during use; may increase the risk of blood clots upon discontinuation
Zolpidem (Ambien)	May cause memory loss of events and activities that take place shortly after consuming a dose

Temperature-Controlled Storage Systems

As you know, failure to store medications properly with the correct temperature, humidity, and light-sensitive conditions may result in loss of drug potency or effects, which can cause serious harm. The following examples illustrate this:

- Inadvertent freezing of certain types of insulin results in changes in the formulation. Once the drug has been thawed and administered, the body absorbs it differently, resulting in a less than desired effect.
- Improper storage of nitroglycerin—a medication used to treat angina or chest pain—results in a loss of therapeutic efficacy. Nitroglycerin molecules adhere to plastics and cotton; therefore, sublingual tablets must be stored in original glass containers under airtight conditions without cotton.
- Dornase alfa inhalation solution (Pulmozyme) is medication for cystic fibrosis that needs to be protected from light and stored under refrigeration. If exposed to light, the medication loses potency. Product stability is compromised if exposed to elevated temperatures for more than 24 hours.

Consistent checking of refrigerator and freezer temperatures in the pharmacy or on the nursing unit must be done frequently and be well-documented. Keeping a computer or written log of temperature checks is often a technician's responsibility. However, any staff member accessing these storage areas should carefully monitor temperature and report any abnormal readings immediately.

If power is lost in any pharmacy setting for an extended period of time, such as after a hurricane, backup generators must be available or the drug inventory will need to be destroyed. Table 14.11 lists the information needed and the resources used to avoid potential errors in the eighth step of the prescription-filling process.

TABLE 14.11 Step 8: Store-Completed Prescription

Information to Check	Resources to Verify Information	Potential Errors Resulting from Failure to Check/ Verify Information
Are storage conditions appropriate for the medication (e.g., humidity, temperature, light exposure)?	Package insert	Medication becomes degraded
Are each patient's medications adequately separated?	Physical review of medications placed in bags, boxes, or bins	Patient receives medication not intended for them; patient fails to receive medication (i.e., omission)
Are storage areas kept neat and orderly?	Use of organizational systems (e.g., bins, boxes, bags, alphabetizing, numbering, consolidation)	Patient receives medication not intended for them; patient fails to receive medication (i.e., omission)

Step 9: Deliver Medication to Patient or Nursing Unit for Administration

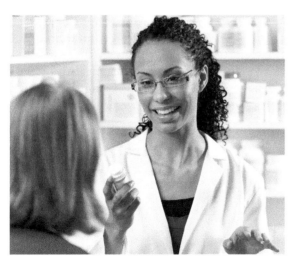

The technician should verify the date of birth and/or the address of the patient and the name of the expected medication before presenting the drug to the patient.

At the point of delivery to a patient or administering nurse, opportunities for mix-ups arise. For instance, there may be medications for both Rachel C. Gonzales and Raquel V. Gonzales in the storage bins. Using a date of birth and/or an address, or a hospital patient bar code ensures that the correct medication is dispensed to the correct patient. Once the patient's identity is reconfirmed, the technician needs to double-check *the number* of medications that the patient or the adminis tering nurse expects to receive.

Patients and nurses often notice something different from their expectations, and verifying the medication with them can serve as a triple-check. Errors—such as receipt of the wrong medications or missing medications (omission of therapy) as well as dosage form and administration errors—can be caught in this way. See Table 14.12 for safety tips for the ninth and final step.

TABLE 14.12 **Step 9: Deliver Medication to Patient or Nursing Unit for Administration**

Information to Check	Resources to Verify Information	Potential Errors Resulting from Failure to Check/ Verify Information
Will the appearance of any of the medications be new to the patient, caregiver, or nurse?	Prescription label, patient, patient education handouts, patient profile	Administration error made; patient nonadherent with medication instructions
Is the patient receiving medications intended for them?	Patient, caregiver, original prescription, patient profile, bar coding identification system	Patient receives medication not intended for them; patient fails to receive medication (omission)
Does the patient or caregiver understand the instructions for use?	Pharmacist, patient education handouts, drug information resources	Administration error made; patient nonadherent with medication instructions; drug interactions, adverse reactions, degradation of medication occurs because of improper handling or storage
Does the patient, caregiver, or nurse know what to expect?	Pharmacist, patient education handouts, drug information resources	Side effects and adverse reactions occur; clinical effect not achieved
Are all of the medications prescribed for the patient included?	Consolidation of medications into one bag, bin, or box; use of organizational systems (e.g., bins, boxes, bags, alphabetizing, consolidation)	Patient fails to receive medication (omission); therapy not completed

Explanation of Medication to Medication Administrator

Before delivering a medication to a patient, be aware that counseling by a pharmacist may be required first. When it is appropriate to hand over the medication, remember to ask basic questions, such as "Do you understand why this medicine is being used and are you comfortable with how this medicine works?" and "Do you know how to take it?" (Most nurses are well aware of how the typical medications work but may be unaware of a new one.) Call attention to auxiliary warnings and caution labels on the medication bottle, and, if a Medication Guide is stapled to the bag, unstaple it and open it up to highlight key pieces of information. (If a required Medication Guide is not distributed, the pharmacy may receive heavy fines during an audit.) If the patient has questions, call the pharmacist over to answer them. The key information a patient must understand is listed on Table 14.13.

Your conversations and questions can uncover key information and provide essential guidance to the patient and the nurse.

TABLE 14.13 Information Patients Must Know About Their Medications

1. Brand and generic name
2. The medication's appearance
3. The purpose of the medication and the duration of treatment
4. The correct dosage and frequency and the best time or circumstances to take a dose
5. How to proceed if they miss a dose
6. Medications or foods that interact with the prescribed medication
7. Whether the prescription is in addition to or replaces a current medication
8. Common side effects and how to handle them
9. Special precautions necessary for each particular drug therapy
10. Proper storage for the medication

"Show-and-Tell" Technique with Patient In some community pharmacies, a "show-and-tell" technique is employed. The technician or pharmacist opens the vial, shows the drug product to the patient, and describes its proper use. This added step not only helps the patient identify the drug, but also provides an extra opportunity to check that the correct drug product was put into the vial. It also shows patients that you and the pharmacist really care, which helps them trust enough to listen carefully, follow directions more closely, and share key information. If the patient notices that a refilled drug looks different from a previously filled drug, the patient has a chance to point this out and have this discrepancy verified.

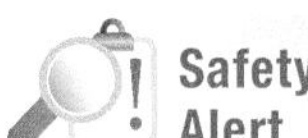
Safety Alert

Pharmacy technicians are only permitted to review information on a medication's label with a patient. If a technician suspects that a patient has questions or is in need of further counseling, the technician should alert the pharmacist.

In many cases, the correct drug was dispensed, but the prescription may have been refilled with a different generic drug, so the shape or color of the tablet or capsule differs, and you can explain this. The "show-and-tell" technique plus counseling will save a later telephone call to the pharmacy.

The technician is encouraged to use the "show-and-tell" followed by the "tell back" system to minimize patient administration errors. This process also ensures that the proper medication is being dispensed, as the patient will generally correct the technician if not.

"Tell Back" System Similar to the "show-and-tell" technique, the "tell back" system is recommended by the Institute for Safe Medication Practices. **Tell back** is a collaborative approach that uses patient-centered, open-ended questions to encourage the patient to repeat back what he or she understands. This method is especially useful for dispensing new medications or when providing medications to a new patient.

For example, you could say something like "Ms. Rodriguez, you are taking several medications for high blood pressure and cholesterol. I have given you a lot of information on the attached medication information sheets, including these Medication Guides. It would be helpful for me to hear your understanding of these medications and their side effects." This line of questioning is preferred over the more common, closed-ended questioning like "Do you have any questions?" If you sense any lack of understanding, the pharmacist should be notified and the patient counseled.

Hospital Prevention Procedures

Upon delivery of medications to a nursing unit, you should determine if the appropriate nurse knows about newly prescribed medications and if the delivered medications were all that were expected. When medication carts are returned with unused, regularly scheduled medications, follow up to determine whether errors of omission occurred. Also, note any discrepancies in the nursing units' automated drug dispensing machines between quantity counts of what should be present and what actually is present. Then you or the pharmacist can discuss the gaps with the nurses to discover the reasons and resolve them.

In the treatment of certain diseases, such as cancer, multiple drug therapy combinations are prescribed together because they work in concert to treat the disease. If a particular drug is missing from the drug therapy combination, treatment is incomplete, so each drug should be verified separately, not as a set. In addition, many of these drugs are extremely toxic, and any dosing error could be fatal. So all chemotherapy and hazardous substances must be triple-checked by the technician, the pharmacist, and the nurse.

Beyond the Pharmacy—Patient Self-Administration

Even with labels and a great deal of printed information handed to them, patients often make errors in the self-administration of their drug therapies for various reasons. Patients often contribute to medication errors by doing the following:

- forgetting to take a dose or doses
- taking too many doses
- dosing at the wrong time
- not getting a prescription filled or refilled in a timely manner
- not following directions on how to take the doses and what behaviors to avoid with them (such as not eating certain foods or avoiding alcohol)
- terminating the drug regimen too soon (which can be problematic with antibiotics)

Any of these actions may result in an adverse drug reaction or a subtherapeutic (less than desired effect)—or even toxic—dose. Not taking a prescribed medication could result in the progression of a chronic disease. Any of these circumstances could result in short-term or long-term harm, depending on the drug and the disease being treated.

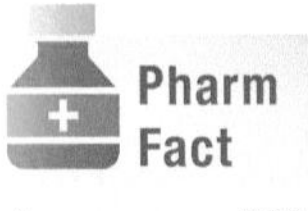

As many as 50% of patients on essential long-term medications no longer take their medication after one year.

Patient failure to follow medication therapy as the physician instructs is **medication nonadherence**, and it occurs because of many different personal and financial reasons. These include not having had medication information explained well, misunderstanding the instructions (perhaps because of inattentiveness, language barriers, or cultural barriers), not taking the instructions seriously, or not remembering to follow the directions.

If there are cultural or language barriers, some actions can be taken to overcome these obstacles, which will be addressed in the next chapter. If forgetting may be an issue, you can suggest daily or weekly medication boxes and refrigerator magnet reminders. In cases where memory problems exist, educating the caregiver in addition to the patient is important. If other issues are present, alert the pharmacist or guide the patient to counseling.

When refilling a prescription, take note of the history from the computer profile. If the patient appears to be nonadherent with the prescribed medication, perhaps having gaps in refill timing, it is helpful to ask some questions to gain more information. Tactfully inquire if prescriptions have been filled at another pharmacy or via mail order, and, if so, add this to the medication profile.

However, all patients should be strongly encouraged to use only one pharmacy to lower the risks of serious medication interactions and errors because of lack of shared medication information. Patients should also be encouraged to talk to the pharmacist or call later if questions on proper medication use or unexpected or serious side effects arise after leaving the pharmacy. If using multiple pharmacies, problems with memory, or an improper understanding of label directions *are not the causes* of medication nonadherence (or you cannot help the patient resolve these issues), the gap(s) or problems in therapy should be brought to the attention of the pharmacist for follow-through counseling intervention.

Cost is often an issue for patients when they are not seeing their doctors, filling, or refilling their medications. If cost is an issue, technicians can help them find coupons, assistance, or insurance coverage, as noted in Chapter 8. If cost is a concern, the pharmacist should discuss less costly therapy options with the prescriber so that the illness or disease can be adequately treated.

14.4 Manufacturers' Innovations to Promote Safety

Drug manufacturers and retail packagers also have a role in improving medication safety in the ways they design and package their drug products. Many companies manufacture formulations and packaging with unique colors, shapes, or markings to assist in distinguishing between different types and dosages or competitor products. They are also including more patient educational materials. Technicians and pharmacists can take advantage of these safety innovations and offer them to their patients, especially to those who are vulnerable.

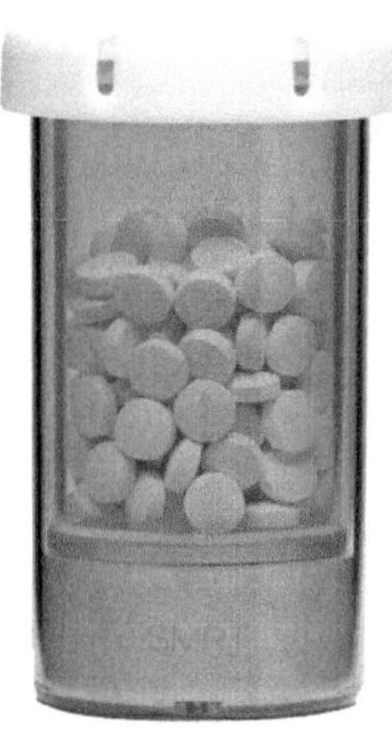

Advances in technology—such as SMRxT's Nomi pill bottles fitted with cellular technology that takes a weight reading every time the bottle is moved—are helping patients with medication adherence.

Some pharmaceutical manufacturers have the middle four numbers of the NDC or the middle letters of the drug name either in a larger font or boldface type to minimize selection errors. This can be helpful for patients and technicians with declining vision. Otherwise, without magnifying glasses, they could reach for the wrong medication. The ISMP has been recommending the use of "**tall man lettering**" warning statements on the stock labels of high-risk medications and other labeling changes to better differentiate products and dosages to reduce medication errors. "Tall man" is larger, bold lettering to distinguish similar medications, such as hydrOXYzine and hydrALAzine—two products that are available in similar doses. A list of other medications in the community and hospital pharmacy settings with "tall man" lettering is available at https://PharmPractice7e.ParadigmEducation.com/TallmanLetters.

For other products, such as generic levothyroxine, different doses of the same medication have different colors printed on the front of the stock bottle. OTC drugs like Coricidin have varying colored packaging for the different formulations that address various indications. For some products, special markings on the tablet or capsule verify the drug and dose.

An innovation in packaging design for patients taking multiple medications comes from the mail-order PillPack Pharmacy. The PillPack provides an individualized packet of all medications that a patient needs to take at a given time. This makes taking drugs much easier and safer for elderly people. Medications are individually packaged in a time-of-day strip per each day that rolls out of a disposable dispenser (see Figure 14.3). The medications are also delivered to the patient's home in all 50 states every two weeks, insurance is billed, and there is no additional cost.

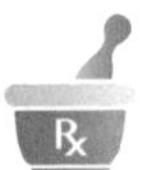

Practice Tip

Since community pharmacies do not generally create their own packaging solutions, they depend upon the personal touch of technicians and pharmacists to know their customers well and individualized help and counsel to ensure customer safety.

FIGURE 14.3 PillPack Dispensing

PillPack provides an innovative packaging design to minimize patient medication errors.

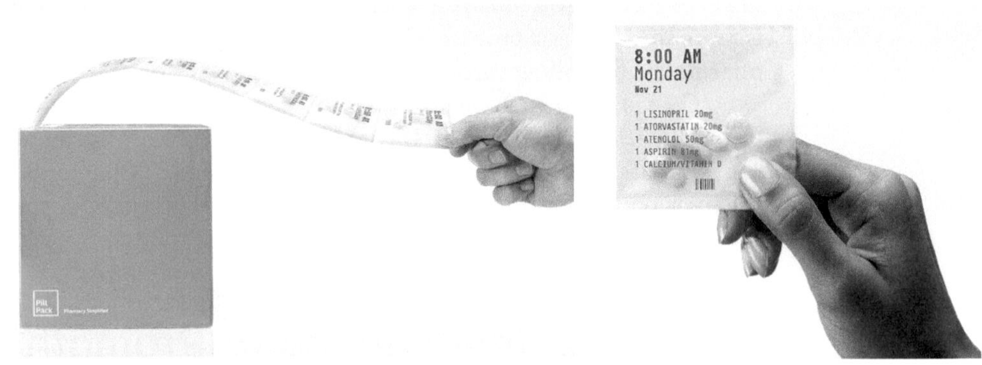

Technology is being used to improve patient safety and medication adherence. AdhereTech's Smart Pill Bottle system can send reminder text messages or phone calls for missed doses. The Smart Pill Bottle can also communicate with the dispensing pharmacy. SMRxT's Nomi is a pill bottle that senses and records if and when a dose of a certain medication is taken. Missed dose reminders can be sent to the patient, as well as their families and caregivers.

14.5 Medication Error Reporting Systems

In most pharmacy settings, errors are reported internally and analyzed within the organization rather than being reported to a centralized external national database. Fear of punishment, of course, is always a concern when an error arises. As a result, healthcare professionals admit to not reporting an error when it is discovered, leaving the door open for the same error to occur again. For this reason, anonymous or no-fault systems of reporting have been established. The focus of no-fault reporting is on fixing the problem rather than on assigning blame.

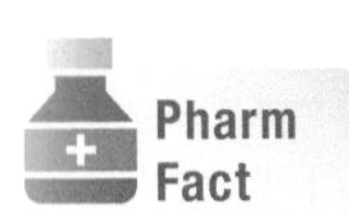

Pharm Fact

The error rate for chain pharmacy personnel is generally less than 5 in 10,000 prescriptions. If a pharmacist or a technician is at or exceeds this rate, they are counseled and put on notice. If this error rate is repeated, termination may result.

The task of error reporting is generally performed by the pharmacist. However, pharmacy technicians are an integral part of the process of error identification, documentation, and prevention. An understanding of the *what*, *when*, *where*, and *why* of error reporting is important for pharmacy technicians as well as for pharmacists.

Telling Patients about Errors

An important piece of medication error reporting is the delicate task of informing the patient that a medication error has taken place to avoid a problematic drug reaction or stop the continuation of the medication problem. This is typically the pharmacist's responsibility.

The circumstances leading to the error should be explained completely and honestly. Patients should understand the nature of the error, what (if any) effects the error may have, and how they can become actively involved in preventing errors in the future. If the medication error will lead to a side effect or adverse drug reaction or impact on the disease or illness being treated, the pharmacist must also contact the prescriber.

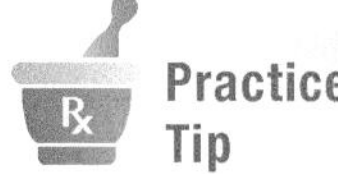

Practice Tip

Generally speaking, people are more likely to forgive an honest error reported immediately upon recognizing it, but rarely accept concealment of the truth.

Pharmacy Safety Organizations

Several efforts have been made to create a safe and comfortable atmosphere for individuals to report medication errors. In 2005, Congress passed the **Patient Safety and Quality Improvement (PSQI) Act** dedicated to promoting a culture of patient safety and continuous quality improvement (CQI) in healthcare facilities, provider organizations, and pharmacies. The act promoted the creation of certified **patient safety organizations (PSOs)** that systematically and confidentially collect error information from various providers, analyze it, and sort it for trends. Then the PSOs communicate the information through a network of medication error databases along with recommendations for improvement. PSOs may be nonprofit or business entities, within healthcare systems or insurance companies.

Hospitals have internal CQI programs for accreditation. Some community pharmacies work with outside companies such as Pharmacy Quality Commitment (PQC™). This company offers a quality improvement system specifically for community pharmacies to integrate error logging and analysis software and other resources to:

- establish a quality-conscious work flow;
- encourage adoption of a fair and positive safety culture;
- identify, collect, and report **quality related events (QREs)**—medication errors that harm the patient, "near misses," and unsafe conditions;
- analyze the pharmacy's QREs to identify process improvement opportunities;
- improve work flow to decrease harmful QREs.

According to the PSQI, any information gathered in a PSO for the purpose of improving pharmacy patient safety is not admissible in criminal, civil, or administrative proceedings.

Many states have mandatory error-reporting systems, but most officials admit that medication errors are still underreported, mostly because of fear of punishment and liability. State boards of pharmacy do not punish pharmacists for errors as long as a good-faith effort was made to fill the prescription correctly. States such as Virginia, Florida, Texas, and California regulate, require, or recommend a CQI program to detect, document, and assess medication errors to determine the causes and to develop an appropriate response to prevent future errors. To avoid censure for self-reported errors, pharmacists in these states must indicate the steps that are being taken to eliminate weaknesses that might allow such errors to continue. Federally sponsored pharmacy programs encourage or require CQI programs for reimbursement.

Programs of the Institute for Safe Medication Practices

The **Institute for Safe Medication Practices (ISMP)** has been mentioned often as a leader in patient safety initiatives. It is a nonprofit healthcare agency whose membership is primarily composed of physicians, pharmacists, and nurses. The ISMP does not set standards but analyzes the causes of medication errors to communicate critical error-reduction strategies to the healthcare community, policy makers, and the public.

It is a federally certified patient safety organization (PSO), providing legal protection and confidentiality for submitted patient safety data and error reports in its programs.

The ISMP has sponsored national forums on medication errors, recommended the addition of labeling or special hazard warnings on potentially toxic drugs, and encouraged revisions of potentially dangerous prescription writing practices. For example, the ISMP first promoted the now common practice of using the leading zero in pharmacy calculations. The Joint Commission has adopted many ISMP recommendations, including avoiding the use of common abbreviations such as "U" for unit or "IU" instead of international unit (which should be fully spelled out instead) and avoiding the use of the trailing zero when possible (such as lisinopril 5 mg, not 5.0 mg).

The ISMP disseminates information through email newsletters, journal articles, and video training exercises. In addition, the ISMP has both FDA safety and hazard alerts posted on its website at https://PharmPractice7e.ParadigmEducation.com/FDASafetyAlerts.

Medication Error Reporting Programs

The ISMP provides the national error-tracking programs called the **Medication Errors Reporting Program (MERP)** and the **Vaccine Errors Reporting Program (VERP)**. These programs are designed to encourage healthcare professionals to voluntarily and anonymously report medication and vaccine errors (or near errors) directly. The ISMP shares all information and error-prevention strategies with the FDA. Reports can be completed confidentially online.

When reporting an error or hazard, include these key elements:

- Tell the story of what went wrong or could go wrong, the causes or contributing factors, how the event or condition was discovered or intercepted, and the actual or potential outcome of the involved patient(s).
- Be sure to include the names, dosage forms, and dose/strength of all involved products. For product-specific concerns (such as labeling and packaging risks), please include the manufacturer.
- Share your recommendations for error prevention.
- If possible, submit associated materials (such as photographs of products, containers, labels, prescription orders without the patients' personal information) that help support the report being submitted.

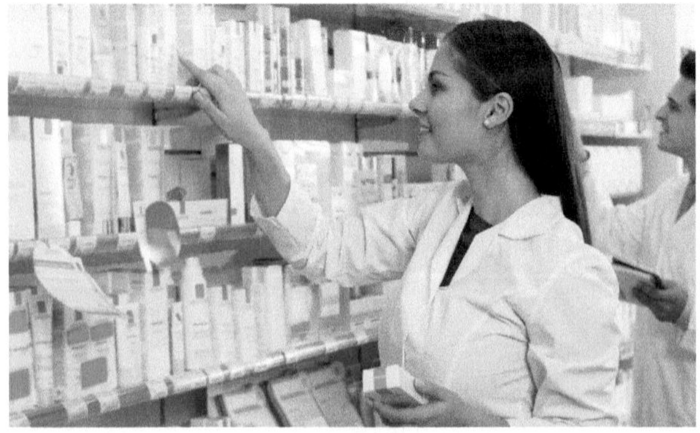

Pharmacies have to consider their own systems for staffing, training, dispensing, organizing, storing, and controlling drugs to look for flaws in the systems and opportunities for improvements. The ISMP self-assessment safety checklists and HAMMERS can help.

Safety Assessment Initiative

The ISMP has also published an extensive report with a checklist of system-based safety strategies for pharmacy-related corporations, healthcare facilities, and community pharmacies, called "ISMP Medication Safety Self-Assessment for Community/ Ambulatory Pharmacy." The report's recommendations include the following:

- adequate pharmacist and technician staffing and training
- appropriate ratios of pharmacists and technicians
- review and verification by pharmacists of all information input by technicians

- review of all medication alerts on dosing and frequency as well as contraindications or warnings about potential drug interactions

The report also emphasizes the importance of a nonpunitive internal reporting system to minimize future medication errors. The reporting system should include the following:

- The order entry person should differ from the one who fills the order, thus adding an independent validation, or additional checks, to the order-entry process.
- Pharmacy personnel should not prepare prescriptions from the computer-generated label in case an error occurred at order entry; they should use the original (or scanned copy) prescription.
- Pharmacy personnel should keep the original prescription, stock bottle, computer label, and medication container together during the filling process; the pharmacist should verify dispensing accuracy by comparing all these with the NDC and/or bar code scan.

High-Alert Medication Modeling and Error-Reduction Scorecards

In addition to free safety assessment tools for institutional pharmacies, the ISMP also offers the **High-Alert Medication Modeling and Error-Reduction Scorecards (HAMMERS™)**, which are free scorecard-based tools designed to help community pharmacies:

- identify their own particular system and procedure/behavior risks related to dispensing certain high-alert medications
- estimate how often the pharmacies commit an error or contribute to patients' adverse drug events

HAMMERS can provide the most benefit when used to assess the risk errors of high-alert medications, which are those that have a high incidence of errors in all settings. Some high-alert medications include blood thinners (warfarin, enoxaparin), pain medications (hydro- and oxycodone with acetaminophen, fentanyl patch), the potent arthritis drug methotrexate, and several kinds of insulin. All chemotherapy and HIV drugs also fall into this category. These medications can produce serious injury or death to a patient if misused. Due to potential declines in diabetic patients' blood glucose levels, insulin and oral hypoglycemics must also be carefully monitored.

The tool provides five scorecards, each assessing a type of error:

- prescribing errors (such as wrong drug, dose, or directions)
- data entry errors on patient (wrong patient)
- data entry errors on drug (such as wrong drug, dose, or directions)
- medication container selection errors (wrong drug or dose)
- point-of-sale (POS) errors (medication dispensed to wrong patient)

By using the scorecards, pharmacies can estimate how often prescribing and dispensing errors reach patients and how the frequency will change if certain interventions are implemented. The scorecards can be found at https://PharmPractice7e.ParadigmEducation.com/HAMMERS.

The ISMP also publishes a list of common look-alike and sound-alike drugs that often contribute to medication errors—for example, Reminyl versus Amaryl. Reminyl is used to treat Alzheimer's disease whereas Amaryl is used to lower blood glucose levels. The ISMP stresses awareness of such drugs and promotes adding a medical indication for each drug, as well as encouraging e-prescribing. To see the list, go to: https://PharmPractice7e.ParadigmEducation.com/ConfusedDrugNames.

Joint Commission Safety Initiatives and Reporting

Accreditation by the Joint Commission is, in part, dependent upon hospitals demonstrating a Sentinel Event Policy—an effective medical and medication error-reporting system through which all healthcare members may channel information confidentially. A **sentinel event** is an unexpected occurrence involving death, serious physical or psychological injury, or the potential for such occurrences to happen. When a sentinel event is reported, the organization (for example, a hospital, infusion pharmacy, or managed-care company) is expected to analyze the cause of the error

FIGURE 14.4 The SPEAK UP Program

SPEAK UP is an acronym that stands for the following:

S **peak up** if you have questions or concerns. If you still don't understand, ask again. It's your body, and you have a right to know.

P **ay attention** to the care you get. Always make sure that you're getting the right treatments and medications from the right healthcare professionals. Don't assume anything.

E **ducate yourself** about your illness. Learn about the medical tests you get and your treatment plan.

A **sk for an advocate**—a trusted family member or friend to listen to the medical information, ask questions, and speak up on your behalf.

K **now the medications** you take and why you take them. Medication errors are the most common healthcare mistakes.

U **se a certified facility**—hospital, clinic, surgery center, or other type of healthcare organization.

P **articipate** in all treatment decisions. You are the center of the healthcare team.

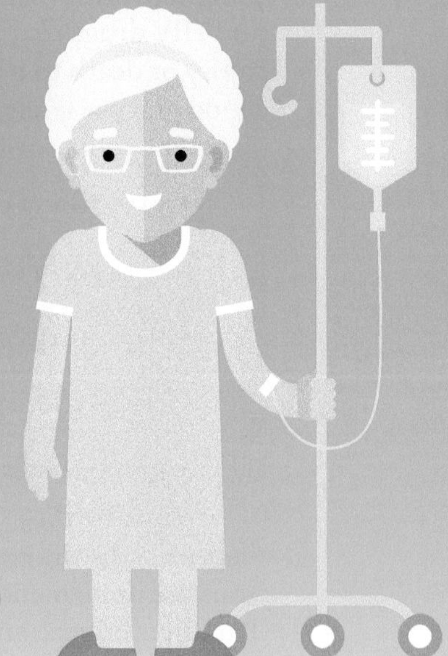

(i.e., perform a root-cause analysis), take action to correct the cause, monitor the changes made, and determine whether the cause of the error has been eliminated.

The Joint Commission's safety-related standards are based on the assumption that when a preventable medication error occurs, investigating the cause and making necessary corrections in policy or procedure are much more important than placing blame on an individual. Once the cause of the error is identified, a repeat medication error may be prevented in the future. Joint Commission standards also require that the hospital outline its responsibility to advise a patient about any adverse outcomes from the medical or medication error.

SPEAK UP Campaign for Patients

In concert with the Centers for Medicare and Medicaid Services (CMS), the Joint Commission has developed an educational series of written brochures and videos for patients called the **SPEAK UP** campaign (see Figure 14.4). This program urges consumers to take a more active role in their health care and minimize misunderstandings that may lead to medication errors. The program has been adopted by many healthcare facilities for their patient education programs.

ASHP Initiatives

In response to health system medication errors leading to serious patient injuries and deaths, the American Society of Health-System Pharmacists (ASHP) advocates for state laws to standardize technician certification. The organization emphasizes the need for pharmacy technicians to be trained in ASHP-accredited training programs and to be certified by the Pharmacy Technician Certification Board (PTCB).

US Pharmacopeial Convention (USP) Safety Initiatives

Many other professional organizations support patient safety efforts by gathering medical error information and using the data to create tools to support healthcare professionals in specific settings or situations. The USP supports two types of reporting systems for the data collection of adverse events and medication errors: the ISMP's MERP (the national reporting program discussed earlier) and MEDMARX, an international reporting system.

MEDMARX Reporting System

The internet-based program **MEDMARX** allows institutions and healthcare professionals around the globe to anonymously document, analyze, and track adverse events such as medication errors and adverse drug events specific to an institution.

In a study of 26,604 medication errors reported to MEDMARX, the analysis found that:

- more than 60% of these errors occurred during the dispensing process;
- pharmacy technicians were involved in nearly 40% (38.5%) of the occurrences;
- 1.4% caused significant patient harm, including the deaths of seven patients.

Major contributing factors to the errors included *distraction in the workplace*, *excessive workload*, and *inexperience*.

Analyzing other trends in the error reports, the USP has addressed error prevention through medication labeling recommendations. For example, the organization established a new labeling standard to improve the safety of neuromuscular blockers in the surgical suites of hospitals. Such drugs now carry the label: "Warning—Paralyzing Agent." For the chemotherapy drug vincristine, administered in the hospital and outpatient cancer clinics, the medication label now reads: "For Intravenous Use Only—Fatal if Given by Other Routes." These labeling changes were a direct result of an analysis of voluntary reports of medication errors in MEDMARX.

14.6 FDA Adverse Reaction Reporting Systems

Even if no medication errors occur, drug risks are still present. Though every US drug goes through a rigorous approval process, consumers need to remember that all drugs—prescription, OTC, and diet supplements—have some toxicity risks and a potential for adverse drug reactions. So the FDA established a nationwide post-marketing surveillance system to serve as a conduit for reporting serious adverse effects of certain medications. This FDA Adverse Event Reporting System (FAERS) is a centralized database that stores information from two separate federally sponsored reporting programs: MedWatch and the Vaccine Adverse Event Reporting System (VAERS). The VAERS database (discussed later) publishes a quarterly newsletter that can be accessed online at https://PharmPractice7e.ParadigmEducation.com/MedWatch.

MedWatch

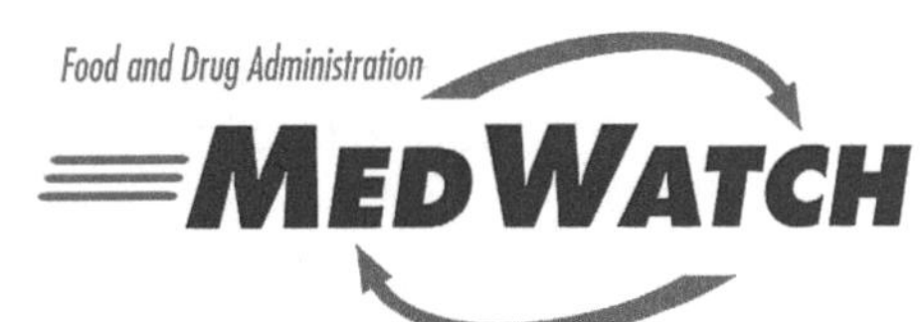

MedWatch gives consumers a way to make anonymous reports on adverse drug effects.

MedWatch is a voluntary program (run in collaboration with the ISMP) that offers healthcare professionals *and consumers* an avenue to anonymously report a serious adverse event associated with any specific drug, biological device, or dietary supplement. From 1969 to 2012, the FDA received over nine million reports of medication problems of many types (reports from MedWatch began in 2000), with incidents rising each year. In 2014 (the latest posted FDA statistics), 1,289,133 reports were received. Reports may be filed online or by phone. Yet only those who actually recognize that their reaction was connected to a specific drug *and* are aware of the MedWatch program (listed in Medication Guides and on labels) *and* elect to report them online are tabulated. Clearly, these numbers are far lower than the actual incidents of ADRs per each medication. Even so, the FDA uses this information to track problems or issues that were not apparent when the medication was initially approved. In fact, the occurrence of some side effects may only be detected in a large population after the drug comes to market.

The recognition of a potential problem does not always mean that the product will be recalled to be removed from the market, as explained in Chapter 3. The FDA may respond in two other ways:

1. Issue safety alerts to healthcare professionals or consumers for drugs (including drug recalls), biologicals, dietary supplements, and counterfeit drugs
2. Request medication-labeling changes to the product package information (PI), including contraindications, warnings, boxed warnings, precautions, and adverse reactions

Safety alerts and labeling changes are published in a monthly MedWatch newsletter.

Risk Evaluation and Mitigation Strategies

As noted in earlier chapters, some drugs that are more dangerous require even more than a Medication Guide for communication before administration. As part of the **risk evaluation and mitigation strategy (REMS)** for certain drugs, community pharmacies (and prescribers) must register with the drug manufacturer (or official wholesaler) and receive drug-specific REMS training. The pharmacist must pledge to not only go over the Medication Guide with patients, but do other counseling and monitoring activities. REMS programs are designed to closely track patients on these high-risk drugs and make periodic assessment reports to the FDA on their status.

REMS are required and developed for new or existing drugs each year. Over 80 REMS drugs were posted in 2019 on the FDA's website. You can become familiar with some of these drugs at https://PharmPractice7e.ParadigmEducation.com/REMS.

Some of the more common REMS drugs are discussed below.

Isotretinoin and the iPLEDGE Program

Isotretinoin (and isotroin, a derivative) is a common generic drug for intense acne and other skin problems that has a very high incidence of harm to the fetus, or **teratogenicity**. Common brands of this drug are Accutane and Claravis (see Table 14.14 for others). The **iPLEDGE Program** is a REMS that was designed for isotretinoin and related drugs to prevent fetal exposure and the resulting birth defects and to educate all patients (both female and male) on the drugs' risks and how to use the medication safely.

TABLE 14.14 Isotretinoin and Isotroin Drugs in the iPledge Program

The generic drugs isotretinoin and isotroin come in the following brand names:

- Absorica
- Accutane
- Amnesteem
- Claravis
- Epuris
- Myorisan
- Sotret
- Zenatane

Pharmacists who dispense these drugs and patients who use them must agree to the terms of the iPledge Program as part of the REMS for these drugs.

All prescribers, pharmacies, and drug wholesalers must be enrolled annually and certified to participate in this program; all patients must be registered and agree to meet all conditions required during treatment. Pharmacies may receive the drug only from a certified wholesaler and can only dispense written prescriptions authorized by a certified prescriber. An assigned Risk Management Association (RMA) number must be placed on each prescription, and prescribers must agree to provide contraception counseling to patients prior to and during treatment with this drug.

If patients are sexually active, prescribers must document the forms of contraception the patients are currently using. Women of childbearing potential must agree to monthly pregnancy tests, and they must have a negative result prior to prescribers issuing a new or refill prescription. If sexually active, they must commit to two forms of contraception while on the drug and for one month after drug discontinuation. In addition, they must agree to pick up the prescription within a specified period (usually within seven days) or the prescription is void.

The quantity is limited to a 30-day supply with no refills. All pregnancies while on this drug must be reported. Patients must also agree not to share their medication with anyone or donate blood while on the medication and for one month after drug discontinuation.

IN THE REAL WORLD

Accutane has caused huge controversy since it was first introduced to the market in 1982. After the patent ran out, other manufacturers followed with the generic drug isotretinoin. Dermatologists have praised it as a drug of choice for severe acne, yet some physicians compare the drug to thalidomide because of the extensive documentation on isotretinoin in connection to severe birth defects and miscarriages.

What is less discussed are the incidents in patients of both genders of inflammatory bowel diseases and severe depression, with some cases leading to suicide. The most frequent population for this acne drug is teens, an age group already at a higher risk of suicide. The Swiss drug manufacturer Roche has lost numerous lawsuits about these connections with Accutane and has paid a significant amount in damages.

Though the FDA has received case reports of increased suicide risk with isotretinoin, it has not deemed that there has been sufficient accumulated concrete evidence to make a definite causal relation sufficient to recall it. However, due to serious side effects, the FDA recommends that the drug be reserved for severe refractory cases of acne unresponsive to conventional therapies, stating:

"All patients treated with isotretinoin should be observed closely for symptoms of depression or suicidal thoughts, such as sad mood, irritability, acting on dangerous impulses, anger, loss of pleasure or interest in social or sports activities, sleeping too much or too little, changes in weight or appetite, school or work performance going down, or trouble concentrating, or for mood disturbance, psychosis, or aggression. . . . Patients taking isotretinoin may experience side effects including bad headaches, blurred vision, dizziness, nausea, vomiting, seizures, stroke, diarrhea, and muscle weakness. Additionally, serious mental health problems, such as depression and suicide, have been reported with isotretinoin use."

Transmucosal Immediate-Release Fentanyl

The pain medication skin patches of transmucosal immediate-release fentanyl (TIRF) have a REMS program designed to mitigate the risk of misuse, abuse, addiction, overdose, or severe complications. The strategies seek to:

1. limit the medication only to appropriate opioid-dependent cancer patients tolerant of around-the-clock opioid therapy;
2. prevent inappropriate dosage conversion from similar narcotics;
3. promote safe storage to prevent accidental exposure in children;
4. educate prescribers, pharmacists, and patients on the safe and appropriate use of fentanyl.

As with isotretinoin, prescribers, pharmacies (both hospital and retail), and wholesalers must enroll and complete an education program to be certified to handle this medication (brand and generic). Renewal is every two years. Prescribers must agree to initiate therapy with the lowest dose, follow up on efficacy of dose titration, and document any signs of misuse or abuse. Pharmacies are also responsible for training all staff, including pharmacy technicians; hospital pharmacies can dispense TIRF to inpatients only.

Patients must review and study the Medication Guide, sign an agreement with the prescriber, and follow prescribed instructions exactly. There can be no medication transfer to others, and if, for any reason, the opioid therapy is discontinued, the TIRF therapy must also be stopped. Patients must also agree to safely store and discard the medication to prevent harm to children and pets.

Subutex and Suboxone

Sublingual (under the tongue) buprenorphine (Subutex, Suboxone) are used to treat opioid dependence. Certified physicians have DEA numbers that start with an "x," indicating their ability to prescribe these medications. Subutex is commonly prescribed to initiate treatment and Suboxone to maintain it. The REMS goals are to prevent accidental overdose, misuse, and abuse, and to inform patients of serious risks. Prescribers must use low doses, conduct frequent follow-up visits to assess efficacy, and provide counseling and psychosocial support for the patient.

Pharmacists who are certified to dispense Subutex and Suboxone agree to counsel the patient on safe use, including potential drug interactions with alcohol, anxiety/sleep medications (such as benzodiazepines), and antidepressants. The pharmacist must also counsel patients on securely and safely storing their medication to deter theft or access by children.

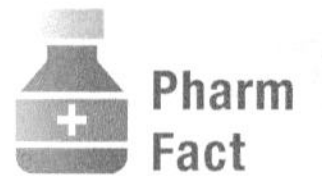

A social controversy exists over whether or not the MMR (measles, mumps, rubella) vaccine or receiving numerous vaccines at very young ages can result in autism (a developmental disorder) or other health issues. Viewing the body of existing scientific study, the CDC stated in 2015 that there is insufficient scientific evidence to establish a relationship between autism and any particular childhood vaccination.

Mycophenolate

Mycophenolate is an immunosuppresant medicine used to help prevent organ rejection in transplant patients and for autoimmune diseases. The REMS goals are to prevent miscarriage and birth defects when used in pregnancy. The prescriber, pharmacy, and patient all must participate in this REMS. Before starting mycophenolate, patients of childbearing potential require education on the risks of exposure during pregnancy. Pregnancy planning education must also occur. Women of childbearing potential must either abstain from intercourse or use acceptable contraception during their entire treatment course of mycophenolate, as well as six weeks after discontinuing therapy. Pregnancy testing must occur twice before starting mycophenolate (the second test occurs 8 to 10 days after the first). Repeat pregnancy tests must occur at all routine follow-up visits. Any pregnancies that occur while a patient is using mycophenolate should be reported.

Vaccine Adverse Event Reporting System

A separate national reporting system, called the **Vaccine Adverse Event Reporting System (VAERS)**, is run by the FDA and the Centers for Disease Control and Prevention (CDC) to collect and analyze information on adverse events that occur after immunizations. This is not a vaccine error-reporting system but rather a system for tracking dangers caused by the vaccines themselves. Since 1990, VAERS has received over 200,000 reports, most of which describe mild side effects, such as a fever. As with medications, hundreds of thousands of vaccine administrations often need to occur before being able to statistically detect a problem. In fact, it may take more than a million doses of a vaccine for a few adverse effects to occur and be investigated.

The FDA and the CDC use VAERS information to ensure the safest strategies of vaccine use and reduce the rare risks associated with vaccines. Healthcare personnel are mandated by the National Childhood Vaccine Injury Act of 1986 to report serious adverse reactions from vaccines. With pharmacists and their technicians becoming more involved in vaccine administration, it is important to report any adverse effects. Patients can report any problems with a vaccine as well. A VAERS report can be made via an 800 number (1-800-822-7967), by mail or fax on a downloaded form, or online at https://PharmPractice7e.ParadigmEducation.com/VAERS.

14.7 Safety and Controlled Substances

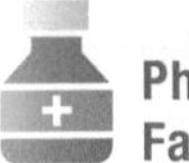

Pharm Fact

According to the Agency for Healthcare Research and Quality, the highest death rate from prescription drug overdose is for patients ages 45 to 54, and the fastest growing rate of overdose deaths is from ages 55 to 64. It is expected that the death rate among this group is underreported.

Not all safety issues are about personal injuries. Many safety issues affect families and communities, such as prescription drug abuse. Prescription and illegal drug abuse are growing national problems that need to be addressed by the pharmacy field. The abuse of prescription pain medication *is the fastest-growing drug problem in the United States.*

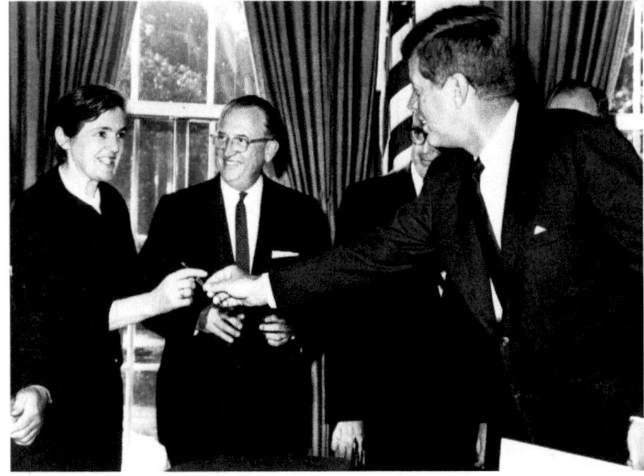

President Kennedy hands a pen to Dr. Frances O. Kelsey after passing the Kefauver-Harris Amendments, establishing safeguards now used by the FDA.

The statistics speak for themselves. According to the Drug Enforcement Administration (DEA), more than seven million Americans abuse pain and anxiety medications every year, and the numbers are increasing at a fast rate. More than 130 people die every day from opioid overdose. The NIH has declared the opioid abuse problem a crisis.

Physical and Psychological Dangers of Dependence

Understanding drug dependence can give pharmacy personnel a healthy caution in dispensing drugs. It is a complex and difficult mental health and biological problem that drastically affects individuals, families, and communities, contributing to crime and violence. As with alcohol, prescription drug and controlled substance dependence often begin with drug tolerance and progressively escalate to dependence, both psychological and physical, and then to completely controlling addiction:

- **Drug tolerance** is when the body adapts to a drug so that higher doses are needed to produce the same pharmacological effect. For example, a patient who is taking a Schedule II narcotic for pain relief may build up a drug tolerance, resulting in less pain relief. Consequently, that patient must take higher doses or more frequent doses to achieve the same degree of pain relief they once had at a lower dose. Long-term drug tolerance can lead to psychological and physical dependence, and addiction.

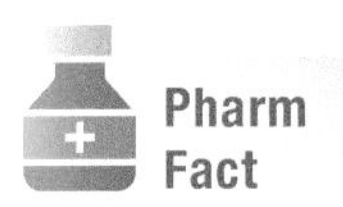

2013 research estimates found that prescription opiod abuse cost the healthcare system $78.5 billion annually. These costs have grown extensively as the prescription drug problem has reached epidemic proportions.

- **Psychological dependence** is when the patient takes a drug on a regular basis because it produces a sense of well-being that the patient does not want to consider being without. If the patient stops taking the drug, they experience anxiety or withdrawal symptoms due to the psychological security that the drug offered. For example, a patient who takes sleeping medication every night may experience fear of going off the drug because it may mean no sleep or a disruptive sleep pattern. The patient has associated getting a good night's sleep with taking the medication and has a hard time imagining doing without it.
- **Physical dependence** is defined as taking a drug continuously so that when the medication is stopped, physical withdrawal symptoms occur, such as restlessness, anxiety, insomnia, diarrhea, vomiting, and goosebumps. Withdrawal symptoms commonly occur with high doses of Schedule II drugs, and, for some patients, may occur after four weeks of many high doses. In some cases, the physical dependence on one drug such as Suboxone can substitute for the physical dependence on another drug, such as narcotic pain relievers.
- **Addiction** is defined as a chronic disease marked by compulsive and uncontrollable use of a drug substance. Addiction is characterized by a powerful, compulsive urge to use a drug or substance when it is not required medically. Those with addiction may prioritize getting and using drugs over other activities in their lives. Addiction builds on a spectrum of increasing severity the longer it goes unchecked. Addiction can be harmful to the patient and the public at large. That is why the DEA controls substances that are highly addictive like the Schedule II drugs.

IN THE REAL WORLD

In the United States alone, more than 18 million people misused opioids, central nervous system depressants, and stimulants in 2017, according to the 2017 NIH. The US Substance Abuse and Mental Health Services Administration (SAMHSA) reports that, after marijuana, nonmedical or recreational use of painkillers is the second most common form of illicit drug use in the United States. Prescription opioid painkillers (such as hydrocodone/acetaminophen Vicodin, oxycodone/acetaminophen [Percocet], and oxycodone hydrochloride [OxyContin]) have caused more deaths than illegal substances such as heroin.

Prescription Strategies to Fight Abuse

Hydrocodone (Vicodin), oxycodone (OxyContin), and oxymorphone (Opana) are prescription opioids that are popularly misused recreationally. Because of the high rates of abuse and death from prescription opioids, pain clinics at the Mayo Clinic and other major health facilities aim to get chronic pain sufferers (especially older patients) to avoid or get off of opioid medications. The pain counselors recommend the following:

- Start at a low dose, perhaps half the usual, and go slowly with dosage increases.
- Avoid mixing with alcohol or any other medications.
- Monitor medications and follow up with the doctor often.

- Be realistic and don't expect a medication to take away all aches and pains.
- Try to find nonpharmaceutical ways to reduce pain, such as yoga, rehabilitation therapies, meditation, and others.
- Keep prescriptions in a locked drawer or cabinet.

Pharmacy Techniques for Abuse Prevention

Dispensing controlled substances requires a great deal more documentation and checking throughout the filling, dispensing, delivery, purchasing, and inventory processes, as has been explained throughout other chapters. Stay alert for forged prescriptions and drug-seeking behaviors of patients and also coworkers. This can be difficult, especially during a busy pharmacy workday. However, there are some telltale signs and trends to watch for (see Table 14.15).

Be on the Lookout for Drug Seekers

As a technician, you need to be on the lookout for the behavioral red flags of **drug seekers**, those patients who constantly request "early refills" or receive prescriptions for the same or similar controlled drugs from several physicians. They are also known as "doctor shoppers." Drug seekers often use more than one physician, dentist, and pharmacy and pay with cash to minimize insurance tracking. Pay close attention to prescription dates. The original prescription date for all controlled drugs must be entered into the profile rather than the prescription *filling* date so that customer trends can be seen by checking the medication history. If you see any of these signs or have a gut feeling, consult the pharmacist.

A drug seeker is most likely psychologically or physically dependent or addicted to the medication—or may be illegally selling the drugs. Many are very skilled and may try to flatter you and the pharmacists to gain trust and allay any concerns about drug abuse or diversion. If these individuals have been dispensed a narcotic and an antibiotic from an ER, they may request that only the pain medication be filled. The policy for most emergency rooms is "all or nothing" on the prescriptions written. Again, if you suspect that a patient may have illegal intentions, seek the professional judgment of the pharmacist.

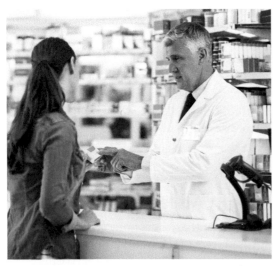
Pharmacists and technicians have to be on the lookout for drug seekers and forged prescriptions without jumping to conclusions and offending customers. Look patients in the eyes and at the trends in their profile to get to know them as much as possible and watch for warning signs of abuse.

Also exercise caution when another person (other than the patient or a family member) attempts to call in a refill or pick up a prescription for a controlled substance. When in doubt, call the patient to relay the situation and verify approval for medication pickup, documenting everything. Pharmacies generally request a photo ID (such as a driver's license) to confirm the identity of the person picking up a controlled substance prescription. Federal law requires a name, signature, and physical address (not a post office box) for patients with all controlled substance prescriptions and for those picking them up. If another individual picks up the prescription, ask for the patient's address and/or date of birth.

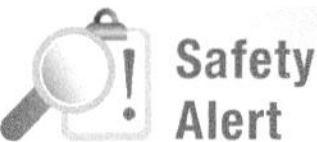

Abuse of prescription drugs accounts for 45% (and growing) of drug overdose deaths, according to the CDC. Pharmacy technicians must be thoroughly familiar with regulations concerning scheduled substances for the state in which they practice.

TABLE 14.15 Indicators of a Potentially Forged Prescription or Drug-Seeking Behavior

- The prescription is altered (for example, a change in quantity).
- Prescription pads have been reported missing from local doctors' offices.
- The prescription is presented as a clever computerized fax on non-tamper-proof safety paper.
- There are misspellings on the prescription.
- A refill is indicated for a Schedule II drug.
- A prescription from the emergency department is written for more than a #30 count or a seven-day supply.
- A prescription is cut and pasted from a preprinted, signed prescription.
- A second or third prescription is added to a legal prescription written by a physician.
- A patient presents a prescription containing several medications, but wants the pharmacy to fill only the narcotic prescription.
- The prescription is signed with different handwriting or in different ink, or the prescription is not signed by the physician.
- The DEA number is missing, illegible, or incorrect.
- The prescription is written by an out-of-state physician or a physician practicing in an area far from the pharmacy. This event is particularly suspicious if the prescription is received at night or on the weekend, when it would be difficult to confirm.
- An individual other than the patient drops off the prescription. Pharmacy personnel should require a photo ID such as a driver's license and document this information.
- A new patient specifies a brand name narcotic.
- A new patient wants to pay for the prescription with cash even though they have insurance. Doing so avoids a paper trail.

Watch for Prescription Forgeries

A key way to catch illegal drug activity is to detect a falsified prescription. E-prescriptions for controlled substances have double authentication protocols, so they are considered more difficult to forge, but it is not impossible. Paper prescriptions are easier to forge but also easier to detect. Problematic DEA numbers are a first sign.

DEA Number Check Most pharmacies have a computerized physician database containing DEA, NPI, state license numbers, and contact information. Pharmacy technicians should learn to recognize the names and legal signatures of the local prescribers who send prescriptions to the pharmacy, especially for controlled substances. Insurance plans require a pharmacy to have a physician's DEA number on file to be reimbursed for prescriptions for all controlled medications. The validity of the prescriber can be checked by adding the numerals of the DEA number combined with the first letter of the physician's last name (see Table 14.16).

Other Signs of Forgeries Wrong DEA numbers are not the only signs. Caution must be used when accepting prescriptions from out-of-state patients, especially at night or on weekends when the prescription authenticity cannot be proven by calling the prescribing office or prescriber. Some pharmacies fill controlled substances only for patients residing in their immediate geographical area and for prescribers who practice in their community and write their prescriptions with tamper-proof paper.

TABLE 14.16 Steps for Checking a DEA Number

1. Add the first, third, and fifth digits of the DEA number.
2. Add the second, fourth, and sixth digits of the number, and multiply the sum by two.
3. Add the results of steps 1 and 2. The last digit of this sum should be the same as the last digit of the DEA number.
4. The second letter of the DEA number should be the same as the first letter of the physician's last name.

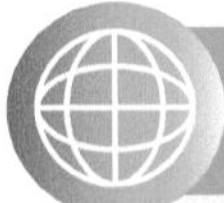

IN THE REAL WORLD

Child actor Corey Haim was a "doctor shopper" under the care of seven different doctors, using seven different pharmacies, and obtaining 553 tablets of Vicodin, Valium, Xanax, and Soma in the 32 days before his death. He had enough money to pay cash to avoid the insurance DURs. Sadly, he died of a drug overdose in 2010 at the age of 38. Similar drug shopping and/or prescription drug abuse are considered to have contributed to the deaths of Prince, Michael Jackson, Heath Ledger, Anna Nicole Smith, and Whitney Houston. One must also remember the thousands who are not famous who die each year from similar addictions and abuses of prescription medications.

Response to Potential Forgery If a forgery or drug-seeking behavior is suspected, retain the prescription (in case of forgery), try to detain the individual, and notify the police. To allow time to consult the pharmacist without offending the patient (who may not be guilty), simply say, "This prescription may take some time to fill. Can you come back in one hour?" Always keep the name and phone number of the local DEA agent handy. A new DEA-sponsored anonymous texting tip line may be also available in your area as it is being gradually implemented across the nation.

In addition, most pharmacists will usually make some sort of notation on the prescription to alert other pharmacists to a potential problem in filling the prescription. Many local pharmacies activate a "calling tree list" or email to alert other pharmacies of a potential problem prescription circulating in the community. If there is concern that the patient is abusing a legal prescription or receiving controlled substances from more than one prescriber or more than one pharmacy, the pharmacist has the professional responsibility to contact the prescriber.

The Right of Refusal

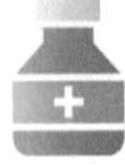

Pharm Fact

A pharmacist has the right to refuse to fill a prescription for any drug, including a controlled substance.

A pharmacist always has the **right of refusal**, declining with cause to fill *any* prescription, especially those for controlled substances. For example, it does not make sense to fill a narcotic prescription for severe pain three months after the date it was written; or a patient may request a three-month supply of a narcotic medication when only one month is covered by insurance and the patient is willing to pay with cash. The patient's medication profile may also show numerous pain medications from different prescribers. The pharmacist often directs the technician to express concern for the patient but also state that the pharmacy does not have the prescribed drug or prescribed quantity in stock.

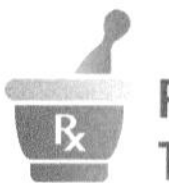

Practice Tip

The DEA launched a texting tip line in some areas to anonymously report suspicious prescription drug activity. Type TIP411 (847-411) for the phone number, then type DEADRUGS or PILLTIP. Text a description of the suspicion or send an image. The DEA cannot see the texter's phone number (100% anonymous) but can assign an investigator to respond. Various cities and states are encouraging its use in their area.

What if a prescriber orders an excessive amount of a narcotic that could do harm to a patient, and the prescriber verifies it? The pharmacist can still elect not to fill it and most likely should do so unless there are extenuating medical reasons that make sense. Perhaps the provider is not qualified in pain management but is writing prescriptions outside the scope of their practice. If that is the case, the prescription also should not be filled. However, if the diagnosis is cancer or the patient is under care of a hospice team or oncologist (cancer physician), the use of high-dose narcotics for comfort and pain relief is generally considered medically necessary.

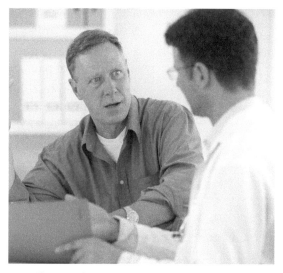

Prescribers are becoming more aware of and proactive about preventing prescription drug abuse by discussing the drugs and their effects, checking the patient's prescription data with other healthcare providers, and being more cautious about their prescribing.

State and Federal Efforts for Prevention

Most states have authorized their state drugs and narcotic agencies to establish a **Prescription Drug Monitoring Program (PDMP)** or a similar program to gather data for monitoring, tracking, and analyzing trends and sharing information on drug dispensing. As of 2019, 49 states had operational PDMPs. These data networking programs have been designed to offer healthcare professionals access to a regional multi-state database of prescription data. This access helps professionals:

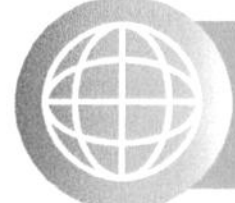

IN THE REAL WORLD

A technician in Colorado was working at one Safeway Pharmacy but also serving as a substitute at other nearby locations. A customer came in once a week to the technician's home store for hydromorphone, a controlled substance. "The prescription did not look fraudulent, and the customer was always friendly." However, the technician noticed the same customer coming into other pharmacies with different names and the same prescription. "I informed the pharmacy manager, but he did not believe me. . . . I insisted that he needed to call and verify the prescription, and he finally did."

It turns out that the customer had stolen the doctor's prescription pads with DEA number and was filling fake prescriptions all throughout the state of Colorado under different names. Because of the technician's alert, the person was caught. The technician concluded, "It is important to always be persistent and speak up for what you believe in. It never hurts to double-check and make sure a prescription is real."

- share information and work together to make informed decisions about dispensing controlled substances and reducing abuse,
- improve the quality of health care by limiting the use of medications to proper treatment of pain and terminal illness, and
- reduce overprescribing and duplication in controlled substance prescriptions.

If you are presented with a suspicious prescription, you can ask the pharmacist to access the database to see if the patient is receiving controlled drugs from other pharmacies.

Pharmacy personnel should also be aware that each state has its own requirements and definitions for a "tamper-resistant" prescription (TRP). Consequently, a prescription for a Schedule II drug that was written out of state will probably not meet in-state requirements and thus can only be filled in the state in which it was written.

Prescribers and Pharmacists Work to Prevent Opioid Abuse

A 2015 Boston Medical Center study showed that over 90% of patients who nearly died of opioid overdose received a refill or new opioid prescription immediately afterwards. Part of the problem is that there has been no system to alert the physicians of the overdose.

In light of the public health epidemic of overprescribing opioid medications, the CDC published guidelines in 2016 for healthcare prescribers of these drugs for pain. The guidelines encourage prescribers to favor nondrug and non-opioid therapy, using opioid therapy as a last resort. There are 12 recommendations that focus on criteria for when and why to begin opioid therapy for chronic pain; guidelines on opioid selection, dosages, duration, follow-up, and situations for discontinuation; and methods to assess the risk and harm of opioid use for each patient. The guidelines include recommendations for how to ease patients off opioid therapies too. For the complete guidelines and background, visit: https://PharmPractice7e.Paradigm Education.com/CDCGuidelines2019.

Prescribers are encouraged to use e-prescriptions for controlled substances instead of written ones. If using paper, they should carry their tamper-proof and other prescription pads with them or lock them in the drawers of the examination rooms. These measures prevent patients and other healthcare personnel from accessing blank prescriptions for illegal use. Prescribers are also encouraged to write out the numeral names of quantities so that 12 tablets of a narcotic cannot be altered by adding a zero, thus creating 120.

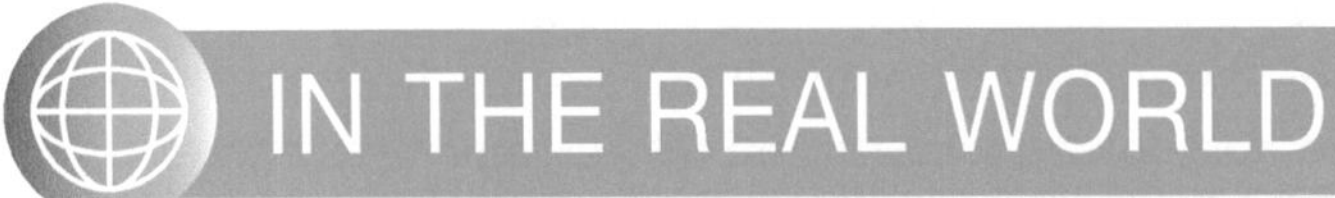

In 2015, because of the growing numbers of drug overdose deaths, Minnesota and Wisconsin approved the ability of CVS pharmacies and certified responders to provide the drug naloxone (Narcan) without a prescription. This drug is an antidote for those experiencing an overdose, and reverses respiratory depression. First responders and certified citizens may now use naloxone on those they see overdosing. Many doctors say that it is safe to use naloxone to address the symptoms of heroin or prescription pain drug overdose. Other states and pharmacies are watching to see the outcomes. Now the majority of states permit naloxone to be distributed via standing orders, collaborative practice agreements, or pharmacist prescriptive authority.

IN THE REAL WORLD

In 2015, Drug Enforcement Administration officials arrested 22 doctors and pharmacists involved in a prescription drug ring that was illegally providing people with controlled prescription drugs, including oxycodone, hydrocodone, and alprazolam (Xanax). Nearly 260 other individuals across four states were also arrested in "Operation Pilluted," the biggest prescription drug bust ever. This was part of the DEA's increased effort to crack down on prescription drug abuse trafficking.

DEA Special Agent in Charge Keith Brown publicly stated, "The doctors and pharmacists arrested in Operation Pilluted are nothing more than drug traffickers who prey on the addiction of others while abandoning the Hippocratic Oath adhered to faithfully by thousands of doctors and pharmacists each day across this country."

It is illegal for a physician to write a prescription for a Schedule II drug for a family member, and it is considered unethical for a prescriber to write a Schedule III or IV prescription for themselves or a family member. Circumstances vary, and it will be up to the professional judgment of the pharmacist to fill or refuse to fill such a prescription. If a pharmacist or a technician has a prescription for a controlled substance, it should be filled by another pharmacist or technician. Professional drug abuse signs and responses are handled in the next chapter, Chapter 15.

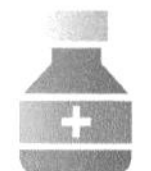

Pharm Fact

While marijuana is legal for prescribed medical and/or recreational use in several states, it is still classified as a Schedule I drug under federal law. General pharmacies cannot dispense medical marijuana, or they will lose their DEA registration.

The Complex Case of Medical Marijuana

As some states are legalizing **marijuana**, or cannabis, pharmacies are left in a strange zone. They cannot legally sell the drug (which is an illegal Schedule I controlled substance, according to the DEA), but in some states where it has been legalized for some or all uses, other vendors can sell within restrictions. Many state-legalized dispensaries are becoming marijuana medication therapy clinical offices, with patient education and high security. Yet the drug can interact with other medications, so ideally it should be overseen by a pharmacist and have a DUR to check interactions with other drugs.

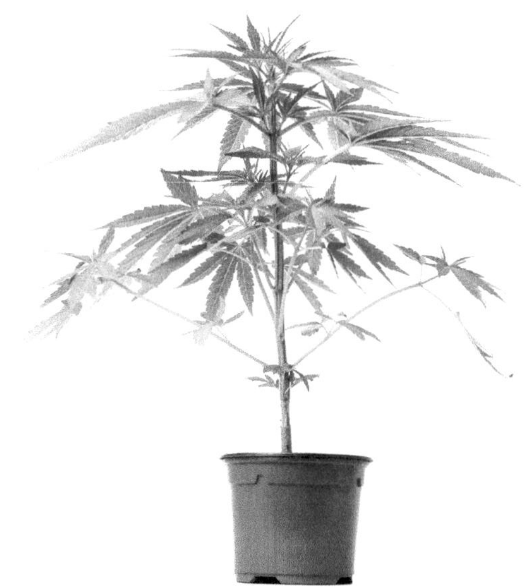

The legalization of marijuana in some states has led to questions about how to address the need to check interactions with other medications, as federal law prohibits pharmacists from dispensing the drug.

How are states with legalized medical marijuana addressing this problem? Through its 2012 law legalizing medical cannabis, Connecticut requires that the medical marijuana dispensaries have a board-certified pharmacist on-site. As with other prescription drugs, the pharmacists (and technicians) must check the patient medication profiles before dispensing the marijuana medication. Patients and the physicians licensed to prescribe the drug count on the pharmacists for counsel on type, dosages, and drug interactions. Minnesota has followed Connecticut's lead of involving pharmacists in its medical marijuana law. Pennsylvania requires either a pharmacist or a physician be on-site at a dispensary.

Connecticut's pharmacy law that requires one pharmacist for every three technicians is the same for marijuana dispensaries. The medications come in prepackaged dosages from licensed state growers, and four of the first six state dispensaries have been owned by pharmacists. Medical marijuana was at first restricted to treat only eleven conditions: cancer, Parkinson's disease, multiple sclerosis, spinal cord nerve damage, glaucoma, Crohn's disease, epilepsy, post-traumatic stress disorder, wasting disease, HIV/AIDS, and cachexia. More conditions have been added. Each state has its own list of covered medical conditions.

Patients in Connecticut must have a physician's diagnosis of a qualifying condition, and be registered with a medical marijuana card. No more than 2.5 ounces can be dispensed within 30 days. The medication comes in tablets, capsules, oils for vaporization and vape pens (personal oil vaporizing devices), topical creams and oils, strips that melt in the mouth, dried leaves and flowers for cooking or smoking (heat releases the active ingredients), and some consumable food products such as pastries with the medical dosage incorporated.

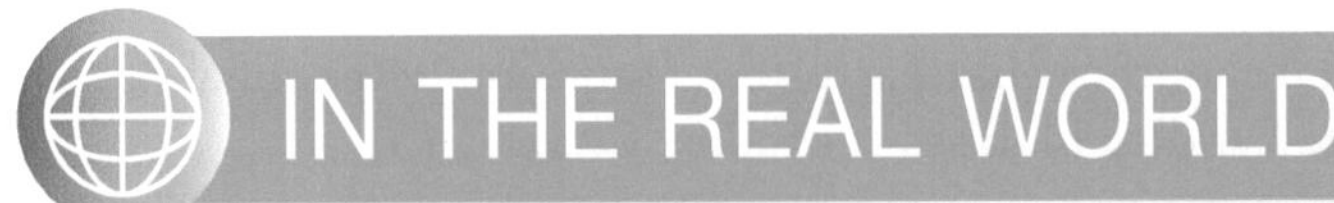

Medical marijuana is commonly indicated for nausea and vomiting from chemotherapy, severe pain, epilepsy (especially in children), and glaucoma. By spring 2019, 34 states and the District of Columbia had legalized the medical use of marijuana. Ten states and the District of Columbia have legalized recreational use, with more considering it in their legislature.

14.8 Pharmaceutical Temptations for Abuse and Theft

Drug abuse is an enormous problem, not only for patients, but also for pharmacy and medical personnel who are tempted into illegal behaviors due to access. According to *USA Today* in April 2014, more than 100,000 healthcare practitioners are abusing legal drugs, which affects not only themselves and their families but also the quality of the care they give patients.

Drug Abuse in Health Professionals

Health professionals, like physicians, nurses, pharmacists, and others, often fall victim to drug abuse and controlled substances diversion. It is not uncommon for a pharmacy technician to succumb to the temptation to pilfer prescription drugs. It is estimated that more than 10% of healthcare professionals have a drug or alcohol

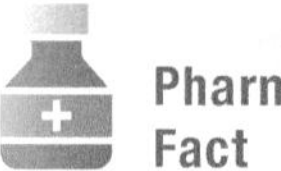

Pharm Fact

In 2018, the *Salem News* released an investigative report on a pharmacy technician charged with stealing 18,000 pills and vials of medication. Medications taken include oxycodone, fentanyl, and hydrocodone. The thefts took place over a 13-month period in a hospital is Massachusetts.

abuse problem—a statistic that is similar to substance abuse in the general population. Access to controlled drugs offers a temptation to healthcare workers who are drug seekers. Some will divert and abuse these drugs for reasons such as self-medication to relieve stress or pain, improve work performance and alertness, or to sell and make money.

When the prescriber, pharmacist, or technician is caught, it can mean loss of job, license, and registration, and embarrassment to the family and profession. In addition, a drug-impaired pharmacist or technician is more likely to make medication errors and be subject to criminal prosecution.

Prevention

Criminal background checks and urine drug screening tests have become an essential component of prescreening for pharmacy technician and pharmacist education programs and employment opportunities. Due to risk of abuse and easy access to controlled drugs, pharmacies have also implemented measures to prevent drug theft, including cameras, tablet-by-tablet inventories, and staff in-service training. Such training includes recognizing the signs and symptoms of substance abuse and knowing the course of action to take if you suspect a colleague has a substance abuse problem.

Signs and Symptoms of Substance Abuse Substance abuse is difficult to spot because it is a behavior most people cleverly learn to hide. Possible signs and symptoms include changes in appearance (such as bloodshot eyes) and changes in behavior (such as abrupt mood swings, slurred speech, poor listening skills, belligerence, overconfidence, lying, absenteeism, and forgetfulness). While anyone can have a "bad day," sudden and consistent behavioral changes may indicate a serious problem. The problem may also stem from personal or relationship issues, economic issues, health issues, stress, or other causative factors.

Course of Action If you are aware that a technician or a pharmacist has a problem, you have a legal and ethical responsibility to uphold the law and protect society. There is a natural reluctance to getting involved with a colleague's problems. Anyone would want to avoid retribution or contributing to a technician's termination or a pharmacist's loss of licensure. Even so, encourage your coworker to seek professional drug treatment. By getting help for your colleague, you are protecting not only their safety and welfare but also that of the other employees and patients.

Rehabilitation

Pharmacists, pharmacy students, or pharmacy technicians who are impaired from alcohol or drug abuse can be referred (or volunteer to be admitted) to a drug rehabilitation counseling program offered through their state pharmacy organization. Most state boards of pharmacy have a **Pharmacists Recovery Network (PRN)** or similar organization to provide assistance and treatment for impaired colleagues without the risk of losing their license or registration.

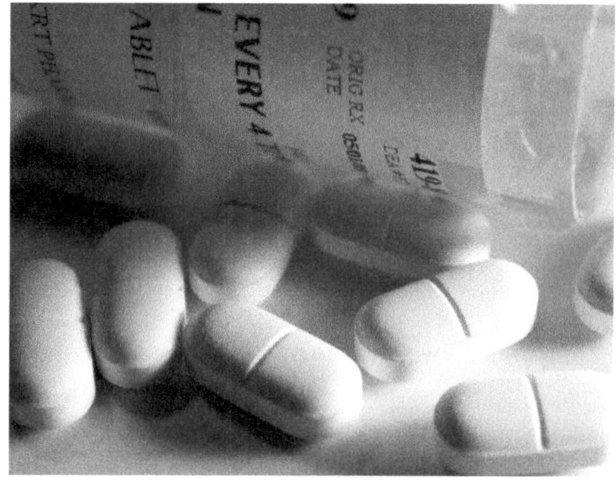

One commonly abused drug is a combination of hydrocodone and acetaminophen.

Contact information for each state may be found at https://PharmPractice7e.ParadigmEducation.com/StateContact. The successful completion of such a program may result in reinstatement of registration or license.

Prescription Drug Theft

Certainly, drug tolerance and addiction are major reasons for prescription drug abuse, but drug diversion for money, especially in challenging economic times, is also a major cause of abuse. Each dose of a prescription drug may command a high price among recreational users. Sadly, some Medicare and Medicaid patients give their legal prescriptions for narcotics to drug dealers for cash. National and regional databases share information about the prescribing and dispensing of these drugs between states to better identify drug seekers and traffickers.

Preventing Pharmacy Robberies

Retail pharmacies, due to the presence of money and especially drugs, are targets for robberies from criminals and addicts. In 2015 there were over 800 armed robberies of retail pharmacies in the United States. Hopefully, you will never encounter such an event, but if you do have such an emergency, do you know the right and wrong things to do?

Purdue Pharma, in conjunction with the National Community Pharmacists Association (NCPA), has developed a crime prevention and training program called **RxPatrol**. This is a collaborative effort between industry and law enforcement designed to collect, collate, analyze, and disseminate pharmacy theft information. The RxPatrol website has training videos and a security checklist to help make your pharmacy safer from robbers. There is also a national database of pharmacy robberies. If you have an incident at your pharmacy, you can report it, or you can review the robberies in your geographic area and alert other staff members.

During a robbery, the acronym to remember is **REACT**:

R - **Remain calm**, comply, and do not resist.

E - **Eyewitness**; remember all you can, such as age, height, weight, race, gender, body markings, and clothing.

A - **Activate** your panic alarm when safe.

C - **Call police**; describe incident, robber, and their mode and direction of travel.

T - **Take charge**; lock the door so the robber cannot return, protect the crime scene, keep customers calm, and have them remain in the store as witnesses when police arrive.

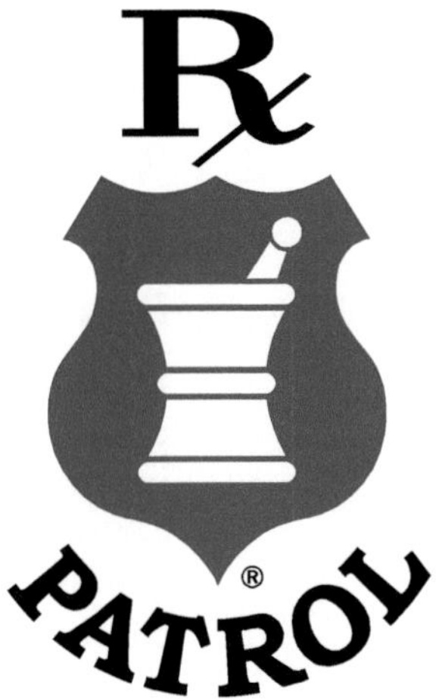

RxPatrol is an acronym for Pattern Analysis Tracking Robberies and Other Losses.

Practice Tip

Post decals at the front door—"This Pharmacy belongs to RxPatrol"—or signs near the pharmacy that read "Controlled drugs in limited supply in time-release safe."

Prevention strategies are also important to deter potential robberies. Keep an eye on customers you do not recognize; many times they may be scoping out the pharmacy. Keep security cameras visible and functional. Have more than one panic alarm button and have an escape plan with your staff. Keep the phone number of your local police precinct readily available.

The National Association of Boards of Pharmacies (NABP) and the Drug Enforcement Agency (DEA) recommend that both C-II *and* C-III drugs be locked in a steel cabinet with access limited to the pharmacist. This is not always practical, though C-II drugs must legally be locked. To prevent night robberies, a good alarm system plus the locked cabinets is a prudent prevention strategy.

14.9 Not Only Do No Harm, But Do Much Good

As a pharmacy technician, you have a career based on helping people live healthier lives. As you have seen, that is a challenging task. The incidence, adverse effects, and economic impact of medication errors remains too high in all pharmacy settings. As part of a healthcare team, technicians and pharmacists working together have roles in the identification, resolution, and prevention of medication errors and prescription drug abuse. Most errors are preventable with training, experience, and careful attention to detail. Personal and professional distractions must be minimized during each step of the dispensing process, and patient safety can never be compromised for expediency.

If you do spot problems, yours or those of others, they should be reported to the pharmacist and documented. The emphasis must be on identifying what went wrong so as not to repeat the error rather than placing blame for any punitive action. The use of automation will minimize but not eliminate the risk of medication errors. Reporting the medication error to a central database may prevent a similar error from occurring in the future at your pharmacy as well as at another pharmacy or a hospital.

As a technician, you must also have a healthy respect for the dangers of accidental misuse or deliberate abuse of the drugs and supplements you work with and sell over the counter. Providing patient education materials and referring patients to the pharmacist when needed are essential safety tasks, and the pharmacist will depend on you to do them well when working with customers. You also will be on the front line of spotting prescription forgeries and drug seekers and seeking help for coworkers if needed. In addition, you need to know how to react in case of a drug theft or pharmacy robbery.

In all of these ways, you and your pharmacy are working to help promote the safety and well-being of your patients, your coworkers and yourself, and your community.

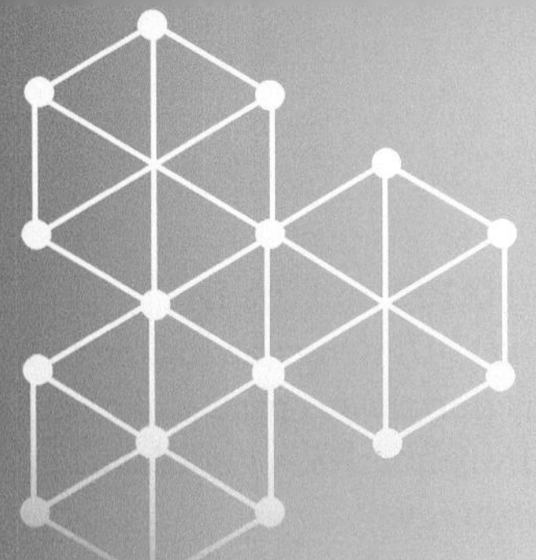

Review and Assessment

CHAPTER SUMMARY

- It is estimated that over 400,000 medical errors occur in the hospital each year.
- Almost 2% of all prescriptions dispensed in a retail pharmacy result in a medication error, causing an estimated 7,000 deaths per year (as most go unreported).
- The economic impact of medication errors is substantial each year.
- Specific practices, careful work habits, and a clean work environment promote patient safety and decrease illness and injury caused by medication errors.
- Pharmacy technicians play a crucial role in the prevention of medication errors, and knowing the potential causes and categories of medication errors is the first step in preventing them from occurring.
- Patients depend upon receiving the seven "rights" in medications, which a technician should know, as they are also the areas where there are often errors.
- Errors can occur because of failures in the various levels of pharmacy systems: organizational, technical, and human.
- Organizations and supervising pharmacists have the responsibility to foster a culture, policies, and facilities that emphasize safety first.
- Automation and technological advances, including e-prescribing and bar code scanning, can minimize medication errors.
- Medication error prevention must be emphasized by all healthcare team members.
- There are numerous psychosocial reasons for human errors, including incomplete information, incorrect assumption, selection error, capture error, rushing, distraction, and fear.
- Typical medication errors can be specifically categorized as wrong drug, adverse drug, wrong amount, mislabeling, wrong formulation, documentation, medication education, and contaminated product.
- Once errors are identified by root-cause analysis, corrective measures should be put in place, and permanent elimination of the source of error should be the goal.
- Each step of the medication-filling process has the potential to produce a medication error or to catch an earlier error, so it is important to know the informational resources, automation resources, and human resources available at each step to help prevent an error.
- Although pharmacy technicians cannot counsel patients concerning their medications, they can encourage them to ask questions of the pharmacist.
- Helping patients become more informed also empowers them to be advocates for their own safety and health.

- The pharmacy technician should adopt effective personal prevention strategies to minimize human errors.
- Several medication error reporting systems exist. Pharmacy personnel should be familiar with these organizations, initiatives, and resources, and use them to confidentially report errors so that the errors do not occur again.
- The Joint Commission has published an "unapproved abbreviations" list to minimize medication errors.
- There are levels of progressively unhealthy/harmful relationships with prescription and illegal drugs, including tolerance, psychological dependence, physical dependence, and addiction. All are risks with the long-term use of controlled substances.
- The pharmacy technician must be aware of a forged prescription or "drug-seeking" behavior.
- Technicians need to keep up to date on the regulations about dispensing medical marijuana, as they are different in each state and changing rapidly.
- Prescription drug abuse continues to be a major problem in health care and pharmacy today.
- It is important that community pharmacy technicians know how to act during a robbery.

CHECK YOUR UNDERSTANDING

To ensure that you recall and understand the key chapter concepts, please read the question or statement and select the appropriate lettered option.

1. Research studies indicate that, for every 250 prescriptions dispensed in a community pharmacy, how many contain a medication error of some type?
   a. 0
   b. 1
   c. 4
   d. 25
2. Root-cause analysis is a systematic approach to identifying the deep causes of why a medication error happened in order to prevent its recurrence. Inadequate staffing in the pharmacy is an example of what kind of failure?
   a. technical failure
   b. government failure
   c. organizational failure
   d. human failure
3. Filling a prescription with generic bupropion SR when the drug requested was bupropion XL is an example of which type of error?
   a. assumption error
   b. selection error
   c. capture error
   d. omission error
4. When a prescribed dose is due but not taken by the patient or administered by the nurse, it is considered what kind of error?
   a. wrong time error
   b. omission error
   c. extra dose error
   d. mislabeling error

5. What is the correct way a prescriber should write five milligrams to prevent a medication error?
   a. 5.0 mg
   b. 5 mg
   c. .5 mg
   d. 0.05 g

6. To avoid a medication error, if a prescription is written or electronically prescribed as "DAW," the pharmacy technician should enter the prescription in the computer software as the
   a. generic drug.
   b. brand name drug.
   c. generic or brand name drug.
   d. lowest cost generic drug available.

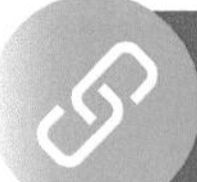

MAKE CONNECTIONS

Take a moment to consider what you have learned in this chapter and respond thoughtfully to the following prompts. Note that some of these activities will require internet access.

1. You receive a prescription for Wellbutrin 150 mg XL 1 po q 12 hours #60 with two refills. No DAW is noted on the prescription. You enter the prescription into the computer exactly as it was written on the prescription with the generic bupropion (Watson brand), but the pharmacist said you may have missed a potential medication error. In a short essay, identify the error and how you would resolve it? Would bar code scanning of the NDC have prevented this error?
2. Drug abuse is a major problem in the US not only with recreational, but also with prescription drugs. Describe the extent of drug abuse in the US today by addressing the following points:
   a. What is the most abused class of medications?
   b. List at least three ways that a pharmacy technician may detect a forged prescription.
   c. List three ways a technician may identify a drug abuser.
   d. What program tracks Schedule II controlled substance use within the state and the region in which you live to better identify "drug shoppers"?
   e. What are the restrictions on filling out-of-state Schedule II controlled substance prescriptions?

The online course includes additional review and assessment resources.

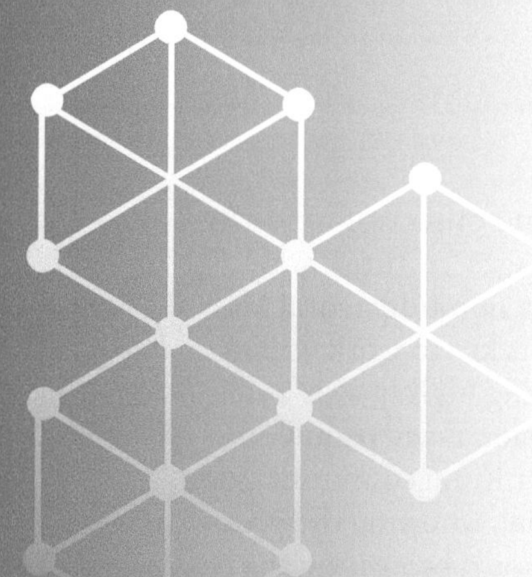

15 Professional Performance, Communications, and Ethics

Learning Objectives

1. Explain the important role of the pharmacy technician as a member of the customer care team and discuss the concepts of professionalism and teamwork in the pharmacy. (Section 15.1)
2. Identify and discuss desirable personal characteristics and attitudes of a pharmacy technician. (Section 15.2)
3. Differentiate verbal and nonverbal communication skills. (Section 15.2)
4. Identify and resolve cultural and other differences in working with a customer. (Section 15.2, 15.3)
5. Identify and resolve challenges related to working with a customer with disabilities. (Section 15.3)
6. Define *discrimination* and *harassment*, and explain the proper procedures for dealing with these issues in the workplace. (Section 15.4)
7. Identify and discuss the important areas of HIPAA. (Section 15.5)
8. Define ethics and discuss characteristics of ethical behavior and dilemmas in the workplace and provide examples of corporate integrity in a community pharmacy. (Section 15.6)
9. Provide an overview of corporate ethics and the consequences of medical identity theft and fraud. (Section 15.7)
10. Identify several green pharmacy and public health initiatives, including take-back medications and sharps collection programs. (Section 15.8)
11. Explain why emergency preparedness is a pharmacy responsibility requiring planning. (Section 15.9)

ASHP/ACPE Accreditation Standards
To view the *ASHP/ACPE Accreditation Standards* addressed in this chapter, refer to Appendix B.

All the knowledge of drugs and skills of dispensing, preparing, or compounding medications would be without merit if a pharmacy technician is not effective in working with colleagues and providing good, professional customer care. In the community pharmacy, the customer is most often the patient. In the hospital pharmacy, the customer may also be a physician or a nurse. Good interpersonal and communication skills are necessary to have a long and successful career as a pharmacy technician.

As has been seen throughout the chapters, the pharmacy profession has been evolving into greater emphasis on patient-oriented clinical practice, with a focus on the pharmacist offering medication therapy management and other services. Technicians have made this shift possible by handling more of the prescription filling and customer service functions. Dealing with concerns of

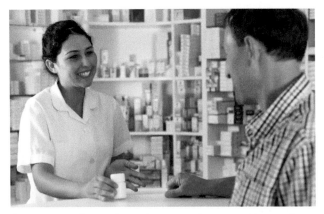
Courteous and attentive assistance makes a good impression on customers and influences their decision to return to your pharmacy.

patients, pharmacists, and other staff of different ages, abilities, languages, cultures, and beliefs must be done in a nonjudgmental and professional manner. It is key to work well as a cohesive team in providing high-quality care. The soft skills of professionalism, teamwork, interpersonal and intercultural communication, and ethics are all essential. Knowing the pharmacy's responsibility toward protecting the environment and emergency preparedness are also needed. This chapter provides guidance and examples to help you be successful on professional and personal levels, get along well with colleagues, and provide first-rate customer service.

15.1 Professional Attributes and Practices

A successful pharmacy technician must possess a wide range of knowledge and skills and certain personal characteristics. Besides accumulating a broad knowledge of pharmacy practice and drugs, technicians must have an eagerness to learn, a sense of responsibility toward patients and healthcare colleagues, a willingness to follow instructions, an eye for detail, confidence in basic mathematics, good research skills, and the ability to perform accurately and calmly in hectic or stressful situations.

Healthcare professionals at all levels are expected to act maturely, project a positive and inviting physical appearance and attitude, and be willing to work hard, get the job done, and serve the customer. This requires attention to both written and unwritten rules of personal and professional behavior, and getting into good habits of mind, body, and professional practice.

Knowledge of Policies and Procedures

It is important to get to know the ins and outs of pharmacy practice in any particular facility. Most pharmacies spell out policies in online or written materials during initial job orientation and training. In large-scale pharmacies, a **policy and procedure (P&P) manual** outlines the roles and responsibilities of staff members as well as the procedures of the facility. The implementation of a P&P manual is particularly important to the smooth operation of large, more complex chain and hospital pharmacies.

Make sure that you are thoroughly familiar with your pharmacy's guidelines and abide by them in your routine practice. Below are some sample questions that may be addressed in a P&P manual or may be accepted pharmacy practice:

- *Can employees fill their own prescriptions or the prescriptions of family members?* Store or hospital policy may dictate that an employee cannot fill their own prescriptions or those belonging to a family member. Violations could result in job termination.

- *Is compensation available if you have to work late?* In some practice settings, you will need to use a time clock to punch in and out for both your breaks and your shift. Overtime pay may need to be approved by the lead technician, the supervising pharmacist, or the vstore manager.

- *Are pharmacy technicians allowed to add auxiliary labels to medication vials?* Some pharmacy practice settings dictate that only the pharmacist can affix auxiliary labels to medication vials; in others, the technician is required to add all auxiliary labels.

- *Can a technician retrieve and fill a C-II prescription or medication order?* At some pharmacies, only the pharmacist is allowed to retrieve and count C-II drugs; in others, the technician may retrieve and count, but initialing and double-counting by the pharmacist is always required as part of the final check.

- *What is the process for prescription verification at time of pickup?* Some pharmacies will require a signature by the person picking up the medication or a driver's license number if it is a C-II drug. Some pharmacies will require verification by address, telephone number, or date of birth.

Guidelines such as these are not always written, so you will have to ask questions because these unwritten rules will need to be learned and followed just as will the state pharmacy laws. It may take as long as three months or more in the community or hospital pharmacy setting to fully learn the roles and responsibilities expected of you. Technicians are often trained to assume different roles in the department to increase scheduling flexibility. As new policies and procedures are implemented, you will have to read and document your understanding of these changes. If you deviate from written procedures, it could result in a medication error leading to harm to the patient and a legal case against the pharmacy, the pharmacist, and perhaps you as well.

Professional Standards of Behavior

Some of the unwritten, assumed standards of professional behavior in a pharmacy include appearance, decorum, etiquette, direct address, timeliness, dependability, cooperation, positive attitude, and restraint.

Professional Appearance

Appearance is the overall outward look of an employee on the job, which may be different from the outward look of the same person outside of work. How you look on the job affects how other people perceive you—your boss, colleagues, and customers. So your choices in dress and grooming need to help encourage people to trust you, which means projecting a sense of official responsibility, precision, and cleanliness, as this is a career in the healthcare field.

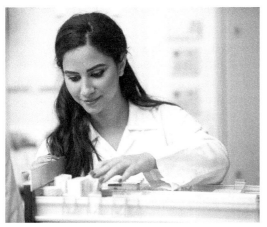

Pharmacy technicians need to dress neatly and professionally.

In many pharmacies, the technicians may be required to wear a certain color lab coat or scrubs to differentiate them from the pharmacist. You will need to wear a name tag at all times for easy identification and follow the pharmacy's dress code, which may be crisp and professional or more relaxed and casual. Having unkempt hair or a uniform smock thrown over a pair of jeans will not help colleagues or customers trust you. The customer may not consciously register these observations, yet could leave with a vague impression that the pharmacy is not a professional operation. Proper attire, impeccable grooming, and good personal hygiene are important ways to convey a positive, professional atmosphere.

Decorum and Etiquette

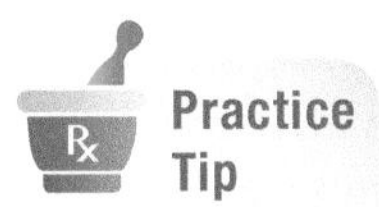

Practice Tip

As part of personal hygiene, it is important to consider body and breath odor and how to prevent them, as they can also affect professional impressions.

Decorum means proper and polite behavior, acting in good taste with civility. Arguing with your boss, colleagues, or patients is an example of impropriety, or a lack of decorum and civility. Health care is a demanding industry, often requiring long hours and involving stressful emergency situations and unrealistic patient demands. As a result, practitioners in the industry often suffer from fatigue and stress. Sometimes this stress shows itself in unintentional rudeness or in abrupt behavior toward coworkers, including pharmacists, physicians, nurses, medical assistants, administrators, store managers, sales representatives, insurance personnel, and other technicians.

For example, busy healthcare professionals may sometimes speak to subordinates in an inappropriate and unprofessional manner. The degree to which you maintain courtesy and respect even in the face of rudeness is a measure of your decorum and professionalism. If you return rudeness with kindness, then you often find that, immediately or over time, the quality of your interactions improves. If you answer the telephone and someone barks a command at you, then demonstrate your professionalism by attending to the content of the message and not to its tone.

Another set of social mores to be followed is often referred to as etiquette. **Etiquette**, defined as rules of good manners, is often recognized most easily when it is not being followed. For example, being disrespectful to a physician, a nurse, or a colleague is an obvious breach of the proper etiquette of being respectful of those in authority or with whom you work.

Proper Direct Address

In the presence of patients, refer to the pharmacist as "Doctor" if they have a Doctor of Pharmacy degree. Some states have designated all pharmacists as "Doctors" in recognition of their professional experience. Referring to the pharmacist as "Doctor" raises the level of customer respect toward the pharmacist and also toward the technician, who is the "Doctor's Assistant." It is also important to refer to physicians, chiropractors, osteopathic professionals, and dentists using the title "Doctor" and to other supervisors using appropriate courtesy titles, such as "Ms.," "Mrs.," or "Mr.," plus the last name, or "Sir," "Madam," or "Ma'am."

Customers deserve the same form of address. A degree of formality in day-to-day operations is always in order until you are requested to use more informal modes of address.

Ensuring Timeliness

Whenever you are in a work situation, your employer and colleagues depend upon you. Therefore, showing up a little early for each of your work shifts so that you can put away your belongings and prepare your mind for work is necessary. It is disconcerting to the pharmacist and other technicians if you come rushing into work just in the nick of time, or, even worse, late as they do not know for sure that you will be there.

Consider your habits and build in extra time before work, always allotting a little more than you think you will need so that you can arrive and breathe easily, enjoying a measure of mental space rather than feeling rushed and stressed. Problems usually arise when people are rushed, and things inevitably go wrong.

When planning how you will get to work to make your shifts, have a "Plan A": the ideal way for you to get there that will work most days. But also have a "Plan B" in case you miss the bus or your car or your bike breaks down. Who could you call to get a ride?

Could you get a taxi? Who could take care of your children if your childcare falls through? Think through the various pieces of your life that need to be in place for you to come to your shifts ready and able to work.

Being Dependable

If you cannot make a shift because of being ill or some major issue with transportation or family issues, make sure that you inform your employer immediately when you know this and offer a "Plan B" to have your shift covered.

Understand that when you commit to a work schedule, you are important to that workplace; people depend upon you, and you need to show up or find a replacement or some other solution. Also, it is unacceptable behavior to sleep in and miss a work shift. If you are a person who stays up late at night with friends, then plan your social life to happen on evenings when you don't have an early shift at work.

Work Wise

No one is perfect, and we all have bad days. If this occurs, understand that you are human and try to focus on something that you are grateful for to get through the shift. Or do something nice for someone else to make their day. Then start fresh the next day.

Exhibiting Cooperation and a Positive Attitude

Cooperation is that sense that everyone in the pharmacy is working together for the same goals of serving the patients and customers, providing accurate and safe prescriptions. In the community pharmacy, there are the additional goals of providing other health aids and retail items, and of being profitable. In the institutional pharmacy, there are the additional goals of working efficiently and effectively within the larger mission of the hospital or long-term care facility, responding as part of the in-house medical teams. Your supervising pharmacist needs to have a clear sense that you are aware of the larger responsibilities of the pharmacy operation and are willing to do what is asked of you to assist in the pharmacy's goals and mission to serve. No one wants to hire someone with whom they will have to argue about getting a task done or who resents helping others in their work.

Attitude is the overall emotional stance or disposition that workers adopt toward their job duties, customers, coworkers, and employers. Attitude is extremely important in professionalism and customer relations. In a community pharmacy, the technician is on the front line of customer service. In the hospital setting, technicians often conduct their jobs behind the scenes, ordering and stocking items in the pharmacy or the nursing unit, retrieving stock for compounding operations, maintaining records, filling prescriptions or unit dose carts, preparing compounded sterile preparations in the cleanroom, and performing general housekeeping tasks to maintain cleanliness in the pharmacy environment. Whether up front or behind the scenes, in all your tasks, you must be listening and communicating well with the pharmacist, other technicians, and hospital staff. You must maintain a positive attitude even on those days that are hectic or understaffed or during times when you are not feeling 100%.

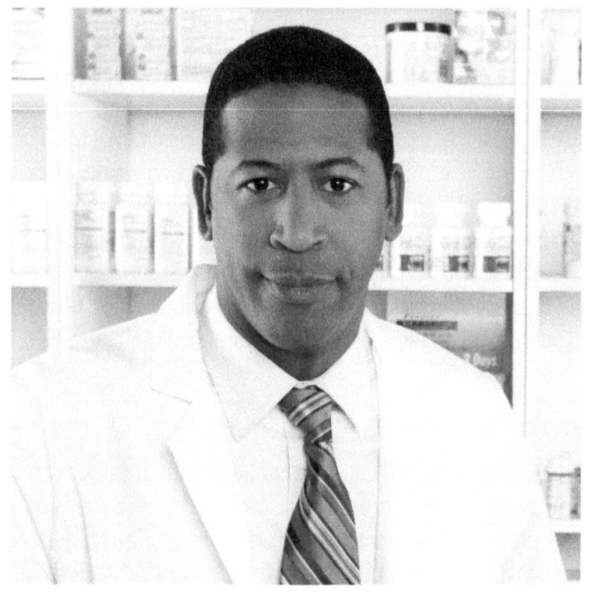

A person's attitude is reflected in the eyes, smile, posture, and other nonverbal and verbal communication.

Having a good attitude also means taking pride in your workplace. You may need to provide feedback or offer suggestions to the supervising pharmacist or store manager on ways to improve operations and customer service. Examples include suggestions for more efficient or effective processing of medical orders, stocking of prescription or OTC (over-the-counter) products, managing customer drop-off or pickup lines, handling insurance issues, ordering from wholesalers, juggling work schedules, and so on. You should not criticize management but instead offer thoughtful, constructive solutions. Being an invaluable asset to the overall pharmacy operation can assist you in advancement and in negotiating a pay raise in the future.

Professional Restraint

Some employees like to gossip or speak badly about their supervisor, coworkers, or customers. Never engage in this type of behavior because it undermines trust and goodwill. In addition, customers may speak poorly of or inquire about physicians, specialists, and other healthcare professionals. General information and positive recommendations may be given, but opinions on the competence of a particular physician or healthcare provider should not be given out by anyone in the pharmacy. At all times, avoid making disparaging comments about other healthcare providers. If such comments are made and the person's professional reputation is questioned, then you could be sued for slander.

Managing Change

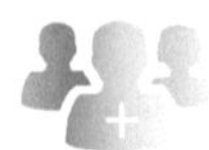

Work Wise

One of the ways to manage change is to stay flexible in mind and habit and take the perspective of wanting to be a lifelong learner who is eager or open to new knowledge and ways of doing things.

Working in a professional setting also means managing change. By definition, health care is dynamic—always changing—as are the medications and treatments being provided: new generics, new formulations, new dosages, and so on. The pharmacy work environment also flows with dynamic small changes, such as shifts in customer service approaches, last-minute switches in work or vacation schedules, revising of insurance plan coverage, or updates to government policies.

During training in a community pharmacy, you will learn how to use the prescription software, the cash register, pricing procedures, credit card scanners, and inventory management tools. You will also gain an understanding of prescription insurance plans and the processing of claims—these, too, will be changed on a regular basis.

Similarly, in the hospital pharmacy, you will have to learn the ins and outs of the pharmacy and hospital software and medical order transmissions. Mastery will also be needed of the various automated tools used in the pharmacy, including bar code scanners, dispensing units in the pharmacy and the nursing unit, compounding devices, repackaging and dispensing machines, digital balances, and primary engineering control (PEC) workstations in the IV cleanroom. Confidence in running the pharmacy's equipment will take time, but you can begin in classroom simulations, externships, and internships. Since the technology and procedures will be updated often, you have to be ready to always be a learner. However, you will be able to handle it because you have learned the basics.

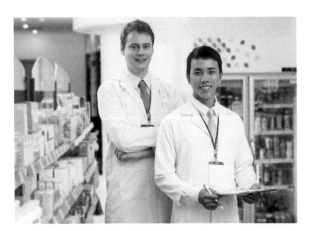

Technicians need to work with pharmacists as part of a pharmacy team wherever they work.

Teamwork

For eight hours or longer per day, technicians and pharmacists must work together along with others as a cohesive healthcare team to provide quality care and to process prescriptions for patients efficiently and safely. Each member must establish collegial relationships built upon respect for others, an appreciation of others' workplace contributions, and a willingness to help one another during busy times or in times of change. You also need to be honest about your own capabilities. *If you feel overwhelmed on the job, do not be afraid to ask for help.* For example, have a colleague double-check your filling, compounding, or dosage calculations.

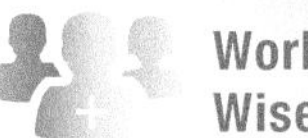

Work Wise

Knowing when you need help and being able to ask for it are signs of wisdom rather than weakness.

Respecting Differences

In any pharmacy, you will work with personnel from varied age groups, genders, ethnicities, and religious backgrounds. Personalities differ and sometimes clash. Is someone too talkative or loud, or too quiet and passive? Are some personnel too obsessive and compulsive? Do some seek patient contact and communication primary engineering control (PEC) whereas others would rather fill prescriptions and minimize patient contact?

These differences cannot be allowed to interfere with the work at hand. There must be respect for other personnel, both individually and with regard to their roles in the pharmacy. Unresolved issues should be brought to the attention of the supervising pharmacist privately. Any criticism of an individual's quality of work should be viewed as a constructive learning experience. Problems may range from a small typo to a larger medication error, but personal differences should never be a factor in addressing a problem in the workplace. Remember, you are part of a team with a role and mission much larger than yourself.

Appreciating the Contributions of Colleagues

Being aware and appreciative of each team member's contributions is essential to the smooth operation of a pharmacy. Seek out those who are more knowledgeable or skilled to obtain information or learn how to handle a difficult situation. For example, oftentimes pharmacists consult technicians about insurance issues because technicians are well versed in the nuances of various plans. At other times, technicians rely on the guidance of pharmacists to manage a difficult patient.

Recognizing these contributions with common courtesies, such as "Thanks for staying late to help out during this busy time" or "Thank you for helping me locate that OTC medication for the customer," can build rapport among team members. You can also build rapport by showing an interest in coworkers' personal lives. On breaks, simple questions like "Where did you go on vacation?" or "Did you have a fun weekend?" contribute to team building.

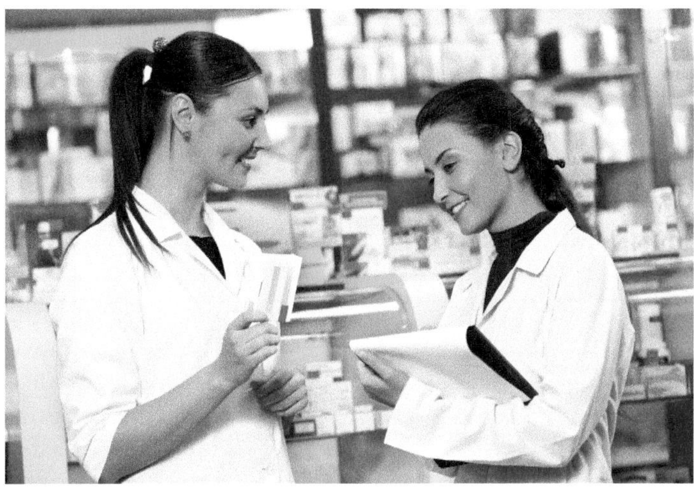

A pharmacy technician should seek guidance from a pharmacist on how to handle a challenging situation.

Good Communication Skills

The glue that holds all teams together is communication. Communicating effectively takes practice and involves both verbal and nonverbal communication strategies. Model yourself after someone whom you admire, and keep in mind that some of your coworkers have different roles and thus different communication needs and styles.

Work Wise

To learn to listen well, you must not interrupt. Ask questions, wait silently in a conversation for the responses, and care about what someone else says.

Listening and Verbal Communication Skills

The heart of verbal communication is, of course, listening. Paying close attention to the words and the voice that you are hearing is important. Maintain eye contact with the person speaking, and send the speaker other nonverbal signals of being attentive to indicate that you are genuinely interested in what they are saying. Ask questions to clarify issues, and repeat portions of the conversation to confirm that you have correctly heard what was said.

There is the additional challenge of hearing the correct drug name and term when there are so many similar ones that are very difficult to say and remember. Learning the correct pronunciations and definitions is one hurdle you can overcome with study. Listening and asking a coworker to carefully repeat and pronounce difficult words are the best ways to learn on the job. Repeat difficult words to yourself several times. You may also find it helpful to acquire pocket-sized reference guide on drug names handy and make notes in it regarding pronunciation and usage.

Nonverbal Communication Skills

Facial expression, posture, hand gestures, and of course eye contact are all methods of communicating without using words. As small children, we learn quickly how to interpret **nonverbal communication**. Mannerisms and gestures often indicate agreement or disagreement.

Watch colleagues and customers carefully. Their attitudes and reactions to information can often be determined through their nonverbal communication. Technicians need to learn how to interpret nonverbal communication, clarify it, and respond accordingly. The goodwill that you communicate always comes back to you in one way or another.

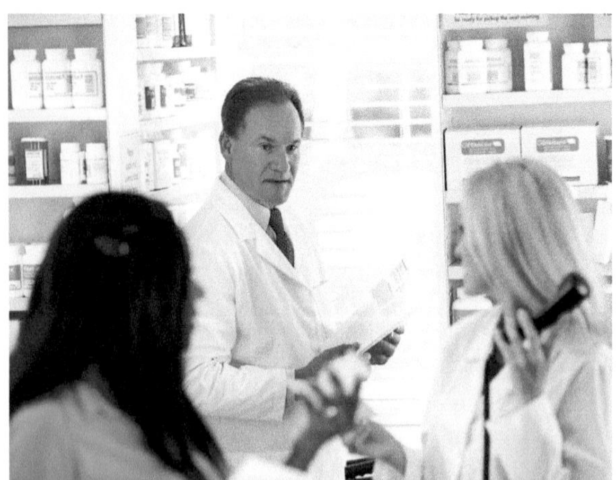

Pharmacy technicians should always interact with other professionals respectfully.

Personal Conduct and Lifestyle

Personal telephone calls, texting, and visits should be conducted only during breaks. Telling offensive or off-color jokes is not acceptable and can make colleagues and patients feel uncomfortable. When in doubt as to the expected behavior in a situation, watch and learn from someone else in the pharmacy who is a suitable model, and perform your assigned task. If you are not sure, ask questions of the senior pharmacy technician or the supervising pharmacist.

Appropriate workplace behavior also demands that you do not let your personal life interfere with your work performance. You must be "on top of your game" to safely and efficiently input, fill, and dispense prescriptions and interact with customers and healthcare personnel for hours-long shifts. If you bring your personal problems to the workplace, you may not have the concentration needed to perform your job responsibilities accurately and safely. Interpersonal issues, such as family obligations, personal health, dating, and the need for more flexible work hours, may cause tension and adversely affect job performance. Intimate personal relationships with coworkers or pharmacists are discouraged or not allowed in most practice settings. A transfer to another pharmacy may be appropriate if you plan to carry on a relationship with a colleague.

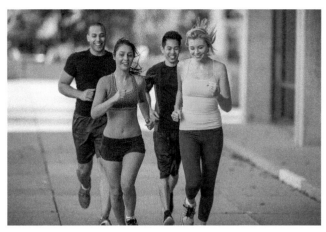

De-stressing and exercising off the job mean that you can be more attentive on the job.

Technicians must take care of themselves as well as their patients. Although refusing to work a long shift or overtime is not always a realistic option, technicians can heed the recommendations of the Healthcare Provider Service Organization (HPSO) to help combat fatigue and, therefore, prevent medication errors. These include getting enough sleep and exercise, eating healthy foods, and avoiding illegal drugs and too much caffeine or alcohol (see Table 15.1).

TABLE 15.1 Healthy Lifestyle Choices Conducive to Job Professionalism

Pharmacy technicians should be mindful of the following lifestyle recommendations offered by the Healthcare Provider Service Organization (HPSO) and summarized here:

- Get enough sleep. Experts say that eight hours of sleep a night is best, so go to bed early enough. Avoid staying up until you cannot keep your eyes open any longer; as soon as you feel sleepy, turn out the lights and turn in.
- Exercise regularly. You may feel more tired at first, but regular exercise should eventually help boost your energy level. Plan to do your workout several hours before bedtime so that you are not keyed up when it is time to sleep.
- Take breaks at work. Even when things are busy, take short or longer breaks (for lunch/dinner) to relax and revitalize yourself even if it means going outside to clear your head for a couple of minutes. You will not be much help if you cannot think clearly.
- Be wise about food. Eat a well-balanced diet for optimal energy. During your scheduled break, avoid sugar-laden snacks and choose complex carbohydrates for stamina.
- Avoid excessive alcohol. A nightcap or two at home may relax you at first, but as the alcohol wears off, it disrupts your normal sleep patterns.
- Cut the caffeine. Coffee, tea, and other drinks that contain caffeine do not prevent fatigue; they just hide it. Limit your caffeine intake, especially near bedtime, as it can interfere with a restful sleep.
- Avoid illegal drug use. Most pharmacies require drug tests before hiring and periodically after employment. So besides being personally detrimental, illegal drug use can get you fired. This is true even in states where marijuana use is legal. The effects of the drug can linger in your body and interfere with your performance at work.

15.2 Providing Professional Customer Service

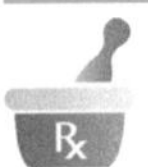

Practice Tip

In a *Consumer Reports* survey, 90% have rated independent pharmacies as "excellent" or "very good" for pharmacists' knowledge about drugs and other products, helpfulness and courtesy, speed and accuracy, and personal service.

Other written and unwritten standards that come into play in the community pharmacy have to do with professional customer service. In the 1960s and 1970s, mass merchandising was an innovative retail marketing strategy, and customers became accustomed to large impersonal drug stores with numbered aisles of merchandise, price tags, and cash registers. By the 1980s, however, customers missed the days of personal service attending to an individual customer's needs associated with the small, independent neighborhood pharmacy of the past, where everyone affectionately called the pharmacist "Doc." Surveys have indicated that customer service and accessible location are the most important aspects consumers consider when choosing a pharmacy.

In the institutional pharmacy, some operations also view nurses and the other healthcare professionals as their clients or customers to keep satisfied. So many of these customer service principles also apply to the institutional pharmacy in hospitals and long-term care facilities.

Customer Attentiveness

Among small businesses, pharmacies (and banks) have received the highest marks for in-person customer service from Gallup surveys. A little personal attention pays off. A courteous voice, a welcoming smile, a moment of assistance finding merchandise, or holding a door can go a long way toward making customers think of your pharmacy as a pleasant place to visit and do business. Greeting patients by name is especially important. Patients are far more likely to return to a pharmacy where someone knows their name and they have received personal attention than to one where they have not.

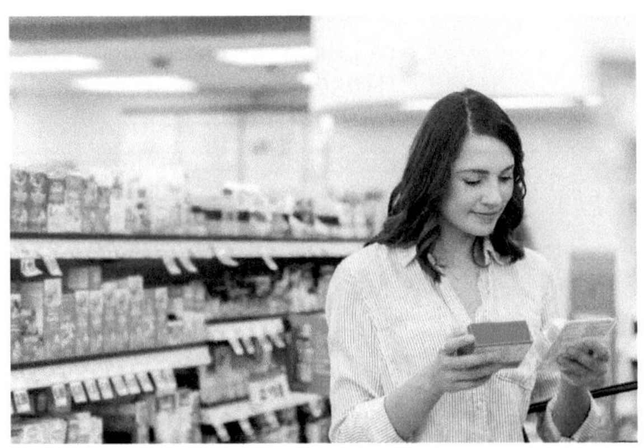

Pharmacy technicians can help customers read labels to compare brand and generic OTC labels.

Often a customer is reluctant to ask for help to avoid imposing on the pharmacy staff member's time. Approach any customer who has an uncertain look or is wandering the OTC aisles and ask courteously, "May I help you?" Then after the customer's response, ask some clarifying questions. For example, if a customer is looking for aspirin, then they may need to know not only where the OTC analgesic products are located, but also where to find a specific analgesic such as baby aspirin, aspirin for a migraine, Goody's powders, or an enteric-coated form for those whose stomachs cannot tolerate conventional analgesic dosage forms. If possible, escort customers to the place where the desired merchandise is shelved and then help them find it. Point out items that may be on sale this week.

Similar principles apply in the institutional setting. If a nonemployee looks lost or confused, offer assistance. A friendly "May I help you?" can make a difference in someone's experience. If they ask for directions to a certain unit or area of the hospital, try to take them there if possible. While the layout of a hospital may be familiar to someone who works there, hospitals can be extremely confusing for patients and their visitors.

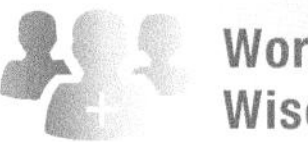

Work Wise

Asking the pharmacist how they would like to prioritize the different types of demands can help you triage many tasks.

Juggling Demands

In the community pharmacy, many things may be happening at once: you are making a sale; the phone is ringing; a customer is waiting for help in the OTC aisle; and five patients are waiting to pick up prescriptions. Here, a good pharmacy technician will **triage**, or sort out the various types of requests, and handle those that are appropriate to specified duties and leave others that apply only to the pharmacist. This involves strategizing about available resources to attend to the varying customer needs.

First, acknowledge each customer's request for service by a simple statement like "I will be right with you." Focus attention on each customer one by one for a moment and then on getting their needs met—this helps make them feel it was worth the wait. If possible, request help from other technicians, the pharmacist, or the store manager. During the wait or after providing the needed service, acknowledge their inconvenience by saying, "Thank you for waiting," or "I appreciate your patience."

If a customer requests an OTC product outside of the immediate pharmacy department area, assist them by providing the aisle number and location, or page a store manager if you are busy. When a product is out of stock, apologize to the customer and offer a rain check. If a customer requests a unique product not typically in stock, then check with the manager or consult the wholesaler log to see whether a special order can be made. If so, let the customer know when the product should be received (usually the next business day), and get their name and phone number for a courtesy call. Making the extra effort to provide customer service pays off in long-term dividends and return business for any retail operation.

In the institutional setting, technicians may also be required to triage and prioritize. For example, this might involve being asked to restock medications in an automated dispensing machine and deliver a compounded sterile product for a patient in critical care. Consider the urgency of both requests and respond appropriately. In the example provided, delivering the compounded sterile product to the patient in critical care would be the higher priority. After delivery is completed, the automated dispensing machine can be restocked. Best practice is to communicate prioritization plans to any colleagues that may be affected, if feasible.

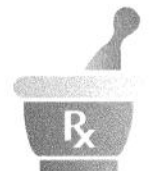

Practice Tip

When trying to engage a patient or draw out information, use open-ended questions instead of closed-ended ones.

Gathering Information

To triage well, gather information from the customers to help discern their needs and assist the pharmacist in arranging medication therapy management or counseling sessions. Ask well-phrased questions that are appropriate to the type of information needed. A **closed-ended question** is one asked in a yes-or-no format, such as "Do you have a headache?" or "Have you tried aspirin?"

An **open-ended question** allows the patient to share more information about their illness and provides more helpful information to the pharmacist for recommending the best treatment. Asking the patient open-ended questions like "Can you please describe your headache pain for me?" is always preferable. Gathering this information and relaying it to the pharmacist will expedite customer service.

When speaking, work to enunciate clearly while looking someone in the eyes, especially when conversing with older adults who may have trouble hearing. People in a rush also tend to slow down and hear more effectively when eye contact is established. Eye contact and a smile help people be more receptive and attentive, which is essential if you are trying to communicate drug administration directions. Tone of voice also matters: is it friendly, warm, and appealing? Or stern, grouchy, crisp, dismissive, or absentminded? Always use a nonjudgmental expression and tone of voice. Never let patients feel that they are imposing or that they are being scolded.

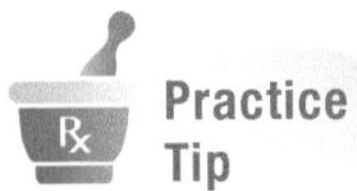

Practice Tip

Remembering to make eye contact ensures that you have the customer's attention. At the same time, it is always good to be aware that in some cultures it is a sign of respect to lower one's eyes. So do not be offended if this occurs.

In many cultures, eye contact is often associated with honesty, sincerity, and respect. Older patients and those who are hard of hearing sometimes need to lip-read to supplement the words that they cannot make out. Speak with your head facing the patient to make what is being said easier to understand. This is true for all patients at a community pharmacy with a drive-through window. It is already difficult to communicate over engine and ambient noise. Be ready to repeat the customer request—whether it is verifying patient name, date of birth, address, or other information.

Providing Empathy

While gathering information or serving a patient, it is important to act with **empathy**, which is the ability to share and understand another person's feelings. Perhaps the customer has recently lost a loved one, or a loved one has become seriously ill, or the patient may just have been recently diagnosed with a serious illness. Perhaps the person has just been discharged from the hospital or spent the better part of a day or night at the emergency room. Whatever the customer's circumstances, try to be consistently open and receptive and not make any assumptions or rash judgments so it's easier to serve the patient's needs as well as possible.

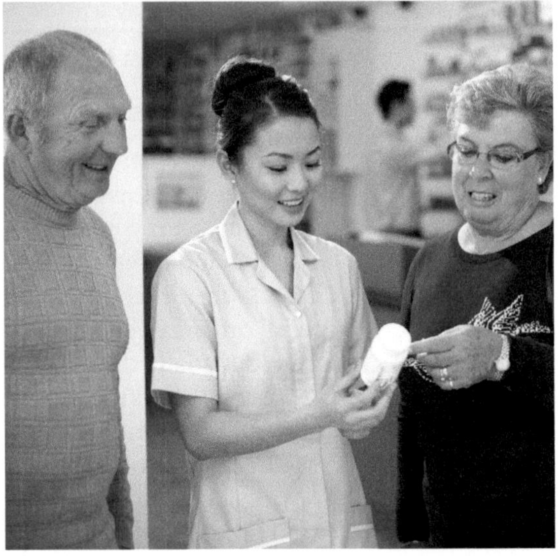

Applying old-fashioned manners never goes out of style and is the way to success with customers in the ever-changing world of pharmacy.

Being Courteous

In every interaction with a customer, sprinkle the conversation with courteous words and phrases because they show respect and provide openings for empathy and service. Memorize names and faces to greet people by name. Get to know local and cultural pleasantries, such as talking about the weather, how someone is doing, the news of the local team winning, and other common ways of building a connection. Ask about people's children and pets. Get to know your clientele.

Common Phrases of Courtesy

To ensure that your customer has a good experience and will want to come back, use respectful expressions of address like "Ma'am" and "Sir" to those you do not know. Begin and end customer interactions, even the briefest ones, with formal courtesies such as, "Good afternoon" and "Have a nice day." "Please" and "Thank you" should become a part of your regular vocabulary. Offer a sense of hospitality by practicing courteous speech, as demonstrated in these examples.

Unwelcoming: What do you need?
Welcoming: May I help you?

Unwelcoming: It's over there.
Welcoming: That item is in aisle three. Follow me, and I'll show you.

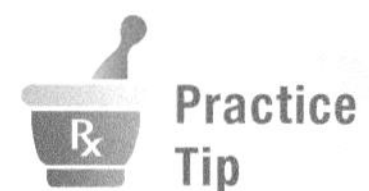

It is important to remember at the end of every transaction to thank the customer.

Unwelcoming: It's $8.39.

Welcoming: That will be $8.39, please.

Unwelcoming: Next?

Welcoming: May I help who is next?

Or even better: Hello, Mr. Fibich. Are you here to pick up or drop off a prescription?

Sometimes mistakes are made. Customers will call attention to things that may or may not be a problem or the pharmacy's fault. Thank them for making you aware of the problems, and bring the issues to the attention of the pharmacist. If a mistake is yours, make eye contact with the pharmacist and admit to making an honest mistake. The pharmacist will decide how to handle it. If no mistake was made by the pharmacy, then you should be as understanding as possible and try to address the customer's concerns to find a solution. If there is a delay in filling the prescription, then apologize to the customer for the inconvenience.

Nonverbal Courtesies

As with colleagues, nonverbal gestures, expressions, or movements can help or hinder communications, so you need to be very aware of them. If not, you can communicate exactly the opposite message from the professional one that you would like. Consider these scenarios:

Unprofessional: Talking to a customer while filling a prescription or answering the phone.

Professional: Asking the customer to wait a moment, then completing the prescription or placing the telephone caller on hold (or have another staff member take the call), and going down to the front counter or private counseling area to talk to the customer.

Unprofessional: Showing surprise through an open-mouthed facial expression when a customer shares a diagnosis with you (such as HIV, gonorrhea, syphilis, or depression).

Professional: Being nonjudgmental, mirroring their facial expressions or exhibiting minimal facial expressions other than kindness, and then assisting the customer with the information or products that they need. Be empathetic and show genuine concern. Remember that all patient medical information is confidential and protected by law.

Unprofessional: Answering a customer's question about an OTC recommendation with your arms crossed at some distance from the patient.

Professional: Smiling and making eye contact, letting the customer know with your body language that you welcome the opportunity to help them. Move closer to the customer, ask open-ended questions, listen carefully, and be aware of both your body movements and those of the customer. Crossed arms often convey some barrier to communication, such as that you are too busy to be helpful.

Pharmacists' Patient Care Process

Strong patient care isn't limited to being pleasant and helpful during face-to-face interactions. It requires far-reaching communication skills to make sure that patients, families, and caregivers are engaged as much as possible, whenever possible. In 2014, the Joint Commission of Pharmacy Practitioners identified the steps of the **Pharmacists' Patient Care Process**, a method of collaborating with prescribers, other pharmacists, and pertinent health care professionals to provide "safe, effective, and coordinated care." As members of a team, pharmacy technicians will play an important role in assisting pharmacists with each step of this process.

Using principles of evidence-based practice, the Patient Care Process guides pharmacists to:

- **Collect**–The pharmacist oversees the collection of relevant information about the patient to create a comprehensive medical/ medication history.
- **Assess**–The pharmacist assesses the information collected and accounts for the patient's overall health goals, identifying problems and evaluating solutions.
- **Plan**–The pharmacist creates an individualized, cost-effective, and evidence-based care plan tailored to the individual patient.
- **Implement**–The pharmacist implements the care plan while collaborating with other health care professionals and the patient or caregiver.
- **Follow-up: Monitor and Evaluate**–The pharmacist monitors and evaluates how effective the care plan is and adjusts in collaboration with other health care professionals and the patient or caregiver as needed.

For more information on the Patient Care Process, see: https://PharmPractice7e.paradigmeducation.com/PatientCareProcess

15.3 Telephone Courtesies

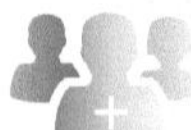

Work Wise

Try to smile while talking on the phone to customers and make them feel that their call was welcomed.

Customers and healthcare professionals often contact pharmacies by telephone. They may be calling in refills, inquiring as to whether a new prescription has been received or filled, asking about the cost of medications, and verifying insurance coverage for certain prescriptions in the community setting. In the institutional setting, nurses may be calling to locate a missing medication, pharmacists may be calling to request delivery of an item, or an outside hospital may be calling to ask to borrow medication. These are all requests the technician can easily address. The following are some guidelines for using the telephone properly:

- When you answer the phone, identify yourself and the pharmacy, as in "Good morning, Reinhardt's Pharmacy. My name is Jess. How may I help you?" or "Good evening. Inpatient pharmacy. Pharmacy technician Katherine speaking. How may I help you?"
- Always begin and close the conversation with a conventional courtesy like "Good morning" and "Thank you for calling." Stay alert to what the caller is saying and use a natural, conversational voice. You should be friendly but not too familiar with the caller. When speaking to patients who are hard of

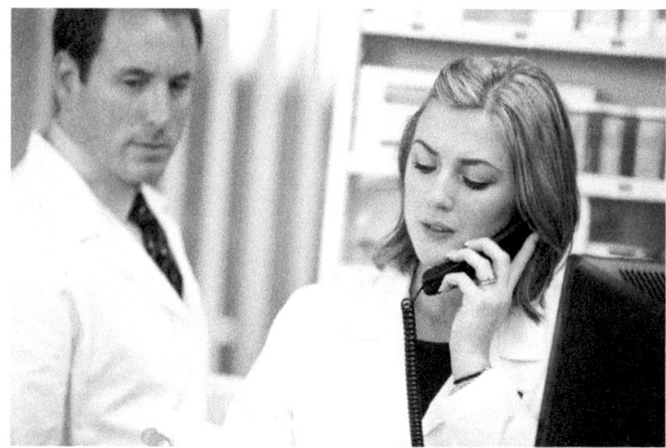

Pharmacy technicians need to be able to communicate professionally with patients and healthcare professionals, even when on the telephone. Studies say that listeners can tell if people speaking on the phone are smiling when they speak or not.

hearing, speak clearly, pronounce each word distinctly, and be prepared to repeat yourself without frustration.

- If a prescriber is calling in or ordering a new prescription, you may need to turn over the phone to a pharmacist. In most states, technicians by law are not allowed to take prescriptions over the telephone. Be sure that you are aware of the regulations in your state.
- If the caller has questions about the administration or effects of a medication or about a medical condition, adverse reaction, or drug interaction, place the customer on hold and refer the call to the pharmacist on duty.
- Make sure that any information you provide is accurate. Giving incorrect directions to a customer in need of a prescription can be a life-threatening mistake.
- In the community setting, if the caller is requesting a refill, then politely ask for their name and date of birth and/or prescription number. After verifying that the prescription can be refilled and dispensed, give the caller an approximate time when it will be ready for pickup, and thank them for calling ahead.
- Depending on the regulations in your state and the procedures of your community pharmacy, you may be authorized to handle prescription transfers or to provide information related to prescription refills. Follow the procedures outlined by your supervising pharmacist.
- If a customer is calling about a medical emergency or a prescription error, refer the call to your supervising pharmacist.

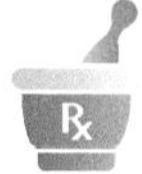

Practice Tip

Refer to a pharmacist any questions involving:

(1) patient assessment;

(2) proper administration, dosage, uses, or effects not noted on directions or packaging; and

(3) the need for a pharmaceutical opinion or judgment.

Respecting Professional Boundaries

Queries involving pharmacy location, printed product directions, availability, or price can be handled by the technician. As you know, questions that involve professional medical or medication information, judgment, or counseling must be referred to the pharmacist. So use common sense to determine whether a given query from a customer exceeds the bounds of common knowledge. The customer may want to know whether to take aspirin or another OTC analgesic such as ibuprofen, or they may ask whether it is acceptable to take ibuprofen with a prescribed blood pressure medication. You may say to the customer, "That is a good question; let me have you speak with the pharmacist."

Exhibiting Patience

The pharmacy technician must have patience when working with customers. In the community setting, insurance issues in particular can be complicated and frustrating for patients and technicians—and resolving these issues can be time-consuming, especially for an inexperienced pharmacy technician. It takes time and experience to learn the ins and outs of the numerous prescription drug insurance plans, so if you

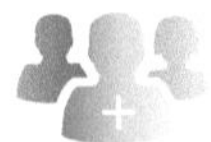

Work Wise

Five tips for best customer interactions:

(1) face the patient and speak slowly;

(2) avoid slang or medical terms, putting information in clear, everyday language;

(3) be a good listener;

(4) keep the conversation succinct and focused;

(5) rephrase and summarize to make sure you understand information correctly.

cannot adequately address the patient's questions or concerns, don't be embarrassed or anxious. Check with a senior technician or the pharmacist to better understand the issue and how it can be resolved within a reasonable time period. Inform the patient of the outcome, and learn from the encounter to better serve a future customer.

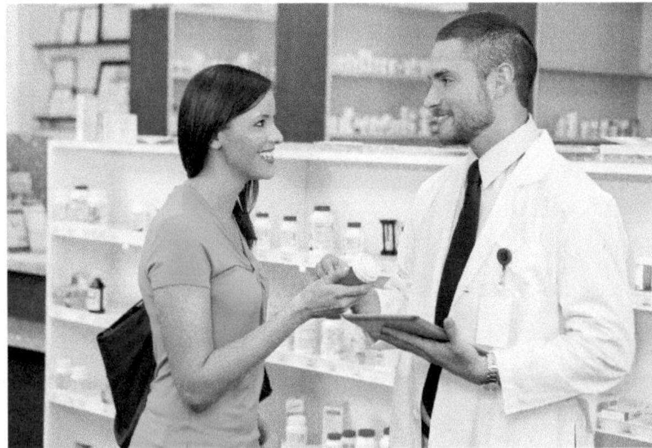

Pharmacy technicians must learn patience and friendliness in their interactions with their colleagues and customers.

Working in a customer service-oriented position can be difficult and tiring. Therefore, it is common in larger pharmacies to rotate responsibilities so that every two to four hours the technician may have different duties. In the community pharmacy setting, collecting payments and dealing with the public, entering new prescriptions and refill requests, resolving insurance claims, filling prescriptions, ordering medications, and checking inventory may all occur in one shift. Preparing sterile compounded products, refilling automated dispensing machines, and delivering medications and supplies are duties that you may be asked to perform.

Being Sensitive to Diverse Patient Populations

As a technician, you will run into a great range of cultural backgrounds of customers, patients, and coworkers in a community or institutional pharmacy. Be sensitive to and respectful of differences in culture, religion, language, abilities, and other backgrounds. Do not assume that everyone thinks as you do, or should think and act as you do. Try to become aware of differences while understanding that everyone has similar human hopes and needs, though expressed differently.

Work Wise

US population projections show that America will grow even more diverse every year because of differing birth rates between majority and minority groups, and immigration. This diversity has increased the nation's variety of foods and restaurants, arts, and culture, and Americans' love for travel.

Awareness of Cultural, Religious, Gender, and Ethnic Differences

We live in an increasingly culturally and ethnically diverse society. According to 2014 US Census Bureau estimates, the majority (60.7%) of the US population was non-Hispanic white Americans, which is a diverse group encompassing individuals of many cultural Slavic and European backgrounds. Latin Americans (or Latinx) made up 18.1% of the population, followed by African Americans at a little over 13%, Asian Americans at nearly 6%, and 2.7% multiracial Americans. Within the Asian community there are diverse cultural differences among the Chinese, Japanese, Vietnamese, Korean, Filipino, East Indian, and other populations. The non-Hispanic white populations are trending down while the other population sectors are trending upward.

Cultural Identity The term "**culture**" is commonly defined as the customs, beliefs, art, food, traditions, religious practices, marriage and family structures, and attitudes that are learned and shared to varying degrees by members of a group. Our cultural values influence our behavior and response to medications. According to studies, cultural differences affect patient attitudes about medical care and treatment. For example, in some Asian countries, mental illness is considered a dishonor to the family. Consequently, the number of patients seeking psychiatric care in these countries is small. This stigma continues in several immigrant communities and in the general populace of the United States, though not as intensely. This may affect how these patients feel as they come to pick up mental health medications.

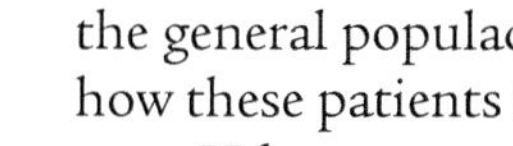

Work Wise

To successfully understand someone else's iceberg of cultural beliefs, it is very helpful to explore one's own.

Urban community pharmacies and hospitals are usually located in areas catering to diverse customers. Differences in age, gender, sexual orientation, ethnicity, language, culture, economic status, educational background, and disability will be part of your everyday practice in the pharmacy. To serve varied customers, **cultural sensitivity** is a valuable skill. Cultural sensitivity is defined as awareness, knowledge of, and respect for cultural beliefs that differ from your own. Knowing more about a customer's culture helps you provide higher-quality service and shows a customer that you care about them. Working to overcome any cultural barriers will help you make every patient and coworker feel at ease to trust you and vice versa.

Iceberg Metaphor of Cultural Identity The social scientist Edward T. Hall compared culture to an iceberg. On the surface, we may perceive differences in physical features, manner of dress, native language, accent in speaking English, traditional foods, and neighborhood composition and location. These are the visible top layers of a person's cultural iceberg. Underneath the visible level are the beliefs, attitudes, values, and perceptions that consciously and often subconsciously guide a person's decisions and actions (see Figure 15.1). Being knowledgeable about the unseen aspects of cultural identity can help create empathy toward cultural barriers.

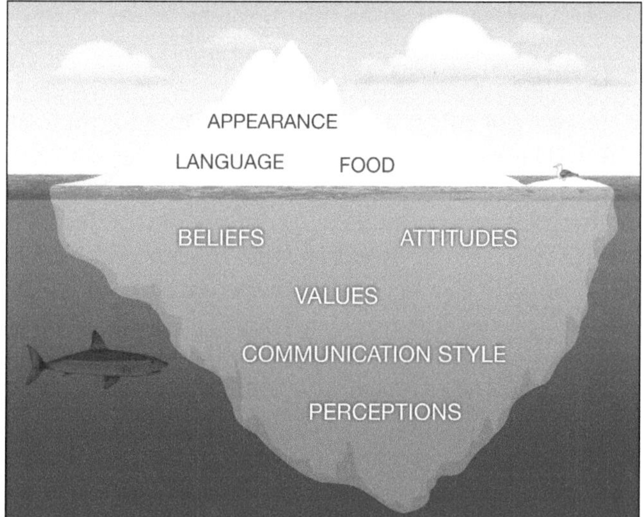

FIGURE 15.1 **The Iceberg Metaphor of Cultural Identity**

Multiple Levels of Influence on Identity Each individual is influenced by many levels of culture and identity. We each have a family of origin with its own history, traditions, and beliefs that exists within a larger community culture, neighborhood, or identity group (such as high school teenagers), which is often part of a larger group in the United States of mixed ethnic and cultural backgrounds. This local community culture exists within the larger culture of American media, infrastructure, and politics.

Then there are the layers of socioeconomic status, religious identity, educational influences, and work. Each person is a complex mix, as is each community. People and communities exhibit a spectrum of behaviors and beliefs. In America, political affiliations or leanings can also have a huge defining effect and are connected often to media preferences, religious identity, and socioeconomic status, so politics is another aspect of culture that can grow out of other elements. Gender also has a huge influence because of differences in perceptions of, expectations for, and treatment of the genders in various cultural contexts (see Figure 15.2).

FIGURE 15.2 The Multicomponent Cultural Identities of Individuals

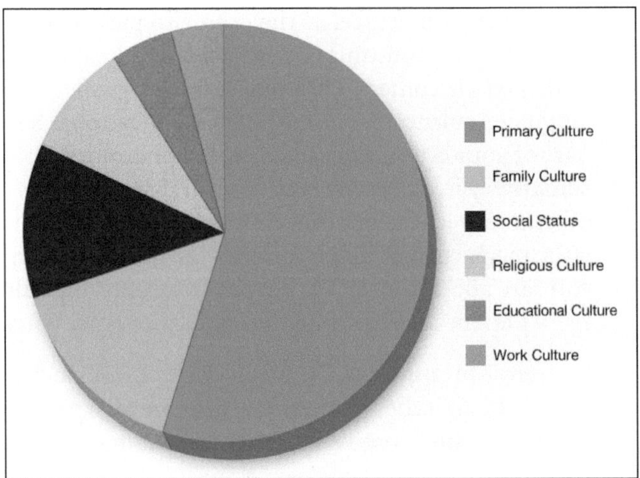

Source: *What Language Does Your Patient Hurt In? 3e*

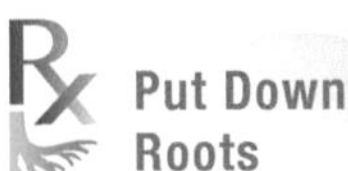

Put Down Roots

Cultural competence in the pharmacy refers to having the capacity to serve effectively and respectfully the diverse individuals and communities of pharmacy patients and customers in the context of their varied cultural beliefs, needs, and behaviors.

Accommodating Cultural Trends

It is helpful to be aware of cultural trends when striving for understanding and overcoming cultural barriers and communicating with respect. You may perceive them in yourself, colleagues, and customers. If you understand the potential origin of some trends, you can both understand and communicate more effectively in addressing concerns. However, it is very important to avoid in your mind letting observation of simple trends solidify into flat stereotypes. A **stereotype** is an oversimplified characteristic of a group of people. It is a generic image of a group of people based on patterns, word-of-mouth stories, prejudiced attitudes, opinions, or uncritical judgments about isolated incidents blown into sweeping generalizations.

It is essential that trends you encounter or are presented with do not fall into stereotypes or fixed images of anyone from a certain background. The interesting part about humans is that they rarely fit well into a static definition, even when they try to. Because there are so many levels to every person that make up their history, genetic and cultural makeup, experiences, and many aspects of cultural identity, each person is as individualized as their fingerprint.

Work to discover the individualized and deeper aspects of each person: their beliefs, attitudes, values, perceptions, and everyday interests. Completing an inventory of your own influences can help you understand yourself and why you may react in one way or another to things you encounter.

For greater understanding, read Paradigm's *What Language Does Your Patient Hurt In? (Third Edition)*. It has essential counsel for how to develop cultural and linguistic competence and handle cross-cultural communication. It has chapters with special counsel and awareness for health care for patients of African American, Native American, Hispanic and Latinx, Asian, Middle Eastern, Eastern European, and specific religious backgrounds.

Mistrust of Western Medical Practice Considering the complex history of race relations in the United States, it is not surprising that many minority cultures do not always accept or trust current medical practice or recommendations. For example, some African American patients may mistrust conventional medicine due to systemic mistreatment of their communities, such as the infamous Tuskegee study, an unethical experiment conducted between 1932 and 1972 in which the effects of untreated syphilis were studied in black men without their knowledge.

Similarly, Native Americans have endured unspeakable hardships at the hands of Western medicine and are often understandably reluctant to seek care. Pharmacy personnel need to be sensitive to these long-standing cultural memories and belief systems.

Reliance on Self-Care Many cultures or communities, especially those that have a history of oppression or poverty, have developed a strong reliance on self-care out of necessity. For example, less affluent people in some neighborhoods may rely more on self-care, OTC medications, and dietary supplements and less on physician visits. They also may be less likely to believe in the benefits of long-term treatments, as they may have fewer models of successful health treatments in their neighborhoods and less ability to pay for them than more financially stable patients. Therefore, they may discontinue their drug therapy before it has run its course. In Japanese and Vietnamese cultures, patients often self-regulate their medications with lower-than-recommended doses due to concerns about side effects.

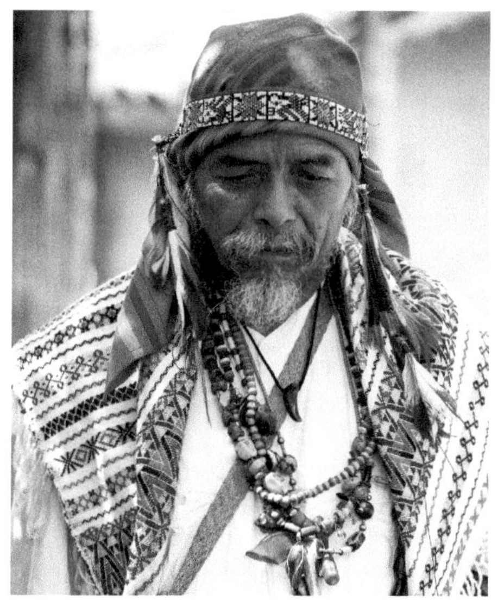
Non-Western medical practices may involve shamans, herbalists, and healers to provide primary care to patients.

Reliance on Herbalists and Healers Traditional healers have a nearly universal presence in indigenous and folk cultures. If you practice in the rural United States, then you may hear more about home remedies. In Native American communities, patients tend to place more belief in family and spiritual values and treatments than in contemporary Western medicine. Within the diverse US tribal populations, illness is often considered to be due to an unhealthy imbalance in one's life within the body but also within interpersonal and spiritual relationships. All things are seen as connected, so healing does not just involve the body but is placed within a more holistic context. Traditional healers may believe that prescription drugs cannot work alone; they encourage spiritual and social therapies too.

In Mexican American communities, primary care is often provided by *curanderas*, or spiritual healers. They employ a rich mix of herbal remedies and rituals to encourage healing and drive off bad spiritual practices and forces, and encourage good ones. Root doctors from the American South use prayer rituals and herbs to restore the body to health. Many patients from Asia have stronger cultural beliefs in the healing power of herbs and practices like acupuncture and yoga rather than in prescribed medications and Western surgical practice. In the varied Chinese cultures, the yin (cold) and yang (hot) energies must be placed in harmonious balance for the patient to be at optimal health. Western medicine is beginning to learn from all these cultures as they are learning from Western medicine, which is why there is a marked increase in the integration of alternative holistic practices, herbal medicines, dietary supplements, psychology, and even spirituality into Western medical understanding.

Influence of Religion on Medical Care Religious holidays and customs can also have a great impact on healthcare practices. For Muslims, the monthlong fast of Ramadan may interfere with the ability to take prescribed medications on their usual time schedules. During this holy month, Muslims do not drink or eat until after sundown. They also may prefer a healthcare practitioner of their same gender, as do many people in Orthodox Jewish communities. Religious faith and prayer also have a major impact on health attitudes within many Christian communities, with prayer groups offering healing support. Fasting is a recommended practice for certain seasons among Catholics, Muslims, and others. Christian Scientists and Jehovah's Witnesses generally do not believe in any source of healing other than prayer and the revising of wrong thinking that leads to wrong actions, which they believe leads to illness.

Influence of Gender and Sexuality Often people prefer to discuss personal medical issues with pharmacists or technicians of the same gender. For example, some male customers may feel more comfortable discussing questions on condom use or erectile dysfunction drugs with a male technician or pharmacist. Similar issues may arise in the case of a female customer with issues regarding menstruation or menopause. Be sensitive to this; if you sense that a patient would like to talk about a sex- or gender-related issue, or is from a traditionally orthodox religion, then it would be wise to call over someone of that person's same gender to offer that person service.

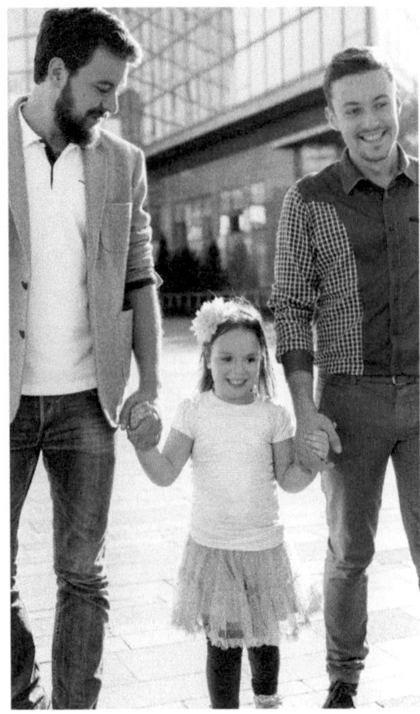

Patients and colleagues come from a wide variety of backgrounds, and all deserve respect.

The pharmacy technician should also be understanding of the unique health concerns and needs of the gay, lesbian, bisexual, and transgender populations in the communities they serve. By establishing a comfortable, nonjudgmental environment for the discussion of gender and sexuality issues as they relate to healthcare needs, pharmacy personnel can establish rapport and provide effective treatments for all patients.

Diseases that Disproportionately Affect Certain Ethnic and Socioeconomic Communities Certain diseases are on the rise among specific ethnic groups for a mixture of many different reasons. These health concerns can, in part, be attributed to the unhealthful eating habits of many individuals living in poverty in the United States, due to the lack of funds and the expense of fresh fruits, vegetables, and meats; the lack of grocery stores and farmers' markets in poor neighborhoods; and the lack of car transportation and gas money to travel to areas that possess them. Poor diet and stress can result in medical issues.

For example, the incidence of diabetes is much higher among Mexican Americans and Native Americans. The African American population has a higher incidence of hypertension, stroke, and kidney disease. Obesity is an issue with many American cultural groups.

All US populations tend to have more reliance than other countries on processed food products and fast foods, both of which tend to be higher in salt, sugar, calories, and numerous additives, and lower in nutritional value. As many Asian immigrants have adopted a more typical US diet, there is now a higher prevalence of diabetes among these American communities. Youth and teens of all American backgrounds have growing rates of obesity and diabetes. These trends are occurring in other countries as well, as they adopt American fast food restaurants and processed foods.

Education level also greatly affects health, with more educated individuals having more access to health information and therefore often putting more of a priority on healthy eating and fitness. More educated individuals often have higher earning levels and more access to healthy foods.

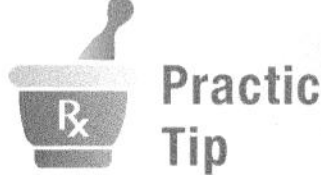

Practice Tip

Many pharmacy software programs can print patient materials in different languages.

Overcoming Language Barriers

Language differences, medical terminology, slang, and accents can create communication barriers with patients. If patients are not native English speakers, they may come in nervous and self-conscious about their language skills and ability to tell you what you need to know. They also may not understand the questions you are asking and simply nod or say yes to avoid embarrassment.

If you cannot understand a customer because of a language difference, then do not speak louder or in an exaggerated slow manner that can seem condescending. Simply enunciate in a clear, slow, but natural way, and avoid using slang terms, medical terms, or abbreviations because the person may not be familiar with them. Use respectful descriptive gestures if they can help. Apologize courteously for your language deficiency if necessary, and utilize translator services. Translators can usually be available within minutes using telephone or teleconferencing capabilties.

If you have a translator available, summarize the key information that you need to obtain from the patient. Keep sentences short, and repeat the questions using gestures and facial expressions if the patient does not understand. Be patient; give the translator time to formulate thoughts in the customer's language; and do not interrupt the exchange.

If a translator is not available, then the pharmacist may have counseling sheets that use drawings, diagrams, and clocks made especially for this purpose. Also, be aware that some computer software programs print medication labels and patient information leaflets in different languages. Many foreign language apps are available for smart phones that may facilitate communication.

Accommodating for Physical and Mental Disabilities

Patients with particular visual, hearing, cognitive, and mental challenges or conditions often require special accommodations by pharmacy personnel.

Visual and Hearing Impairment For patients with visual impairment, a pair of custom reading glasses or large-print or Braille materials can be helpful. Patients may need to number or color code their morning versus evening medications. A family member or pharmacy technician may assist by filling up a drug calendar or a plastic drug organizer with the weeks' or months' worth of medication. Patients who are hard of hearing may benefit from a slow, deliberate, short discourse (for lipreading) or—if they are deaf—from sign language, or written instructions.

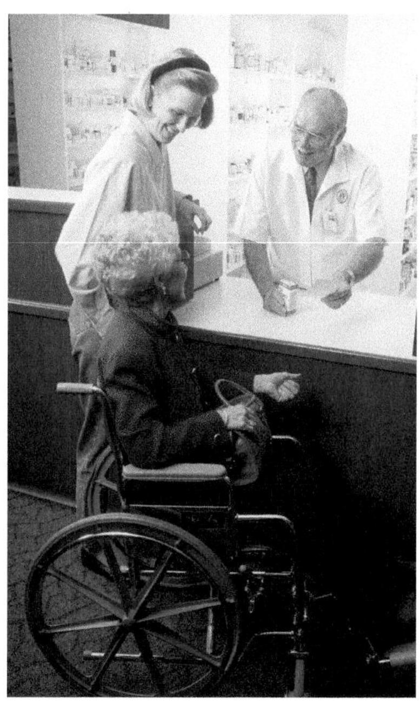

Pharmacy staff must strive to meet customers where they are and accommodate any physical or mental challenges.

Mental and Physical Challenges Some patients may have varying degrees of intellectual or physical barriers to understanding you. If you are interacting with a patient who struggles with understanding or the ability to move easily to where you are, you may need to be particularly understanding and accommodating as you work to obtain necessary demographic, insurance, and health information. Providing directions about medication use or payment should be directed at the appropriate level of understanding. For patients with physical disabilities, pharmacy personnel should make every effort to accommodate their needs. These accommodations may include recommending drive-through service, using non-childproof container lids, providing assistance in obtaining items from shelves, or ensuring their comfort during the medication filling process.

Accommodating for Economic Hardship Hard economic times and rising healthcare costs have made it increasingly difficult for patients to afford medications and other forms of treatment. Pharmacy staff members should be attuned to these patients' needs and offer compassion and creativity in trying the many different strategies for assistance as described in Chapter 8.

15.4 Problem-Solving Abilities

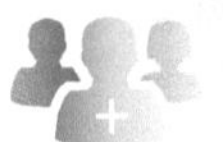

Work Wise

Meeting frustration and anger with anger or outrage escalates the anger in everyone. Meeting the other person's anger with calmness and affirming aspects of the other person's perspective can de-escalate problems and lead to thinking that can offer solutions.

Being a good problem solver for patients or workplace issues is an important asset for a pharmacy technician. You will often be the bearer of bad news to patients, such as an insurance claim denial, an expensive copayment, or an out-of-stock medication. Take the extra time to explain *why* a prescription cannot be filled or *why* it can be filled only partially or *why* it costs so much. Patients can tolerate inconvenient or disheartening news when the reasons are explained and are not personal. Solutions can then be sought.

For example, if a patient needs an out-of-stock medication, check with your supervising pharmacist and then offer to call neighboring pharmacies to find the medication. If another pharmacy has the medication in stock, arrange for the customer to pick up the prescription at that facility. If there is an insurance problem, offer to call the patient's insurance company to find a resolution or—if you are busy—attempt an insurance override, or call the company later and advise the patient of the outcome (more counsel on solving insurance problems can be found in Chapter 8).

Following written or unwritten policies and procedures in the pharmacy can assist in problem solving, but there are still many situations where you will have to respond with a creative application of the strategies you have learned and with a willingness to help. You will also need such a frame of mind for resolving potential conflicts with fellow employees, supervisors, or management.

Handling Angry Customers

It is not uncommon to encounter angry customers. They may be angry prior to even coming into the pharmacy, for reasons unrelated to the pharmacy visit. A patient may have received a "bad" new diagnosis or prognosis on an existing disease for themselves or their child. Perhaps they have spent the last 16 hours at the emergency room at the hospital or have just been discharged from the hospital and had to drive 50 miles home through rush-hour traffic. Perhaps a couple has recently lost their jobs and health insurance. Or maybe they are just having a bad day—we have all been there.

A pharmacy technician overreacting to this situation may escalate tensions and worsen the situation in the presence of other customers. If you can remain level-headed when dealing with difficult patients and stressful situations, it will be beneficial to all concerned. See Table 15.2 for tips on handling angry customers.

TABLE 15.2 LEAD Is the Way to Handle Angry People

Use the acronym LEAD when dealing with an angry customer or patient or colleagues:

L-Listen

E-Explain why it happened

A-Acknowledge that it is a legitimate problem

D-Discuss to decide how to resolve the issue, and thank the customer

Studies have demonstrated a 20% increase in employee productivity when using a similar protocol to handle an angry or unsatisfied customer.

Handling Conflicts with Coworkers

Differences of opinion and frustrations will arise with coworkers and even supervisors. They may come to you with issues, and a similar procedure can work as with an angry customer. You may, however, need more of a discussion. If that is the case, use the acronym LEAD to let each side respond alternatively: **L**isten, **E**xplain why it happened, **A**cknowledge the issues involved, and then **D**iscuss to decide or at least come to consensus on possible options based on more shared knowledge.

It also helps to try to avoid taking issues personally and getting defensive, sarcastic, or impatient or raising your voice. Using empathy and trying to understand the other person's side and repeating key issues can show that you have heard them, even if you don't agree with all the points or would like to offer alternative scenarios or options.

When someone tells you ways you can improve, do not resent the messenger. Professionals take criticism as counsel that can help them do better. You will find this kind of advice a gift to you in the long run, despite it being a hassle now. You will have job reviews where you will be given a list of expectations and suggestions. If handled well by both your reviewer and you, these reviews can help you grow and succeed in your career goals. This openness to the opinions of others or different viewpoints will also help you in customer service and other professional interactions.

Handling Discrimination and Harassment

If you find yourself the object of discrimination or harassment, first try to resolve the issue with the person or persons involved. **Discrimination** is preferential treatment or mistreatment for reasons of age, gender, ethnicity, sexual orientation, religion, or other factors, and **harassment** is aggressive mistreatment, pressure, or intimidation that can be sexual or otherwise. These activities, particularly if they are of an ongoing or persistent nature, are not only unethical but also illegal.

Do your best to maintain your composure and to express your discomfort calmly and rationally. If possible, have a witness present to verify your communication. If discrimination or harassment persists, discuss the matter with a supervisor or with human resources. The law requires all businesses, pharmacies included, to post information related to workplace discrimination and harassment.

In the past, *sexual harassment* was defined as unwanted physical contact or as the act of making sexual conduct a condition for advancement, preferential treatment, or other work-related outcomes. However, the Supreme Court has since redefined *sexual harassment* more generally as the creation of an unpleasant or uncomfortable work environment through sexual action, innuendo, or related means. Thus, you do not have to put up with off-color or crude jokes if you do not wish to hear them. Be aware that you must not contribute in any way to creating an environment that is uncomfortable for your coworkers. One person's remark made in the spirit of fun can be the basis for another person's legal action.

If the problem is not resolved, follow up first with store management or the human resources department and then, if necessary, with upper-level management. If you are unsuccessful you can make inquiries regarding the discrimination and harassment laws and procedures in your state. Most community and hospital pharmacies have written policies and procedures to address such matters; follow the established protocol. If a facility's hiring or promotion practices fail to follow proper written procedures and guidelines, then the facility may be subject to a lawsuit.

15.5 Adhering to the Health Insurance Portability and Accountability Act

As discussed in Chapter 2, the **Health Insurance Portability and Accountability Act (HIPAA)** is a comprehensive federal law passed in 1996 to, among other goals, protect patients' private health information. Obviously, though, a physician, a nurse, a pharmacist, and a pharmacy technician must have access to medical information to serve the needs of each patient. For this reason, all healthcare professionals are bound by law and ethics not to disclose information about consultations, diagnoses, tests, services, and medications, as well as any personal identifiers, outside the immediate pharmacy workplace. This is all considered **protected health information (PHI)**.

All healthcare facilities (including pharmacies in all practice settings) that access, store, maintain, or transmit patient-identifiable medical information must comply with HIPAA regulations. Failure to do so can result in severe civil and criminal penalties.

Both state and federal laws govern patient confidentiality. Some states may have more stringent requirements than the federal law. As with controlled drugs, the more stringent policy generally takes precedence. Pharmacy technicians should know the laws in the state where they are practicing. If the technician moves to another state, it is important to learn the regulations and laws of the new state.

Notice of Privacy Practices and Permissions

Confidentiality is defined as keeping privileged information about customers from being disclosed without their consent. Therefore, each pharmacy is required to have a policy statement that defines patient privacy rights and protections and how patient information will be used by the pharmacy, which must be presented to the patient for signed consent. This policy statement is called a **notice of privacy practices**. It must be presented and explained at someone's first time as a new pharmacy customer. Patients may list others whom they allow to have access to their information. The signed notice is kept on file for six years.

Sharing with Family Members and Friends

Even for sharing healthcare information with other family members, permission is important. Parents or legal guardians of minor children are considered their dependents' personal care representatives and *can* sign for their children up to an age determined by the state. For instance, in some states, adolescents at age 16 can receive mental health and/or reproductive counsel and pharmaceuticals, such as birth control

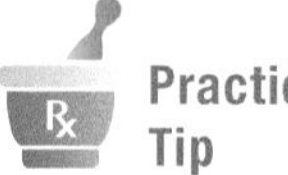

Each state determines the age at which a teenager can receive health care (in specific situations or in general) without parental knowledge or permission. So it is essential to know your state's HIPAA guidelines.

or prescriptions for sexually transmitted infections, without their parents' knowledge or approval. This occurs even if the parents are paying for their coverage via billing or insurance. These are not the only situations where teenage minors may be treated as adults with respect to access and disclosure of health information records.

Teens, however, may list their parents and others as able to access their health records. Elderly parents often list their sons and daughters as having permission to access their records and pick up their prescriptions. Spouses, too, often give permission in order to access each other's care information. Patients may ask you to print their annual prescription records (for income tax preparation) as well as those of their spouses or of-age dependents, but you may not do this without the written permission from the others involved.

Protecting Patient Identifiers

A community pharmacy depends upon protected health information to dispense medications and have them covered by insurance. To be in HIPAA compliance, pharmacy personnel must therefore remove or conceal from public view the PHI while they are working. Computer screens should be aimed away from the public and/or protected from over-the-shoulder scanning. One of the many reasons only authorized personnel are allowed entrance into the pharmacy area is to safeguard patients' private health information stored in the computers and files.

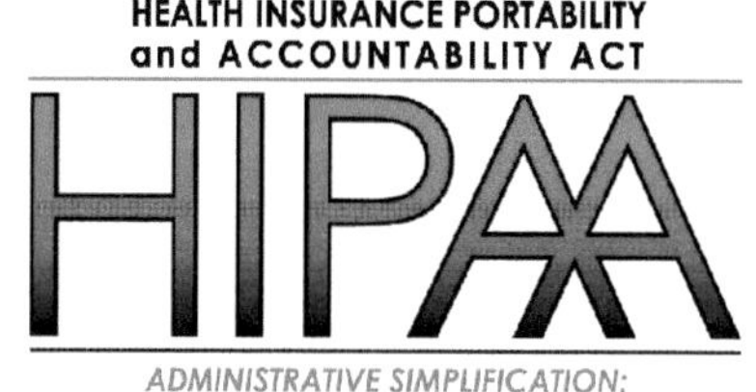

Always stay up to date on the latest standards to be in HIPAA compliance.

Examples of **patient identifiers** that must be protected are listed in Table 15.3. In addition, pharmacy personnel must take measures to conceal the medication itself. To this end, an FDA-required Medication Guide should be stapled underneath the cover sheet and placed inside the patient's bag for pickup, so that the medication cannot be seen by anyone other than the patient.

The medical information that a patient shares in a discussion with a pharmacy staff member is confidential and protected by law.

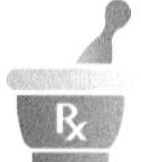

Practice Tip

Patient confidentiality of electronic transmissions includes email correspondence that includes PHI. It must be secure, without a patient identifier in the subject line, and sent only to those allowed access to treat the patient and for this purpose.

TABLE 15.3 Protected Health Information Patient Identifiers

- Name
- Address and ZIP code
- Relatives
- Employer
- Date of birth
- Telephone number or fax number
- Email address
- Social Security number
- Medical record number
- Health plan identification number
- Account number
- Vehicle identification
- Certificate or license number
- Uniform resource locator (URL) or internet protocol (IP) address
- Fingerprint or voiceprint
- Photo

Patient identifiers may be used legally for billing and credit card processing, and are occasionally used for sending out quality assurance surveys by the pharmacy or prescriber. They may also be provided by the pharmacy or prescriber in response to a lawsuit. In most legal cases, the lawyer obtains written approvals from the patient to release their prescription records, or the pharmacy gets the approval directly from the patient. PHI may be released without permission in the case of a court order or evidence of a crime or fraudulent activity. All requests for PHI other than by the patient should be directed to the pharmacist.

Permitted Protected Health Information Sharing

Medical necessity dictates professional PHI sharing regulations. *Who* must have access to *what* information inside or outside the pharmacy for the best medical service to the patient, and who does not have that access? How can unnecessary access to patient health information be limited, especially in large organizations such as hospitals, chain pharmacies, research sponsors, or insurance providers?

Sharing Among Healthcare Personnel In the process of diagnosing or treating a patient, the physician and the pharmacist (or their agents, on their behalf) may exchange information without restriction, or without the expressed written permission of the patient. For example, if a patient is receiving controlled narcotic prescriptions from several physicians, the pharmacist may notify these physicians.

In addition, some insurance reimbursement requires diagnostic codes from the physician for select diabetic and respiratory drugs, and this information can be provided to the pharmacy without explicit patient permission. Also a pharmacist may need to see a copy of a patient's hospital discharge summary or recent laboratory results for insurance coverage of the follow-through drugs. These documents, however, cannot be viewed without the patient's permission, so this permission must be asked for in written form.

PHI Sharing Between Insurance Providers and Employers A patient's insurance provider or pharmacy benefit manager is also bound to privacy and may not pass on an employee's information to their employer. Nor can a technician discuss such information or pass it on to an employer. An insurance processor requires a great deal of personal medical and medication information, including which drug and dosage was dispensed, but they may not share this information. In the past, insurance companies occasionally shared medical information with an employer, resulting in illegal employment termination for the patient. This situation is outlawed by HIPAA.

PHI Sharing Among Investigational Drug Personnel How much information does an investigational drug study (often by a pharmaceutical company) need to know about the patients? Some—but not all—health information is shared with investigational drug studies, according to the limits outlined for the study and agreed to by the patient before the study begins. Studies must be designed so that patients cannot be individually identified. A minimum amount of information that directly relates to the study is exchanged with the sponsor, according to protocols approved by the Institutional Review Board or the Human Use Committee.

Security and Electronic Transmission

The electronic transmission of PHI data is a necessity at the pharmacy and involves several parties, including healthcare practitioners, pharmacy personnel, and third-party insurance companies. All such transmissions are protected by state and federal laws and must have built-in software encryption and security systems that fit HIPAA standards to be legal. Other safeguards include limited access of certain healthcare professionals to fields of information and frequent password changes to limit access to patient information. Patient data privacy laws also extend to email correspondence. Never send any emails containing patient identifiers in the subject line. Some employers do not allow email transmission of PHI or require special precautions be taken (such as using a unique acronym in the message) before sending.

Sending medical or prescription information via fax has been a common pharmacy practice, especially for refill authorization from a physician's office. Like other types of electronic submissions, a fax must be carefully monitored. Faxes to and from the pharmacy and medical offices are in an encrypted format. The receipt of faxed information is intended only for personnel of the medical office or pharmacy to which it was sent. This information should be filed or securely disposed of (shredded) after it has been reviewed. If an inadvertent fax was transmitted to the wrong number, the sender must be notified and the protected information returned or destroyed immediately.

Protecting Operational Records

Though individual patient information is considered the property of the patient, the prescriber's medical records themselves are considered the property of the facility that generates them. Patients, however, are entitled to a copy of their personal records at any time through a written request. While a patient and a provider have a right to review and add to the records as appropriate, medical records belong to the facility, but they are still protected information and may not be sold or distributed without authorization.

Pharmacy medication dispensing records are similar. You must keep your employer's proprietary information protected from competitors, including individual records, but also operational records. This includes prescription volume, pricing issues, and pharmacy policies and procedures. If you are not sure, ask a senior pharmacy technician or pharmacist. You must also protect your customers' private billing information to avoid any issues of identity theft.

Pharmacy Strategies for HIPAA Compliance

Each pharmacy develops its own mechanisms to implement, communicate, audit, and document compliance with HIPAA regulations. This may include the layout of the pharmacy customer area, its lines, pickup stations, and counseling areas. Each pharmacy has a set of policies and procedures in its manual to cover the HIPAA regulations. Depending on the size of the pharmacy, formal training programs with annual refresher courses may be used.

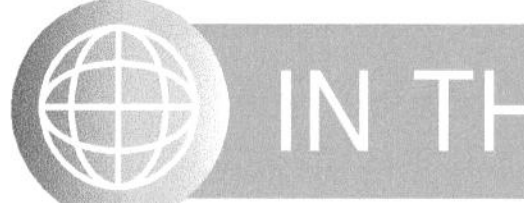

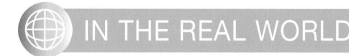

IN THE REAL WORLD

If you knowingly obtain or use protected health information in violation of the law, you can be fined up to $50,000 and sentenced to up to one year in prison. If you obtain information under "false pretenses," it climbs to a fine of up to $100,000 and up to five years in prison. Someone who obtains health information with the intent to sell, transfer, or use it for commercial purposes or personal gain can be fined up to $250,000 and sentenced to up to 10 years in prison.

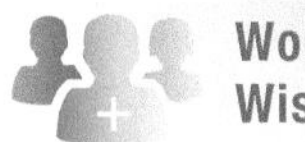

Work Wise

Remember that sharing any patient information on social media, whether on the job or off, is illegal, and sufficient reason for immediate termination of your job. If you have trouble keeping secrets or being discreet, being a pharmacy technician is not the job for you.

Pharmacies are held liable for any problems with privacy, and can be sued or have legal sanctions for any confidentiality leak. Casually mentioning or passing on any patient information in conversation in the pharmacy or outside of it or on social media is illegal in every sense, as well as a professional and ethical breach of judgment. You will face legal consequences and may lose your job immediately.

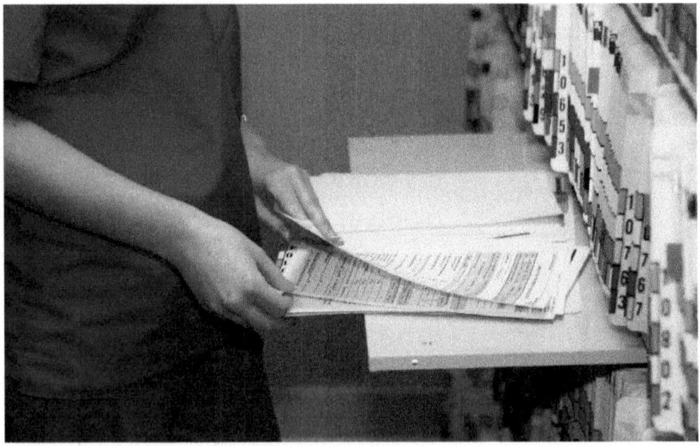

The information contained in both medical and pharmacy records is protected under HIPAA laws.

Since the PHI belongs to the patient and not to the pharmacy, it is best to always err on the side of caution when it comes to releasing or discussing patient information. Follow the golden rule of HIPAA: treat every person's information with *at least* the same caution and respect you would want for your own information, if not more. That requires great discretion in pharmacy conversations.

Maintaining Privacy in Patient Discussions

When a patient requests a private consult with a pharmacist, both the technician and the pharmacist should conduct these discussions quietly and discreetly. When using the telephone, pharmacy personnel should not use speakerphone when talking with a patient, and should not leave a message for a patient that divulges any medical or drug information unless given express written permission to do so by the patient. Maintaining the security and privacy of a patient's medical information must remain a high priority.

In addition, be careful about discussing sensitive medical issues while other customers are waiting in line. As you update customer records, make sure that you maintain privacy. If, for example, you are stationed at the pharmacy window and need patient profile information, use a written form for the patient to fill in or find space for the customer to answer your questions away from the customer line. Some pharmacies have a waiting area for the line that is a few paces from the counter to give the person being served some privacy.

Outside of the immediate pharmacy work area, such as in the lunch break room, at home, or with friends, avoid any discussion of patients and their medications. No PHI can leave the pharmacy premises.

Prescription Pickup

A patient's illness can often be determined by their medication history. A patient receiving antiviral prescriptions for HIV, antibiotics for gonorrhea, antivirals for herpes, antidepressants, erectile dysfunction drugs, or chemotherapy requires the same amount of privacy as in a physician's office or the hospital. Many states have specific laws protecting patients with HIV or acquired immune deficiency syndrome (AIDS).

Because of this, when a patient is picking up a prescription, speak in a low voice when confirming their identity and what medication is being picked up, so as not to broadcast to nearby customers what the patient is receiving. If someone else is picking up a medication, especially for a controlled substance, many pharmacies have a policy of requesting and recording a photo ID, such as a driver's license. Many pharmacies now have a separate area for prescription pickup and counseling, where the patient can have a higher degree of privacy.

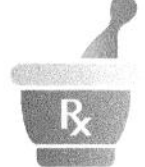

Practice Tip

As a part of the healthcare profession, you must adopt a helpful, no-nonsense, professional attitude toward the body and its functions.

Customer Retail Sales Privacy

If a patient cannot trust the pharmacist or the pharmacy technician with personal health information, then a good customer will be lost. That is why, in addition to HIPAA regulations, the pharmacy technician needs to be sensitive and respectful of customer privacy regarding retail health purchases and information. Pharmacies sell many products related to private bodily functions and conditions (e.g., condoms and other contraceptives, feminine hygiene and menstrual products, suppositories, hemorrhoid remedies, enemas, adult diapers, catheters, bed pans, pediculocides). Customers often are embarrassed to ask about such products and have to work up the nerve to request assistance.

Responding to an inquiry about such a product with efficiency, courtesy, respect, and a certain degree of nonchalance often relieves your customer's embarrassment and demonstrates your professionalism. Speak in a clear voice but not so loudly that other customers or employees are privy to your private exchange with the customer. For patients who request specific product information that requires expertise or counseling, technicians should refer these patients to the pharmacist.

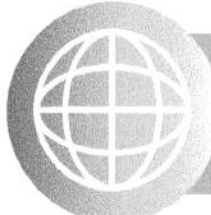

IN THE REAL WORLD

In 2015, a Denver pharmacy was fined $125,000 for a HIPAA violation for improperly disposing of protected health information on 1,600 patients in an unlocked container. The information was not shredded but was simply discarded in general trash. The pharmacy was also required to develop written policies and procedures and institute a staff training program.

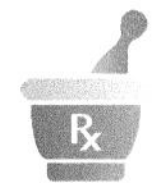

Practice Tip

Per HIPAA, personal information on the labels of medication containers (including IV bags and other compounded sterile preparations [CSPs]) must be removed or covered before disposal. Many are incinerated rather than being thrown in the trash.

Disposal of Patient Protected Information per HIPAA Guidelines

PHI must never be thrown in the general trash. If patient-identifying information is discarded in the trash by mistake and recovered, the pharmacy would be subject to a considerable fine from the federal government.

In the pharmacy, shredding (or burning) of all printed patient-related information is common practice, where it denotes the patient name, address, date of birth, prescription number, or other personal identifiers. This encompasses the whole range of medication container labels, information sheets, insurance information, prescription vials, patient profiles, insurance or Drug Utilization Reviews, and so on. All must be discarded appropriately for privacy protection. If not shredded, this information must be discarded in a special designated container (not accessible to the public) that is incinerated or sealed and mailed for incineration. Electronic PHI must be regularly purged or destroyed per pharmacy policy to prevent misuse.

As a technician, you must be vigilant about following HIPAA regulations. If you see potential violations, bring them to the attention of your pharmacy supervisor. Maintaining the privacy and security of health information is an extremely important ethical and legal issue.

15.6 Personal Professional Ethics

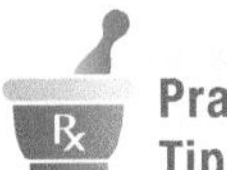

Printed labels and documents containing patient-related information must be shredded or incinerated for proper disposal.

Not all behaviors in pharmacy practice are done solely because of the law. Moral obligations exist that are not legal obligations, and vice versa. Laws and regulations governing the practice of pharmacy do not always dictate the proper behavior in every situation. **Ethics** puts communal values into **standards** (measures) of conduct and moral judgment based on accepted rights and wrongs of behavior and character. Ethics requires a process of reflection and analysis of options of behavior when the proper course of action is unclear. It is the basis on which to make judgments. In addition, particular individuals, groups, and professions have their own specialized codes of ethics based on their goals and values. Religion often has an influence on personal ethics, but it is not necessarily inherent to religious belief; those who subscribe to no religion also have a sense of right and wrong conduct.

The most important aspect of studying ethics is to internalize a framework or a set of guidelines based on high professional standards to guide your decision making and actions. The old saying is "Forewarned is forearmed." Be aware of the variety of situations you could find yourself in, and discuss them with your professors, colleagues, and the pharmacists with whom you work. You want to act thoughtfully, not react on the spur of the moment. By thinking through your ethical options of response ahead of time, you can avoid the paralyzing quandary of being confronted with questionable circumstances and not knowing what to do.

Professional codes of ethics regarding professional behavior are often written as formal documents (see Figure 15.3) and supported by professional organizations. These statements provide language to aid in the decision-making process when an ethical issue presents itself in pharmacy practice.

Codes of Behavior

Ethical codes of behavior in pharmacy are based on a trusting relationship. Patients have to put their trust in the knowledge, competency, honesty, and integrity of the pharmacist and the technician each time they request a prescription. There are two reasons for this. First, the service and product provided are not standardized; they are unique and personal to the patient's situation and condition. Second, the patient is very vulnerable and can be either physically helped or harmed by the service provided, and the patient does not possess the professional knowledge to oversee the outcome.

For these reasons, pharmacy personnel must be held to high standards of conduct and meet selected criteria. First, pharmacists must know well their specialized body of knowledge, and this enables them to perform their highly useful profession. Pharmacy technicians, as paraprofessionals, are also, by extension, held to higher standards of knowledge and conduct in their everyday practice, compared to cashiers or warehouse clerks. Pharmacy technicians who are certified and/or registered are held to an even higher level of expectations. Technicians, like pharmacists, have a duty to maintain their competence and continually enhance their knowledge through continuing education.

Second, the attitude you possess also influences your workplace behavior and the patient's trust in you. The basic attitude needed is an unselfish concern for the welfare of others called **altruism**. Because many patients on a daily basis feel ill or have serious diseases, technicians and pharmacists can better serve if they can feel and express empathy with the patients and understand them.

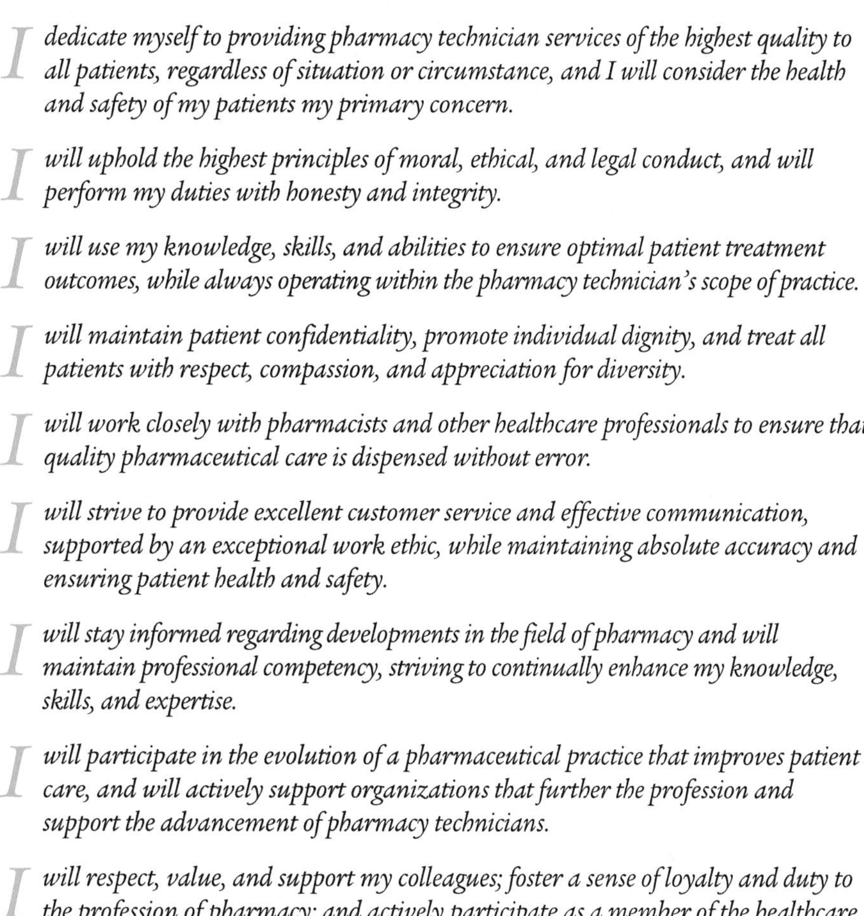

Oath of a Pharmacy Technician

I dedicate myself to providing pharmacy technician services of the highest quality to all patients, regardless of situation or circumstance, and I will consider the health and safety of my patients my primary concern.

I will uphold the highest principles of moral, ethical, and legal conduct, and will perform my duties with honesty and integrity.

I will use my knowledge, skills, and abilities to ensure optimal patient treatment outcomes, while always operating within the pharmacy technician's scope of practice.

I will maintain patient confidentiality, promote individual dignity, and treat all patients with respect, compassion, and appreciation for diversity.

I will work closely with pharmacists and other healthcare professionals to ensure that quality pharmaceutical care is dispensed without error.

I will strive to provide excellent customer service and effective communication, supported by an exceptional work ethic, while maintaining absolute accuracy and ensuring patient health and safety.

I will stay informed regarding developments in the field of pharmacy and will maintain professional competency, striving to continually enhance my knowledge, skills, and expertise.

I will participate in the evolution of a pharmaceutical practice that improves patient care, and will actively support organizations that further the profession and support the advancement of pharmacy technicians.

I will respect, value, and support my colleagues; foster a sense of loyalty and duty to the profession of pharmacy; and actively participate as a member of the healthcare team.

I will strive to conduct myself with professionalism and integrity and maintain a full appreciation of the responsibility that the public entrusts to me.

FIGURE 15.3 Oath of a Pharmacy Technician

Third, knowing that there are consequences for bad behavior helps build trust in the profession. **Social sanctions** are negative repercussions provided by the profession and/or society if trust is broken. Social sanctions come in the form of disapproval of pharmacy colleagues; fines; loss of your job, license, or registration to practice; and legal repercussions.

Because pharmacists and technicians work together so closely and the pharmacist is legally bound for all prescriptions dispensed, society's trust in the pharmacist is being transferred more and more by extension to the pharmacy technician. It is important, therefore, to honor that trust and always seek to do what is right for the patient—at times, that may mean helping the pharmacist fill a few doses of a prescription for a heart or blood pressure medicine for a patient in the middle of the night or on the weekends while awaiting refill permission.

Ethical Dilemmas Facing Technicians

A code of ethics assists healthcare professionals in choosing the most appropriate course of action when they are faced with an ethical dilemma. An **ethical dilemma** is a situation that calls for a judgment between two or more solutions, not all of which are necessarily wrong. Deciding which action to take in the pharmacy requires considering the circumstances, choosing an action, and justifying the action. To do this, you should ask questions such as:

- What is the dilemma?
- What options are available?
- What is the best action or pharmaceutical alternative, and can it be justified on moral grounds?

Pharmacy technicians must recognize and accept the ethical standards of pharmacy practice and apply them when working side by side with pharmacists. They must also understand decision-making processes and become personally involved in obtaining facts that are relevant to a dilemma, evaluating the alternatives, and determining the correct solutions. The following scenarios and the ethical dilemmas that they pose are commonly seen in the pharmacy setting and are worth discussing:

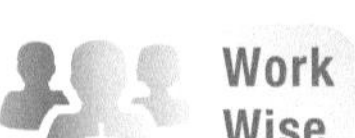

Each community and hospital pharmacy must have policies and procedures in place for such situations. For legal reasons, any refusal to fill must be documented by the pharmacist.

- A prescription or medication order is issued for an abortifacient drug (that is, a drug designed specifically to terminate a pregnancy). You are uncomfortable with meeting that request because you consider the action morally or ethically unsound based on your religious beliefs. Do you have the right to refuse dispensing the drug based on your beliefs? What are your options of action?
- You do not have problems dispensing a drug but the pharmacist does. Does the pharmacist have the right to refuse to fill the drug? What are the options you have, and what do you consider to be the pharmacy's responsibility to the patient in this case? If a pharmacist elects not to fill and dispense the substance, should you refer the patient to another pharmacist who is "on call" to come in and fill the prescription? Or to another local pharmacy?
- Although the physician wrote a prescription for three tablets a day of a blood pressure medication, after conferring with the patient you find out that they are is taking only one tablet a day as directed by the pharmacist. Is this endangering the patient? Was the prescription deliberately written so that the patient can stockpile the medication to last for a longer time to reduce prescription costs? What steps would you take to inquire further into this situation and to work with the pharmacist and the physician about this issue?
- You notice that the technician with whom you work has made numerous errors in calculations of days' supply and dilutions. You don't want to get him in trouble, but you are afraid for patients' health. What do you when you see an error? What do you do when you see a trend? What are your options?
- A friend who is a technician with you boasts about how good her memory is and how all the extra safety checks are a waste of time and she is far more productive than anyone else by cutting just a few unnecessary corners. How do you respond to her? Do you take any additional actions and, if so, why and which ones?

- A patient confides that she has asked the prescriber for several prescriptions that are not needed, because she is giving the extra doses of the prescription to a friend with a similar medical condition who cannot afford insurance or is agoraphobic and is afraid of going out of her home to see a doctor. Are you bound by patient confidentiality and HIPAA regulations not to reveal this confidence? What are the legal (and ethical—later in this chapter) ramifications of this scenario? What are the options and best course of action?

- An out-of-town customer is requesting that you sell him some insulin syringes. Since you do not have a medication profile on this patient, you do not know if the syringes are for the treatment of diabetes or if he is requesting the needles for illegal drug use. What are the legal issues in this situation? What are the ethical considerations?

- An out-of-state customer comes in saying that she is on vacation and her whole family has come down with severe colds, so she is buying a variety of OTC pseudoephedrine products. She does not appear to have a cold herself. What are your options, and how would you respond?

- Someone who has hurt someone you love comes in for a prescription, and now you know that he is being prescribed mental health drugs. You could shame this person for what he did by posting on Facebook that rumor has it that this person is under the care of a psychiatrist and that is why he is so mean. This would make your friend look better and make up for some of what has happened to her. Is this legal, even if you never mention any drugs he is on? What would you do if you found out a colleague had posted something like this?

Other ethical dilemmas with narcotics to consider:

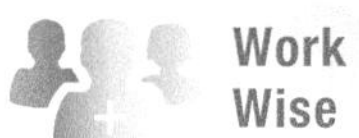

Work Wise

If a pharmacist declines to fill a prescription, the technician should work out ahead of time with the pharmacist the right language to use to communicate this information to the customer to reduce frustration.

- You receive a legal narcotic prescription from an individual who you are fairly certain is selling the drugs on the street. What are some of your options? Do you tell the pharmacist and refuse to fill the prescription or contact the physician?

- You are asked to fill narcotic or sedative prescriptions for a patient who is slurring words and appears to be physically dependent on the drugs. Is intervention necessary or ethically sound? How would you and the pharmacist proceed to intervene? Have the pharmacist check the regional database? Contact the physician? The police? A family member?

- A patient receives three prescriptions from a "pain clinic" but elects to get only the narcotic filled, leaving the other drugs "on profile" for future use. A review of the profile indicates that the patient has not filled any profile drugs for the past six months. What are your options for action? Which is the best one and why?

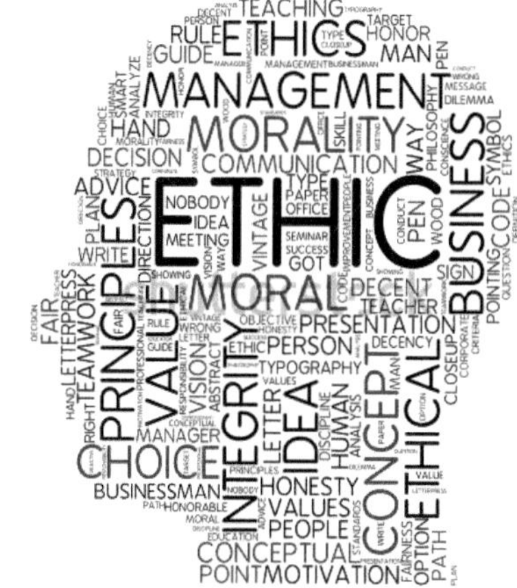

Ethical problems can come up unexpectedly. When unsure how to respond to an ethical problem, consult a supervisor.

- A patient is receiving the same or similar narcotic from two physicians and a dentist. Do you alert the prescribers? Why or why not?

- A specific prescriber seems to be consistently prescribing opioids, not seeming to follow the stair-step approach to analgesics and painkillers. You've heard about the problems of overprescribing these drugs leading to addiction and transferal to heroin. Is this your concern? What options do you have, and which is the best one?

- A patient on Medicaid has received five narcotic prescriptions from three different doctors in the past four weeks. Insurance will not pay for the sixth prescription until next month, but the patient is willing to pay cash. What would you do?

- Your partner is pressuring you as the technician to take just "a few" select drugs because they know you work at a pharmacy. You know that you could probably steal a few tablets of hydrocodone or alprazolam without anyone noticing. Do you keep your relationship or your job?

Each state has its own laws to address ethical dilemmas that come up in pharmacy practice. Be sure that you understand these laws and any internal policies that may cover gaps in the law.

As modern pharmacy practice continues to evolve, new questions will arise that challenge pharmacy personnel in new decision-making deliberations. The answers to such ethical practice questions should certainly come under scrutiny by pharmacy personnel and professional pharmacy organizations. As with any politically, professionally, and emotionally charged topic, a variety of opinions will surface.

15.7 Corporate Ethics/Medical Identity Theft and Fraud

In addition to a personal code of ethics, many organizations have a code of business (or pharmacy) conduct policy that all employees agree to maintain. This policy spells out the highest standards of ethical behavior and professional conduct. For example, personnel cannot take even one dose of a prescription medication without a legal prescription or medication order, even for something as simple as a headache. Any unauthorized sale, possession, use, or diversion of controlled drugs results in termination of employment.

Pharmacies must also abide by state and federal laws, such as the Red Flags Rule (having software systems that set up red flags when potential identity theft or fraudulent activities occur) and the False Claims Act (which imposes penalties on trying to defraud government programs with made-up claims). These laws are meant to protect customers, staff, and the pharmacy itself from identity theft and fraud. The pharmacy must have in place store policies and agreements in which all employees must agree to avoid any pretense of participation in any fraudulent activity or identity information theft.

Besides regular retail billing issues with customer credit and identity information, pharmacies may be subject to medical identity theft—that is, a person who seeks health care (or retail purchases) using someone else's name, credit card, or insurance information. An example of medical identity theft would be a person submitting an altered or forged driver's license for identification. Each healthcare provider is required by federal law to have a policy and a training program in place to help employees spot warning signs or "red flags" to prevent medical identity theft.

Any pharmacy organization that submits claims to a government insurance provider such as Medicare, Medicaid, or Tricare is required by the Department of Health and Human Services to have a training program for all employees on corporate integrity. Any pharmacy organization's billing practices are subject to an annual independent review of compliance. **Compliance** is defined as adherence to a required set of standards, regulations, laws, and practices. The **Corporate Integrity Agreement** is defined as the obligation to report all fraudulent activities under "whistle-blower protection." Such activities may occur in the purchasing of pharmaceuticals or the insurance billing and reimbursement policies.

In terms of billing in a community pharmacy practice, all prepared submissions for online adjudication must be accurate. In light of that, a pharmacy technician *cannot*:

- enter or dispense a false prescription;
- enter an incorrect days' supply;
- backdate an order if a patient's refill prescription has already expired;
- dispense a medication and wait to bill the insurance company until three days later when insurance for the prescription will be approved;
- change a 30-days' supply order to a 90-days' supply order without documented approval from the medical office (in most states);
- dispense an ordered days' supply of medication (such as 10 days) and change the days' supply to five days because the patient's insurance whistle-blower a five-day supply;
- dispense a refill of a drug if the prescription is more than one year old or if a controlled drug prescription is more than six months old;
- add a refill and bill insurance if the patient is out of refills without the prescriber's authorization;
- accept a store or drug discount card or a manufacturer's coupon from a patient who uses a government insurance program–including Medicare Part D;
- bill insurance for a brand name drug and dispense a generic drug;
- dispense a controlled drug, unless the prescription is written on security paper and is being used for a legitimate medical purpose.

Violations of any of these policies could result in disciplinary action that may include termination. If independent audits demonstrate inaccurate billing, the claim will be denied, and the pharmacy will lose both the cost of the drug and the money required to reimburse the government agency for the amount that was submitted. In addition, the pharmacy may be subject to criminal and/or civil monetary penalties if repeated or flagrant fraudulent activity has occurred.

15.8 Safe, Green Pharmacy

What to do with unused medications is also a matter of corporate and professional ethics as well as public safety. Safe disposal in the home, pharmacy, and institutional settings helps to control drug abuse and prevent environmental pollution. Proper recycling of the many plastic and glass drug stock bottles is also best practice for the environmentally sensitive pharmacy.

The issue of disposal is such an important one that the International Pharmaceutical Federation (FIP) has a publication dedicated to the topic. FIP has published the "Green Pharmacy Practice Report for Pharmacists," which recommends increased awareness and education of both pharmacy personnel and consumers. For a view of the initial study report, go to https://PharmPractice7e.ParadigmEducation.com/FIP.

Work Wise

If your pharmacy does not have the capabilities to take back medications, you can help patients find a disposal site by directing them to the locator on AWARxE site: https://PharmPractice7e.ParadigmEducation.com/Disposal.

Take Back the Medications

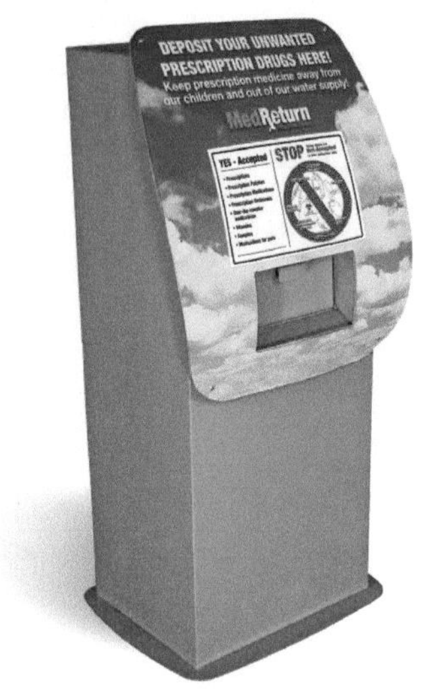

DEPOSIT YOUR UNWANTED
PRESCRIPTION DRUGS HERE!
Keep prescription medicine away from our children and out of our water supply.
MedReturn
STOP

The DEA is helping communities sponsor drug take-back days and location sites.

Pharmacy personnel can educate consumers and help them dispose of their unused medications. Experts say that the first, best option for consumers handling unused or expired medications is to return them to the pharmacy where they were dispensed. Each pharmacy can establish its own safe medication return container. The National Community Pharmacists Association (NCPA) offers a Dispose My Meds program for over 1,600 participating independent pharmacy members. The object is to protect patients and the environment while potentially attracting new patients through this low-cost return program. Pharmacy containers to collect medications are available in either 10- or 20-gallon drop boxes, or pharmacies can give patients convenient postage pre-paid envelopes. Other methods for drug disposal can be found at https://PharmPractice7e.ParadigmEducation.com/Disposal.

If your pharmacy does not yet have such a program, the DEA sponsors a National Prescription Drug Take Back Day event in the spring or fall, and pharmacies can get involved. More information can be found at https://PharmPractice7e.ParadigmEducation.com/TakeBack.

In some communities, local fire departments, hospitals, university pharmacy departments, and/or waste management facilities assist in disposing of medications in an environmentally friendly and safe manner as well. Unused drugs and samples in sealed packaging that have not been tampered with can at times be donated to charity pharmacy clinics.

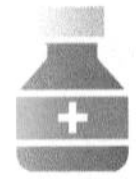

Pharm Fact

By the beginning of 2016, the FDA had reported at least 26 cases of accidental exposure to fentanyl transdermal patches; most of the cases were of toddlers less than two years of age. Sadly, 10 children died and 12 required hospitalization.

Home Drug Disposal

Proper disposal of expired or unused medications at home is also important to the safety of patients, children and young adults, and the environment. Therefore, pharmacy personnel need to discuss options for proper disposal of medications with their patients.

Flushing medications down the toilet is no longer recommended due to adverse effects on the environment. Studies have demonstrated that pharmaceuticals are present in our nation's waterways, and further research suggests that drug traces are appearing in our drinking water and also causing harm to aquatic species in our rivers, lakes, and oceans. These flushed medications include prescription drugs, samples, OTC drugs, and diet supplements. One option for the home disposal of medications is to mix them with some undesirable material like coffee grounds or kitty litter, then put them in a sealed plastic bag or can and place them in the trash.

Scratch out the label's prescription information, and recycle the container.

Patients also need to be counseled on the safe disposal of used transdermal patches that contain medications, especially for the narcotic fentanyl or nicotine (for smoking cessation therapies). Medication remains in the patches, causing serious adverse effects and even death in young children and pets if used or ingested. The patches must be kept out of their reach, so patients should not simply toss them in the trash. Patients can safely discard used patches by folding the sticky sides together and also placing them in coffee grounds or kitty litter, sealing them in a bag or unmarked container, and immediately putting them into a sealed, pet- and child-proof trash receptacle. As noted, flushing used patches down the toilet removes the patches but causes other problems. Unused nicotine patches (as well as nicotine gum and lozenges) are considered hazardous waste and must be discarded per state regulations.

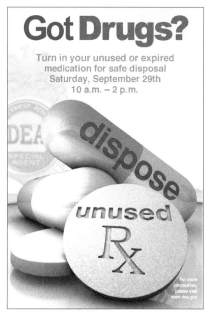

Ask if the pharmacy participates in National Prescription Drug Take Back Day.

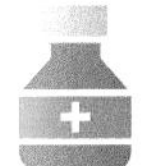

Pharm Fact

More than 100 different pharmaceuticals have been detected in lakes, rivers, streams, and reservoirs. The drinking water of 41 million Americans also has traces of medications that can affect their health.

Community Pharmacy and Institutional Drug Disposal

Proper disposal of all expired or unused pharmacy inventory—medications and syringes—is an important corporate responsibility In the past, liquid drugs (even hazardous agents) were discarded in the sink, drain, or toilet. The Environmental Protection Agency (EPA) has studied the problems of pharmaceutical waste. As a result of those studies, new mandates were issued that declared all expired drugs—of any dosage form—to be hazardous waste. The EPA rules require all healthcare facilities (including hospitals, clinics, physician and dental offices, long-term care facilities, and community pharmacies) to implement an effective plan for the disposal of hazardous pharmaceutical waste, instead of using the drain or trash disposal. Returning expired or unused medications to the wholesaler is the preferred method. The new rules simplify requirements for shipping hazardous drug waste to disposal facilities.

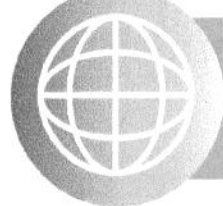

IN THE REAL WORLD

In Tulsa, Oklahoma, a network of over 20 retired physicians go on rotational visits to 68 long-term care facilities to pick up unused medications. They transport these to Tulsa County's low-cost pharmacy clinic to be dispensed for free to those who cannot afford the medications they need. The program started in 2004. As of June 2019, over 241,260 prescriptions have been filled, with a value of over $24 million. Because the program is run with volunteer help, it has cost only $6,000 of administration time to accomplish this, putting these medications to good use for poor county residents and keeping the medications from the detrimental waste stream, saving safe disposal costs.

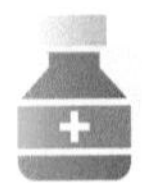

Pharm Fact

Over four billion prescriptions are filled in the United States every year, and it has been estimated that as much as a third of the dispensed medication goes unused—leading to potentially 200 million pounds of pharmaceuticals that can be abused or adversely affect the environment if disposed of improperly.

Medications Recovered for the Less Fortunate

It is estimated that between 10% and 30% of prescribed drugs are never used. In some areas, networks of retired physicians and pharmacists are collecting unused, unopened medications from nursing homes and other long-term care facilities to redistribute at low-cost or charity pharmacies. In these situations, the institutional facility must ensure that no tampering has happened to the medications unused by the patients. These programs are run in ways to ensure that controlled substance protocols and documentation rules are met.

Sharps Disposal

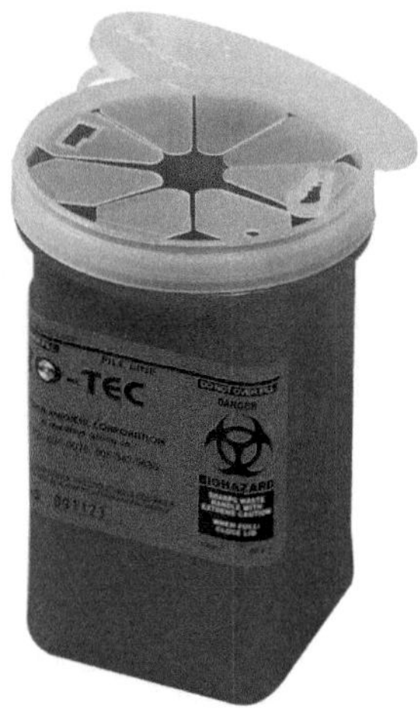

All vaccine and insulin syringes and needles must be disposed of in a sharps container.

As explained in earlier chapters, syringes, needles, and lancets are considered "sharps" and should not be discarded in common trash receptacles, whether at the pharmacy or at home. Since community pharmacies are more and more frequently administering vaccines, they are generating sharps waste. Hospitals and long-term care facilities abound in used sharps. Proper disposal of all sharps is critical not only to the safety of individuals, but also to the prevention of communicable diseases, such as hepatitis or HIV. It is mandatory that all of these items be thrown away in a sharps container. The sharps container should be placed in the pharmacy in a secure location away from children, and when nearly full (75%), it should be sealed, labeled, and mailed to a designated vendor according to pharmacy protocol.

More than eight million patients every year are self-administering injections (such as insulin, allergy shots, vitamin B12, blood thinners, and hormones) while at home. Unfortunately, this increased patient use of sharps has resulted in an increase in improper waste disposal. According to the US Environmental Protection Agency, over three billion needles, syringes, and lancets are improperly disposed of each year.

A vast majority of these are from diabetic patients. All diabetic patients on insulin or checking their blood sugar at home should be encouraged by technicians and pharmacists to purchase a rigid, puncture-resistant, hard plastic sharps container from their community pharmacy to dispose of all sharps safely. Proper disposal of sharps protects everyone–family members as well as garbage disposal workers–from the risk of injury or infection that comes with contact with the trash. Sharps, including needles, lancets, and razor blades, can also be placed in the hard plastic containers that once held oral tablets for safe disposal in the trash.

For more information, "Community Options for Safe Needle Disposal" can be found at https://PharmPractice7e.ParadigmEducation.com/SharpsDisposal.

Waste and Recycling

During the day, a typical pharmacy as a business will accumulate a great deal of waste. Several times during the day a pharmacy technician may need to empty the trash baskets, seal the trash bags, and bring them to a trash bin for pickup or incineration. No syringes, needles, medications, or protected patient information should be discarded in the common trash receptacles. Responsible pharmacies participate in a store- and hospital-wide recycling program, making available appropriate receptacles for correct disposal of each different type of recyclable material, from plastics to paper. If your pharmacy is not yet doing so, a query or suggestion can be made about this.

Every pharmacy also accumulates hundreds of empty plastic drug stock bottles each day. Most are eligible for recycling. Many pharmacies allow patients to bring their empty medication bottles back for a refill of the exact same medication rather than starting a new one. So it is a good practice to ask patients if they brought their old container and would like it refilled.

Developing countries are in desperate need of medication containers! Many patients in places such as Malawi have to leave a rural clinic or hospital with their pills wrapped in torn pieces of paper. Patients in the United States can collect their containers, wash them in dishwater or with boiling water to clean them and remove the labels, and then send to collection groups for those in need. Some charity organizations in the United States accept them as well, such as free medical clinics and homeless shelters, veterinary clinics, and hospitals.

Also, it is a good idea to remind patients (in person or with posters or flyers) that, after being washed, medication containers can be useful around the house for storage of many small items, such as buttons, fishing hooks, or bobby pins.

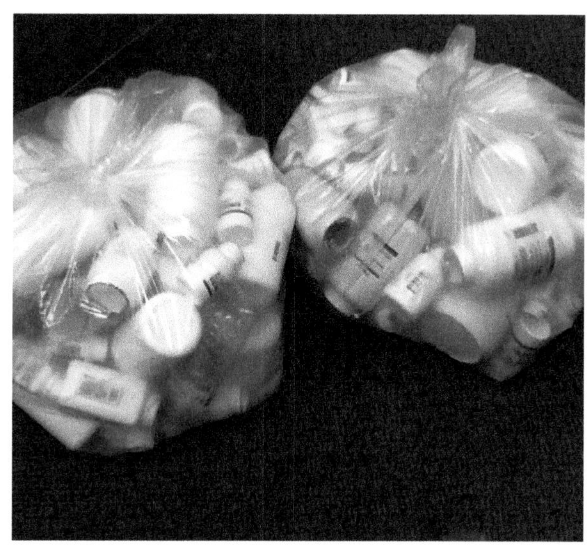

Most empty drug stock bottles are eligible for recycling.

15.9 Emergency Preparedness

In other emergencies, such as epidemics or natural disasters, all pharmacy personnel may be called into action to help support the community. Many personnel may be out sick, and transportation and distribution networks may be seriously compromised. How can your wholesale vendor get medications to you? How can patients from your pharmacy, displaced by floods, tornadoes, or hurricanes, get needed medication? What role can the pharmacy best serve in the community?

Your retail or hospital pharmacy may be asked by the regional health department to volunteer and participate in emergency preparedness drills or real-life emergencies in your local community. In addition to attending planning meetings, all staff must complete educational programs for the pharmacy to prepare and participate fully. An interested technician could assist in planning and serve as a liaison with the health department.

Epidemic Preparedness

If there is a serious epidemic, what is the plan for your pharmacy? Can it be a source of information and education for patients? Can the pharmacy share personnel with the department of public health? What type of protective gear will be available, and which personnel will receive vaccines or antiviral medications if dealing with the public?

Pharmacies, by working with community healthcare resources and emergency planning, can be particularly significant in preserving health and saving lives during times of crisis.

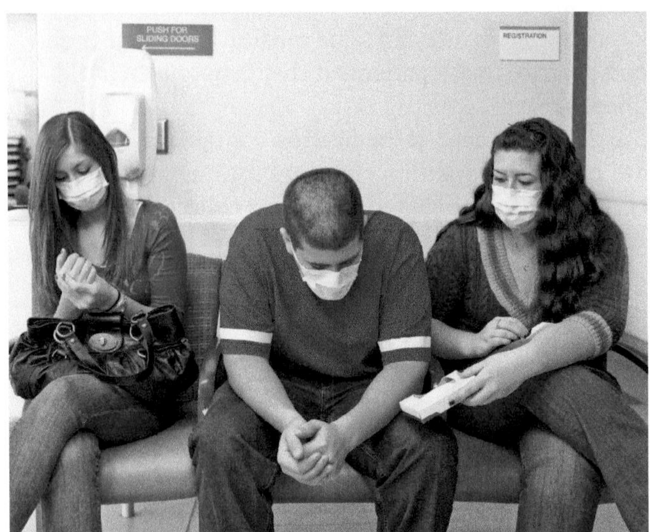

During an outbreak of an easily communicable disease or illness, such as the flu, many healthcare facilities may ask patients waiting for treatment to wear masks to avoid spreading the contagion to others.

If you have specialized lifesaving credentials, such as cardiopulmonary resuscitation (CPR), advanced cardiovascular life support (ACLS) certification, or experience as an emergency medical technician (EMT) or as a medic in the military, then you are a particularly valuable asset to your pharmacy at any time and to your whole community in the time of a health crisis. **Credentialing** is the process for validating the qualifications of licensed professionals and may define what functions and roles pharmacists and pharmacy technicians can perform. Depending on your training and experience and the extent of the crisis, you may be triaging or screening injuries or illnesses in the field, performing CPR, providing necessary medications and supplies to medical personnel, or administering vaccines in times of a regional pandemic or epidemic.

Natural Disaster Preparedness

Natural disasters, such as hurricanes, floods, earthquakes, blizzards, and fires, can be devastating to both a business and a community. If the disaster is more than just a temporary power outage, the pharmacy could lose and not recover customers. An extended power outage affects not only lights, but also heating and air conditioning (and phones) and may have an adverse impact on the integrity of the drug inventory. The alarm systems at the store may not be functional. As covered in Chapter 9, all computer data should be backed up daily preferably, off-site.

If you reside in a high-risk area, it is even more important to have a well-thought-out and well-written disaster plan. That plan should be communicated to employees and followed up with training programs and drills. A pharmacy technician can offer to work with the owner of the pharmacy to develop this plan. Some potential disasters allow some time for advance preparation. Monitoring the National Weather Service may allow the pharmacy to stock up on inventory from its wholesaler, or phone customers to come early to pick up refills. A particularly useful web resource for emergency planning may be found at https://PharmPractice7e.ParadigmEducation.com/Disaster.

The plan should also consider a time to restore and reopen the pharmacy to fill emergency prescriptions, perhaps at a temporary location. The pharmacy should always keep ice chests and coolers readily available, to store refrigerated items such as insulins and high-cost biotechnology drugs.

Communication plans must be thought through ahead of time, before any disaster is pending. How will the pharmacy communicate with its employees and customers? Does it have sufficient information to text on cell phones? Or develop a phone tree? A hard copy of important phone numbers should be readily available. A current list of inventory should be accessible in the event of later liability or insurance claims.

A community pharmacy could collaborate with other local small businesses and serve as a communications hub during a time of emergency. The devastation of natural disasters cannot be prevented, but an effective disaster plan may minimize its adverse impact on a small business and the community.

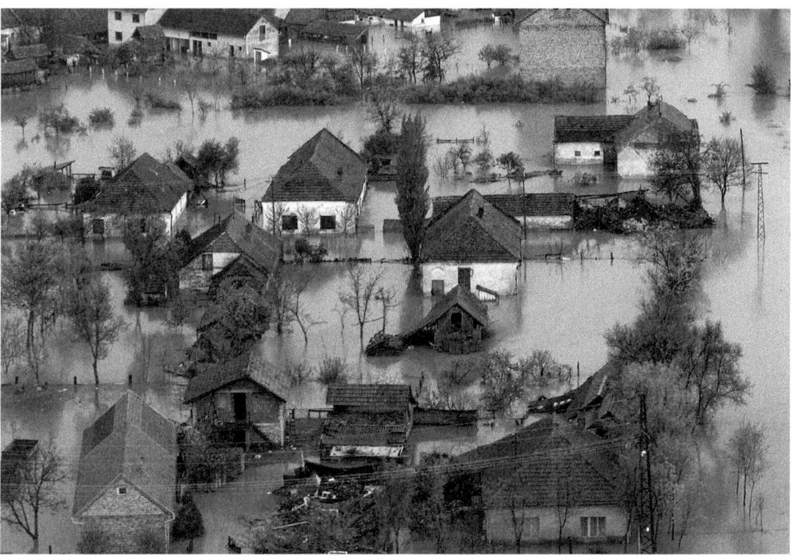

Disasters come in different forms, such as flooding, and though no one knows when they may happen or what they will fully involve, community pharmacies and hospitals have to plan for them.

15.10 The Power of Professionalism

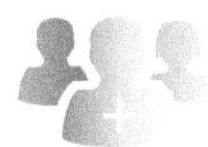

Work Wise

We must be kind and courteous and patient with ourselves, too, in order to be so to others. We all have a learning curve and bad days, and we need to come to work fresh each day, growing from our past mistakes but not carrying them with us into the new day.

Now that you've learned about the ideal criteria for the professional technician, you may be overwhelmed and think, "I would have to be perfect to do this job." We all know no one is perfect, and this is a job where everyone must be constantly learning. It will take time and experience before you feel confident in what you do and have built the work habits that will help you succeed. That is the same for everyone. So you will need to be patient with yourself as you learn skills and professional habits. You will have bad days. You will have challenging tasks, colleagues, decisions, coworkers, bosses, workplaces, schedules, and opportunities. Challenges, though, are good and help us grow, even when we make mistakes, as everyone does.

So the professional rule of thumb is to follow procedures so that the safety checks in place help others catch any errors you make and help you catch the errors that your colleagues, pharmacists, and prescribers make. You are a healthcare team. Expect challenges and rise to meet them. Tell yourself that you can do it, and see the stress of the challenge as the energy to help you meet your goals.

Some workplace infractions, however, will not be tolerated, such as discrimination, harassment, privacy violations, and abuse and theft of drugs. As a trained and certified pharmacy technician, you are entrusted with much responsibility; as such, much will be expected of you. The pharmacy is an essential component of any community; in the case of epidemics and natural disasters, pharmacy personnel will be needed to provide drugs, vaccines, and medical supplies to their community. A pharmacist and by extension the pharmacy technician remain high in the public trust of all professions in all Gallup surveys. Be sure to keep that trust.

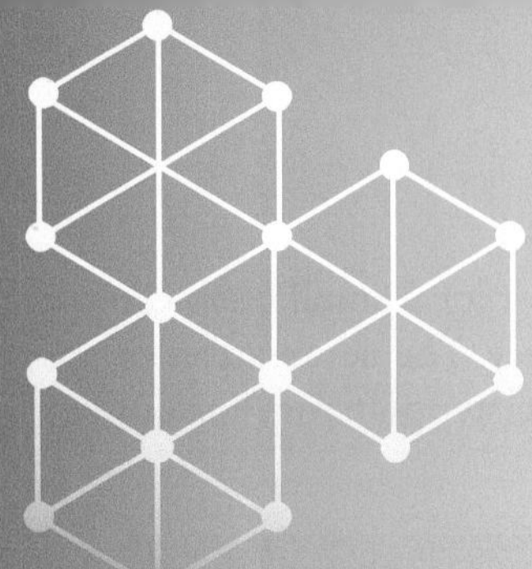

Review and Assessment

CHAPTER SUMMARY

- Community pharmacies are returning to the concept of personalized customer-oriented services.
- Customer service involves appearance, such as professional attire, grooming, and personal hygiene.
- Customer service also involves coming to work with the right attitude to be empathetic and helpful to the needs of the patient.
- Skills in both verbal and nonverbal communications are necessary to obtain information and provide good customer service.
- Extending common courtesies in person and over the telephone contributes to an overall good impression of the pharmacy.
- The pharmacy technician should be helpful, understanding, and sensitive to language, gender, religious, cultural, and other differences.
- Providing customer care to a patient with a mental or physical disability may provide a challenge to the technician.
- Problem solving with insurance issues or calming down an angry patient are important skills for a technician working in a community setting.
- Teamwork is an essential quality to providing good customer care.
- A pharmacy technician must be sensitive to maintaining patient privacy, confidentiality of medical information, and compliance with all state and federal HIPAA regulations.
- A pharmacy technician must exhibit ethical personal behavior and act in accordance with both a personal and a corporate code of ethics.
- Ethical dilemmas exist in pharmacy practice and must be resolved following pertinent state laws and the policies and procedures of the pharmacy.
- Technicians should be aware of the green pharmacy practices available in their practice setting and locale, and should implement them wherever possible to protect themselves, the patients, and the environment.
- Technicians can educate patients on how to properly dispose of their medications, sharps, and medicine containers at home, and how to take advantage of take-back programs and events for unused medications.
- Pharmacies need to plan for emergencies and natural disasters so they can continue, if possible, to serve patients through troubled times.

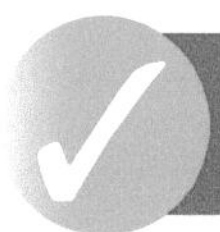

CHECK YOUR UNDERSTANDING

Take a moment to review what you have learned in this chapter and answer the following questions.

1. *Decorum* can be defined as
   a. proper or polite behavior, or behavior that is in good taste.
   b. dissatisfaction with services provided.
   c. lack of understanding of the options available.
   d. the ability to negotiate for goods and services.

2. Lifestyle changes conducive to job professionalism include all the following except:
   a. avoid illegal drugs.
   b. avoid taking breaks.
   c. get sufficient sleep.
   d. exercise regularly.

3. The best way for a pharmacy technician to gather information from the patients to help discern their needs is to ask
   a. the pharmacist to help the patient.
   b. "closed-ended" questions.
   c. "open-ended" questions.
   d. the store manager to help the patient.

4. We live in an increasingly culturally and ethnically diverse society. Identify the incorrect statement on ethnic diversity in the US as discussed in Chapter 15.
   a. Non-Hispanic white populations are trending down.
   b. There are diverse cultural differences within the Asian community.
   c. Hispanic Americans make up 15% of the US population.
   d. The largest minority group, according to the 2014 US census, is African Americans.

5. A *stereotype* can be defined as
   a. an oversimplified characteristic of a group of people.
   b. an open-minded view of individuals.
   c. mistrust of Western medical practice.
   d. the underlying beliefs, attitudes, values, and perceptions that guide a person's choices.

6. A drive-through service would be most beneficial to a patient with a
   a. mental disability.
   b. physical disability.
   c. visual impairment.
   d. hearing impairment.

MAKE CONNECTIONS

Take a moment to consider what you have learned in this chapter and respond thoughtfully to the following prompts. Note that some of these activities will require internet access.

1. Natural disasters, such as hurricanes, floods, earthquakes, blizzards, and fires, can be devastating to both a business and a community. Prepare a 10-15 slide PowerPoint presentation on emergency preparedness recommendations. If you live in a "high risk" area, what is essential? What is the potential impact on Schedule II drugs and drug inventory in general? Use the internet to lookup information on "emergency preparedness in the pharmacy," and share the Rx Response experience developed by PhRMA to assist pharmacies and patients during various natural disasters such as the Sandy and Katrina hurricanes.
2. *Confidentiality* is defined as keeping privileged information about a customer from being disclosed without their consent. Therefore, each pharmacy is required to have a policy statement that defines patient privacy rights and protections and how patient information will be used by the pharmacy, which must be presented to the patient for signed consent. This policy statement is called a notice of privacy practices. In a short essay, describe with whom the pharmacy can share information and what kind of information can be shared without violating HIPAA—family members, health professionals, PBMs? Can a family member request "end of year" tax records for himself and his spouse? Why or why not? What is required? What information can be requested from the prescriber with and without permission of the patient?

 The online course includes additional review and assessment resources.

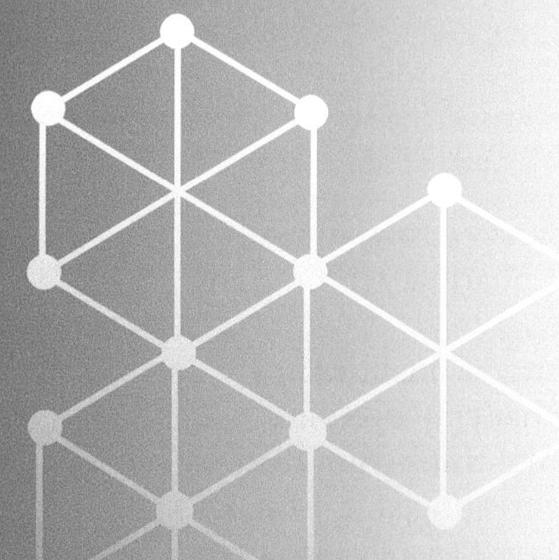

16 Your Future in Pharmacy Practice

Learning Objectives

1. Give an overview of gaining experience as a pharmacy technician, including externships and internships. (Section 16.1)
2. Describe the preparation and application process for taking the certification examinations.
3. Compare and contrast the format and content of the PTCE and ExCPT certification examinations. (Section 16.2)
4. Identify the criteria for recertification of pharmacy technicians. (Section 16.2)
5. Outline a plan for a successful job search using networking and social media. (Section 16.3)
6. Write an effective résumé and a cover letter. (Section 16.3)
7. Prepare for a job interview. (Section 16.3)
8. Identify desirable characteristics and skills that employers are seeking. (Section 16.3)
9. Describe the performance review process. (Section 16.3)
10. Identify future advanced roles and career paths within pharmacy and other healthcare professions for a technician. (Section 16.4)
11. Discuss the importance of technician involvement in professional organizations and networking with colleagues. (Section 16.5)

ASHP/ACPE Accreditation Standards
To view the *ASHP/ACPE Accreditation Standards* addressed in this chapter, refer to Appendix B.

The past 50 years have seen dramatic changes in the pharmacy profession, especially as the roles of pharmacists and technicians have expanded. More exciting changes are afoot as states and pharmacies are requiring standardized and more formalized (and ASHP-accredited) education and training of pharmacy technicians along with national certification. State boards of pharmacy, community pharmacies, and hospitals are seeing how necessary these standards are to safely and efficiently fill prescriptions and assist pharmacists in the ASHP's Practice Advancement Initiative.

Technicians in the field are also finding that they can advance more quickly in their careers if they pursue continuing education, garnering more healthcare certificates, such as for sterile compounding, Basic Life Support (or CPR), or phlebotomy. These certificates lead to greater responsibilities, recognition, pay, and placement opportunities in various employment settings, including community pharmacies, hospitals, long-term geriatric care and home healthcare pharmacies, and specialty practices such as sterile infusion and nuclear pharmacies. There

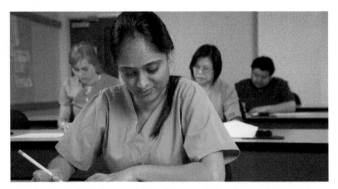
Continuing education and learning new job-related skills are key to career advancement.

are also a variety of advanced roles in management functions for pharmacy technicians to consider.

What are the desirable qualities in a pharmacy technician that employers are seeking? You will learn to think from their point of view. Tips for creating an eye-catching cover letter and résumé as well as ways to prepare yourself for a job interview are covered. You will also learn how to get your foot in the door and stay current and active in the pharmacy profession as a whole.

16.1 Gaining Experience

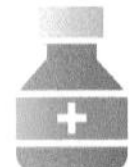
Pharm Fact

Students who are part of a CTE (career and technical education) program have an honor society they can 7 that offers support and scholarships. Membership may be attractive to potential employers. To learn more about the National Technical Honor Society (NTHS), go to: https://PharmPractice7e.ParadigmEducation.com/NTHS.

Today's employers often tend to expect more of their technician applicants than they have in the past, including experience and certification. Since you are in the midst of an academic and formalized training program, you are already on your way toward a career as a pharmacy technician and perhaps eventually positions in medically related fields. Since experience counts greatly, more and more educational programs are requiring hands-on laboratory experience and externships, and encouraging internships.

Externships

An **externship** is a temporary, short-term student work experience, usually arranged by the school as part of the program. Schools typically want students to have two externships—one at a community (ambulatory, outpatient) pharmacy and one at an institutional pharmacy, preferably a hospital. At the externship, students are assigned to a **preceptor**—an experienced practitioner from the externship facility who instructs and supervises at the site. The preceptor facilitates the practical learning experiences. Ideally, you will perform specific tasks in these externships that fit ASHP-based objectives. You will be assessed for skills competence and areas of strength and weakness. Some of the areas to be assessed include the following:

- dispensing (and insurance in community pharmacy settings)
- inventory (and billing in community pharmacy settings)
- storage and control
- communication
- documentation
- error prevention and quality control
- work ethic

In addition, the ambulatory pharmacy offers learning and assessment in community dispensing and retail practice, while the institutional pharmacy focuses on the medication order and unit-dose cart filling practice of hospital pharmacy practice. Most schools arrange these experiences, but, if yours does not, you may approach pharmacists and these types of institutions to see if you can arrange an externship with them, scheduled during their less busy hours.

Internships

Internships are different from externships in that they are official positions where a trained or semi-trained person is hired to handle entry-level duties and work as an apprentice in training. These positions may come with payment or not. Pharmacy technician internships are usually paid and are generally competitive and have to be applied for, as with any job.

For most pharmacy technicians, an entryway to an unofficial internship is to work part-time in the retail area of a community pharmacy or in a hospital nursing assistant, maintenance, or volunteer position. All of these positions, though they are unskilled labor, provide you with valuable experience in the pharmacy work setting and offer you connections and references that could lead to jobs later.

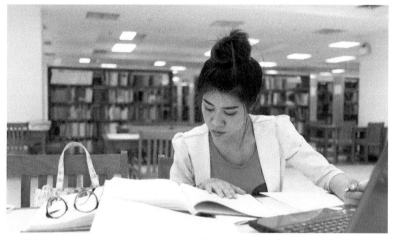

Studying to pass one of the national certification exams is well worth the time.

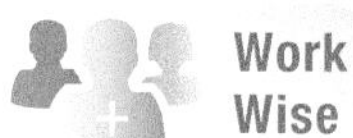

Work Wise

Getting involved in the volunteer activities of pharmacy organizations and doing legislative lobbying with your state board of pharmacy are great ways to meet colleagues and potential employers.

Professional Involvement

Another way to gain valuable experience is to become involved in your school pharmacy club, state professional pharmacy organizations, and local chapters of national pharmacy organizations, such as the ASHP and the APhA. They often have volunteer projects or committees. At first, you may just observe, but you will learn how **professionals** in your field are thinking and planning for the future. Attending meetings can be a good way to meet people for future job contacts. Not only that, it is a way to affirm the importance of the field you are in and your own commitment to it. You can make valuable friends and swap experiences with other technicians in the field.

Subscribing to *Pharmacy Times* can also provide you with ideas about settings to seek positions in the field while keeping you abreast of the latest news.

16.2 Preparing for the Certification Exam

As explained in Chapter 1, each state has its own requirements for registration, licensure, and certification for practice. More than half the states have made national certification either mandatory or preferred for licensure or practice, and the number of states making this a requirement continues to grow. In states with fewer requirements, employers are often making this requirement on their own to increase their business or facility rates of medication safety and efficiency. The certification requirement is especially common in hospitals, as they desire ongoing accreditation.

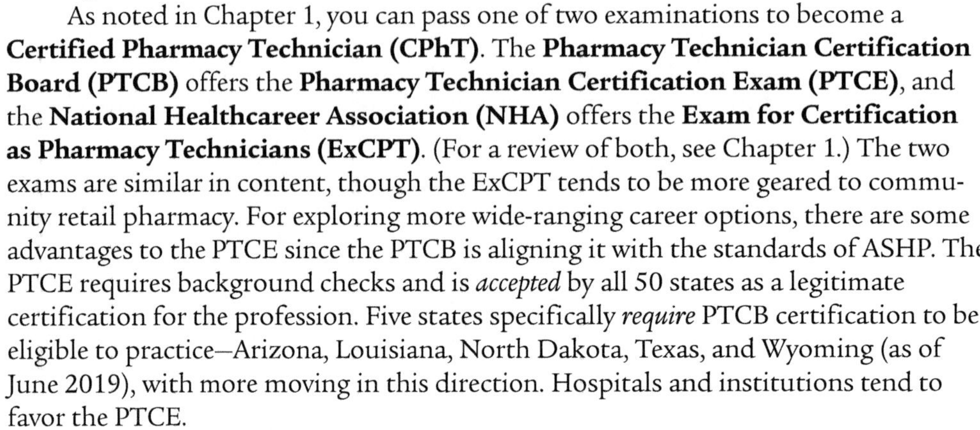

The American Society of Health-System Pharmacists (ASHP) has provided a **model curriculum** and standards for an accredited pharmacy technician education and training program that mandates a minimum of 600 hours—including 160 hours of classroom coursework, 80 hours of laboratory training, and 360+ hours of hands-on practice site experience. A task force of the National Association of Boards of Pharmacy (NABP) has recommended that state boards of pharmacy license or register pharmacy technicians, requiring standardized guidelines for education and training.

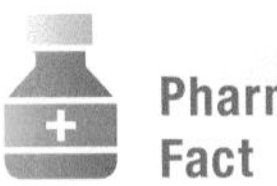

Pharm Fact

The ExCPT is not nationally recognized.

As noted in Chapter 1, you can pass one of two examinations to become a **Certified Pharmacy Technician (CPhT)**. The **Pharmacy Technician Certification Board (PTCB)** offers the **Pharmacy Technician Certification Exam (PTCE)**, and the **National Healthcareer Association (NHA)** offers the **Exam for Certification as Pharmacy Technicians (ExCPT)**. (For a review of both, see Chapter 1.) The two exams are similar in content, though the ExCPT tends to be more geared to community retail pharmacy. For exploring more wide-ranging career options, there are some advantages to the PTCE since the PTCB is aligning it with the standards of ASHP. The PTCE requires background checks and is *accepted* by all 50 states as a legitimate certification for the profession. Five states specifically *require* PTCB certification to be eligible to practice—Arizona, Louisiana, North Dakota, Texas, and Wyoming (as of June 2019), with more moving in this direction. Hospitals and institutions tend to favor the PTCE.

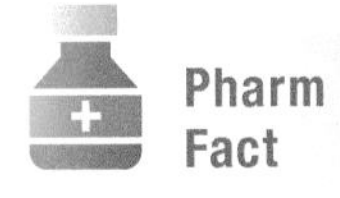

Pharm Fact

Many hospitals favor or require PTCB certification.

The PTCB's executive director, William Schimmel, explained to an interviewer for *Pharmacy Times* that national certification becomes a "portable credential" that can travel from state to state and job to job. "Employers place a considerable value on certification because it demonstrates your knowledge as a technician and your commitment to your role in the pharmacy. As we see things change in the profession and advanced roles for technicians open up, certification will open a number of new opportunities."

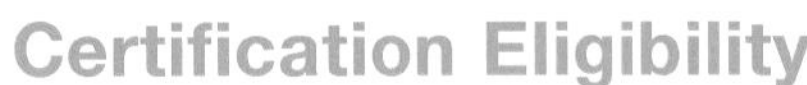

Certification Eligibility

Both certification exams require the applicant to be a high school graduate or to have passed the General Education Development (GED) test or some other equivalency test. You may also have achieved a foreign or alternative diploma recognized by your state and the American Association of Collegiate Registrars and Admissions Officers as indicating sufficient secondary education proficiency. If this has not yet been attained but will be in the next 60 days, you are allowed to sit for either exam. Eligibility requirements for the two national certification tests differ slightly.

PTCE Eligibility

PTCB certification requires a disclosure of all criminal and state board of pharmacy violations. Many academic pharmacy technician programs do a screening of students and also have them complete a drug screening test. As of 2020, the PTCB offers two eligibility pathways for technicians seeking certification. One is the completion of a PTCB-recognized education program. The other pathway is through equivalent work experience.

The PTCB also requires all exam certification applicants and certified personnel to be in compliance with all its policies, including its Code of Conduct, summarized in Table 16.1. The PTCB standards and expectations are outlined on its website and include following all PTCB, federal, state, local, and employer rules and

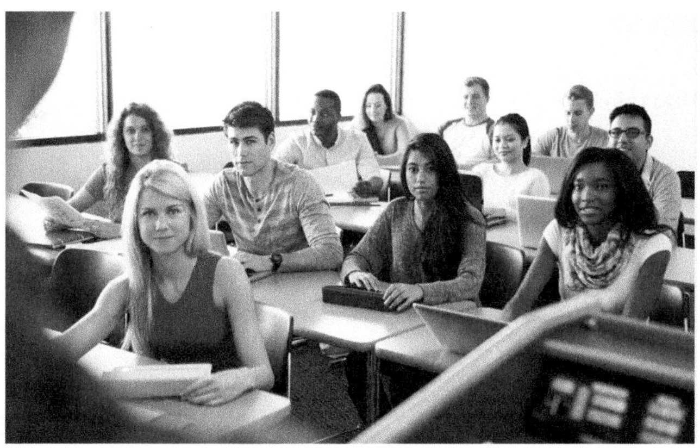
A PTCB-recognized education program can help pharmacy technicians on the path to achieving certification.

laws; upholding professional standards; delivering safe medications and recognizing practice limitations in deference to the pharmacist; maintaining and respecting patient and professional confidentiality; providing truthful representation of one's actions and credentials; following appropriate safety procedures and standards; and avoiding conflicts between patients and employers, among other standards. For more information, visit https://PharmPractice7e.ParadigmEducation.com/PTCB and its code of conduct page: https://PharmPractice7e.ParadigmEducation.com/Conduct.

TABLE 16.1 Code of Conduct and Ethical Expectations for Pharmacy Technicians

The **PTCB Code of Conduct** expects its certified technicians to:

- maintain high standards of integrity and conduct
- accept responsibility for their actions
- continually seek to improve their performance in the workplace
- practice with fairness and honesty
- encourage others to act in an ethical manner consistent with PTCB standards and responsibilities

Source: Pharmacy Technician Certification Board website at https://PharmPractice7e.ParadigmEducation.com/Conduct

The **NHA Code of Ethics** expects its certified professionals to:

- use their efforts for the betterment of society, the profession, and the members of the profession
- uphold the standards of professionalism and be honest in all professional interactions
- continue to learn, apply, and advance scientific and practical knowledge and skills, staying up-to-date on the latest research and its practical application
- participate in activities contributing to the improvement of personal health, our society, and the betterment of the allied health industry
- continuously act in the best interests of the general public
- protect and respect the dignity, privacy, and safety of all patients

Source: *National Healthcareer Association Certification Candidate Handbook* at 6https://PharmPractice7e.ParadigmEducation.com/NHAHandbook

ExCPT Eligibility

In addition to the secondary education requirement, all ExCPT candidates must have completed a pharmacy technician training program from a state-recognized institution within the past five years. In lieu of this, you can have passed an employer-based academic training program that has been approved by the state board of pharmacy or have 1,200 hours of employer-supervised pharmacy-related experience within any one year of the past three years. Those with pharmacy-related training in the military are also eligible. The student must prepare a "candidate profile" and agree to an **attestation statement**, a statement by a witness who verifies that they observed that correct individuals put their signatures on a given document, before sitting for the exam.

The NHA also sets out a high standard of expectations for all its allied health certifications in its NHA Code of Ethics, and it further outlines specifics of behaviors expected for pharmacy technicians to attain and maintain certification. These include, among many other standards, that pharmacy technicians "assist and support pharmacists in the safe and efficacious and cost effective distribution of health services and healthcare resources," "continually enhance professional knowledge and expertise," and "respect and support the patient's individuality, dignity and confidentiality." The list is longer and has been adapted from the American Association of Pharmacy Technicians' Code of Ethics. For more information, go to the NHA website at https://PharmPractice7e.ParadigmEducation.com/NHA.

Preparing for the Exams

Students taking the PTCB exam are encouraged to review *Certification Guidelines and Requirements: A Candidate Guidebook*, which is available online. The NHA suggests that the candidate download its *Candidate Handbook*. Paradigm Education Solutions offers a *Certification Exam Review for Pharmacy Technicians* (in its most current edition), which has an extensive number of up-to-date practice exam questions and has been recommended by many instructors. Practice exams and study guides are also available from the American Pharmacists Association (APhA), *The Pharmacy Technician Workbook & Certification Review*, and other commercial sources.

Both the PTCB and the NHA also offer online study guides and practice exams for a fee. There are other sites that offer them as well. The purpose of the practice exams is to provide the applicant with familiarity with the content, format, and structure of the exam. Schools and other educational groups offer practice tests as well. Instructors have found that the students who take practice tests gain confidence and understanding of what to expect and do better on their exams.

Scheduling and Taking the PTCE

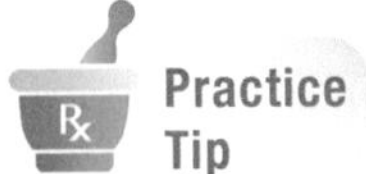

Many employers may pay or reimburse you for taking the PTCE or ExCPT.

There are a few steps involved in scheduling to take the PTCE. First, you must apply online at https://PharmPractice7e.ParadigmEducation.com/Application1.

If the application is accepted, authorization to schedule an exam will arrive via email and be valid for 90 days. Because the test must be taken at a computer-based testing site at one of the Pearson Professional Centers or military testing centers, you must schedule with Pearson VUE via telephone at (866) 902-0593 or online at https://PharmPractice7e.ParadigmEducation.com/Application2.

Be prepared to pay the testing fee (which in 2019 was $129). A confirmation of the test date and place will be sent via email within 24 hours. Candidates who need special testing accommodations must call (800) 466-0450.

You will be given one hour and fifty minutes to complete the 90-question examination. The PTCE is organized into four domains or sections, each of which is weighted differently. Skills and knowledge from both the community and institutional settings are required to pass this examination, including basic compounding knowledge and skills. Table 16.2 details the exam content as specified by the PTCB. Out of the 90 multiple-choice questions, only 80 are scored, and each comes with four possible choices. Only one answer is correct. You should answer every question whether you are sure of the answer or not, because the final score is based on the total number of questions answered correctly rather than the percentage of correct answers. Educated guesses are encouraged. In the final 10 minutes, you will take a post-exam survey and receive your unofficial results on-site.

TABLE 16.2 PTCE Content

1.	**Medications**	**40%**
1.1	Generic names, brand names, and classifications of medications	
1.2	Therapeutic equivalence	
1.3	Common and life-threatening drug interactions and contraindications (e.g., drug-disease, drug-drug, drug-dietary supplement, drug-laboratory, drug-nutrient)	
1.4*	Strengths/dose, dosage forms, routes of administration, special handling and administration instructions, and duration of drug therapy	
1.5	Common and severe medication side effects, adverse effects, and allergies	
1.6	Indications of medications and dietary supplements	
1.7*	Drug stability (e.g., oral suspensions, insulin, reconstitutables, injectables, vaccinations)	
1.8	Narrow therapeutic index (NTI) medications	
1.9	Physical and chemical incompatibilities related to non-sterile compounding and reconstitution	
1.10	Proper storage of medications (e.g., temperature ranges, light sensitivity, restricted access)	
2.	**Federal Requirements**	**12.5%**
2.1	Federal requirements for handling and disposal of nonhazardous, hazardous, and pharmaceutical substances and waste	
2.2*	Federal requirements for controlled substance prescriptions (i.e., new, refill, transfer) and DEA controlled substance schedules	
2.3	Federal requirements (e.g., DEA, FDA) for controlled substances (i.e., receiving, storing, ordering, labeling, dispensing, reverse distribution, take-back programs, and loss or theft of)	
2.4*	Federal requirements for restricted drug programs and related medication processing (e.g., pseudoephedrine, Risk Evaluation and Mitigation Strategies [REMS])	
2.5	FDA recall requirements (e.g., medications, devices, supplies, supplements, classifications)	
3.	**Patient Safety and Quality Assurance**	**26.25%**
3.1	High-alert/risk medications and look-alike/sound-alike (LASA) medications	
3.2	Error prevention strategies (e.g., prescription or medication order to correct patient, Tall Man lettering, separating inventory, leading and trailing zeros, bar code usage, limited use of error-prone abbreviations)	
3.3*	Issues that require pharmacist intervention (e.g., Drug Utilization Review [DUR], adverse drug event [ADE], OTC recommendation, therapeutic substitution, misuse, adherence, post-immunization follow-up, allergies, drug interactions)	
3.4	Event reporting procedures (e.g., medication errors, adverse effects, and product integrity, MedWatch, near miss, root-cause analysis [RCA])	
3.5*	Types of prescription errors (e.g., abnormal doses, early refill, incorrect quantity, incorrect patient, incorrect drug)	
3.6	Hygiene and cleaning standards (e.g., handwashing; personal protective equipment [PPE]; cleaning counting trays, countertop, and equipment)	

continues

TABLE 16.2 PTCE Content—*Continued*

4.	**Order Entry and Processing**	**21.25%**
4.1*	Procedures to compound non-sterile products (e.g., ointments, mixtures, liquids, emulsions, suppositories, enemas)	
4.2*	Formulas, calculations, ratios, proportions, alligations, conversions, Sig codes (e.g., b.i.d., t.i.d., Roman numerals), abbreviations, medical terminology, and symbols for days' supply, quantity, dose, concentration, dilutions	
4.3*	Equipment/supplies required for drug administration (e.g., package size, unit dose, diabetic supplies, spacers, oral and injectable syringes)	
4.4*	Lot numbers, expiration dates, and National Drug Code (NDC) numbers	
4.5	Procedures for identifying and returning dispensable, non-dispensable, and expired medications and supplies (e.g., credit return, return to stock, reverse distribution)	

*Some or all of this statement reflects calculation-based knowledge.

Scheduling and Taking the ExCPT

To schedule your ExCPT, you also need to apply online at https://PharmPractice7e.ParadigmEducation.com/Application3.

Once you receive approval to schedule, you can schedule at your school if it is an NHA-affiliated school offering the test or schedule the date at the nearest PSI Testing Center (PSI is an international company specializing in testing). Call (800) 733-9267 or schedule online at https://PharmPractice7e.ParadigmEducation.com /Application4.

The NHA test fee (which in 2019 was $117) may be accompanied by additional PSI fees. NHA-affiliated schools often include the fee for the exam in the costs of the school program. If special testing accommodations are needed, you must fill out a form at the NHA website: https://Pharm Practice7e.ParadigmEducation.com /Application5.

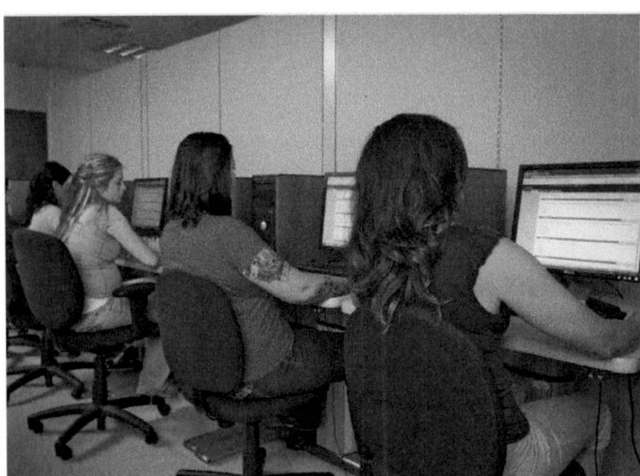

Both the PTCE and the ExCPT are offered at computer testing sites.

Though the ExCPT can also be taken as a paper test at some sites (bring two number 2 pencils and an eraser), it is generally offered as a computer-based examination. The ExCPT seeks to ensure that you can properly assist pharmacists in dispensing medications by receiving and processing prescriptions from patients and from doctors' offices, establishing and maintaining patient records, accurately measuring medication amounts, packaging and labeling the medications, accepting payments and processing insurance claims, and managing inventory. Test takers are given two hours and ten minutes to complete the 100 multiple-choice questions (and 20 pretest questions) from a large test bank. The content for the graded exam is weighted approximately as follows:

- 25 questions on regulations (including controlled substances) and technician duties
- 15 questions on drugs and drug products (Top 200 Rx and Top 100 OTC products)

- 45 questions on the dispensing process (including calculations and compounding)
- 15 questions on medication safety and quality assurance

A detailed breakdown of each of these categories can be downloaded under the ExCPT Test Plan at https://PharmPractice7e.ParadigmEducation.com/TestPlan.

Taking the Exams

The night before you take the test, get a good night's sleep, and have something to eat in the morning before the test. Don't be afraid of test-taking stress. It is not a bad sign, but it shows instead that your body and mind are recognizing a challenge and preparing to meet it. Use the sense of stress to motivate yourself to study ahead of time, and understand that stress is a natural part of the process and should not be feared but applied to help you focus.

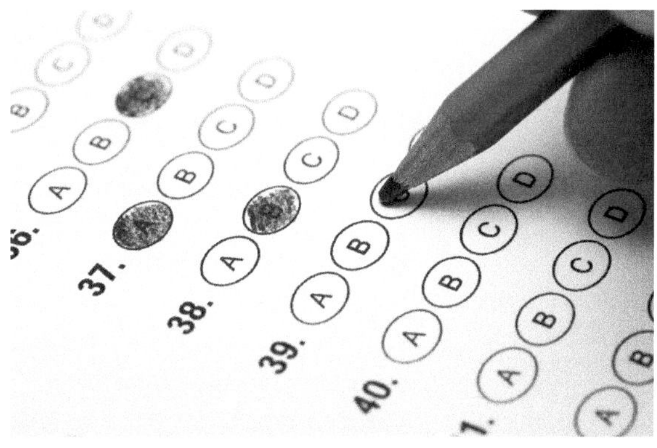

Both the PTCE and ExCPT are offered by computer. For a paper exam, students must go to a special site or make a request for accommodation.

On the day of the scheduled exam, you should arrive at least 30 minutes early (having made sure ahead of time that you have the directions and know where to park). Be sure to bring valid identification, which is defined as an unexpired, government-issued ID with photograph *and signature*. Common valid IDs include a driver's license, a passport, or a military ID. If the identification does not include a signature, a secondary ID will be required. This could be a Social Security card, a credit/debit/ATM card, or an employee/school ID.

Personal items will be stored in a provided locker. No electronic devices such as cell phones, tablets, or calculators are allowed in the testing room. Calculators will be provided online or will be available upon request from the testing monitor. The applicant must agree to all PTCB or NHA testing policies prior to starting the appropriate exam.

Grading of the PTCE

As noted, before leaving the test site, you will receive unofficial results, with the official results being emailed to you and/or posted on the PTCE website in two to three weeks. According to the PTCE scoring blueprint, the range of possible scores is 1,000 to 1,600, and 1,400 or higher is passing. The PTCB reports that, since its inception, the test has been rigorous, with numerous math and drug questions—an average of 57% of the scored exams qualified the test taker for certification. With the new ASHP standards, the test has become even more rigorous. You can take it four times, though you must wait 60 days between attempts (you must reapply and pay the fee each time). The official certificate that recognizes you as a Certified Pharmacy Technician (CPhT) will arrive in the mail in four to six weeks.

Grading of the ExCPT

The ExCPT is immediately graded, and students at the PSI testing centers find out whether they passed or not. The scores are confidentially posted on the NHA website within two days. The scores range from 200 to 500, converted from the raw test scores and weighted question system. A passing score is 390 or above. Those who successfully pass the ExCPT will receive a formal CPhT certificate and wallet card within 7 to 10 business days of the exam date. Candidates who do not pass the ExCPT are allowed to retake the exam after four weeks. You can log into your account at the NHAnow.com website for a diagnostic of your test and recommendations for improvement.

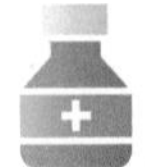

Pharm Fact

For PTCB recertification, 10 credits may be related college courses but 10 must be pharmacy specific, with 1 credit in medication safety and 1 credit in pharmacy law. Free credits can be found at Power Pak C.E. For registration, go to https://PharmPractice7e.Paradigm.Education.com/Powerpak.

Recertification

Recertification is required by both the PTCB and NHA every two years to maintain certification status. To be recertified, you must earn 20 hours of credit in pharmacy-related, approved continuing education (CE). Both ExCPT and PTCB recertification requires one hour of continuing education in medication or patient safety and one hour in pharmacy law. Acceptable CE topics include drug distribution, inventory control, managed health care, drug products, therapeutic issues, patient interaction, communication, interpersonal skills, pharmacy operations, prescription compounding, calculations, pharmacy law, preparation of sterile products, and drug repackaging.

Certificates of participation must be obtained for each CE program. Pharmacy-related continuing education may be provided by professional organization meetings and websites, employers, and professional journals. In some cases, applicable college courses where students received a grade of C or better may also be eligible for CE credit.

16.3 Preparing for the Job Search

Job applicants with pharmacy experience, formalized training, *and certification* are considered to be more qualified than other applicants without such credentials. These, then, are the best base credentials. However, other elements, such as additional allied health certifications and varied job, volunteer, and leadership experiences, are all elements considered by employers when choosing whom to hire.

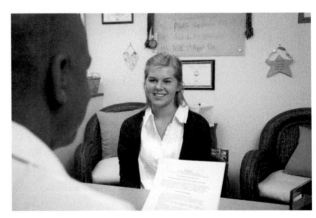

Job candidates with a wide arrange of experience fare the best when it comes to finding choice positions.

How can you get the one job you really want? Many people find the prospect of job hunting overwhelming. Try to avoid such negative thinking. Break the process into smaller steps, each one very doable. The following suggestions will help you on the path to a new job, and hopefully one you like.

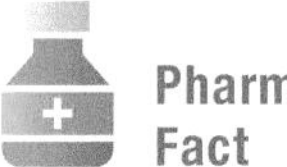

Pharm Fact

According to the National Pharmacy Technician Association, there are more than 39,000 jobs for technicians available every year.

Identifying Your Career Goals

Finding a job is difficult if you are not sure what you are looking for. Do you want to work in a community pharmacy? Do you want to work in a hospital, a compounding pharmacy, or a home infusion pharmacy?

Consider your externship experiences. What were the pros and cons of the different settings? If you were not able to gain experiences in some of the settings you may find attractive, approach a pharmacist or a technician in one of these work environments and ask politely if you might interview them. Make sure that you approach the individual at a downtime when there is little pressure or stress, such as "on break" or at lunch. Other technicians and previous graduates of your educational program can also provide valuable information about job settings and hiring practices.

Personal Survey

Think about what you want out of a job. Do you love dispensing and customer care and want to focus on these skills? Are you interested in jobs with opportunities for advancement in management, such as store manager in a chain pharmacy or as a senior pharmacy technician in the hospital? Do you want to eventually master the preparation of sterile products or the compounding of nonsterile products or specialize in ordering, inventory, and billing? Later in this chapter various career paths within and outside the profession will be discussed.

Consider how you would like your work life to fit with your personal life in terms of location, family responsibilities (including child care if appropriate), pay scale, and schedule. For instance, you often may be working nights and weekends, especially if working in a 24/7 hospital environment. Will that work for you and your family?

Creating a career is a gradual, step-by-step, experience-by-experience, position-by-position process, with each one building on the last or giving you more information about what you like and what you don't, what you are good at and what you aren't, where you are strong and where you need more learning and development.

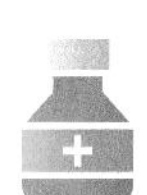

Pharm Fact

Job opportunities for certified technicians are predicted to grow by 12% between 2016 and 2026.

Create some options for the types of jobs that may suit your ambitions, talents, acquired skills and knowledge, and life situation. Be open. Something that may seem different from what you desire, but is currently available, may turn out to be the very position you would have wanted if you had known what it was really like. When you are starting out, you may need to try tasks that you may not like but may open doors that can start you on the path toward a position that you want long term.

Many schools have career counselors who can help you explore such questions. Check with your instructor or make an appointment to visit and talk to a career counselor. You may also want to use the internet or the library to obtain more background information.

Informational Interview

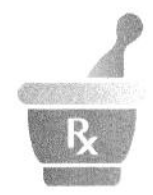

Practice Tip

Handwritten thank-you notes help people remember you well. Lack of a formal thank-you does the opposite.

Once you know more about what you are looking for, start to look for professionals you know or can meet in those settings. People are often very willing to meet for an informational interview, a meeting where you are not directly seeking a job but are desiring to know more about the position. If possible, select a pharmacist or a technician you have met or observed and admire. This will allow you to offer genuine positive comments about their professional manner and show your interest and powers of observation. Such actions may encourage them to go out of their way to share time with you.

IN THE REAL WORLD

Using a combination of data sets, Timothy O'Shea, PharmD, reported in *Pharmacy Times* that the 10 US cities for best work and life opportunities for pharmacy technicians are the following:

- Memphis, TN
- Spokane, WA
- Ogden-Clearfield, UT
- Burlington, NC
- Yakima, WA
- Iowa City, IA
- Santa Cruz, CA
- Edison-New Brunswick, NJ
- Stockton, CA
- Yuba City, CA

Rankings were calculated using weighted percentages of mean annual salary, number of jobs, cost of living, location quotient, and placement in Livability's 2016 Top 100 Best Places to Live list. For the full article and additional data, go to https://PharmPractice7e.ParadigmEducation.com/BestOpportunities.

Set up a time that fits the pharmacist's or the technician's schedule and preferences rather than yours. Make sure that you prepare for the informational interview by brainstorming questions ahead of time and writing them down. For instance, "What aspects of your job in this setting do you like most?" "What aspects make it the most difficult?" "What is a typical day like?" "A typical hour?" "What aspects are the most stressful?" "How do you handle this stress?" "What are you looking for in a technician in this position?" "What advice would you offer someone like me?"

Hearing the answers to some of these questions and others you have thought of will help narrow down your interests. Make sure that you follow up with a handwritten thank-you note and perhaps a gift or gift card to thank the individual for the time and effort.

Identifying and Researching Potential Employers

If your school has a career placement office, you can find out where it posts job openings registered by local employers. You can also use its career search engines and look up employers in directories.

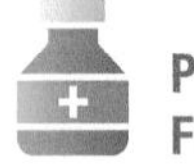

Pharm Fact

Without certification and experience, it will be difficult to land a position in a hospital pharmacy.

You can also explore career opportunities posted on websites and job search websites; most chain pharmacies (Walgreens, CVS, Kroger, Publix, Walmart) require an online application. Your application may be kept on file for job openings at more than one pharmacy in your regional geographic area. Many local hospitals also have websites that are used to post job vacancies; you may apply online or visit the human resources department to complete a written application and complete a screening interview. The classified ads of newspapers in print and online are also good sources of job postings.

Your state board of pharmacy as well as state community pharmacy and hospital pharmacy association offices also often post technician position vacancies. Many have offices or career centers that allow employers to post job openings and a job seeker to search for and browse available positions or post their résumé online. Examples would be the American Association of Pharmacy Technicians (AAPT) and the National Pharmacy Technician Association (NPTA). These associations may be especially valuable if you are relocating to a pharmacy in another state.

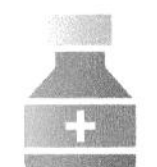

Pharm Fact

Did you know that over 70% of all job openings are never advertised? Employers have their own networks to identify potential candidates for hiring from family, friends, other employees, or business associates.

Thinking Like an Employer

Once you have zeroed in on some jobs you may want, you need to take the steps to apply. The first step is to try to put yourself into the mindset of that employer. What characteristics do you imagine that a pharmacy or human resources manager is looking for in a pharmacy technician? In a retail pharmacy, managers consider customer service. As discussed in Chapter 15, good communication and interpersonal skills are essential for the technician, who interacts with pharmacy coworkers, patients, and other healthcare professionals on a daily basis. In a hospital pharmacy, one must be content having fewer patient interactions but take satisfaction in the organization and efficiency in unit-dose filling or aseptic technique in sterile compounding.

The pharmacy technician in any setting must enjoy performing precise work (math calculations, computer prescription entry) where accuracy can be a matter of life or death. Pharmacy technicians must also be able to maintain this accuracy even in stressful situations or while working on multiple tasks. Finally, all employers want dependable employees who show up for work on time and who are also willing to be flexible in their work schedules and take shifts for others when needed.

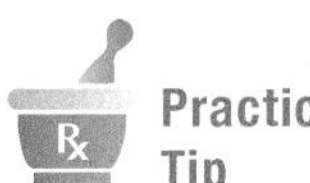

Practice Tip

In the general job market, most people find jobs through someone they know. That is why making a good impression in externships and internships might lead to job offers after graduation and passing a certification exam.

Establishing a Network

Networking is defined as reaching out to meet people with the specific purpose of identifying job leads. Talk to friends in person, give them a call on the telephone, or email them to let everyone know what kind of job you are looking for. Tell everyone you know that you are looking for a job. Identify faculty, pharmacists, acquaintances, friends, and relatives who may be able to assist you in your job search.

Make sure that you dress professionally (suit and tie for men, and modest skirt and jacket or pants and jacket for women). As a technician is unlikely to need a suit for everyday work but will need one for networking and job interviews, remember that consignment and Goodwill shops often have very nice professional clothing at affordable prices.

Be prepared to give an organized, short (less than 30 seconds) sales pitch about yourself, such as your name, occupation, current status, job opportunity you are seeking, and what you can offer. Networking may allow you to learn about a position prior to its posting or advertising.

If you complete any practical on-the-job experiences as part of your training, ask your supervisors and coworkers about anticipated openings. If there are no openings, they may be willing to serve as references for you. If you perform well as a student-in-training, then you will be viewed as a good potential employee at that site or at another pharmacy. If anyone says yes to any request, get their business card, and always follow up with a handwritten thank-you note. This is not only a courtesy, but it helps people remember you and keep their promises. Also, be willing to offer similar job-hunting help to others.

Practice Tip

Social media can be helpful in your job search if you present yourself professionally. Ensure that your online presence is appropriate and something you are comfortable with potential employers viewing. Consider your posts carefully, particularly when addressing controversial topics.

If you are new to the geographic area, check career centers at the state Department of Labor or local churches or civic organizations. A local pharmacist may know of openings in other area pharmacies. Alumni from your school program can be good connections as well. This is one of the advantages of joining in school, local, state, and national professional associations and attending meetings. These are perfect opportunities for networking with colleagues and potential employers.

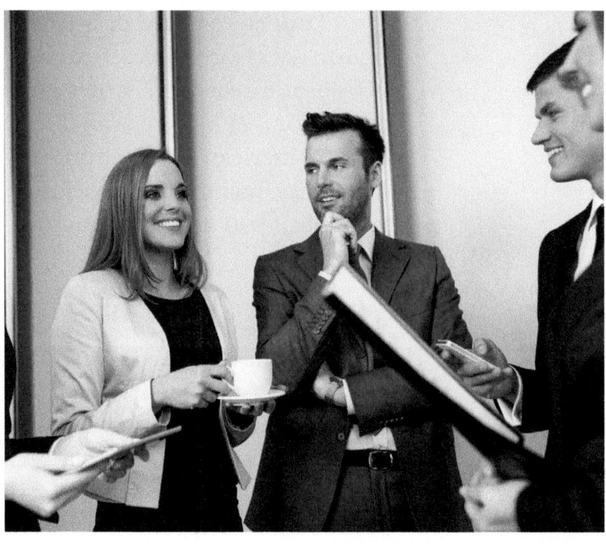

Networking is a powerful tool in your job search.

If you have hospital experience or are seeking an advanced technician pharmacy role, **social media** outlets such as Facebook, Twitter, CareerBuilder, and LinkedIn can provide worthwhile online tools for networking. (They may not be as useful for entry-level positions.) Many of these require posting your job experiences and skills in a short form, with precise language to highlight the experiences desired by potential employers. *Money* magazine reported that 95% of recruiters use or plan to use social media to find and vet candidates for available positions.

Career experts recommend that you include your area of expertise, level of experience, hobbies, and a link to your LinkedIn page so that recruiters can access your résumé. Show your expertise by sharing any web links to news or information in pharmacy that is relevant to your target audience.

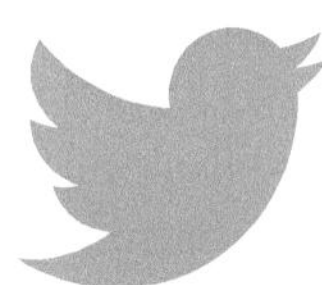

If you are reading *Pharmacy Times* or are involved in professional organizations, you will have more access to interesting news to pass on. If you use Twitter, you are allotted only 280 characters—use them wisely. First impressions count, so include a professional headshot and include your name in your handle, such as "@DonnaTaylor_pharmacy tech." Be careful, however, and consider this tool with your instructor first as it may not be appropriate for entry-level positions and may even be considered annoying. Always use tools that most suit the type of job you are seeking.

Writing a Strong Résumé

Employers and human resource specialists are likely reviewing multiple candidates and need to have a quick, eye-catching overview of each potential hire. You may need to simply fill out an online application for the position you want, or you may need a résumé. A **résumé** is a brief, concise, vivid written summary of what you have to offer an employer. A résumé is an opportunity to present your work experience, your skills, your background, and your education (and certification) to an employer. Even if you only need to fill out an online application with a template, building a résumé is helpful because you can copy and paste the information in—and you won't need to go looking for the information. Table 16.3 outlines the general topics to be included in a chronological résumé.

TABLE 16.3 The Parts of a Chronological Résumé

Heading	Provide your full name, address, and telephone number. Include your ZIP code in the address, area code in the phone number (and cell phone number), and your email address so that a potential employer can contact you.
Education	Provide your high school or college, city, state, degree, major, date of graduation, and additional course work related to the job, to the profession, or to business in general. State your cumulative grade point average (GPA) if it helps to sell you (3.0 or higher). List any honors or recognitions received in high school or college.
Professional Certifications	Provide any professional certifications/licenses, such as your pharmacy technician certification, registration, CPR/first aid, and so on. You may optionally list your certification or registration number, but it is not required—simply state "available upon request."
Experience	In reverse chronological order, list your work experience, including on-campus and off-campus work. Do not include jobs that would be unimpressive to your employer. Be sure to include cooperative education experience. For each job, indicate your position, employer's name, the location of the employment, the dates employed, and a brief description of your duties. Always list any advancements, promotions, or supervisory responsibilities. Be sure to include any certifications, registrations, or licensures on your résumé.
Skills	If you do not have a lot of relevant work experience, then include a skills section that details the skills that you can use on the job. Doing so is a way of saying, "I'm really capable. I just haven't had much opportunity to show it yet." If you have foreign language or computer software skills, be sure to emphasize them.
Related Activities	Include any activities that show leadership, teamwork, or good communication skills. Include any club or organizational memberships as well as professional or volunteer community activities that may help sell your skills. Hobbies and interests may be listed to demonstrate your more personal side.
References	State that these are available on request. Speak to former employers about using them as a reference, and then have a list of references available when an interview is granted.

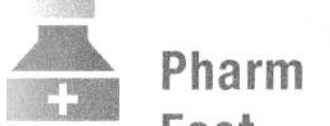

Pharm Fact

October is National Pharmacy Month. Celebrate your key role in health care the whole month by thinking of a way each day that you help people heal, stay healthy, and be safe in their drug therapies.

Collecting Your Information

Building a résumé is intimidating for some people, but try to look at it as a good recap of your achievements. You may be surprised to find out that you have more to offer than you think; one way to start is by brainstorming and free-writing—sketch out on a piece of paper all the jobs you have had even if they were not directly related to pharmacy (include name of company, address, phone, supervisor, dates of employment, and title of your position[s]).

Ask yourself for each position, what did I do each day and bring to the job that was significant? You may have cheerfully and efficiently filled orders at a restaurant. This could be a transferable skill to pharmacy dispensing. Did you get promoted? Gain new responsibilities with time? If so, write these achievements down. Use vivid action words (verbs) to describe what you did, the title, which skills you used there that may be applied to your work in the pharmacy, and what you achieved. For instance, if you worked as a warehouse clerk, then you know how to work with inventory. Or perhaps you were a maintenance worker at a hospital—you learned how the hospital works and the importance of cleanliness and infection control. Or perhaps you worked at a clothing shop; you can highlight your customer service skills and ability to select products unique to the needs of each customer.

Do not forget to consider any volunteer or leadership experiences you have had. Just because you did not get paid does not mean that these experiences are not important. They tell key things about who you are, what you care about, your initiative, and how responsible and self-initiating you can be. Sketch those experiences as "positions" (include name of organization, address, phone, key contact, dates of engagement and leadership, and title of what you did). For instance, you may have been in a club and organized a coat drive for needy children and helped make signs to get the word out to others. This shows drive, compassion for potential community pharmacy customers, and the ability to market an event. These skills could be applied to getting the word out about a flu-shot promotion.

Writing the Résumé

Résumés often follow a consistent, standard format, such as the one shown in Figure 16.1. It always starts with your name in bold and your contact information in slightly smaller type or unbolded type below, generally centered at the top. The next line, which is often listed as the "Objective" but does not have to be, is your first line or two to grab the employer's attention and get them to keep reading. It is also like your thesis statement about yourself—it sums up what you have to offer and highlights the key points you want employers to notice. So make it fit what the employer is looking for. Make sure that it communicates what you have to offer and does not only focus on what you want.

If you are a strong writer, you can choose a format and write your own résumé, but always have a few people read it to give you feedback for revision for format, appeal, readability, and grammatical errors. You can use the Purdue Online Writing Lab, or OWL, for more résumé-writing tips at https://PharmPractice7e.ParadigmEducation.com/ResumeWriting.

There is also some excellent résumé-writing software now available, or you can contact a résumé-writing service. Your résumé is your ad or marketing tool, and the product you are selling is yourself, so you want it to be great.

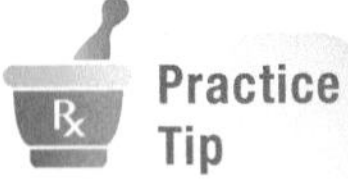

Practice Tip

Mistakes on your résumé may affect your prospective employer's confidence in the accuracy of your work. Consider having several trusted reviewers edit your résumé before submitting it to a potential employer.

Entry-level résumés are best limited to a single page. You can write a base résumé, and use it as the template. Tweak and tailor each résumé and its accompanying cover letter to the specific job and company you are contacting. For each company, do a quick online search (or better yet, visit) so that you know something about the organization and the specific position. Pay attention to the key words used in any job postings, and use a few of those in your résumé if you can do so naturally. You want your résumé to stand out in the crowd of résumés and job applications. You can do this by knowing something about your audience and tailoring your appeal to their needs. For instance, if you are applying to a hospital, emphasize the section in your résumé that has to do with hospital experiences.

If you are sending your résumé by mail or delivering it in person, print it out on high-quality 8½ × 11-inch paper. Special résumé paper is available from stationery and office supply shops. Remain conservative when selecting stationery to convey a professional image.

FIGURE 16.1
Sample Résumé

Kelly Nettleton
1700 Beltline Blvd.
Tate, GA 30107
knettleton@ppi-edu.net; 706-868-XXXX

Objective: As a pharmacy technician, to use my academic knowledge and hands-on skills in pharmacy, attention to detail, and fluency in Spanish to serve customers effectively as a part of a pharmacy team

Education

Diploma, Pharmacy Technician Program August 202X–May 202X
Appalachian Technical College, Tate, GA
Dean's List

Certification

Pharmacy Technician Certification Exam July 202X

Experience

Pharmacy Retail Clerk September 202X to Present
Waleska Pharmacy, Tate, GA
Attend to needs of customers, operate cash register, and stock inventory (part-time job while attending school)

Pharmacy Technician Extern January 202X to May 202X
Waleska Pharmacy, Tate, GA
Assisted the pharmacist and pharmacy technicians in preparing prescriptions and refills, performed inventory management and control, processed and troubleshot third-party insurance claims, provided exceptional customer service to patients and healthcare providers, and performed clerical duties (answering telephones, operating the cash register, filing paperwork, and helping to manage work flow)

Sales Associate March 202X–September 202X
Tommy's Sporting Goods, Canton, GA
Achieved high sales while serving customers and operating cash register

Pertinent Skills

- Proper dispensing skills and insurance processing procedures
- Pharmacy calculation, including conversions, basic formulas, ratio and proportion methods, and alligation
- Careful interpretation of prescriptions and physician's orders
- Compiling and updating patient prescription and allergy histories
- Operation of pharmacy computer systems and software
- Ordering and inventory procedures (both retail and pharmaceutical)
- Preparation of nonsterile compounded prescription products
- Conversational Spanish
- CPR training

Activities

Member, National Pharmacy Technician Association

References available on request.

Be sure to read your résumé aloud word by word to see how it sounds to an employer. Check it numerous times for errors in spelling, grammar, usage, punctuation, capitalization, and form. Once your résumé is complete, always have another person (or a few people) proof it for any typos or final overall impact. Polished résumé in hand, visit retail and hospital pharmacies in the area. If they do not have a current opening, leave the résumé on file for future contact. Introducing yourself in person and handing it to someone is best (if you dress appropriately). If you do this, potential employers see your personal touch and determination, and they are likely to remember you.

If you are submitting your résumé online, be careful to cut and paste your polished résumé into the correct slots. Read it over and proof each section before clicking "send," as you cannot get it back! Online job applications and résumés are convenient but not always the preferred route. The disadvantages of online applications are that they are less personal, the employers have no face to match with a name, there is an increased number of applicants, less room for creative expression, and, occasionally, some fees at the job search website.

Curriculum Vitae

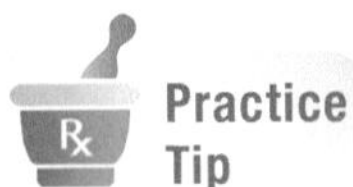

Practice Tip

The cover letter is especially important for online job applications, as the employer may not have the time to review all résumés but will scan the letter to screen for qualifications.

Another form of summing up one's experiences is the **curriculum vitae (CV or vitae)**, also known as an academic vita. This format is used when more detail is needed. It often uses paragraphs to communicate specific themes and is commonly used in academic service. If someday you decide to teach future pharmacy technicians, then you may want to use a CV. Otherwise, it is best to stick to a résumé or an online submission based on a fine-tuned résumé.

Writing a Strong Cover Letter

A **cover letter**, or letter of introduction and application, usually needs to accompany your résumé and set the scene for reading it. It is your first communication to the prospective employer, often in response to a specific job advertisement or postingv , but also for unposted jobs to businesses you would like to work for.

Overview of the Letter

Pharm Fact

Pharmacists may have various degrees or titles: Registered Pharmacist (RPh), Bachelor of Science in Pharmacy (BS Pharm), Doctor of Pharmacy (PharmD). Make sure to get the right one!

The cover letter should highlight your knowledge of the business and suitable qualifications, calling attention to your résumé, preferably in a one-page format. It should be in a business format and have margins of at least one inch on all edges. The cover letter is especially important for online job applications, as the employer will scan the letter for qualifications and personality to decide whether the résumé is worth reading. The cover letter is where your research on the company and position will really come to the forefront.

Hand-delivered or mailed, the cover letter should be printed on the same kind of paper as the résumé, and both should be placed in a matching business envelope. The letter should be single-spaced, using a block or modified block style. In the block style, all text begins at the left margin. (See Figure 16.2 for a sample cover letter and Table 16.4 for the content and format.) In the modified block style, the sender's address, the complementary close, and the signature are left-aligned in the center of the paper, and all other parts of the letter begin at the left margin.

Greeting Line Address the letter, whenever possible, to a particular person by name and by title, and make sure to identify the position for which you are applying. Sometimes it takes extra investigation to find out these details, but it shows initiative and professionalism when the letter is addressed to the specific person (with their

FIGURE 16.2 Sample Cover Letter in Block Style

Diane Stamey, PharmD
Pharmacy Manager
Main Street Pharmacy
1500 Main Street
Tate, GA 30107

February 1, 202X

Dear Dr. Stamey:

Through the placement office at Appalachian Technical College. I was pleased to learn of an opening for a technician at the very pharmacy that my family has frequented for years.

In May, I graduated from Appalachian Technical College's pharmacy technician training program, and I just took the Pharmacy Technician Certification Examination. The preliminary results say that I passed with a high ranking (confirmation will come in two weeks). I would welcome the opportunity to apply what I have learned to a career with your pharmacy. I bring a number of strengths, including a 3.4 grade point average, a commitment to the continuing development of my skills as a technician, a willingness to work diligently and accurately, and a desire to be of service. My fluency in Spanish would also be of use for serving the many Hispanic patients who come to the Main Street Pharmacy.

As you can see from my enclosed résumé, I have experience in the pharmacy and retail sides of a drug store. In these settings, I gained knowledge of business operations and exceptional customer service, which I am eager to apply to my hometown pharmacy.
I will call next week to inquire about a convenient meeting time, or you may reach me at 706-868-XXXX or knettleton@ppi-edu.net. I am most easily reached evenings and weekends. Thank you for considering my application.

Sincerely,

Kelly Nettleton

Kelly Nettleton
1700 Beltline Blvd.
Tate, GA 30107

Enc.: résumé

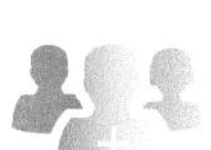

Work Wise

Call the pharmacy, receptionist, or secretary at the employer's office to confirm the correct spelling of the recipient's name and their title. No one likes to receive correspondence with their name or that of the business spelled wrong. That could lose you the job opportunity.

correct degree and title) doing the hiring—for example, the director of pharmacy, the pharmacist supervisor, or the human resources or store manager. Some business letter formats now simply put the person's name with the title and a colon to open the letter instead of including "Dear." For instance, "Pharmacy Director Sean Casey:" might work. Make sure that you spell the person's and business's names correctly.

Opening Paragraph In your initial paragraph, you must attract the employer's attention and demonstrate that you understand the business's mission and have something the company needs to meet its goals. This may take some investigation, but it shows desire and thoroughness. Make clear what specific position or type of work you are seeking, and whether you are interested in full- or part-time work. If you learned of the opening through someone in your network and that of the pharmacy, mention who told you about the position. It may help get the employer's attention. Describe how you would fit within the organization and its goals with your skills.

TABLE 16.4 Suggested Format for Cover Letters

First Paragraph	Catch the employer's attention with qualities that make you uniquely qualified for the position. Make clear the specific position or work you are seeking and what you have to offer that will further the business's mission.
Second Paragraph	Explain why you are interested in the position, the organization, or the organization's products and services. State how your academic background makes you a qualified candidate for the position. If you have had some practical experience, then point out your specific achievements.
Third Paragraph	Refer the reader to the enclosed or attached résumé: a summary of your qualifications, training, and experience. If specific items on your résumé require an explanation, then tactfully and positively point them out. You can include work experience from outside the pharmacy field, but be sure that it relates to skills that you will use as a technician.
Fourth Paragraph	Indicate your desire for a personal interview and your flexibility as to the time and place. Repeat your telephone number (and cell phone number), as well as the best times to reach you in the letter. If you use email as a preferred method of communication, then let the employer know that. Close your letter with a statement or question to encourage a response, or take the initiative by indicating a day and date on which you will contact the employer to set up a convenient time for a personal meeting. Express gratitude for their time and consideration.

Imagine yourself as the employer: wouldn't you rather hire someone who knows something about your company and already has a sense of your goals than someone who does not? Each cover letter should be unique and tailored, though it will have similar content for each similar position.

Body Paragraphs The next two or three short paragraphs should explain why you want the position and highlight qualities about yourself (practical pharmacy skills, experience, personality, leadership) the company could use, as well as qualities unique to you. This is your opportunity to share what makes you an attractive candidate. If you have graduated from an ASHP-accredited training program and achieved CPhT certification, be sure to emphasize those qualifications, as they may separate you from other applicants in states that do not require these as standard.

Highlight skills, initiative, or responsibilities that can carry over from the experiences on your résumé to your work as a technician. Perhaps you learned how to work well with people in a retail job, or how to help someone handle money and insurance while in a high school accounting internship experience, or how to do careful measurements and conversions in a landscaping or catering job. All of these qualities can be called out as preparing you to help customers in a community pharmacy. Or perhaps you were a hospital volunteer or worked with patients in a residential care unit and saw how important the medications were to the seniors you worked with. If you have hospital-related experience and are applying for a hospital position, be sure to mention that in your cover letter.

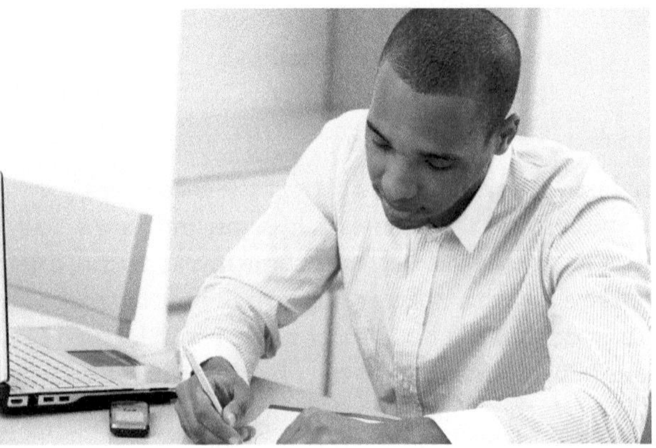

Taking the time to draft a personal cover letter that fits the job and you is important. Always get someone else's impression of it, revise it, and then read it out loud.

If specific items on your résumé require an explanation, then tactfully and positively point them out. This might include taking time out of the workforce to raise children or care for an elderly parent, or it may be related to a health issue like a surgery. Put a positive spin on the reasons.

TABLE 16.6 Guidelines for Job Interviews

1. Find out the exact place and time of the interview. Get directions or information about parking if necessary.
2. Know the full name of the company and its address (and directions to get there), and the interviewer's full name with its correct pronunciation. Call the employer, if necessary, to get this information.
3. Know something about the company's operations.
4. Pay close attention to your personal appearance. Be sure that your appearance reflects good hygiene and that your clothing and shoes are clean, neat, and appropriate for the job.
5. Bring to the interview your résumé and the names, addresses, and telephone numbers of at least three people who have agreed to provide references.
6. Arrive 10 to 15 minutes before the scheduled time for the interview.
7. Be courteous to the sales clerk, technician, or hospital receptionist (if one is present), and to other employees. Any person with whom you meet or speak may be in a position to influence your employment.
8. Greet the interviewer and call them by name. Introduce yourself at once. Remain standing until invited to sit down.
9. Be confident, polite, poised, and enthusiastic.
10. Look the interviewer in the eye while talking and listening.
11. Speak clearly and loudly enough to be understood. Be positive and concise in your comments. Do not exaggerate, but remember that an interview is not an occasion for either modesty or for boasting. Confident truth is the best path.
12. Focus on your strengths. Be prepared to enumerate these qualities, using specific examples to support the claims that you make about yourself.
13. Do not hesitate to ask about the specific duties associated with the job. Show keen interest as the interviewer tells you about these responsibilities.
14. Avoid bringing up hourly rate or salary requirements until the employer broaches the subject.
15. Do not chew gum or smoke.
16. Do not criticize former employers, coworkers, or working conditions.
17. At the close of the interview, thank the interviewer for their time and for the opportunity to learn about the company.
18. Send a personal note the next day to thank the interviewer for their time and consideration. Feel free to remind them what you have to offer the job and say that you look forward to hearing from them.

What did you learn from these experiences that helps make you a better pharmacy technician? Perhaps you helped your diabetic grandfather with his injections and were trained in how to do this by a kind pharmacist and that made you want to be a pharmacy technician. In a short sentence, note this. If your grades are average (you don't mention this!), state instead how you have received consistently high recommendations from your professors and preceptors at your externships. For instance, you could mention that Pharmacist Darlene Casey at Walgreens said you were "a quick learner, dependable, easy to work with, and accurate."

Closing Paragraph Refer the reader to any letters of reference from your instructors, preceptors, and former employers. Indicate your desire for a personal interview and your flexibility as to the time and place. Repeat your cell phone or contact telephone number from the top of your résumé, as well as the best times to reach you, in the letter. Also include your email address, and check your inbox regularly. IIt's always nice to end by thanking the prospective employer for their consideration. You might also mention a date and time in the future when you plan to follow up with them.

Professionally Polishing the Letter

As with your résumé, read your cover letter out loud so that you can hear it many times. Have others read it and make any corrections needed. Proofread the cover letter carefully for errors in spelling, grammar, usage, punctuation, capitalization, and form. A poorly written cover letter detracts from even the most professional résumé.

Preparing for the Interview

Review your research on the employer and role-play an interview situation. Again, put yourself in the position of the employer. Brainstorm questions they may ask, and make a list. Consider those and the questions in Table 16.5, and prepare the wording of your answers.

Be prepared for questions like, "What do you consider your greatest strength for this position?" "What do you consider your greatest weakness in this job?" Consider these questions carefully and come up with strategies to overcome your weaknesses or turn them into a strength. Remember that every strength can become a weakness when taken to an extreme or out of context. Perhaps you are good at speaking up about what things can be improved. But this is a weakness if you do it too often, too soon, too brashly, or without gratitude or thought for those who set up the current system.

Perhaps you feel you are too shy. Being shy can make you very observant of people, and so you know better how to serve them and speak up when you need to. Think about your strengths and weaknesses, what the "other side" of them can be, and how to use them to serve the pharmacy so you can be prepared for this question.

Preparing for Questions

Some interviewers pose hypothetical situations and ask for your response, or they may ask you to describe a past experience and how you handled it. These types of questions require you to *think on your feet* and talk about your problem-solving skills. At the least, be ready to describe a situation or two from your past where you had to deal with a difficult coworker or member of the public. Choose a situation where you were pleased with how you responded, and describe the measures you took to improve the end result.

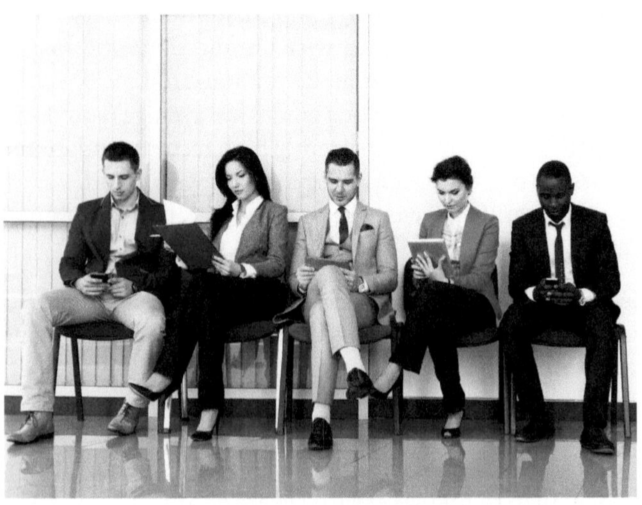

Before an interview, it's always a good idea to research a company and, if possible, the people you'll be interviewing with.

Interviewers should not ask you questions about your religion, marital status, or if you have or plan to have children. You are not obligated to answer questions such as these.

After you have brainstormed some questions that you may be asked, come up with some strong questions you can ask the interviewer, such as "How would you describe the patient base of this pharmacy in terms of types of most common prescriptions?" "Do technicians work here in a team setting or more independently?" "What qualities are you looking for most in a technician?" "What is a typical shift like?" and "What do you see as the most challenging aspects of the position?"

TABLE 16.5 Potential Interview Questions

1. Why did you apply for a job with this company?
2. What part of the job interests you most and why?
3. What do you know about this company?
4. What are your qualifications?
5. What did you like the most and the least about your work experience?
(Note: Explaining what you liked least should be done in as positive a manner as possible. For example, you might say that you wish that the job had provided more opportunity for learning and then explain that you made up the deficiency by studying on your own. Such an answer indicates your desire to learn and grow and does not cast your former employer in an unduly negative light.)
6. Why did you leave your previous job? (Avoid negative responses. Find a positive reason for leaving, such as returning to school or pursuing an opportunity, or moving from part-time to full-time to be eligible for benefits for your family.)
7. What would you like to be doing in five years? What are your money expectations? (Keep your answer reasonable, and show that you have ambitions consistent with the employer's needs.)
8. What are your weak points? (Say something positive such as, "I am an extremely conscientious person. Sometimes I worry too much about whether I have done something absolutely correctly, but that can also be a positive trait.")
9. Why do you think that you are qualified for this position?
10. Would you mind working on the weekends or putting in overtime? How do you feel about traveling to work in other pharmacies?
11. Do you prefer working with others or by yourself? Do you prefer a quiet or a noisy environment?
12. If you could have any job you wanted, what would you choose, and why?
13. What information would you like to share about yourself?
14. What are your hobbies and interests?
15. Why did you attend the college (or training program) that you attended?
16. Why did you choose this field of study?
17. What courses did you like best? What courses did you like least?
(State your responses to both questions in positive ways.)
18. Do you plan to continue your education?
19. What have you learned from your mistakes?
20. What motivates you to put forth your greatest efforts?

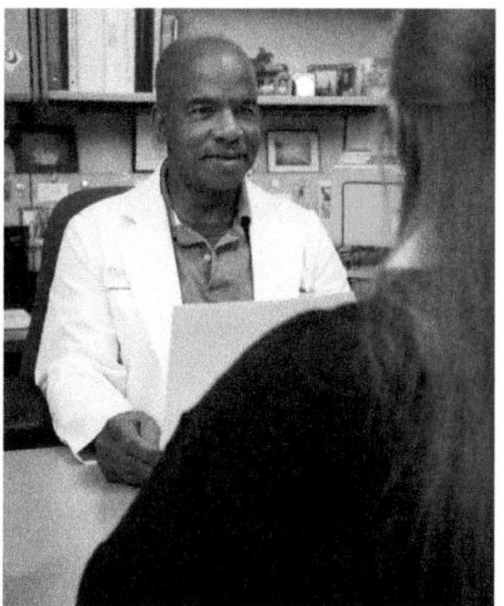

If possible, find someone with knowledge of your field to role-play an interview with you.

If the opportunity arises toward the end of the interview, then be sure to ask any questions that you may have—such as typical work schedule, weekends, vacation, benefits, orientation schedule, and so on. Some employers will cover the cost of annual registration, the PTCB exam, and continuing education. These questions, though, should come towards the end of the interview if the employer has not already explained them. You need to find out about the nature of the job first.

Role-Playing the Interview

Once you have written down the questions you may be asked and all your answers, and you are prepared with some you can ask, have different people play your interviewer so you can practice. Ask them to come up with questions you have not thought. Rehearsing out loud can help you identify wording choices and avoid mixing up words during the actual interview. When coming up with your responses, bear in mind the employer's point of view. Imagine what you would want if you were the employer, and then take the initiative during the interview to explain to the employer how you can meet those needs.

You can do this role-playing with a study group. This may be a great group activity in your training program.

Handling the Interview Well

You should plot out how to get to the interview location the day before, and have a backup to get there if something falls through. (It's best to do a test run to get to the pharmacy a day or two before, and perhaps observe it to get ideas for questions you may want to ask.) Get plenty of sleep, eat well, dress professionally, leave with plenty of time in case of a delay in traffic or transportation, and don't be afraid of the stress of excitement. Tell a joke or have someone else tell you some so you can laugh ahead of time and be at ease and let your self shine through naturally. The guidelines provided in Table 16.6 can serve as reminders of key tips.

TABLE 16.6 Guidelines for Job Interviews

1. Find out the exact place and time of the interview. Get directions or information about parking if necessary.
2. Know the full name of the company and its address (and directions to get there), and the interviewer's full name with its correct pronunciation. Call the employer, if necessary, to get this information.
3. Know something about the company's operations.
4. Pay close attention to your personal appearance. Be sure that your appearance reflects good hygiene and that your clothing and shoes are clean, neat, and appropriate for the job.
5. Bring to the interview your résumé and the names, addresses, and telephone numbers of at least three people who have agreed to provide references.
6. Arrive 10 to 15 minutes before the scheduled time for the interview.
7. Be courteous to the sales clerk, technician, or hospital receptionist (if one is present), and to other employees. Any person with whom you meet or speak may be in a position to influence your employment.
8. Greet the interviewer and call them by name. Introduce yourself at once. Remain standing until invited to sit down.
9. Be confident, polite, poised, and enthusiastic.
10. Look the interviewer in the eye while talking and listening.
11. Speak clearly and loudly enough to be understood. Be positive and concise in your comments. Do not exaggerate, but remember that an interview is not an occasion for either modesty or for boasting. Confident truth is the best path.
12. Focus on your strengths. Be prepared to enumerate these qualities, using specific examples to support the claims that you make about yourself.
13. Do not hesitate to ask about the specific duties associated with the job. Show keen interest as the interviewer tells you about these responsibilities.
14. Avoid bringing up hourly rate or salary requirements until the employer broaches the subject.
15. Do not chew gum or smoke.
16. Do not criticize former employers, coworkers, or working conditions.
17. At the close of the interview, thank the interviewer for their time and for the opportunity to learn about the company.
18. Send a personal note the next day to thank the interviewer for their time and consideration. Feel free to remind them what you have to offer the job and say that you look forward to hearing from them.

Avoid the Pitfalls

According to a *USA Today* poll of more than 1,900 job interviewers, the following are the most important factors in how to "blow your interview":

- Not learning about the job or organization (26%)
- Being arrogant (21%)
- Showing up late (15%)
- Not asking any questions (12%)
- Not speaking professionally (6%)

Be cognizant of these pitfalls and come to the interview interested and prepared.

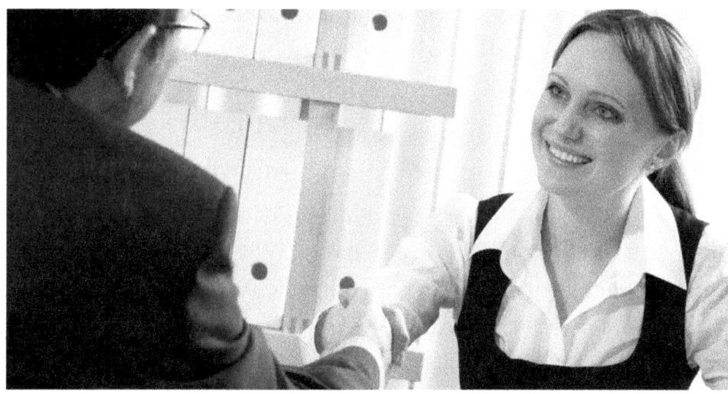

Always express gratitude for the opportunity to interview, both in person and (later) in writing.

Following Up

After the interview, follow up with a written note thanking the interviewer for seeing you and (within an appropriate time) follow up with a telephone call. Be persistent but not pushy. If you did not get the position, then thank the employer for the opportunity to interview and request that the company keep your cover letter and résumé on file for consideration of future positions.

Handling Performance Reviews

Congratulations, you got the job! If you have not worked before or if your work experience has been sporadic, then getting used to your job as a technician might seem like acclimating to life in a foreign country. You have to adjust to a new work culture, different behaviors, responsibilities and expectations, unfamiliar customs, and even a new language—the technical scientific jargon of the profession.

Your orientation will include experience and self-study on the computer of pertinent policies and procedures specific to your organization. Then you will begin your work as a technician. If you are not certified yet, your organization may require you to be within the next 6 to 12 months.

Many pharmacy technicians may be hired on a contingency basis. A **performance review** is completed by your pharmacy supervisor initially after three to six months, then annually thereafter.

Practice Tip

Unreliable employees in the healthcare industry do not keep their jobs for long, so make sure that your employer can always depend on you to arrive at work on time.

You will be evaluated in many different concrete, measurable areas such as:

- attendance and timeliness (versus tardiness)
- dress code compliance
- computer skills and accuracy
- adherence to pharmacy policy and procedures
- processing of insurance claims
- efficiency and accuracy in filling of prescriptions
- completion of assignments

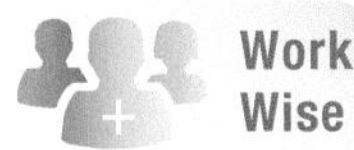
Work Wise

Surprisingly, attitude is one of the greatest predictors of job success. Be positive, cooperative, self-confident, and enthusiastic.

In addition to concrete, measurable skills, reviews also cover significant but less objectively measurable aspects of your performance, including the following:

- customer service and phone etiquette
- teamwork and ability to take correction
- motivation and self-direction
- improvement in learning and job skills
- relationships with colleagues
- relationship with supervisor

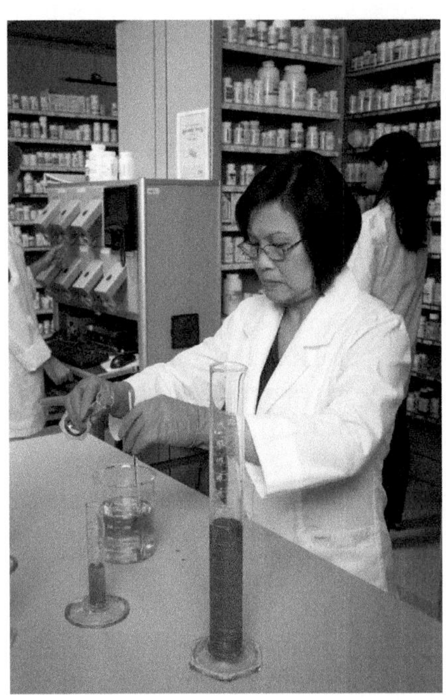
The best way to receive a good job performance review is to remain diligent in your duties.

These or similar job responsibilities, skills, and competencies are often evaluated on some sort of scale similar to exceeding, meeting, or falling short of expectations. It is common for an employer to ask you to self-evaluate your performance in each category. Your supervising pharmacist will independently evaluate your performance on the same categories. Then you will discuss your ratings, where you see things similarly, and where they are different. Accept criticism gracefully.

With determination and commitment, you will likely have met or exceeded expectations. But there is always room for growth. Most performance reviews have a process to help you determine areas that could use improvement or where you can gain greater learning and responsibility. Supervisors often ask employees to write down a personal goal or two to achieve in the upcoming months. They may then ask what things they might do to help you in your goal. After fully discussing your performance and goals, you and your supervising pharmacist may sign your review for documentation of the meeting and future reference.

After your first performance review, if you do well and stay on the job, you will likely meet with your supervisor on a quarterly, semiannual, or annual basis per policy to compare performance evaluations.

16.4 Advancing Your Career

There will never be a time in your career in health care to coast and relax. Good career opportunities can arise unexpectedly, so make a habit of reviewing your career path and career goals regularly. Planning lends structure and substance to your career management. Many pharmacy technicians use their experiences as springboards into careers as pharmacists or nurses, or other related healthcare disciplines. As noted, there are chances to attain specialized training and certificates in sterile, hazardous, and nuclear compounding, among others. However there are other opportunities, many of which do not require new certifications but do require initiative.

Consider the decades of experiences Nicole Blades, CPhT, in Ann Arbor, Michigan, has had. She told the PTCB in a CPhT Spotlight interview: “I have 10 years retail experience, 7 years in an IV outsourcing facility, 2 years in a small hospital, 2 years in long-term care, and 14 years in compounding, non-sterile and sterile. I have been a trainer, inventory specialist, and lab manager.” Ms. Blades represents the career movement that can occur within the field.

The Effects of the ASHP Practice Advancement Initiative

Traditionally, less than 10% of technician time was spent in nontraditional or advanced roles, but these percentages are changing as pharmacists' roles are expanding. With the multiplication of new drugs, drug interactions, drug studies of old drugs, and prescription drug abuse, doctors and physicians and other healthcare providers simply are not equipped with the time or resources to keep up with all this drug information as well as pharmacists are.

The ASHP is promoting its **Practice Advancement Initiative (PAI)** to help things change even more rapidly, but also consistently and effectively. The goal of the PAI is to advance the health and well-being of patients by supporting futuristic practice models that support the most effective use of pharmacy professionals in direct patient care. The PAI states that the desired healthcare team model "urges technicians to handle nontraditional and advanced responsibilities to allow pharmacists to take greater responsibility for direct patient care."

In the past, about 70% of pharmacy technician positions have been in community pharmacies, but these pharmacies are changing in nature with the rise of mail-order pharmacies and more tech-check-tech positions. Hospital pharmacy positions and clinical office positions are diversifying as well. Pharmacists are specializing more, which affects technician opportunities. Some home healthcare and community pharmacists choose to focus their practice on pain management for hospice patients or on oncology to treat cancer patients. Managed care pharmacists may select areas like anticoagulation control and cholesterol management for patients with high risk for heart disease. In the hospital, pharmacists are specializing in nutrition, pharmacokinetics, infectious disease, oncology, critical care, pediatrics, neonatology, and so on. This shift has led to groups of physicians opening their own pharmacies to accompany their practices, which opens up specialty areas for the technicians as well. Technicians who work with specializing pharmacists also become specialized in the same fields.

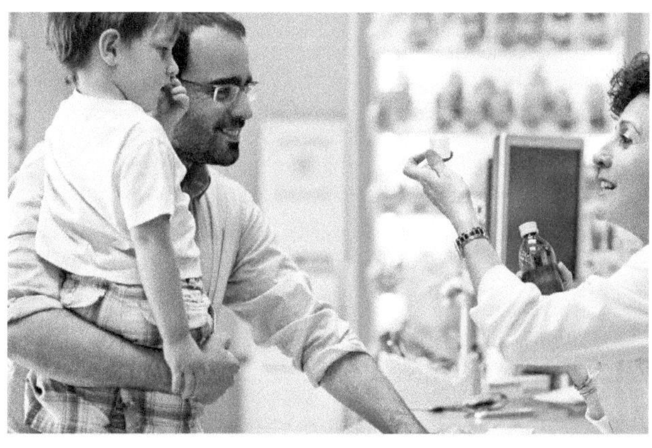
Pharmacists are doing more and more direct patient care and medication counseling.

Advancement Opportunities

As technicians become more indispensable to the pharmacy team, there will be an increase in salary and benefits. The average salary in retail pharmacy is about $30K per year; in the hospital pharmacy it is slightly higher at $35K per year. Salaries depend highly on the state, region of the country, certification, and experience. Most technicians who assume supervisory or advanced roles are eligible for salaries in the range of $40K to $50K or more per year, again depending on experience and geographical location. To follow are some of the many advancement opportunities that exist.

Tech-Check-Tech and Dispensing Management Positions

In many high-volume institutional, community, and mail-order pharmacies, a hierarchy or "career ladder" of pharmacy technician jobs has evolved, especially in institutional settings. If certification is not yet required for an entry-level technician, then it is

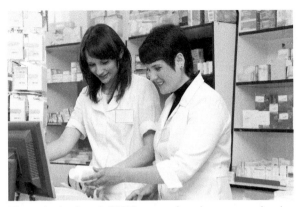

The tech-check-tech (TCT) system has demonstrated to be as or more accurate than a sole pharmacist check and has been approved by several state boards of pharmacy.

generally required for the higher levels. Corresponding job titles are Technician I and II or Entry-Level Technician and Technician Specialist or Senior Technician. The difference in responsibility (and reward) grows and expands as the technician moves up the department ladder and with the number of technicians that the individual handles with tech-check-tech. Research studies have demonstrated that a **tech-check-tech** system (that is, a senior technician checking another technician before the final pharmacist check) is likely to catch more errors than simply a pharmacist checking.

Strong leadership and management skills are necessary to be a successful senior technician. You may be involved in the interviewing and hiring of technician personnel, orientation and training of new employees, and performance review, as well as designing schedules and assigning workloads.

Controlled Substances Specialist

The controlled substance technician is responsible for ensuring facility compliance with all applicable laws, regulations, directives, policies, and procedures applying to the dispensing, storage, transfer, inventory, and accountability of controlled substances. This technician serves as the narcotic control and accountability agent for the department under the supervision of the pharmacist or the director of pharmacy. In this type of position, you would be responsible for maintaining all the necessary records for a perpetual inventory and for security of all narcotic and controlled drugs in the vault. Part of this responsibility is to perform random audits and resolve any discrepancies in inventory. You would also train new employees and update existing employees on all policies relating to controlled substances in the central or outpatient pharmacy and nursing units.

Pharmacy Benefits/Insurance Liaison

As was discussed in Chapter 8, in the retail pharmacy environment, it is important to have an experienced technician who is extremely knowledgeable about the nuances of insurance eligibility, verification, and claims processing. If a claim cannot be processed, the reason must be identified and resolved, and often the insurance liaison handles the cases the other technicians could not or did not have time to resolve, including situations requiring prior authorization (PA), charge-backs, or claims rejected in an audit. You may also be responsible for gathering information and submitting claims for medication therapy management services, which are less straightforward than the drug claims, as they may entail counseling and immunizations. As a technician, you could work from the other end, too, employed by the pharmacy benefit manager to work with pharmacies since you understand the intricacies of medications and dispensing.

In addition, as a payment specialist, you may handle or specialize in any medication assistance programs for patients of the community pharmacy or those preparing for discharge from the hospital. If the patient does not have drug insurance, you would provide the patient some options for ACA (Affordable Care Act) health insurance, visiting a community health center, seeking medication assistance online from the pharmaceutical manufacturer, or using available drug coupons. You may also advocate with the pharmacist or prescriber for a change to a lower-cost generic drug. Though this position is common in community pharmacies, medical billing departments have an emerging role in medication assistance advocacy as well.

IN THE REAL WORLD

A pilot study at Wake Forest Baptist Medical Center revealed that there was only one error in 265,000 orders in a "tech-check-tech" system, which was a better safety record than without the system. The North Carolina Board of Pharmacy formally approved this role after reviewing the results of the pilot study. Similar results were demonstrated in Texas and Idaho with tech-check-tech being used to check cart fills and floor stock refills. Now more than 19 states have approved or are allowing some form of this tech supervision. This role will increase the availability of pharmacist time to provide medication therapy management (MTM) services to provide better care and lower hospital costs.

Drug Distribution and Inventory Specialist

In community and institutional pharmacies, technicians can often move up the ladder of responsibility by gaining the position of manager of inventory. You may be responsible for preparing requests for proposals (RFPs) during the competitive drug bidding process for medications and intravenous solutions, and in some cases medical supplies. You would monitor **stock par levels** (the minimum amount of inventory needed on hand to meet known customer demand and a small surplus in case of unexpected demand) and oversee proactive ordering to ensure that neither shortages nor expensive overstocks occur.

This position is important to community pharmacies as they do not have enormous storage space or budgets for the high overhead costs of overstocking. In the hospital, this position is essential as well, because the cost of drugs and supplies generally is 60% to 70% of the total pharmacy operating costs. The budget must be continuously monitored as newer and more expensive drugs are prescribed or added to the drug formulary. The tech must assign minimum and maximum inventory levels that might need to be seasonally adjusted. The person in this position is responsible for checking any drug recalls, pulling these drugs from the shelf, as well as checking and returning any medications that are due to expire soon.

Medication Therapy Management Assistant

In the community pharmacy, pilot projects have utilized technicians to assist pharmacists in making telephone calls and gathering information on medication effectiveness and concerns from patients with diabetes, hypertension, asthma, chronic obstructive pulmonary disease (COPD), and heart failure (HF) in preparation for medication therapy management (MTM) counseling. This could be an area where you can specialize and then learn to process and submit MTM interventions from pharmacists for reimbursement. These targeted intervention programs (TIPs) are initiated by pharmacy benefit managers (PBMs) and are pharmacy- and patient-specific. TIPs include such cost-saving strategies as patient education on nonadherence to prescribed therapy, therapeutic duplications or potential drug interactions, under- and overdosing, and switching from nonformulary to formulary medications. As a specialist in this area, you could also be called upon to help monitor patient progress by checking in with the patients to track therapy adherence.

Pharmacists in the retail setting or clinics administer nearly every CDC-approved vaccine to patients upon request (influenza vaccine) or by written or verbal prescription to anyone over the age of 13 years (eligibility varies by state). You can focus on assistance by reminding patients about the importance of receiving vaccines, setting up and reminding patients about appointments, and helping them complete all the necessary forms (including the CDC-required VIS, or Vaccine Information Sheet). You can assemble all the supplies (vaccine, diluent, syringes, alcohol wipes, etc.) and draw up the vaccine (allowed in many states) for the pharmacist. You would also update the patient's primary care clinician on the vaccinations for more effective record keeping.

To specialize in this area, you should get certification from the American Heart Association or American Red Cross in **Basic Life Support/Cardiopulmonary Resuscitation (BLS/CPR)**. A certification as a phlebotomist (to draw blood) and various types of Occupational Safety and Health Administration (OSHA) certifications are helpful for specializing in immunization and blood testing medication therapy services.

In the future, with specialized training and certifications, technicians may be allowed to administer the vaccines and administer blood tests, especially during an emergency.

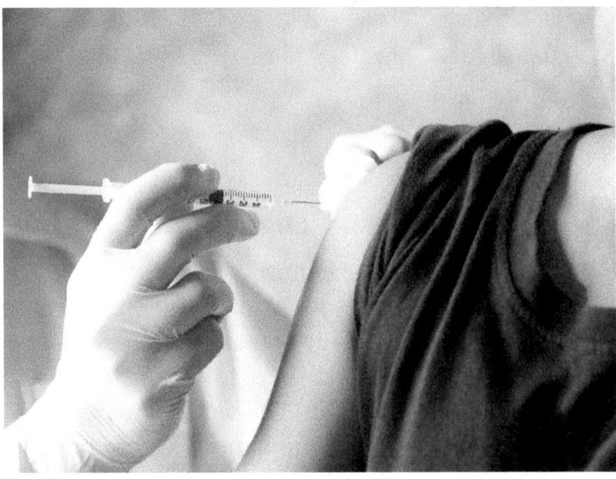

Though technicians can assist with vaccinations, they cannot administer them. But with appropriate training and certifications, they may be able to do so in the future.

Ambulatory Clinical Pharmacy Services Specialist

The pharmacist role has expanded to providing patient care services in ambulatory care clinics. In this role, pharmacists provide medication management for patients with chronic disease such as diabetes and hypertension. Pharmacy technicians are needed to assist in the ambulatory clinical pharmacy setting. Technicians serve as a point of contact for both patients and clinic staff. They also are able to increase efficiency of interactions between patients, pharmacists, and other clinic staff to help maximize the number of pharmacist appointments while minimizing communication errors. Additionally, ambulatory clinical pharmacy services technicians can help pharmacists by decreasing administrative responsibilities, allowing the pharmacist to dedicate more time to direct patient care.

Healthcare Device Patient Education Specialist

Patient counseling on prescription and OTC medications in most states may be offered only by the pharmacist. But there are no restrictions on technicians educating patients about how to monitor their disease and choose proper disease control devices. Such a role requires further preparation and home study. A motivated and experienced technician could consider focusing their efforts on learning about the available devices for treating common chronic conditions such as diabetes. With such information, you could help patients locate home aids for their drug therapy, trouble-shoot blood glucose monitoring equipment and instrument-specific test strips, and provide information about where to find no/low-sugar OTC products and diabetic skin care products in the store. You could also encourage patients to attend programs on diabetes education, including the advantages of various insulins and oral therapies.

In the future, with advanced training and certification, it is possible that pharmacy technicians may be allowed also to do limited counseling on OTC drugs and dietary supplements.

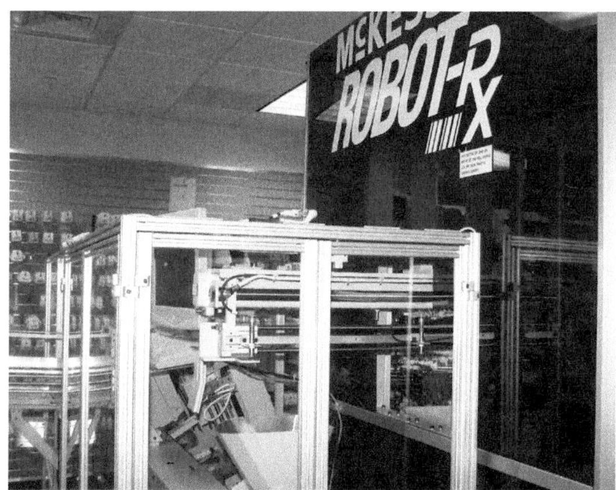

Specialists are needed who know the automated pharmacy equipment well enough to train others and maintain it.

Automation Specialist

As you have seen, automation plays an increasing role in both central pharmacy and nursing-unit drug distribution systems. The need exists for a pharmacy technician to oversee the operating system and keep technicians and pharmacists up to date on the automated technology. You may specialize in-house or gain special training and certification from the manufacturer on the automation systems your pharmacy or institution uses. You would then be in charge of troubleshooting and managing the systems you oversee, keeping the automation up to date and maintained, and training others in the use and maintenance of the equipment. You would research and make recommendations for the installation of new innovative technology.

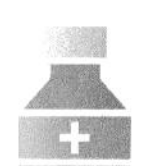
Pharm Fact

Some studies indicate that, when hospital staff compile patient medication histories without a technician, one or more errors occur 15% of the time.

Informatics Specialist

If you have an aptitude for working with computers, you may be assigned as a **pharmacy informatics** technician to work with the pharmacy software. Effective use and overseeing (and sometimes tailoring) of the interconnecting pharmacy software in either the retail or hospital setting are key to improving medication safety and health outcomes and lowering healthcare costs. In managing these software systems, you would be responsible for keeping up to date with the newest technology, handling updates and upgrades, virus and hacking prevention, and data backups. Training other pharmacy personnel in software use might also be your responsibility. You would compile and analyze various departmental data reports.

Hospital Admissions Medication History Specialist

During the hospital admissions process, it is important to determine all the medications and doses (including OTC drugs and dietary supplements) that a patient is taking, as well as drug allergies, *prior* to the admitting physician writing medication orders. Studies have found that medication histories are more accurately done by a pharmacy technician. As a medication history specialist, you would interview the patients, their guardians or those admitting them, their physicians, and others to collect crucial information about patients' current drug and alcohol use and allergies. With knowledge of medications, you can help collect and verify the correct names and dosage levels. You would also do internet research through the medical records systems to collect any accessible information. In addition to your knowledge as a technician, you would be utilizing a great deal of communication and people skills.

IN THE REAL WORLD

In a pilot study in a Wisconsin hospital emergency department, trained pharmacy technicians were put to work compiling patient medication and allergy histories. The trained technician conducted about 13 medication histories per day, and there were few errors and discrepancies. The pharmacist was still required to review the histories before placement in the medical chart. Prior to the study, the hospital admission team reviewed only 10% of the patients' medication and allergy histories before the admitting physician wrote the medication orders. In the study, technicians reviewed 98%. The cost savings from reduced errors were estimated at greater than $100K per year, and the role of medication history specialist was officially implemented after the study's completion.

Similar results were reported in a study from Connecticut. Over 25,000 emergency department reconciliations over a 12-month period of time demonstrated 96% accuracy when collected by the technicians and checked by a pharmacist. This change provided a 66% increase in accuracy over the previous process. In Florida, the accuracy of medication histories increased from 65% (from nurses) to 93% (with techs). Similar results were identified in hospitals in New Jersey, Maryland, California, and Utah.

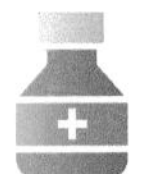

Pharm Fact

Over 80% of hospital stays involve drug therapy. The most prescribed drug types are to address pain; vertigo, nausea, and vomiting; dehydration, and mineral or electrolyte deprivation/imbalance. Many drugs need to be continued after discharge.

Hospital Discharge Care Transition Specialist

This discharge specialist role includes easing the transition from acute care in the hospital to follow-up care in the community with the local pharmacy and primary care physician. Several pilot programs have demonstrated that an experienced pharmacy technician can facilitate the discharge prescription process. You would facilitate insurance verification and claims processing, identification and resolution of any prior authorizations, and referral to medication assistance programs if necessary. If the patient transfers to a rehabilitation center, long-term care center, hospice, or nursing home, you may help transition the medication information and discharge plans to the facility and to the relatives and caregivers.

For certain high-risk patients on anticoagulants or transplant drugs, you would telephone and set up important follow-up visits with the laboratory or primary care physician or specialist in the community. If the patient needs a special injectable anticoagulant, you may call their community pharmacy to ensure that it is available in the inventory before discharge. During the exit interview with the patient, you would identify any discrepancies in the discharge prescriptions or patient education on the prescribed therapy, checking with the pharmacist or prescriber to address any problems. In one study, the percentage of readmissions to the hospital was reduced by 50% after this technician-based patient medication education program was implemented.

Hospital Pharmacy Satellite Pharmacy Managers

Some hospital pharmacies have elected to decentralize their pharmacies by creating smaller satellite pharmacies serving various wings or units. Common satellite pharmacy stations include pediatrics, neonatology, surgery, and the emergency department. Most satellite pharmacies provide both administrative drug distribution

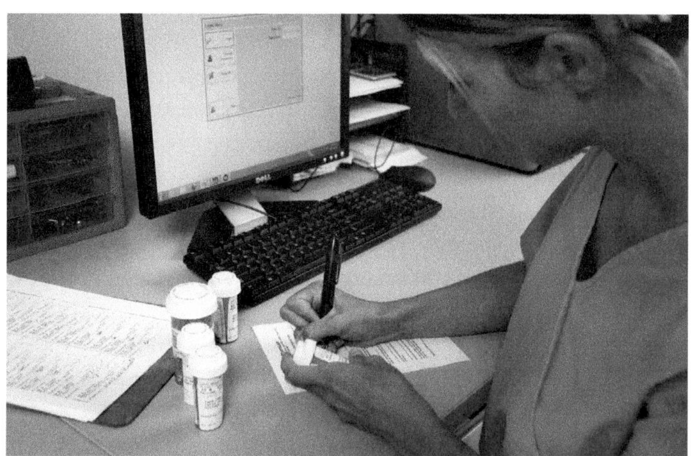

Having technicians compile hospital patient medication and allergy histories *before* the admitting physician writes the first medication orders greatly aids in accurate medication reconciliation and reduces medication errors.

and clinical services. In this situation, a specialized technician can advance to become the manager of the satellite's inventory and/or a key member of the clinical pharmacy team.

The specialized pharmacist and technician team in a satellite pharmacy can provide better quality and continuity of care and be more readily available to the hospital units' physicians, surgeons, and nurses. The pharmacist rounds with the medical teams to better monitor drug therapy for side effects, adverse reactions, or drug interactions.

As part of the unit team, you would serve as a liaison with the central pharmacy and the assigned clinical pharmacist and monitor floor stock inventory. You would become a specialist in the drug therapies prescribed in those units, such as birth and neonatal, heart, or oncology medications. You and the pharmacist may also be responsible for participating and assisting in any "codes" called on this hospital floor to provide **stat** (immediate, high-priority) **medications**. Checking the automated dispensing cabinets (ADCs)—such as Pyxis—on each nursing unit, optimizing and adjusting the drug inventory, monitoring for any drug diversion (especially controlled drugs), and troubleshooting any failures of the units' ADCs would also be your responsibilities.

With a decentralized hospital pharmacy model, there is usually an improvement in the drug distribution system on the unit, a shorter turnaround time for stat medications, a reduction in missing doses from the unit dose cart, an improvement in nursing satisfaction, and an increase in time available for pharmacists to perform MTM services. The pharmacist would develop guidelines and protocols, and write medication orders following approved drug protocols, as well as teaching students and residents in both pharmacy and medicine.

Hospital Clinical Services Assistants

Expanded roles exist for pharmacy technicians in clinical services as well, including medication safety, patient education, immunization assistance, transitions of care, and medication therapy management services. These services have improved the quality of care provided to patients, especially in bridging therapies upon admission and discharge from the hospital.

Telepharmacy Technicians

Over 4,000 hospitals in the United States do not have 24-hour pharmacist services coverage, leading at times to problems for after-hours medication orders. Services can be provided around the clock when technicians remain to take night shifts, supported by on-call pharmacists. The off-site pharmacists can then provide services through FaceTime, Skype, and other wireless and internet audiovisual technology. These shifts or locations serviced by a remote pharmacist are called **telepharmacies**.

Alaska, North Dakota, Washington, California, Iowa, Montana, Texas, Vermont, Wisconsin, Utah, and other states and numerous naval bases are among the places that operate telepharmacies without a pharmacist physically present. These

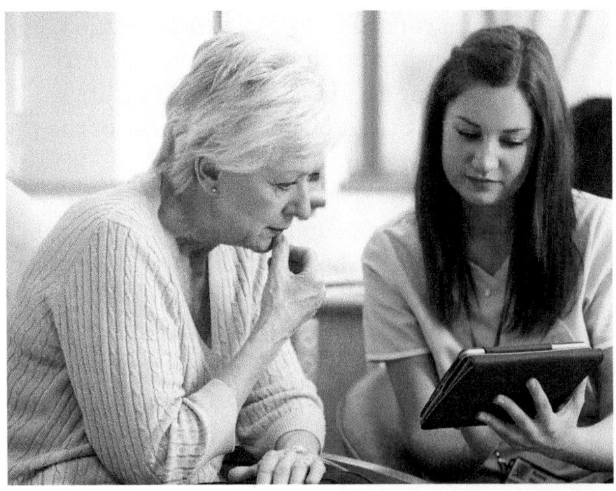

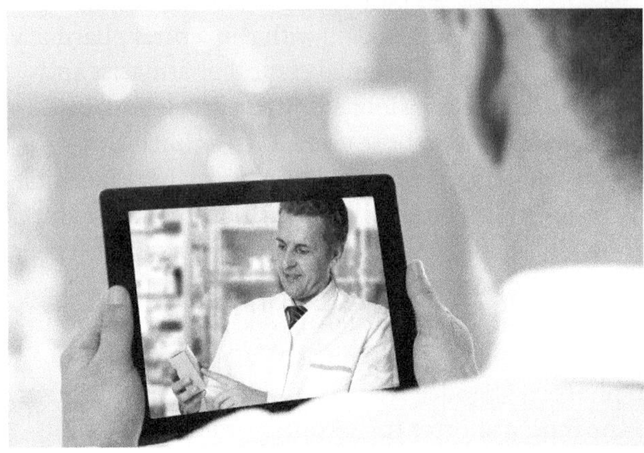

Pharmacy personnel may work inside a satellite unit. A technician could get direction from a pharmacist at a remote location.

telepharmacies use state-of-the-art telecommunication and audiovisual software from multiple vendors to provide pharmacy services at a distance. Communications are via a HIPAA-privacy secured line. Pharmacists remotely enter and review all medication orders or prescriptions prior to technicians, nurses, and physicians dispensing or removing medications from floor stock or from an automated storage and distribution device.

Studies have demonstrated that telepharmacies provide patients with increased access to necessary medications, especially in rural hospitals and clinics, and that error rates do not increase with the use of telepharmacies. Software for telepharmacies has received the approval of both Centers for Medicare and Medicaid Services (CMS) and the Joint Commission. You can see an example of a telepharmacy services company, Telnet-Rx, at https://PharmPractice7e.ParadigmEducation.com/Telnetrx.

Training to set up telepharmacies becomes essential in emergency preparedness—to be ready to deal with natural-disaster situations when traditional community and institutional pharmacy infrastructures have been harmed and pharmacists are unable to travel to the makeshift dispensing locations or are unavailable for mobile dispensing units.

Investigational Drugs Specialist

The experienced and certified pharmacy technician may also be involved in other expanded roles, depending on the size and location of the university or healthcare facility. The tech may be involved in investigational drug control in a large university and/or teaching hospital where several drug research studies are being conducted. Surveys have shown that some institutions allow technicians to perform a number of key tasks without direct pharmacist supervision, primarily in the areas of inventory management, communicating with clinical monitors (personnel that provide "on-site" monitoring of adherence to investigational drug studies), and auditing. Keeping track of each investigational drug administered to each patient is an important and necessary task for the technician. Many institutions have also reported technician involvement in teaching activities.

If you have experience as an investigational drug technician, you may be eligible for a position in the pharmaceutical industry working under the direction of a health professional or a scientist. Job responsibilities include supervising ongoing experiments, recording laboratory results, keeping records, testing for various compounds, and maintaining laboratory cleanliness. More responsibilities are typically given as the technician gains experience in laboratory techniques and proper research methodology.

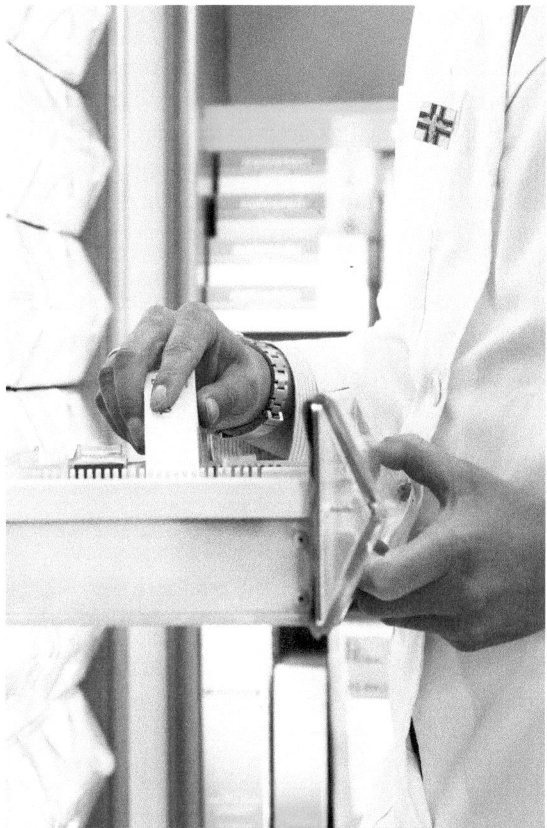

Taking inventory and doing the record keeping for investigational drugs in university and teaching hospital drug research studies can be part of a new advanced role for the pharmacy technician.

Compounding and Infusion Specialist

With advanced practice certifications in sterile, hazardous, and/or nuclear pharmacy, technicians have the additional ability to specialize within these fields. They may hold positions in compounding facilities that specialize in neonatal and pediatric medications, oncology, gerontology, or parenteral nutrition for specialized cases, among other areas of focus. Within these facilities, technicians may also gain advancement in tech-check-tech, quality assurance, inventory, and automation.

Quality Assurance Specialist

Every retail pharmacy is required by the state board of pharmacy and CMS to have a **quality assurance (QA)** program to investigate and correct medication errors. The QA specialist oversees the implementation of improvement programs, error tracking and analysis, awareness building, and training. Hospitals and institutions also require such programs for Joint Commission accreditation. If a program does not exist, it may affect accreditation and reimbursement from government and private insurance.

Many pharmacies are reluctant to keep records on medication errors for fear of liability, but these records are exempt from legal requisition. The purpose of a QA program is not to penalize the pharmacist or the technician, but to identify the cause of the error and to implement policies to prevent a reoccurrence.

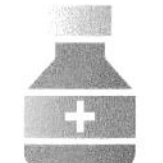

Pharm Fact

Medication error records are exempt from legal action in order to encourage pharmacies to keep accurate records and analyze them.

A compounding pharmacy must also have a QA program that includes:

1. written procedures for verification, monitoring, and review of the adequacy of the compounding processes;
2. written standards for qualitative and quantitative integrity, potency, quality, and labeled strength analysis of compounded drug products;
3. written procedures for scheduled action in the event that a compounded drug is below minimum standards for integrity, potency, quality, or labeled strength. Such a program is required by law, especially after recent deaths from contaminated steroid injections by a compounding pharmacy in Massachusetts.

In hospitals, the manager of quality assurance must implement programs to improve departmental and employee performance and productivity as well as investigate relevant information on medication errors. Pharmacy technicians have also been utilized by drug information pharmacists to gather information on adverse drug interactions as well as medication errors; this information is then reviewed by the pharmacist before it is submitted to the Pharmacy and Therapeutics Committee.

A QA program may also include testing for aseptic technique and product sampling from the hospital's IV cleanroom environment. As a quality assurance specialist, you would work closely with the cleanroom director to verify the stability, integrity, and safety of the medications compounded in the pharmacy.

Systematic Barriers to Technician Advancement

For the advanced practice roles for technicians to fully develop, the state boards of pharmacy have to advocate to their legislatures to write laws allowing these expanded roles. The National Association of Boards of Pharmacy has drafted language that each state board of pharmacy can use for a Pharmacy Practice Act that encourages the advancement of both the pharmacists and the technicians. The *Model State Pharmacy Act and Model Rules of the National Association of Boards of Pharmacy (Model Act)* can be accessed at https://PharmPractice7e.ParadigmEducation.com/ModelAct.

Currently, there are several barriers to accelerating these advanced roles for the pharmacy technician:

- the lack of standardization in education and training programs
- professional liability
- concerns for patient safety and incidence of medication errors
- regulations and restrictions by the state boards of pharmacy
- pharmacist resistance to change as a threat to job security
- lack of funding to support pilot projects to demonstrate the benefits of several of these advanced roles for technicians

Once the study results are completed, state boards of pharmacy have been receptive to allowing expanded technician roles in the Pharmacy Practice Act.

16.5 Career Building Counsel

The secret to success with almost any job is to identify and seize opportunities that arise. However, if you find that these aren't always apparent or readily available, you may need to make your own. There are specific ways that you can cultivate opportunities, both within your current company and outside of it.

Achieving Career Goals

Defining solid goals can help you visualize what you hope to accomplish on your career trajectory. Climbing the ladder at work may require you to marshal skills and demonstrate qualities that supervisors can easily recognize as efforts to foster opportunity. Some suggestions include:

Build a Good Relationship with Your Supervisor

Always show your supervisor (pharmacist or senior technician) a reasonable degree of deference and respect. Ask your supervisor how they prefer to be addressed. Be personable and respectful of your supervisor's experience and knowledge. Learn about their preferences, hobbies, or interests so that you can ask about them when appropriate to build a trusting relationship, though do not get too personal. Avoid any romantic relationships at work. If tensions arise between you and your supervisor, take positive steps to ease them. Your supervisor has power over your raises, promotions, benefits, and references for future employment. When you disagree, discuss these differences in private.

Foster a Positive Attitude Under Stress

Be an encourager rather than a complainer, and do not give in to the temptation to behave in ways that are elitist or superior. Remember that you are part of a healthcare team, and cooperation is extremely important.

Reflect a Desire for Self-Improvement

Get in the habit of asking questions respectfully and listening to the answers. Sometimes people are afraid to ask questions because doing so might make them appear less intelligent or less knowledgeable. Nothing could be further from the truth. Listen to the advice of others who have been on the job longer. If you make a mistake, own up to it. If you are criticized unfairly, adopt a non-defensive tone of voice and explain your view of the matter calmly and rationally. This behavior is key to performing with integrity, an important part of being a professional.

Become Known for Reliability

Health care, like education, is one of those industries in which standards for reliability are very high. You cannot, for example, show up late for work or take days off arbitrarily without good reason and prior supervisor approval. Unreliable employees in the healthcare industry do not keep their jobs for long, so make sure that your employer can always depend on you to arrive at work on time. Staying late does not make up for a tardy arrival. Tardiness can play havoc with other people's work schedules and workloads and lead to preventable medication errors. Finish dressing, grooming, and eating before you enter your work area.

Excel in Your Performance

Demonstrate that you can get things done and that you put the job first. Develop work habits to ensure accuracy, and expect to be held responsible for what you do on the job. Work steadily and methodically. Employers expect you to devote your full attention to your responsibilities for the entire length of your shift. Rushing through a task because it is close to the end of your shift places patient care at risk. Keep your attention focused on the task at hand, and always double-check everything you do, even close to quitting time.

Turn Problems into Opportunities to Develop and Implement Solutions

Instead of complaining about problems, look for creative fixes that improve systems and situations. This can earn you recognition and new responsibilities, and often a new title and an increase in benefits. When a crisis occurs, do not overreact, but keep looking for solutions. Take time to think and then act, and do not keep the crisis a secret from your supervisor.

Nurture Healthy Professional Alliances

In all organizations, two kinds of power systems exist: (1) formal, or structural, hierarchies; and (2) informal collegial relationships, or alliances. Cultivate friendships on the job, but make sure that you are not seen as part of a clique or an exclusive group. Even as a new employee, begin to build power through trusting, supportive connections with your colleagues and in professional organizations outside of the job. If a problem or an opportunity arises, then you will probably hear about it first through your allies. If an impending change in the workplace affects you, advance notice may give you the necessary time to plan a strategic response. Most of the big lucky breaks in life come through knowing the right people at the right time. By cultivating alliances, you can control your luck more than you might expect.

Develop Specialized Expertise

How can you become a person who makes things happen? Become highly knowledgeable about a specialty within your company or field, inventory control, insurance billing, non-sterile compounding, and so on. Be the most expert technician that you can be in that area, then move on and master another area. Soon, others will be asking for your advice, and your reputation (and your salary) will grow. You can also choose to pursue additional certifications in pharmacy or in allied health to create more opportunities.

Build an Active Professional Reputation

Many people assume that if they work hard and are loyal, they will be rewarded. This is often but not always true. Management personnel may be so involved with their own concerns that you remain little more than a face in the crowd. Being pleasant to others helps you to be noticed, as does making helpful or useful suggestions. Volunteer to serve on committees within the institution. Make yourself indispensable to the organization. Be open and flexible to learning new positions, and be proactive, accepting new responsibilities within the pharmacy. When you have won an award or achieved some other success, see that your name is publicized in institutional newsletters, community newspapers, or the publications of professional organizations. Give presentations at professional meetings, civic groups, churches, or synagogues. Write or contribute to articles for publication in professional journals.

Commit to Ongoing Continuing Education

Pharmacy is a rapidly changing field. Staying current on new drugs, dosage forms, medication safety, laws, and regulations is important. Accept the idea of continuing education (CE) as a way of life. CE may include reading pharmacy journals and newsletters or attending workshops at professional meetings. You may need to take formal course work (in person or online) or attend CE programs every year to maintain your certification and keep current on the latest trends. Think of your job-related learning as a regular "information workout," as necessary to your employment fitness as aerobic workouts are to your physical fitness. Reading *Pharmacy Times* on an ongoing basis will help you keep abreast of new drugs. For a taste of this excellent source for ongoing news, visit https://PharmPractice7e.Paradigm Education.com/PharmacyTimes.

Practice Tip

There are many options for attaining the useful Basic Life Support (BLS)/CPR certification first aid, or other healthcare training. You can go to the American Red Cross for a session near you. Visit https://PharmPractice7e.Paradigmeducation.com/CPRclass to learn more.

Develop Depth and Breadth in Operational Skills

Higher-level positions require initiative and the ability to work independently, efficiently, and without procrastination. They generally integrate skills beyond those of basic competence for an entry-level technician in one or more of the following areas:

- advanced calculations
- ability to precisely check work of other technicians
- advanced communication and public relations/marketing skills
- advanced knowledge of computer and automation applications
- billing and documentation procedures
- inventory ordering and purchasing
- leadership, organizing, and management skills
- staff training responsibilities
- supervision skills and ability to build cooperation among team members

Acquire Additional Certifications, Diplomas, and Degrees

Advanced technician positions (sterile, hazardous, and nuclear certifications), first aid, BLS/CPR, phlebotomist, emergency medical services (EMS), and OSHA certifications provide a range of skills and greater job opportunities and pay. Look at as stepping stones or stackable skills that help advance your career in many ways, offering you unforeseen opportunities to move both laterally into more rewarding areas for you personally, and vertically, into greater supervision and management positions.

Additionally, graduate degrees, such as an MBA or a degree in human resources or health system management, offer you even wider-ranging opportunities in pharmacy and health care. They assist your marketability as an employee by always building on the extensive pharmaceutical education, training, understanding, and experience you received as a CPhT.

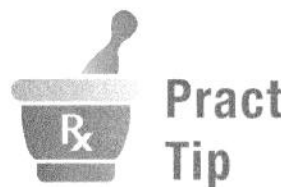

Do not keep your professional qualifications a secret. Join professional organizations and volunteer to serve on committees within the organization.

Become Active in Professional Pharmacy Organizations

Being part of a profession means taking an active role in advancing the profession, especially if you are seriously considering taking on one or more advanced roles. As **paraprofessionals** in pharmacy practice, technicians have an obligation and a vested interest to make their ideas heard in the local, state, and national forums that discuss issues facing their field. The future of the technician role is in the hands of those within the profession. This self-governance, something that is increasing for technicians, is one characteristic of a professional. As the status and role of pharmacy technicians increase, those within the profession should get involved in the decisions and movements affecting it. Apply for membership in the **American Association of Pharmacy Technicians (AAPT)** or the National Pharmacy Technician Association, and get involved.

American Association of Pharmacy Technicians

The AAPT was the first professional organization for pharmacy technicians. It was organized in 1979 and is still run today by volunteer pharmacy technicians. The mission statement is as follows:

- Provides leadership and represents the interests of its members to the public as well as healthcare organizations
- Promotes the safe, efficacious, and cost-effective dispensing, distribution, and use of medications
- Provides continuing education programs and services to help technicians update their skills to keep pace with changes in pharmacy services
- Promotes pharmacy technicians as an integral part of the patient care team

There are low membership rates, especially for students and those entering their first year of practice. All members are eligible to take necessary continuing education courses online at no cost, and the organization also has blogs run and written by peers, current information updates, and a career center. Several states have local chapters for networking, CE, and involvement. For more information, visit https://PharmPractice7e.ParadigmEducation.com/PharmacyTech.

Attending and actively participating in professional organizations is an excellent strategy for networking and job advancement.

The ASHP encourages membership of pharmacy technicians, especially those practicing in hospitals.

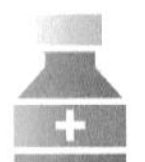

Pharm Fact

Pharmacy Technician Day is October 20. It is a good day for gathering with other technicians and lobbying your state pharmacy board or legislature for greater recognition of technicians, certification requirements, pay, and benefits.

National Pharmacy Technician Association

The **National Pharmacy Technician Association (NPTA)** is the largest professional society for pharmacy technicians. Low-cost membership is offered to technicians, students, and educators. NPTA is an advocacy organization that updates its members on relevant news and provides online continuing education courses.

Get Involved

There are several ways to get involved in your professional network to help advance within the profession:

- Serve on AAPT or NPTA committees, participate in state and national conferences, and run for office in your local chapter of these organizations, as appropriate.
- Attend the meetings of your state pharmacy board and state chapter of the National Association of Boards of Pharmacy (NABP) and volunteer on committees if allowed; each state NABP chapter welcomes technician input and participation.
- Apply for membership in the American Society of Health-System Pharmacists (ASHP) and/or the National Community Pharmacists Association (NCPA); volunteer to serve on local chapter committees and eventually the Pharmacy Technician Advisory Group of the ASHP, which is charged with advising the ASHP's staff and Board of Directors about actions, products, and services pertaining to pharmacy technicians.
- Explore opportunities with the Pharmacy Technician Certification Board (PTCB) Certification Councils at the national level.
- Participate in your state pharmacy association's annual pharmacy legislative day activities.

After attending local, state, or national meetings, report what you learn to your employer and fellow technicians. Learning about and voicing concern about issues facing technicians and taking ownership in decisions made to advance their roles give you a sense of control over your own destiny, especially when you do this with others. Participating in professional organizations can also provide needed CE credits for recertification.

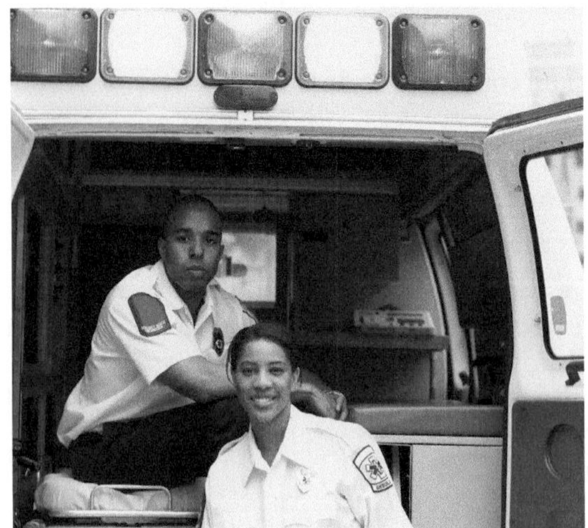

Training and experience as a pharmacy technician can lead to other health-related jobs, such as EMT.

Current issues that face technicians are standardization of technician training and education programs; expansion of technician responsibilities to assist with the projected shortages in pharmacy workforces; salary and benefits enhancements; and implementation of state requirements for national certification. Contact your local technician organizations and inquire about how you can participate in decisions affecting the future practice of pharmacy in your state.

Springboard to Other Healthcare Disciplines

Some pharmacy technicians use their training and experience in customer service and knowledge of drug therapy as a springboard to other associated careers or higher-paying health professions. In the allied health field, many healthcare-related assistant or technician positions may require only one or two years of study. Examples of such rewarding occupations include technician positions in emergency medical treatment (an EMT), anesthesia, chemotherapy, electrocardiology, emergency room, endoscopy, health information, home health (assistant/aide), magnetic resonance imaging (MRI), medical billing and coding, medical laboratory, nuclear medicine, operating room (OR), radiology, respiratory technology, or certain kinds of surgery.

Some pharmacy technicians like the profession so much that they want to advance into a career as a pharmacist. Some of the most successful practicing pharmacists started out as pharmacy technicians. If your grades in prerequisite course work are above average and you do well on the standardized Pharmacy College Admission Test (PCAT) (like a science-related SAT), this may be a good plan, and the experience of working in a pharmacy (with good references and letters of recommendation from your supervisor) will be a big bonus. This experience will allow you easier admission than inexperienced applicants. You may still be able to work as a pharmacy technician some nights or weekends as you attend pharmacy school, and many chain pharmacies offer scholarship help and loan forgiveness if you elect to take a job with them for a set number of years after graduation and receiving your certification.

Other students may use their technician experience to pursue a higher-paying career in nursing, physical therapy, or clinical nutrition. However, these careers, as well as pharmacy, will take four to six years of full-time study to complete. You may be able to work as a technician part-time while taking courses.

16.6 Claim Your Future, the Opportunities Are There

The increasing number of prescriptions dispensed to the American population, along with a rising proportion of seniors and the expanding roles of both pharmacists and technicians, translates into an increase in needs in the pharmacy workforce. According to the Bureau of Labor Statistics, the demand for pharmacy technicians is expected to continue to increase faster than that of the average job in the next decade. In addition to dispensing more prescriptions, pharmacists will be expected to play a more prominent role in controlling drug costs and abuse through more effective counseling of patients as well as monitoring disease outcomes with the most cost-effective therapies. This shift offers more and more opportunities for you as you enter this exciting and ever-changing field.

With a commitment to excellence, improvement, problem solving, leadership, and continuing education, you will be able to grasp many varied opportunities, and develop a satisfying and rewarding career with many exciting steps, turns, and leaps into a fulfilling future.

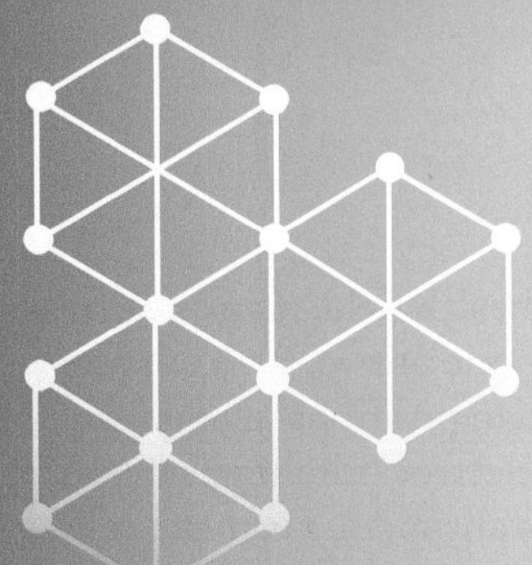

Review and Assessment

CHAPTER SUMMARY

- Society and pharmacy professional organizations hold the pharmacy technician (as a paraprofessional) to a strict code of ethics.
- Certification for pharmacy technicians is offered through the exams of the Pharmacy Technician Certification Board (PTCB)—the PTCE—and the National Healthcareer Association (NHA)—the ExCPT.
- More states are requiring national certification and a standardized formal education for pharmacy technicians.
- Specialty certifications and experience may be required in select areas of pharmacy practice.
- Clarifying your career goals, networking, using social media, and researching the job market are crucial first steps to starting your career.
- Writing a comprehensive, attractive résumé and cover letter is an important part of a carefully planned job search.
- Preparing for a job interview is integral to obtaining a desirable pharmacy technician position.
- Preparing to work in an institutional or community-based pharmacy requires serious thought about one's attitude, reliability, accuracy, responsibility, personal appearance, organizational skills, and ability to relate to others.
- Technicians will have increasing opportunities for job advancement as requirements for certification and training increase.
- A hierarchy of pharmacy technician positions has evolved to reflect training, credentials (including certification), experience, and specializations.
- Advanced roles in pharmacy management and provision of clinical experience are available for the self-motivated, experienced, and certified pharmacy technician.
- Active involvement in professional organizations is important for establishing a network of colleagues and for professional advancement.
- The short- and long-term occupational outlooks for pharmacy technicians are promising.

CHECK YOUR UNDERSTANDING

To ensure that you recall and understand the key chapter concepts, please read the question or statement and select the appropriate lettered option.

1. Eligibility for certification by the PTCB includes all of the following *except*
   a. urine drug screen.
   b. high school diploma or GED.
   c. disclosure of any criminal violations.
   d. compliance with Code of Conduct.
2. Which of the following statements about PTCE pharmacy technician certification is correct?
   a. It is granted by a governmental body.
   b. It is mandatory in all states.
   c. It is transferrable to all states.
   d. It requires college course work.
3. The format for the PTCE and ExCPT is
   a. essay.
   b. multiple choice.
   c. true or false.
   d. on-site laboratory assessment.
4. Which category of the PTCE carries the highest weighted percentage?
   a. Pharmacology for Technicians; Order Entry and Processing
   b. Medication Safety; Patient Safety and Quality Assurance
   c. Pharmacy Laws and Regulations; Federal Requirements
   d. Medications; Order Entry and Fill Process
5. Once a pharmacy technician becomes certified, they must become recertified every
   a. six months.
   b. year.
   c. two years.
   d. five years.
6. Which social media platform is recommended by career experts so that interested recruiters can access your résumé online?
   a. Facebook
   b. Twitter
   c. LinkedIn
   d. Instagram

MAKE CONNECTIONS

Take a moment to consider what you have learned in this chapter and respond thoughtfully to the following prompts. Note that some of these activities will require internet access.

1. Many pharmacy technicians may be hired on a contingency basis—contingent upon a favorable performance evaluation. Write a short essay about the evaluation process that answers the following questions: When is the first evaluation typically held and how often are evaluations completed after initial hire? What measurable and nonmeasurable areas are covered in an initial evaluation? What kind of evaluation scale is used and how is it critiqued?
2. Traditionally, less than 10% of pharmacy technician time is spent in nontraditional or advanced roles, but these percentages are changing as pharmacists' roles are expanding. With the manufacturing of new drugs, plausible drug interactions, drug studies of old drugs, and prescription drug abuse, doctors and physicians and other healthcare providers simply cannot find the time or resources to keep up with all this drug information as thoroughly as pharmacists. In the community pharmacy, pilot projects have utilized pharmacy technicians to assist pharmacists. In a short essay, describe some advanced roles for the pharmacy technician as they assist the pharmacist in providing MTM. What advanced roles for the pharmacy technician may be feasible in this area in the future?

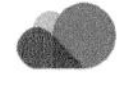
The online course includes additional review and assessment resources.

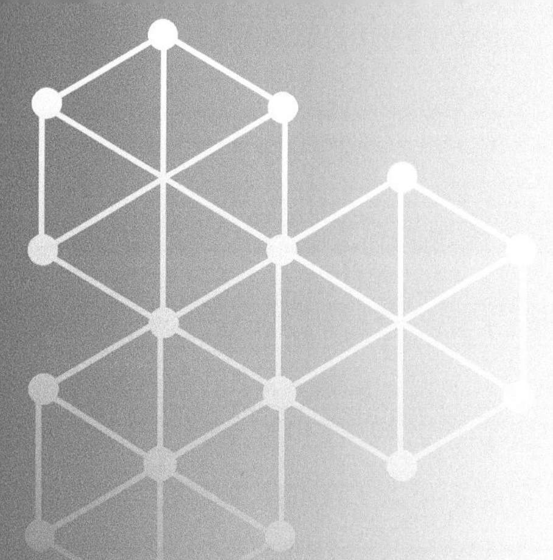

Appendix A

Common Pharmacy Abbreviations and Acronyms

The abbreviations with red lines through them are ones that are still in use but are discouraged by Institute for Safe Medication Practices (ISMP). The ISMP recommends the use of the correct words instead. Many of these discouraged abbreviations are also on the Joint Commission's Official "Do Not Use" List of Abbreviations.

Abbreviation	Meaning
A-B-C	
aaa	apply to affected area
ACA	Affordable Care Act (Patient Protection and Affordable Care Act)
~~ac~~; ~~a.c.~~; ~~AC~~	before meals
ACE	angiotensin-converting enzyme inhibitors
ad; a.d.; AD	right ear
ADD	attention-deficit disorder
ADH	antidiuretic hormone
ADHD	attention-deficit hyperactivity disorder
ADME	absorption, distribution, metabolism, and elimination
ADR	adverse drug reaction
AIDS	acquired immune deficiency syndrome
AM; a.m.	morning
ANDA	Abbreviated New Drug Application
APAP	acetaminophen; Tylenol
AphA	American Pharmacy Association
ARBs	angiotensin receptor blockers
~~as~~; ~~a.s.~~; ~~AS~~	left ear
ASA	aspirin
~~au~~; ~~a.u.~~; ~~AU~~	both ears; each ear
b.i.d.; BID	twice daily
BMI	Body Mass Index
BP	blood pressure
BUD	beyond-use date
°C	degrees centigrade; temperature in degrees centigrade
Ca^{++}	calcium

Abbreviation	Meaning
Cap, cap	capsule
CDC	Centers for Disease Control and Prevention
CF	cystic fibrosis
CHF	congestive heart failure
CNS	Central Nervous System
COPD	chronic obstructive pulmonary disease
CPR	cardio pulminary resuscitation
CSP	compounded sterile preparation
CV	cardiovascular
D-E-F	
D_5; D_5W; D5W	dextrose 5% in water
D_5 ¼; D5 1/4	dextrose 5% in ¼ normal saline; dextrose 5% in 0.225% sodium chloride
D_5 ½; D5 1/3	dextrose 5% in ⅓ normal saline; dextrose 5% in 0.33% sodium chloride
D_5 ½; D5 1/2	dextrose 5% in ½ normal saline; dextrose 5% in 0.45% sodium chloride
D_5LR; D5LR	dextrose 5% in lactated Ringer's solution
D_5NS; D5NS	dextrose 5% in normal saline; dextrose 5% in 0.9% sodium chloride
DAW	dispense as written
~~DC~~; ~~d/c~~	discontinue
D/C	discharge
DCA	direct compounding area
Dig	digoxin
disp	dispense
EC	enteric-coated
Elix	elixir
eMAR	electronic medication administration record
EPO	epoetin alfa; erythropoietin
ER; XR; XL	extended-release
°F	degrees Fahrenheit; temperature in degrees Fahrenheit
$FeSO_4$	ferrous sulfate; iron
G-H-I	
g, G	gram
gr	grain
GI	gastrointestinal
GMP	good manufacturing practice
gtt	drops
h; hr	hour
HC	hydrocortisone
HCTZ	hydrochlorothiazide
HIPAA	Health Insurance Portability and Accountability Act
HIV	human immunodeficiency virus
HMO	Health Maintenance Organization
HRT	hormone replacement therapy

Abbreviation	Meaning
~~h.s.~~; ~~HS~~	bedtime (comes from Latin hora somni <italic hora somni> meaning "hour of sleep")
IBU	ibuprofen; Motrin
ICU	intensive care unit
IM	intramuscular
IND	Investigational New Drug Application
Inj	injection
IPA	isopropyl alcohol
ISDN	isosorbide dinitrate
ISMO	isosorbide mononitrate
ISMP	Institute for Safe Medication Practices
IV	intravenous
IVF	intravenous fluid
IVP	intravenous push
IVPB	intravenous piggyback
J-K-L	
K; K+	potassium
KCl	potassium chloride
kg	kilogram
L	liter
LAFW	laminar airflow workbench; hood
lb	pound
LD	loading dose
LVP	large-volume parenteral
JCAHO	Joint Commission on the Accreditation of Healthcare Organizations
M-N-O	
Mag; Mg; MAG	magnesium
MAR	medication administration record
mcg	microgram
MDI	metered-dose inhaler
MDV	multiple-dose vial
mEq	milliequivalent
mg	milligram
~~Mg~~SO_4	magnesium sulfate; magnesium
mL	milliliter
mL/hr	milliliters per hour
mL/min	milliliters per minute

Abbreviation	Meaning
MMR	measles, mumps, and rubella vaccine
MRSA	methiciliin-resistant S. aureaus
MOM; M.O.M.	milk of magnesia
~~M.S.~~	morphine sulfate (save MS for multiple sclerosis)
~~MU~~†; ~~mu~~	million units
MVI; MVI-12	multiple vitamin injection; multivitamins for parenteral administration
Na^+	sodium
NABP	National Association of Boards of Pharmacy
NaCl	sodium chloride; salt
NDA	New Drug App
NDC	National Drug Code
NF; non-form	nonformulary
NKA	no known allergies
NKDA	no known drug allergies
NPO, npo	nothing by mouth
NR; d.n.r.	no refills; do not repeat
NS	normal saline; 0.9% sodium chloride
½ NS	one-half normal saline; 0.45% sodium chloride
¼ NS	one-quarter normal saline; 0.225% sodium chloride
NSAID	nonsteroidal anti-inflammatory drug
NTG	nitroglycerin
OC	oral contraceptive
~~od~~; ~~o.d.~~; ~~OD~~	right eye
ODT	orally disintegrating tablet
OPTH; OPHTH; Opth	ophthalmic
~~os~~; ~~o.s.~~; ~~OS~~	left eye
OTC	over the counter; no prescription required
~~ou~~; ~~o.u.~~; ~~OU~~	both eyes; each eye
oz	ounce
P-Q-R	
p.c.; PC	after meals
PCA	patient-controlled anesthesia
PCN	penicillin
pH	acid-base balance
PHI	protected health information
PM; p.m.	afternoon; evening
PN	paternal nutrition

Abbreviation	Meaning
PNS	peripheral nervous system
PO; po	orally; by mouth
PPE	personal protective equipment
PPI	proton pump inhibitor
PR	per rectum; rectally
PRN; p.r.n.	as needed; as occasion requires
PTSD	Post Traumatic Stress Disorder
PV	per vagina; vaginally
PVC	polyvinyl chloride
q	every
q.h.; qhour	every hour
q2h	every 2 hours
q4h	every 4 hours
q6h	every 6 hours
q8h	every 8 hours
q12h	every 12 hours
q24h	every 24 hours
q48h	every 48 hours
QA	quality assurance
QAM; qam	every morning
qDay; QD	every day
q.i.d.; QID	four times daily
QOD; Q other day; Q.O. Day	every other day
QPM; qpm	every evening
qs; qsad	quantity sufficient; a sufficient quantity to make
QTY; qty	quantity
qwk; qweek	every week
RA	rheumatoid arthritis
RDA	recommended daily allowance
Rx	prescription; pharmacy; medication; drug; recipe; take
S-T	
sig	write on label; signa; directions
SL; sub-L	sublingual
SMZ-TMP	sulfamethoxazole and trimethoprim; Bactrim
SNRI	serotonin nonrepinephrine reuptake inhibitor
SPF	sunburn protection factor

Abbreviation	Meaning
SR	sustained-release
~~SS~~; ~~ss~~	one-half
SSRI	selective serotonin reuptake inhibitor (don't use for sliding scale insulins)
STAT, Stat	immediately; now
STD	sexually transmitted disease
~~Sub-Q~~; ~~SC~~; ~~SQ~~; ~~sq~~, subcut, SUBCUT	subcutaneous
SUPP; Supp	suppository
susp	suspension
SVP	small-volume parenteral
SW	sterile water
SWFI	sterile water for injection
Tab; tab	tablet
TB	tuberculosis
TBSP; tbsp	tablespoon; tablespoonful; 15 mL
TDS	transdermal delivery system
~~t.i.d.~~; ~~TID~~	three times daily
~~t.i.w.~~; ~~TIW~~	three times a week
TKO; TKVO; KO; KVO	to keep open; to keep vein open; keep open; keep vein open (a slow IV flow rate)
TNA	Total Nutrition Admixture
TPN	total parenteral nutrition
TSP; tsp	teaspoon; teaspoonful; 5 mL
U-V-W	
~~U~~ or ~~u~~	unit
~~u.d.~~, ~~UD~~, ~~ut dictum~~	as directed
ung	ointment
USP	U.S. Pharmacopoeial Convention
USP-NF	U.S. Pharmacopoeia-National Forumulary <italics>
UTI	urinary tract infection
UV	ultraviolet light
VAG; vag	vagina; vaginally
Vanco	vancomycin
VO; V.O.; V/O	verbal order
w/o	without
X-Y-Z	
Zn	zinc
Z-Pak	azithromycin; Zithromax

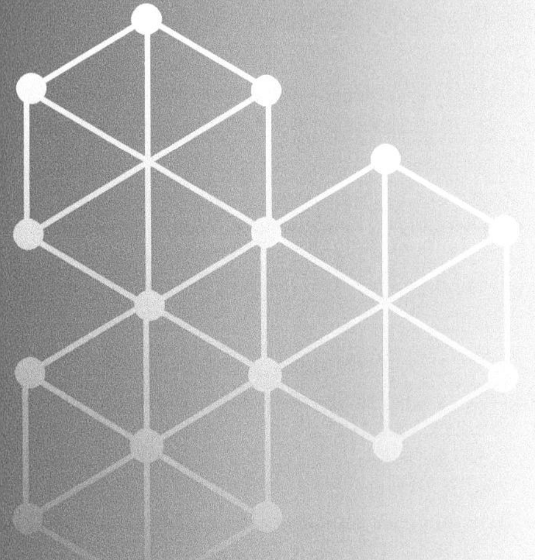

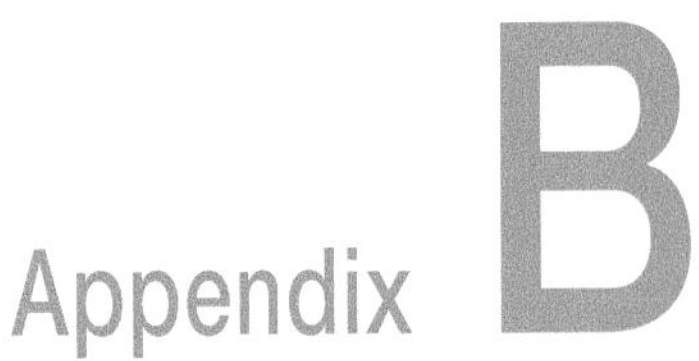

Appendix B

ASHP/ACPE Accreditation Standards

The following identifies the *ASHP/ACPE Accreditation Standards* addressed in each chapter of Paradigm's *Pharmacy Practice for Technicians*. This appendix identifies the *ASHP/ACPE Standards* associated with the module content. This list is meant for guidance purposes only. Neither ASHP nor ACPE has participated in or had any role in creating the list of standards or any other content that is included in this book.

Chapter 1
Entry-Level: 2.1, 2.2, 2.3, 2.7, 4.1, 4.2, 4.7, 5.1, 5.2, 5.3, 5.4, 5.5, 5.6
Advanced-Level: 4.9, 4.11, 4.13, 5.9, 5.10

Chapter 2
Entry-Level: 2.2, 3.10, 3.12, 4.1, 4.2, 4.3, 5.1, 5.2, 5.3, 5.4, 5.5, 5.6, 5.7
Advanced-Level: 4.12, 5.9, 5.10

Chapter 3
Entry-Level: 2.5, 3.10, 4.1, 4.2,
Advanced-Level: 2.9, 3.30,

Chapter 4
Entry-Level: 2.5, 4.1, 4.2, 5.1, 5.2, 5.3, 5.4, 5.5, 5.6
Advanced-Level: 2.9, 4.9, 5.9, 5.10

Chapter 5
Entry-Level: 2.5, 3.9, 4.2
Advanced-Level: 2.9

Chapter 6
Entry-Level: 2.6, 3.20, 5.5, 5.6
Advanced-Level: 5.9

Chapter 7
Entry-Level: 1.4, 2.2, 2.3, 2.4, 2.6, 2.7, 3.1, 3.2, 3.3, 3.4, 3.6, 3.7, 3.8, 3.11, 3.12, 3.13, 3.14, 3.18, 3.19, 3.22, 4.1, 4.2, 4.3, 4.5, 4.6, 4.7, 5.1, 5.2, 5.3, 5.4, 5.5, 5.6, 5.7
Advanced-Level: 1.10, 2.11, 3.27, 3.28, 3.31, 4.9, 4.10, 4.11, 4.12, 5.9, 5.10

Chapter 8
Entry-Level: 1.4, 2.2, 2.3 2.6, 3.1, 3.2, 3.3, 3.13, 3.14, 3.21, 4.1, 4.2, 4.5, 4.7, 5.1, 5.2, 5.3, 5.4, 5.5, 5.6
Advanced-Level: 1.10, 3.26, 3.29, 3.31, 4.9, 4.11, 5.9, 5.10

Chapter 9
Entry-Level: 1.4, 2.2, 2.3, 2.4, 2.6, 3.1, 3.3, 3.8, 3.10, 3.11, 3.13, 3.14, 3.18, 3.19, 3.22, 4.1, 4.2, 4.4, 4.5, 4.7, 5.1, 5.2, 5.3, 5.4, 5.5, 5.6
Advanced-Level: 1.10, 2.11, 3.26, 3.27, 3.28, 3.31, 4.11, 4.13, 5.9, 5.10

Chapter 10
Entry-Level: 3.4, 3.5, 3.6, 3.9, 3.10, 3.13, 3.15, 3.16, 3.17, 3.20, 4.1, 4.2, 4.8
Advanced-Level: 2.10, 3.24, 3.25, 3.26

Chapter 11
Entry-Level: 1.4, 2.2, 2.3, 2.7, 3.1, 3.2, 3.4, 3.6, 3.7, 3.8, 3.13, 3.15, 3.18, 3.19, 3.22, 4.1, 4.2, 4.3, 4.5, 4.7, 4.8, 5.1, 5.2, 5.3, 5.4, 5.5, 5.6
Advanced-Level: 3.26, 3.27, 3.30, 3.31, 4.11, 4.12, 5.9, 5.10

Chapter 12
Entry-Level: 1.1, 2.1, 2.2, 2.3, 2.4, 2.8, 3.4, 3.5, 3.6, 3.8, 3.11, 3.13, 3.15, 3.20, 3.21, 4.1, 4.2, 4.8, 5.1, 5.2, 5.3, 5.4, 5.5, 5.6, 5.7
Advanced-Level: 2.10, 2.11, 3.23, 3.25, 3.26, 3.29, 5.9, 5.10

Chapter 13
Entry-Level: 2.1, 2.2, 2.3, 2.6, 2.8, 3.1, 3.2, 3.4, 3.5, 3.6, 3.8, 3.9, 3.11, 3.13, 4.1, 4.2, 5.1, 5.2, 5.3, 5.4, 5.5, 5.6, 5.8
Advanced-Level: 2.10, 3.23, 3.25, 3.30, 3.31, 4.9, 5.9, 5.10

Chapter 14
Entry-Level: 1.1, 1.3, 2.2, 2.4, 2.7, 2.8, 3.1, 3.2, 3.6, 3.7, 3.1, 3.12, 3.13, 3.21, 4.1, 4.2, 4.3, 4.4, 4.5, 4.7, 5.1, 5.2, 5.3, 5.4, 5.5, 5.6
Advanced-Level: 1.11, 1.12, 2.11, 3.29, 3.31, 4.9, 4.11, 4.12, 4.13, 5.9., 5.10

Chapter 15
Entry-Level: 1.1, 1.2, 1.3, 1.4, 1.5, 1.6, 1.7, 1.8, 2.1, 2.2, 2.3, 2.4, 2.7, 3.3, 3.12, 3.1, 4.2, 4.4, 5.1, 5.2, 5.3, 5.4, 5.5, 5.6
Advanced-Level: 1.9, 1.10, 1.11, 1.12, 2.11, 5.9, 5.10

Chapter 16
Entry-Level: 1.2, 1.4, 1.6, 1.7 1.8, 2.1, 2.2, 2.3, 4.5, 4.7
Advanced-Level: 1.9, 1.10, 1.11, 1.12, 3.30, 4.11, 4.13

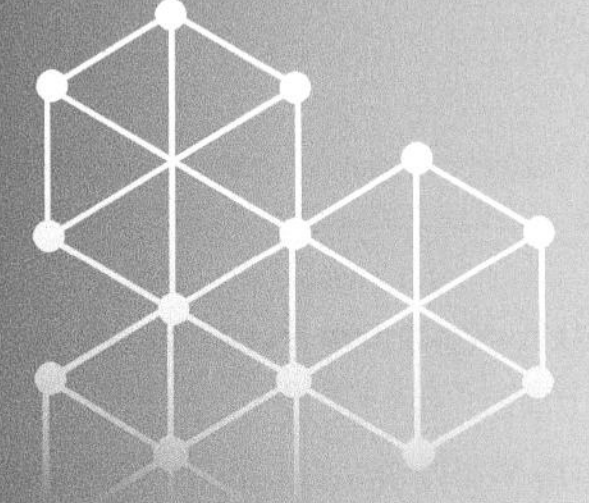

Glossary

2-in-1 solution a parenteral nutrition solution that contains a formulation of dextrose and amino acids with the lipid emulsion administered via piggyback in a separate bag

3-in-1 solution a parenteral nutrition solution that contains dextrose, amino acids, and lipids in one bottle

abbreviated new drug application the process by which applicants must scientifically demonstrate to the FDA that their generic product is bioequivalent to or performs similarly to the innovator (brand name) drug

abortifacient drug drug designed specifically to terminate a pregnancy

Accountable Care Organizations (ACOs) groups of prescribers, pharmacists, and other providers, hospitals, and healthcare facilities that work together in a coordinated manner to seek out measurable improvements in patient outcomes

Accreditation Commission for Health Care (ACHC) an organization that sponsors the Pharmacy Compounding Accreditation Board (PCAB), which certifies compounding pharmacies in quality and safety standards

accreditation the status achieved by meeting the quality standards and requirements designated by the accrediting organization

acquisition cost the net price paid by the pharmacy to acquire a product from a wholesaler or supplier, including the adjustments such as discounts and rebates

active ingredient the biochemically active component of a drug that exerts the desired therapeutic effect

active pharmaceutical ingredient any substance in a compounded preparation that confers pharmacological activity

added substances ingredients that are necessary to a preparation but do not confer pharmacological activity; inactive ingredients

addiction compulsive and uncontrollable use of a drug substance for reasons other than prescribed

adjuvant medications medications that assist another drug to offer more effective or long-lasting pain relief

admitting order a request for specific medications and medical procedures written by the admitting physician

adulterated product a product that differs in drug strength, quality, and purity from the original

adverse drug error a medication error that occurs when the prescribed drug initiates an allergy or an adverse drug interaction because a flag was missed

adverse drug events (ADEs) injuries or harmful responses due to the use of a drug

adverse drug reaction (ADR) an unexpected negative consequence from taking a particular drug

Adverse Event Reporting System (AERS) a post-surveillance centralized database maintained by the FDA for all reported adverse events from drugs and vaccines

aerosol a pressurized container with a propellant that is used to administer a drug through oral inhalation into the lungs

Affordable Care Act (ACA) mandated healthcare coverage under threat of personal penalties for all US citizens

agglomerations clusters, lumps, clumps, or globs of ingredients in a liquid, semiliquid, or powdered vehicle, which are undesired in compounding

air exchange replacement of air

alchemy the European practice during the Middle Ages that combined elements of chemistry, metallurgy, physics, and medicine with astrology, mysticism, and spiritualism to turn a common item into something special or extraordinary; an example would be the transmutation of a base metal into silver or gold

alcoholic solutions alcohol-based solutions for oral dosage forms

alert fatigue fatigue that arises and causes the technician and/or the pharmacist to have a relaxed attitude and bypass drug utilization warnings

allergy a state of heightened sensitivity as a result of exposure to a particular substance

alligation alternate method method of calculating the proportions of two different substances to be combined in a new product to create a different concentration of the active ingredient

alternative medicine the use of medical products and practices that are not part of standard care

altruism an unselfish concern for the welfare of others

American Association of Pharmacy Technicians (AAPT) the first professional organization for pharmacy technicians that was organized in 1979 and is still run today by volunteer pharmacy technicians

American Botanical Council (ABC) a nonprofit organization, started in 1988, dedicated to educating consumers, healthcare professionals, researchers, educators, industry, and media about proper and safe use of herbs and medicinal plants

American Herbal Pharmacopoeia (AHP) a nonprofit organization, started in 1995, that has the mission of promoting responsible use of herbal products and medicines with scientific research, quality testing, and education

American Pharmacists Association (APhA) an organization that helped establish professional practice standards for drug ingredients, compounding, and dosages; it also encouraged regulation for pharmacy apprentices to pass formal certification exams before becoming full pharmacists

American Society of Health-System Pharmacists (ASHP) represents the interests of pharmacists and pharmacy technicians who practice in hospitals, health maintenance organizations, long-term care facilities, home care, and other components of healthcare; formerly called the American Society of Hospital Pharmacists, an organization that developed formalized technician training programs and a model curriculum

ampule a small, hermetically sealed sterile container made of glass

anabolic steroids synthetic, performance enhancing drugs that mimic the human hormone testosterone; because of abuse by athletes, this drug has been reclassified by the DEA as a controlled substance

analgesia substance used to relieve pain

angioedema swelling under the skin that can be a life-threatening allergic reaction; manifests by swelling of the tongue, lips, or eyes

angiotensin-converting enzyme (ACE) inhibitors medications that lower blood pressure by blocking the liver's production of an enzyme that constricts blood vessels

angiotensin receptor blockers (ARBs) a family of drugs that lowers blood pressure by blocking the absorption of the enzyme that constricts blood vessels

anteroom an ISO Class 8 or cleaner room with fixed walls and doors where personnel hand hygiene, garbing procedures, and other activities that generate high particulate levels may be performed. The ante-room is the transition room between the unclassified area of the facility and the buffer room

anti-inflammatory drugs drugs that reduce swelling in skin and internal organs

antibiotics chemical substances with the ability to kill or inhibit the growth of bacteria by interfering with bacteria life processes

antibodies the part of the immune system that neutralizes antigens or foreign substances in the body

anticipatory compounding the preparation of excess product (in excess of a compounded prescription) in reasonable quantities; these preparations must be labeled with lot numbers and beyond-use dates

anticonvulsant acting in a manner that controls seizures

antidepressants drugs that work to lift moods and/or change perceptions

antidiabetic drugs drugs that supply insulin to lower sugar or stimulate the pancreas to produce more insulin

antigen a foreign substance or toxin introduced into the body that stimulates an immune response

antihistamines drugs that block certain histamine receptors and are used to treat and lesson the symptoms of allergies

antihyperlipidemic drugs cardiovascular drugs used to treat high cholesterol and triglycerides

antihypertensive agents drugs that lower high blood pressure

antipsychotic drugs medications used to manage disordered thought and personality behaviors, such as depression, delusions, hallucinations, mania, and severe agitation

antiseptic refers to a substance that kills or inhibits the growth of microorganisms on the outside of the body to reduce the possibility of infection, sepsis, or putrefaction

antiviral drug a drug that kills viruses, such as HIV

apothecary a shop where medicines are gathered, stored, and compounded by skilled artisans using herbs and other natural ingredients

apothecary system a measurement system developed by the Romans

appearance the overall outward look of an employee on the job, including dress and grooming

apyrogenicity not causing a fever

aqueous solutions water-based solutions for oral dosage forms

Arabic numeral system a mathematical system using numbers, fractions, and decimals to indicate numerical values

aromatic water a solution of water containing oils or other substances that has a pungent, and usually pleasing, smell and is easily released into the air

arrest to lock balancing pans on a balance scale

aseptic handwashing a more aggressive soap and water hand-washing procedure, followed by use of an antiseptic agent before donning sterile attire

aseptic technique a set of methods used to keep objects and areas free of microorganisms and thereby minimize infection risk to the. patient; accomplished through practices that maintain the microbe count at an irreducible minimum

atomic weight the weight of a single atom of an element compared with the weight of one atom of hydrogen

attention deficit hyperactivity disorder (ADHD) a disorder that manifests itself in difficulty focusing or concentrating, over-activity, and difficulty with impulse control

attenuated virus a weakened virus contained in some vaccines, as opposed to a live or inactive virus

attestation statement a statement by a witness who verifies that they observed the correct individuals put their signatures on a given document

attitude the emotional stance or disposition that a worker adopts toward job duties, customers, employer, and coworkers

atypical antipsychotic drugs first-line therapy for schizophrenia and other psychoses to manage dysfunction in specific neurotransmitters

audit a challenge on a reimbursement from a PBM or insurance provider on a prescription claim that has been previously processed

audit log a report listing the various prescription transactions with prices, discounts, payments, and reimbursements that occurred in a set time period, categorizing them in different ways for tracking and analysis

autoclave a device that generates heat and pressure to sterilize objects and instrumentsautomated compounding device (ACD) a programmable, automated device to make complex IV preparations such as TPNs

automated dispensing cabinet (ADC) mobile and secured cart that houses the automated medication dispensing system for floor stock on each nursing unit

automated medication dispensing system (AMDS) software that works with an ADC and is integrated into the hospital's patient management system to track the dispensing and administration of each patient's medication

auxiliary clamp slide clamp used to completely stop the IV solution from flowing

average wholesale price (AWP) the average price that wholesalers charge the pharmacy for a drug, serving as the benchmark price to estimate reimbursement rates and retail price without insurance

avoirdupois system a system of measurement that originated in France and is used for common measurements in the United States, including the foot, mile, grain, pound, and ounce

Ayurvedic medicine an ancient, holistic, Indian approach to medicine that includes a patient's spiritual well-being

backups copies of prescription record data and software that is downloaded for remote storage, typically done by the main pharmacy computer(s) on a daily basis

bactericidal agent a drug that kills bacteria

bacterium a small, single-celled microorganism that can exist in three main forms, depending on type: spherical (i.e., cocci), rod-shaped (i.e., bacilli), and spiral (i.e., spirochetes)

bank identification number (BIN) the information located on most drug insurance cards to identify the correct pharmacy benefit manager (PBM); the BIN, processor control number (PCN), group, and patient ID number are all necessary to process the drug claim

bar code point-of-care (BPOC) technology where the bar code on the wrist of the patient is compared to the bar code on the medication before the drug is administered to minimize medication administration errors

Basic Life Support/Cardiopulmonary Resuscitation (BLS/CPR) emergency first aid procedures that include ongoing chest compression and breaths

batch a 24-hour supply of every CSP for each patient in a unit, wing, or the hospital

benefit the services and products of health and drug insurance coverage by an employer

benzodiazepines (BZDs) a class of drugs that acts as a sedative, hypnotic, antianxiety medication, and anticonvulsant

beta-adrenergic blockers (beta blockers) drugs that slow the fight or flight response to stress and make the heart beat slower with less force by blocking the hormone epinephrine, also known as adrenaline

beyond-use date (BUD) the last recommended date for administration; provided by a compounding facility

bioaccumulate to collect in a biological system over time, often with harmful effect

bioavailability range the percentage of how much of the active ingredient in the drug is absorbed by the body

bioavailability the rate and extent to which a drug reaches the bloodstream after administration

biochemistry applying chemistry to biological processes

bioequivalence having similar strength and outcomes to a brand name product

biogenetically engineered drugs substances derived from the biotechnology to produce specific therapeutic effects

biological reference product the original patented biological drug or bioengineered drug upon which biosimilars and interchangeables are modeled

biological safety cabinets (BSCs) shielded, enclosed, or sealed PECs (with HEPA filtering and exhausting) that work to contain hazardous substances from the personnel and rest of the facility; come in classes (I, II, III—with some subclasses)

biosimilar drugs (biosimilars) drugs deemed by the FDA as biologically comparable and very much like the original biological drug reference product (but not necessarily equivalent or interchangeable)

biotechnology the field of study that combines the sciences of biology, chemistry, and immunology to produce unique synthetic drugs with specific therapeutic effects

bipolar disorder referring to a condition having two extremes, depression (low mood and energy) and mania (high mood and energy)

bisphosphonates agents used with estrogen to reduce osteoporosis by slowing down the cells that reabsorb the calcium and dissolve the bone

blending the act of combining two substances by using nongrinding techniques such as spatulation, sifting, and tumbling

body surface area (BSA) a measurement related to a patient's weight and height, expressed in meters squared (m2), and used to calculate patient-specific dosages of medications

boxed warning a warning that appears on the package insert and in other drug materials that highlights dangerous side effects

brand name the name under which the manufacturer markets a patented drug; also known as the trade name

break ring a scored area on the neck of an ampule that marks the site where a technician will break the glass to access the ampule's contents

bridging therapy a drug that serves as a transition to another drug when moving a patient from one treatment to the next; commonly used in clotting disorders

buccal route of administration a transmucosal route of administration in which a drug is placed between the gums and the inner lining of the cheek

buffered tablet a medication, such as "buffered aspirin," that has the additive of an antacid, such as calcium carbonate, that reduces the acid from the medication to make it easier on the stomach

buffer room an ISO Class 7 or cleaner room with fixed walls and doors where PEC(s) that generate and maintain an ISO Class 5 environment are physically located. The buffer room may only be accessed through the ante-room

bulk counterbalance a large two-pan scale used for weighing bulk ingredients and material up to 5 kg, with a sensitivity rating of +/− 100 mg

burden of proof the obligation of a person or party filing a lawsuit to provide enough evidence to prove a case

calcium channel blockers (CCBs) drugs that treat hypertension by blocking calcium from entering the cells of the blood vessels to prevent then from gaining rigidity

calculation by cancellation another name for the dimensional analysis method of setting up a conversion from one measurement system to another by using the conversion rate as a fractional unit (desired measure on top and current on bottom) and multiplying the existing amount by it, then canceling out the known measure in the numerator and denominator

calibrate to gauge a measuring instrument with a standard scale of reading

cannula the barrel of a syringe or the bore area inside the syringe that correlates with the volume of solution

caplet an oral, solid dosage form sharing characteristics of both a tablet and a capsule

capsule an oral dosage form containing powder, liquid, or granules in a gelatin covering

capture error a medication error that occurs when focus on a task is diverted elsewhere and, therefore, the error goes undetected

capture the claim successfully process the prescription through drug utilization review (DUR) and online adjudication to receive confirmation of reimbursement from the pharmacy benefit manager (PBM)

cardiovascular pertaining to the heart and blood vessels

cart fill list a daily printout of all patient medication orders

catastrophic insurance a plan that is aimed at protecting oneself from the high costs of a severe accident or unexpected, debilitating illness or disease; has low monthly premium payments in exchange for a very high deductible (i.e., $5,000–$10,000) and is also referred to as catastrophic coverage

Celsius temperature scale the temperature scale that uses 0°C as the temperature at which water freezes at sea level and 100°C as the temperature at which it boils

central venous catheter (CVC) a catheter placed into a large vein deep in the body, often used for TPN solutions; also called a *central line*

cephalosporin antibiotics drugs developed to act like penicillin against bacteria

certificate of medical necessity (CMN) documentation, including diagnosis codes, needed for Medicare Part B coverage of durable medical equipment (DME)

certification the process by which a professional organization grants recognition to an individual who has met certain predetermined qualifications

Certified Pharmacy Technician (CPhT) a pharmacy technician who has passed the Pharmacy Technician Certification Exam (PTCE) or the Exam for Certification of Pharmacy Technicians (ExCPT)

charge-back a rejection of a prior prescription claim by a PBM or an insurance provider that must be investigated and resolved

chemical compatibility the ability of two or more base components to combine in solution or with other solutions (such as another IV solution or blood serum) without resulting in physical or chemical property changes to any of them

chemotherapy dispensing pin a small plastic device used to relieve (vent) the negative pressure within a drug vial safely while its built-in HEPA filter traps any drug particles or escaping fluid from the vial

chemotherapy gloves medical gloves that meet the ASTM Standard Practice for Assessment of Resistance of Medical Gloves to Permeation by Chemotherapy Drugs

chewable tablet a solid oral dosage form meant to be chewed that is readily absorbed; commonly prescribed for school-age children

child-resistant container a medication container with a special lid that cannot be opened by 80% of children under age 5 but can be opened by 90% of adults; designed to prevent child access to drugs to reduce the number of accidental poisonings

Children's Health Insurance Program (CHIP) a low-cost to free healthcare insurance program run jointly by the states and federal government aimed at uninsured children from ages 0 to 19 whose parents (including pregnant women) earn over the federal poverty line but too little to cover healthcare insurance for their children

civil law the category of the law that concerns citizens and the crimes they commit against one another

Class III prescription balance a two-pan balance used to weigh material (between 120 mg and 120 g) with a sensitivity rating of +/− 6 mg; also known as a Class A prescription balance

cleanroom a system of rooms in which the concentration of airborne particles is controlled to meet a specified airborne-particulate cleanliness class to prevent particle and microbial contamination of CSPs

closed-ended question a question that requires a yes-or-no answer

closed-system transfer devices (CSTDs) a drug transfer device that mechanically prohibits the transfer of environmental contaminants into the system and the escape of HD or vapor concentrations outside of the system; these devices protect the worker from exposure to hazardous drugs

COBRA insurance insurance policy when a former employer is required to keep a former employee on the employee insurance plan at full premium cost for 18 to 36 months; the ACA guarantees such patients cannot lose coverage with job changes

code blue an emergency call for personnel and equipment to resuscitate a patient, especially when suffering from respiratory failure or cardiac arrest

coinsurance a percentage-based insurance plan in which the patient must pay a certain percentage of the prescription price; commonly used in high-cost specialty drugs

collaborative practice agreement (CPA) a formal agreement that allows providers to see the patient, make a diagnosis and care plan, and refer the patient, under specific protocol, to the pharmacist to discuss and manage drug therapy

collodions syrupy topical emulsion where the thick liquid is dissolved in a mixture of alcohol and ether; after application, the alcohol and ether solvent vaporizes, leaving a medicated film coating on the skin

colloid the dispersion of ultrafine particles in a liquid formulation

colony community of microorganisms

commercial insurance coverage for medical or prescription costs provided by an employer or purchased by an individual; also called private insurance

comminution the act of reducing a substance to small, fine particles using particle-reducing techniques like trituration, levigation, and pulverization

community pharmacy any independent or chain pharmacy that dispenses prescription medications to outpatients; also called a *retail pharmacy*

complementary medicine a nonconventional treatment that is used together with conventional medicine

compliance adherence to a required set of standards, regulations, laws, and practices

component an ingredient in a compounded product

compound (used as a verb) the action of hand-preparing a new pharmaceutical product by mixing, combining, or integrating ingredients; (used as noun) the resulting prepared product, which can be sterile or nonsterile

compounded preparations patient-specific medications prepared on-site from individual ingredients, often by a technician under the direct supervision of the pharmacist

compounded sterile preparation (CSP) a preparation intended to be sterile that is created by combining, admixing, diluting, pooling, reconstituting, repackaging, or otherwise altering a drug product or bulk drug substance

compounding the process of preparing a medication for an individual patient from bulk ingredients according to a prescription from a licensed prescriber

compounding aseptic containment isolator (CACI) A specific type of CAI that is designed for the compounding of sterile HDs. The CACI is designed to provide worker protection from exposure to undesirable levels of airborne drugs throughout the compounding and material transfer processes and to provide an aseptic environment with unidirectional airflow for compounding sterile preparations

compounding aseptic isolator (CAI) An isolator specifically designed for compounding sterile, non-hazardous pharmaceutical ingredients or preparations. The CAI is designed to maintain an aseptic compounding environment throughout the compounding and material transfer processes

compounding pharmacy a pharmacy that specializes in the compounding of nonsterile (and sometimes sterile) preparations that are not commercially available

Compounding Record a printout for a specific patient, including the amounts or weights of all ingredients with national drug code calculations and instructions for compounding; used by the technician to document a compounded medication for a patient

compression tablet a tablet consisting of an active ingredient and inactive dry ingredients pressed together under great pressure to form a solid

computerized prescriber order entry (CPOE) the process of having a prescriber use a handheld device (or mobile PC) at a patient's bedside to enter and send medication orders to the pharmacy

confidentiality keeping privileged information about customers from being disclosed without their consent

containment primary engineering control (C-PEC) A ventilated device designed and operated to minimize worker and environmental exposures to HDs by controlling emissions of airborne contaminants through the following: the full or partial enclosure of a potential contaminant source; the use of airflow capture velocities to trap and remove airborne contaminants near their point of generation; the use of air pressure relationships that define the direction of airflow into the cabinet; and the use of HEPA filtration on all potentially contaminated exhaust streams

containment quality control measured steps to ensure the containment of HDs

containment secondary engineering controls (C-SECs) The room with fixed walls in which the C-PEC is placed. It incorporates specific design and operational parameters required to contain the potential hazard within the compounding room

contaminated product error a medication error that occurs when aseptic technique is not followed in compounding, and the drug is no longer sterile and causes a microorganism infection

continuation order a medication order in which a physician must review, approve, rewrite, and renew all daily medication orders at least weekly

continuous quality improvement (CQI) a process of written procedures designed to identify quality and safety problems and recommend solutions

contraindication a disease, condition, or symptom for which a drug should not be used because it may be harmful

controlled-release (CR) formulation a dosage form that releases medication over a long duration

controlled substance a drug with potential for abuse; organized into five schedules of restriction that specify the way the drug must be stored, dispensed, recorded, and inventoried

Controlled Substance Ordering System (CSOS) a DEA-approved online system that some pharmaceutical suppliers have set up that replaces the paper DEA Form 222

Controlled Substances Act (CSA) a federal law created to combat and control drug abuse

coordination of benefits (COB) online billing of both a primary and a secondary insurer

copayment (copay) the amount that the patient is to pay for each prescription as determined by the insurance carrier

coring an inadvertent introduction of a small piece of the rubber closure into the solution while removing medication from a vial

Corporate Integrity Agreement the obligation to report all fraudulent activities under "whistle-blower protection"

corrosivity the potential to damage or destroy other substances through an intense acidic, base, or other chemical composition

corticosteroids steroid hormones produced by the adrenal cortex often used to reduce inflammation and pain

cortisol a hormone that the adrenal glands naturally produce that helps the body deal with stress

Cosmas and Damian (ca. 270–303 CE) a physician and a pharmacist who were Syrian Christians dedicated to healing the poor and rich alike, never accepting money for services. For their ethics and Christian martyrdom, they were widely considered the models and patron saints of all pharmacists and physicians in the Middle East and Europe for centuries and are considered so today by Roman Catholics

cost-benefit analysis spreadsheet an extensive table that itemizes the costs of business versus the income generated for the same time period

cover letter a letter of introduction to a potential employer that accompanies a résumé

crash cart a mobile cart that holds necessary drugs for an emergency code

cream a cosmetically acceptable oil-in-water (O/W) emulsion for topical use on the skin

credential a documented piece of evidence of one's qualifications

credentialing the process for validating the qualifications of licensed professionals; may define what functions and roles pharmacists and pharmacy technicians can perform

criminal law the category of law that addresses broken laws and regulations—offenses against the government as it represents the public

critical site a location that includes any component or fluid pathway surfaces (e.g., vial septa, injection ports, and beakers) or openings (e.g., opened ampules and needle hubs) that are exposed and at risk of direct contact with air (e.g., ambient room or HEPA filtered), moisture (e.g., oral and mucosal secretions), or touch contamination.

cultural sensitivity an awareness, knowledge of, and respect for cultural beliefs that differ from your own

culture the customs, beliefs, art, food, traditions, religious practices, marriage and family structures, and attitudes that are learned and shared to varying degrees by members of a group

current good manufacturing practices (CGMPs) the regulations and main regulatory standards enforced by the FDA for the manufacturing of drug products in the United States

Current Procedural Terminology (CPT) a standardized coding system to report procedures and services for healthcare providers; an example would be medication therapy management (MTM) services by the pharmacist

curriculum vitae (CV or vitae) a résumé format that uses paragraphs to communicate specific themes; used in academic service; it is also known as an academic vita, or vita

D_5W an abbreviation for the solution dextrose 5% in water, a common IV solution

daily order an initial (or new) medication order written by a physician

daily value (DV) the recommended level of intake of a certain vitamin or mineral

database management system (DBMS) the administrative software system that integrates the many different pharmacy software programs and the online transmissions

days' supply the time that a given amount of prescribed medication lasts a patient until the next refill; required on drug claims submitted for online insurance billing

deactivation treatment of an HD with another chemical, heat, ultraviolet light, or other agent to create a less hazardous agentDEA number an identification number assigned by the Drug Enforcement Administration (DEA) to identify someone authorized to handle or prescribe controlled substances within the United States

decimal any number written using a decimal point to separate whole numbers from their accompanying fractions in tenths; the whole numbers are on the left side of the point and the fractions are on the right (e.g., 10.25 is equal to 10 and 25/100)

decontamination inactivation, neutralization, or removal of HDs, usually by chemical means

decorum proper or polite behavior that is in good taste

deductible an amount on some insurance plans that must be paid by the insured person before the insurance company considers paying its portion of a medical or drug cost

defendant one who defends against accusations brought forward in a lawsuit

Defense Health Agency (DHA) administers Tricare, a federal governmental health insurance program for active and retired military personnel and their dependents

delayed-release (DR) formulation a dosage form, such as an enteric-coated aspirin tablet, that contains a special coating designed to delay absorption of the medication and to resist breakdown by acidic gastric fluids

denominator the number on the bottom part of a fraction that represents the total number of pieces in the whole

deoxyribonucleic acid (DNA) the helix-shaped molecule that carries the genetic code that direct the growth of the cell

depot injection an injection where a drug is administered into an internal pool or reservoir so surrounding tissue can gradually absorb the pool

depressant drug meant to reduce functional or nervous activity; includes sedatives, tranquilizers, hypnotics, and opiates

depression a common but serious disorder that can affect mood, thinking, or ability to engage in daily activities, such as working, eating, or sleeping

dermal route of administration application of a topical drug directly to a specific place of skin surface; has a localized effect

destructive agent a drug that kills bacteria, fungi, viruses, or even normal or cancer cells

diagnostic agent a drug that helps a provider determine the correct diagnosis; may contain tracer radioactive isotopes or dyes used to help visualize problems

dietary supplement a category of nonprescription substances, which includes vitamins, minerals, and herbs, that is not considered drugs but is regulated by the FDA

diluent an inactive fluid or chemical substance that is added to the active drug in compounding a tablet, capsule, solution, or topical formulation

diluent volume (dv) the volume that a diluent takes up in a solution

dimensional analysis calculation method of setting up a conversion from one measurement system by multiplying the known measurement by the conversion rate as a fraction (with the known measure as the denominator), also known as calculation by cancellation

Dioscorides, Pedanius (40–90 CE) An early Greek physician credited with writing one of the world's greatest pharmaceutical texts: *De Materia Medica* (*On Medical Matters*)

direct compounding area (DCA) a critical area within the ISO Class 5 PEC where critical sites are exposed to unidirectional HEPA-filtered air, also known as first air

director of pharmacy the chief executive officer of the hospital pharmacy department; also known as the pharmacist in charge (PIC)

discharge order an order written by a physician that provides take-home instructions, including prescribed medications and doses, for a discharged patient

discount card a manufacturer's card for those without traditional coverage or to lower the cost of a prescription drug; patients on any government insurance program are not eligible for coordination of benefits

discounted acquisition cost the discounted price that a pharmacy pays when the wholesaler offers a discount

discrimination preferential treatment or mistreatment for reasons of age, gender, ethnicity, sexual orientation, religion, or other factors

disinfectant a chemical or physical agent used on inanimate surfaces and objects to destroy fungi, viruses, and bacteria; sporicidal disinfectant agents are considered a special class of disinfectants that also are effective against bacterial and fungal spores

dispense as written (DAW) on a prescription, DAW1 indicates that a brand name drug is necessary or that a generic substitution is not allowed; DAW2 is often used to indicate patient preference for a brand name drug

dispersion a liquid dosage form in which undissolved ingredients are mixed throughout a liquid vehicle

distillation process of boiling a liquid and capturing the condensed gases or vapor back into a purified liquid form

distraction error a medication error that occurs when a technician or pharmacist is interrupted in the middle of a filling process and forgets a portion of key information or train of thought, and some information or a safety decision gets missed

diuretic a drug that rids the body of excess fluid and electrolytes by increasing the urine output

dock a device used to assemble the vial-and-bag IV unit within PEC to prepare for activation by the nurse at the patient bedside

documentation error a medication error that occurs when essential information is not properly noted, such as a prescription, allergy, patient request, or other information in the medication profile, or when insurance or billing claims are not properly processed

dopamine a neurotransmitter that is associated with catalyzing pleasure, motivation, action, and enjoyment

dosage form the physical manifestation of a drug (for example, a capsule or a tablet)

double gloving wearing two sets of gloves at once for HD sterile compounding

drip chamber the small, open space just below the spike adapter where the drops of fluid from the IV bag into the tubing are counted by the nurse to determine the flow rate of the IV solution

drop factor the number of drops that an IV tubing delivers to provide 1 mL; this number may be used by nurses to calculate the IV flow rate when using certain types of primary IV tubing; also called *drop set* or *drip set*

droppers glass or plastic pipettes with suction bulbs on one end used to transfer small amounts of liquid; often used to administer accurate medication dosage for infants

drug any substance taken into or applied to the body for the specific purpose of altering the body's biochemical functions and physiological processes; also called a medication

drug delivery system a design feature of the dosage form that affects the timing of delivery of the drug, such as delaying or extending the release of the active drug

Drug Enforcement Administration (DEA) the branch of the US Justice Department that is responsible for regulating the sale and use of drugs with abuse potential

drug formulary a list of approved medications for use within the hospital; this list is approved by the P&T Committee

drug interaction a reaction when a drug interacts with another medication, including prescription, over-the-counter, and homeopathic drugs, as well as vitamin, herbal, and nutritional supplements

Drug Quality and Security Act (DQSA) an act to create regulatory oversight over smallbatch medication compounding

drug recall the process of withdrawing a drug from the market by the FDA or the drug manufacturer for serious adverse effects or other defects in the product

drug seeker a patient who is dependent on or addicted to drugs, who may receive prescriptions for the same or similar controlled drugs from several physicians and pharmacies

drug tolerance when the body adapts to a drug so that higher doses are needed to produce the same pharmacological effect

drug utilization review (DUR) a procedure built into pharmacy software that alerts pharmacists to check for potential medication errors in dosage, drug interactions, allergies, etc.

dual copay insurance coverage in which a patient pays one copay for brand name drugs and a lower copay for generic drugs; also known as two-tier

dual eligible refers to a patient who has both a primary and secondary insurance plan

dumb terminal computer device with a monitor and keyboard that doesn't contain storage and processing capabilities

durable medical equipment (DME) medically necessary, reusable equipment such as nebulizers, hospital beds, wheelchairs, and walkers that may be purchased in a community pharmacy or billed to Medicare Part B

dysphoria state of anxiety, hyperfear, restlessness, malaise, or hallucinations

e-prescription a computer-generated digital prescription processed online

effervescent salt granular salts that release gas and dispense active ingredients into solution when placed in water

elastomeric device sterile delivery device; a small, solution-filled sterile plastic ball attached to a sterile catheter line

electrolyte solution dissolved mineral salts in a fluid

electronic digital balance a single-pan scale that is more accurate than Class III balances or counterbalances; has a capacity of 100 g and sensitivity as low as +/- 2 mg

electronic health record (EHR) computerized health information record used to share patient information among authorized healthcare providers to better coordinate health care

electronic medication administration record (eMAR) an online record that documents the administration time of each drug to each patient by a nurse using bar code technology

elixir a clear, sweetened, flavored solution containing water and ethanol

embolism blockage of a blood vessel from a blood clot or inadvertent injection of an air bubble

emollient base an ointment with the ability to soften skin, such as with bath oils

empathy demonstration of the ability to share and understand another person's feelings

emulsifying agent an inactive ingredient that makes the emulsion stable, binding the two substances so that they are less prone to separation

emulsion a mixture of two unblendable substances; the dispersion of a liquid in another liquid differing in viscosity

EMV chip new technology of digital data chips with integrated circuits embedded in credit cards to decrease fraudulent use

end-of-the-day report a tally of the day's sales receipts and prescriptions filled that is generated at the end of the business day

endocrine having to do with the hormonal system and glands

enema a solution administered into the rectum to evacuate or retain the colon's contents

enteral route of administration delivery of a drug via the digestive tract in oral form or through a feeing tube; enteral forms generally provide systemic therapeutic effects

enteric-coated tablet (ECT) a tablet with a coating designed to resist destruction by the acidic pH of the gastric fluids and to delay the release of the active ingredient

epidemic a regional widespread contagious disease

equivalent ratios two ratios that have the same value; for example, 1/2 and 4/8

equivalent weight (Eq) equal to one mole divided by its valence, or the number of grams of solute dissolved in 1 mL of solution

estrogen hormones important for reproduction; found in higher concentrations in females than males

estrogen replacement therapy (ERT) treatment consisting of replacing one or more female hormones in oral or topical formulations

ethical dilemma a situation that calls for a judgment between two or more solutions, not all of which are necessarily wrong

ethics standards of behavior that all professionals are encouraged to follow

etiquette rules of good manners

euphoria state of extreme high mood and energy

Exam for Certification as Pharmacy Technicians (ExCPT) an examination offered by the National Healthcareer Association (NHA) that technicians can pass to be certified and receive the title of CPhT

Exam for the Certification of Pharmacy Technicians (ExCPT) an examination developed by the National Healthcareer Association (NHA) that technicians can pass to be certified and receive the title of CPhT

excipients inactive ingredients

express pay option a payment option where the customer does not need to present payment because the customer has a credit card on file that is automatically charged (an option set up earlier by the customer)

extemporaneous compounding compounding products that are done for a specific patient's immediate need but not commercially available; a common form of nonsterile compounding in a community pharmacy

extended-release (XL) formulation a tablet or capsule that releases medication gradually to reduce frequency of dosing compared with immediate-release and most sustained-release formulations

externship a temporary, short-term student work experience, usually arranged by a school as a part of its program

extra dose error a medication error that occurs when more doses are received by a patient than were prescribed by the physician

extremes the first and fourth numbers in an equal proportion

Fahrenheit temperature scale the temperature scale that uses 32°F as the temperature at which water freezes at sea level and 212°F as the temperature at which it boils

Failure Mode Effects Analysis (FMEA) an analysis procedure that breaks larger processes down into levels and tasks to find the root causes of failures (problems) and the rate or probability of failure occurrences, the consequences, and ways to fix the failures

FDA Orange Book (The Orange Book) (also known as the Approved Drug Products with Therapeutic Equivalence Evaluations) the official legal source for information on generic and pharmaceutical alternative drugs

fear error a medication error that occurs when a technician fears the consequences of speaking up and asking the pharmacist or the prescriber to double-check an element of the prescription

Federal Trade Commission (FTC) a federal agency created to protect the consumer from deceptive advertising, as with dietary supplements

film-coated tablet (FCT) a tablet coated with a thin outer layer that prevents serious GI side effects

filter needle a needle that is equipped with a 5-micron (or finer) filter within its core to catch any microscopic glass shards and impurities to prevent them from entering the CSP

filter straw a syringe attachment similar to a filter needle, only instead of a needle, this is a thin tube with a filter

filtration funneling of a liquid or gas through filters or mesh screens with minute holes too small for biological and chemical contaminants to pass through

first party payer the person (or their parent, guardian, or other responsible party) who directly receives the benefits of a service or product and is responsible for paying for it

flex card a medical and prescription insurance debit card

flexible spending account an account which patients, through their employer, can place pretax dollars for medical expenses and child and dependent care; these dollars must be carefully predicted and typically spent within the year

floor stock medications stocked in a secured area at each nursing patient care station or floor

fluidextract a liquid dosage form prepared by extraction from plant sources and commonly used in the formulation of syrups

Food and Drug Administration (FDA) the agency of the federal government that is responsible for ensuring the safety and efficacy of food and drugs prepared for the market

Food and Drug Modernization Act the federal law that improved the regulation of small-batch compounding, biological products, medical devices, and food

forceps a stainless steel pincher instrument like a large tweezer used to pick up small objects, such as pharmacy weights

four Ds of negligence duty, dereliction, damages, and direct cause; these factors must be proven by a plaintiff in cases of negligence or malpractice

fraction a portion of a whole that is represented as a ratio with a numerator (number of parts) on the top and the denominator (total in one whole) on the bottom

fungus an organism, which may be single-celled, that lives on organisms by feeding on living or dead organic material

Galen, Claudius (130–210 CE) prominent Greek physician and medical author in the Roman Empire who dissected animals and gathered herbs and medications, and wrote about their properties; considered the "Father of Pharmacy"

galenical pharmacy herbal and vegetable extracts and medicinal preparations

gastroesophageal reflux disease (GERD) a GI disease characterized by radiating burning or pain in the chest and an acid taste; caused by backflow of acidic stomach contents across an incompetent lower esophageal sphincter; also referred to as heartburn

gastrointestinal (GI) relating to the stomach and intestines

gelatin shell a protein substance that is easily dissolved in the stomach; encloses granular powder or liquid gel in a capsule that is meant to be ingested

gene a distinct segment of DNA that determines an organism's specific individual characteristics, like blue eyes or brown hair

generic drug a drug that contains the same active ingredients as the brand name product and delivers the same amount of medication to the body for a similar medicinal effect; acetaminophen is the generic drug for the brand Tylenol

genetically engineered the process of using DNA biotechnology to create a variety of drugs or biological products

genitourinary having to do with the urinary tract, reproductive system, and genitals

geometric dilution method a process that uses a mortar and pestle to gradually combine several active ingredients (drugs) with inactive ingredients (diluent) to produce a more homogenous product

germ theory of disease the scientific concept that microorganisms cause disease

gloved fingertip sampling a quality control procedure in the IV compounding area to detect touch contamination from improper aseptic technique

glucometer a blood sugar measuring device

glycerogelatin a topical preparation made with gelatin, glycerin, water, and medicinal substances

good compounding practices (GCPs) USP standards in many areas of practice to ensure high-quality compounded preparations

graduated cylinder a conical or cylindrical flask used for accurately measuring liquids

grain (gr) a small dry-weight unit of measurement in the apothecary system (e.g., 5 grains [5 gr] of aspirin are equivalent to approximately 325 mg)

gram base unit of the metric system for measuring weight

Greenwich mean time the international civil time standard based at the Royal Observatory, Greenwich, in London

gross profit the accumulation of all sales receipts before deducting expenses

group number an important piece of information on the insurance card that identifies the employer sponsor of the drug insurance program

harassment aggressive mistreatment, pressure, or intimidation that can be sexual or otherwise

hazardous communication standard (HCS) a US government regulation designed to ensure that the hazards of all chemicals produced or imported are evaluated and that details regarding their hazards are transmitted to employers and employees

hazardous compounding pharmacies a pharmacy that specializes in toxic substances that are chemical, biological, or radioactive

hazardous drug (HD) any drug identified by at least one of the following six criteria: carcinogenicity; teratogenicity or developmental toxicity; reproductive toxicity in humans; organ toxicity at low doses in humans or animals; genotoxicity; new drugs that mimic existing hazardous drugs in structure or toxicity

HCPCS the Healthcare Common Procedure Coding System, used to report supplies, equipment, and devices supplied for medical purposes

healthcare-associated infections (HAIs) infections that patients acquire as a result of treatment in a healthcare facility; also called nosocomial infections

healthcare exchange an online shopping tool to find insurance for the uninsured or self-insured; made possible by the Affordable Care Act

healthcare interface network an online healthcare information and processing server that connects providers, pharmacists, electronic records, and national healthcare and pharmaceutical information sources; examples include Surescripts and RxHub

health insurance coverage of incurred medical costs, such as physician and emergency room visits, laboratory costs, and hospitalization

Health Insurance Portability and Accountability Act (HIPAA) a law passed by Congress that addressed the confidentiality of patient medical records as well as prescription records

health maintenance organizations (HMOs) a managed care insurance plan that requires members to get services and products only through their staff or contracted providers and facilities

health savings accounts (HSAs) savings accounts that can be started by patients or their employers to set aside tax-deferred money specifically for healthcare costs not covered by insurance

hematologic having to do with the blood

herbal medicine the use of natural plant products to maintain health by preventing or curing certain illnesses

herbals natural dietary supplements made of medicinal plant matter

High-Alert Medication Modeling and Error-Reduction Scorecards (HAMMERS™) a free tool from ISMP designed to help community pharmacies identify the unique set of system and behavioral risks associated with dispensing certain high-alert medications and to estimate how often an error or adverse drug event reaches a patient

high-density lipoprotein (HDL) the "good cholesterol" that picks up floating low-density lipoproteins (the "bad cholesterol") and sweeps them away through the bloodstream

high-efficiency particulate airflow (HEPA) filter a filter designed to remove 99.97% of airborne particles measuring 0.3-micron or greater in diameter passing through it

Hippocrates (ca. 460–370 BCE) an early Greek physician who not only observed medical states and wrote about methods to cure illness, but also wrote a code of ethics for physicians. He is considered the "Father of Modern Medicine"

histamine-2 antagonists a class of drugs that work to slow the release of stomach acid

home healthcare the delivery of medical, nursing, and pharmaceutical services and supplies to patients at home

home infusion pharmacy a specialty pharmacy set up particularly to serve home healthcare dispensing

home medications (home meds) a patient's medications brought from home to continue using while in hospital

homeopathic a class of drugs in which minute dilutions of natural substances purportedly stimulate the body's immune system

***Homeopathic Pharmacopeia of the United States/ Revision Service* (*HPRS*)** a compendium of standards and research created by the American Institute of Homeopathy

horizontal laminar airflow workbench (H-LAFW) a type of laminar airflow system that provides an ISO Class 5 or better air quality environment for sterile compounding; also provides a unidirectional HEPA-filtered airflow

hormone replacement therapy (HRT) therapy consisting of some combination of estrogen, progestin (female), and androgen (male) hormones

hormones secretions released by glands into the circulatory system that have specific regulatory effects on organs and other tissues; for instance, insulin is secreted from the pancreas to lower blood sugar

hospice care home healthcare services typically involving pain management of a terminally ill patient

hospital pharmacy an institutional pharmacy that dispenses and prepares drugs and provides clinical services in a hospital setting

household system a system of measurement based on the apothecary system; units of measure include the ounce, pound, drop, teaspoon, tablespoon, and cup

human failure a medication error generated by failure that occurs at an individual level

hydroalcoholic solutions water- and alcohol-based solutions for oral dosage forms

hydrogel an injectable gel drug form that is pliable and offers extended release of the drug

hyperthyroidism a condition caused by excessive thyroid hormone and marked by increased metabolic rate; also called thyrotoxicosis

hypertonic solution a parenteral solution with a greater number of particles than the number of particles found in blood

hypnotic drugs medications that induce sleep

hypothyroidism an underactive thyroid, producing too little thyroid hormone

hypotonic solution a parenteral solution with a lower number of particles than the number of particles found in blood

iatrogenic condition an illness that is caused by a physician or medication

ICD-10 the International Classification of Diseases, 10th revision; a coding system used by prescribers and insurance companies to offer billing codes for specific diagnoses and diseases

ignitability the potential for sparking and causing flames when meeting air, water, other chemicals, or environmental triggers

immunity bodily processes that provide protection against disease

imperial system (also known as the British imperial system) a system of measurements used historically across the British Empire with inches, feet, yards, furlongs, and miles, as well as fathoms and nautical miles, fluid ounces, drams, pints, quarts, and gallons; grains, pounds, stones, and tons

in-line filters devices used in the IV line to remove contaminants such as glass, fibers, bits of rubber, and bacteria from IV fluids

in-network providers prescribers and pharmacies that have a contract with the insurance provider

incomplete information error a medication error that a medication error that occurs when full information is not available because the patient was not asked sufficient or proper questions, or the answers were somehow not recorded in the profile, or the patient withheld information deliberately or by accident of memory

incorrect assumption error occurs when an essential piece of information cannot be verified, and an assumption is made

indications the common intended uses of drug to treat specific diseases, symptoms, or conditions

inert ingredient an inactive chemical—such as a filler, preservative, coloring, or flavoring—that is added to one or more active ingredients to improve drug formulations while causing *little or* no physiological effect; also called an inactive ingredient

Infection Control Committee (ICC) a hospital committee that provides leadership in relation to infection control policies

informed consent form a document that states, in easily understandable terms, the purpose and risks of the drug research that someone volunteers to take part in

infusion rate the speed of administration of IV fluids and/or medication, commonly expressed in mL per hour

inhalation route of administration delivery of a drug by inhalation into the lungs; also called *intrarespiratory route of administration*

injection port a connector on the IV tubing that allows the injection of IV fluid or medication other than that in the current IV bag to be infused into the patient's vein

inscription part of a prescription that identifies the name of the drug, the dose, and the quantities of the ingredients

instillation the application of drops to the skin or eyes

Institute for Safe Medication Practices (ISMP) a nonprofit healthcare agency whose primary mission is to understand the causes of medication errors and to provide time-critical error-reduction strategies to the healthcare community, policy makers, and the public

institutional pharmacy a pharmacy that is organized under a corporate structure, following specific rules and regulations for accreditation

Institutional Review Board (IRB) a committee of the hospital that ensures that appropriate protection is provided to patients using investigational drugs; sometimes referred to as the Human Use Committee

insulin a hormone secreted by the pancreas, or an injected drug that helps cells the body regulate sugar levels

insulin pen a portable device in which the dose of insulin can be easily dialed up before administration

insurance fraud intentionally filing an insurance claim under false pretenses; subject to civil and criminal law and employment termination

insurance policy the plan that outlines the processes, rates, rules, and restrictions of what is covered by the insurance company and what is covered by the patient

intake record documentation by the nurse upon admission to the hospital

integrative medicine a combination of conventional treatments with alternative medicine

interchangeable biological drugs drugs deemed by the FDA as exerting the same therapeutic effects as each other in similar pharmaceutical and safe ways and may be substituted without prior approval of prescriber

interchangeables biosimilar drugs that are deemed as legal substitutions for biologically based brand drugs, many created through genetic engineering

international normalized ratio (INR) a standardized measurement for how long it takes blood to clot; especially important when taking blood thinner medication

International Organization for Standardization (ISO) an air quality classification from the International Organization for Standardization measures the amount of particulate matter in room air; the lower the ISO number, the less particulate matter is present in the air

internship official positions where a trained or semi-trained person is hired to handle entry-level duties and work as an apprentice in training

interoperability the interactive communication and operation between internal record programs, software and hardware systems, and external information sources

intradermal (ID) route of administration injection into the top layer of skin

intramuscular (IM) route of administration injection of a drug directly into the muscle

intranasal route of administration the placement of sprays or solutions into the nose

intrarespiratory route of administration delivery of a drug by inhalation into the lungs; also called inhalation route of administration

intrathecal injection into protective membrane around the spinal cord

intrauterine device (IUD) a device that is inserted into the uterus to prevent conception

intravenous (IV) admixture service a centralized pharmacy service that prepares IV, TPN, and hazardous preparations in a sterile, cleanroom work environment

intravenous (IV) route of administration injection of fluid or medication into the veins, usually over a prolonged period of time

intravenous (IV) solutions liquid medications administered directly into a patient's vein

inventory range a maximum and a minimum number of stock units of each product to have on hand in the inventory

inventory the entire stock of products on hand for sale at a given time

inventory turnover rate the amount of time the average drug inventory will be replaced during a 12-month period; most pharmacies replace inventory every two to four weeks

inventory value the total value of the entire stock of products on hand for sale on a given day

investigational drug a drug used in clinical trials that has not yet been approved by the FDA for use in the general population, or a drug used for non-approved indications

investigational new drug (IND) application the process by which a manufacturer submits research results from animal studies to the FDA to gain approval to gather data and test a new drug on humans

iPLEDGE program a specific risk assessment program for isotretinoin, which can cause a high incidence of birth defects if not properly monitored

irrigating solution any solution used for cleansing or bathing an area of the body, such as the eyes or ears

iso-osmotic term that describes a solution that should have the same number of particles per unit volume and the same osmotic pressure as blood; similar to isotonic

isotonic solution a parenteral solution with an equal number of particles as blood cells; 0.9% normal saline is isotonic

IV administration set a sterile, disposable device of many components (including the tubing and ports) used to deliver IV fluids to patients

IV bolus injection an injection in which a drug is administered intravenously all at once

IV infusion an infusion in which a drug is slowly administered directly into a vein over a given period

IV piggyback (IVPB) a small-volume parenteral (SVP) infusion (50 mL, 100 mL, 250 mL) containing medications attached to a primary LVP IV solution

jelly a gel that contains a higher proportion of water in combination with a drug substance as well as a thickening agent

Joint Commission an independent governing body that sets standards for quality patient care and safety in hospitals and other healthcare facilities; responsible for the accreditation of hospitals

just-in-time (JIT) purchasing frequent purchasing in quantities that just meet supply needs until the next ordering time

lactated Ringer's solution (LR) a common specially formulated mix of minerals and electrolytes (includes sodium chloride, sodium lactate, potassium chloride, and calcium chloride) used often for fluid restoration after blood loss from injury, surgery, or burns

large-volume parenteral (LVP) solutions IV solutions of more than 250 mL that may contain medications, nutrients, or electrolytes

law a rule that is designed to protect the public and is usually enforced through federal, state, or local governments; also known as statutory law

law of agency and contracts the general principle that allows an employee to enter into contracts on the employer's behalf

leading zero a zero that is placed in the ones place in a number less than zero that is being represented by a decimal value

least weighable quantity (LWQ) percentage of the sensitivity range over the error range

legend drug a drug that requires a prescription; labeled "Rx only" on medication stock bottle

levigation a process usually used to reduce the particle size of a solid during the preparation of an ointment

licensure the granting of a license by a state board, usually to allow work in a profession, to protect the public; all pharmacists must be licensed to practice by their state boards of pharmacy

liniment a medicated topical preparation, such as Bengay, that is applied to the skin

lipids fatty molecules that are an important constituent of cell membranes; includes natural oils, waxes, and steroids

liposome a bubble-like sphere made of organic cell membrane-like material generally holding a watery fluid sac

liter the base unit of the metric system for measuring volume

localized effect when an applied drug's benefits are limited to site-specific areas of the body

low-density lipoprotein (LDL) the "bad cholesterol" that circulates in the blood and attaches itself to the lining of the blood vessels, clogging them

lozenge a solid medication in a sweet-tasting formulation that is absorbed in the mouth; also known as a *troche*

lyophilized refers to a medication available as a freeze-dried powder

macrodrip tubing sets IV tubing sets that have a sufficient diameter to deliver 10, 15, 20 per milliliter (10 gtt/mL, 15 gtt/mL, 20 gtt/mL), used for adult patients

magma a milk-like liquid colloidal dispersion, such as Milk of Magnesia, in which particles remain distinct in a two-phase system

Maimon, Moses ben (1135–1204 CE) a Jewish-Arab physician in the sultan's court in Cairo who wrote extensively on illnesses and on ethical treatment of poor and rich alike in pharmacy and healing. His pharmacist's prayer was recited for centuries

malpractice a form of negligence in which improper, illegal, or neglectful professional activity is in evidence

managed care a type of health insurance system (HMO) that emphasizes keeping the patient healthy or diseases controlled to reduce healthcare costs

managed care organizations (MCOs) healthcare insurance programs that cut costs by limiting choices to those considered most cost-efficient and effective for the most people

mania excessively high mood, energy, and activity

manufactured drug products medications or ingredients prepared off-site by a large-scale drug manufacturer in a production facility

marijuana a Schedule I controlled drug that cannot be dispensed in pharmacies due to federal law restrictions though it is legal for prescribed medical and/or recreational use in multiple states

markup percentage the percentage by which the acquisition price is marked up to secure a gross profit

markup rate the ratio by which the acquisition price is marked up for customer sale to secure a gross profit

markup the difference between the acquisition cost and the selling price; also called *gross profit*

Master Formulation Record a recipe for a compound preparation that lists the name, strength, dosage form, ingredients and their quantities, mixing instructions, and beyond-use dating; many recipes are available from the Professional Compounding Centers of America (PCCA)

masticated chewed

means the second and third numbers in an equal proportion

Medicaid a state governmental health insurance program for low-income and disabled citizens

medical chart a hard copy or digital legal document that contains the clinical information that a hospital collects in-house and consists of patient-identifying demographics, hospital room number, physician notes, problem list, medication orders and list, nursing assessments, and discharge

medical surveillance collected and interpreted data on workers who handle HDs to detect any changes in their health status due to potential exposure

Medicare government-provided health insurance primarily for patients over age 65

Medicare Modernization Act (MMA) the federal law called the Medicare Prescription Drug, Improvement, and Modernization Act, which updated Medicare, added Medicare Parts C and D, and required the offer of annual medication management therapy (MTM) reviews for Medicare patients, especially on high-cost drugs or with chronic conditions

Medicare Part A federally sponsored insurance plan that covers 80% of the cost of hospital stays, as well as limited coverage of skilled nursing facilities, rehabilitation, and home health care; drugs are not covered under this plan

Medicare Part B federally sponsored insurance that partially covers the cost of outpatient doctor visits; may cover the cost of nebulizer, nebulizer medication, and diabetes supplies

Medicare Part C federal- and state-sponsored insurance that covers both health and prescription insurance from the same insurance provider; also called a Medicare Advantage plan; may include coverage for eye and hearing examinations, glasses, hearing aids, etc.

Medicare Part D a federal- and state-partnered insurance program that provides partial coverage of prescriptions, primarily for patients who are eligible for Medicare

medication container label a label containing the dosage directions from the prescriber that is affixed to the container of the dispensed medication; the pharmacy technician may use this copy to select the correct stock drug bottle and to fill the prescription

medication education error a medication error that occurs when the proper medication education materials and counsel are not passed on to the patient or medication administrator

medication error any preventable event that may cause or lead to inappropriate medication use or patient harm while the medication is in the control of the healthcare professional, patient, or consumer

Medication Errors Reporting Program (MERP) national a program designed to allow healthcare professionals to report medication errors directly to the Institute for Safe Medication Practices (ISMP)

Medication Guide printed information in which the FDA communicates side effects, adverse reactions, and boxed warnings for high-risk drugs

medication information sheet a leaflet printed from the prescription software and provided to patients on select medications dispensed; a Medication Guide serves as a required medication information sheet on high-risk drugs

medication nonadherence failure to take medication therapy as the physician instructs; may also be called *noncompliance*

medication order a prescription written in the hospital setting

medication special a single-dose preparation not commercially available that is repackaged and made for a particular patient

medication therapy management (MTM) a service that optimizes therapeutic outcomes for individual patients; includes five core elements: medication therapy review, personal medication record, medication-related action plan, intervention and/or referral, and documentation and follow-up

Medigap insurance private insurance coverage in addition to Medicare Part B that covers a portion of the costs for outpatient physician visits as well as laboratory and x-ray fees not covered by Medicare Part B

MEDMARX an international internet-based program of the USP for use by hospitals and healthcare systems for documenting, tracking, and identifying trends for adverse events and medication errors

MedWatch a voluntary program by the FDA that allows any healthcare professional or consumer to report a serious adverse event associated with the use of any drug, biological device, or dietary supplement

meniscus the crescent-shaped or concave appearance of a liquid in a graduated cylinder; used during the volume measurement process, with the center being the accepted level

metabolism the transformation of food into energy; consists of the buildup and breakdown of substances

metabolizing transforming food into energy by building up and breaking down its core constituents

metered-dose inhaler (MDI) a device used to administer a drug in the form of compressed gas through the mouth and into the lungs

meter the base unit of the metric system for measuring distance, length, or body surface area

methamphetamine (meth) a highly addictive illegal stimulant made from specific OTC drug ingredients

methicillin-resistant *Staphylococcus aureus* (MRSA) potentially lethal bacteria that causes infections on the skin and requires antibiotics to treat

metric system a measurement system based on subdivisions and multiples of 10; made up of three basic units: meter, gram, and liter

microbiology the study of microorganisms

microdrip tubing sets IV tubing sets that have a smaller diameter and provide smaller drops and more drops per milliliter, such as 60 gtt/mL; used for pediatric patients and others who need more gradual dosing

microemulsion a clear formulation, such as Haley's M-O, that contains a liquid composed of tiny droplets dispersed in another liquid

micrometer (micron) a particle measurement unit that is used with air filters; one millionth of a meter, or 0.001 mm

microorganisms one-celled or multicelled microscopic organisms, including bacteria, viruses, fungi, and protozoa

military time (similar to international time) a measure of time based on a 24-hour clock in which midnight is 0000, noon is 1200, and the minute before midnight is 2359; also referred to as 24-hour time

milking the technique of inserting a little air pressure and withdrawing a little fluid into a syringe

milliequivalent (mEq) equal to 1 mM divided by its valence

millimole (mM) one thousandth of a mole

misbranded product a product whose label includes false statements about the identity or ingredients of the container's contents

mislabeling error a medication error that occurs when a medication has incorrect information on it leading to the wrong use of it, or the wrong patient receiving it

model curriculum ASHP standards for an accredited program mandating a minimum of 600 hours, including 160 hours of classroom training, 80 hours of laboratory training and 360+ hours in practice site experiences

mole a unit of measurement based on the number of particles in a given substance

molecular weight the sum of the atomic weights of all the atoms in one molecule of a compound

monthly premium the cost a patient pays each month for health and/or drug insurance

mortar and pestle a bowl and club-like implement, often glass or porcelain, used for mixing and grinding pharmaceutical ingredients

multiple-dose vials (MDVs) containers of sterile medication (water or saline) with preservatives; used to reconstitute medication powders

multiple compression tablet (MCT) a tablet formulation on top of a tablet or a tablet within a tablet produced by multiple compressions in manufacturing

muscle relaxants drugs that reduce or prevent skeletal muscle contraction and pain

narcotic class of drugs that numb or blunt the senses, induce sleep, or have other psychoactive properties; includes the opium-based and opium-like drugs

narrow therapeutic index drugs medications where small differences in dose or blood concentration may lead to adverse reactions or therapeutic failures

National Association of Boards of Pharmacy (NABP) an organization that represents the practice of pharmacy in each state and develops pharmacist licensure examinations and Model State Pharmacy Act/Rules

National Council for Prescription Drug Programs (NCPDP) a not-for-profit organization that issues an NCPDP Provider ID Number to pharmacies and providers of pharmaceuticals who make online transactions

National Drug Code (NDC) number a unique number assigned to any brand name or generic drug products to identify the manufacturer, drug, and packaging size

National Healthcareer Association (NHA) an allied health careers accreditation organization that offers the Exam for Certification as Pharmacy Technicians (ExCPT)

National Institute for Occupational Safety and Health (NIOSH) a federal agency that establishes policies to protect workers from exposure to hazardous agents

National Pharmacy Technician Association (NPTA) the largest professional society for pharmacy technicians

National Provider Identifier (NPI) the unique number assigned to the provider by the federal government to allow authorized healthcare providers to process insurance claims for pharmacy reimbursement

nebulizer a device used to deliver medication in a fine mist form to the lungs; often used in treating asthma

negative pressure refers to air pressure that is lower than adjacent rooms because air is suctioned out into an external filtered exhaust system to protect the compounding personnel from the hazardous agents

negligence a tort civil case about carelessness that led to harm to someone else

net profit gross profit minus all expenses

networking reaching out to meet people with the specific purpose of identifying job leads

neurons specialized nerve cells that transmit nerve impulses

neurotransmitters the group of chemical substances emitted by neurons to communicate with each other, such as serotonin, dopamine, and norepinephrine

new drug application (NDA) the process through which drug sponsors formally propose that the FDA approve a new pharmaceutical for sale and marketing in the United States

nonformulary drug a drug not included on the hospital's drug formulary

noninjected CSPs miscellaneous sterile solutions

nonpathogenic not related to disease

nonsterile compounding compounding noninjectable, not commerically available products in a community pharmacy for a specific patient's immediate needs; also known as extemporaneous compounding

nonsteroidal anti-inflammatory drugs (NSAIDs) a class of drugs that reduce pain, swelling, and fever

nontaxable items products for purchase that do not have sales tax because of restrictions based on federal or state laws

nonverbal communication communicating without words—through facial expression, body language, posture, and tone of voice

nonvolumetric glassware a beaker or flask that is not calibrated and cannot be used to accurately measure liquids; limited to storing, containing, and mixing liquids with other bulk ingredients

norepinephrine a neurotransmitter that is associated with responding to challenges by raising blood pressure and increasing breathing and sugar levels; known as the "stress hormone"

normal saline (NS) a sterile solution containing a concentration of 0.9% sodium chloride in water

notice of privacy practices a written policy of the pharmacy to protect patient confidentiality, as required by HIPAA

nuclear pharmacy a specialized practice that compounds and dispenses sterile radioactive pharmaceuticals

nuclear pharmacy technician (NPT) one who has received specialized training to prepare radioactive pharmaceuticals

numerator the number on the upper part of a fraction that represents the part of the whole

occlusive refers to an ointment base that has the ability to hold moisture in the skin; best used when additional hydration is needed

Occupational Safety and Health Administration (OSHA) an agency of the Department of Labor, whose primary mission is to ensure the safety and health of US workers by setting and enforcing regulations and standards

ocular route of administration application of sterile ophthalmic medications into the eye

oil-in-water (O/W) emulsion an emulsion containing a small amount of oil dispersed in water, as in a cream

ointment a semisolid emulsion for topical use on the skin

ointment slab a flat, hard, nonabsorbent surface used for mixing compounds; also known as a compounding slab

omission error an administration error in which a prescribed dose is not given

online adjudication real-time insurance claims processing via electronic wireless telecommunications

open-ended question a question that requires a descriptive answer, not merely yes or no

ophthalmics solutions that pertain to the eye

opiate a narcotic that is either derived from opium or synthetically produced to resemble opium derivatives chemically

opioids opium-like drugs that exert similar effects

oral disintegrating tablet (ODT) a solid oral dosage form designed to dissolve quickly on the tongue for oral absorption and ease of administration without water

oral route of administration delivery of medication through swallowing for absorption along the GI tract into systemic circulation

oral syringe a needleless device used for administering medication to pediatric or older adult patients unable to swallow tablets or capsules

organizational failure an error generated by failure of organizational rules, policies, or procedures

orphan drug a medication approved by the FDA to treat a rare disease

osmolarity the concentration of all molecules in a volume of fluid

osmosis the natural flow of molecules in a solution through semi-permeable cell walls

osmotic pressure system a drug delivery system in which the drug is slowly "pushed out" into the bloodstream

osmotic pressure the pressure required to maintain equilibrium, with no net movement of solvent

otic route of administration application of solutions or suspensions into the ear

out-of-network providers prescribers and pharmacies that do not have a contract with the insurance provider; the cost of services is generally higher

out of stock (OOS) a situation in which the pharmacy does not have the prescribed drug in inventory

over-the-counter (OTC) a drug that may be sold without a prescription

overfill the amount of solution manufacturers add to make up for the loss of water due to evaporation through plastic

package insert (PI) a drug information sheet or pamphlet provided by the drug manufacturer with the drug stock; required by law for certain drug products

palliative care focuses on pain relief and quality of life for those with serious, ongoing painful debilitating illnesses

pandemic a globally widespread contagious disease, or an epidemic that has reached enormous international effect

paradoxical drug reactions side effects that are the opposite of the intended effects of the drug or its indication

paraprofessionals trained personnel who assist a professional person

parenteral intravenous fat emulsions (IVFEs) IV solutions that include a fatty nutritious additive

Parenteral nutrition (PN) specialized LVP solutions that provide nutrition and nutrient requirements to patients who require a long-term alternative to oral and digestive feeding

parenteral route of administration the injection or infusion of fluids and/or medications into the body bypassing the GI tract

parenteral solutions products that are prepared in a sterile environment for administration by injection

PAR levels the minimum restock and maximum reorder levels for each drug on each nursing unit; PAR stands for Periodic Automatic Replenishment

partial fill a situation in which the pharmacy cannot completely fill the prescribed quantity written on the prescription, so a starter amount of the medication has been offered to the patient until the remainder arrives

paste a water-in-oil (W/O) emulsion containing more solid material than an ointment

patent drug another name for an over-the-counter (OTC) medication

pathogenic that which is harmful

pathophysiology the study of disease and illnesses affecting the normal functions of the body

patient-controlled analgesia (PCA) (also known as Patient Controlled System [PCS]) a method for the delivery of a pain medication that gives the patient more management of the rate of administration

patient identification (ID) number identifies the primary drug insurance card holder and may identify other dependents on the policy

patient identifiers any demographic information that can identify the patient, such as name, address, phone number, Social Security number, or medical identification number

patient profile a confidential computerized record kept by the pharmacy that lists a patient's contact information, insurance information, medical and prescription history, and prescription preferences

Patient Safety and Quality Improvement (PSQI) Act a federal law passed in 2005 dedicated to promoting a culture of patient safety and quality assurance; created a network of safety databases and the ability to create PSOs

Patient Safety Organizations (PSOs) groups designed to collect and analyze error data from more than one health provider and offer quality improvement counsel

peak flow meter a device used to measure a patient's expirations and assess severity of asthma symptoms or benefits of therapy; usually used twice a day by asthma patients

percentage of error the acceptable range of variation above and below the target measurement; used in compounding and manufacturing

percentage the number or ratio per 100

performance review assessment of quality of work by a supervisor initially after three to six months, then annually thereafter

periodic automatic replenishment (PAR) levels when an item of stock goes below an established minimum inventory level, new stock is automatically ordered

peripheral IV line an IV line that is connected to a catheter inserted in a peripheral vein in a limb rather than in a main blood vein leading to the heart

peripheral parenteral nutrition (PPN) short-term parenteral nutrition with carbohydrates and/or lipids

perpetual inventory record a record that accounts for each unit of Schedule II drug dispensed or received

person code a two- or three-digit number added to the patient identification number listing family members covered by the insurance plan

pharmaceutical alternative a drug that is similar to another drug but not equivalent per the FDA and therefore not substitutable without provider's approval

pharmaceutically elegant a product that is aesthetically pleasing, both in appearance and application

pharmaceutically equivalent referring to a drug that contains the same amount of active ingredient in the same form to meet the same standards for strength, purity, and identity as the original FDA-approved patented drug product

pharmaceutical mechanism of action the precise way that a drug exerts its influence on the body

pharmaceutical weights measures of various sizes of full gram and of fractional grams (mg) often used with a two-pan prescription balance; available in both metric and apothecary weights

pharmaceutics the study of the release characteristics of various dosage forms or drug formulations

pharmacist one who is licensed by the state to prepare and sell or dispense drugs and compounds and to fill prescriptions

Pharmacists' Patient Care Process a method of collaborating with prescribers, other pharmacists, and pertinent health care professionals to provide safe, effective, and coordinated care.

Pharmacists Recovery Network (PRN) an organization to provide assistance and treatment for impaired colleagues who seek help without the risk of losing their license or registration

pharmacodynamic agent a drug that alters body functions in a desired way

pharmacodynamics biochemical, physiologic, and molecular effects of drugs on the body

pharmacogenomics a field of study that blends two scientific areas: pharmacology and genomics and examines the relationship between an individual's genes and their body's response to drugs

pharmacognosy the study and identification of natural sources of drugs

pharmacokinetics branch of pharmacology pertaining to absorption, distribution, metabolism, and elimination of drugs from the body

pharmacology the science of drugs and their interactions with the organ systems of living animals

pharmacopeia an official listing of medicinal preparations; also called a *formulary or dispensatory*

Pharmacy and Therapeutics (P&T) Committee a committee of the hospital that reviews, approves, and revises the hospital's formulary of drugs and maintains the drug use policies of the hospital

pharmacy benefit manager (PBM) a company that administers drug benefits for many insurance companies

Pharmacy Compounding Accreditation Board (PCAB) the organization responsible for accreditation for nonsterile (and sterile) compounding, working through the Accreditation Commission for Health Care (ACHC)

pharmacy informatics the use of computer systems and software, online processing, and technology for the integration of pharmacy-related data, information, expertise, and automation

Pharmacy Practice Model Initiative (PPMI) required the education and certification of pharmacy technicians and encouraged implementation of pharmacy practices

Pharmacy Technician Accreditation Commission (PTAC) a collaboration between the ASHP and the American Council on Pharmaceutical Education (ACPE), formed to review and accredit all future pharmacy technician education and training programs

pharmacy technician an individual working in a pharmacy who, under the supervision of a licensed pharmacist, assists in activities not requiring the professional judgment of a pharmacist

Pharmacy Technician Certification Board (PTCB) a national organization that develops pharmacy technician standards and serves as a credentialing agency for pharmacy technicians

Pharmacy Technician Certification Exam (PTCE) an examination developed by the Pharmacy Technician Certification Board (PTCB) that technicians must pass to be certified and receive the title of CPhT

Pharmacy Technician Educators Council (PTEC) an organization of instructors dedicated to developing and sharing pharmacy technician program curricula, educational materials, and instructional materials, advocating for greater education, training, certification, and responsibilities for technicians across the states

Pharmacy Technician Initiative an ASHP lobbying initiative done in partnership with individual state affiliates that advocates for state laws that require all pharmacy technicians be trained in an ASHP-accredited program and be certified by the Pharmacy Technician Certification Board (PTCB)

phlebitis an inflammation of the vein caused by administration of drugs

pH value the degree of acidity or alkalinity of a solution; less than 7 is acidic and more than 7 is alkaline; the pH of blood is 7.4

physical dependence taking a drug continuously so that when the medication is stopped, physical withdrawal symptoms occur

pick station an area of the inpatient pharmacy that houses frequently prescribed formulary drugs in commercially available unit dose packaging, thus allowing efficient medication cart filling by more than one technician

pipette a long, thin, calibrated, hollow tube used for measuring small volumes of liquids

plaintiff one who files a lawsuit for the courts to decide upon

plaster a solid or semisolid, medicated or nonmedicated preparation that adheres to the skin

point-of-care testing (POCT) diagnostic testing completed at or near the time and place of the patient

point-of-sale (POS) cash register a computerized register that is part of a larger automated system that includes a barcode scanner and credit-checking technology

Policy and Procedure (P&P) Manual an online or written, step-by-step set of instructions for pharmacists and technicians alike on all operations within the pharmacy department

positive pressure created when air is blown into a room and therefore has higher pressure than the adjacent spaces so the net airflow is out of the area

positron emission tomography (PET) an imaging test that uses a radioactive drug as a tracer to help reveal the function of tissues and organs

posting the process of reconciling an invoice and updating inventory at time of receipt of stock delivery

powder fine particles of medication used in tablets and capsules

powder volume (pv) the amount of space occupied by a medication in a sterile vial; used for reconstitution; equal to the difference between the total volume (tv) and the volume of the diluting ingredient, or the diluent volume (dv)

Practice Advancement Initiative (PAI) an ASHP-driven effort to expand the scope and quality of professional pharmacy practicepreceptor an experienced practitioner from the externship facility that instructs and supervises at the site

preferred drug list a formulary provided by an insurance company that indicates preferred prescription generic and brand name drugs and their corresponding copays

preferred provider organization (PPO) private practice prescriber that has signed a contract with the health insurer to provide services at a discounted rate

prescription (script) a direction for medication to be dispensed to a patient; written by a physician or a qualified licensed practitioner and filled by a pharmacist; referred to as an order when the medication is requested in a hospital setting

prescription drug a drug that requires a prescription from a licensed provider for a valid medical purpose; also known as a legend drug

prescription drug insurance insurance that specifically covers some of the cost for medications

Prescription Drug Monitoring Program (PDMP) a program, generally state-sponsored, to gather data to monitor controlled drug dispensing

prescription on profile a prescription to be filled at a future date

preservatives substances added in multiple-dose containers to inhibit microbial growth and promote a longer shelf-life

primary engineering controls (PECs) a device or zone that provides an ISO Class 5 air quality environment for sterile compounding

primary health insurance plan the plan that pays first, up to its limits of coverage

primary tubing IV tubing that is attached to the primary IV bag of solution

primary wholesaler purchasing the ordering of the majority of drugs and supplies from a single local or regional vendor who delivers the products to the pharmacy on a daily basis

prime vendor purchasing contract an agreement made by a pharmacy with a wholesaler or warehouse for a specified percentage or dollar amount of purchases

priming the act of running fluid through IV tubing to flush out small particles and expel air from the tubing before medication administration

prior authorization (PA) approval for coverage of a high-cost medication or a medication not on the insurer's approved formulary obtained after a prescriber calls the insurer to justify the use of the drug; must be obtained before the drug is dispensed by the pharmacy to be covered by insurance

prn the abbreviation for a common Latin phrase, *pro re nata*, or "in circumstances," directing patients to "take as needed" rather than a routinely scheduled dosage

probiotic live bacteria and yeasts that are good for a healthy digestive system; probiotic treatments are common after or during an antibiotic prescription; live acidophilus culture in yogurt is considered a probiotic

processor control number (PCN) an important piece of information located on most drug insurance cards to identify the correct PBM in order to process a prescription claim

productivity reports measurements of labor hours worked versus prescriptions filled and/or income generated

product line extension a marketing strategy by which a brand-name product is brought to market with different combinations of active ingredients and different indications, leading to potential consumer errors

Professional Compounding Centers of America (PCCA) an international organization that networks compounding pharmacists and technicians in the United States, Canada, Australia, and other countries of the world; a source for training, chemicals, software, and other compounding resources

professionals individuals with recognized expertise in a field who are expected to use their knowledge and skills to benefit others and to operate ethically with some autonomy

professional standards guidelines of acceptable behavior and performance established by professional associations

profit the amount of revenue received that exceeds the expenses of the sold product, services, and overhead

progesterone the hormone that prepares the uterus for the reception and development of the fertilized ovum

prophylactic agent a drug used to prevent disease, such as aspirin to prevent heart attacks

proportion a comparison of equal ratios; the product of the means equals the product of the extremes

protected health information (PHI) medical information that is protected by HIPAA, such as medical diagnoses, medication profiles, and results of laboratory tests

proton pump inhibitors (PPIs) a class of drugs that stops stomach acid production by blocking gastric acid secretion by inhibiting the enzyme that pumps hydrogen ions into the stomach

protozoan a single-celled organism that inhabits water and soil

psychoactive drugs medications targeted to modify the brain functions to influence mood, perception, and/or consciousness

psychological dependence when the patient takes a drug on a regular basis because it produces a sense of well-being that the patient does not want to consider being without

psychopharmaceutical drugs used to treat mental health diseases, such as depression

pulverization by intervention the process of reducing particle size by adding an evaporative agent to allow for greater grinding into smaller, softer elements

punch method a method for filling capsules in which the body of a capsule is repeatedly punched into a cake of medication until the capsule is full

purchasing the ordering of products for use or sale by the pharmacy

pyrogen a fever-producing by-product of microbial metabolism

quality assurance (QA) a system of procedures, activities, feedback, and oversight that ensures that operational and quality standards are consistently met

quality control (QC) procedures to measure quality and progress on quality initiatives that involve the sampling, testing, and documentation of results that, taken together, ensure that specifications have been met

quality related events (QREs) medication errors that reach the patient; this includes "near misses" and unsafe conditions

radiopharmaceuticals radioactive compounded drugs like irradiated iodine that are created in a nuclear compounding facility

radiopharmacy isolators lead-encased C-PECs designed specifically for handling radioactive diagnostic and therapeutic agents

rapid-dissolving tablet (RDT) a tablet that disintegrates rapidly (within 30 seconds) on the tongue

ratio a comparison of numeric values

ratio strength the portion, or ratio, of the active strength ingredient to the whole drug product

REACT an acronym for what to do in the case of a robbery: **R**emain calm, **E**yewitness, **A**ctivate alarm, **C**all police, **T**ake charge

reactivity the potential to cause chemical reactions when encountering other chemicals, molecules, or substances

reasonable doubt a doubt about the guilt of a defendant that arises or remains after thorough consideration of the evidence or lack thereof

receipt a printout that is a proof of purchase

receiving a series of procedures for accepting the delivery of products to the pharmacy from a wholesaler or centralized warehouse

recertification the periodic updating of certification

reciprocal ratio switching the numerator with the denominator in a ratio

reconcile to match the cash, credit card receipts, personal checks, coupons, rebates, voided sales, and patient charges with the tape printout from each cash register

reconstitute the process of adding distilled water to a powder formulation like an antibiotic; requires a "shake well" and expiration date on the label

rectal route of administration the delivery of medication via the rectum

rectum the final section of the intestines ending in the anus

referral a primary healthcare provider's recommendation that a patient go to a specialist or receive additional services

registration the process of becoming enrolled on a list created by the state board of pharmacy in order to practice

regulation a set of written rules and procedures that exist to carry out a law

release testing visual assessment performed to ensure that a final CSP meets appropriate quality characteristics

remote computer a minicomputer or a mainframe that stores and processes data sent from a dumb terminal

renal having to do with the kidneys

repackaging control log a form used in the pharmacy when drugs are repackaged from manufacturer stock bottles to unit doses; the log contains the name of the drug, dose, dosage form, quantity, manufacturer, lot number, expiration date, and the initials of the pharmacy technician and pharmacist

resistant something that is immune to an antibiotic that bacterial cells can develop after encountering antibiotics but not being fully eradicated

restricted access barrier system (RABS) an enclosure that provides HEPA-filtered ISO Class 5 unidirectional air

right of refusal the ability of a pharmacist to decline with cause to fill any prescription, especially those for controlled substances

risk evaluation and mitigation strategy (REMS) a program designed by the FDA for prescribers, pharmacies, and patients to more closely monitor selected high-risk drugs

robotic dispensing system automation in the central pharmacy to more accurately and efficiently fill unit dose orders for frequently used oral medications

roller clamp the hard plastic device that provides compression on the tubing, thereby controlling the flow rate of the IV solution

Roman numeral system a mathematical system in which numerical values are expressed in either capital or lowercase letters

root-cause analysis a logical and systematic process used to help identify what, how, and why something happened to prevent recurrence

rotating the stock positioning the units of product with the shortest expiration dates where they will be the first units selected for use; usually the most recent products will be used last

rounded off simplified by adding a little to the number to the left (rounding up) or taking a little away (rounding down)

route of administration a method of delivering a drug to the body, such as orally, topically, or parenterally

rushed error a medication error that occurs because of the pressure of meeting corporate or self-imposed time constraints, resulting in not fully checking and double-checking information by the technician and pharmacist

℞ Patrol a collaborative effort between industry and law enforcement designed to collect, collate, analyze, and disseminate pharmacy theft information

℞ prescription; stands for Latin verb recipere, meaning "to take"

résumé a brief, concise, vivid written summary of what you have to offer an employer

Safety Data Sheet (SDS) formerly Material Safety Data Sheet (MSDS); a document that contains important technical information on the hazards of chemicals used in compounding and procedures for the treatment of accidental ingestion or exposure

schedule a listing of controlled substances categorized for a specific level of restriction by the DEA according to their potential for abuse and physical or psychological dependence

Schedule II drug administration record a manual or electronic form on the patient care unit to account for each dose of each Schedule II narcotic administered to a patient

Schedule V drug a medication with a low potential for abuse and a limited potential for creating physical or psychological dependence; available in most states without a prescription

schizophrenia chronic mental health disorder with mental and emotional fragmentation and retreat from reality, hallucinations, ambivalence, and bizarre or regressive behavior

scoop method placement of the needle tip into the inside of the cap and scooping it up before putting pressure on the cap to secure it

scoring indenting of a tablet by the manufacturer to encourage easier breaking or cutting along the indented lines for proportional dosages

secondary engineering controls (SECs) area where the PEC is placed (e.g., a cleanroom suite or an SCA); incorporates specific design and operational parameters required to minimize the risk of contamination within the compounding area

secondary health insurance plan the plan that pays what the primary insurer does not—if the service is covered

secondary tubing IV tubing for another medication that is attached to the primary tubing at a Y-site injection port

second party payer the person or entity that provided healthcare services

sedation a state of induced calm, drowsiness, or sleep

segregated compounding area (SCA) a designated, unclassified space, area, or room with a defined perimeter that contains a PEC and is suitable for preparation of Category 1 CSPs only

seizures spasms caused by overfiring of the neurons of the brain and nervous system

selection error a medication error that occurs when two or more options exist, and the incorrect option is chosen

selective serotonin reuptake inhibitor (SSRI) an antidepressant drug that blocks the reabsorption of serotonin, with little effect on norepinephrine and fewer side effects than other antidepressant drugs

semisynthetic drug a drug that contains both natural and synthetic components

sensitivity range the potential range of error for a measuring device

sentinel event an unexpected occurrence involving death or serious physical or psychological injury or the potential for such events to occur

sepsis a toxic condition that occurs when an infection is so threatening to the body that the immune system begins to attack the body's own blood vessels and organs causing inflammation, leaky vessels, organ failure, and septic shock

serotonin a neurotransmitter that affects mood, sexual desire, appetite, sleep, and memory

shadowing when a supply item, hand position, or action gets in the way of the first air from the PEC over the direct compounding area and process

sharps container container to dispose of any needle, lancet, scalpel blade, or other medical equipment that can be a source of infection

side effect a secondary response to a drug other than the primary therapeutic effect for which the drug was intended

sifting a process used to blend powders through the use of a sieve

signa (sig) the part of the prescription that indicates the directions for the patient to follow when taking the medication

signa code directions part of a prescription that provides directions to be included on the label for the patient to follow in taking the medication

single-dose vials (SDVs) containers of sterile medication for parenteral administration (e.g., injection or infusion) that are designed for use with a single patient as a single injection/infusion; a single-dose container does not contain a preservative

small-volume parenteral (SVP) preparations IV solutions of generally 25 to 250 mL, typically administered as an IV piggyback (infusing into the LVP)

smart terminal computer containing its own storage and processing capabilities

smurfing when someone pays others to purchase restricted OTC medications, such as those containing pseudoephedrine, for the purpose of making illegal drugs

social media internet outlets such as Facebook, Twitter, CareerBuilder, and LinkedIn that can provide a worthwhile online tool for networking

social sanctions negative repercussions imposed in social or professional situations for inappropriate or wrong behavior

software update transmission of programming and data to make the software current

software upgrade new edition of a software product with improved and enhanced capabilities; sold as a separate product or as an upgrade to a current version

solid extract a potent dosage form where most or all liquid has been evaporated to produce powder or solid matter

solute an activeingredient dissolved in a solution or dispersed in a suspension

solution a liquid dosage form in which the active ingredients are completely dissolved in a liquid vehicle

solvent the larger amount in a solution into which the ingredients are dissolved

spacer device a device commonly prescribed for children and older adults to assist in the administration of drugs from MDIs; medication can be inhaled at will rather than through timed, coordinated breathing movements

Spanish flu a disease caused by the H1N1 virus

spatula a stainless steel, plastic, or hard rubber instrument used for transferring or mixing solid pharmaceutical ingredients

spatulation a process used to blend ingredients with a spatula; often used in the preparation of creams and ointments

SPEAK UP an acronym for advice for hospital patients to get the safest, best health care, promoted by the Joint Commission and Centers for Medicare and Medicaid Services

specific gravity the ratio of the weight of a substance compared to an equal volume of water when both are the same temperature at sea level

sphygmomanometer an arm or wrist cuff with a gauge monitor to measure blood pressure

spike adapter the sharp plastic end of IV tubing that is attached to an IV bag of fluid

spill kit a container of supplies, warning signage, and related materials used to contain the spill of an HD

spirit an alcoholic or hydroalcoholic solution containing volatile, aromatic ingredients

spray the dosage form that consists of a container with a valve assembly that, when activated, emits a fine dispersion of liquid, solid, or gaseous material

stability the ability of a drug to maintain its potency and integrity in its compounded form

staging area the assembly space of the compounding work surface

standard a guideline, benchmark, or desired level of quality to serve as the expected norm for a product or professional performance

standard of care the usual and customary level of practice in the community

standard operating procedures (SOPs) written guidelines that integrate the guidelines in *USP* <797> (rev. 2019) to bring consistency of sterility, accuracy, and quality for sterile compounding facilities

standards measures of acceptable behavior of a professional or paraprofessional

standing order a preapproved list of instructions, including specific medications and doses, commonly written after a surgery or procedure

state board of pharmacy governing body responsible for the regulation of the practice of pharmacy within the state

statins (HMG-CoA reductase inhibitors) family of drugs that prevents the production of "bad cholesterol" or LDL by blocking a key enzyme in the liver that makes it

stat medications medications that require immediate high-priority filling and administration

stat order a medication order that is to be filled and sent to the patient care unit immediately

stereotype an oversimplified characteristic of a group of people

sterile compounding pharmacies pharmacies that specialize in sterile compounds, such as IV solutions, parenteral nutrition, and injections

sterile compounding the preparation of a parenteral product in the hospital, infusion, nuclear, or compounding pharmacy, an example is an intravenous antibiotic or an ophthalmic solution

Sterile Hazardous drugs (HD) any drug identified by at least one of the following six criteria: carcinogenicity, teratogenicity or developmental toxicity, reproductive toxicity in humans, organ toxicity at low dose in humans or animals, genotoxicity, or new drugs that mimic existing HDs in structure or toxicity and are administered via a pathway that requires the drug to be sterile

Sterile Nuclear drug products radioactive compounded drugs that diagnose and treat various diseases, primarily administered by the IV route

sterile the absence of all viable microorganisms

sterility testing a documented and established laboratory procedure for detecting viable microbial contamination in a sample or preparation

sterilization the process of using chemicals, heat, cold, pressure, or other forces to kill microorganisms on exposed surfaces

steroids complex synthetic drug substances that resemble human hormones

stock bottle the original pharmaceutical manufacturer's container of medication stored on the pharmacy shelf for dispensing individual prescriptions

stock par levels the minimum amount of inventory needed on hand to meet known customer demand and a small surplus in case of unexpected demand

subcutaneous (subq) route of administration injection of a drug into the layer of fat under the skin

sublingual route of administration oral administration in which a drug is placed under the tongue and is rapidly absorbed into the bloodstream

subpoena a legal order

subscription the part of the prescription that lists instructions to the pharmacist about dispensing the medication, including compounding or packaging instructions, labeling instructions, refill information, and information about the appropriateness of dispensing drug equivalencies

sugar-coated tablet (SCT) a tablet coated with an outside layer of sugar that protects the medication and improves both appearance and flavor

sulfa drugs sulphur-based drugs used to fight microbial infections

sulfonylureas antidiabetic drugs that stimulate the pancreas to produce more insulin

superbugs microorganisms that are resistant to antibiotic therapies

supplemental engineering controls special supplies used within the DCAs during transfers to keep toxic agents from escaping into the air, onto the technician, or onto work surfaces

suppository a solid formulation containing a drug for rectal, urethral, or vaginal administration

suspendibility ability to become and remain suspended in a dissolving liquid

suspension a liquid dosage form with the dispersion of a solid in a liquid

sustained-release (SR) formulation an extended-release dosage form that allows less frequent dosing than an immediate-release dosage form

synthesized drug a drug created artificially in the laboratory but in imitation of a naturally occurring drug

synthetic drug a drug that has been created from a series of chemical reactions to produce a specific pharmacological effect

syringe a device used to inject a parenteral solution into the bloodstream, muscle, or under the skin

syringe injections smaller volume sterile solutions administered via a syringe

syrup an aqueous solution thickened with a large amount of sugar (generally sucrose) or a sugar substitute, such as sorbitol or propylene glycol

systemic effect the distribution of a drug throughout the body by absorption into the bloodstream

tablet splitter a device used to manually split or score tablets

tablet the solid dosage form produced by compression of dry ingredients and containing one or more active and inactive ingredients

tall man lettering enhanced lettering on the stock labels of similar-sounding high-risk medications, or other labeling changes to help better differentiate products and dosages and reduce medication errors

tamper-resistant prescription (TRP) a prescription that is written on secure paper that is specifically designed to prevent copying, erasure, or alteration

tare weight the weight of the empty container, such as the weighing paper or boat that must be figured in or "tared" out to make the weighed measurement accurate

targeted drug delivery system technology to deliver high concentrations of drugs to the diseased organ rather than expose the whole body to adverse side effects; commonly designed for cancer chemotherapy

taxable items products that must have a sales tax due to state law

tech-check-tech (TCT) function a senior pharmacy technician checks another pharmacy technician's work to add another layer of verification of the medication order prior to drug administration

technical failure an error generated by failure of equipment

telepharmacies shifts or locations serviced by a remote pharmacist that can accept new prescriptions from a physician's office without a pharmacist physically present

tell back a collaborative approach that uses patient-centered, open-ended questions to encourage the patient to tell back what he or she understands; an especially useful method for new patients and/or new prescriptions

teratogenicity high potential of a drug to cause harm to a fetus

tetracycline antibiotics complex antibiotics that are particularly dangerous for pregnant or nursing patients

thalidomide a drug prescribed for pregnant women in mostly European countries in the 1960s, causing birth defects, but the FDA refused approval, saving many children from these effects

therapeutic agent a drug that targets a specific need in the body and maintains health, relieves symptoms, combats illness, and reverses disease processes

therapeutically equivalent referring to a substitution drug that has the same or equal therapeutic (medicinal) effect

therapeutics the study of the appropriate use of drugs for targeted medicinal purposes

third party payer an organization other than the patient or healthcare provider who is responsible for covering costs; typically insurance companies, government agencies, or individual employers

tiered copayment insurance coverage in which the patient has an escalating copay, depending on whether the filled prescription is a generic drug, a preferred brand name drug, or a non-preferred brand name drug; higher tiers may include expensive specialty drugs

tincture an alcoholic or hydroalcoholic solution of extractions from plants

tonicity is the directional flow pattern of water in cells based on concentrations and osmotic pressure within their environments

topical route of administration the administration of a drug on the skin or to a mucous membrane; can be dermal or transdermal

tort the legal term used in lawsuits for personal injuries that one citizen commits against another

total parenteral nutrition (TPN) an IV infusion therapy that supplies a patient with all the nutrition needed by the body

total volume (tv) the full amount of the final volume in a drug product with all ingredients, the solutes and diluent solution

totes plastic containers that contain medications sent from the wholesaler, including those for controlled substances and refrigerated items (in cold packs); these containers are sealed at the warehouse for security until delivery to the pharmacy

toxicology scientific discipline that studies symptoms, detection and treatment of poisonous effects and side effects

trace hazardous waste small amounts of HDs remaining on used HD vials, ampules, IV bags, needles, straws, and syringes

traditional Eastern medicine herbal-based treatments based on ancient East Indian and other Asian philosophies that blend various healing modalities to bring balance and harmony to the body

transdermal route of administration delivery of a continuous supply of drug into the bloodstream by absorption through the skin via an ointment, gel, lotion, a patch or disk

transfer in a prescription that is transferred in from another pharmacy

transfer out a prescription that is transferred out to another pharmacy

transmucosal supplying drugs across any mucous membrane of the body, including the mouth, eyes, ears, nose, rectum, vagina, and urethra

triage the assessment and prioritization by the pharmacist of patients' illnesses or symptoms; outcome may be to recommend an OTC product or to refer the patient to a physician or emergency room; also used to assess and prioritize technician responsibilities within the pharmacy

Tricare government insurance program for active and retired military and their families

triglycerides three lipids combined; a type of fat that contributes to artery blockage

trituration the process of rubbing, grinding, or pulverizing a substance to create finer particles

troche a small lozenge that contains active medication

tumbling a process used to combine powders by placing them in a bag or container and rotating or shaking it

turbulence an irregular type of airflow that results whenever anything blocks or interrupts or meets the unidirectional airflow

ultraviolet (UV) radiation energy from the short, intense wavelengths of the light rays of the blue end of the light spectrum that can be used to kill microorganisms in sterilization

underinsured patient insufficiently covered by health insurance

unidirectional airflow air within a PEC moving in a single direction in a uniform manner and at sufficient velocity to sweep particles away from the DCA

uninsured patient patient with no insurance who must pay out of pocket for medical and/or prescription costs

unit dose an amount of a drug that has been prepackaged or repackaged for a particular patient for a single administration at a particular time

unit dose cart a mobile storage unit that contains individual patient drawers of medication for all patients on a given nursing unit

unit dose product label contains product information on drug labels: drug name, dose, strength, manufacturer, expiration date, and bar code

unit of use a fixed number of dose units in a stock drug container, usually consisting of a month's supply of tablets or capsules, such as 30 tablets or capsules

universal precautions for preventing transmission of blood-borne infections procedures followed in healthcare settings to prevent transmission of infection-causing agents as a result of exposure to blood or other bodily fluids

urethral route of administration delivery of a drug by insertion into the urethra

USP Dietary Supplement Verification Program a seal of approval from USP assuring the quality of a dietary supplement

US Pharmacopeial Convention (USP) the independent, scientific organization responsible for setting official quality standards for all drugs sold in the United States, as well as standards for practice

US Pharmacopeia–National Formulary (USP–NF) a resource published by the USP Convention that contains USP standards for best practices, medicines, dosage forms, drug substances, inactive ingredients, medical devices, and dietary supplements

usual and customary (U&C) the reimbursement rate from PBMs to pharmacies for the cost of drugs, plus a pharmacy dispensing fee

Vaccine Adverse Event Reporting System (VAERS) a postmarketing surveillance system operated by the FDA and CDC that collects information on adverse events that occur after immunization

vaccine a substance used to stimulate the production of antibodies and provide immunity

Vaccine Errors Reporting Program (VERP) a national program designed to allow healthcare professionals to report vaccine errors directly to the Institute for Safe Medication Practices (ISMP)

vaginal route of administration delivery of a drug by application of a cream or insertion of a tablet into the vagina

valence a number that represents the capacity of a chemical element to combine with others to form a molecule of a stable new compound, based on the number and activity of the exterior electrons

vehicle the substance that is the carrier of the active ingredients or is the solution in which the active ingredients in liquid, semisolid, or solid form are dissolved or suspended

vented needle a special needle with a hole in the lumen that allows fluid to be injected into a vial while simultaneously allowing the air, or positive pressure, from the vial to escape

Verified Internet Pharmacy Practice Sites (VIPPS) an accreditation of quality for internet pharmacies that is recognized by 17 US states

vertical airflow HEPA-filtered air that projects downward onto the DCA to offer additional protection for both the compounding technician and the environment when aseptically compounding hazardous chemicals; examples of vertical airflow hoods include biological safety cabinets (BSCs) and the compounding aseptic containment isolator (CACI)

vertical laminar airflow workbenches (V-LAFWs) a type of Class II BSC

Veterans Health Administration (VHA) a healthcare system, under the US Department of Veterans Affairs, serving more than 8.76 million veterans and operating over 1,700 care sites

vial-and-bag system a type of SVP in which a specially designed vial and diluent IVPB bag screw or snap together and are activated by the nurse just before patient administration of the medication

vial sealed glass or plastic sterile container with a rubber seal and hard plastic cap

virus a minute infectious agent that does not have all of the components of a cell and thus can replicate only within a living host cell

viscosity the thickness and flow characteristics of a fluid

volume-in-volume (v/v) the volume of active ingredient in the volume of the total solution, such as 3 milliliters (mL) per 100 mL (3 mL/100 mL)

volumetric measurement the act of or result of using a calibrated graduated, conical cylinder, or pipette dropper, to accurately measure liquid volume

water-in-oil (W/O) emulsion an emulsion containing a small amount of water dispersed in an oil, such as an ointment

wax matrix system a drug delivery system where the drug is embedded in an inner chamber surrounded by a waxy substance, and a portion of the drug is partitioned in the inner core of the tablet by the waxy matrix (material surrounding it) for later release using osmotic pressure or an ion exchange resin

weighing boat a plastic container used to weigh large quantities of chemicals

weighing paper a nonabsorbent paper, also called powder paper, that is placed on a weighing balance pan to avoid contact between pharmaceutical ingredients and the balance tray; used to weigh small quantities of chemicals

weight-in-volume (w/v) the weight of the active ingredient (usually in mg or g) within the total volume of a solution, such as 1 mg per 100 mL of solution (1 mg/100 mL)

weight-in-weight (w/w) the weight of the active ingredient as part of the total weight of a compound or solutions, such as 2 mg per 100 grams of total weight (2 mg/100 g)

Western medicine medical treatment by a licensed professional who identifies the cause of an illness by physical examination and then treats the illness with various natural and synthetic medicinal products or drugs

withdrawal symptoms effects as the body struggles to adjust to the lack of the substance to which it is accustomed; includes agitation, muscle aches, nausea and vomiting, sweating, depression, and insomnia

workers' compensation insurance provided for a patient with a medical injury from a job-related accident; also called workers' comp or workman's comp

wrong amount error a medication error that occurs when a dose is either above or below the correct amount by more than 5%

wrong drug error a medication error that occurs when the incorrect drug is substituted for the one prescribed

wrong formulation error a medication error that occurs when the dosage form or formulation is not the accepted interpretation of the physician order

wrong time error a medication error that occurs when a drug is given 30 minutes or more before or after it was prescribed, up to the time of the next dose, not including "as needed" orders

Zika a virus causing a pandemic that may cause birth defects in pregnant women

zone of turbulence when using an H-LAFW, the area the unidirectional filtered air meets resistance or blockage, particularly between the DCA and compounding technician; also the area at the edges of the compounding counter where the horizontal airflow meets the buffer room air

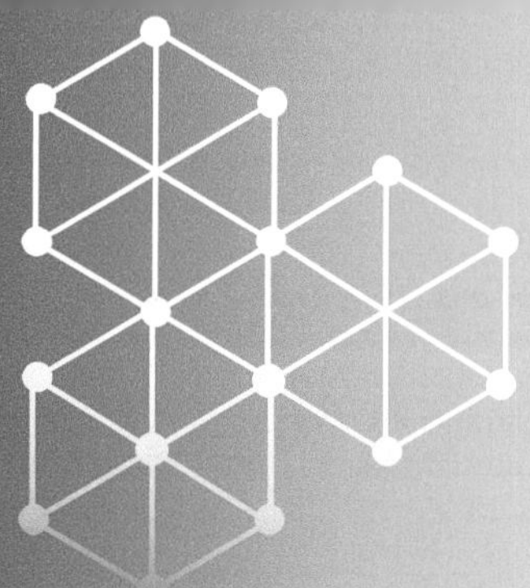

Index

When the letters *t*, *f*, or *p* follow a page number, the reference relates to either a *table*, *figure*, or *photo*.

B

C

D

E

G

H

J

K

L

M

N

O

P

Q

R

S

T

U

V

W

X

Y

Z

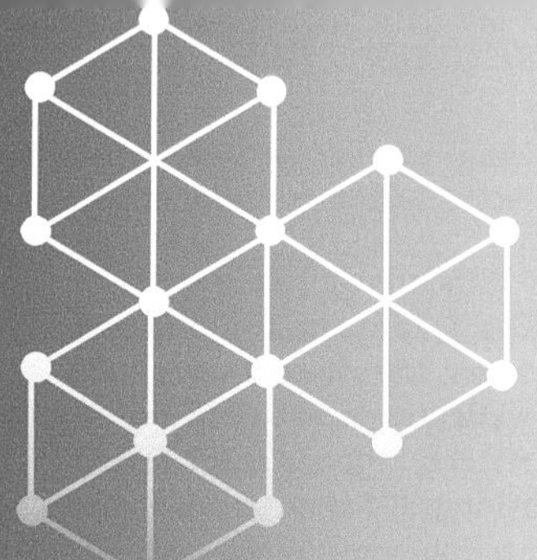

PHOTO CREDITS

1 © iStock/andresr; **4** courtesy of Wikipedia/Public Domain; **5** Lithograph by Pierre Roche Vigneron/Public Domain; **6** Printed with Permission of American Pharmacists Associate Foundation. Copyright 2009 APhA Foundation; **7** (top and bottom) Courtesy of the National Library of Medicine; **8** (top) courtesy of Bob Andersion (bottom) © iStockphoto/AntiMartina; **9** (top) courtesy of Bob Andersion (bottom) Courtesy of Philadelphia College of Pharmacy University of the Sciences in Philadelphia; **10** courtesy of the FDA Photostream; **11** © iStockphoto/HultonArchive; **12** (top) courtesy of US Army Office of Medical History (bottom) Courtesy of the Indiana Historical Society; **13** Courtesy of The Royal London Hospital Archives; **14** (top) © University of Arizona College of Pharmacy (bottom) courtesy of the US Navy; **15** © iStockphoto/asiseeit; **16** © iStockphoto/jcarillet; **19** © iStockphoto/3bugsmom; **21** (top) © Paradigm Publishing (bottom) © iStockphoto/sshepard; **22** © George Brainard; **23** © Shutterstock/Dmitry Kalinovsky; **24** © Paradigm Publishing**;** **25** Image provided courtesy of Laura Humphrey PTCB; **26** courtesy of Lincoln Technical Institute; **27** © Paradigm Publishing; **28** Photograph provided courtesy of Kara Duncan Weatherman PharmD BCNP Purdue University Nuclear Pharmacy Programs. Copyright (2008) Purdue University; **29** Shutterstock/Sura Nualpradid. **36** Chromolithograph by Hughes Lithographers Chicago; **37** courtesy of US Department of Justice; **39** (top) Courtesy of the FDA Photostream (bottom) © Paradigm Publishing; **40** (top) Courtesy of the FDA Photostream (bottom) Otis Historical Archives National Museum of Health and Medicine; **42** © Shutterstock/Iakov Filimonov; **43** © iStockphoto/christine Glade; **44** courtesy of Mallinckrodt LLC; **45** courtesy of Robert Anderson; **47** (top) courtesy of the FDA Photostream (bottom) courtesy of Kevin Rushforth; **50** courtesy of Robert Anderson; **52** (top) courtesy of Assistant Secretary of Public Affairs (bottom) CBS News; **54** (top) Courtesy of the FDA Photostream (bottom) Used with permission of The United States Pharmacopeial Convention (USP); **55** (top) Courtesy of the FDA Photostream (bottom) © VIPPS National Association Boards of Pharmacy; **57** © iStockphoto/sshepard; **58** (top) Courtesy of US Army Office of Medical History (bottom left) US Pharmacopeial Convention (bottom right) © Paradigm Pulblishing; **59** © iStockphoto/Neustockimages. **70** (top and bottom) © Paradigm Publishing; **71** © iStockphoto/sjlocke; **72** © iStockphoto/fluxfoto; **73** (top) © iStockphoto/monkeybusinessimages (bottom) © Shutterstock/Fedorov Oleksiy; **74** (top) Ed Hamman (bottom) Jim Lambert; **75** Courtesy of the National Library of Medicine; **77** (top) Courtesy of the FDA Photostream (bottom) Courtesy of the FDA Photostream; **78** Courtesy of the FDA Photostream; **79** Courtesy of the Thomas Fisher Rare Book Library University of Toronto; **80** (top) © iStockphoto/FrankRitchie (bottom) Courtesy of Wikipedia/Public Domain; **81** (both) Courtesy of Wikipedia/Public Domain; **82** © Shutterstock/dencg; **83** Courtesy of Wikipedia/Public Domain; **84** © iStockphoto/mafoto; **85** © iStock.com/Roel Smart; **86** courtesy of the FDA Photostream; **88** courtesy of the FDA Photostream; **89** © Paradigm Publishing; **90** © Paradigm Publishing; **91** Courtesy of the FDA Photostream; **94** US Food and Drug Administration. **99** © Adobe Stock/Seventyfour; **102** © iStockphoto/asiseeit; **103** © IStock/sevengine sevengine; **104** courtesy of corbis; **110** © Wolter Kluwer; **112** Wikipedia/DiverDave; **115** (top) © Fotolia/WavebreakMediaMicro (bottom) © iStockphoto/mediaphotos; **119** © iStockphoto/Eliza Snow; **121** (both) Custom Medical Stock Photos; **123** ©iStockphoto/YinYang; **125** Warhaftig Associates; **129** © iStockphoto/fluxfoto; **131** Custom Medical Stock Photo Inc.; **132** © iStockphoto/twilightproductions; **134** ©iStockphoto; **136** © Shutterstock/Sebastian Kaulitzki; **138** ©iStockphoto/gokhanilgaz. **146** © Shutterstock/IDAL; **152** (top) © Paradigm (bottom) © Fotolia/enriscapes; **153** © iStock/ruizluquepaz; **155** (top) ©Shutterstock/Keith Homan (bottom) © iStock/CoffeeAndMilk; **156** (top) © iStockphoto/WellfordT (middle) ©Shutterstock/Image Point Fr (bottom) © iStock/JannHuizenga; **158** Courtesy of Tova Wiegand Green; **159** © George Brainard; **162** Courtesy of Tova Wiegand Green; **163** © Shutterstock/BW Folsom; **168** (top) Courtesy of Tova Wiegand Green (bottom) © Shutterstock/Kesu; **173** © iStockphoto/leschnyhan; **175** (top) © Paradigm Paradigm (middle) © Paradigm Publishing (bottom) © iStockphoto/ladyminnie; **176** © Wikipedia/Trainer2a; ©iStock/drawdrawdraw; **179** (top) © iStockphoto/smartstock (bottom) © iStockphoto/CreativeI; **181** courtesy of George Brainard; **182** ©Shutterstock/FedotovAnatoly; **185** © Shutterstock/Dmitry Lobanov; **187** © Shutterstock/Rob Byron; **191** © Shutterstock/Image Point Fr. **199** ©AdobeStock/AnthonyBrown; **208** © Paradigm Publishing; **214** © iStockphoto/Murat Sen; **216** © iStockphoto/malerapaso; **219** © Paradigm Publishing; **220** © Paradigm Publishing; **221** ©iStock/RapidEye; **224** © Paradigm Publishing; **241** Courtesy of Apothecary Products Inc.; **247** ©Shutterstock/MR.LIGHTMAN1975. **260** © Shutterstock/bluecinema; **261** © iStockphoto/kzenon; **262** © iStockphoto/uchar; **264** © George Brainard; **268** © George Brainard; **271** courtesy of ehrscreenshots.com; **272** Courtesy of Health Business System Inc.; **273** © Shutterstock/Stock-Asso; **277** © Paradigm Publishing; **282** © iStockphoto/sjlocke**;** **286** (center) Courtesy of Robert Anderson (bottom) © George Brainard; **287** Courtesy of Robert Anderson; **288** (top) Courtesy of Apothecary Products Inc. (bottom) © iStockphoto/art-4-art; **289** courtesy of Parata Systems LLC; **291** Courtesy of Robert Anderson; **295** (top) Courtesy of Tova Wiegand Green (bottom) © iStockphoto/stevecoleimages; **296** ©iStock/JannHulzenga; **297** © George Brainard. **306** © iStock/spxChrome; **308** © Shutterstock/goddluz; **310** © Shutterstock/robertindiana; **312** © Shutterstock/nelgelpi; **314** (top) courtesy of Social Security History (bottom) courtesy of Medicare; **320** courtesy of Tricare; **322** © iStock/YinYang; **325** © Paradigm Publishing; **327** © Paradigm Publishing; **329**

© George Brainard; **332** courtesy of the NIH; **338** ©Shutterstock/Monkey business Images. **346** © iStock/Peopleimages; **348** (top) © Shutterstock/Tyler Olson (bottom) © Paradigm Publishing; **349** © Shutterstock/Cheryl Casey; **350** Courtesy of Robert Anderson; **351** © Shutterstock/Dean Drobot; **353** © Paradigm Publishing; **355** ©iStock/PeopleImages; **356** Photo courtesy of OraSure Technologies USA; **357** (top) ©Shutterstock/Fotana (bottom) ©Shutterstock/Ugorenkov Aleksandr; **358** Courtesy of Robert Anderson; **359** ©Shutterstock/g215; **360** ©Shutterstock/Dmitry Kalinovsky; **361** ©Shutterstock/Fotocrisis; **362** © iStock/Deklofenak; **364** ©Shutterstock/Marius Pirvu; **365** ©Shutterstock/kadmy; **370** © Paradigm Publishing; **373** Courtesy of Robert Anderson; **375** ©Shutterstock/SofikoS; **377** © iStock/sjlocke; **380** © iStock/SWInsider; **382** Courtesy of Robert Anderson; **383** © iStock/sjlocke; **384** Courtesy of Robert Anderson; **386** ©Fotolia/Katrina Miller. **393** © Shutterstock/Enriscapes; **394** (left) courtesy of NABP (right) © iStockphoto/narxx; **396** George Brainard; **397** (top) courtesy of ACHC (bottom) ©Shutterstock/Jagodka; **399** © Shutterstock/EnolaBrain81; **404** Adobe Stock/trustle; **405** © George Brainard; **406** iStockphoto/DenGuy; **407** (top) Courtesy of Tova Wiegand Green (bottom) © George Brainard; **408** (top) © George Brainard (bottom) ©Fotolia/James Steidl; **414** © George Brainard; **415** (both) Courtesy of Tova Wiegand Green; **416** (both) Courtesy of Tova Wiegand Green; **417** © Paradigm Publishing; **418** courtesy of US National Archives; **419** © Shutterstock/fotohunter; **420** © Paradigm Publishing; **423** (top) © George Brainard (bottom) Courtesy of Torpac Inc. (photographer: Eric Hobaichan); **433** Provided courtesy of Topi-CLICK. Topi-CLICK is a registered trademark. For more information about this product visit www.Topi-Click.com.; **435** Courtesy of Robert Anderson; **436** © iStockphoto/YinYang; **437** © iStockphoto/energy; **438** Courtesy of PK Software a PCCA Company; **439** ©dreamstime.com/Joye Ardyn Durham. **448** Spotmatik Ltd; **450** © Ghislain & Marie Davide de Lossy cultura Jupiterimages; **452** Courtesy of Lisa McCartney; **453** Courtesy of Lisa McCartney; **456** ©Shutterstock/Monkey Business Images; **457** Courtesy of Lisa McCartney; **459** Courtesy of RMS Omega; **463** Courtesy of Lisa McCartney; **464** ©Shutterstock/Stuart Jenner; **465** Courtesy of McKesson Provider Technologies Inc.; p **466** (top) Courtesy of Lisa McCartney (bottom) Medical Packaging Inc; **467** (top) Courtesy of McKesson Provider Technologies Inc (bottom) © George Brainard; **469** (top) Courtesy of Lisa McCartney (bottom) courtesy of Medical inc.; **470** Photo courtesy of the Montreal Gazette; **471** Courtesy of Lisa McCartney; **473** Courtesy of Lisa McCartney; **474** (top) Courtesy of McKesson Provider Technologies Inc. (bottom) ©Shutterstock/ Johan Swanepoel; **477** Courtesy of Lisa McCartney; **478** ©Shutterstock/Minerva Studio; **479** courtesy of Lisa McCartney; **480** (top) Courtesy of BD (bottom) © Shutterstock/bikeriderlondon; **481** ©Shutterstock/Konstantin L. **490** © iStockphoto/sitox; **491** (top) BSIP/SuperStock (middle) Cultura Limited / SuperStock (bottom) ©Fotolia/Wire_man; **493** © Shutterstock/lynea; **495** Courtesy of the CDC; **496** © iStockphoto/Geber86; **498** (top) Library of Congress Archives (bottom) © iStockphoto/dra_schwartz; **500** © iStockphoto/DenGuy; **501** ©Fotolia/thodonal; **502** © Fotolia/Dmitry Vereshchagin; **504** © Paradigm Publishing; **506** Courtesy of Lipscomb University; **507** Courtesy of Wendy Yesenia Almeda; **508** Courtesy of Bioscience International Inc.; **510** (all) © Germfree Laboratories; **511** © George Brainard; **512** (all) © George Brainard; **513** © George Brainard; **517** © iStockphoto/annedde; **520** (top) © Paradigm Publishing (bottom) Courtesy of EastMed; **521** (top) Courtesy of what-when-how.com (bottom) Courtesy of Wendy Yesenia Almeda; **522** (top) Courtesy of ON-Q (bottom) © Paradigm Publishing; **523** (middle) Courtesy of Wendy Yesenia Almeda; **524** Courtesy of Baker Co. **533** © iStockphoto/Eraxion; **535** Courtesy of the American Pharmacists Association; **536** Courtesy of Wendy Yesenia Almeda; **537** © Paradigm Publishing; **542** © iStockphoto.com; **543** (both) © George Brainard; **546** (top) © George Brainard (bottom) © Shutterstock/jomphong; **554** Courtesy of Braun; **557** courtesy of Medline; **558** © George Brainard; **559** © Paradigm Publishing; **560** (left) © George Brainard (right) Courtesy of Wendy Yesenia Almeda; **561** courtesy B. Braun Melsungen AG; **562** Courtesy of BD; **564** Courtesy of the Baxa Corporation; **565** Courtesy of Tova Wiegand Green; **566** © George Brainard; **567** © iStockphoto/annedde; **568** (top) © Paradigm Publishing (bottom) Courtesy of West Pharmaceutical Services; **570** © Shutterstock/frantab; **574** © Paradigm Publishing; **577** © Paradigm Publishing; **579** (both) © Paradigm Publishing; **580** © ICU Medical; **582** Courtesy of United Label; **584** © Shutterstock/Rihardzz; **585** © Paradigm Publishing; **586** Courtesy of Germfree Laboratories Inc. **596** © iStockphoto/sjlocke; **597** (top) © Marharyta Pavliuk (bottom) © Dmitry Kalinovsky; **599** © Paradigm Publishing; **602** © iStock/Steve Cole; **605** Courtesy of MDJunction; **607** © iStock/James Anderson; **608** iStockphoto/sjlocke; **611** © iStock/Steve Cole; **613** courtesy of Lexington VA campaign; **616** Courtesy of Robert Anderson; **619** © Shutterstock/Tyler Olson; **621** iStockphoto/YinYang; **623** iStockphoto/sjlocke; **625** courtesy of SMRxT; **626** courtesy of The Verge/Valentina Palladino; **628** ©Shutterstock/Iakov Fillmonov; **630** ©Shutterstock/Evellean; **632** courtesy of the FDA; **636** courtesy of the FDA; **638** iStock/shapecharge; **641** © Shutterstock/mangostock; **643** © Shutterstock/underworld; **645** © iStockphoto/dptulk; **646** Copyright © 2013 Purdue Pharma L.P. **652** © iStockphoto/energy; **653** ©Shutterstock/diplomedia; **655** © Shutterstock/bikeriderlondon; **656** © iStockphoto/DragonImages; **657** © iStockphoto/kadmy; **658** © iStockphoto/sjlocke; **659** © iStockphoto/Christopher Futcher; **660** © IStock/asiseeit; **662** © iStockphoto/sturti; **664** © iStockphoto/sjlocke; **665** © iStockphoto/asiseeit; **668** © iStockphoto/MickyWiswedel; **669** © iStockphoto/svetikd; **671** © Pixel / Alamy Stock; **674** courtesy of HIPAA; **677** © iStockphoto/spxChrome; **683** © Shutterstock/PlusONE; **685** Courtesy of Northern York County Regional Police; **686** courtesy of the DEA; **687** Courtesy of Apothecary Products Inc; **688** courtesy of RXfitnesslady.com; **689** © iStockphoto/nano; **690** © iStockphoto/SlobodanMilljevic. **696** © Paradigm Publishing; **697** © Shutterstock/Sutichak; **699** © Shutterstock/Monkey Business Images; **702** © Paradigm Publishing; **703** © Shutterstock/B Calkins; **704** © Paradigm Publishing; **708** © Shutterstock/baranq; **714** © Shutterstock/Dean Drobot; **716** © Shutterstock/OPOLJA; **717** © Paradigm Publishing; **719** © Shutterstock/Alexander Raths; **720** © Paradigm Publishing; **721** © iStockphoto/katalinamasQ; **722** © Shutterstock/Novikov Alex; **724** © iStockphoto/Ake Ngiamsanguan; **725** Courtesy of NASH UNC Health Care; **727** © Paradigm Publishing; **728** (top) Shutterstock/Monkey Business Images (bottom) © Shutterstock/Andrey Burmakin; **729** Shutterstock/Diego Cervo; **734** © Shutterstock/Blend Images.

COLUMBIA COLLEGE CHICAGO
3 2711 00166 5458

D1567152

THE

PUBLICATIONS

OF THE

Lincoln Record Society

FOUNDED IN THE YEAR

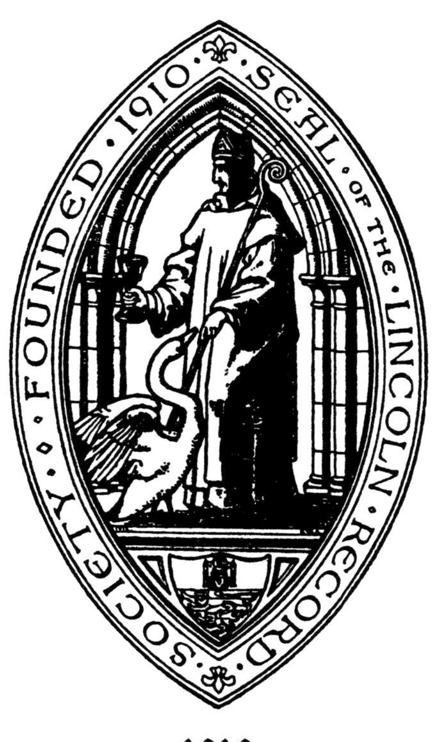

1910

VOLUME 98

ISSN 0267-2634

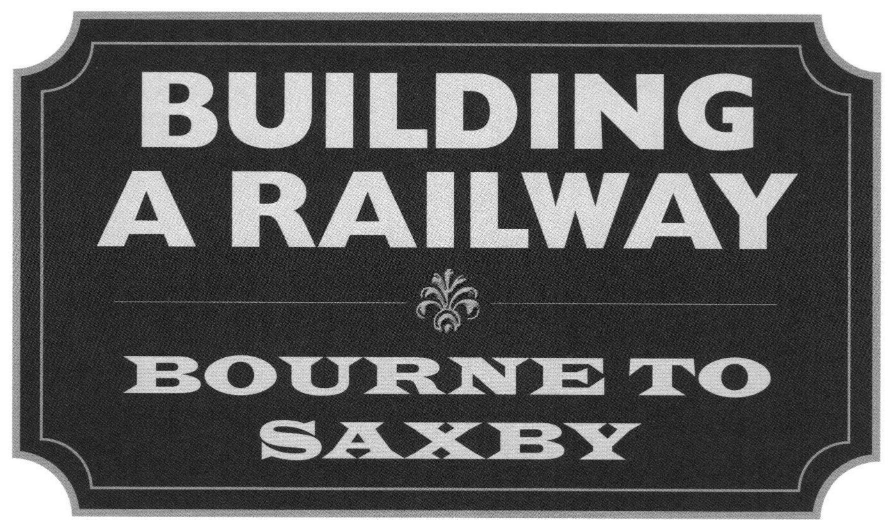

Edited by

Stewart Squires and Ken Hollamby

The Lincoln Record Society
The Society for Lincolnshire
History and Archaeology

The Boydell Press

First published 2009

A Lincoln Record Society Publication
published by The Boydell Press
an imprint of Boydell & Brewer Ltd
PO Box 9, Woodbridge, Suffolk IP12 3DF, UK
668 Mount Hope Avenue, Rochester, NY 14620, USA
website: wwww.boydellandbrewer.com

ISBN 978-0-9015038-62

A CIP catalogue record for this book is available from the British Library

Details of other Lincoln Record Society volumes are available from Boydell & Brewer Ltd

The authors and publishers are grateful to all the institutions and individuals listed for permission to reproduce the materials in which they hold copyright. Every effort has been made to trace the copyright holders; apologies are offered for any omission, and the publishers will be pleased to add any necessary acknowledgement in subsequent editions.

This publication is printed on acid-free paper

Design by Simon Loxley

Printed in Great Britain by PrintWright, Ipswich

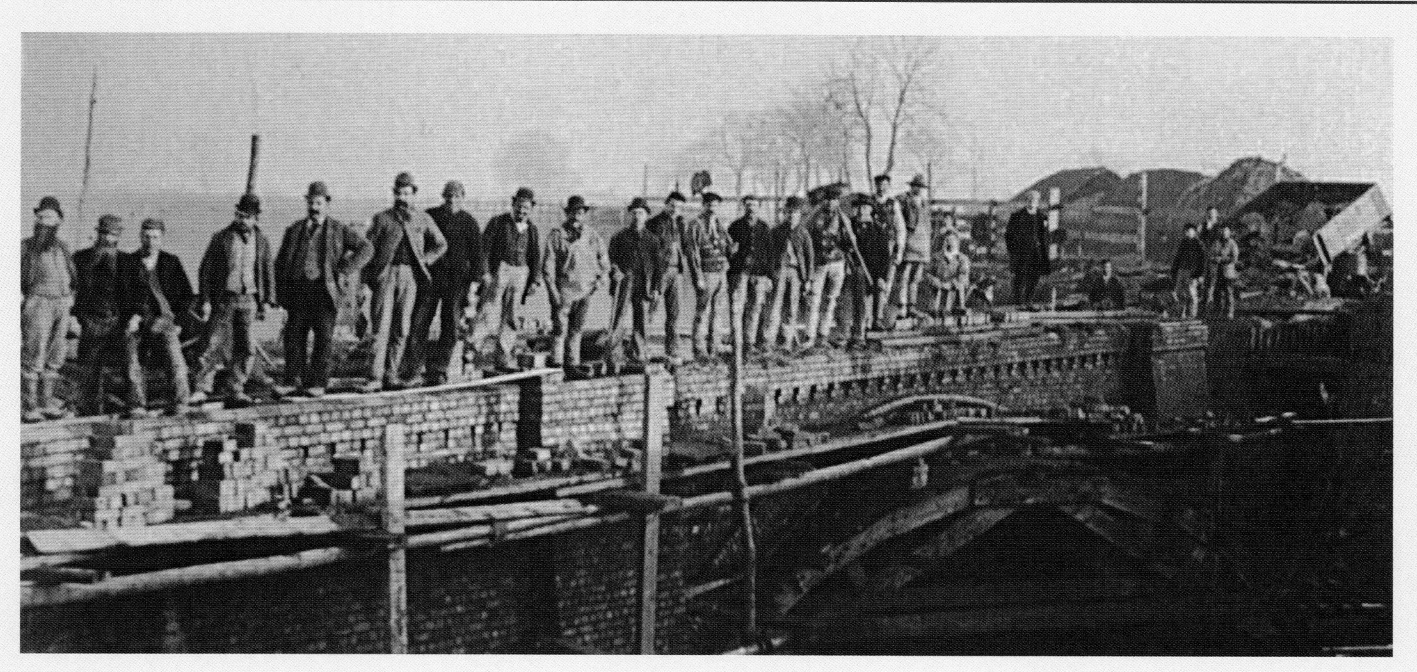

To the memory of Charles Wilson and all those unknown workers who together built the Bourne to Saxby railway.

When the last, long shift will be laboured, and the lying time will be burst,
And we go as picks or shovels, navvies or nabobs, must,
When you go up on the scrap-heap and I go down to the dust.

Will ever a one remember the times our voices rung,
When you were limber and lissome, and I was lusty and young?
Remember the jobs we've laboured, the heartful songs we've sung?

Perhaps some mortal in speaking will give us a kindly thought –
'There is a muck-pile they shifted, here is a place where they wrought,'
But maybe our straining and striving and singing will go for nought.

When you go up in the scrap-heap, and I go down to the dust –
(Little children of labour, food for the worms and the rust,)
When the last long shift will be laboured and the lying time will be burst.

Patrick MacGill, *L'Envoi – To my Pick and Shovel.*
From *Songs of a Navvy* (Windsor, 1911).

Patrick MacGill was born in Donegal in 1890. *Songs of a Navvy* was his second book.

CONTENTS

LIST OF MAPS AND DRAWINGS

Index Maps

Maps within the text

Drawings

Other illustrations

INTRODUCTION

In September 2007 the Society for Lincolnshire History and Archaeology was offered an album of photographs taken of railways being built. The images had no captions but a note on the flyleaf recorded that they had been 'taken by Charles S. Wilson on the Saxby to Bourne Railway'. Their quality was clear as was the fact that while some were on the Saxby to Bourne line others had been taken elsewhere. A little research revealed something of the life of the photographer and the Society's officers soon realised that they had been given something very special.

The interest in railway history never seems to wane. The production of railway literature continues to expand and the aspects covered reach ever further, both into detailed line and area histories as well as into the personalities involved and the effects on society and industry. What is perhaps even more surprising is that historic photographs continue to be discovered. The present book fits into this pattern of expansion: relatively little has been written about the construction of railways and the inspiration for the volume has come from the discovery of a collection of photographs illustrating just that subject.

The Liverpool and Manchester Railway is considered to be the world's first intercity railway designed from the start to carry passengers and goods hauled by steam locomotives. It opened in 1830. While the first photographs were taken by Joseph Nicéphore Nièpce in 1827, the earliest known railway photograph was not taken until 1845.[1] It was not until an easily portable camera and simple film was available in the late 1880s that the art of railway photography could flourish. By that time most of the railway network had been built and the opportunity lost to record the construction phases. The sixty-nine drawings made by J. C. Bourne of the building of the London and Birmingham line (1837–8) provide a visual record to a level never achieved before and rarely after.[2] It was Frank Sutcliffe of Whitby, recording the building of the line from Whitby to Loftus between 1875 and 1881, and S. W. A. Newton, that of the Great Central Main Line from 1894, who were the first to photograph the construction phase.[3] It was in this period that Charles Wilson did likewise and he was taking photographs at the same time as these well known pioneers. The Society, together with the Lincoln Record Society, realised that the photographs deserved to be made available to a wider audience and, with the permission of the donors, Alan and Chris Hogan (Chris being the great-granddaughter of Charles Wilson), the decision to publish was made.

The initial and, as it turned out, rather daunting task was to identify the photograph locations. A railway line, overgrown after fifty years of disuse, with some of its bridges demolished, some of its formation used for landfill and road improvements and almost all in private ownership, is not the easiest stretch of countryside to investigate. However, by concentrating on visits timed for the early months of the year before impenetrable undergrowth restricted both access and photography and with the enthusiastic support of the landowners and local historians met on the way, the work was completed. The locations or sites of fifty-seven bridges, six culverts, two occupation level crossings and the Lound Viaduct and Toft Tunnel were visited, together with some miles of trackbed in between.

Of the seventy-two photographs in the album, sixty-four were taken between Saxby and Bourne and during the construction of the new Saxby curve in the period 1889 and 1893. Of the other eight, two were of Bolton Abbey station and show works on the line between Ilkley and Skipton, in the late 1880s when the work there was almost complete. The photographs are rare in what they depict. What is even more unusual and unique is that they include photographs of the old Saxby curve when it was still in use.

It is the sixty-four Saxby-Bourne photographs that form the core of this book, with three additional photographs Wilson took to illustrate his life when he was living in the area. To these have been added 'after' photographs taken by Ken Hollamby and a narrative of the story they tell in the form of, often extended, captions added by Stewart Squires. Some of the original plans of the bridges on the line are included as these would have been used by Wilson in his work as a Resident Engineer and some extracts from the Ordnance Survey maps of the early years of the twentieth century as these show the line almost as Wilson left it. The 1891 Census Returns were also very fortuitous as these recorded the names of those working on the line, their occupations and where they were living.

Taken together these sources provide a narrow timeframe of activity all helping to put flesh on the bones of the story.

The results of the archaeological survey work undertaken will be collated and deposited with the Lincolnshire HER (Historic Environment Record). Many sites in addition to the photograph locations have been recorded and we consider that the work should be made available for anyone to access. The photograph album itself, together with an index, will be deposited with the Lincolnshire Archives.

The thanks of the Lincoln Record Society and the Society for Lincolnshire History and Archaeology are due to Alan and Chris Hogan (the owners of the photograph album), Chris being the great-granddaughter of Charles Wilson. We would also particularly mention Peter and Aileen Ball of the South Witham Archaeological Group who freely made available the results of all of their relevant local research.

The staff and records of the following have provided valuable assistance: Lincolnshire Archives; Leicestershire Archives; the National Archive at Kew, and the National Railway Museum at York. To these we should add Ian Abram, the Editor of the Midland Railway Society Newsletter; Derek Broughton, the Archivist of the Ruston Bucyrus records; Allen Civil, the Secretary of the Industrial Locomotive Society; John Clark of the British Rail Property Board; Dave Harris at the Midland Railway Study Centre at Derby; Brenda Jones of the Bourne Civic Society; Carol Morgan, Archivist at the Institution of Civil Engineers; Maureen Sibborn of the Lincolnshire Family History Society, Bourne Branch; Allan Sibley, Editor of The Great Northern Railway Society Newsletter; Andrew Watts of the Ceramic Enquiry Team, The Potteries Museum and Art Gallery, and Adrian Whittaker and John Hobden of the Midland and Great Northern Railway Circle.

In addition to this are all of those landowners, local historians and others whose enthusiasm and desire to help has supported and sustained the research and helped to make the work so rewarding to the authors. They are: Gordon Abbot and Mark Buckley of Castle Bytham; G. A. Turner and Ian and Justin Stafford of Little Bytham; Richard Holman, Henry Duffyn and Richard Lamin of the Self Store Centre, all of Saxby; George Geeson and Mick George Ltd, of South Witham; Ruth Genda, Trevor Hickman, Robert and Ben Morgan and Alan Regan and Julie Lockton, all of Wymondham.

Others who have taken an interest are John Musselwhite of Great Coates; Tony Overton of West Bridgford, Chris Squires of Dexthorpe, Tony Wall of Lincoln. Particular thanks are due to Barry Barton for his advice on civil engineering, Nicholas Bennett, our editor, John Rhodes for his earlier history of the line, Dave Watt for drawing the maps and Simon Loxley for designing the book.

We have spoken to others on our travels but without making a record of their names. For that we apologise but we are still grateful for your help.

For those who may wish to follow in our footsteps it must be noted that the land is now all in private ownership and the permission of the landowner should always be sought before any exploration. However, the line is crossed in many places by both roads and public footpaths, clearly shown on present day Ordnance Survey maps, and is readily accessible with their use.

Finally, the year 2009 marks the fiftieth anniversary of the closure of the Midland and Great Northern Joint Railway and its Midland Railway extension from Little Bytham to Saxby. On 28 February 1959 the last passenger trains ran between Saxby and Peterborough in the west to Cromer, Norwich and Great Yarmouth in the east. Trains disappeared from almost 200 miles of track, apart from the use of some short sections for freight which lasted a little longer.[4] The 1950s had seen a number of branch line closures but for the first time a complete network was closed, sending shockwaves through the nation and a portent of what was to come under Beeching. It does seem apt, therefore, to mark this with a look back to the days when one of the last parts of the network was completed and to the time when the Midland and Great Northern Joint Railway was created, in 1893.

1 Robert Pols, *Dating Old Photographs*, 2nd edn (Birmingham, 1995); Jack Simmons, *The Victorian Railway*, new edn (London, 1995), 148.

2 Simmons, *The Victorian Railway*; Marilyn Palmer and Peter Neaverson, *Industry in the Landscape 1700–1900* (London, 1994), 162.

3 Simmons, *The Victorian Railway*, 150-151.

4 John Rhodes, *Bourne to Saxby* (Boston, 1989), 42-43 (see Appendix C); Stewart E. Squires, *The Lost Railways of Lincolnshire* (Ware, 1988), 105-108, 120.

CHARLES STANSFIELD WILSON

1844–1893

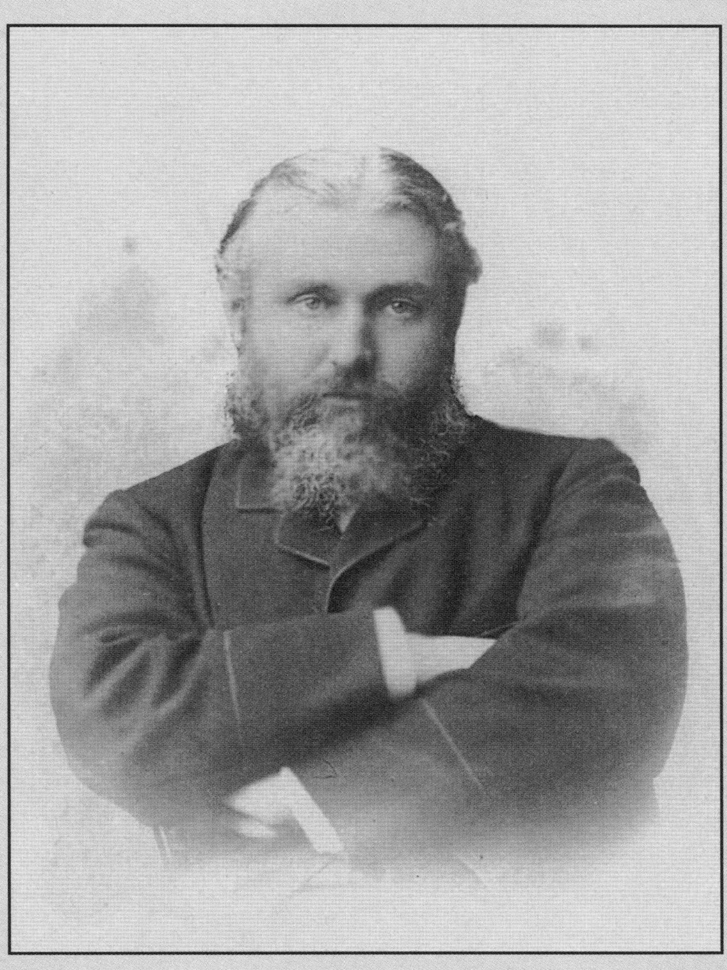

Charles Stansfield Wilson, a studio portrait taken in Ilkley, c.1886

Charles Stansfield Wilson came from a middle class Victorian family. He was born in Bradford on 16 April 1844, the only son and eldest child of Thomas Wilson, a chemist, and Mary Wilson, née Stansfield. In 1848 the family moved to 'Throstle Nest' in Thornton in Craven, in Yorkshire, where he was recorded in the 1851 Census.

Charles was a descendant of a renowned Yorkshire Quaker family and he attended Bootham, a Quaker Boarding School in York, where he was residing at the time of the 1861 Census. There is no record of him again until the 1871 Census, when he is recorded as lodging at Broom House in Mansfield, a hotel owned by the Midland Railway. His occupation is given as a Civil Engineer. The Mansfield and Southwell Railway opened in April 1871 and it is likely that he was involved with the construction of this. The Engineer to the line, John Baylis, is said to have instructed that a set of photographs of this line were to be taken. This was done, in November 1871, by A. W. Cox of Nottingham, and an album of 25 photographs was presented to Mr and Mrs White, the proprietors of the Swan Hotel in Mansfield, 'in testimony of their great kindness and attention to him (John Baylis), during the construction of the Mansfield and Southwell Railway'.[1] Another civil engineer also lodging at Broom House in 1871 was John Argyle, recorded in the Census as 'John Argile', who went on to become the Midland Railway North Division Engineer from 1891 to 1906.

In 1874 Wilson married his cousin, Hannah Wilson, and they moved into their first home, at Baildon, near Shipley in Yorkshire, where he was employed on the construction of the railway line between Shipley and Guisley. Work started on this in 1872 and it opened on 4 December 1876. In May and June 1875 a notebook was compiled by G. Anderson of Nottingham, probably as part of a submission for a professional engineering qualification. This records his involvement with 'the construction of a double line of railway from Shipley forming a junction with the Guisley line' under Mr Wilson CE, Engineer's Office, Baildon, Shipley.[2] It was while the family were living in Baildon that their first child, Edith, was born, on 22 September 1876.

Where he worked immediately after this is not known but in 1878 the family moved south to the Bedfordshire village of Sharnbrook. From the late 1870s the Midland Railway was progressively quadrupling the Midland Main Line south of Kettering.[3] The most important of these works was the Wymington Deviation, a new route to the east of the earlier, and involving the construction of the Sharnbrook Tunnel, 1860 yards in length. This line opened on 4 May 1884. The 1881 Census recorded Wilson as living at Havelock Villa in Sharnbrook. While living here four children were born, Gertrude on 3 September 1878; Thornton on 12 March 1880; Ernest on 7 October 1881; and Mary on 24 December 1882.

In 1883 the family moved back north for Wilson to work on the construction of the Skipton to Ilkley Railway. It was here that we know he was able to develop an interest in photography, as some of the photographs in the album are of this line. He was living in Ilkley when his fourth child, Ernest, died just before his seventh birthday, on 7 July 1886, and his fifth and last child, Reginald, was born on 14 September 1888. The Skipton to Ilkley Railway opened in 1888.

In 1889 the family relocated to Wymondham and moved into The Cottage. The Chief Engineer for the Bourne to Saxby line was J. A. McDonald, the Engineer to the Midland Railway, and his assistants on site were C. S. Wilson, G. C. McDonald and Richard M. Parkinson.[4] As Wilson was living at Wymondham this could account for the proliferation of photographs at the western end.

John Allen McDonald joined the Midland Railway as an Engineer in 1872 and was appointed to the post of Chief Engineer in July 1890.[5] George Champion McDonald was his brother. George McDonald's application for Associate membership of the Institution of Civil Engineers records that he 'was a pupil of Charles S. Wilson, the Resident Engineer on the construction of the Skipton and Ilkley branch of the Midland Railway'. There are no letters after Wilson's name to suggest he was a member of the ICE and he did not second McDonald's application. He would have had to have been a member of the ICE to do this.[6] The application was proposed by his brother John Allen McDonald. There is no record that Wilson was a member or ever applied for membership of the Institute.

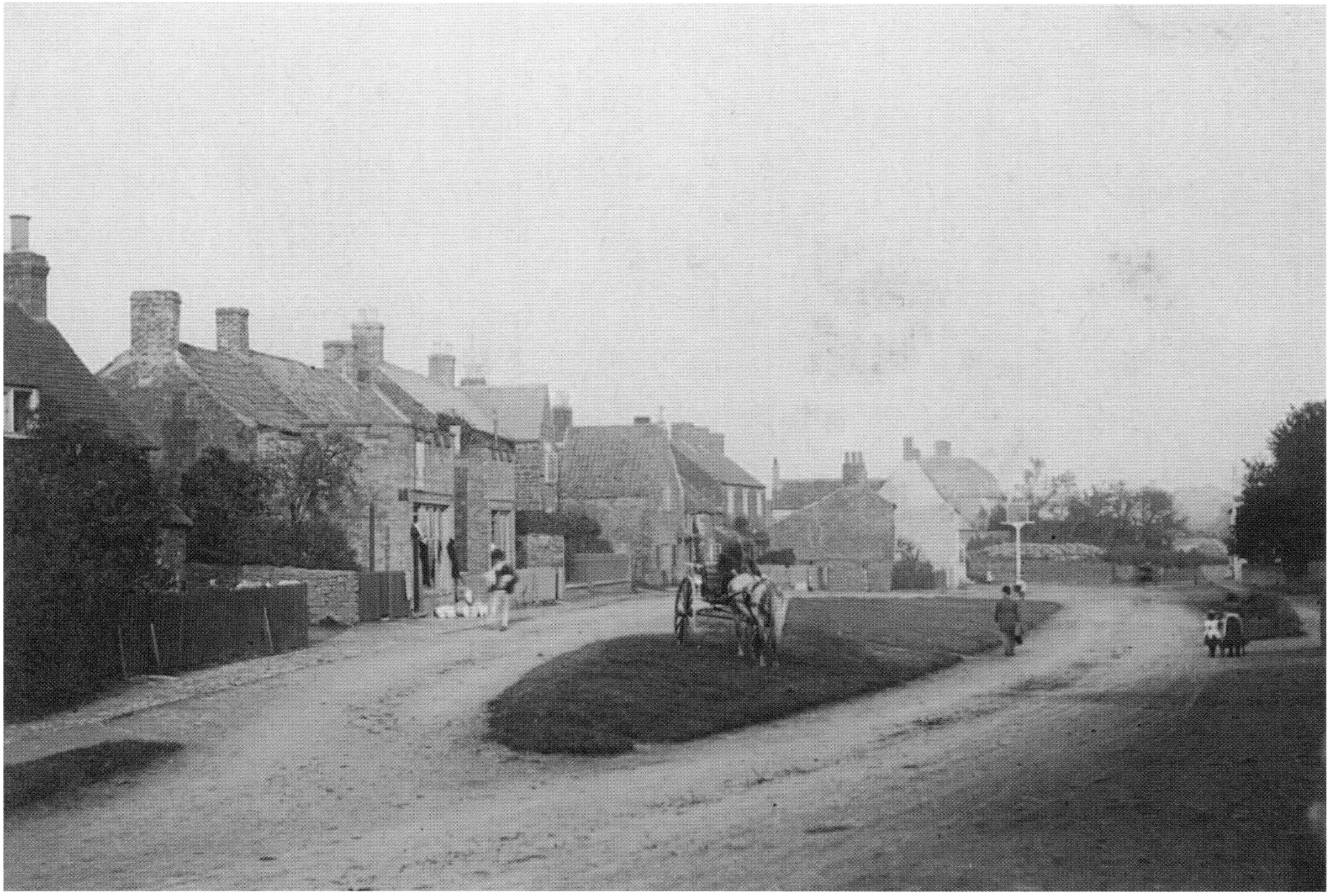

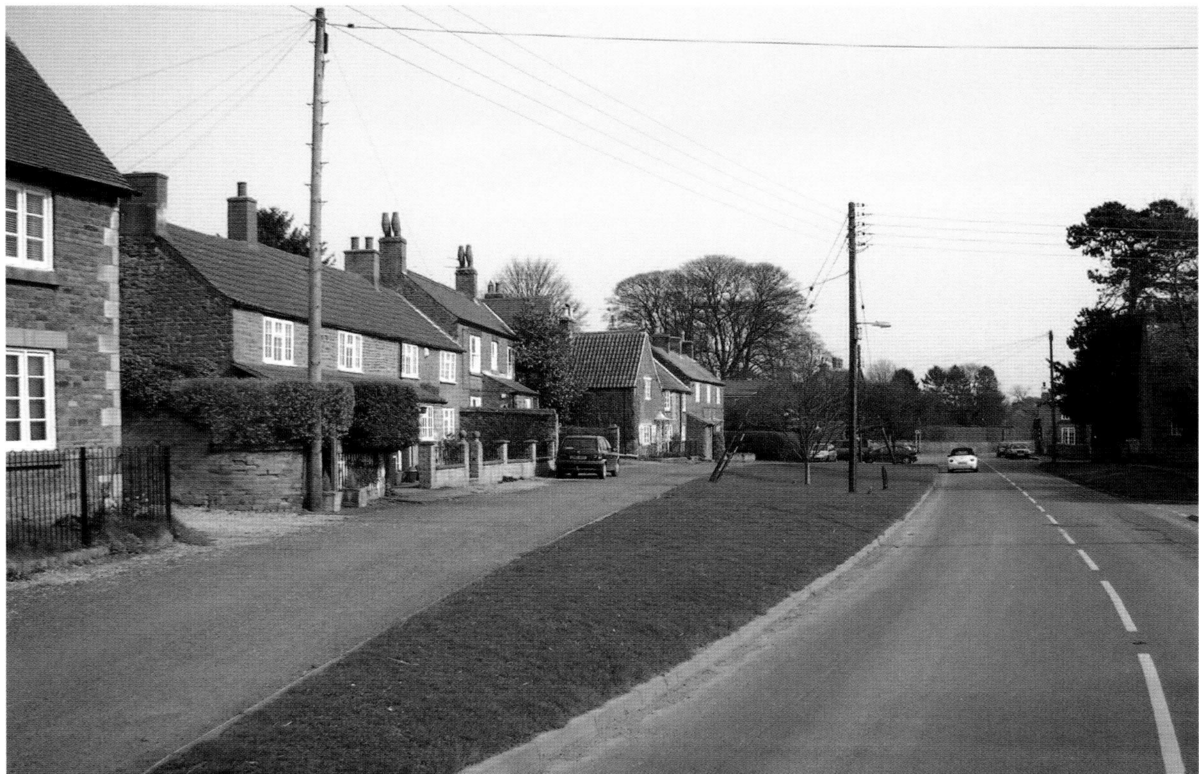

Above: The village green at Wymondham. The Wilson family home, The Cottage, is the house in the centre of the picture, with railings, between the pony and trap to the right and the shop to the left.

Left: The same view in 2009.

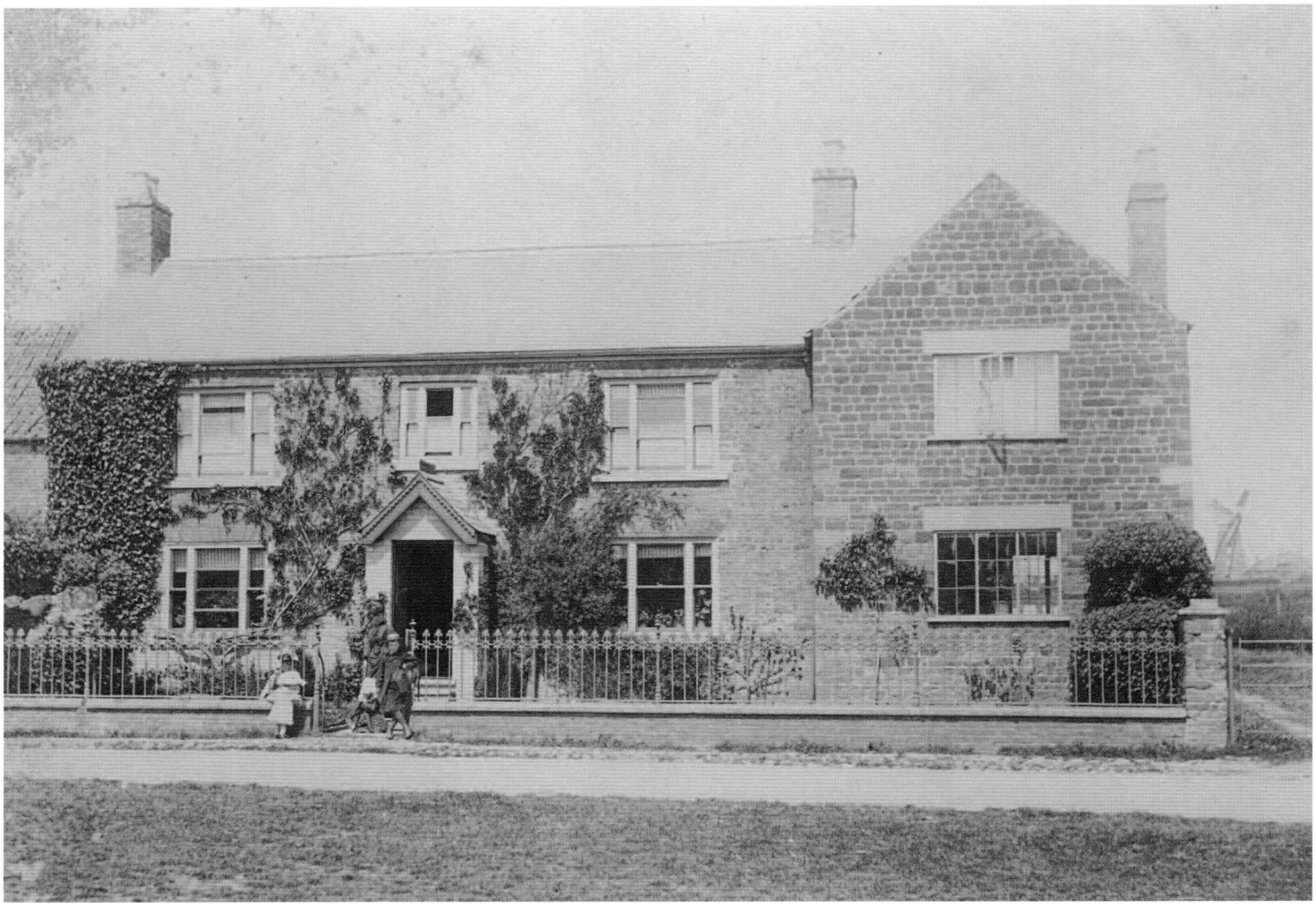

Above: The Cottage, Wymondham. Outside the front door, from the right, the people are believed to be Thornton, the eldest son, born 1880; Miss Jones, the Governess; Reginald, known as Rex, the youngest son, born 1888 and, behind him, crouching down behind the railings, Hannah Wilson, wife of Charles.

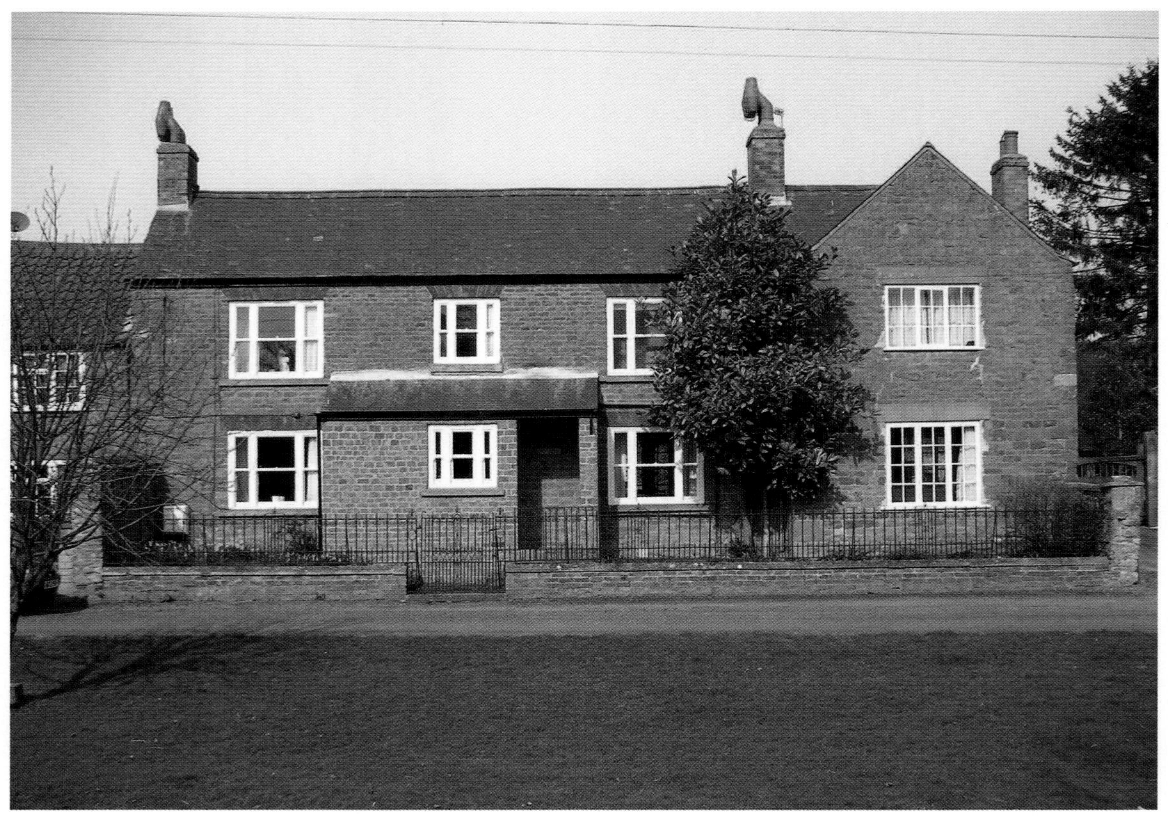

Right: The Cottage, Wymondham, in 2009.

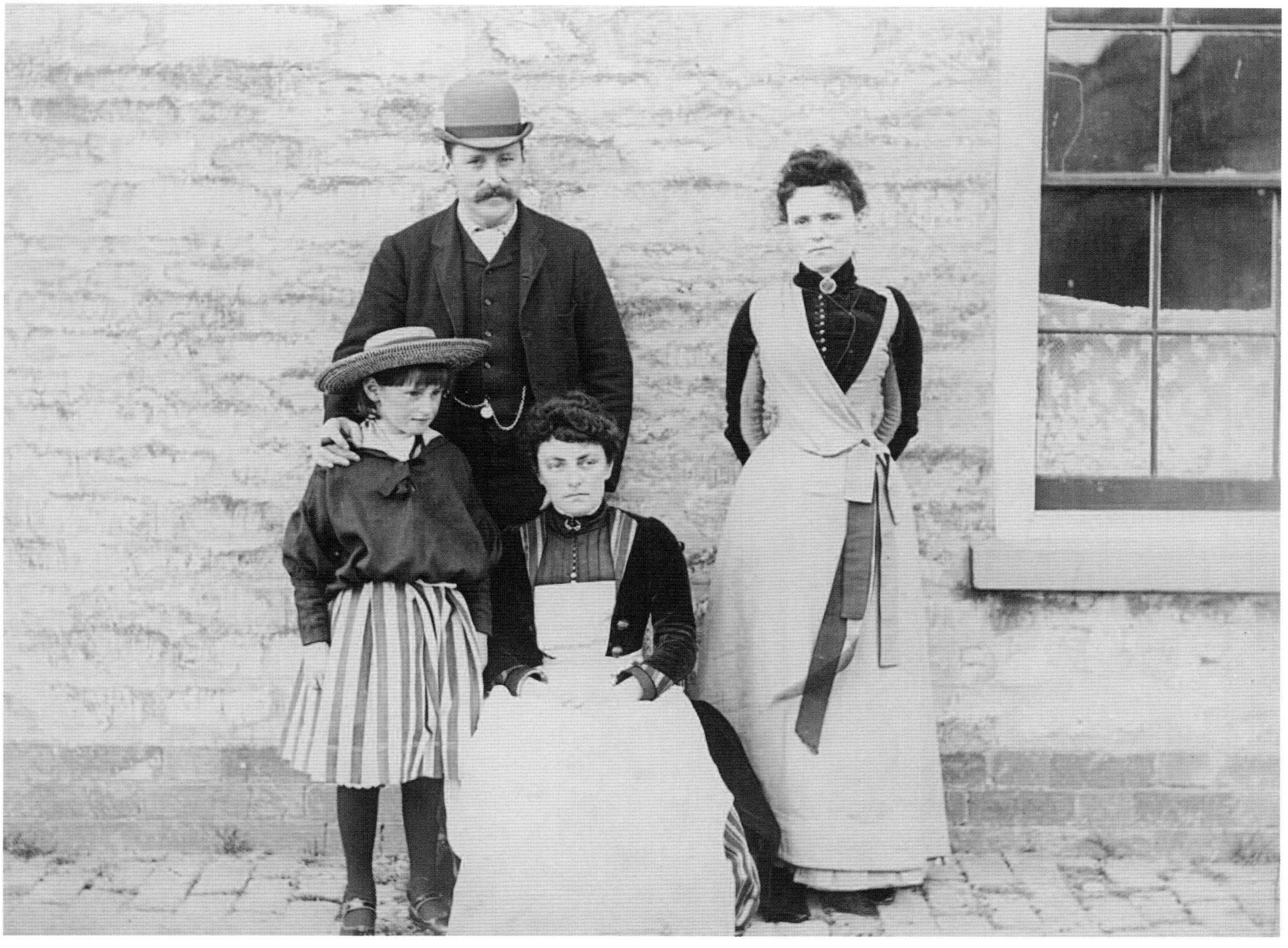

Photograph taken by Charles Wilson and endorsed on the back by a member of the family as 'Enid, Mr and Mrs Noel and Mr N's sister, one of fathers Charles S. Wilson's contractors at S Witham'. The 1891 Census records Herbert E. Nowell and his wife, Alice M. Nowell, living as lodgers at 16 High Street, South Witham. He gave his occupation as a Railway Constructor, from Manchester. The other occupants of the house at that time were the Dunmore family, the father and two sons, all of whom worked as agricultural labourers, with his wife Mary and schoolgirl daughter Minnie.

The 1891 Census recorded that on the night of 5 April Charles, with his wife Hannah and son Thornton, were at the Hydropathic establishment at Matlock in Derbyshire, presumably on holiday and taking the waters. In late 1892 or early 1893 the Wilson family moved on to Millhouses, for the widening of the Midland Main Line south of Sheffield. Following a short illness, however, Charles died of pneumonia on 6 December 1893 at Ingleborough Lodge, Millhouses, aged 49, leaving a widow and five children. He was buried at the Quaker Meeting House at Lothersdale, West Yorkshire.

Charles was a Civil Engineer by profession, even though he did not apply for membership of the Institute of Civil Engineers. Clearly, he was highly regarded for his skills. He was employed by the Midland Railway as a Civil Engineer and the Chief Engineer, John McDonald, was happy for his brother George to train under him.

Charles was working as a Resident Engineer. This was an important role in the construction process and still remains so today. Wilson was responsible for ensuring that the contracts were completed on time and to budget. He lived near to the work and was the first point of contact for the contractor with the Midland Railway. He would attempt to resolve the many problems that inevitably arose during the progress of the works and, if he could not, would ensure that they were referred on to one of his colleagues who could. He had an intimate knowledge of the works under his authority and had considerable responsibility delegated to him.

He would come to know the contractors and their managers very well, probably meeting men on one contract whom he had met on earlier ones. So, for example, W. T. Mousley was the contractor for the Skipton to Ilkley railway when Charles Wilson was Resident Engineer, and was responsible for one of the Bourne to Saxby contracts. He clearly became friendly enough with Herbert Nowell, the manager for the contractor J. D. Nowell, who was living in South Witham, to take a family photograph (see page 17).

Photography was developed in the late 1820s and the 1830s and it is believed that the earliest known railway photograph was taken in Linlithgow, probably in 1845.[7] However, cameras were cumbersome and the development of the exposures complicated, certainly until George Eastman invented a paper backed roll film in 1885 and, in 1889, a box camera to use it in, under the Kodak name.[8] In 1890 he produced the film in rolls giving 12 or 24 prints and, for the first time, photography was truly portable and available to all.

Charles Wilson, therefore, must have been an early amateur photographer as we understand the term today. He may have been influenced by his father's background as early photographers had to have skills in chemistry. He may have been influenced by the photographs taken of the Mansfield to Southwell railway when he was a young engineer in 1871. Or his interest could have been sparked by the Midland Railway's appointment of its first official photographer in 1882. He clearly had a camera by about 1888 but of what type is not known.

Every railway construction contract had its Resident Engineer. Wilson was one of many men who made that vital contribution to the development of the national network. What makes him special is his amateur interest in photography and its application to his everyday work at such an early date. His legacy is the photographs in this book and the story they tell. The irony is that the work he started in about 1888 was cut short by his untimely death in 1893.

Finally, it is interesting to note that the subsequent history of the railway lines Charles Wilson was involved with reflects that of the national network. Some are still open, the Midland Main Line and Shipley to Guisely. Others, Mansfield to Southwell and Saxby to Bourne, have closed. The line from Ilkley to Skipton was closed, but part has been revived as the Embsay and Bolton Abbey Steam Railway.

1 Mansfield Library, L.38.5COX.

2 Midland Railway Study Centre, RFBMCT 13316-1875.

3 Robin Leleux, *A Regional History of the Railways of Great Britain. Volume 9: The East Midlands*, 2nd rev. edn (Newton Abbot, 1984).

4 Ronald H. Clark, *A Short History of the Midland and Great Northern Joint Railway* (Norwich, 1967).

5 Clement E. Stretton, *The History of the Midland Railway* (London, 1901).

6 Correspondence with the Institution of Civil Engineers, June 2008.

7 Jack Simmons, *The Victorian Railway* (London, 1995), 148-151.

8 Robert Pols, *Dating Old Photographs*, 2nd edn (Birmingham, 1995).

THE PHOTOGRAPHS

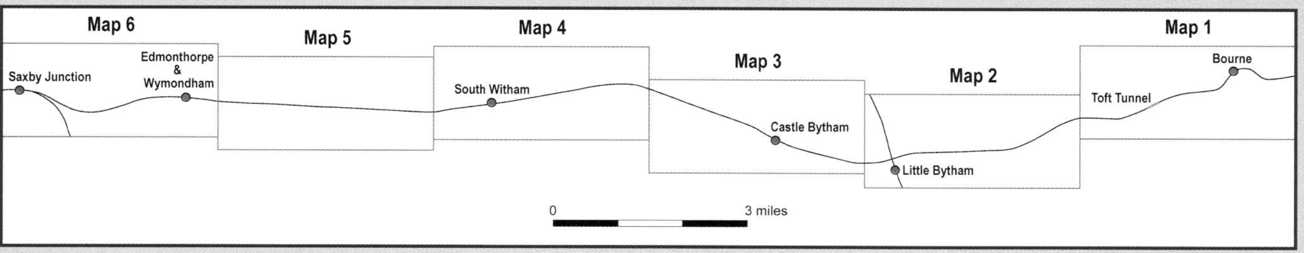

The photographs are described geographically, starting from the Bourne end and working to the west. They end with those of the new Saxby curve and Saxby Station.

The Bridge Numbers used in the text are those used by the railway companies. On the Saxby to Bourne line they are the same today as originally allocated by, to the west, the Midland Railway and to the east, the Midland and Great Northern Railway (M&GN). The British Rail Property Board remains responsible for some of the bridges and identifies them using the same system. These numbers can be seen on some of the bridges to this day. Because of the two ownerships the numbers do not run through in sequence. The Midland Railway bridges start with 1 at Saxby up to 45 at Little Bytham. By contrast the numbering on the Midland and Great Northern Railway starts with 233 at Bourne through to 245 at Little Bytham. Bridge numbering on the M&GN was complicated by the number of companies that came together to eventually combine as the M&GN, the variety of different building dates of the individual sections, and the number of different sections of line.

The line was built at right angles to the grain of the land. The landscape between Bourne and the ancient trackway, The Drift, is that of the Kesteven Uplands and from there to Saxby, the Leicestershire Wolds. Both are cut by a series of river valleys, all flowing generally north to south. From the east to the west these are the East Glen River at Lound Viaduct, West Glen River at Little Bytham, Glen Brook, Castle Bytham, the infant River Witham at South Witham, Wymondham Water at Wymondham and the River Eye at Saxby. This resulted in a succession of embankments and cuttings under and over which it was relatively easy to construct culverts and bridges. In the tradition of railway building, structures were solidly built and built to last. The irony here is that the line only operated in full for sixty-six years, with part of it lingering on for another sixteen. Many of these structures remain as strong today as when they were built.

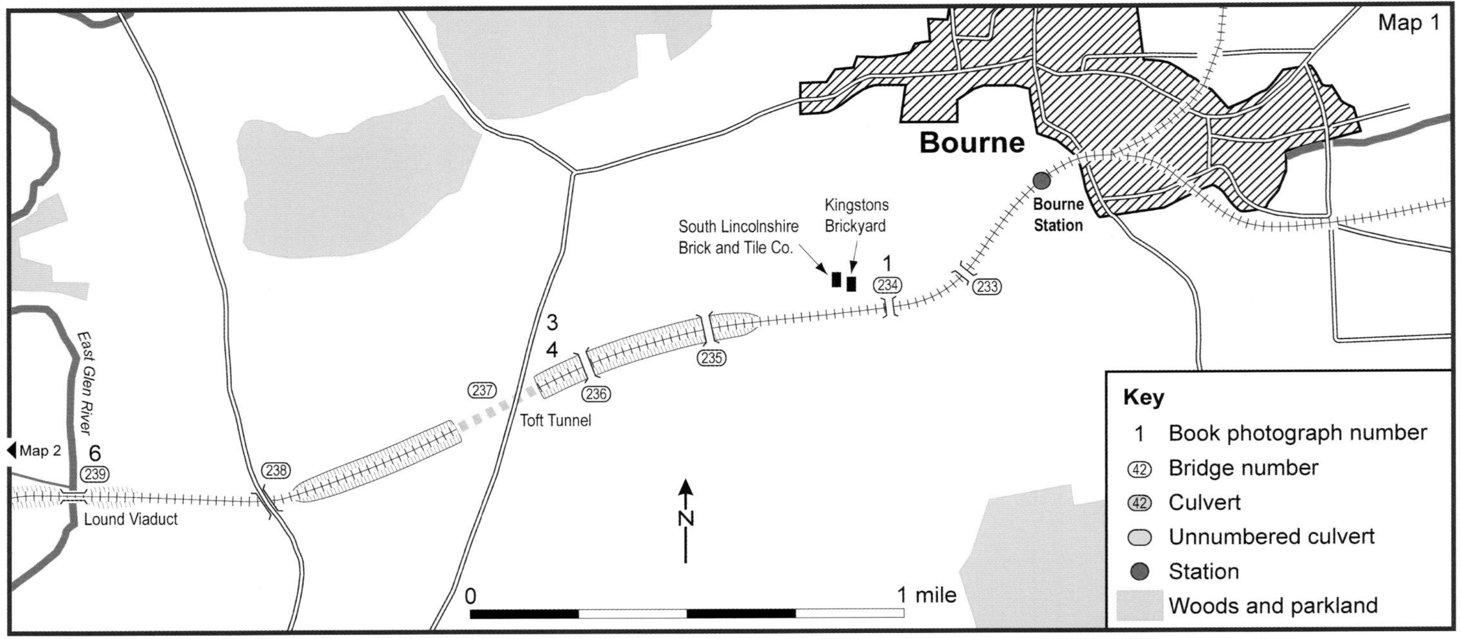
Map 1
Bourne
Bourne Station
Kingstons Brickyard
South Lincolnshire Brick and Tile Co.
1
234
233
235
236
237
3
4
Toft Tunnel
East Glen River
Map 2
6
239
238
Lound Viaduct
N
0
1 mile
Key
1 Book photograph number
42 Bridge number
42 Culvert
Unnumbered culvert
Station
Woods and parkland

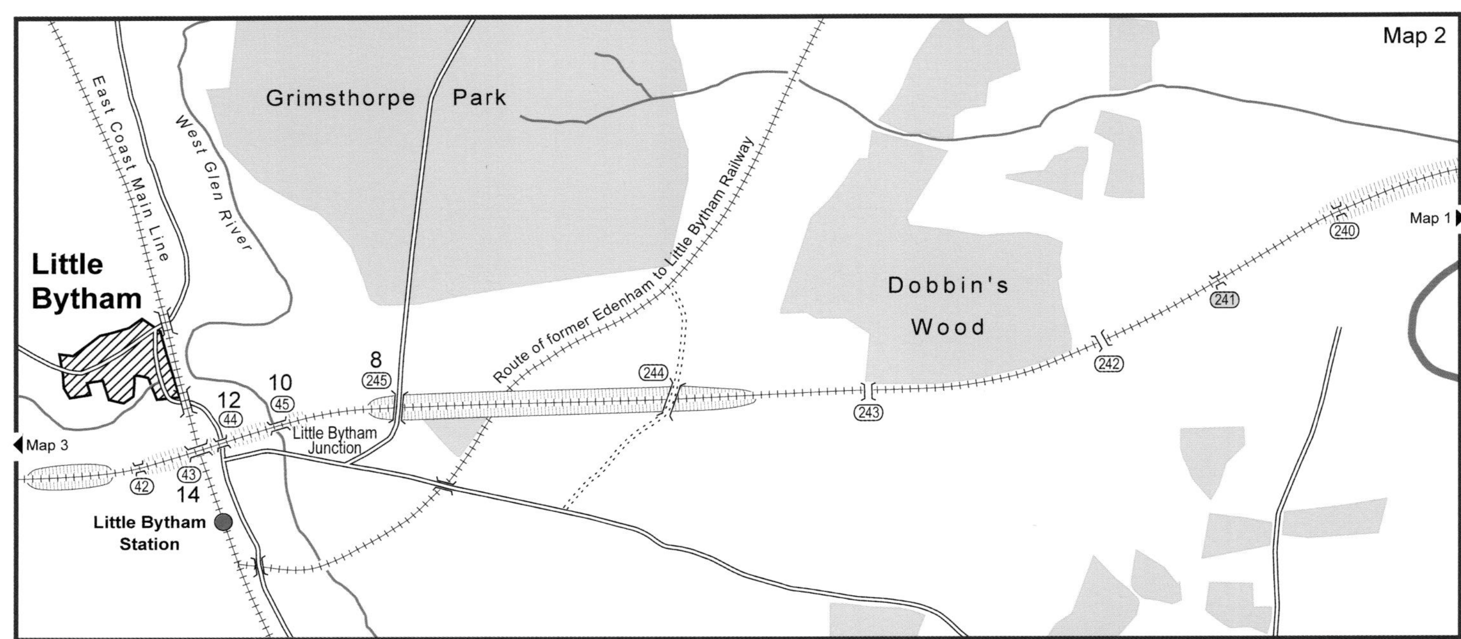
Map 2
Grimsthorpe Park
East Coast Main Line
West Glen River
Little Bytham
Route of former Edenham to Little Bytham Railway
Dobbin's Wood
Map 1
240
241
242
243
244
8
245
10
45
12
44
Little Bytham Junction
Map 3
42
43
14
Little Bytham Station

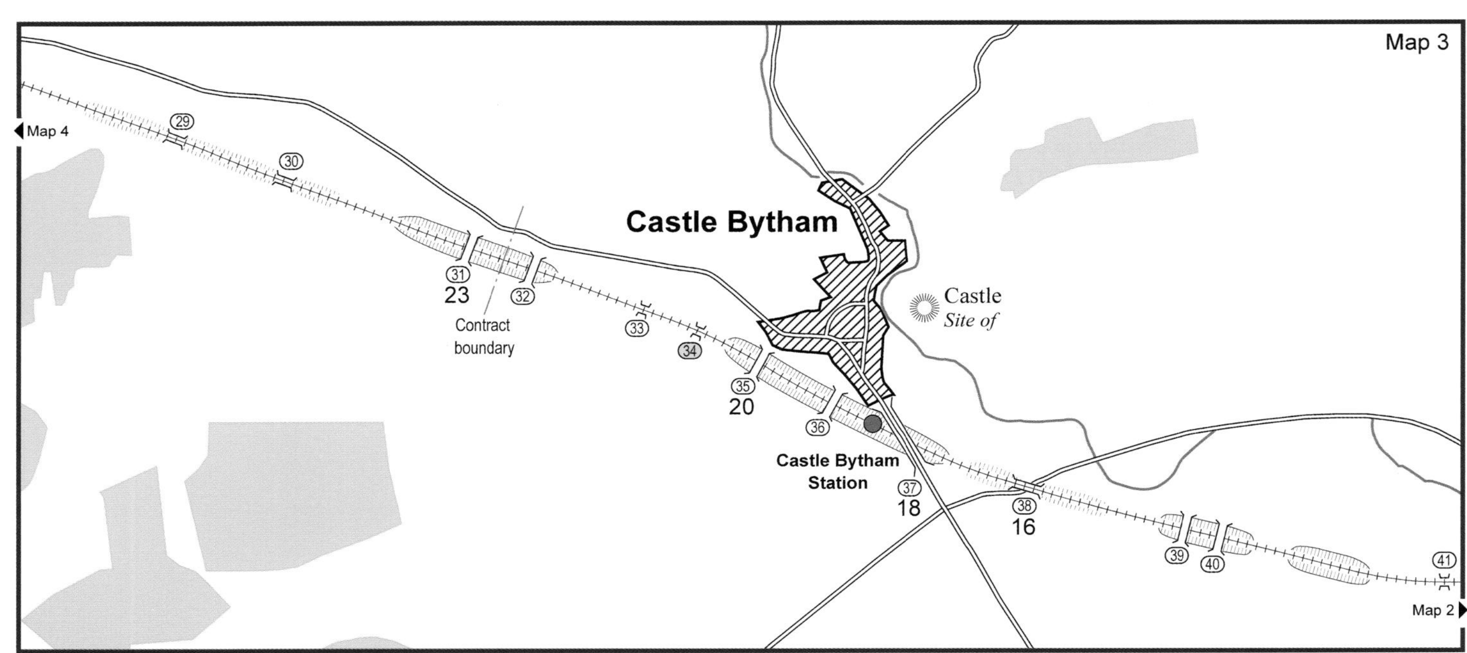
Map 3
Map 4
29
30
Castle Bytham
Castle
Site of
31
23
32
Contract boundary
33
34
35
20
36
Castle Bytham Station
37
18
38
16
39
40
41
Map 2

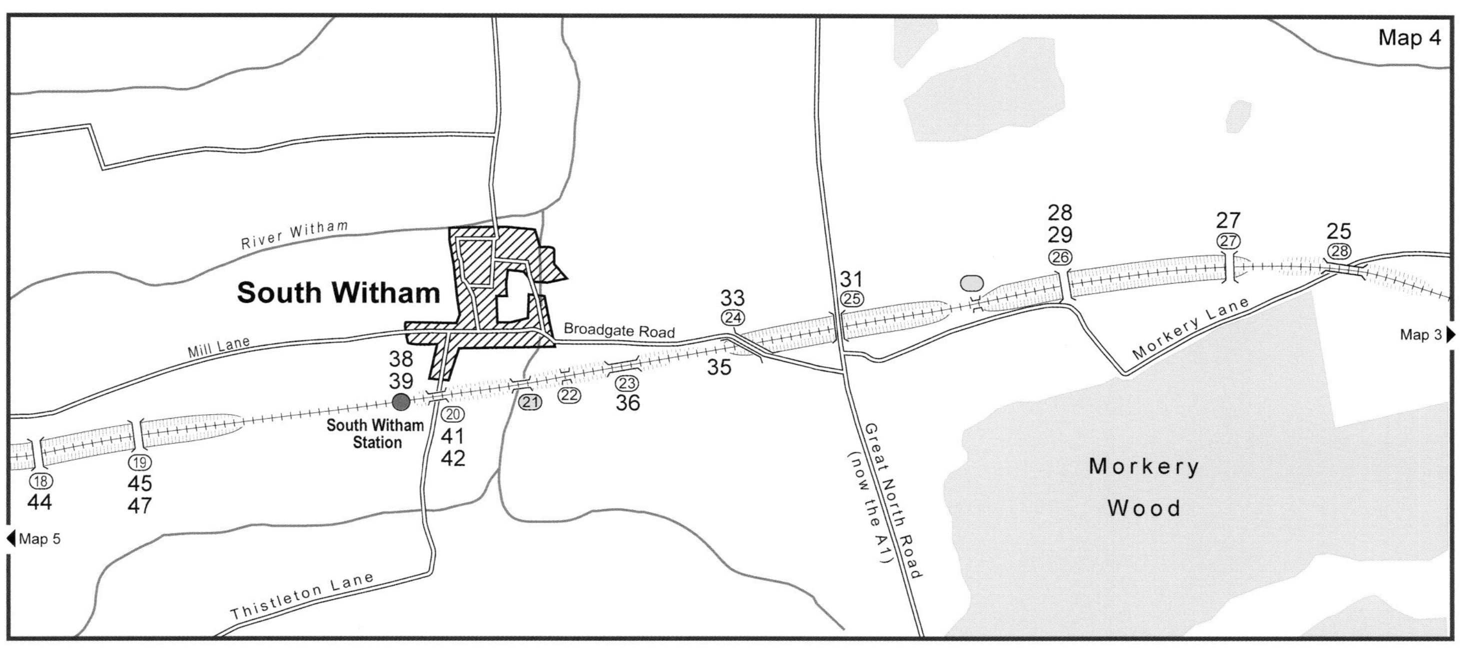
Map 4
River Witham
South Witham
Mill Lane
Broadgate Road
South Witham Station
Morkery Lane
Great North Road (now the A1)
Morkery Wood
Thistleton Lane
Map 3
Map 5

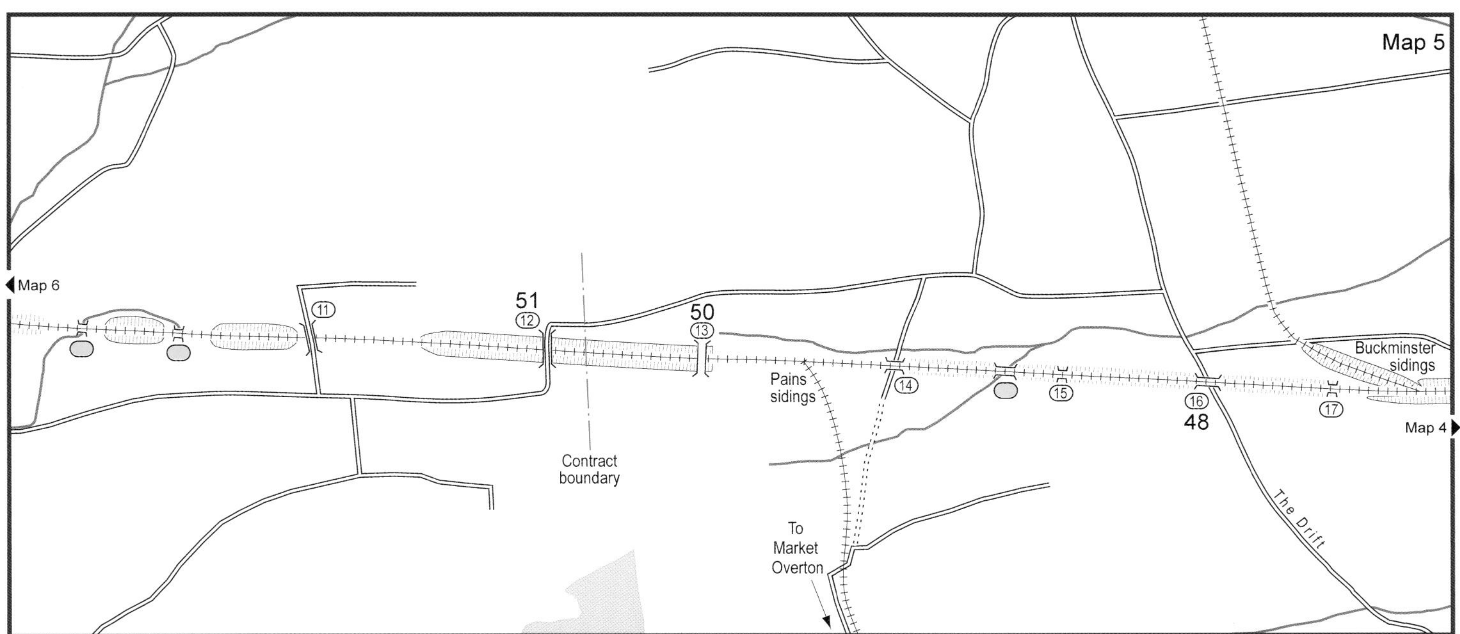
Map 5
Map 6
Map 4
Pains sidings
Contract boundary
To Market Overton
Buckminster sidings
The Drift

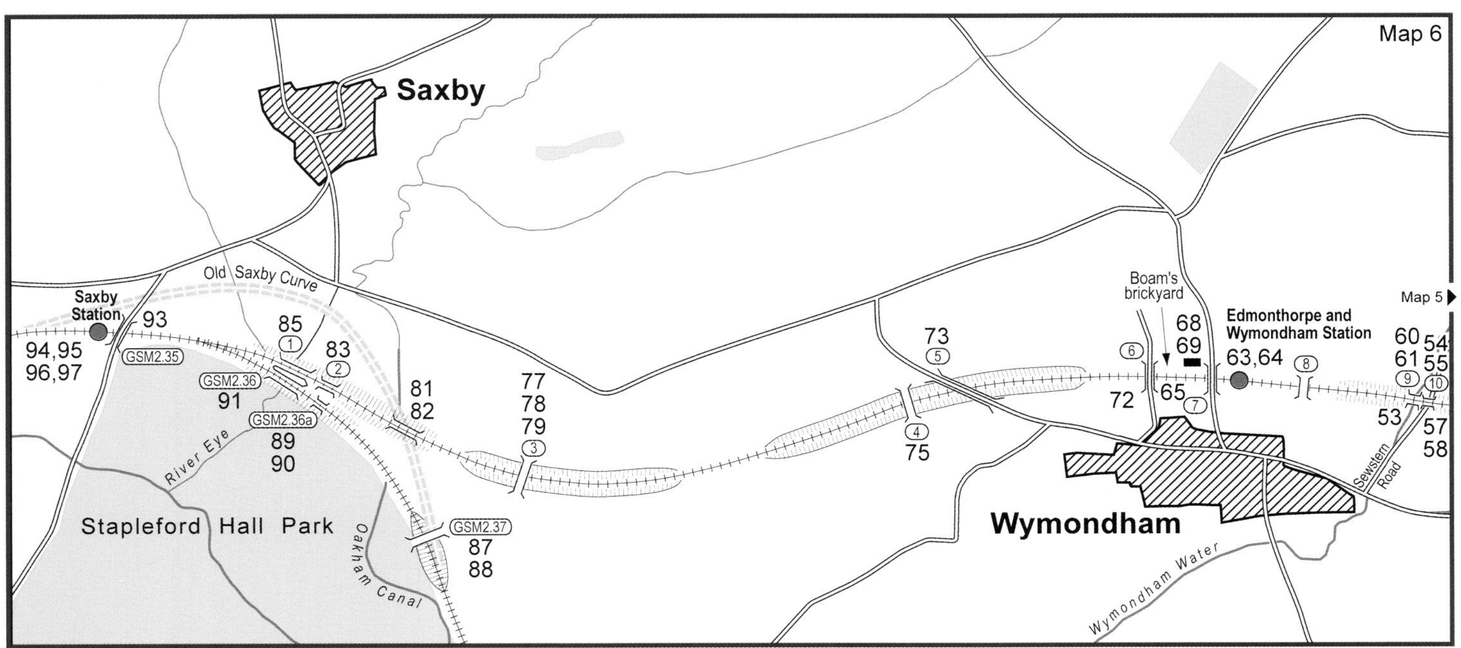
Map 6
Saxby
Saxby Station
Old Saxby Curve
River Eye
Stapleford Hall Park
Oakham Canal
Boam's brickyard
Edmonthorpe and Wymondham Station
Wymondham
Wymondham Water
Sewstern Road
Map 5

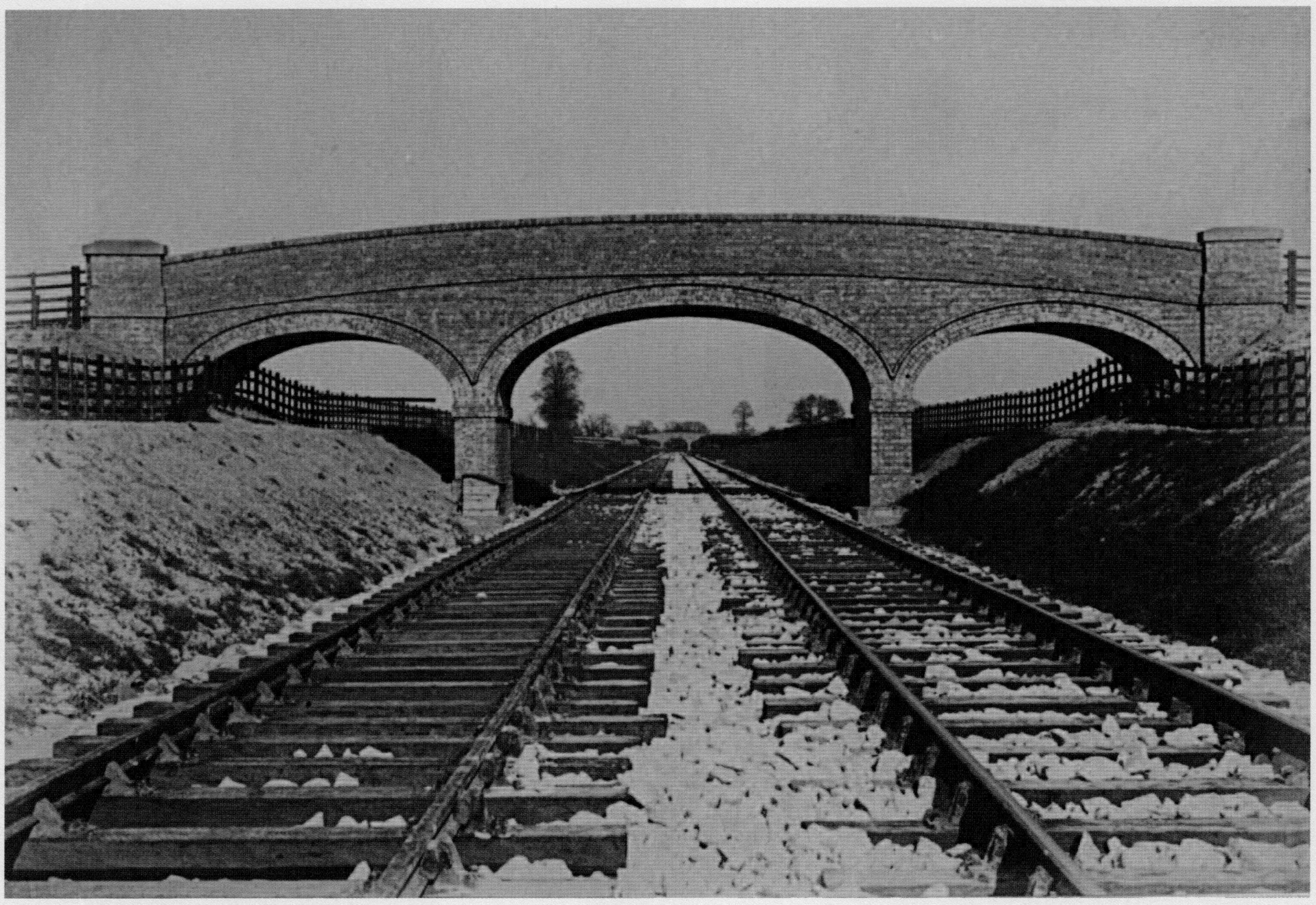

NEAR KINGSTON'S BRIDGE SIDING, BOURNE

PHOTOGRAPH 1

This is the most easterly photograph in the collection and shows Bridge 234 and, in the far distance to the west, Bridge 235. Bridge 234 was only one third of a mile west of the station platform at Bourne. Both of them were occupation bridges and both had substantial earth ramps on either side. From here to Little Bytham the line was built as double track and was to become part of the Midland and Great Northern Railway. It was the first of a series of eight bridges over the line, six of them occupation bridges, with this graceful form of three elliptical arches.

The number of the bridges and the fact that there were no level crossings for public roads is an indication of the expense involved in the construction works. The railway companies clearly did not want the additional expense of the manning costs associated with public level crossings. Level crossings were referred to in the *Grantham Journal* at the time the line was opened[1] and in the tender documents.[2] Those that were provided were farm occupation crossings only. Evidence of two such occupation crossings has been found in the area between South Witham and Wymondham; these and the locations of three others are known from Midland Railway plans of the early twentieth century.[3]

The contract for this section of line between Bourne and Bridge 36 at Castle Bytham was awarded to Messrs W.T. Mousley at a contract price of £84,011.[4] They also had the contracts for the building at the same time of the new station at Bourne and the Spalding Avoiding Line.

In the photograph the rails of the permanent way have been laid but the ballasting has yet to be completed. The stone size used is large, especially when compared with that on the main line at Little Bytham, seen in Photograph 14. According to the specification for the works, the contractor was authorised to run his own trains over the permanent track once it was 'properly laid to assist him in completing the ballasting of the line and for no other purpose'.[5] The permanent way is so called because the earlier track, laid to facilitate the construction of the line, was only temporary.

Two brickworks were established to the right of the line here (see Map 1). Henry Kingston's brickyard had opened in the 1880s and business was enhanced by the need to provide bricks for the line. These were taken by a temporary contractor's line to where they were required.

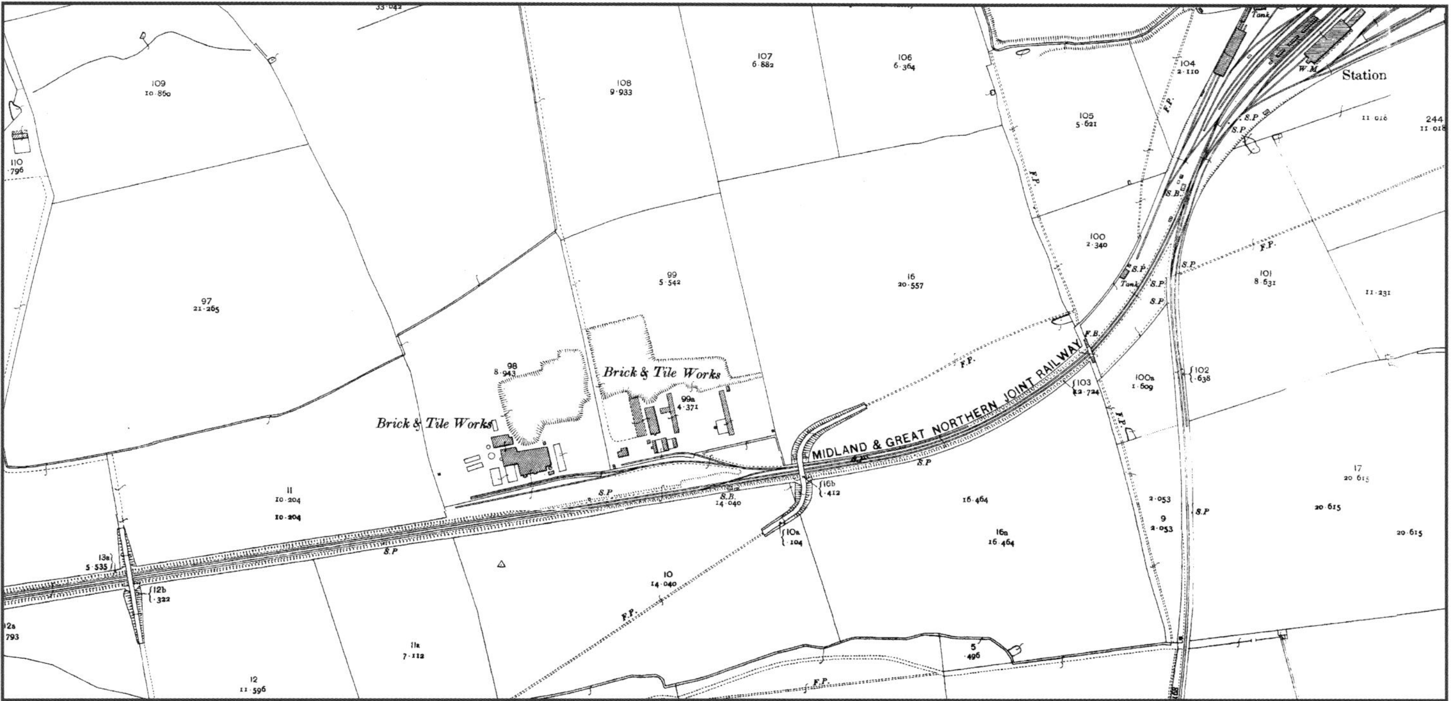

A single siding was laid into the brickyard from the completed line in April 1894.

In 1898 the South Lincolnshire Brick and Tile Company built their brickworks alongside Kingston's.[6] Because of the increased number of sidings a headshunt (that is, a siding which could be used by the engine as it drew loaded wagons out of the sidings and placed empties in them without having to enter the main running lines) had to be provided. This was laid alongside the line and it passed through the right-hand arch of the bridge. A signal box to control the entry to the sidings was built to the left of the line on the far side of the bridge. The headshunt siding was also used by the Midland and Great Northern Railway as a 'lie by'[7] for goods trains. This was a way of increasing line capacity. A slow goods train could reverse into the siding to enable faster trains to pass by without delay to their timetable. The siding was later to be extended to the east to create a refuge siding.

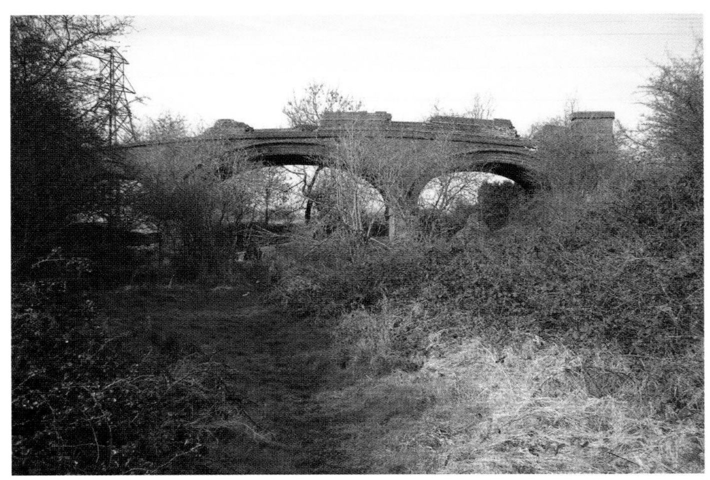

Photograph 2

MAP 1

OS 1/2500 County Series Map, 1904.
Kingston's Siding.

This shows the two Bourne brickworks. Bridge 234 with its very distinctive curved ramps appears just to the left of the M of Midland.

On the north side of the line and passing under the bridge is the siding serving the two brickworks. That to the right was Kingston's which by 1898 had become the Bourne Brick and Tile Company. That on the left was The South Lincolnshire Brick and Tile Company. The latter was bankrupt and sold in 1907.

The letters S.B. identify the location of the Signal Box, known as Kingston's Siding Box. Bridge 235 can be seen on the extreme left.

PHOTOGRAPH 2

Today Bridge 234 is in a poor state of repair. The earth ramps have been removed and bulldozed into the cutting underneath. The bridge is likely to be demolished when this area is redeveloped.

1 *Grantham Journal* (17 June 1893), p. 6, col. 3.
2 National Archives, RAIL 491/548.
3 Midland Railway Study Centre, Item No 00806.
4 John Wrottesley, *The Great Northern Railway, II: Expansion and Competition* (London, 1979).
5 National Archives, RAIL 491/548.
6 National Archives, RAIL 783/352.
7 Ibid.

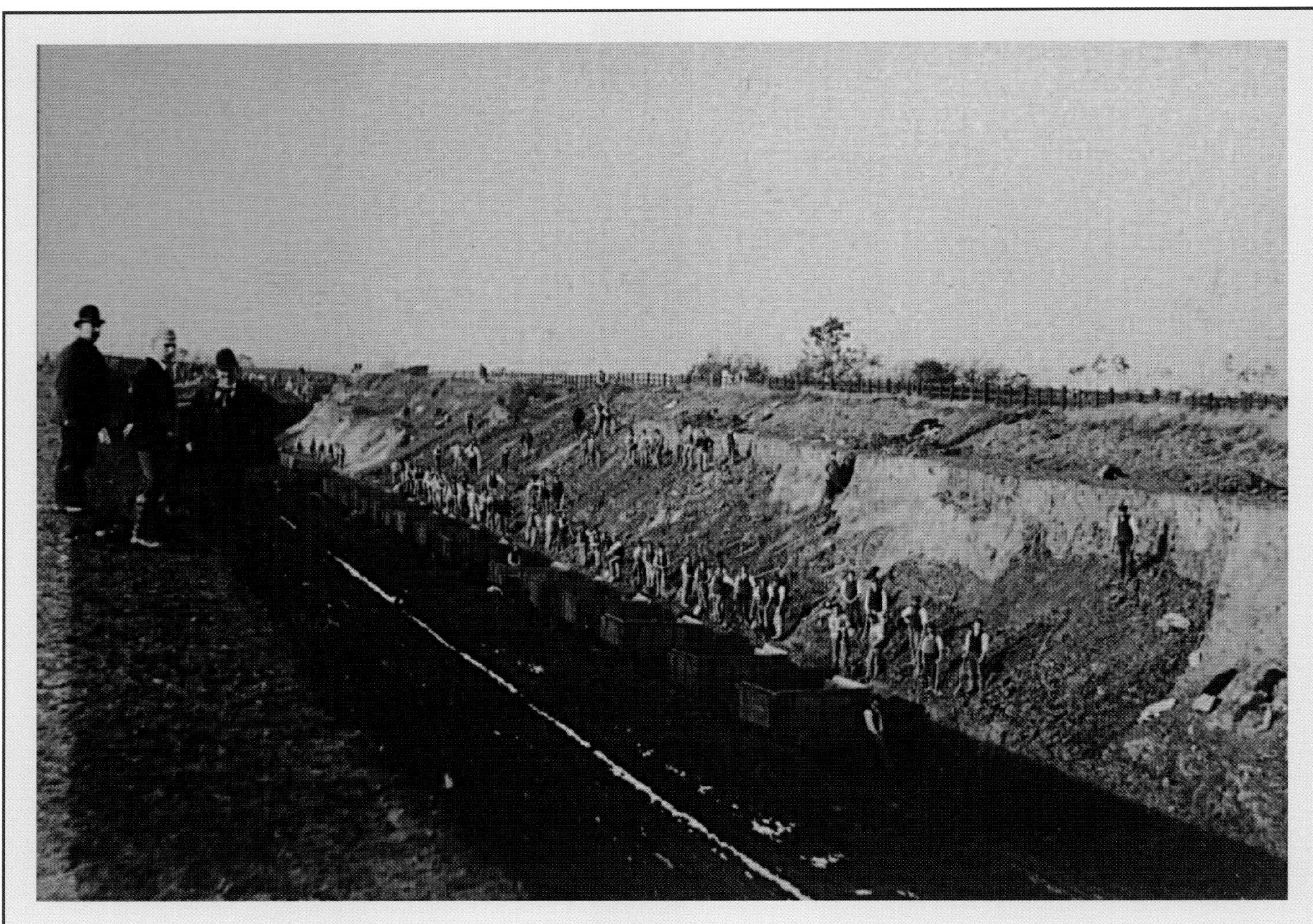

TOFT TUNNEL

PHOTOGRAPH 3

Photograph 3 is believed to be of the length of the cutting immediately to the east of Toft Tunnel, the portal of which is tantalisingly hidden by the men standing on the left.

In this view some sixty-nine men are shown, engaged in profiling the north side of the cutting. The main cut was made by a steam navvy, leaving the conventional curved cutting side with almost a cliff face at the upper part, formed by the path of the bucket moving in an arc of a circle. The men are cutting back the top, towards the fence in the background, and letting the soil fall towards the track to provide a uniform shape. The side to the left has been finished already. (See Photograph 30 for details of steam navvy operation and their ownerships by contractors working on this line.)

The photograph is a reminder that while this line may have been an early example of the mechanisation of civil engineering it was still dependent upon large numbers of workmen. These men were working for W. T. Mousley, the contractor for this section. Some idea of what they were employed to do and how they lived can be gained from the pages of the newspapers, in particular in relation to those men working for Nowell, the contractor for the central section in the South Witham area. (See Photograph 33 for more detail.)

In the bottom of the cutting is a line of tipping wagons waiting to receive the surplus soil and stone. This was taken from the construction works here to Spalding, to form the embankment for the Spalding avoiding line which was being built at the same time. Tipping wagons would normally face the direction in which they were being tipped to empty them. (See Photograph 57 as an example.) The journey to Spalding would not be undertaken by these wagons. They were used within the limits of the construction works simply for moving spoil, a general term for waste material, around to where it was needed. To travel further would require transfer to conventional railway wagons. Here the wagons face to the west and it may be that the tipping arrangements into the transfer wagons required them to face this way. It may also be that the earthwork at Spalding was complete by this time and that the spoil was being taken for use on the embankments of the Lound viaduct or elsewhere.

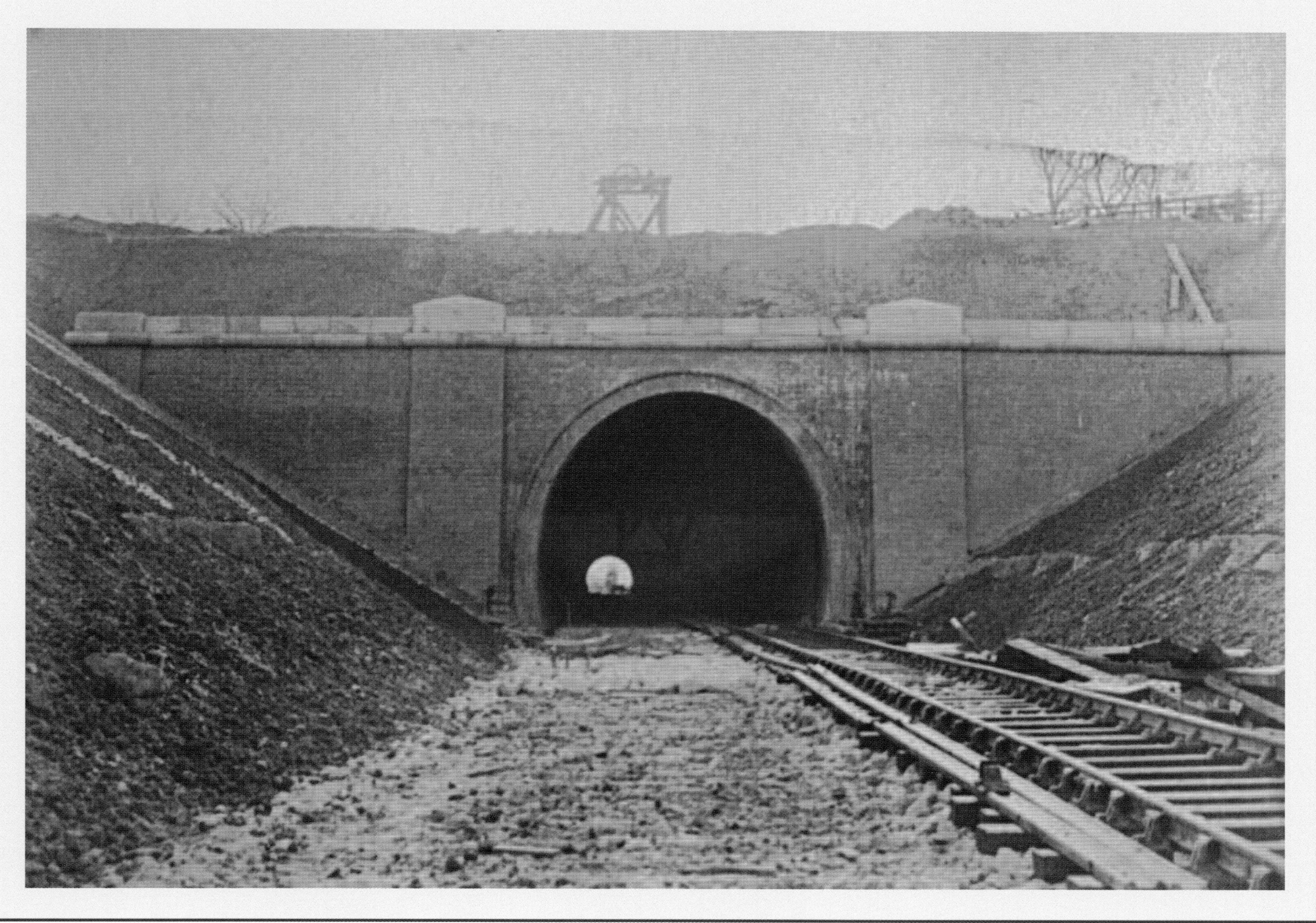

PHOTOGRAPH 4

Toft Tunnel was the only tunnel on the Midland and Great Northern Railway. It is 330 yards long and avoided the need for some steep gradients and a deep cutting to get the line over the ridge west of Bourne. This is the east portal and the elliptical arch form is typical of many similar tunnels as it provides resistance to the thrusts from above and to the sides while, at the same time, providing for the maximum height and width for trains to pass through. The maximum height of the arch above rail level was 21 ft and the maximum width was 26 ft 6 inches.

Adjacent to the tunnel was the work site for this section of line. Its precise location is not known but it is likely to have been at this end. The portal is beneath what is now the A6121 road from Bourne to Stamford and the fence at the top right of the photograph marks its route. Worksites were usually alongside the line where there was also direct road access. John Rhodes records that a collection of workshops – a saw mill, mortar mill, smithies and carpenters shops – grew up around the workings and some four hundred men were employed.[8] These workshops and men would serve the whole of the contract length, not just the tunnel workings.

Tunnels were often cut not only from the ends but also from shafts sunk down to where men worked along the line from the base of the shaft, thereby increasing the number of faces being worked simultaneously. The structure in the centre, above the tunnel, supported the drum around which a rope was wound to raise and lower down the shaft. The shafts were 8 ft x 6 ft x 65 ft deep with a portable steam winding engine at ground level to haul the spoil out. Deep approach cuttings were also needed to each end of the tunnel, and over 300,000 cubic yards of soil were removed.

Kingston's brickyard in Bourne (see Map 1) supplied 2.5 million bricks for the tunnel. These would be used for the lining, with Staffordshire Blue bricks used for the inner, facing, course.[9] (For additional details see also Photographs 20 and 21.) Rabbit burrows nearby reveal large amounts of broken brick and this is evidence that many faulty or damaged bricks were delivered to the site. The Great Central Railway main line from Nottingham to Aylesbury was built in the period 1894 to 1899 and bricks for the construction of Catesby Tunnel were delivered to the site and simply heaped up alongside the contractor's line on the cutting sides.[10] This may have happened here also.

The photograph shows one line of the permanent way built and the cutting sides are complete. The tunnel portal is very plain, relieved only by the brick piers at each side and the arch ring of five courses of brickwork. The tunnel is straight and the western portal can be seen, literally as the light at the end of the tunnel.

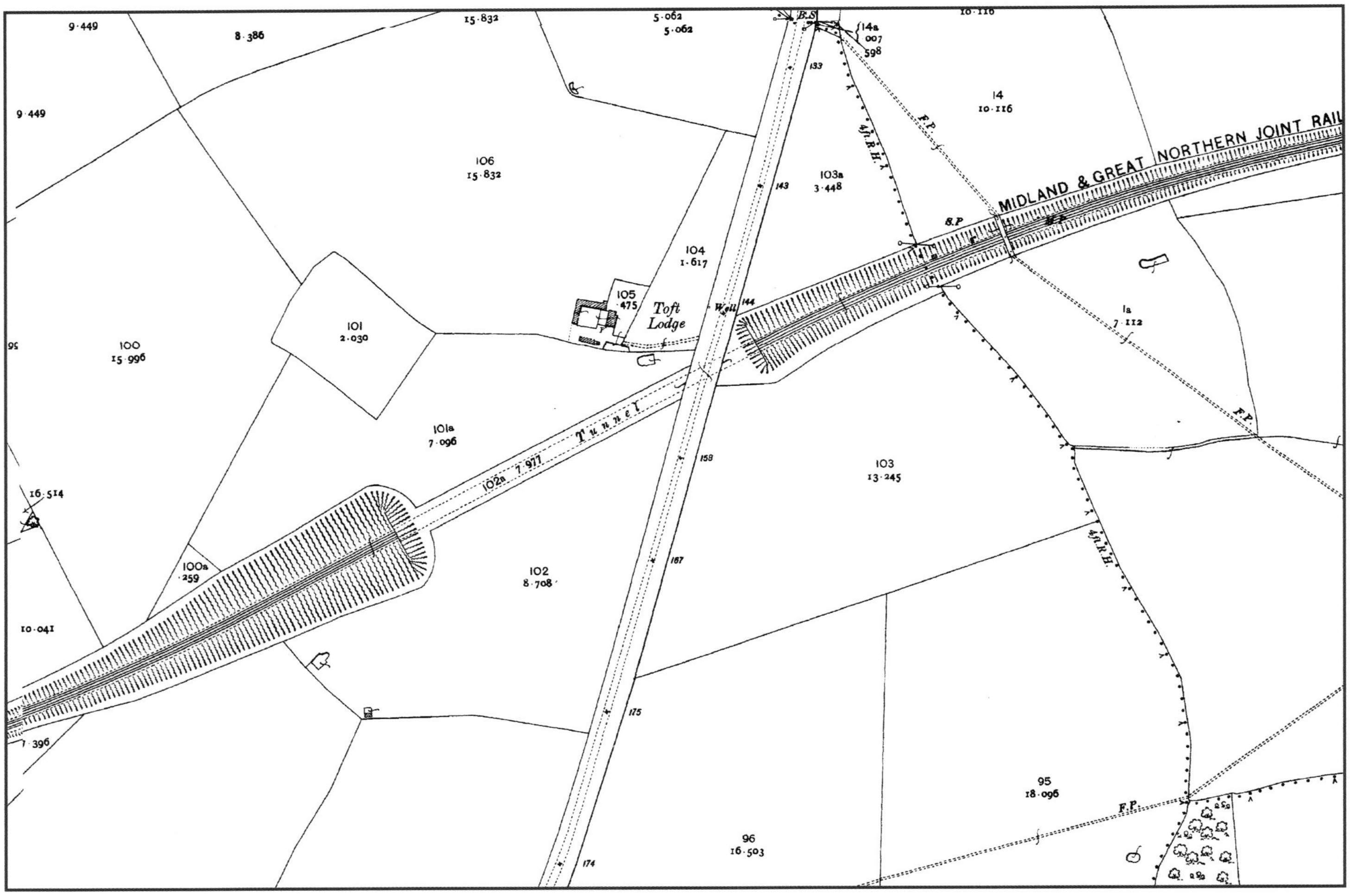

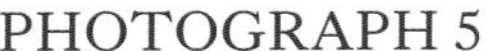

PHOTOGRAPH 5

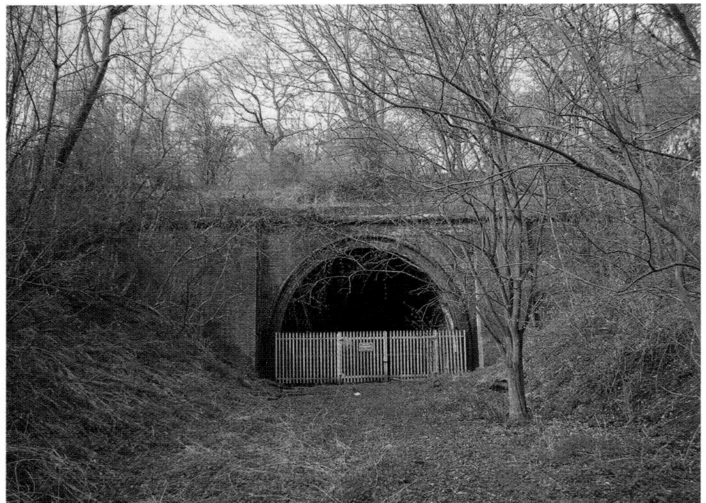

Photograph 5 shows the same view in April 2008. The line here is now a nature reserve under the care of the Lincolnshire Wildlife Trust. The tunnel itself cannot be entered. It is unsafe because of crumbling bricks falling from the roof[11] but a footpath link to the far end follows the line of the tunnel above ground and, on the way, the sites of the two shafts with their attendant spoil heaps, are still clearly visible.

MAP 2

OS 1/2500 County Series Map, 1904. Toft Tunnel.

This shows the route of the tunnel, fenced over the top where the sites of the two shafts were dug and the spoil heaps still exist. There is no evidence of the location of the temporary work camp but it may have been in the triangular field immediately north of the eastern portal, numbered 103a. The well in the hedge alongside the road near to the east portal is not related to the construction of the railway, as it appears on the 1891 map.

The bridge to the east of the tunnel taking a footpath over the line is Bridge No 236. This has been demolished and the Parish Boundary (the line of dots running parallel to the footpath) marks the western limit of the land fill site that has now completely filled the cutting here.

[8] John Rhodes, *Bourne to Saxby* (Boston, 1989), 13. See Appendix C.

[9] *Grantham Journal* (10 June 1893), p. 6, col. 2.

[10] L.T.C. Rolt, *The Making of a Railway* (London, 1971), 71.

[11] Midland and Great Northern Circle Photo Archive, Leicester to South Lynn, catalogue captions for photographs MGM-ME.5330 D and MGN-ME.5331 D.

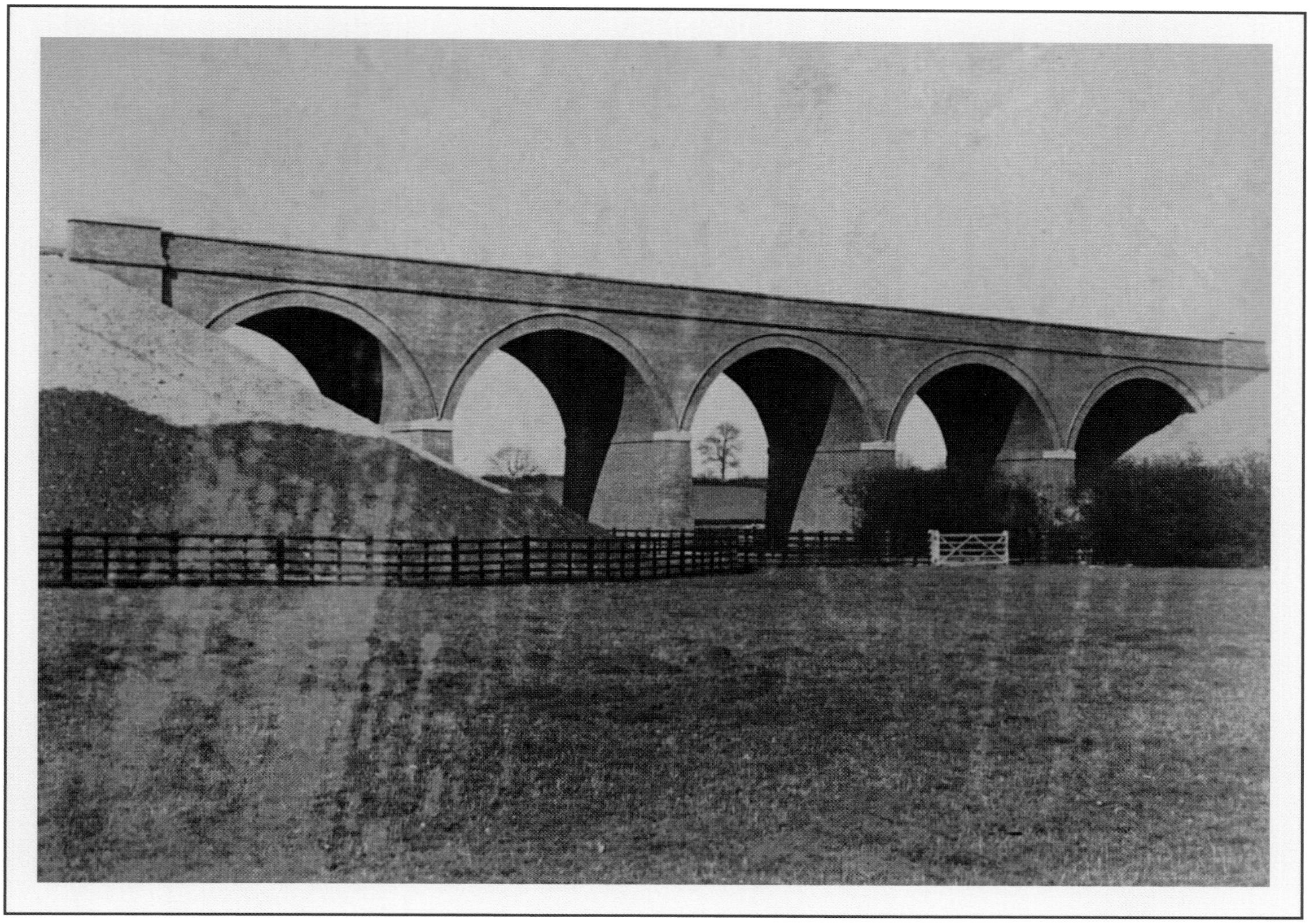

LOUND VIADUCT

PHOTOGRAPH 6

Bridge 239 was the Lound viaduct, built to carry the line over what was the Lound Beck, now known as the East Glen River. It has five semi-circular arches, each with a 40 ft span, 29 ft wide and 44 ft high to the former rail level. The centre arch is over the river with those on either side providing for an occupation road. This graceful structure consumed around 1.5 million bricks, all but the inner arch ring facing of Staffordshire Blue bricks being supplied by Kingston's brickyard in Bourne (see Map 1).[12] It is seen here with some freshly tipped spoil to complete the sides of the embankments.

It was the source of some structural problems and by 1927 there had been clear movement due to the subsidence of one of the piers. The problem was tackled in 1929 and included the provision of new parapets as well as repairs to cracks in the main structure.[13]

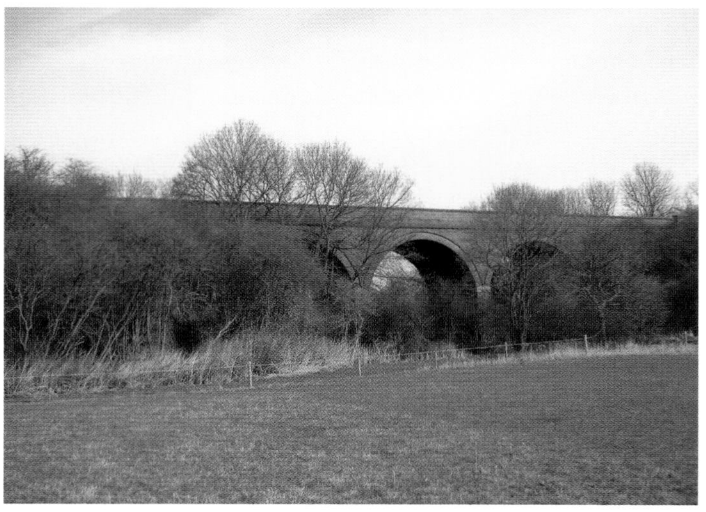

Photograph 7

PHOTOGRAPH 7

Photograph 7 shows the same view in 2008. The viaduct remains in use, now carrying a farm roadway. The parapets are deflected and the brickwork cracked, showing that some structural movement has continued. Presumably, however, this is not such a problem now the structure carries lighter loads than trains.

[12] *Grantham Journal* (10 June 1893), p. 6, col. 3.

[13] Midland and Great Northern Circle Photo Archive, Leicester to South Lynn, catalogue captions for photographs MGM-ME.0177 to MGN-ME.0183 inclusive.

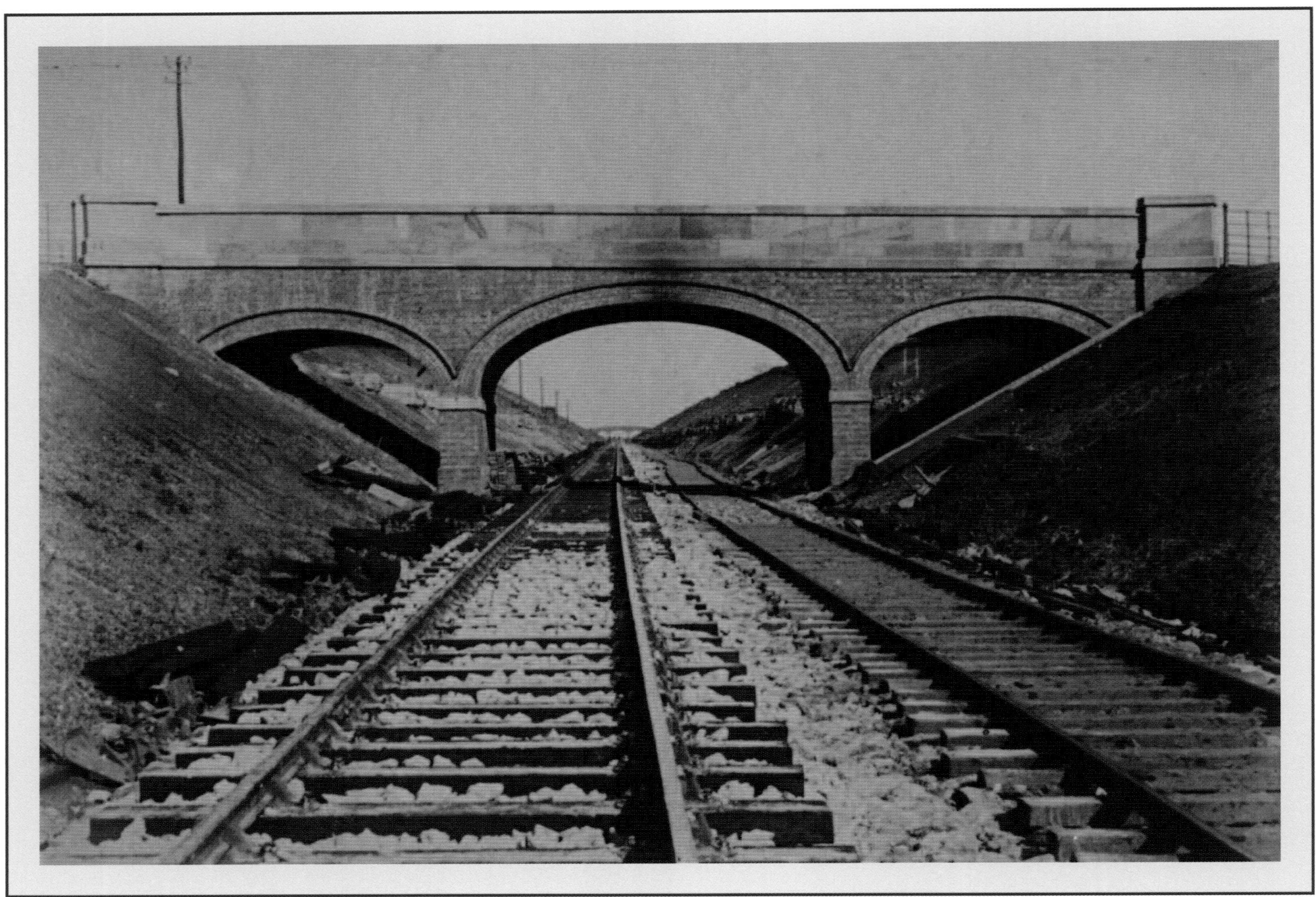

GRIMSTHORPE PARK BRIDGE

PHOTOGRAPH 8

Bridge 245, the subject of Photograph 8, is unique on the line. The arches are the same three ellipses as other bridges on this section but the parapets are of stone. The reason is that this bridge carried the carriage drive from the south end of Grimsthorpe Park up to Grimsthorpe Castle. This view is from the west and Bridge 244 can be seen in the distance.

The land falls steeply here to the West Glen River and the carriage drive followed the contour of the ground as an easy route into the park. However, the former drive would have required a level crossing. To avoid this it was diverted to the east with this bridge built to carry it (see also Map 3).[14] As it was to serve Grimsthorpe Castle it had parapets of stone rather than brick. Note the horizontal line of the parapet wall and the roadway of the bridge, by contrast with the curving wall and roadway of Bridge 234 in Photograph 1. Because the cutting was deeper here the roadway could cross the line on the level.

This was also the last of the bridges on the Midland and Great Northern Railway. The ownership of the line changed one quarter of a mile to the west (behind the photographer) at Little Bytham signal box. The double track became single beyond this point, and remained so all the way to Saxby.

The two lengths of railway line in the photograph show clearly the difference between the contractor's line on the right and the permanent way to the left. The smoke stain on the centre of the bridge shows the use made of the contractor's line, whereas the permanent way could only be used by his locomotives to assist in the ballasting work. (See the caption to Photograph 1 above.) The right-hand line is laid with lighter track and materials, as it had to be transportable and easily handled. Indeed, it appears to have been pushed over, a practice known as 'slewing', to allow the permanent track to be laid. It is not now aligned with the smoke stain. It now meanders slightly to give a maximum height where it passes beneath the bridge. The track was only temporary and the rails were fixed to the wooden sleepers simply by spikes driven in with the use of a sledge hammer. The 'permanent way', by contrast, has sleepers supported by ballast and with the rails held in chairs which are themselves bolted to the sleepers.

Between this bridge and Bridge 244 in the distance, the line severed the route of the former railway line between Little Bytham and Edenham. This was a private railway, built, owned and operated by the 21st Lord Willoughby of Grimsthorpe Castle. The line, four miles in length, opened in 1855. It was last used in 1873, the equipment and the rails being sold by auction in 1890.[15]

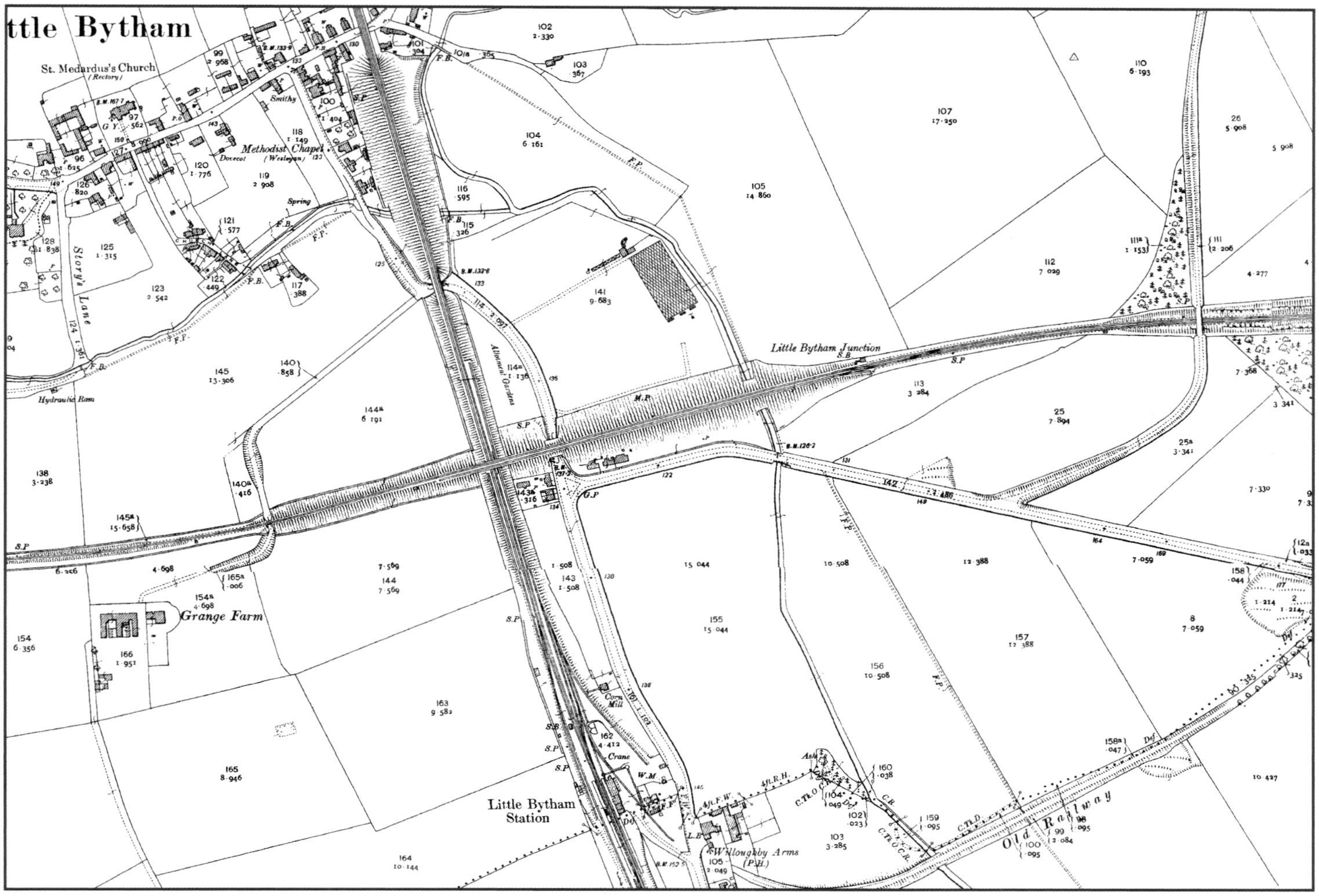

MAP 3

OS 1/2500 County Series Map, 1904. Little Bytham.

Bridge 245, shown in Photograph 8, can be seen at the eastern end of the extract. The former carriage drive followed the western boundary of the woodland to the north west of the bridge, crossed the route of the railway at the end of the cutting and followed the field boundary between Fields No 113 and 25 to the road.

Little Bytham Junction is marked by the signal box (S.B.) This was a rare example of an end-on junction marking a change of ownership rather than the junction of two lines where one branches away from the other.

The bridge taking the river under the embankment next west is Bridge 45 of the Midland Railway (see Photograph 10). Further west again is Bridge 44 (see Photograph 12) and Bridge 43 over what is now the East Coast Main Line (see Photograph 14).

Also of interest is the row of three buildings at the foot of the embankment by the road junction by Bridge 44. These have long been demolished but they were surviving navvy houses left over from the construction phase and subsequently occupied by railway staff. Their plan view indicates that they are likely to have been the same or similar to the one surviving former navvy house shown in Photograph 67. (See also the similar buildings shown on Map 6 and Map 8.)

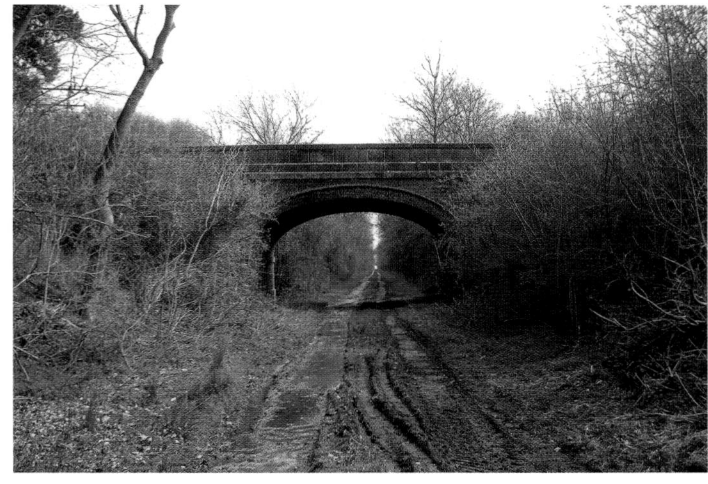

PHOTOGRAPH 9

Photograph 9 shows the same view in April 2008.

[14] R. E. Pearson and J. G. Ruddock, *Lord Willoughby's Railway: The Edenham Branch* (Grimsthorpe: Willoughby Memorial Trust, 1986), 101.

[15] Pearson and Ruddock, *Lord Willoughby's Railway*, 96-102; see also Stewart E. Squires, *The Lost Railways of Lincolnshire* (Ware, 1988), 122-124.

WEST GLEN RIVER BRIDGE, LITTLE BYTHAM

PHOTOGRAPH 10

Photograph 10 is of Bridge 45 which carried the railway over what was then known as the River Glen and is now the West Glen River. Bridge 45 is only about 500 yards west of Bridge 245, shown in Photographs 8 and 9 above. In number sequence it is the last of the Midland Railway bridges and is very near to the end-on junction with the Midland and Great Northern Railway to the east (see Map 3).

This bridge is unusual in that it also carries a footpath, now a public right of way, cantilevered out over the river, the railings of which can be seen within the bridge arch, above the right-hand gatepost. There was no footpath here when the line was built. The Little Bytham Signal Box, which marked the junction of the two ownerships, was built on the north side of the line and the footbridge and its path from the public road were provided to enable the signalmen to reach the box.

The right-hand abutment is adorned by figures, probably Wilson's assistants; the lower of the two has struck a classic pose. The work to the right of the bridge is probably related to track drainage and on the extreme left a chute can be seen running down from the rail level.

PHOTOGRAPH 11

The present day comparison, Photograph 11, had to be taken from a closer viewpoint because of the growth of the trees and shrubs in recent years. In March 2008 the ash tree and the gatepost, shown in the Wilson photograph and here, still survived but shortly after the tree was blown down. The footpath to and across the footbridge is still in use and is a public right of way.

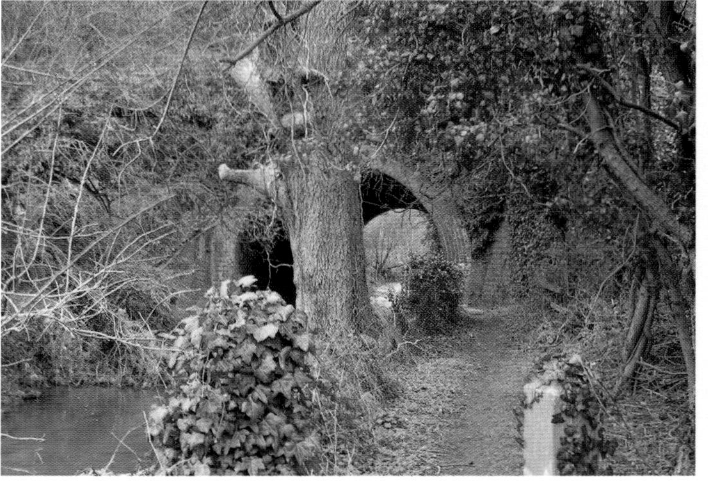

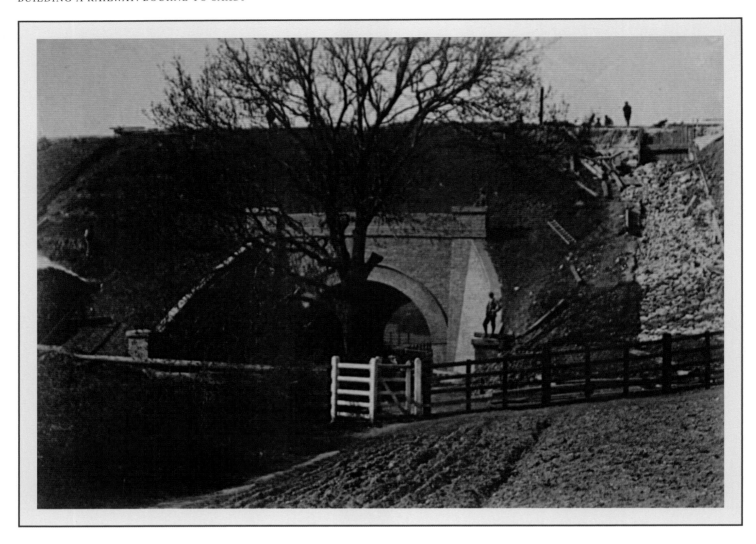

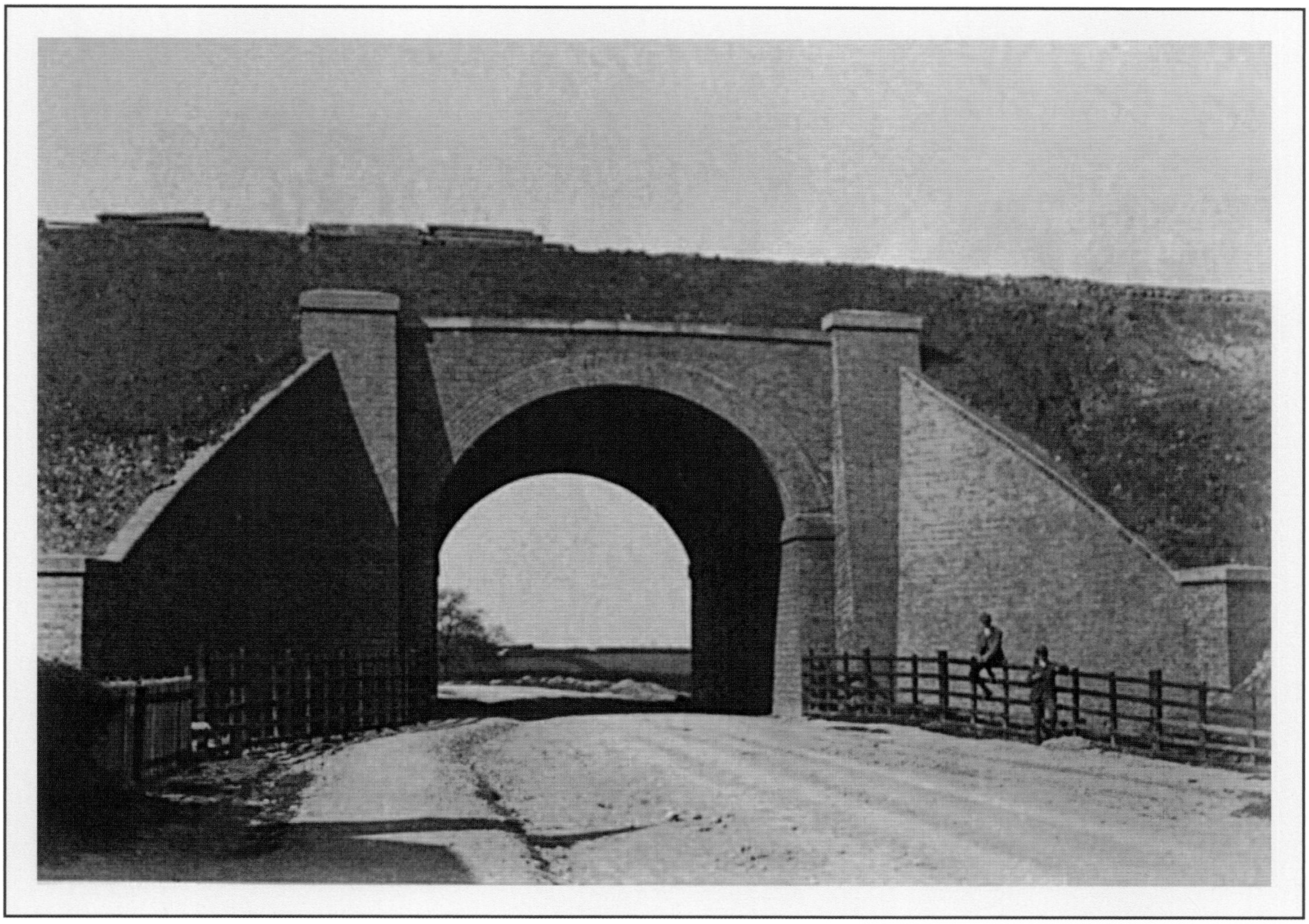

LITTLE BYTHAM ROAD BRIDGE

PHOTOGRAPH 12

Photograph 12 is of Bridge 44, over the road in Little Bytham village, immediately east of the East Coast Main Line. This is the view looking north and the bridge is exactly the same as Bridge 10, over Sewstern Road at Wymondham (see Photographs 57, 58 and 59). The two men to the right may be the same as appear in Photograph 10 above.

In this view the bridge structure looks to have been completed but comparison with Photograph 13 shows that at some time the parapets and piers have been raised by about seven courses of brickwork, probably to contain material eroded by the weather from the trackbed above and stop it dropping onto the road. The depth of fill above the arch, necessitated by the height of the embankment, is unusual. The bridge is also shown on Map 3.

PHOTOGRAPH 13

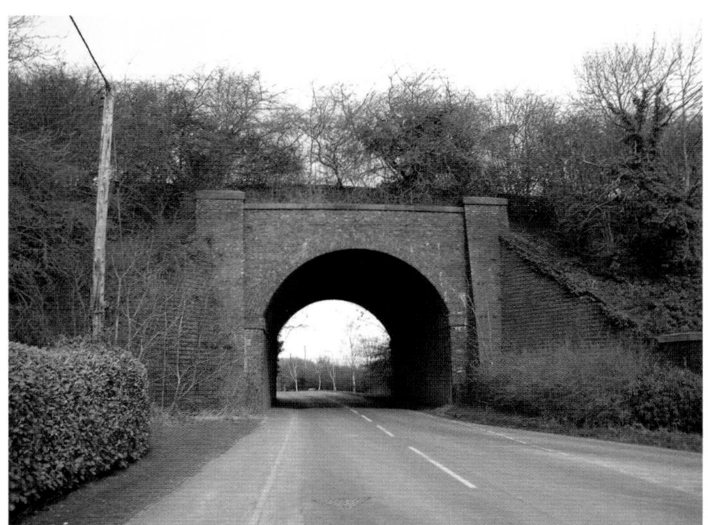

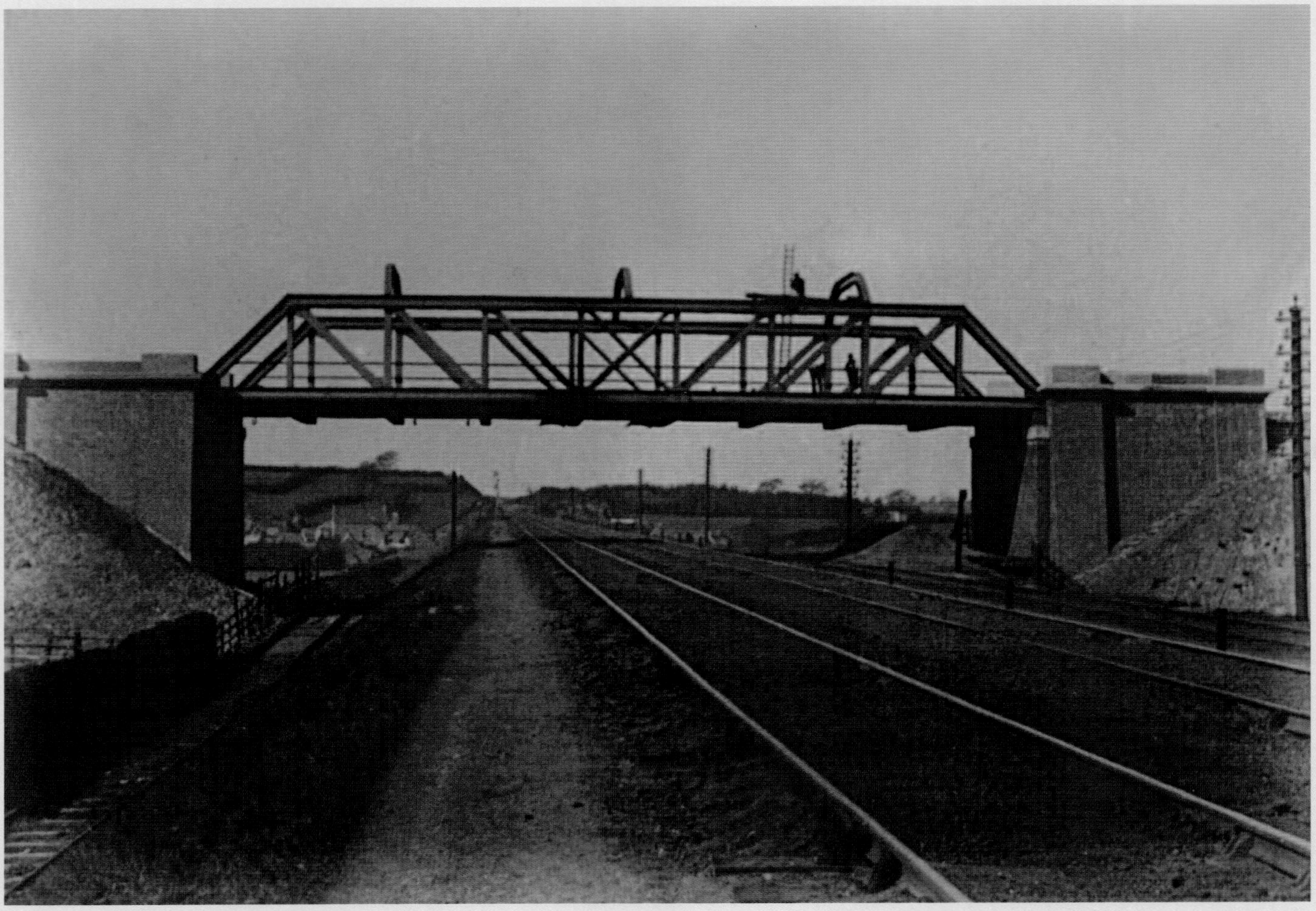

EAST COAST MAIN LINE BRIDGE, LITTLE BYTHAM

PHOTOGRAPH 14

Bridge 43 was a girder bridge that carried the line over what was then the Great Northern Main Line, now the East Coast Main Line. It was the only one of its type between Bourne and Saxby and comprised two open truss main girders, connected by three arched cross girders above and rail bearers beneath. It had a span of 97 feet 6 inches and weighed 152 tons. (See also Map 3 and Drawing 1.)

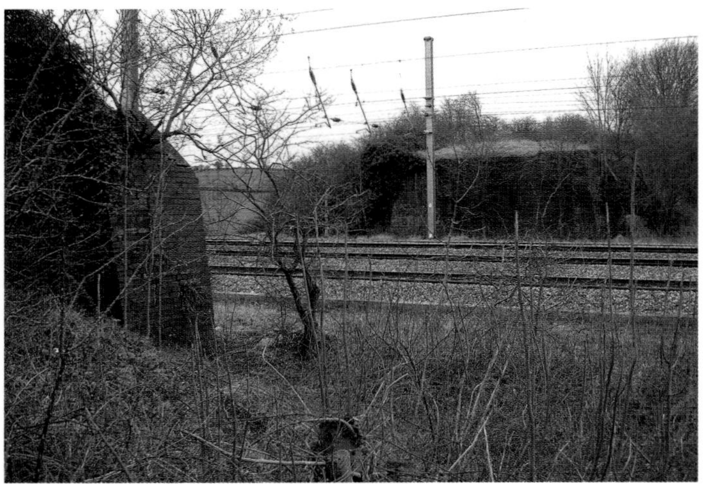

Photograph 15

Note that on the main line the ballast covers the sleepers. This was very typical of the practice on the Great Northern Railway at that time. Three tracks can be seen running under the bridge. The up and down lines to and from London are in the centre, with the headshunt for Little Bytham goods sidings on the extreme right. The line was later widened to the four lines that exist today; indeed, the bridge may have been designed specifically to allow for this. The stations at Corby Glen, Little Bytham and Essendine were rebuilt when the line was widened. The contractor for these works, completed in 1912, was Nowell, the same contractor for the line between South Witham and Castle Bytham. (See photograph on page 17.)

Little Bytham village can be seen beneath the bridge to the left of the line.

PHOTOGRAPH 15

The speed of trains on the East Coast Main Line today means that the same view cannot be taken for comparison. Photograph 15 shows the east and west abutments, the east on the left, with the bridge removed for the erection of the overhead wires.

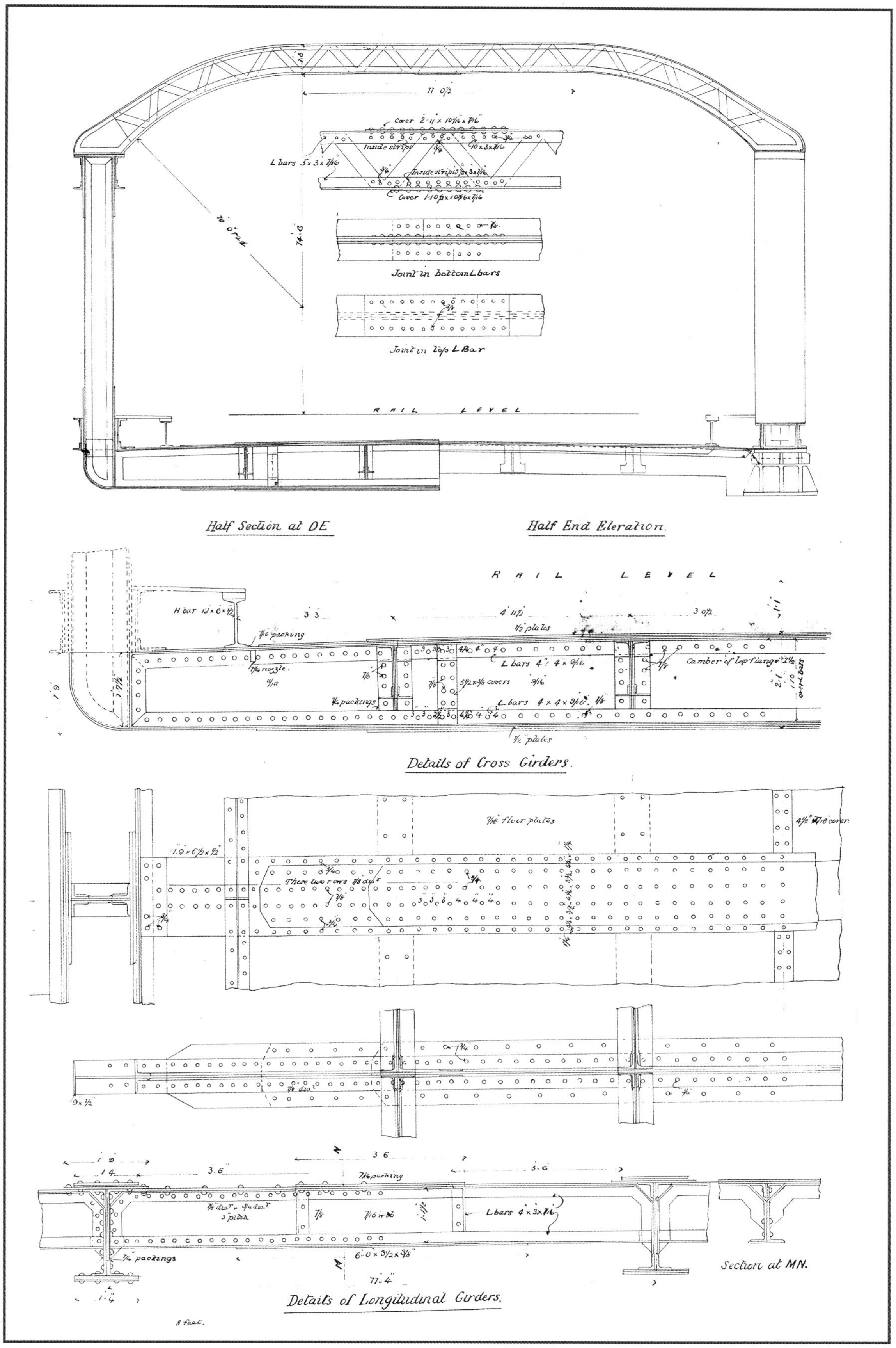

Half Section at DE

Half End Elevation.

Details of Cross Girders.

Section at MN.

Details of Longitudinal Girders.

DRAWING 1

This is an extract from one of the original contract drawings for the construction of Bridge 43. It shows the details of the cross girders. Lettering on this drawing 'CONTRACT No 3', not shown on this extract, has been drawn using a stencil, as was usual at that time, and indeed was a technique still commonly in use until the advent of computers in drawing offices. This drawing was most probably drawn by the contractor as it was standard practice for Midland Railway drawings to have the lettering and the gaps caused by use of the stencil inked in.

This drawing is held within the archive at the Midland Railway Study Centre in Derby (Ref: 1986-1407/11).

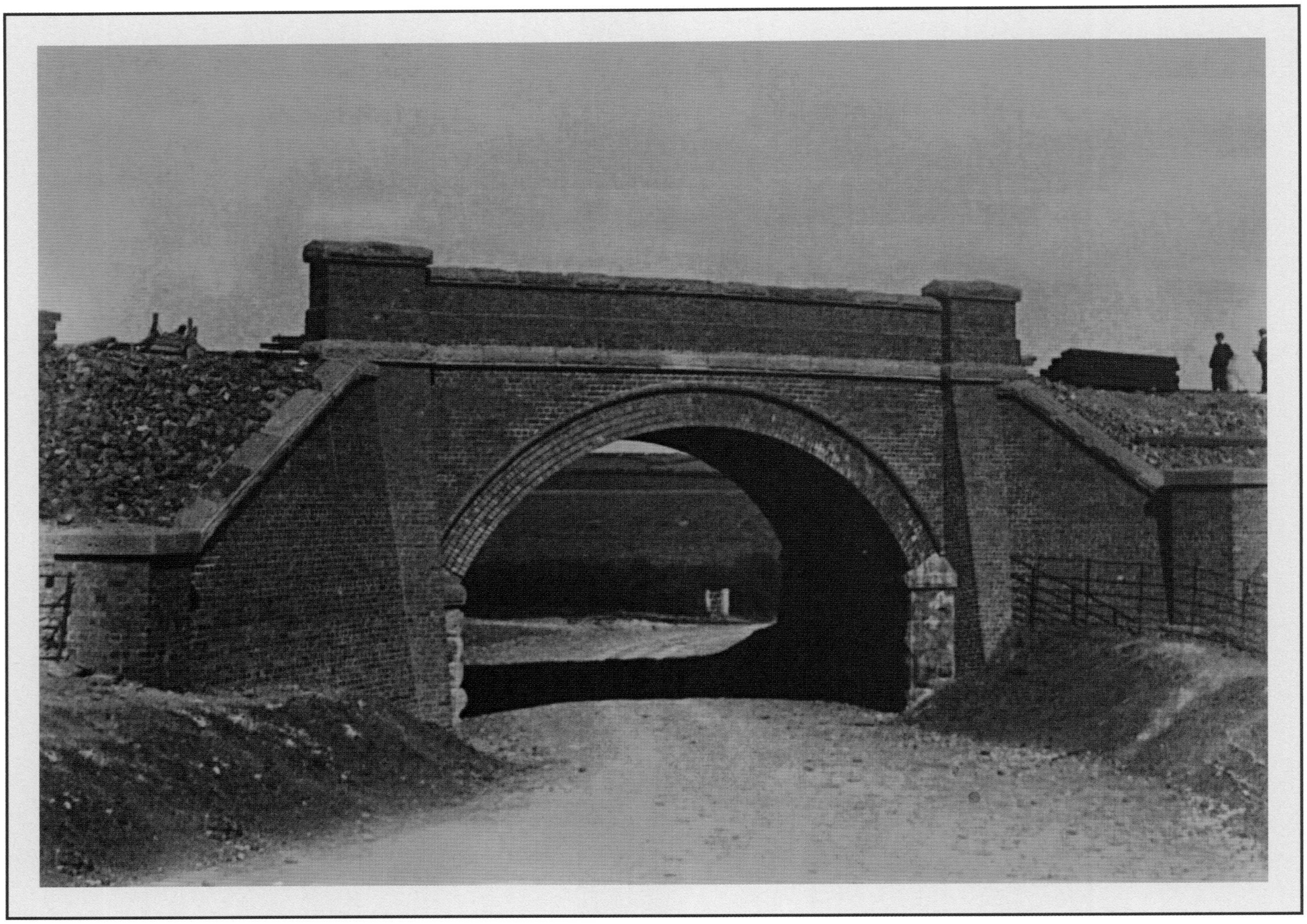

ROAD BRIDGE BETWEEN CASTLE BYTHAM AND LITTLE BYTHAM

PHOTOGRAPH 16

The line crossed the road between Castle Bytham and Little Bytham by Bridge No 38. Similar bridges are in Photographs 10 and 42. This one was built to a slight skew (see Map 4 below) and was unusual for the line in that it had abutment walls of stone below the arch rather than the blue brick used elsewhere.

The surviving contract required all the stone used on the line to be obtained from Derbyshire quarries.[16] The reason can be said to be twofold. First, the suitability and durability of the stone for this use was well known, and secondly, it would have to be transported from the quarries to Saxby by the Midland Railway. The aim of railway companies was to maximise their freight income at all times. From the tracks in the road surface underneath even when it was first built traffic took the central path.

PHOTOGRAPH 17

As Photograph 17 shows, this bridge has since been demolished, in the spring of 1994.

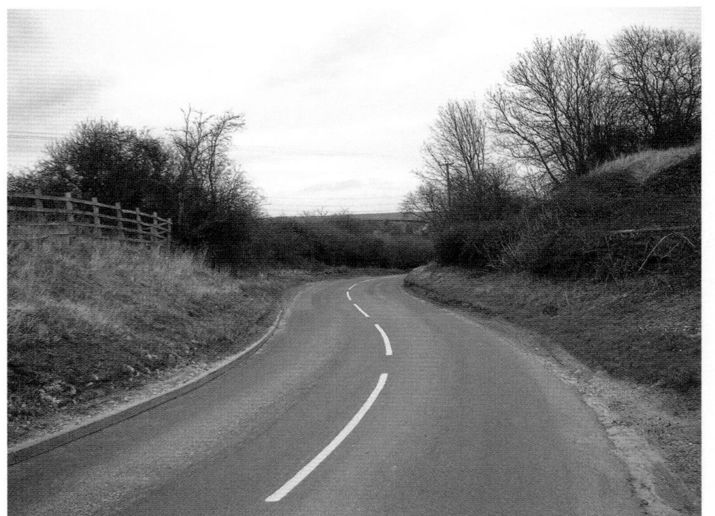

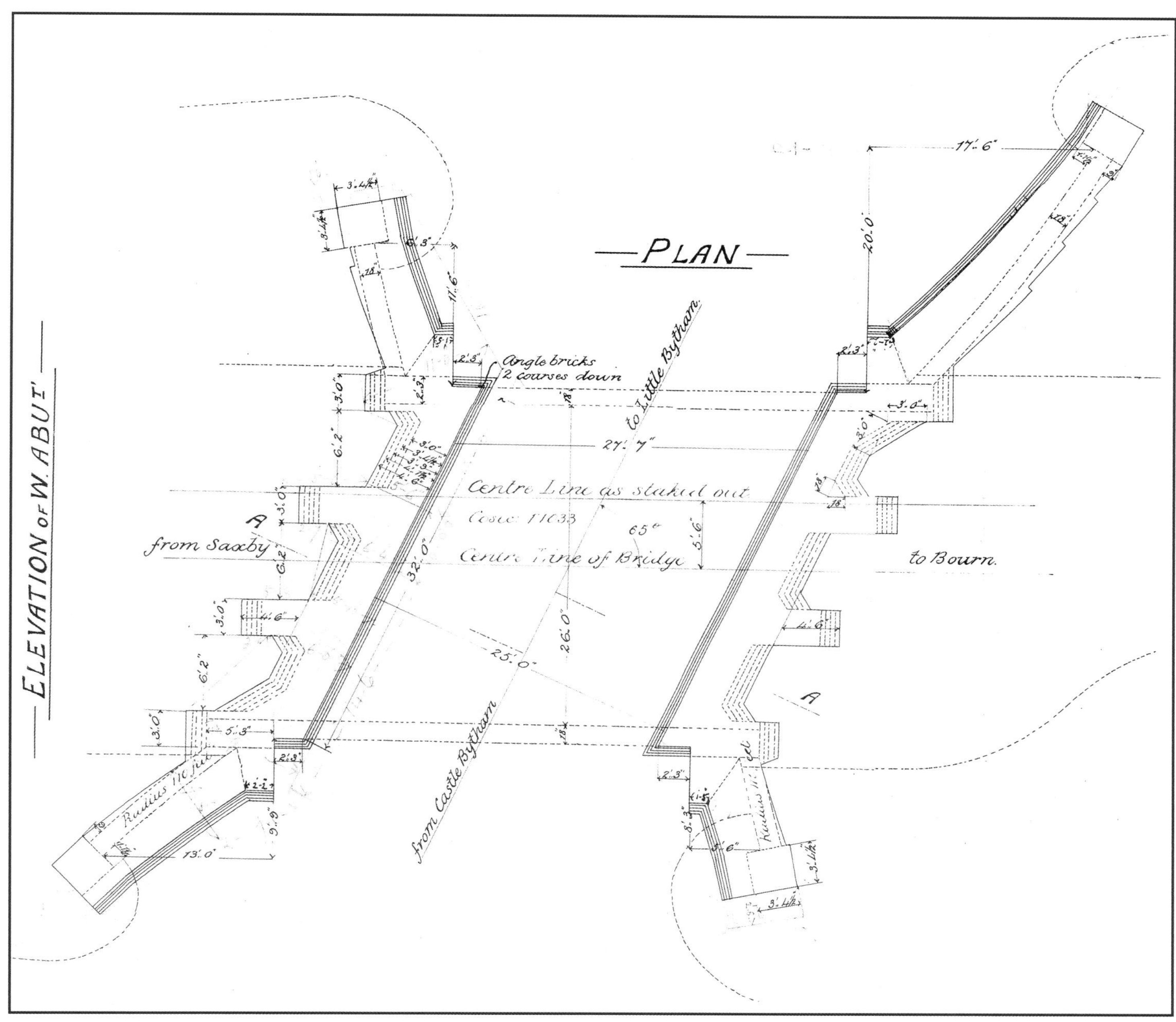

DRAWING OF BRIDGE NO 38

DRAWING 2

This is an extract from a copy of an early drawing for this bridge. At 36 feet between the parapets it was built to be wide enough to carry a double line of rails although only one was laid. The plan does show the trackbed narrowing to the east (right) of the bridge.

The original drawing is held within the archive at the Midland Railway Study Centre at Derby (Ref: 1986-1407/14).

[16] National Archives, RAIL 491/548.

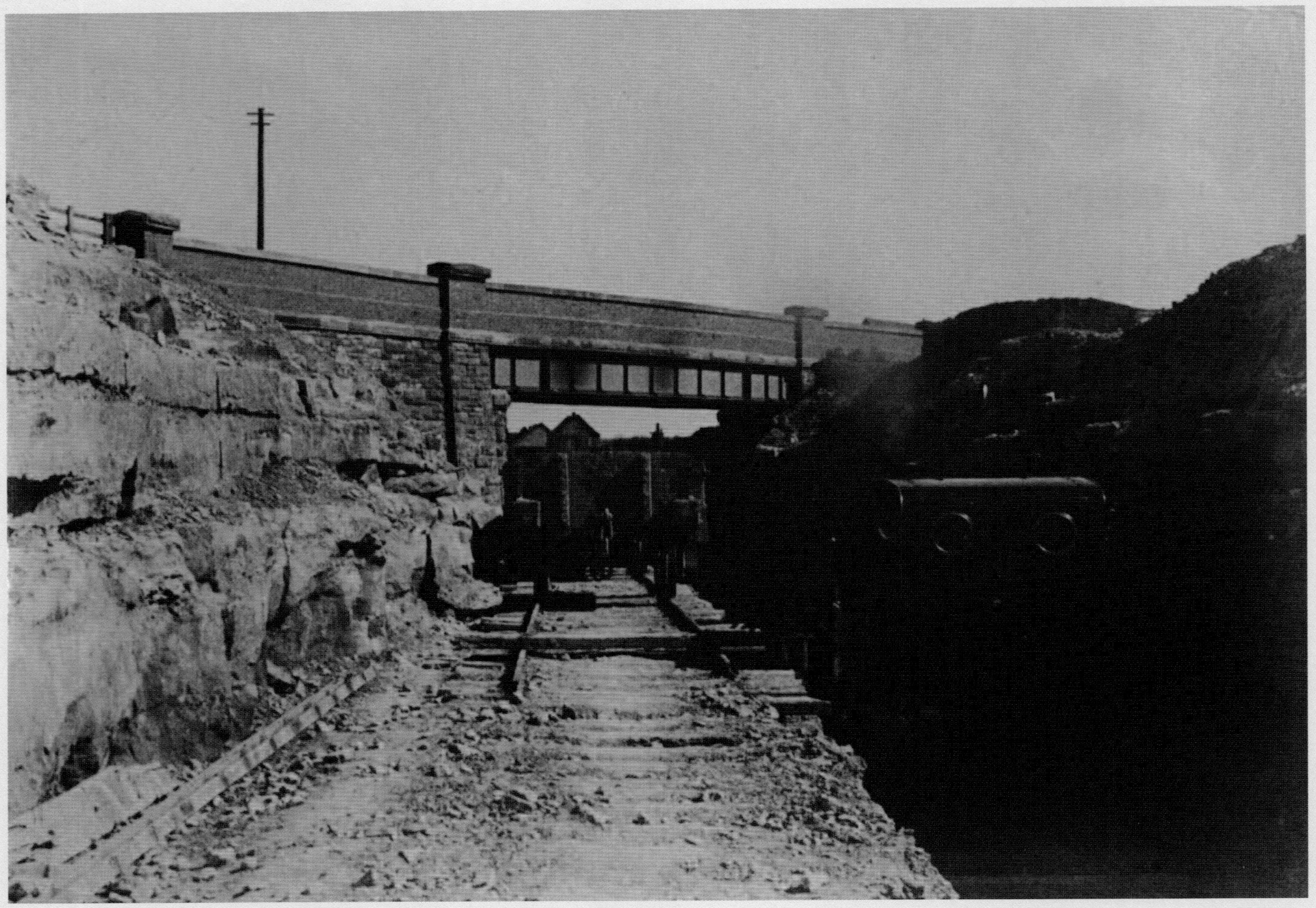

CASTLE BYTHAM, STATION SITE

PHOTOGRAPH 18

Bridge 37 carries the road across the railway on the outskirts of Castle Bytham. Here, a girder bridge with limestone parapets spans a cutting 6.5m (22 ft) deep. The steel beam was probably used here, and not a brick arch, due to problems with achieving adequate headroom across the cutting.

Because the line is cut here into the underlying bedrock the sides are nearly vertical. The photograph shows how this was carried out.

The locomotive, on the right, is at the finished level. On the left, temporary track runs along a bench from which the stone is being excavated from the left-hand side. When this was finished the bench itself would be removed from the lower level. As much as possible would be done working from the side and downwards to make the work quicker and more efficient for the contractor.

It does seem likely that explosives were also used to break up the stone here. The Midland Railway survey of the line shows, within the fenced boundary, a building described as 'Magazine (Disused)' on the south side of the line, east of Bridge 35.[17] No building is shown, however, on the 1904 OS map (see Map 4).

This cutting is the site of Castle Bytham station. No station was proposed in the original plans but it came later in response to local pressure, opening for goods on 3 January 1898 and passengers on 4 April the same year. One thing that is clear from the work here, however, is that ground was cut for a double track from the outset even though only single line was envisaged. Cuttings and bridges over them are invariably wide enough for double track. Embankments and the associated bridges through them are wide enough for a single line but with enough land to enable the embankments and bridges to be widened should this have later proved necessary. This was a prudent balance between initial expenditure and giving options for future development should the traffic warrant.

This is the only photograph that we have of a locomotive within the contract limits of William Mousley. It appears to be a Manning Wardle, two of which Mousley employed on these works. One was a Class K, MW 1221/91, 0-6-0ST, EMPRESS, with inside cylinders, delivered new to W. T. Mousley at Bourne for this contract. The other was a Class F, MW 982/86, STEPHENSON, 0-4-0ST with outside cylinders, delivered new to W. T. Mousley at Ilkley, presumably for a contract there. This locomotive was offered for sale or hire at Bourne on 22 February 1893.[18]

George Bradshaw published his first railway timetable

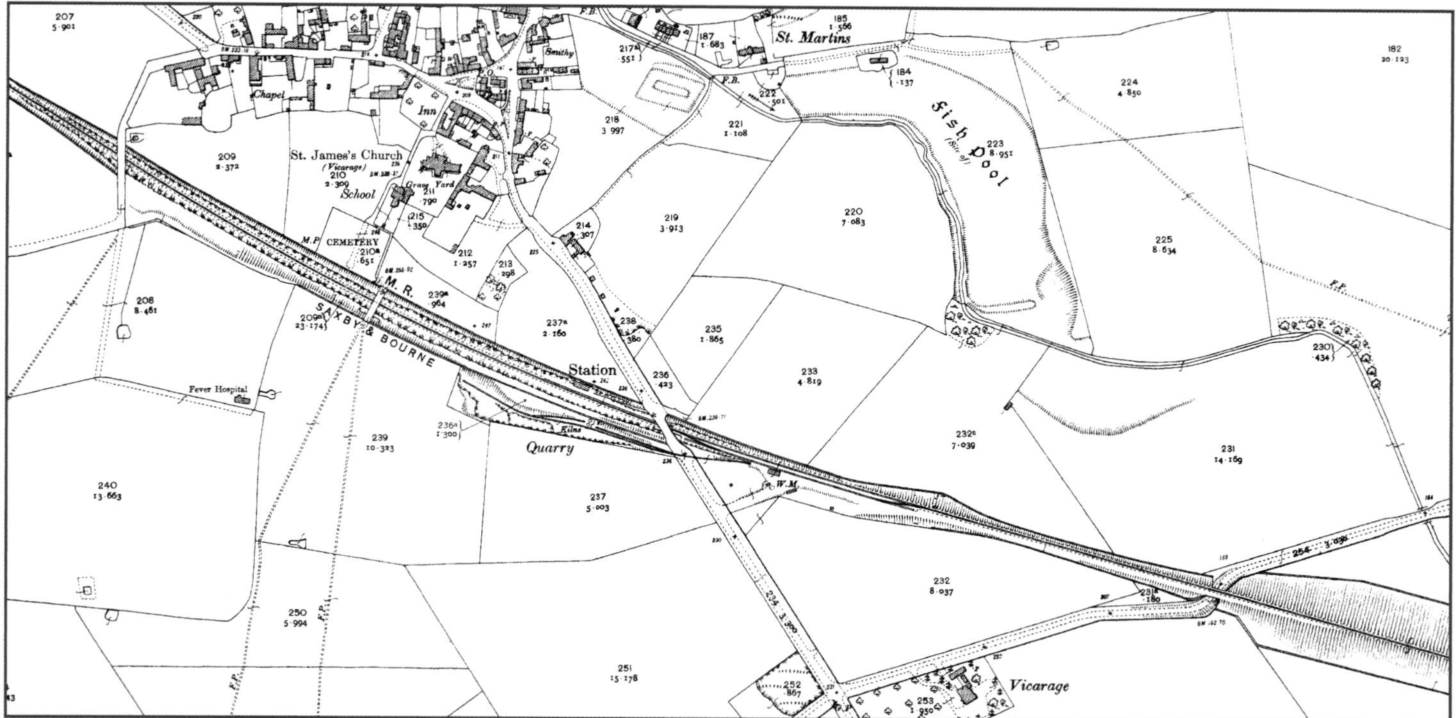

in 1838 and Bradshaw's, as it became known, was a household name right through to the last issue, in 1961.[19] Anyone who wanted to know the times of trains anywhere in the United Kingdom had to have the latest copy and it was trusted for its accuracy. Interestingly, although there is no suggestion that Bradshaw's times for trains between Bourne and Saxby were incorrect, it did include the wrong mileage for Castle Bytham station. The 1904 edition records that Castle Bytham station was 6 miles from South Witham and 5 miles from Bourne, whereas the distance is, in fact, 4 miles and 7 miles respectively.[20]

PHOTOGRAPH 19

This area did change, partly through the completion of the cutting and partly from the building of the station, and since closure has become rather overgrown. The 2008 view in Photograph 19 is taken from a slightly different location.

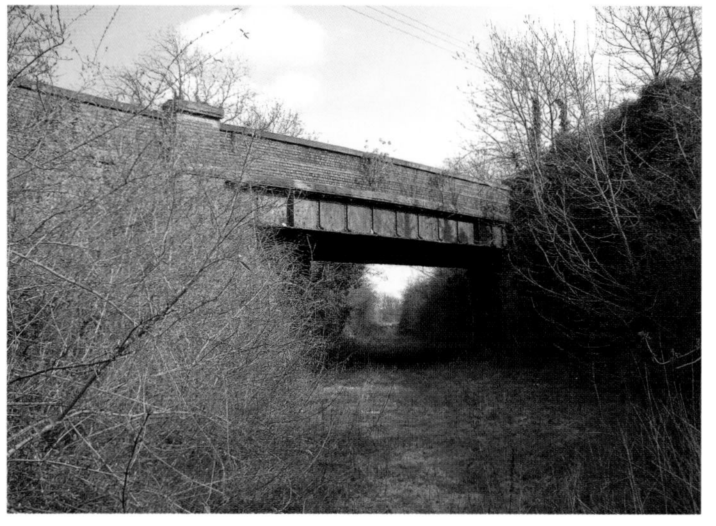

MAP 4

OS 1/2500 County Series Map, 1904. Castle Bytham.

Bridge 37 is in the centre with the passenger station to the west and the single goods siding on a loop to the east. The cliff face cut through the limestone is very distinctive. Although only a single line of rails is shown passing the station platform the goods loop was later extended to the west end of the platform.

With the opening of the railway came the quarry on the south side of the line. Two kilns can be seen, used for burning limestone to make lime for agricultural use. What was most probably a narrow gauge railway is shown running from the quarry, across the road and down to a dock alongside the siding.

The initials 'W.M.' alongside the goods siding access from the road indicates that the small building here was a weighing machine or weighbridge to weigh loads as they were brought to or taken from the station. The bridge to the extreme right of the extract was Bridge 38 shown in Photograph 16. The evidence of the former field boundaries here clearly shows how the road was realigned slightly, creating a double bend, to ensure a reduced skew for the new bridge as it passed under the line.

To the extreme left, on the south side of the line, the widening of the route shows the location of the disused magazine referred to in the caption to Photograph 18.

[17] Midland Railway Study Centre, Item No 00806.

[18] Correspondence from the Industrial Locomotive Society, April 2008.

[19] Jack Simmons, *The Express Train and Other Railway Studies* (Nairn, 1994), Chapter 12.

[20] *Bradshaw's Railway Guide* (November 1904).

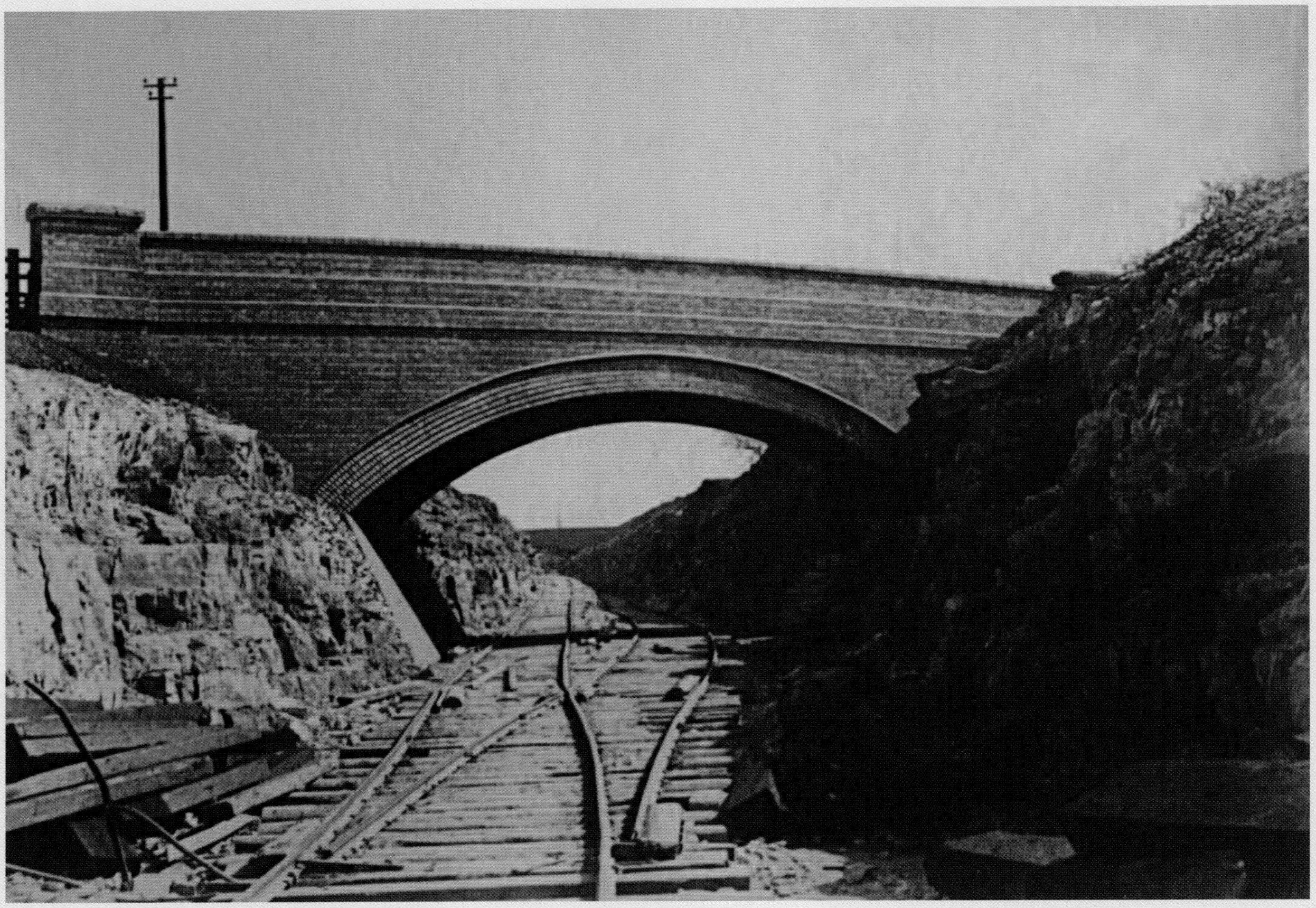

OCCUPATION BRIDGE AT CASTLE BYTHAM

(See also Map 4)

PHOTOGRAPH 20

Bridge 35, an occupation bridge, is seen from the west in Photograph 20. Note the temporary track climbing on to the benching beyond the bridge. The reason for this is discussed in the caption for Photograph 18 and is related to the way the rock was removed to create the cutting.

The contract specified that the 'best brindled Staffordshire District bricks shall be used for all face work'.[21] These dense, hard bricks, produced in Staffordshire, were impervious to penetration by water and damage from frost action. Their use would also ensure that they would be transported from supplier to site by the Midland Railway. One of the main suppliers was Joseph Hamblet of West Bromwich and coping bricks stamped with that name can be found at this bridge. Hamblet owned the largest brickworks in West Bromwich. Blue bricks were one of the specialities of the firm; in 1898, four years after Hamblet's death, it became the Hamblet Blue Brick Co. Ltd. In the mid 1890s the company was producing between 400,000 and 500,000 bricks every week. The works closed in 1915.[22] Similar bricks can be found on Bridge 42 at Little Bytham; Culvert 34 at Castle Bytham; Bridge 31 (Photograph 23); Bridge 12 (Photograph 51); Bridge 10 (Photograph 57); Bridge 7 (Photograph 63); Bridge 5 (Photograph 73); Bridge 4 (Photograph 75) and Bridge 1 (Photograph 85).

Suppliers of similar bricks were Wood and Ivery of West Bromwich, for the platform edgings at Edmondthorpe and Wymondham station (see Photograph 63) and the Haunchwood Brick and Tile Co. Ltd (see Photograph 42). A brick with 'STAFFORD S O T' in the frog at the unnumbered culvert between Bridges 14 and 15 was manufactured by the Stafford Coal and Iron Company at a brickworks at Stoke on Trent, the site of which is close to the Britannia Stadium.[23] (See brick samples on page 40.)

PHOTOGRAPHS 21 AND 22

(opposite)

Here again the cutting is cut through the bedrock which lies very close to the surface. Photograph 20 shows a bench in the side of the cutting giving two levels of working and the side of the ramp on the left can still be seen here today. Photograph 21 is of the same view in 2008 and Photograph 22, taken from under the bridge, shows the

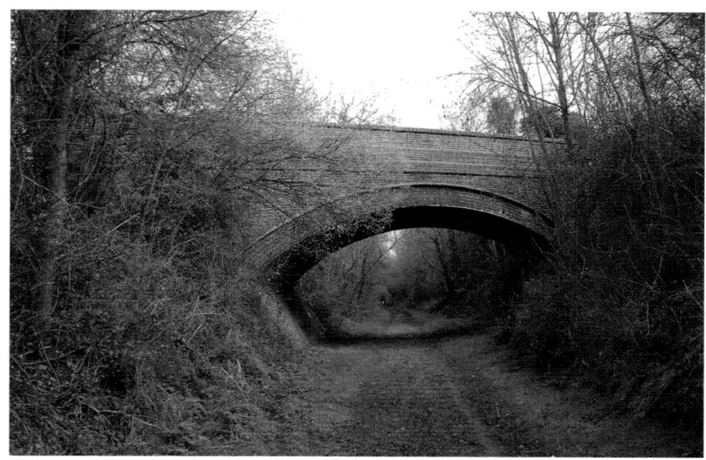

Photograph 21

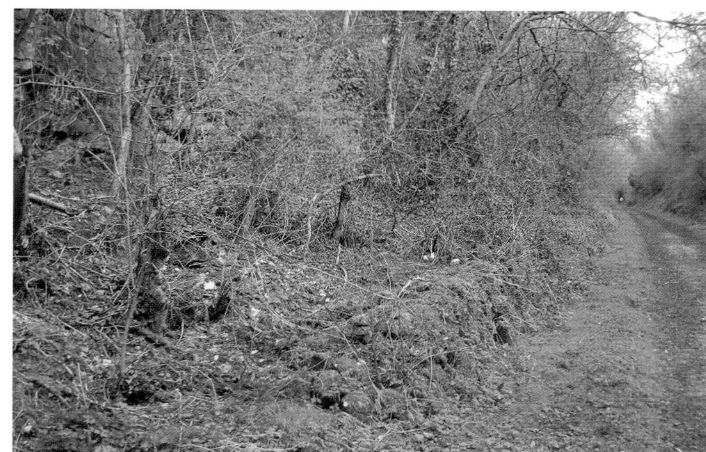

Photograph 22

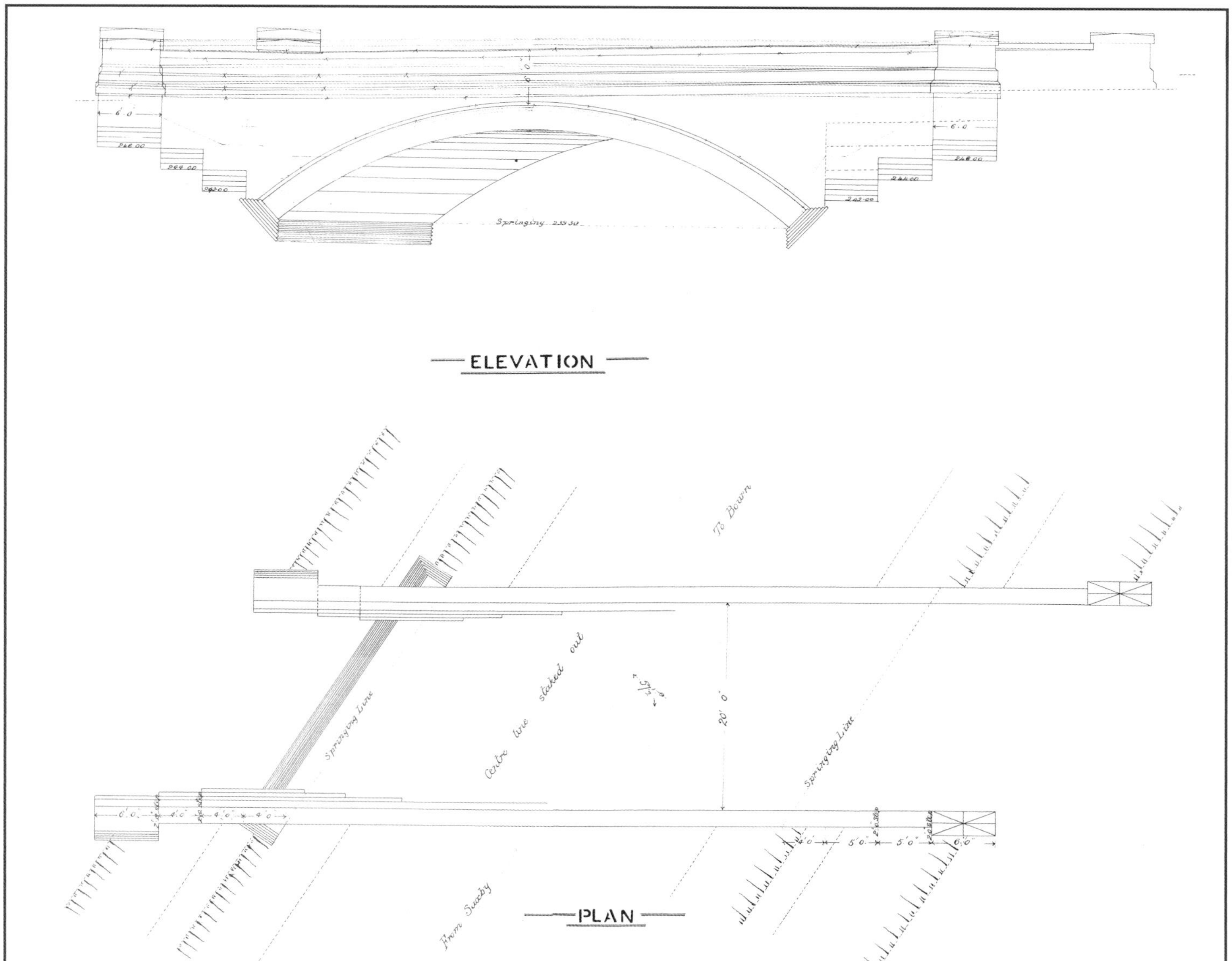

ELEVATION

PLAN

Drawing 3

remnant of the bench in the cutting side. The railway trackbed here shows an unusual new use. It is now used for training racehorses, the white dot in the distance in Photograph 22 being one of the furlong markers.

This is one of the bridges for which the original drawings survive in the archives of the Midland and Great Northern Railway Circle. It was a skew bridge, that is, crossing the line at an angle other than at a right angle. The underside of the arch was 15 ft 6 ins above the level of the trackbed and the width for the roadway between the parapets was 20 ft.

DRAWING 3

(previous page)

Drawing 3 is part of the original drawing for this bridge. Note on the plan how the staking out of the centre line of the single line of rails is shown. This is on the north side of a cutting created for a double line of rails.

The original drawing is held within the archive at the Midland Railway Study Centre at Derby (Ref: 1986-1407/15).

[21] National Archives, RAIL 491/548.

[22] Victoria County History, 'West Bromwich: Economic History' in M. W. Greenslade (ed.), *A History of the County of Stafford 17* (Oxford, 1976), 27-43.

[23] Personal correspondence, Ceramic Enquiries Team, The Potteries Museum and Art Gallery, Stoke on Trent, July 2008.

BRICK SAMPLES

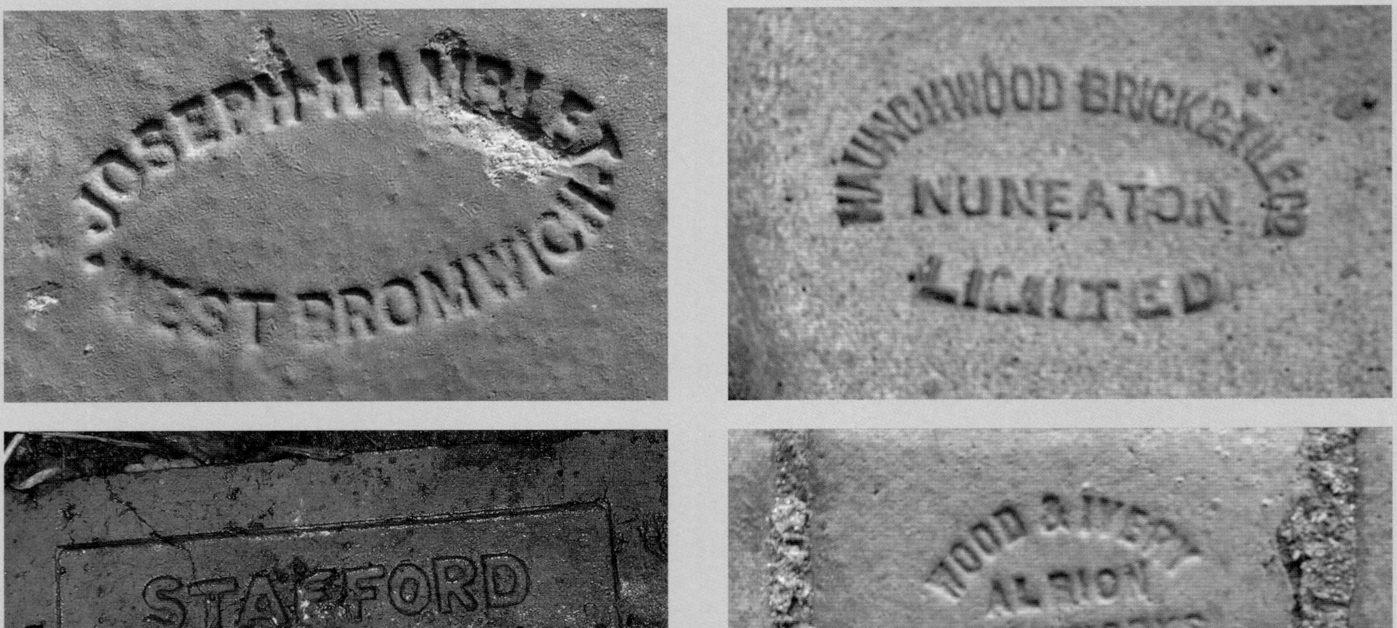

Samples of named bricks. See the caption to Photograph 20 for the details.

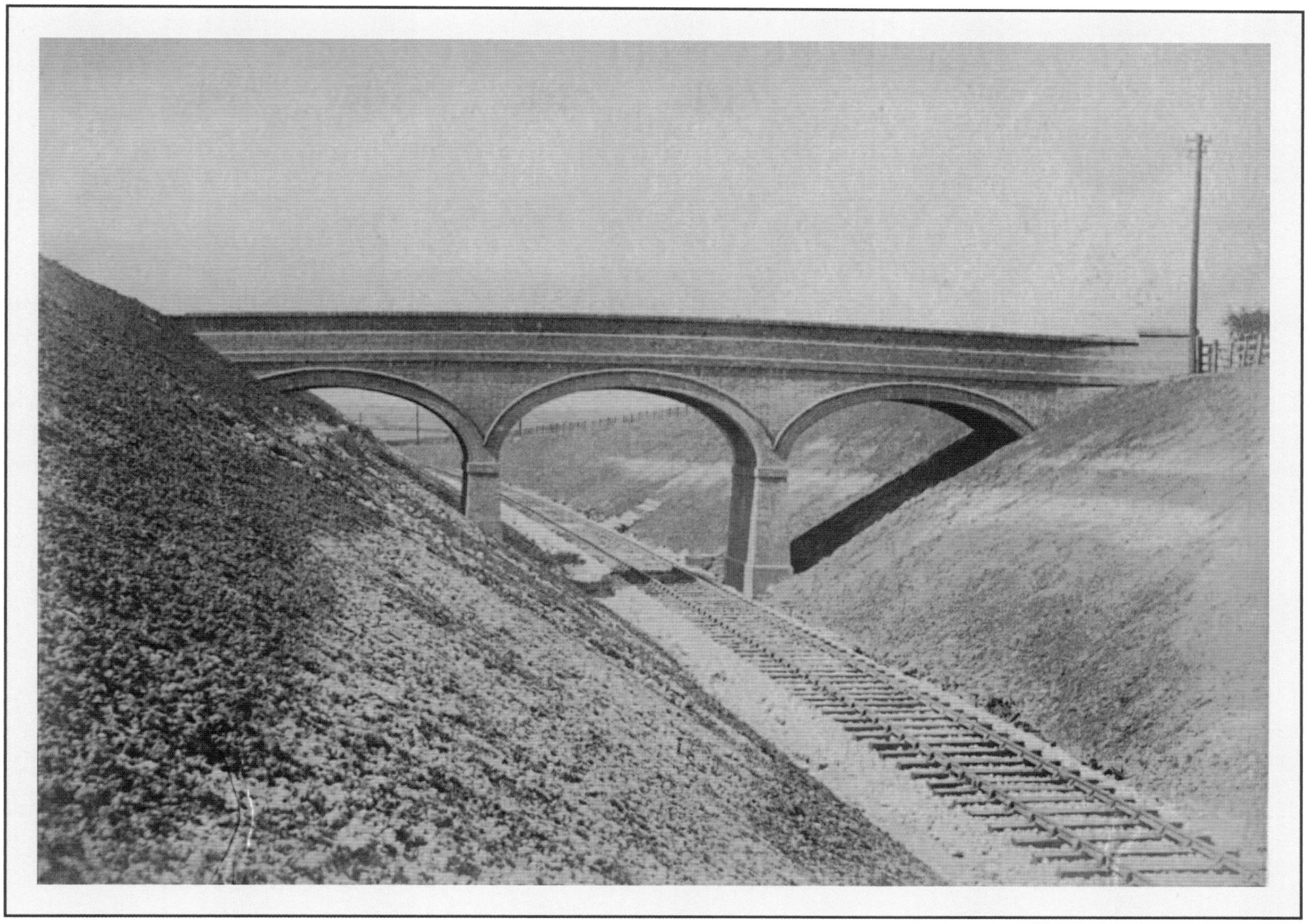

POTTER'S HILL, CASTLE BYTHAM

PHOTOGRAPH 23

Bridge 31 spanned the line in the open countryside almost a mile west of Castle Bytham. With its three elliptical arches it is similar to the bridges east of Little Bytham. It spanned a deeper cutting here, however, and this is possibly the reason for the tapering piers.

When this photograph was taken the permanent way had been laid. On the single line section bridges over the track were wide enough for a second track to be laid if need be, subject only to some widening of the cutting. The track was laid on the north side and the line would be widened to the south. This photograph, of the east elevation of the bridge, shows this clearly. The southerly, left-hand, pier is partially buried in the side of the cutting but was no doubt constructed to full depth with the soil subsequently backfilled round it when the cutting side was profiled.

When Charles Wilson took this photograph, he was standing almost on the junction between two of the construction contracts. This bridge was within the contract awarded to J. D. Nowell, while the route behind the photographer was within that awarded to Mousley. The Nowell family were stonemasons in Dewsbury before becoming railway contractors and they went on to build for at least twenty railway companies.[24] Their contract here, dated 7 October 1890, was for £54,403 12s 3d for the railway between Spalding and 'Bourn'.[25] Bourn station was renamed Bourne from 1 July 1893, the date of the creation of the Midland and Great Northern Joint Railway and almost one month after goods trains first ran between Bourne and Saxby.[26]

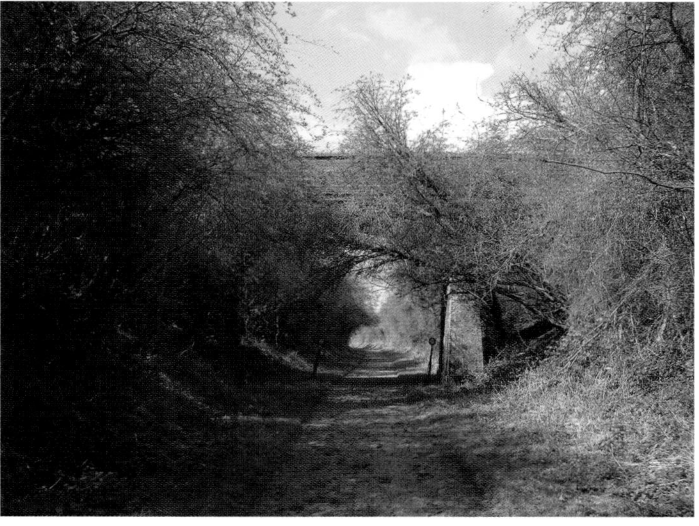

Photograph 24

PHOTOGRAPH 24

(previous page)

The undergrowth that has grown unchecked on the cutting sides since closure has prohibited the same view being taken today. However, Photograph 24, from the track bed, clearly shows the batter to the piers, which identifies the location. The route here is part of the racehorse training gallop (also shown in Photograph 21), which clearly sees much more regular use here.

DRAWING 4

Drawing 4 is one of the original drawings for Bridge 31. What it shows clearly is the grace of the three elliptical arches. This design was used for eight of the bridges between Bourne and Little Bytham, albeit the others all had piers with vertical sides rather than the tapering piers used in this location, possibly due to the cutting here being much deeper. The original drawing is held within the archive at the Midland Railway Study Centre at Derby (Ref 1986-1407/10).

[24] Jack Simmons, *The Victorian Railway* (London, 1995), 116.

[25] National Archives, RAIL 491/548.

[26] C. R. Clinker, *Clinker's Register of Closed Passenger Stations and Goods Depots in England, Scotland and Wales, 1830–1980* (new ed., Weston super Mare, 1988).

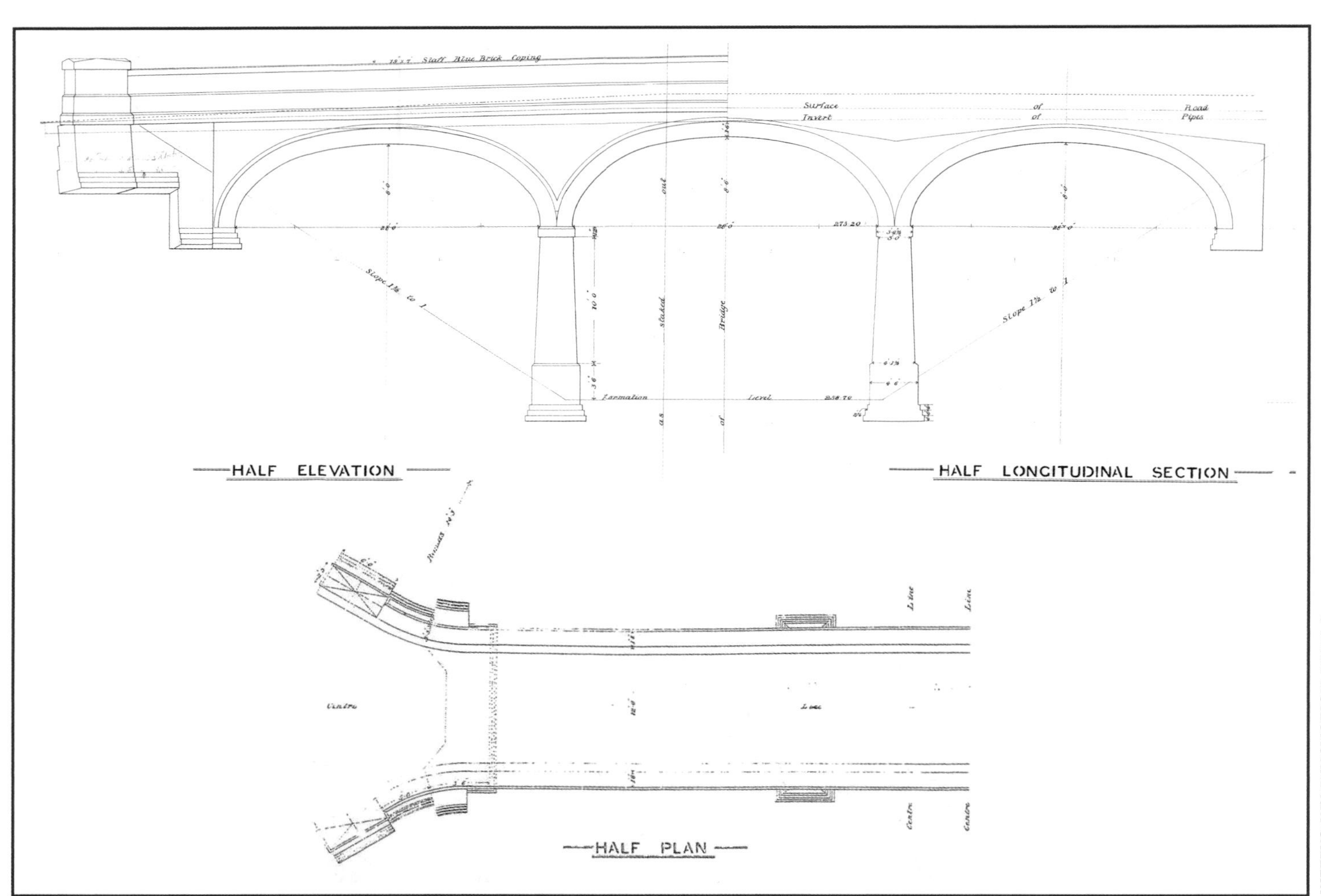

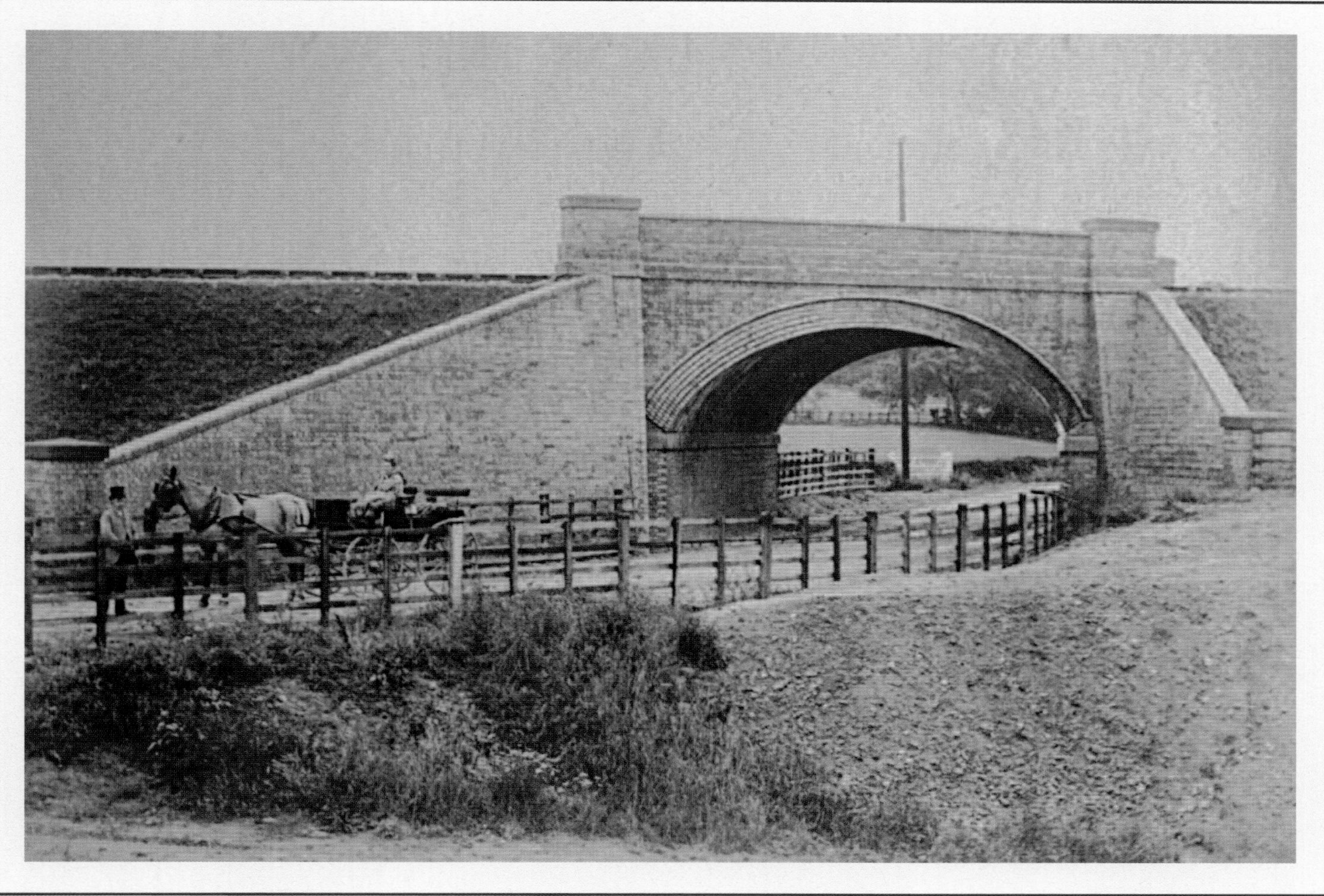

MORKERY LANE BRIDGE, CASTLE BYTHAM

PHOTOGRAPH 25

About half way between Castle Bytham and South Witham, Bridge 28 carries the line over Morkery Lane. This is another example (as with Bridge 38 shown in Photograph 16) where the line of the road was altered to provide a better angle for the railway bridge, creating the double bend in what was previously a straight section of road.

Of particular interest here is the pony and trap, as a copy of this photograph owned by one of Charles Wilson's descendants has the words 'Mother, Charles wife Hannah, in Mr Dockray's wagon near Wymondham' written on the back. So on at least one occasion Charles was accompanied by his wife when he carried out his visits.

A copy of the Contract for this section of the line survives in the National Archives.[27] Included within the Day Work section is the heading 'Allow for providing horse, trap and man for the use of the Resident Engineer or his Assistants whenever required during carrying out of work'. In the 1891 Census a John A. Dockray is recorded as a Civil Engineer and Railway Contractor's Agent, aged 34 and living as a lodger in a house at West End, Wymondham. It is likely that he was the site manager for Holme and King.

PHOTOGRAPH 26

The bridge survives, with a height limit of 4 metres (13 ft), but Photograph 26 had to be taken from a slightly different viewpoint due to tree growth in the intervening years. The retaining wall in the foreground is prominent in both photographs and clearly identifies the location.

[27] National Archives, RAIL 491/548.

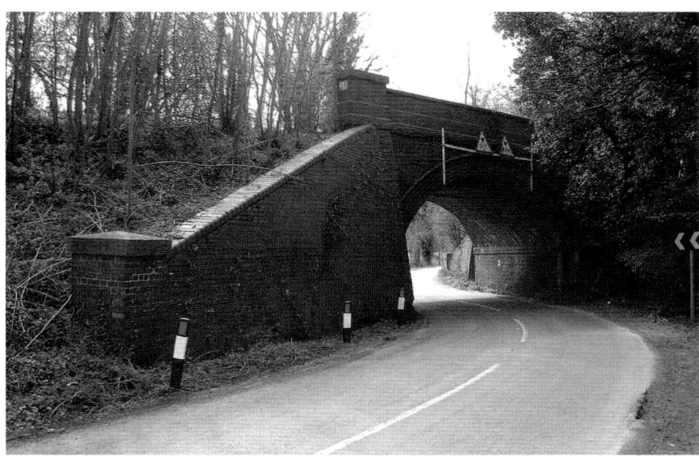

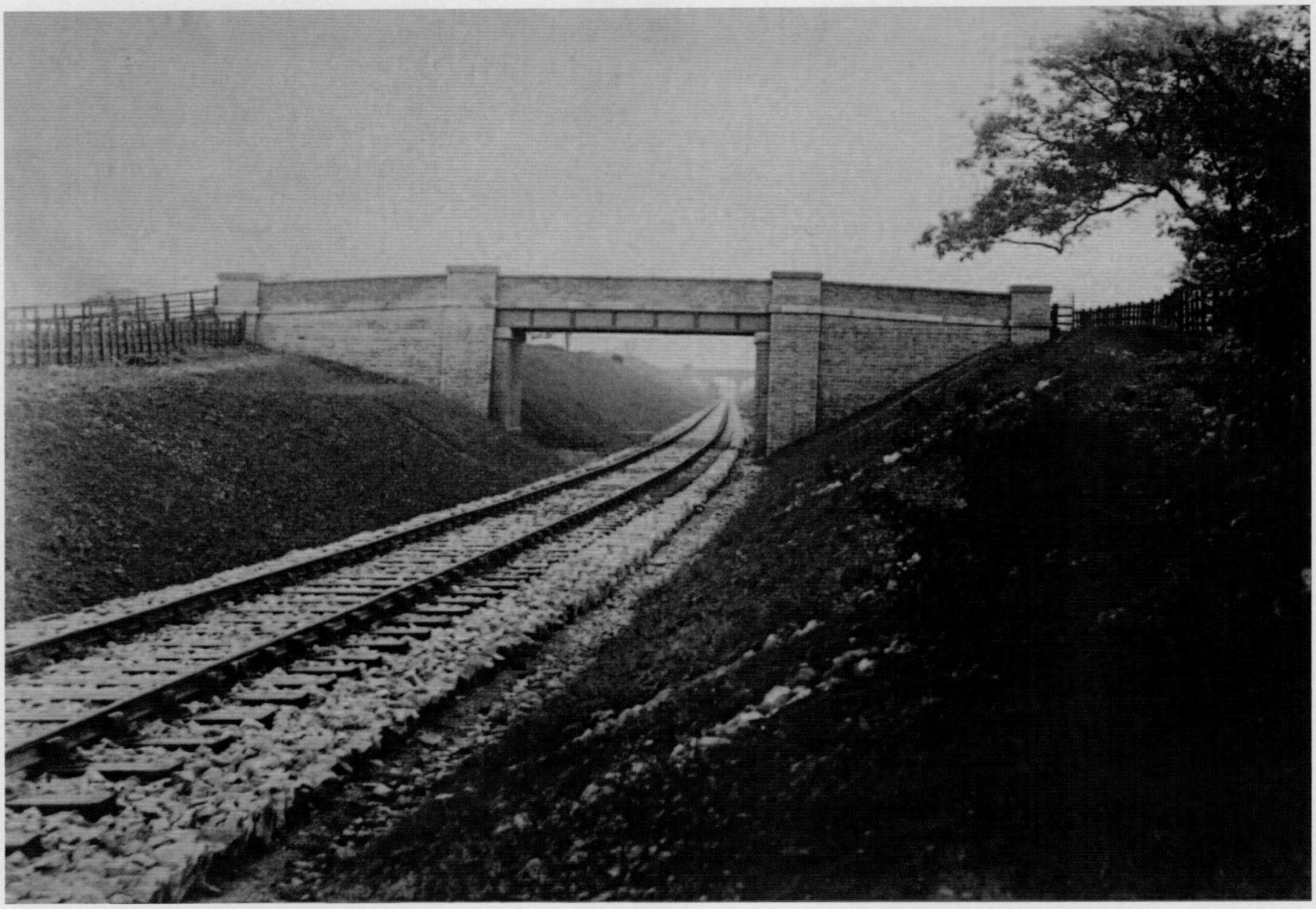

OCCUPATION BRIDGE AT SOUTH WITHAM

PHOTOGRAPH 27

Bridge 27 was an occupation bridge at the east end of the deep cutting through the landscape east of South Witham. Bridge 26 can be seen in the distance through the arch. On the original print the steam navvy shown in Photographs 28 and 29 can be discerned. Note the use here of a steel beam to carry the roadway rather than a brick arch and that the permanent way has been laid and ballasted. This bridge has been demolished and the cutting from here to Bridge 26 has disappeared following its use as a landfill site.

The estimated cost of Bridge 27 in the priced contract was £419 10s and for the larger, three arched, Bridge 26, £494 10s.[28] The estimated costs of all the bridges in this contract are itemised in Appendix A, although it should be noted that not all of the bridges originally allowed for were actually built.

The precise dressing of the cutting sides was achieved with the use of a frame, the dimensions of which are shown on the diagram. This is taken from the notebook compiled by G. Anderson who worked under Charles Wilson in 1875 and referred to on page 14. The long side of the frame would be constructed to fit the required slope. A plumb line ensured that the side of the frame was vertical and if the slope had been correctly dressed the frame would show this clearly.

[28] National Archives, RAIL 491/548

INSTRUMENT FOR DRESSING SLOPES

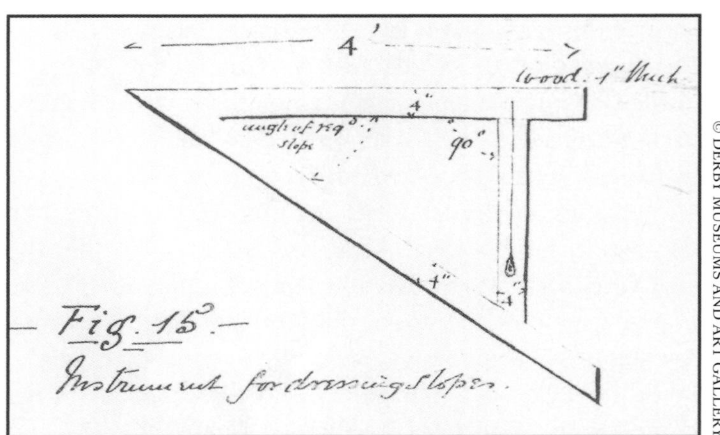

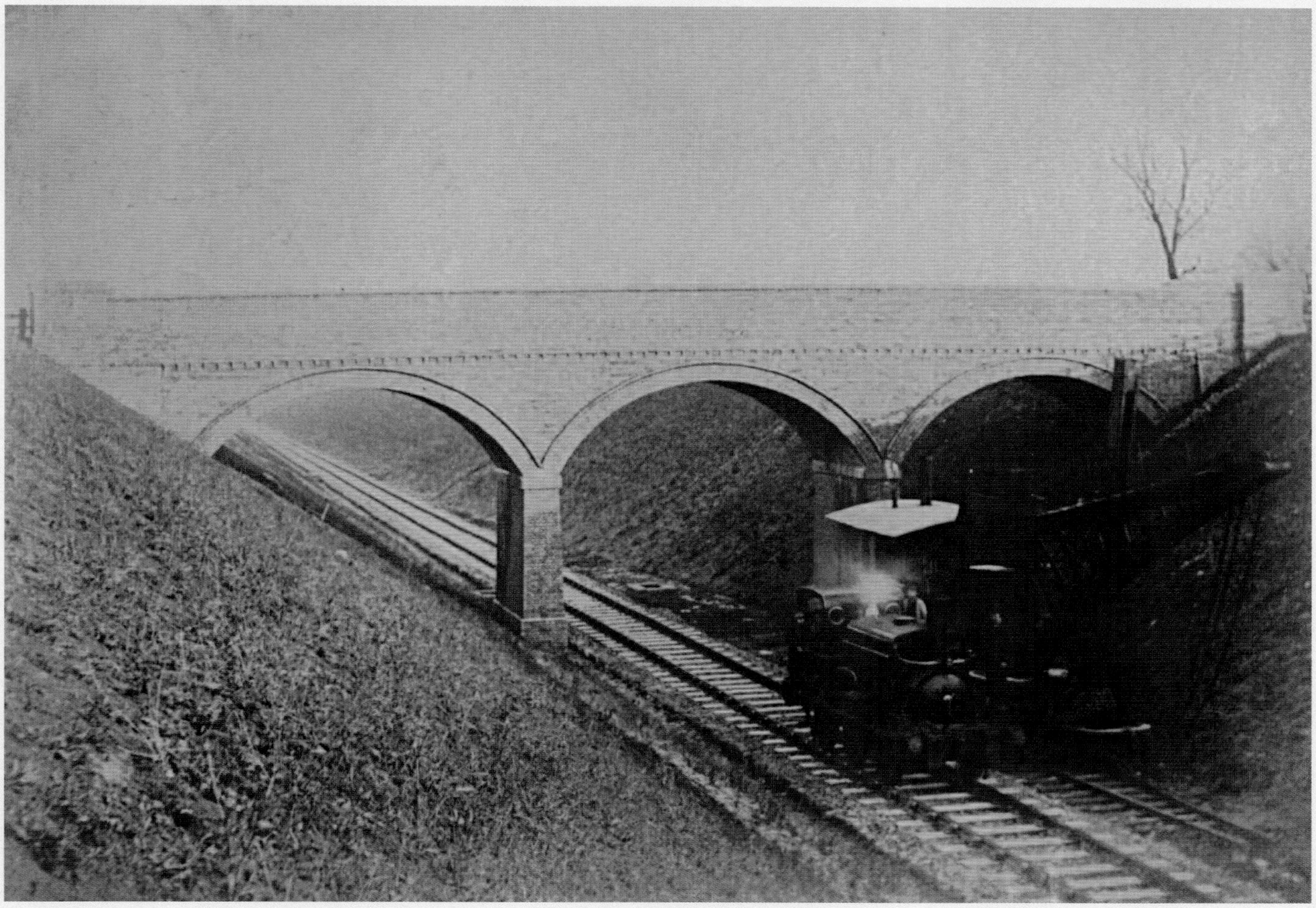

MORKERY LANE, SOUTH WITHAM

PHOTOGRAPHS 28 AND 29

(above and next page, top)

Photographs 28 and 29 both show the same bridge, believed to be Bridge 26. The cutting here has been used for landfill and all that remains of Bridge 26 is the western parapet, the foot of which is now at ground level and, at the time of the recent survey, in the midst of a vast expanse of brambles. Photograph 28 is believed to show the bridge from the west and 29 from the east. The value of these views is in the machinery they show. The locomotive shown in Photograph 28 is probably the same as shown in Photograph 31 and its details are included there. It appears to be a posed shot with the locomotive stationary.

At the side of the track is a Dunbar Ruston Steam Navvy. One of these is shown more clearly in Photograph 30. This is a standard 10 nominal horse power machine; usually know as a 'tower' navvy. Ruston, Proctor and Co of Lincoln was the first European manufacturer of steam excavators. The first model, of which this is one, was built in 1875 and was in production up to 1903. Sales averaged ten per annum but the big boost to their use was the construction of the Manchester Ship Canal between 1888 and 1894. In 1888 the Canal contractor, T. A. Walker, ordered no fewer than forty-two machines from Rustons.[29] The machine here is standing on an isolated section of track, probably awaiting dismantling prior to removal from the site. The jib is facing to the west and this indicates that this machine had been used to construct the cutting from the eastern end, working to the west.

DUNBAR RUSTON STEAM NAVVY

PHOTOGRAPH 30

(page 47)

It is not known exactly where Photograph 30 was taken. All of the three contractors for the line used Ruston steam navvies. One (Works Number 66) was delivered to Holme and King in Liverpool in September 1882. Two were delivered to Nowell and Co: Works Number 156 to Manchester in June 1889, and Works Number 157 to Chorlton cum Hardy in September 1889. Works Number 173 was delivered to W. Mousley in May 1891, despatched to Little Bytham station.[30] The latter must have been used on this line.

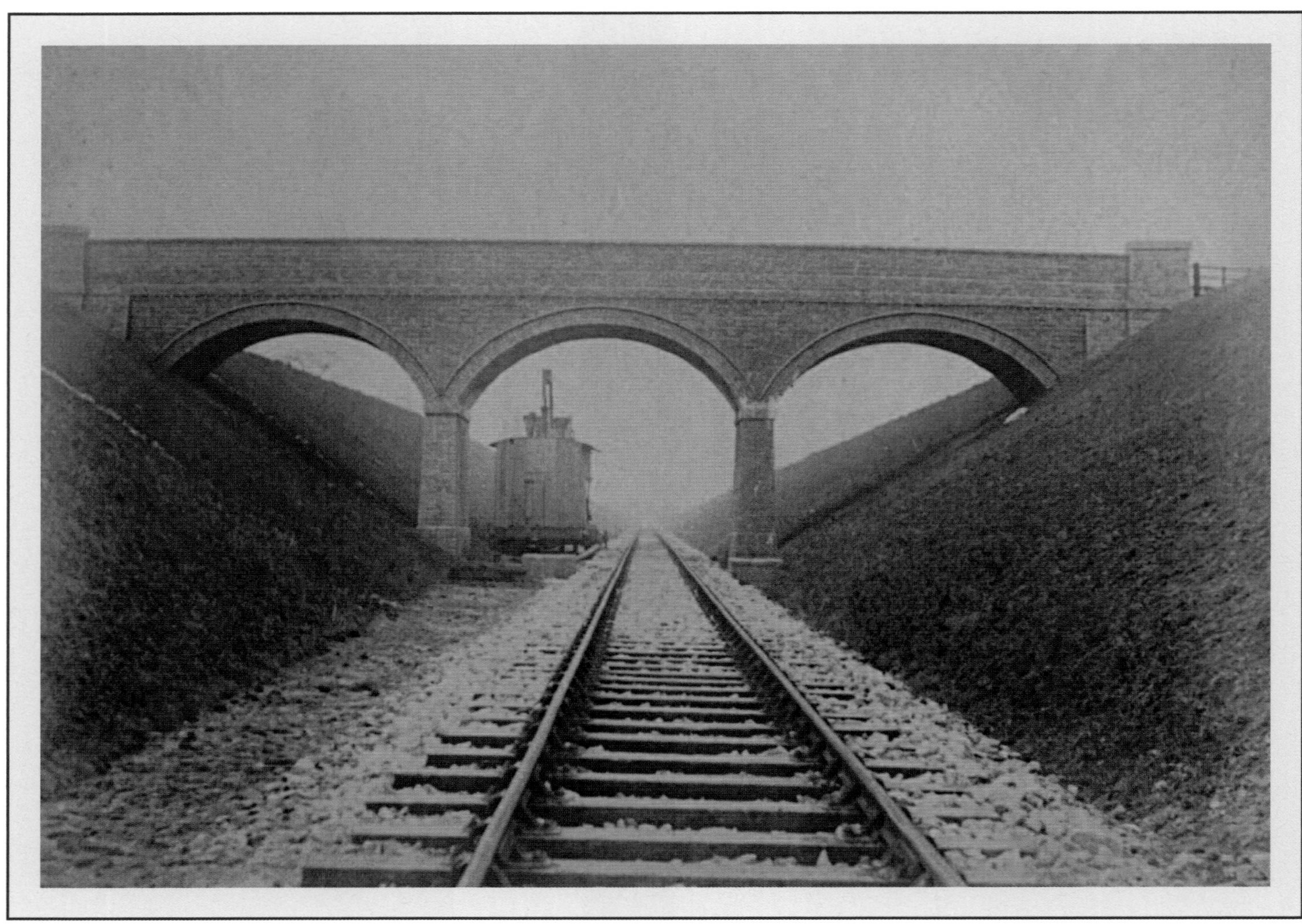

Photograph 29

The *Grantham Journal* reported in December 1890 that a steam navvy, manufacturer unknown, was delivered to Corby station, taken to South Witham, erected by the roadside and put to work on the cutting near to the Blue Bull.[31] Corby must refer to Corby Glen station, six miles away by road, which was renamed as Corby (Lincs.) in 1937 and Corby Glen in 1947 to distinguish it from Corby in Northamptonshire.[32] The steam navvy was being used by Nowell to dig the cutting, about half a mile long and 18 feet deep, over which the Great North Road (now the A1) passes. The paper also reported that at South Witham 'no such piece of machinery having before been seen here, its removal from Corby station to the village and erection by the roadside prior to its being conveyed to the cutting near the Blue Bull, caused much interest among the inhabitants of this and neighbouring parishes.'

Given the transport difficulties of the time, these machines were designed to be dismantled for carriage in railway wagons, and by road haulage, for transport between sites. The machine shown in Photographs 28 and 29 is awaiting this. Economically, it made sense to leave it on site when its work was completed in the hope that it could be delivered direct to its next contract by rail.

The machine was carried on railway wheels. There were two sets. One, inside the frame, was a set of standard gauge railway wheels. The axle on which these were mounted extended outside the frame to a set of double flanged railway wheels. The latter are clearly seen in Photograph 30. The machine was moved backwards and forwards, under its own steam power, on the standard gauge wheels. Once in position to dig, short lengths of rail were laid under the axle wheel ends and these then acted as stabilisers when digging and slewing.

There was a crew of three. A stoker would attend to the firebox and boiler. This is out of sight to the left in Photograph 30. The Driver (the man on the left) stood on a platform in front of the boiler, in charge of the levers controlling forward and reverse movement, the swing of the jib and the lifting and lowering of the bucket. At the front stood the Crowd Man. He had charge of the wheel that operated the 'crowd' action, the forward and back movement of the bucket in relation to the face. In addition to these there might have been an oiler, and two or more men who were responsible for preparing the ground to enable the whole operation to move forward. Photograph 30 shows men who appear to be engaged in laying track alongside the navvy.

The boom could swing through 180 degrees and the machine would cut a semicircular face, semicircular both in plan and elevation, in front of it. Photograph 30 shows a

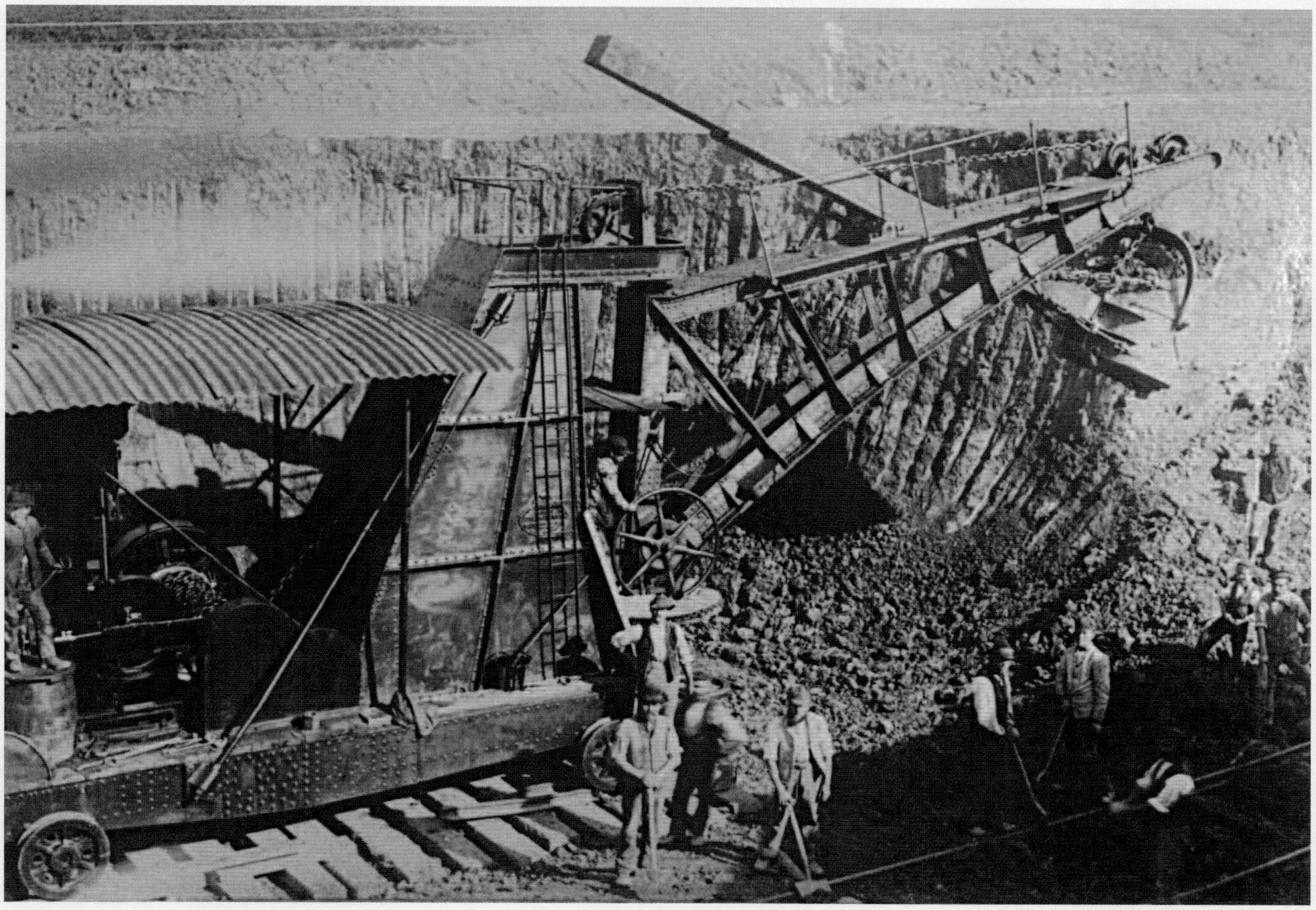

Photograph 30

cutting being created with two parallel cuts. An earlier excavation is in front of the machine which is engaged in widening the cut on the other side. The bucket was emptied into a wagon on a line laid alongside it. Where space permitted a line would be laid on either side to allow empties to be pushed on one side while it was filling on the other. The individual wagons were usually moved by horses.

The corrugated iron roof is a local modification provided to keep the men and machinery dry during wet weather. Note also the use of chain rather than wire rope.

These contracts are an early example of the use of steam navvies on such a scale for the construction of a railway. The little use made prior to this period may have been due to the relatively low cost of labour, which meant that the capital investment was not regarded by contractors as being economic before.[33] The *Grantham Journal* reported in 1891 that in the Broadgate Hill cutting (see Photographs 31 and 33) it was found that they removed 900 or 1000 cubic yards a day.[34] In 1887 it was estimated that a steam navvy could do the work of seventy men. One hundred men were required to excavate by hand 600 yards, the same distance as a machine could do, in a day. Thirty men were required to work with a machine in that length, hence a saving of seventy.[35]

When the cutting under the Great North Road was complete, the *Grantham Journal* reported that a cutting was then being made between the Great North Road and Morkery Lane and, as this was of larger dimensions, two steam navvies had been set to work, one at the east end and one at the west.[36] Photographs 28 and 29 show the one that worked from the east end.

See the extract from the Census on Page 49 which identifies two navvy drivers and one fireman, who were living in South Witham at this time.

[29] Peter Robinson, *Lincoln's Excavators: The Ruston Years, 1875–1930* (Wellington, 2003).

[30] Correspondence with Derek Broughton, Ruston Bucyrus archivist, April 2008.

[31] *Grantham Journal* (20 December 1890), p. 6 col. 4.

[32] Clinker, *Register of Closed Passenger Stations and Goods Depots, 1830–1980* (1988).

[33] Terry Coleman, *The Railway Navvies*, rev. edn (Harmondsworth, 1968), 53-55.

[34] *Grantham Journal* (18 April 1891), p. 6, col. 3.

[35] Coleman, *The Railway Navvies.*

[36] *Grantham Journal* (18 April 1891), p. 6, col. 3.

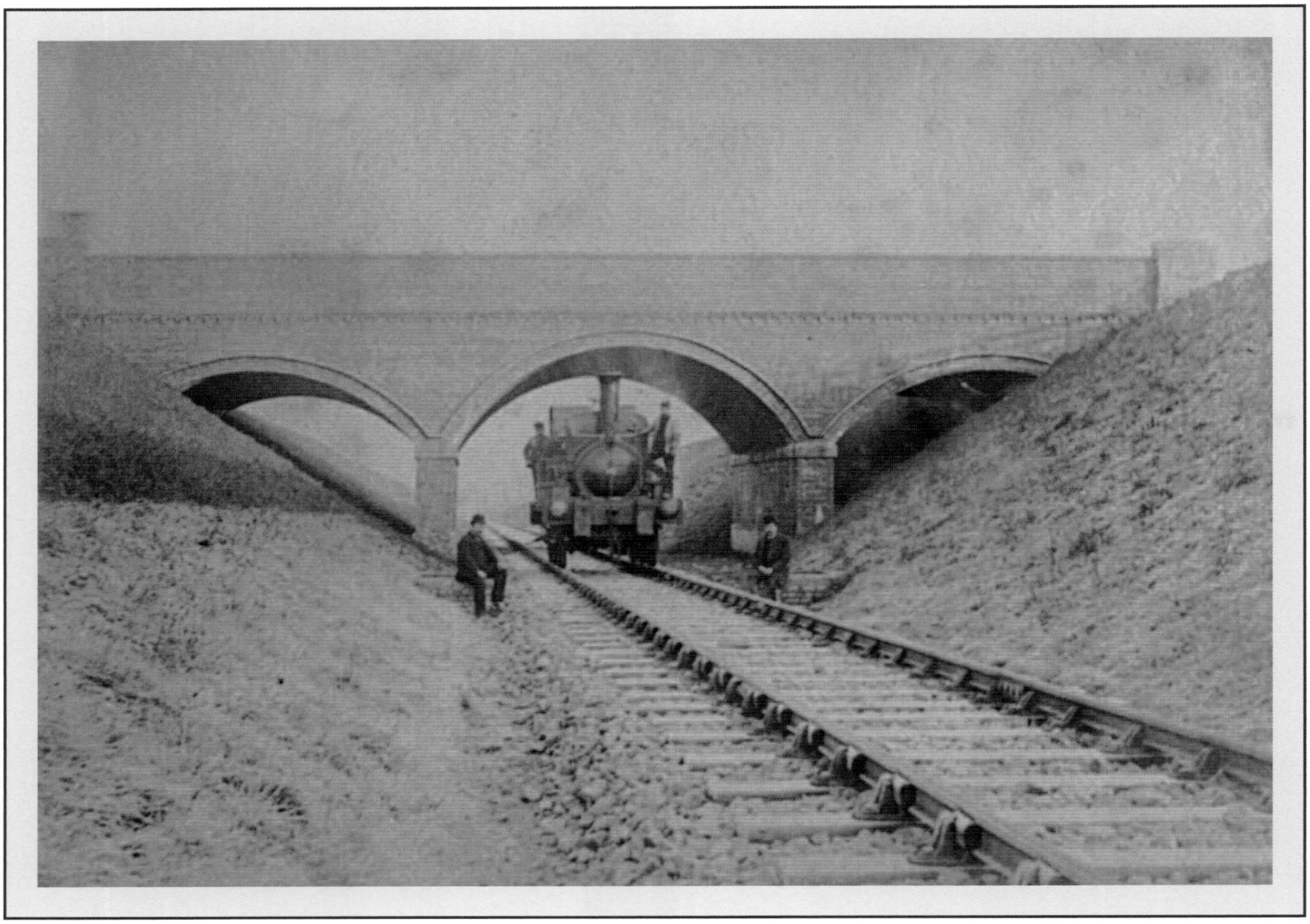

GREAT NORTH ROAD BRIDGE, SOUTH WITHAM

(see also Maps 5 and 6)

PHOTOGRAPH 31

Bridge 25 still carries what is now the southbound carriageway of the A1, the Great North Road, over the railway. Photograph 31 shows it from the west (see Map 6). The works here appear to have been completed. This photograph may show an inspection of the completed works, as it appears to be posed. Photograph 28 may have been taken at a previous stop, a short while earlier. The locomotive is stationary in both photographs and the same four men appear. The two on the engine will be the driver and fireman, with two officials seated here on drainage manholes.

This is on Nowell's contract and the locomotive is an 0-6-0 saddle tank with inside cylinders. It is probably Manning Wardle Class L, Works Number 1121/89, GERTRUDE. This was delivered new to J. D. Nowell at Belle Vue, Manchester, in 1889.[37] The clean state indicates a pride in their engine by the crew and is a feature often seen of such locomotives in their working environment. It may also be that it was cleaned specially for use on this inspection. Note that it has two sets of buffers, normal round and spring loaded for conventional wagons and rectangular dumb buffers for the contractor's tip wagons. GERTRUDE was one of five Manning Wardle locomotives offered for sale in the Contract Journal of 2 November 1892 at Saxby, by G. N. Dixon on behalf of J. D. Nowell.

The cutting sides have been grassed down. The contract required that the sloping faces, after they had been

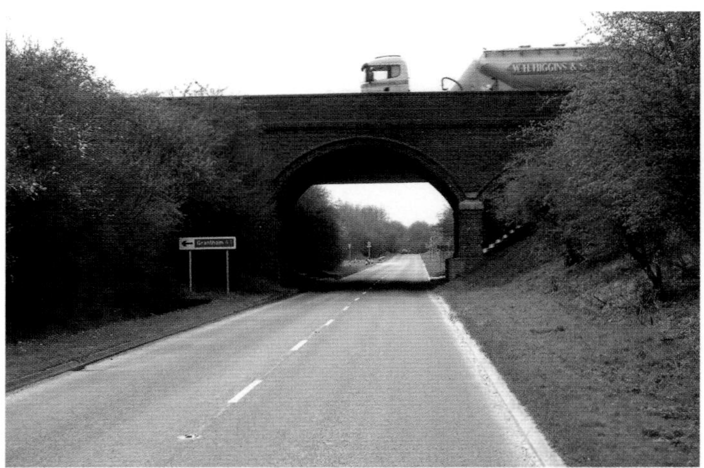

Photograph 32

trimmed to the proper slope, were to be sodded with turf reclaimed from elsewhere on the works, or top soiled, again with reclaimed soil, and sown with an equal mix of rye grass and white clover seed, at 30lbs to the acre.[38]

PHOTOGRAPH 32

(opposite, below)

This section of the line has been utilised to carry the South Witham – Castle Bytham road underneath the A1 for the creation of a grade separated junction with the dual carriageway. The northbound carriageway bridge has been built alongside the earlier bridge. For that reason the comparison, Photograph 32, is a view of the same bridge but from the other direction.

[37] Correspondence from the Industrial Locomotive Society, April 2008.

[38] National Archives, RAIL 491/548.

EXTRACT FROM 1891 CENSUS – SOUTH WITHAM

Administrative County of Lincoln Kesteven — The undermentioned Houses are situate within the Boundaries of the — Page 1 — 121

Civil Parish of South Witham — Municipal Borough of — Municipal Ward of — Urban Sanitary District of — Town or Village or Hamlet of South Witham — Rural Sanitary District of Grantham — Parliamentary Division of Stamford — Ecclesiastical Parish or District of South Witham

1 No. of Schedule	2 ROAD, STREET, &c., and No. or NAME of HOUSE	3 HOUSES Inhabited	4 HOUSES Uninhabited	5 Number of rooms occupied if less than five	6 NAME and Surname of each Person	7 RELATION to Head of Family	8 CONDITION as to Marriage	9 AGE last Birthday of Males	10 AGE last Birthday of Females	11 PROFESSION or OCCUPATION	12 Employer	13 Employed	14 Neither Employer nor Employed	15 WHERE BORN	16 If (1) Deaf-and-Dumb (2) Blind (3) Lunatic, Imbecile or Idiot
1	Poor Row (School House)	1			Frederick Gibson	Head	M	32		Elementary School Teacher		X		Lincolnsh: Market Rasen	
					Alice Gibson	Wife	M		29	Teacher Assistant		X		Berks: Reading	
2	Do Do	1		4	Thomas Tate	Head	M	73		Cottager & Coal Dealer	X			Lincsh: S. Witham	
					Mary Tate	Wife	M		69					Northamptonsh: Easton	
					Thomas W. Sails	Grandson	S	20		Farm Servant		X		Lincsh: S. Witham	
					Samuel Holland	Brother-in-law	Widr	60		Stone Cutter		X		Northamptonsh: Easton	
3	Do Do	1			Joseph Talton	Hd	M	64		Blacksmith		X		Leicestersh: Wymondham	
					Jane Do	Wife	M		69					Rutland: Thistleton	
					Elizabeth Do	Daur	S		27	Dressmaker			X	Do Mkt Overton	
4	High St	1			William Craven	Head	M	60		Grocer, Baker & Provision Dealer	X			Leicestersh: Wymondham	
					Lucy Do	Wife	M		59					Lincolnsh: Lincoln	
					Philip Do	Son	S	26		Grocer and Baker		X		Do South Witham	
					Harry W. Do	Son	M	23		Baker & Confectioner		X		Do Do	
					Albert C. Do	Son	S	21		Fireman Engine Cleaner		X		Do Do	
					Edith M. Do	Daur	S		15	Home Assistant		X		Do Do	
5	Do Do	1			John D. Frisby	Head	M	58		Cottager			X	Lincolnsh: S. Witham	
					Eliza Do	Wife	M		57					Do Swinstead	
					Thomas Batty	Nephew		8		Scholar				Durham: Hartburn	
6	Do Do	1		4	William Heaton	Hd	M	31		Steam Navvy Driver		X		Bucks: Little Woolstone	
					Fanny Do	Wife	M		32					Do Old Bradwell	
					Lillian Do	Daur	S		6					Essex: Grays	
					Alice Do	Daur	S		4					Bucks: Old Bradwell	
					Clara Do	Daur	S		1					Cheshire: Lower Walton	
					Edwin Do	Lodger	S	29		Steam Navvy Driver		X		Bucks: Little Woolstone	
					John Moore	Do	S	27		Navvy Fireman		X		Yorkshire: Sowerby Bridge	
7	Do Do	1		3	John Sharpe	Hd	S	52		Agricultural Labourer		X		Lincs: S. Witham	
					Emma Do	Niece	S		32	Housekeeper		X		Do Do	
8	Do Do	1			Annie Dunmore	Hd	Widow		54	Farmer & Timber Merchant	X			Lincs: Irnham	
					William S. Do	Son	S	26		Farmer's Son		X		Do S. Witham	
					Ada V. Billingham	Daur	M		25					Do Do	
					Annie Dunmore	Daur	S		24	Helper in House		X		Do Do	
8	Total of Houses and of Tenements with less than Five Rooms	8	0	3	Total of Males and Females	16	15								

This is a page from the 1891 Census which includes the names of steam navvy crew members. William Heaton, aged 31, gave his occupation as Steam Navvy Driver. He was living on the High Street with his wife and three daughters, the latter aged 6 and under. Their different birthplaces indicate the peripatetic lifestyle of the railway worker. Lodging with them was Edwin Heaton, aged 29 and also a Steam Navvy Driver. He was born at the same place as William so the two were probably brothers. The final member of the household was another lodger, John Moore, a Navvy Fireman.

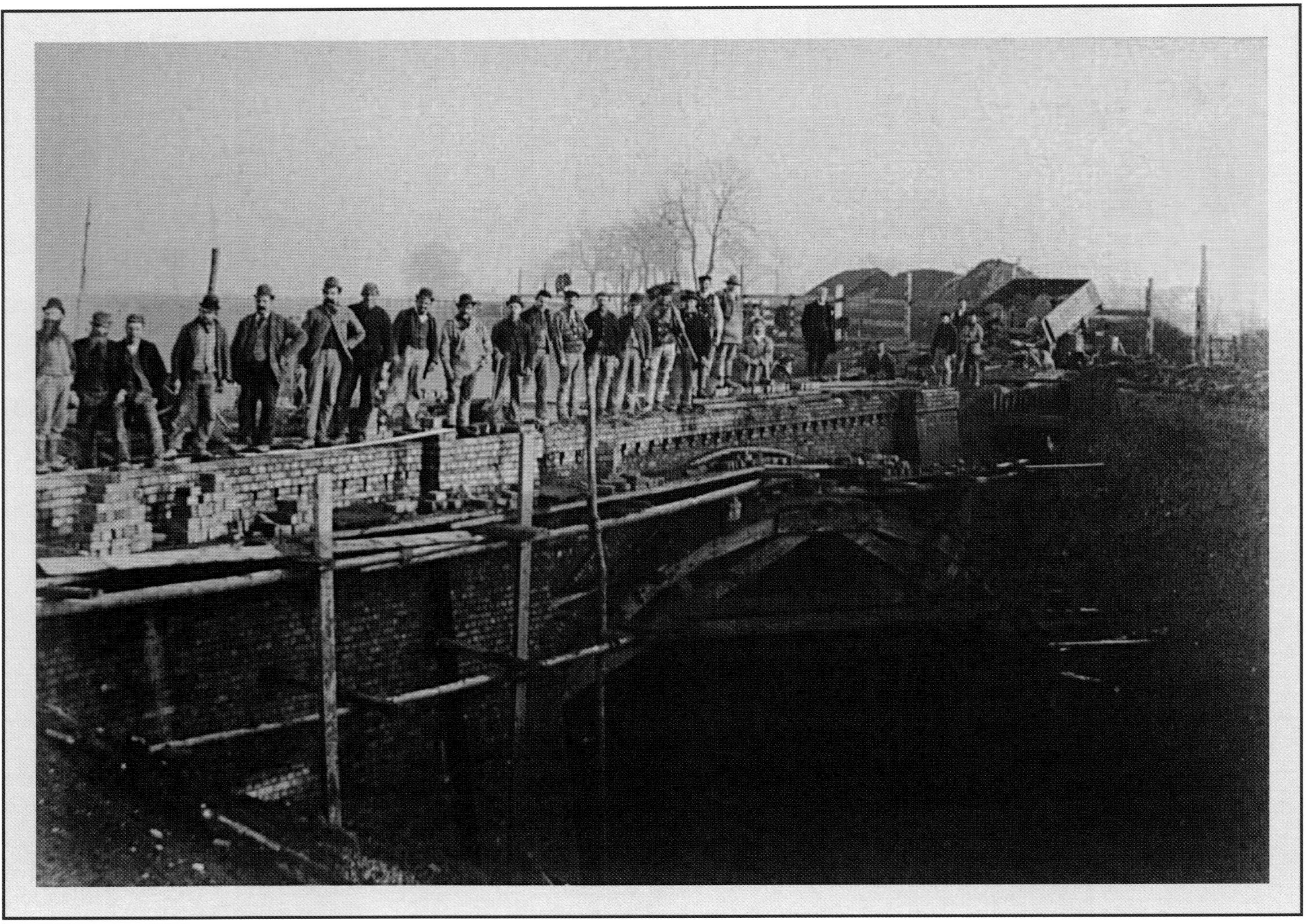

BROADGATE ROAD BRIDGE, SOUTH WITHAM

PHOTOGRAPH 33

Photograph 33 is of Bridge 24 under construction (see Maps 5 and 6). This was just over 400m to the west of the Great North Road bridge. Here the line of the railway and Broadgate Road coincided and, as the railway was in a cutting, the road was diverted for a short length with this skew bridge to carry it over the railway. Note that the timber formwork under the bridge built on the line of the railway clearly indicates the angle of the skew and also that no attempt is made for it to emulate the skew. The scaffolding is also of timber. The trees in the background indicate the line of Broadgate Road on its way to the junction with the Great North Road and the Blue Bull Inn in the south east corner of the crossroads at that point (see Map 5).

There are twenty-four men in the picture. For a bridge such as this they are likely to include bricklayers, stonemasons and carpenters as well as labourers. They are wearing clothes typical of their class at this time: jackets (high buttoned, often worn with the top button done up), waistcoats and tight legged trousers. Almost all of the men wear hats, a mix of caps and bowlers.

Here the *Grantham Journal* reported that 'An embankment is being made past the positions where the operation of "tipping" may be watched, and the skill of the men and horses will be readily acknowledged. About 100 men are at present at work constructing the railway and carting materials to the scene of the operations. They are divided into three gangs, each under the eye of a foreman termed a standing ganger, all again being under the supervision of a skilled workman termed a walking ganger, who goes from one body of labourers to another, seeing that the work is being done thoroughly and in a businesslike manner. One body of men is at work obtaining stone from a quarry situated in Mill Lane; another party is engaged in making a cutting in the hillside of the village on the side and between the village and the Great North Road; whilst a third body may be found at work beyond the Blue Bull, in the direction of Castle Bytham, all working with an energy that bids fair to overcome any difficulty.'[39]

The 1891 Census recorded 128 men living within South Witham Parish who were working on the railway, eighty-five of whom were recorded as Navvies or Railway Labourers. Sixty-one men were described as lodgers or boarders at thirty-two separate addresses. Many were living in navvy houses but significant numbers lodged with local people and provided an additional income for village residents. Of those whose place of birth was recorded, twenty-six came from Lincolnshire (at least ten of these from South Witham), while the remainder originated from twenty other counties.

The contract with Nowell required the workmen to be paid in cash once every fortnight at least.[40] In the early days of railways navvies were sometimes paid in vouchers which were only redeemable at shops owned by the contractor. Unscrupulous contractors charged high prices, especially where men were employed in isolated locations. The requirement of the Midland Railway in this contract is an expression of how steps had been subsequently taken, both by Parliament and responsible agencies such as the railway companies, to treat the man fairly and let them decide how and where their money was to be spent. Despite their hard living and hard drinking reputation there had always been workers, both itinerant and recruited locally, who had families to support. This approach is further reinforced by the more benevolent attitude relating to the navvy housing (see Photograph 65).

On the far side of the bridge is a side tipping wagon. This indicates that there was a siding here, probably running steeply up from the western end of the cutting. This is not surprising as it was at this end of the bridge where, as the *Grantham Journal* reported, 'Offices were erected in a field occupied by Mr Cooper, about half a mile from the Blue Bull ... carpenter's and blacksmith's shops were also erected upon the same site, which also provided accommodation for a circular saw, and a mortar mill, both driven by steam power. Not one hundred yards away a well is being sunk to provide water to feed the engines. The cluster of buildings mentioned above may be said to be the centre of the proposed works.'[41]

The side tipping wagon was known as the Manchester Ship Canal type because they were first used on that project. They had a capacity of 4.5 cubic yards (3.44 cubic metres).[42] The one in the photograph appears to be discharging some large pieces of stone. These are probably for the infilling of the brickwork inside the abutment. The workmen on the bridge, fourth and sixth from the right, are standing at a lower level inside the brickwork, the former up to his waist level, probably on the last load to be delivered. If suitable stone were available from excavations for the railway then it would be used elsewhere within the works (see box on page 60).

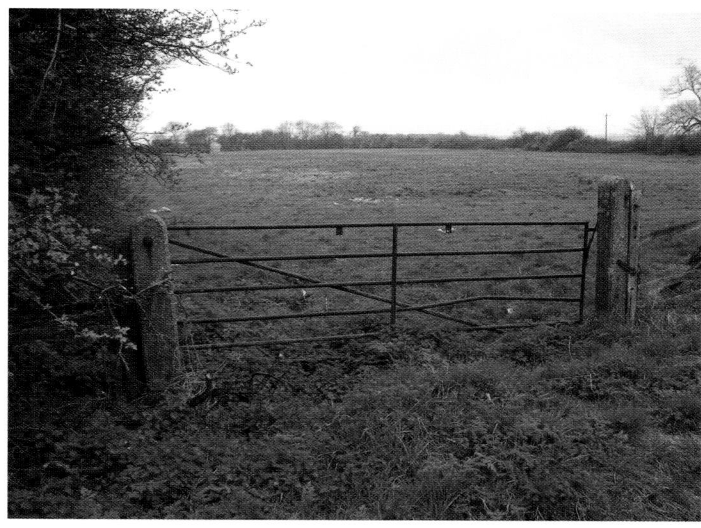

PHOTOGRAPH 34

The contractor for this central section of the line was J. D. Nowell of Manchester and their site agent was Mr H. M. Nowell. His photograph appears in Chapter 2. Their contract length was almost 6¾ miles long, of which this was the midpoint. The field used still today has a railway gate and gate posts, a legacy of the use by the contractor, and the gateway is shown in Photograph 34. The field is identified on Map 5 as that numbered 42, owned by Robert Cecil Cooper and Alice Cooper and as the field numbered 202 on Map 6.

PHOTOGRAPH 35

(overleaf)

Photograph 35 shows the completed Bridge 24 and cutting. In the distance is the Great North Road bridge. Between the two is a steam navvy. This one is facing the opposite way to those in photographs 28 and 34. They can be said, therefore, to be the two steam navvies involved in creating the cuttings here and discussed in detail in the earlier captions.

In 1964 extensive roadworks to create the present grade separated junction with the A1 included the conversion of the railway route into a road (see Photograph 31). As part of this, the cutting was widened and this bridge was demolished.

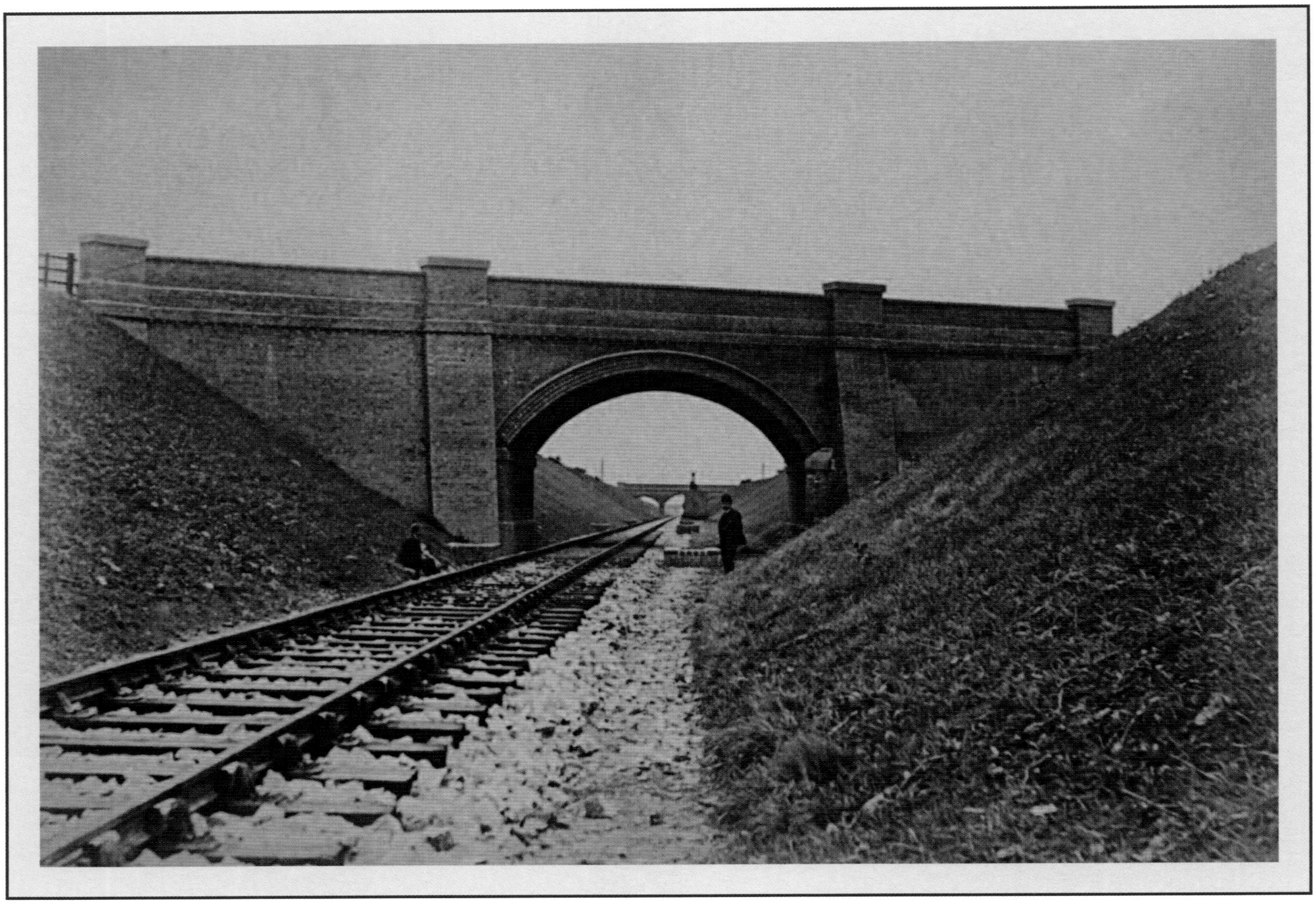

Photograph 35

MAP 5

(opposite, top)
Midland Railway, Saxby and Bourne Line. Extract from Plan showing land taken from the Earl of Dysart. 1891. Great North Road and Broadgate Road, South Witham.[43]

To the lower right the Blue Bull Inn stands at the crossroads of the Great North Road (identified as the North Road on the map) and the road between South Witham, off to the left, and Castle Bytham, off to the right. The lane running west from the crossroads is Broadgate Road. The most efficient way for one route to cross another on a bridge, in terms of construction, is at right angles; the North Road crossing is a perfect example of this. The least efficient is at a very shallow angle, of which the Broadgate Road crossing is another good example.

To reduce the angle of the skew required for the bridge here some additional land was required to realign Broadgate Road. To the north of the line, in field 41 owned by Matthew Cheator Wootten, the slight bulge (identified as having an area of 0 acres 1 rood 12 perches) is the area required for the realigned roadway on the north side of the future bridge. This feature can also be seen on Map 6.

The small triangular area of 26 perches at the north end of field 39, owned by Robert Shilcock, was also taken over by the Midland Railway and used to site a row of three navvy dwellings, with timber boarded walls and a slate roof. These were subsequently converted into two dwellings and used to house railway employees. They survived until after the Second World War and are shown on Map 6.

MAP 6

(opposite, bottom)
OS 1/2500 County Series Map, 1904. Great North Road and Broadgate Road, South Witham.

From the right is the bridge carrying the Great North Road (see Photograph 31) and the skew bridge of Broadgate Road seen in Photographs 33 and 35. Note the former navvy houses in the angle between Broadgate Road and the railway, comparable with those shown on Map 3 and Map 8. Field No 202, to the south of the Broadgate Road bridge, is that in which the contractor's compound was located.

39 *Grantham Journal* (10 November 1890), p. 6, cols 3 and 4.
40 National Archives, RAIL 491/548.
41 *Grantham Journal* (10 November 1890), p. 6, cols 3 and 4.
42 Peter Manktelow, *Steam Shovels* (Princes Risborough, 2004).
43 Map in the ownership of G. Geeson, via the South Witham Archaeological Group. Known as the 'Geeson Map'.

OF RUTLAND
OF LINCOLN
F SOUTH WITHAM
of Dysart
Anne Dunmore
Earl of Dysart
Matthew Cheator Wootten
Earl of Dysart
Betsy Wildman
Earl of Dysart
To Grantham
NORTH ROAD
George Pilkington's Trustees
Parish Boundary
Robert Shilcock
Earl of Dysart
Robert Cecil Cooper and Alice Cooper
Samuel Gambrell
Earl of Dysart
Earl of Dysart
George Skillington
Blue Bull
County and Parish Boundary
OF RUTLAND
3·156 Chains to an Inch.
20 Chains

Map 5

Broadgate Road
F.P.
M.R.
SAXBY & BOURNE
Union & R.D.By
4ft.R.H.

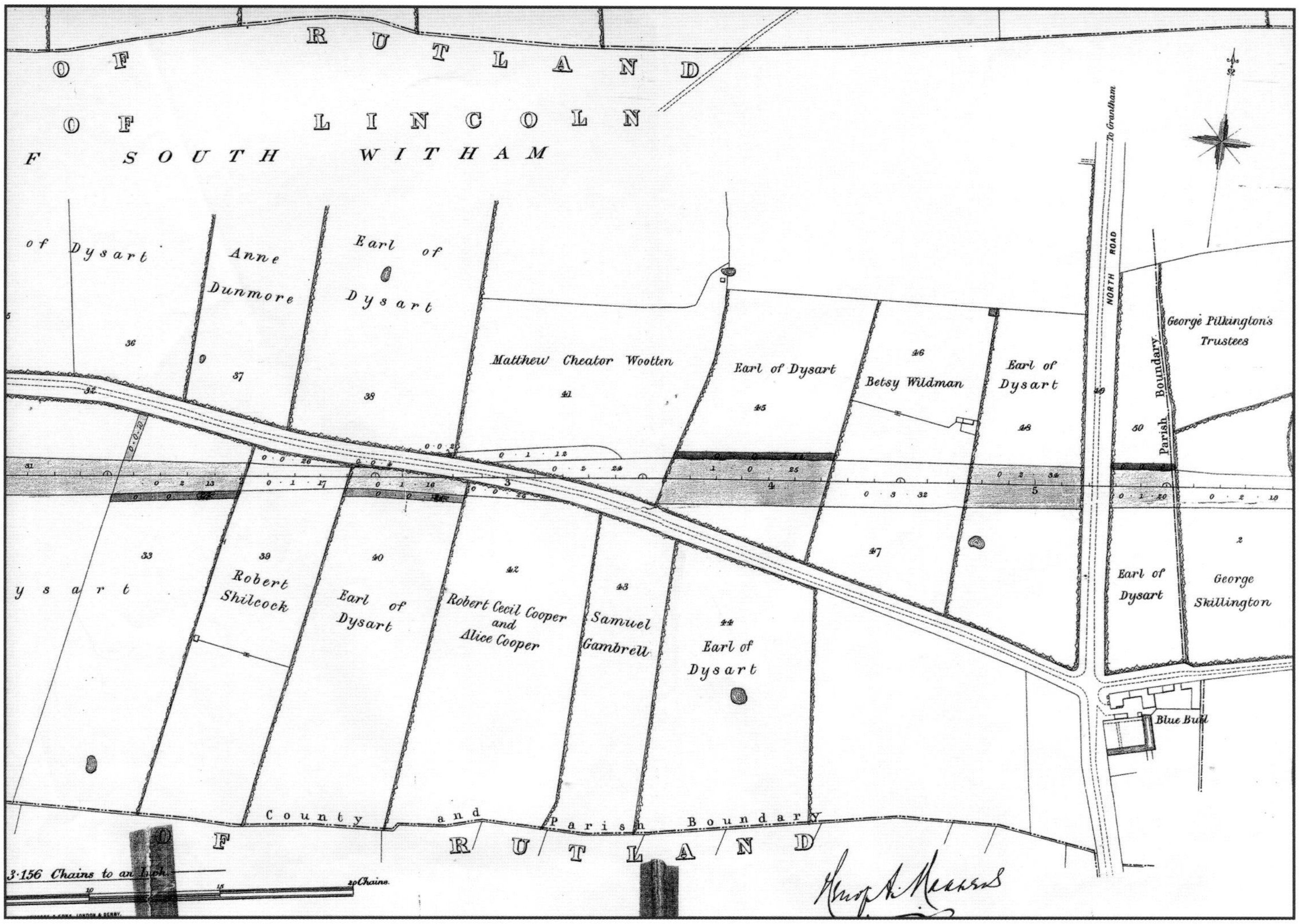

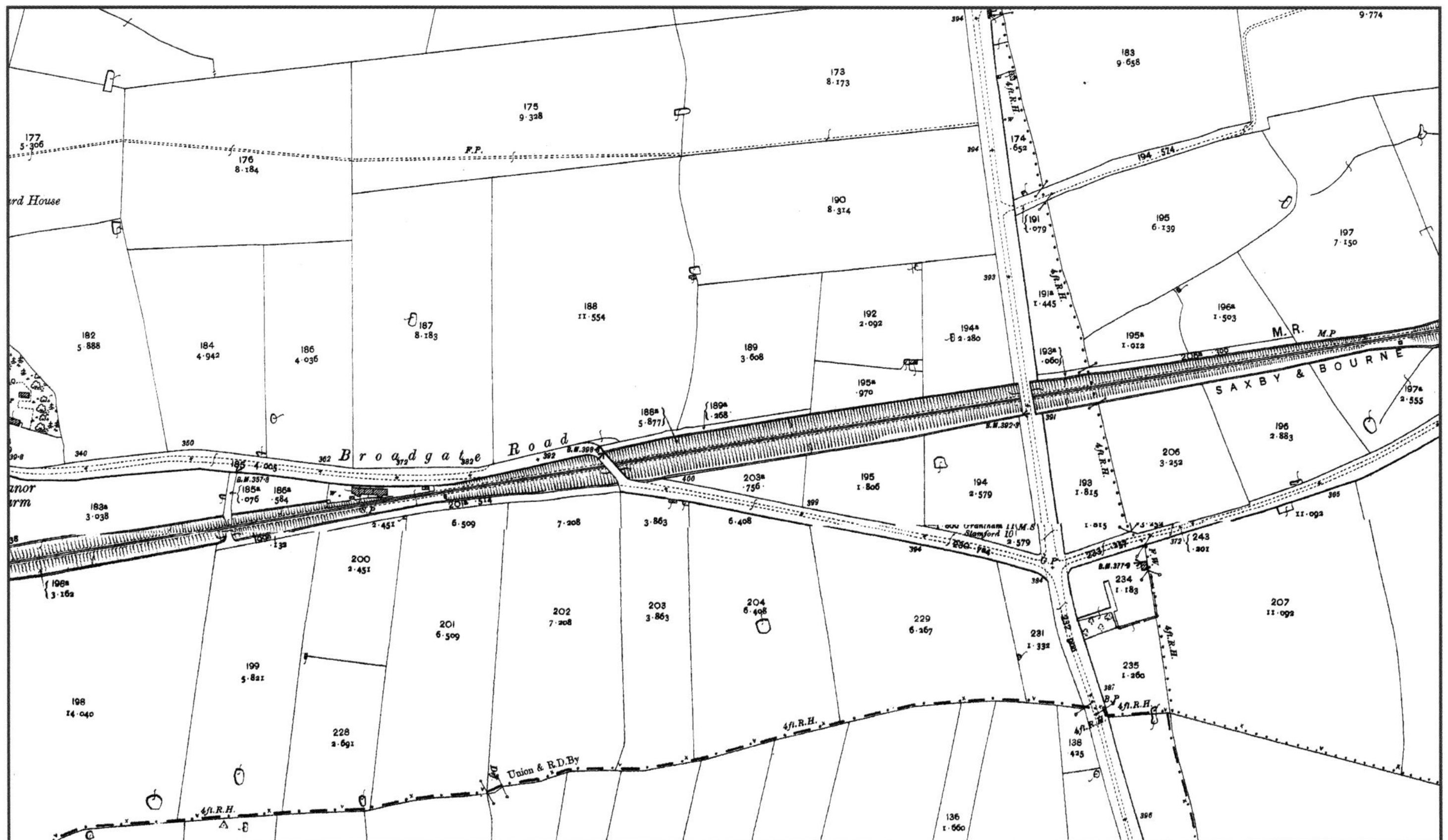

Map 6

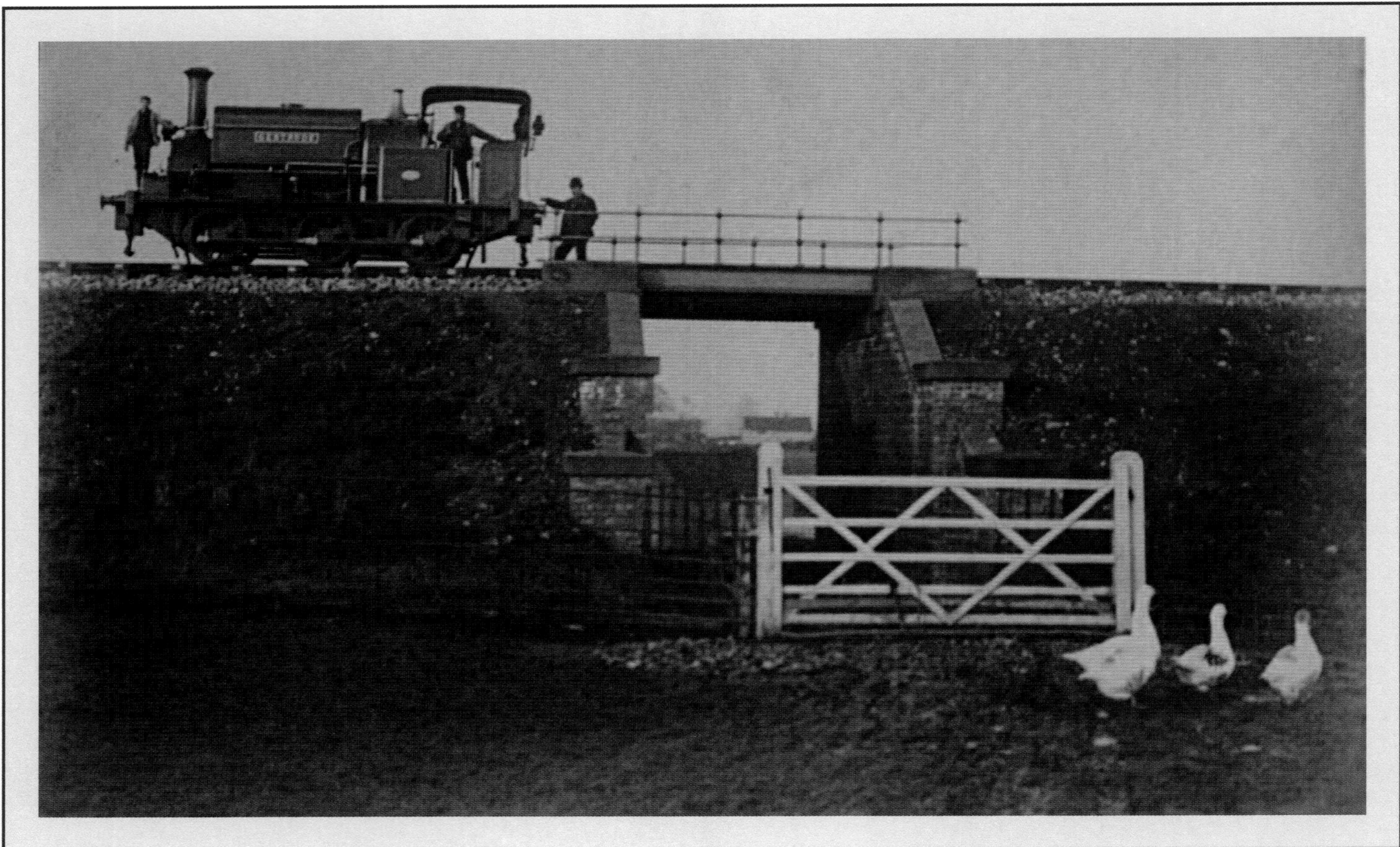

MANOR FARM BRIDGE, SOUTH WITHAM

PHOTOGRAPH 36

There is one contractor's locomotive that can be clearly identified and this is GERTRUDE, shown in Photograph 36 posing alongside Bridge 22 at South Witham. GERTRUDE, owned by the contractor J. D. Nowell, was a Manning Wardle, Class L, 0-6-0 saddle tank, Works Number 1121/1889. Built in 1889, she was delivered to Nowells at Belle Vue in Manchester.[44] She was still relatively new when photographed here but her clean condition is an indication of the pride in their engines of the crews working on these contracts.

Bridge 22 was an occupation bridge built to give the buildings of Manor Farm a link with the fields to the south. Gates were provided at either end to control the movement of livestock. On the single track section, this is a good example of how enough land was taken from the beginning to allow for the line to be doubled in future if needed. The gate and iron fence show the extent of the land taken. While the bridge was built for single track its abutments were also built to allow for extension. On the far side of the line is a vertical face to the abutment. On this side, the brickwork slopes down to intermediate piers. If the line had been doubled, the brickwork and piers on this side would have been extended upwards and the embankment widened.

The contract with Nowell quoted the same price for iron fencing as for timber post and five rail fencing. The price for 8000 linear yards of the former and 8600 yards of the latter was 3s 6d per yard.[45]

PHOTOGRAPH 37

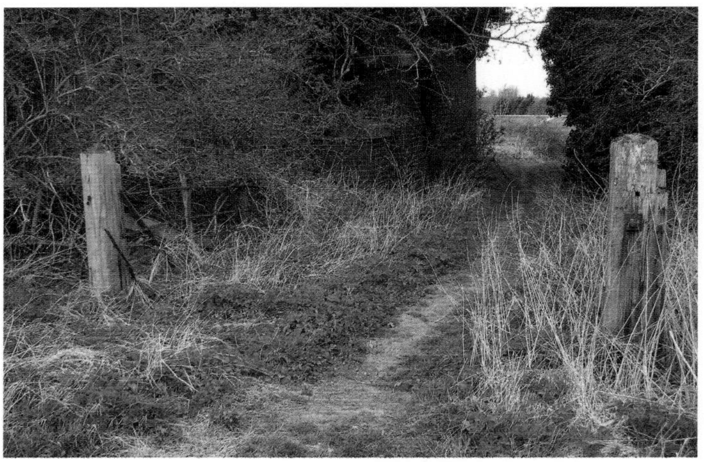

The contrasting photograph was taken from a slightly different viewpoint, as the original would show only rampant overgrowth. Photograph 37 shows that the abutments, gateposts and some of the iron fencing still survive, although the bridge itself has been removed.

[44] Correspondence from the Industrial Locomotive Society, April 2008.

[45] National Archives, RAIL 491/548.

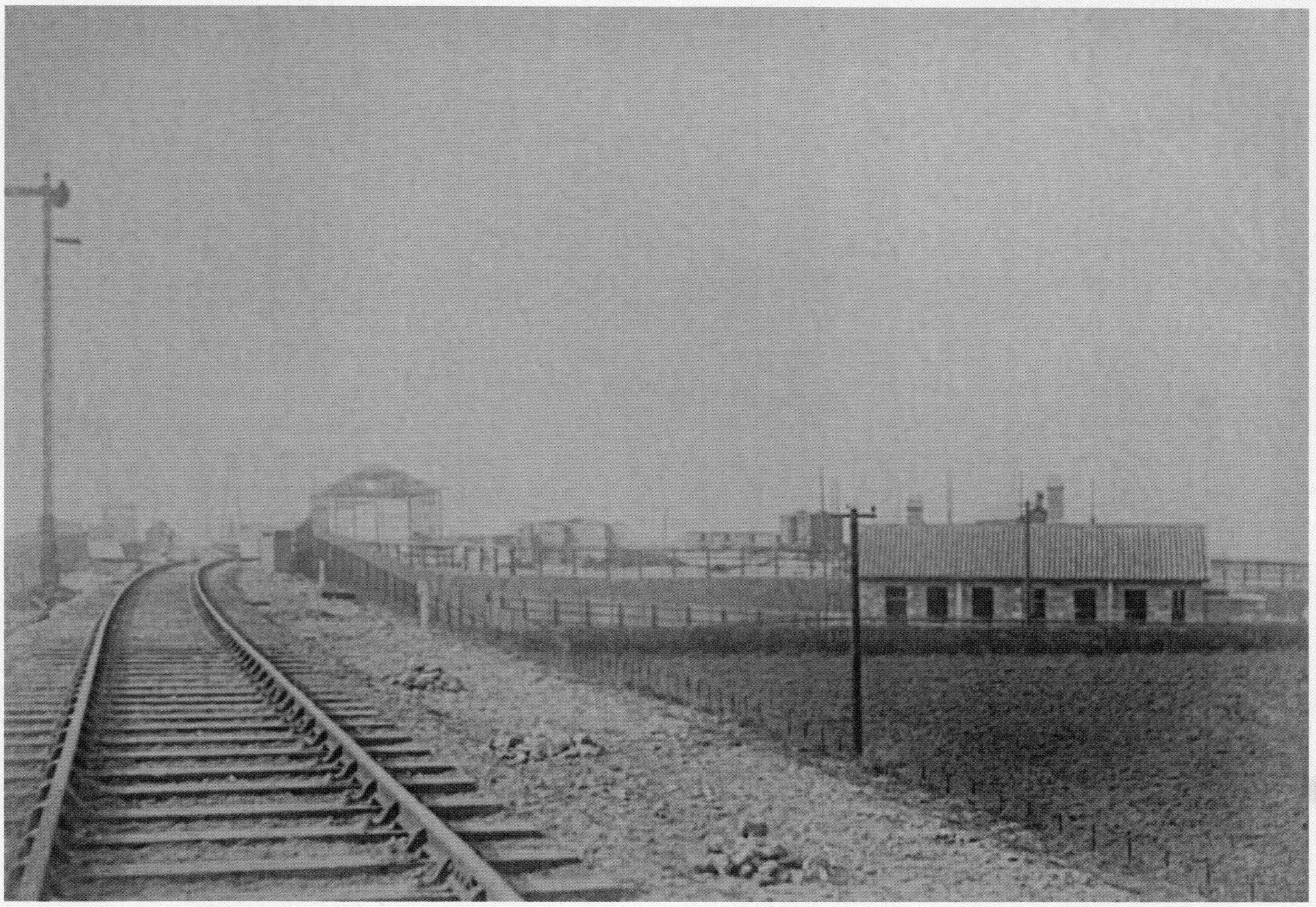

SOUTH WITHAM STATION

(See also Map 7)

PHOTOGRAPH 38

Photograph 38 is taken looking west over Bridge 20 at South Witham to the station beyond. Construction work is ongoing. The station offices to the right (see Photograph 39 below) still have timber scaffolding to the left-hand gable and the goods shed is still a timber frame. Its brick infill walls have yet to be constructed. Its lightweight construction is probably because it was built on ground made up to the level of the railway.

Both platforms are in place, that to the left with its waiting shelter. The line comprised a double track loop through the station but the track on the left-hand side appears not to have been laid. Note also the signal on the tall post to the left of the line, sited to give engine drivers a clear view of it against the sky. At least some goods sidings are in place in the yard, as four wagons can be seen in the centre right rear. When the line opened there were two coal merchants, Messrs Ellis and Everard and Mr T. G. Bennett of Market Overton, operating from here.[46]

What is interesting is what appears to be a lattice tower in the background. It is said that the railway construction revealed at South Witham a bed of Lincolnshire Limestone sixty feet thick, which the Holwell Iron Co. Ltd started to work in 1895, a year after the line opened, for use as a flux in their furnaces near Melton Mowbray. The limestone overlaid a bed of ironstone but it was not until later that this began to be worked.[47]

In 1890 the *Grantham Journal* reported that 'one body of men is at work obtaining stone from a quarry situated in Mill Lane'. The plan of the land take does show a small stone pit on Mill Lane predating the railway.[48] Extensive quarrying has taken place here in the past one hundred years. However, Tonks identifies the site of the earliest stone working as being further west, east of where Buckminster Sidings were eventually built.[49] The Midland Railway survey of the line, undated but believed to have been carried out in the period between 1906 and 1912, shows a disused limestone quarry alongside the line by Bridge 18 but nothing in this field adjacent to the station.[50]

Working of the quarry north of the station commenced about 1907. A hoist was built which raised the stone from the quarry floor and discharged it into railway wagons in a siding at the west end of the goods yard, about in the position of the tower shown in Photograph 38. Map 7 of 1904 has no feature marked at this location, so whatever the use it must have been temporary. The reason for the tower

remains unknown at the time of writing. Nowell's contract specified that stone was to be obtained from Derbyshire quarries and that is to be expected for pier cappings and copings, given the durability of such stone in exposed situations. The local limestone would be very suitable as stone rubble for foundations and the core of embankments and this probably accounts for the evidence of sidings having been laid in the goods yard by this time.

The white post in the centre left, alongside the north side of the line, is a Mile Post, the location of which is shown on Map 7. This recorded a distance of seven miles from the junction Signal Box at Saxby.[51]

Any present day comparison view from this point is obstructed by dense overgrowth that has flourished in the years since closure.

This plan illustrates the uses of the various buildings and structures on the station. It is taken from the Midland Railway Two Chain Plan of the line, dating from about 1911, held in the Midland Railway Archive (Item No 00806). Not all of the references are entirely clear. The lettering on the station building alongside the road and shown in Photographs 38 and 39, reads SM&BO (Station Master's Office and Booking Office) at the south end; GW in the centre (General Waiting) and LWR at the north end (Ladies Waiting Room). WM by the Office is the Weighing Machine; PR on the path from the Booking Office to the platforms will be the Porters Room and WS on both platforms identified the Waiting Shelter.

[46] *Grantham Journal* (10 June 1893), p. 6, col. 4.

[47] Eric Tonks, *The Ironstone Quarries of the Midlands, History, Operation and Railways. Part VIII: South Lincolnshire* (Cheltenham, 1991), 13-16, 81.

[48] *Grantham Journal* (10 November 1890), p. 6, cols 3 and 4; copy of a plan of the land to be taken from the Earl of Dysart, in private ownership.

[49] Tonks, *Ironstone Quarries of the Midlands*, VIII, 81-82.

[50] Midland Railway Study Centre, Item No 00806.

[51] *Ibid.*

SOUTH WITHAM STATION PLAN

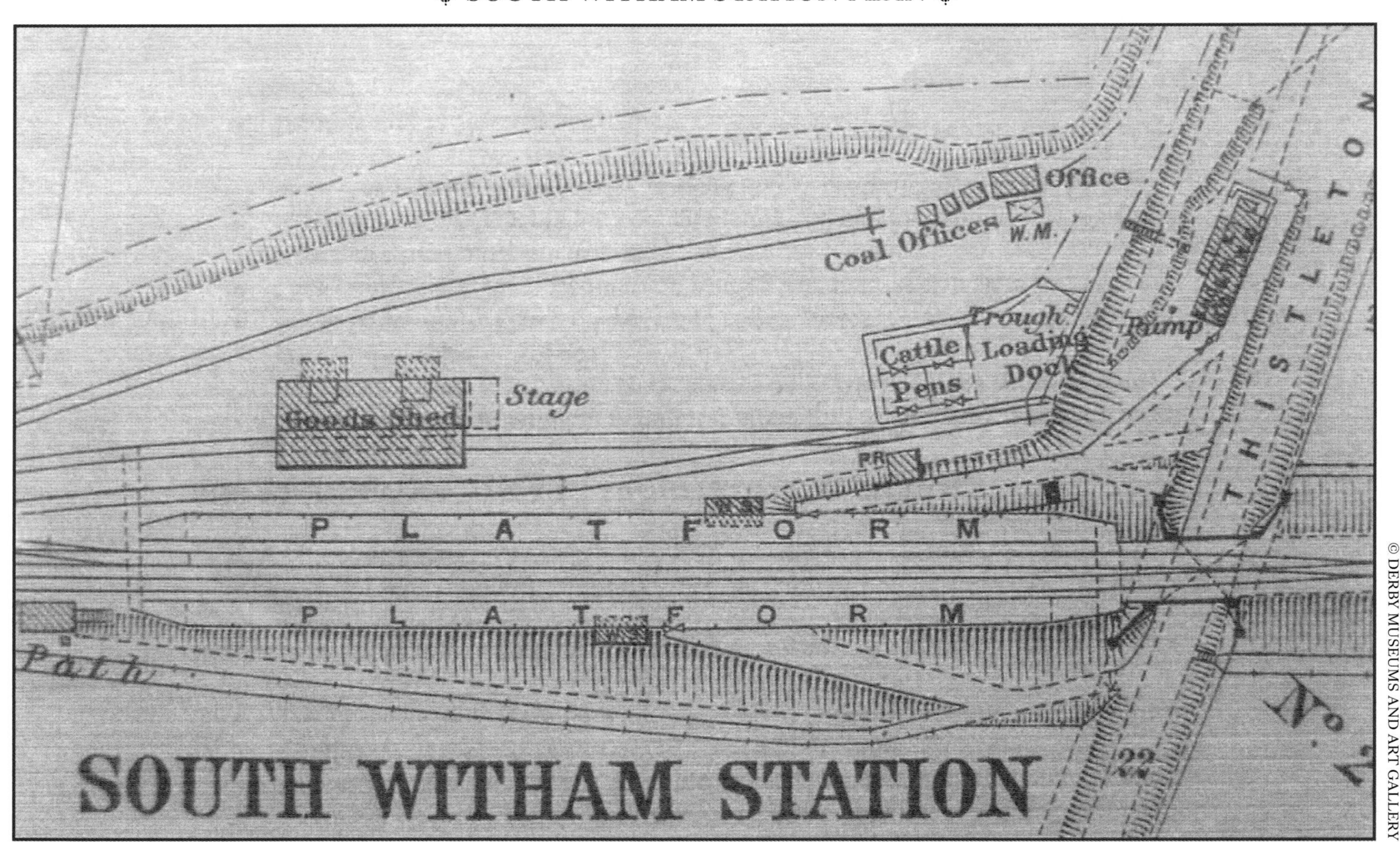

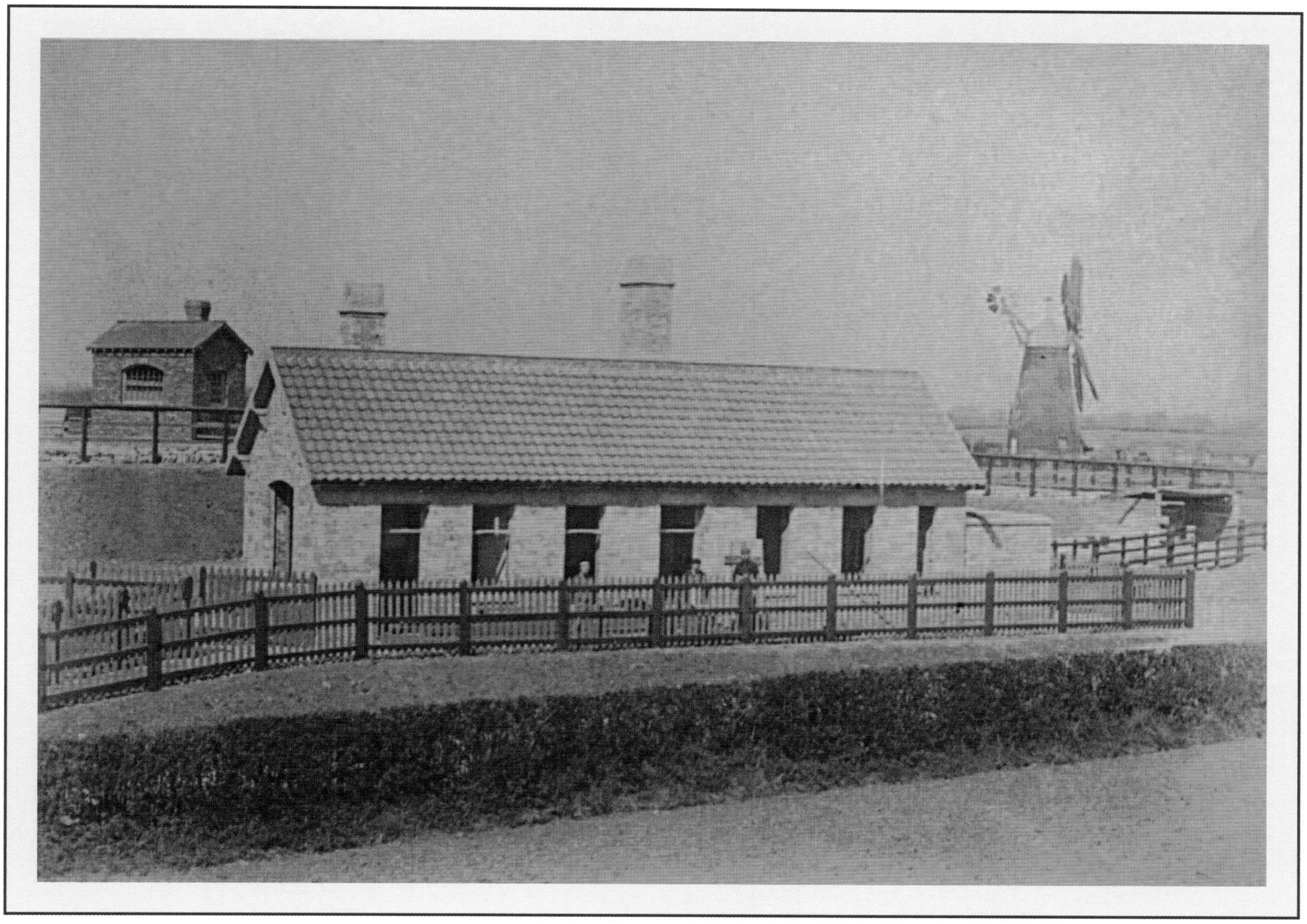

SOUTH WITHAM STATION BOOKING OFFICE

PHOTOGRAPH 39

Because the line crossed Thistleton Lane on an embankment and space was very limited for station buildings, the booking office at South Witham had to be on the station approach rather than with the platforms. Photograph 39 shows the building when first completed, the fenced path to the platforms leading away to the left rear. A house for the Station Master was provided separately on Thistleton Lane immediately north of the goods yard access road.

On the elevation facing the road, the door and window to the left were to the Station Master's Office and Booking Office. The next two openings to the right were to the General Waiting Room, and the next two to the Ladies' Waiting Room. At the right hand end were the Ladies' and Gentlemen's lavatories, the latter, as was usual, without a roof.

The small brick building beyond the booking office probably housed the weighing machine. Most stations had a weighbridge near to the entrance so that goods could be weighed as they entered or left the yard. A similar building can be seen at the entrance to the yard at Wymondham. South Witham windmill can be seen on the right-hand side. Built in 1793, it was out of use in the 1930s and demolished after the Second World War.[52]

PHOTOGRAPH 40

The building, now converted into a house, survives today.

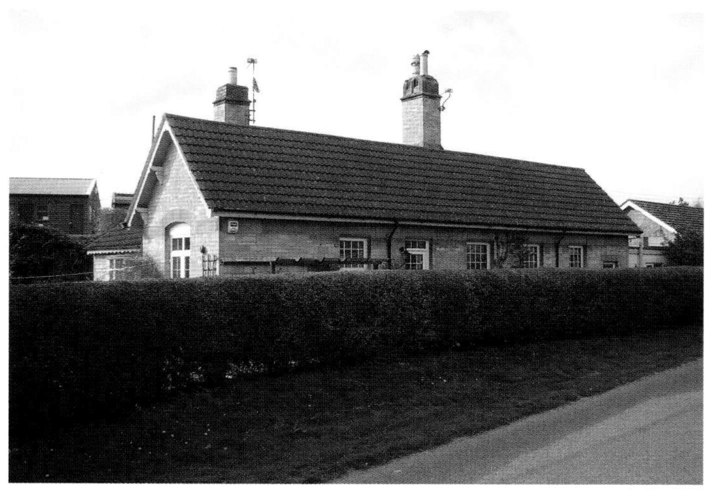

[52] South Witham Archaeological Group, *South Witham Old and New* (Stamford, 2002).

THISTLETON LANE, SOUTH WITHAM

PHOTOGRAPH 41

In South Witham the railway crossed Thistleton Lane by a brick bridge (Bridge 20), shown here in Photographs 41 and 42. In Photograph 41, the bridge has recently been completed but the embankment to either side has yet to be created. This view also shows clearly that the roadway had to be lowered by about eight feet to provide for suitable headroom for road traffic.

PHOTOGRAPH 42

(opposite, top)

Photograph 42 is a similar view but with the embankments built and with one of the station platforms to the left-hand side. The light timber construction of the platform, needed because of the siting on top of the embankment, is evident. The steps on the right-hand side of the road are for a footpath, diverted because of the building of the station, which still runs along the side of the railway embankment here.

Bricks for this bridge and for Bridge 23 at Occupation Road, South Witham, were supplied by the Haunchwood Brick and Tile Co. Ltd, Nuneaton.[53]

PHOTOGRAPH 43

Photograph 43 shows the same view in 2008. The bridge is now too low for present day needs, hence the warning signs. Note also that at some time the parapet of the bridge has been rebuilt and now has a curved, rather than a straight, top and that the remnants of the fencing survive on the left-hand side of the road.

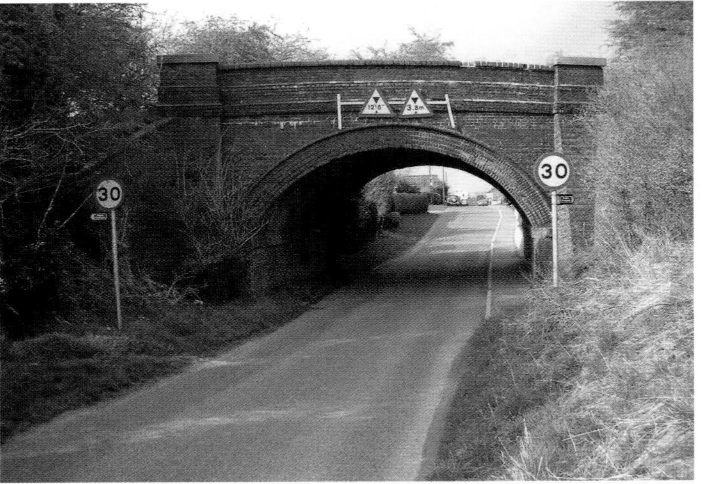

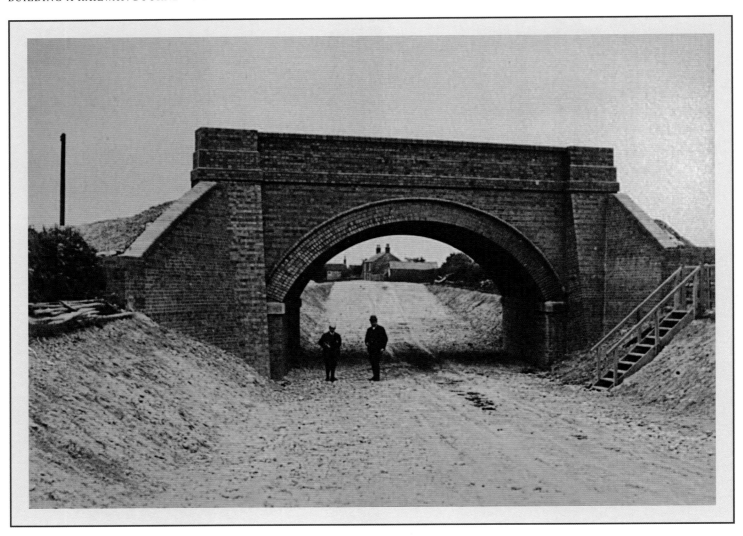

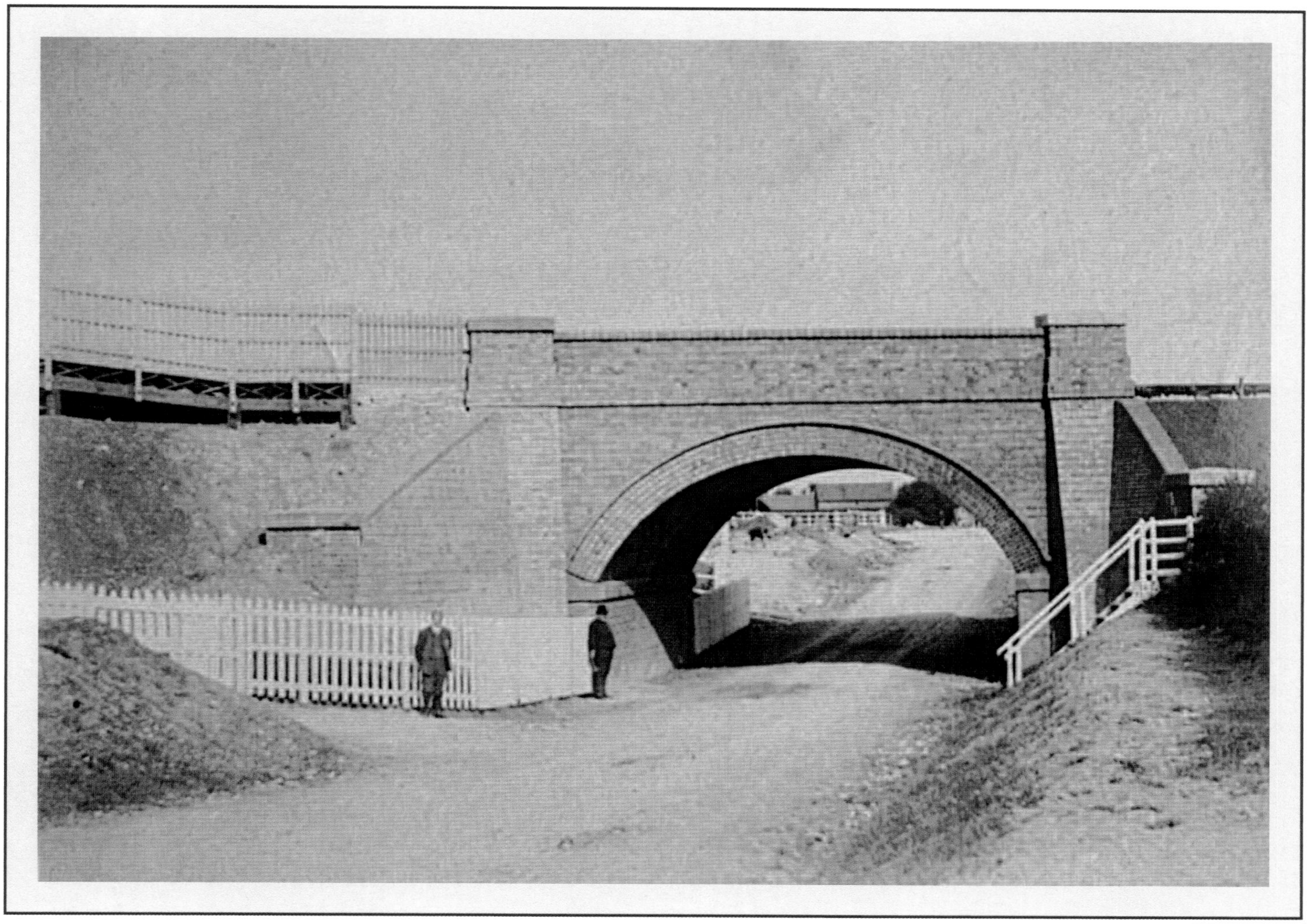

Photograph 42

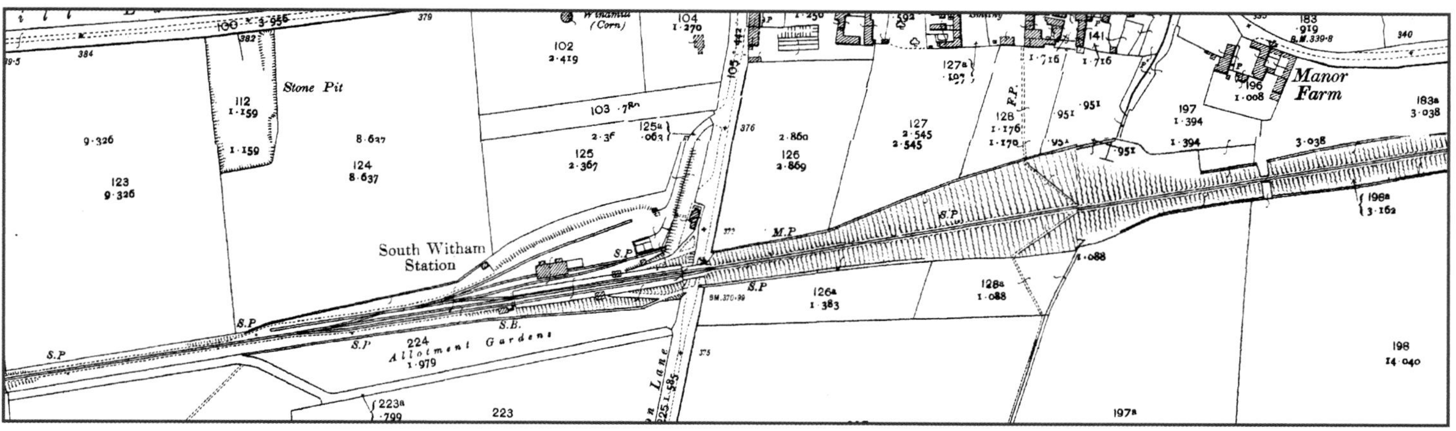

MAP 7

OS 1/2500 County Series Map, 1904.
South Witham Station.

This shows the route of the footpath running along the foot of the embankment to the west of the bridge, between the south side of the line and the allotment gardens. It was diverted here to pass under the Thistleton Lane bridge (seen in Photographs 41 and 42), to avoid the expense of an additional bridge on the original line.[54] Along the side of the station site its route is the double line immediately above the letters S.P. and S.B.

The booking office shown in Photograph 39 is to the west side of the road, north of Bridge No 20, with its fenced footpath link from Thistleton Lane up to the platforms. The letters S.P. indicate the Signal Posts, that to the east of the bridge being the one seen on the left-hand side of Photograph 38. M.P. denotes a Mile Post, this one indicating seven miles from the junction at Saxby (see Photograph 38).

[53] The supply of blue bricks for building works on the line is referred to under Photograph 20 above.

[54] *Grantham Journal* (24 December 1891), p. 6, col. 1.

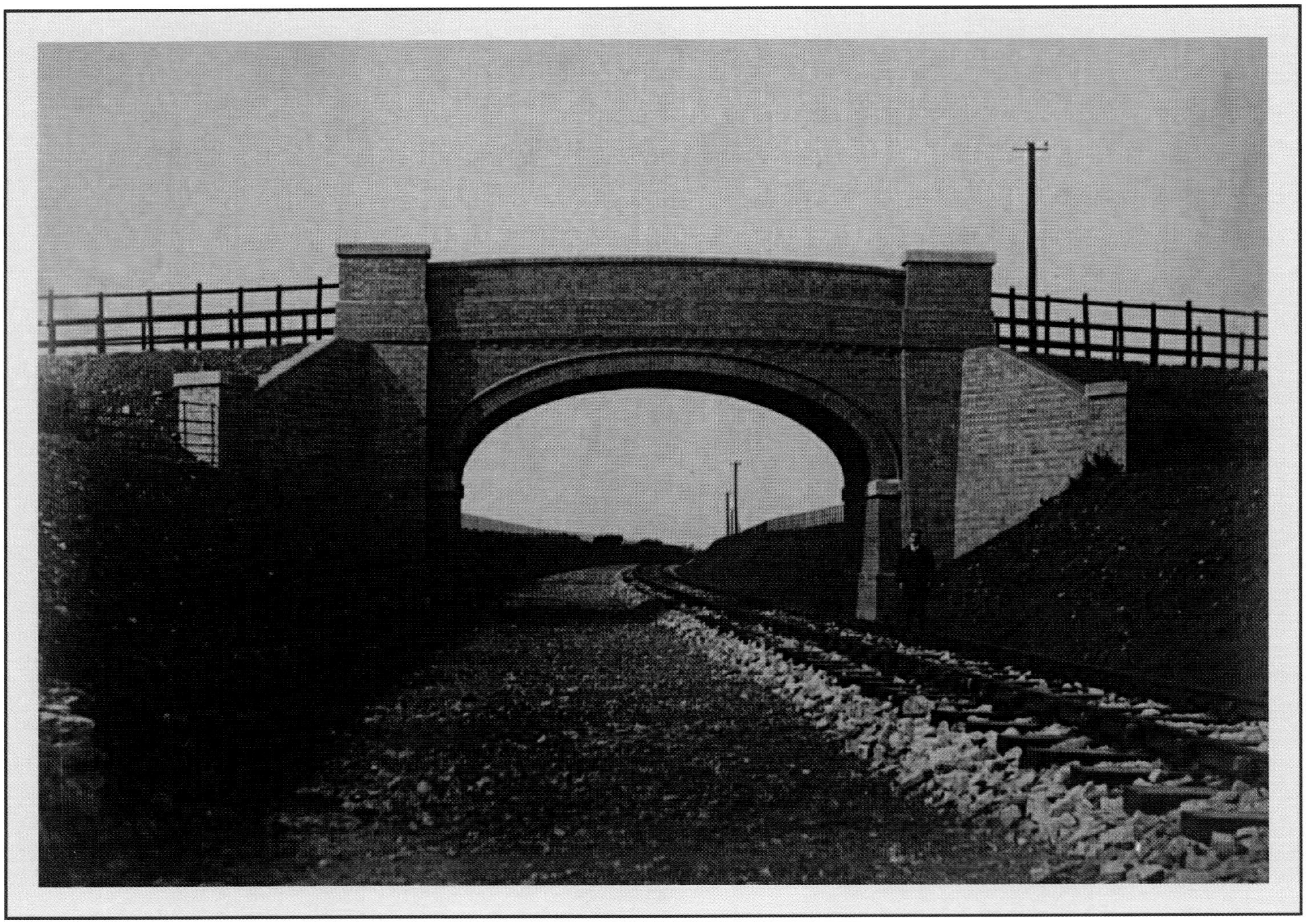

Photograph 44

OCCUPATION BRIDGES WEST OF SOUTH WITHAM

PHOTOGRAPHS 44 AND 45

Photograph 44 is of Bridge 18 and Photograph 45 shows Bridge 19 with 18 in the background. Both have a single elliptical arch and both are occupation bridges with earth approach ramps. The railway fencing here, as opposed to the timber fences to the bridge ramps, is of iron railings; these still survive today alongside the route between the two bridges.

A SIDE TIPPING WAGON

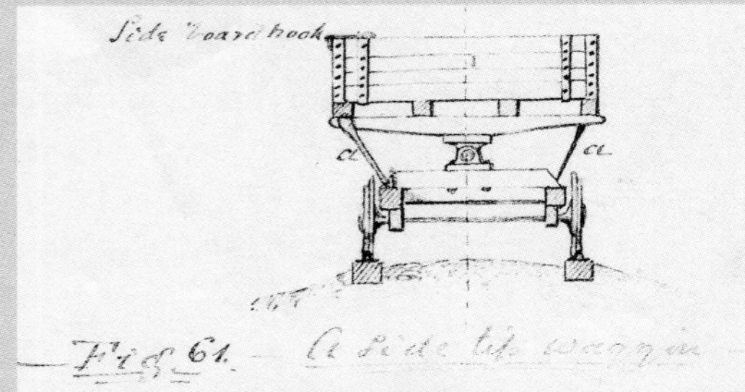

A use of the side tipping wagon is referred to on Page 14, shown on Photograph 33 and described in the text on Page 51. Photograph 47 shows a siding running up alongside what is either Bridge 18 or 19, along which a side tipping wagon will have been used. The sketch of a Side tip waggon (sic) is taken from the notebook compiled by G Anderson who worked under Charles Wilson in 1875.

Anderson describes their use where it would be impossible to make use of an ordinary "end tip". See the caption to Photograph 57 for a description of end tipping. The body of the wagon was supported on a central hinge and kept upright by iron hooks, shown as *aa* on the drawing. The wagon sides were also secured by hooks. When the wagon reached the site where it was to be tipped the hooks would be released to deposit the load where it was required.

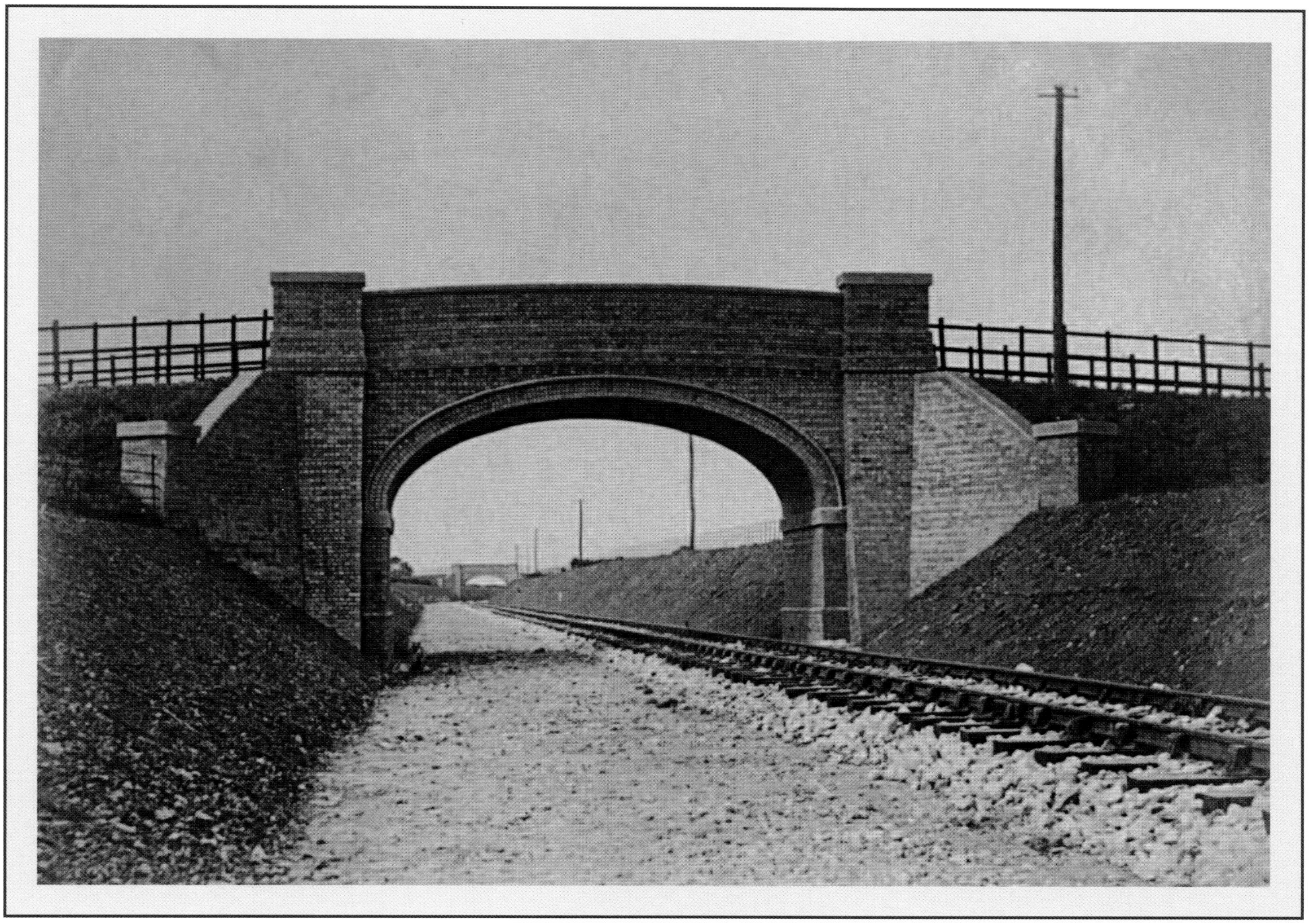

Photograph 45

PHOTOGRAPH 46

What does not survive is Bridge 19. It has been demolished; its site is now within the South Witham limestone quarry. The route of the line between the two bridges survives, although for much of the length the stone has been quarried on either side. This has resulted in the rather bizarre situation of a long, narrow and sheer-sided peninsula running into the quarry, supporting a railway cutting at a high level, still with its iron rail fencing along the edge, as the view in Photograph 46, looking towards the site of Bridge 19, shows.

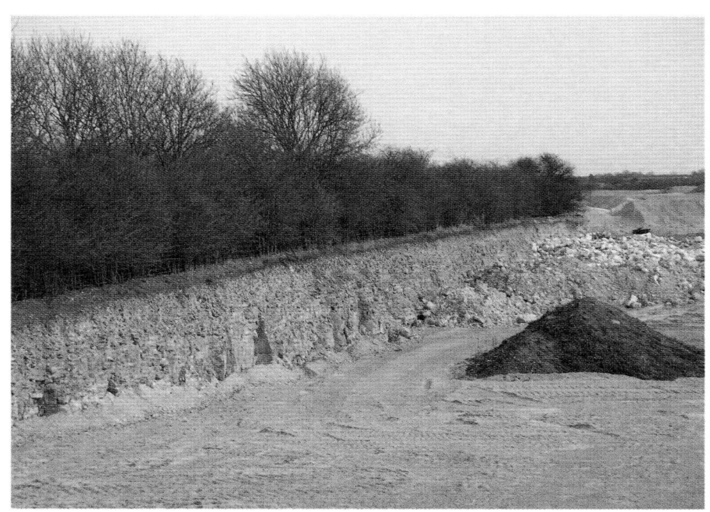

Photograph 46

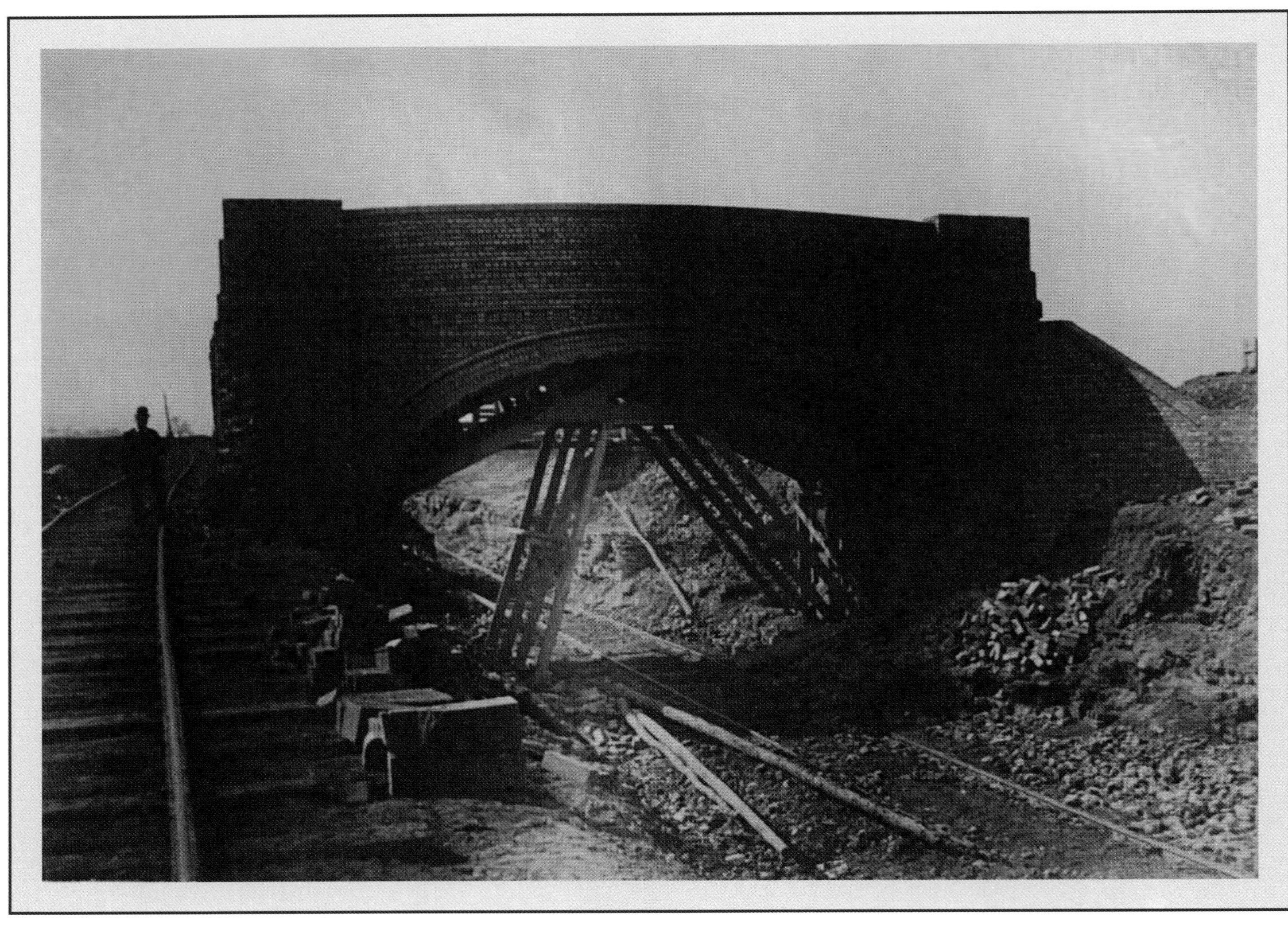

POSSIBLY OCCUPATION BRIDGE NO 19 WEST OF SOUTH WITHAM

PHOTOGRAPH 47

The bridge under construction in Photograph 47 is either Bridge 18 or 19. The cutting sides reveal the rock near to the surface. The bridge will clearly require earth ramps either side to reach the bridge deck level. The siding to the left has risen out of the cutting to enable the soil to create the ramps to be dumped easily. It also appears to have required the demolition of the wing wall to the abutment. It is likely that wagons on sidings such as this would be hauled by horses.

After Bridge 19 was completed, in addition to the earth ramps at right angles to the line shown in Photograph 45 it had a second ramp on the south side running down parallel to the route of the railway. In the latter photograph this is out of sight but immediately off to the left. If Photograph 47 does show Bridge 19 then it may well be that the ramp was the last remaining vestige of the siding shown here.

The construction of the bridge structure in advance of any approach embankments was the conventional method at that time, and remains the approach today, as can be seen along roads and motorways nationwide as road improvements are carried out (see box on page 60).

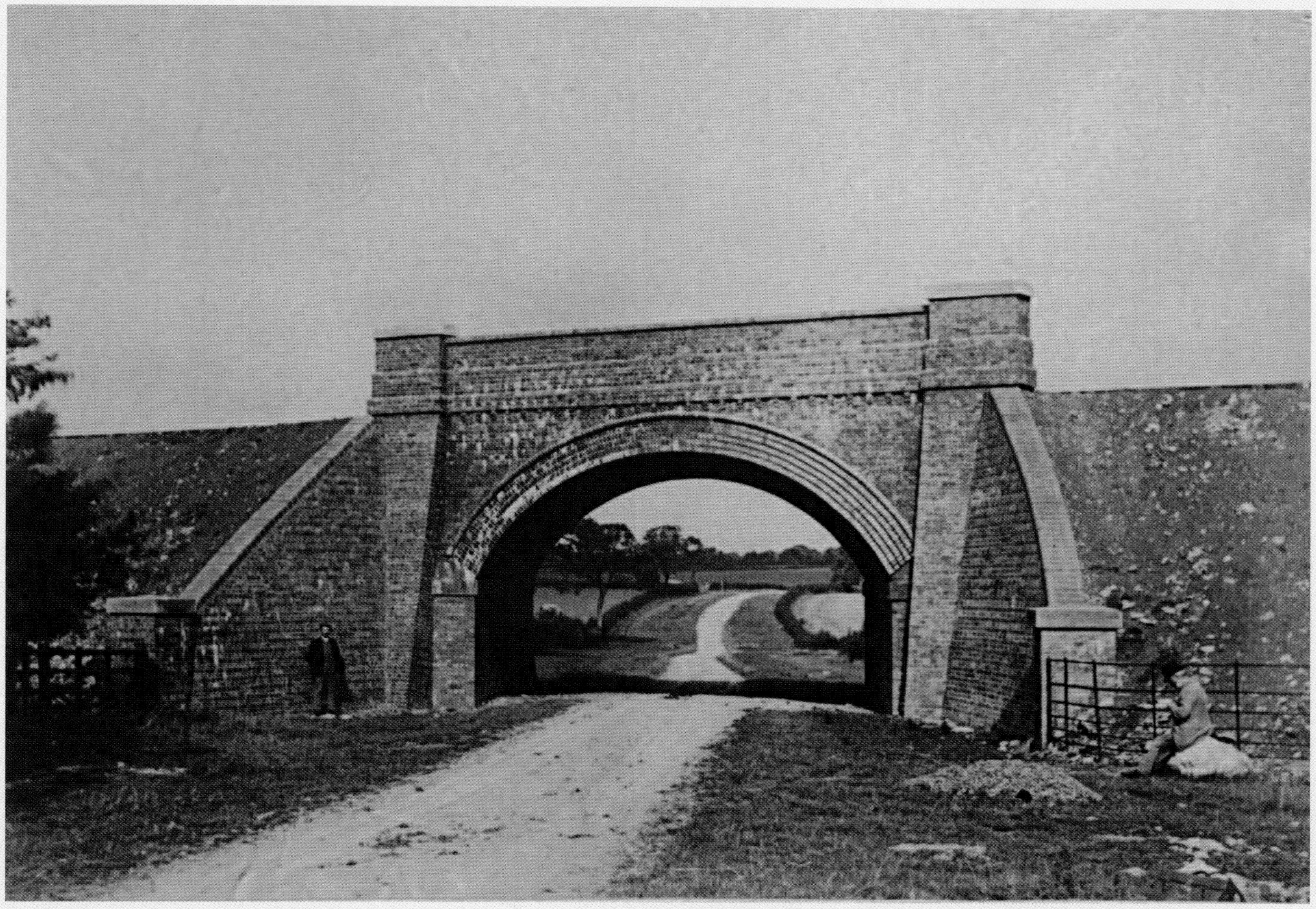

THE DRIFT BRIDGE, SOUTH WITHAM

PHOTOGRAPH 48

Part of an ancient drove road, known as The Drift or Sewstern Lane, runs from Greetham, a few miles north of Stamford to Long Bennington, between Grantham and Newark. It joins with the Great North Road at both ends and it became a useful bypass for cattle drovers and others who wished to avoid paying tolls on the latter in the Turnpike Age. South of Greetham, Sewstern Lane runs on the east side of the A1, crosses the Welland at Uffington and then recrosses the A1 to run on the 'Bullock Road' west of Peterborough.

Photograph 48 shows The Drift, passing under Bridge 16. This is also the point where the line crosses from Leicestershire into Lincolnshire. The County boundary follows the right-hand side of the lane and the point where both counties meet the County of Rutland is only one field away to the south, behind the photographer. This area was famed as a venue for prize fighting in the late eighteenth and early nineteenth centuries.

PHOTOGRAPH 49

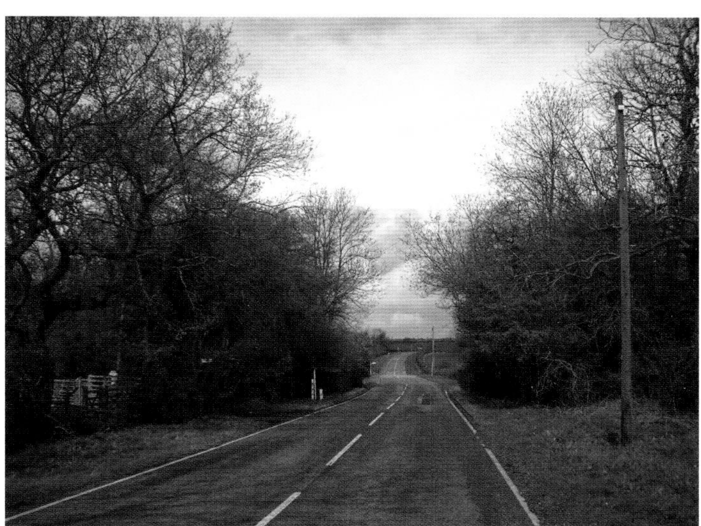

This bridge has been demolished as Photograph 49 shows.The route of the line to the west (left hand) side of the bridge site is now part of the Cribb's Meadow National Nature Reserve. The name commemorates the last bare fist fight in England at Thistleton Gap, two fields to the south, on 28 September 1811, between Tom Cribb and Tom Molineux.

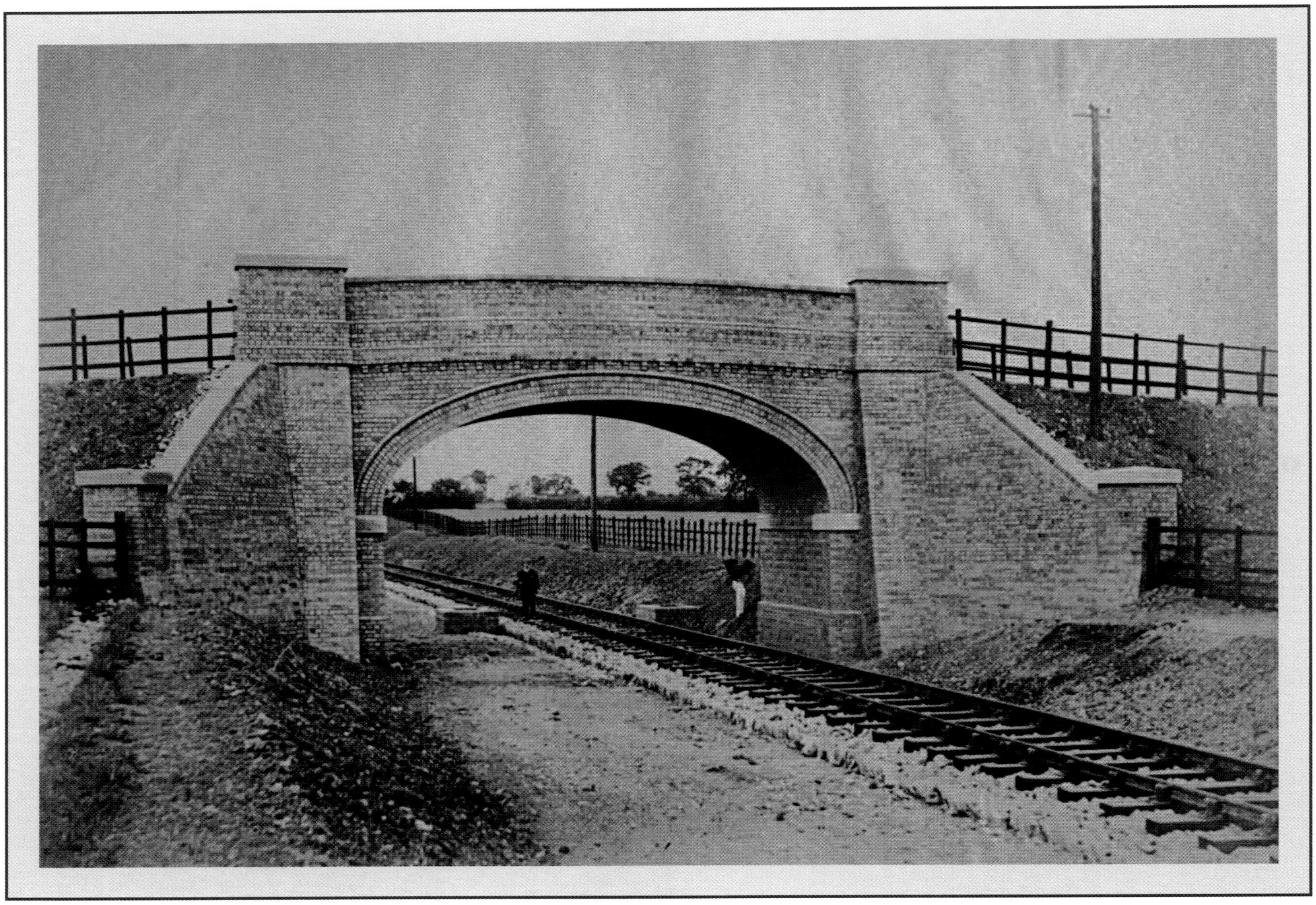

OCCUPATION BRIDGE, WEST OF PAINS SIDINGS, WYMONDHAM

PHOTOGRAPH 50

Photograph 50 is of Bridge 13, an occupation bridge. This is one of three single elliptical arched bridges on the line. The others are Bridges 18 and 19, shown in Photographs 44 and 45. This bridge has been demolished and only remnants of the abutments survive.

The drainage has been constructed alongside the line in the space which could have been occupied by a second track. Comparison with Photograph 51 reveals that this is a contrast with the siting of the drainage at the adjacent Bridge 12, only about 600 yards to the west. Many miles of drainage pipes and their manhole access for cleaning and maintenance had to be constructed. Surface water had to be got rid of quickly, often no mean feat where the line was in a cutting. On the railway the space alongside the track was, and still is, known as the 'cess'. Manholes such as these shown here were known as 'cess pits'. Where the line crossed limestone strata, as opposed to clay, no piped drainage would have been needed as the trackbed would drain freely into the porous rock beneath. Although very significant in terms of man hours and expenditure, as well as the physical need, this element of railway construction is often under-appreciated simply because so much of it is out of sight.

Just beyond the right-hand abutment the white feature is a gradient post. These were installed wherever the gradient changed, the sloping boards at the top indicating the slope in either direction. The figures on this one cannot be read but the Midland Railway survey of the line shows this post as recording a fall towards the photographer of 1 in 132 with the fall easing to 1 in 330 beyond.[55]

Immediately east of this bridge, behind the photographer, was Pains Sidings, the junction with the private line to the ironstone quarries around Market Overton. The quarry line and the sidings opened in 1906. After the ending of the passenger trains in 1959, the line from here, and Buckminster Sidings near South Witham, remained open for ironstone trains. The link to Saxby closed in 1964 but ironstone continued to be mined, and taken out via the link from Pains to Buckminster Sidings and on to the East Coast Main Line until the quarries closed in 1972.[56]

Today the site is heavily overgrown.

[55] Midland Railway Study Centre, Item 00806.

[56] Stewart E. Squires, *The Lost Railways of Lincolnshire* (Ware, 1988), 103-108.

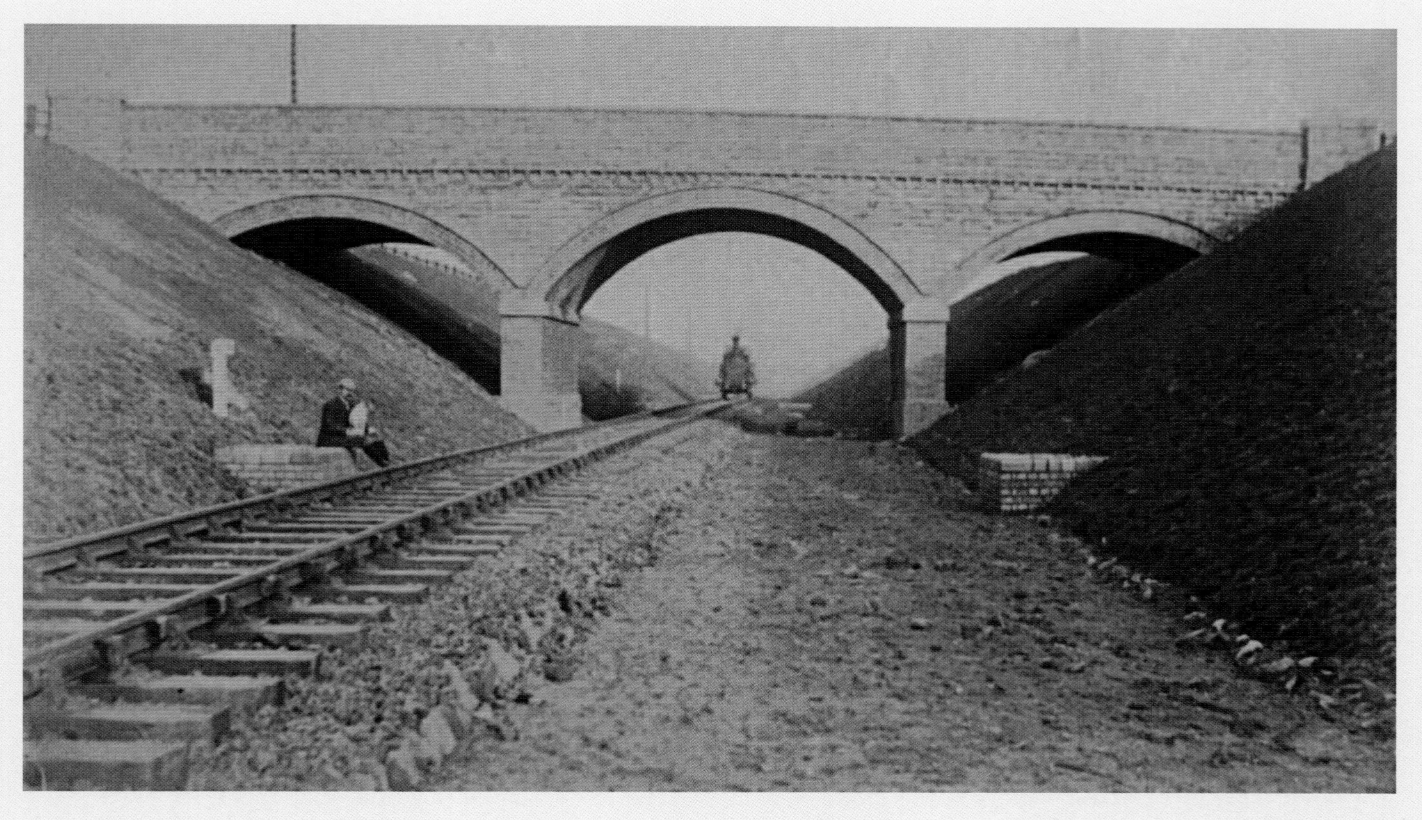

ROAD BRIDGE BETWEEN WYMONDHAM AND SOUTH WITHAM

PHOTOGRAPH 51

This is Bridge 12, which carries the road between Wymondham and South Witham over the railway cutting. This road runs parallel to the railway line, eastwards on the north of the line and westwards on the south. The two were linked by the short stretch of road on the bridge, between two right angled bends. These bends existed before the railway was built and this does not represent a change to the line of the road brought about by the railway.

The man and the dog may be those who appear also in Photographs 58 and 64. The photograph was taken on a misty day but in the original a very ghostly image of Bridge 13 can be made out beyond the contractor's locomotive. The latter cannot be identified. However, its position marks the approximate location of the boundary between the Contract awarded to Holme and King, towards the photographer, and that awarded to J. D. Nowell.

Behind the seated man is a gradient post and beyond the left-hand bridge pier a second similar post can be seen. Between the two the line was level and this level section, at 439 feet above sea level, was the highest point reached by the line.[57]

Of interest in this photograph is the relationship of the trackbed with its drainage. A single line of rails has been laid and this stretch would always be single. However, by contrast with Photographs 50 and 73 the drainage, as indicated by the brick manholes, has been set back to enable any future doubling without disturbance. Compare this with Photograph 50 where the manholes only allow for a single line of rails between them and one manhole appears to be in the centre of the trackbed. The permanent way has been laid here and awaits its final ballasting.

PHOTOGRAPH 52

Photograph 52 shows the overgrown state of the route here in 2008.

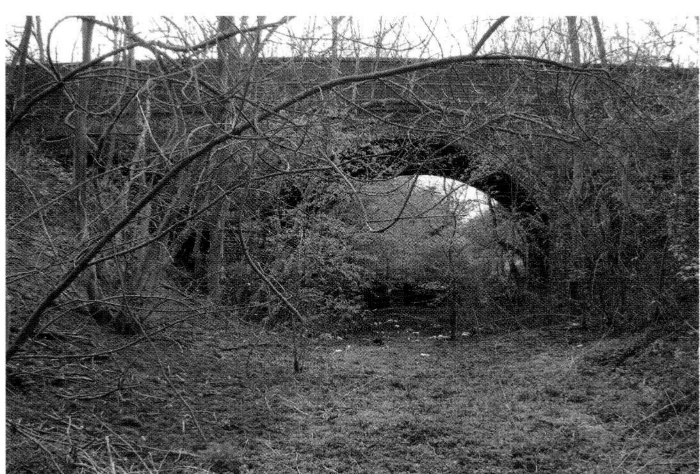

[57] John Rhodes, *Bourne to Saxby* (Boston, 1989), 22. See Appendix C.

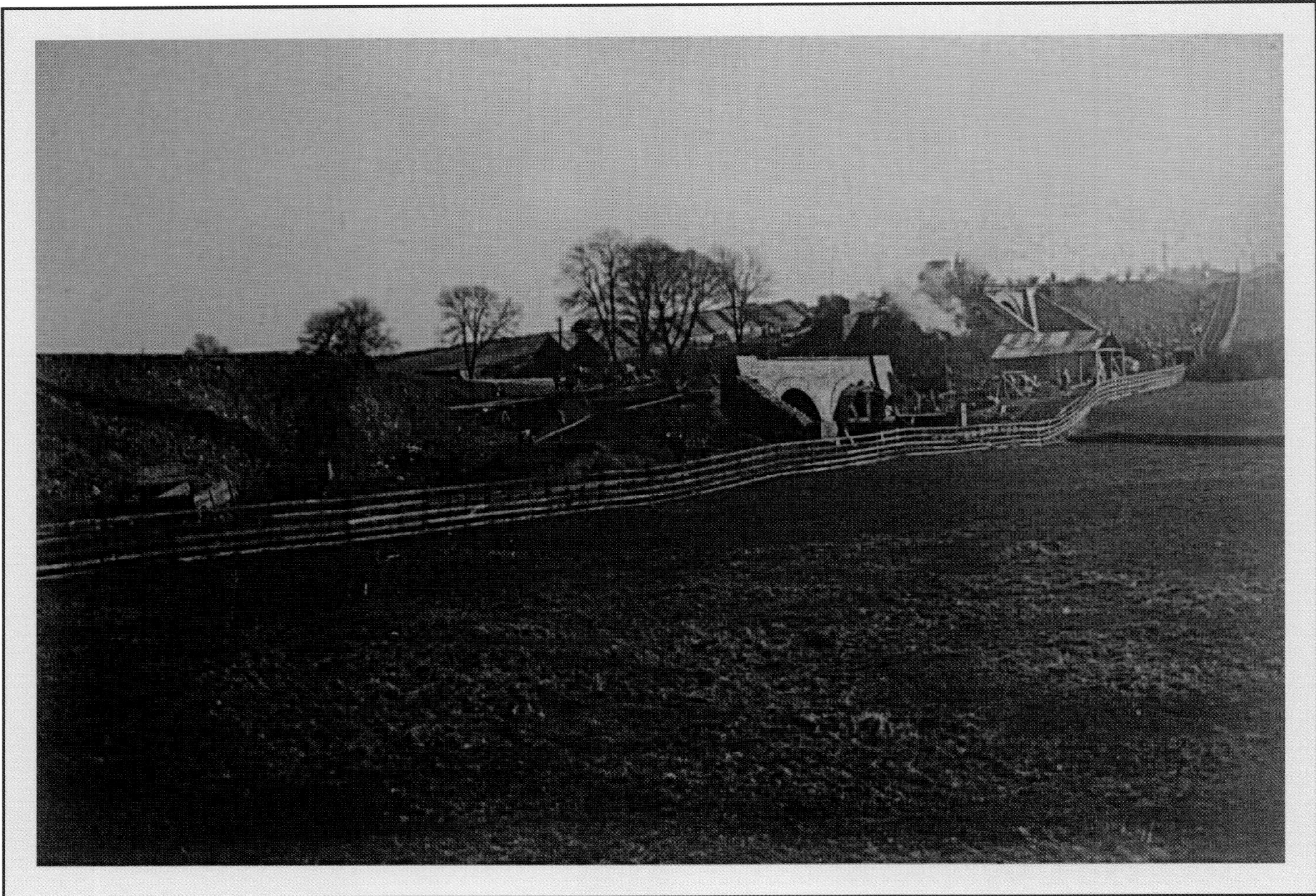

SEWSTERN ROAD AND WYMONDHAM WATER BRIDGES, WYMONDHAM

PHOTOGRAPH 53

Photograph 53 shows both Bridge 9 (in the centre) and Bridge 10 (to the right). The latter crosses Sewstern Road at Wymondham. The embankment at two levels is referred to in the caption to Photograph 54. Photograph 53 is particularly interesting for two reasons: the huts in the background and the activity in front of the embankment.

For each contract the contractor would have to establish a depot where carpenters and blacksmiths shops could be established, and materials delivered, stored and processed (see also Photograph 33). Nearby they would also provide huts for the navvies to live in. Older, more skilled navvies accompanied by their families would live in lodgings or rented houses. The younger, unmarried ones would have been in the huts (see the text with Photographs 65, 66 and 67). The contractor for the section between Saxby and South Witham was Holme and King and this photograph shows the temporary site they established for the construction compound.

The trees in the centre of the photograph mark the route of Sewstern Road. Beyond there is a double row of huts running parallel to the line. Field walking here has revealed evidence of broken bricks and fragments of coal, an indication of occupation by temporary timber buildings, with brick hearths and chimneys. These are likely to have been workshops and storage buildings rather than the homes of many of the men referred to in the text with Photograph 65 below, as the 1891 Census does not record anyone living on the lane to Sewstern.

In the centre Bridge 9 is under construction. The timber framework is still in place to support the right-hand arch. Between it and Bridge 10 beyond is the compound. Little can be determined of the activity here because of the distance, but the machinery between Bridge 9 and the workshop building appears to be a mortar mill, driven by a stationary steam engine with smoke issuing from its chimney.

The fence in the foreground and the wing walls to Bridge 9 give an indication of how the embankment was to rise and spread before it was to reach its completed height. Compare this view with Photographs 60, 61 and 62.

This is one of the few occasions where a horse is pictured, in the centre. Many horses would have been employed on the contracts, engaged in haulage both by road and rail.

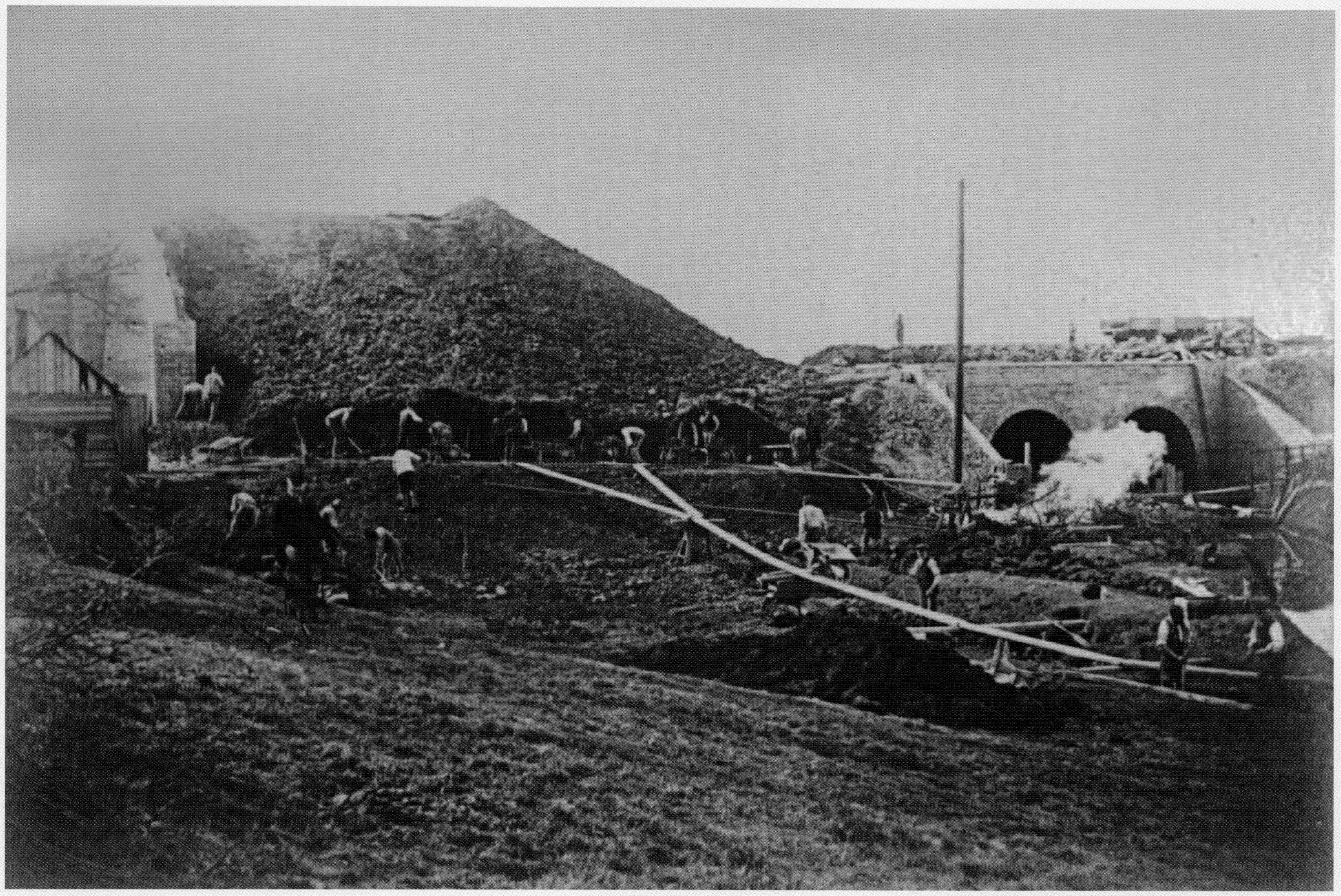

PHOTOGRAPHS 54 AND 55

(above and overleaf)

Immediately to the north of the line, in the field alongside Sewstern Road, Wymondham Water took a sharp right-hand bend. The creation of Bridge 9 to take the stream under the railway also included a diversion of the stream, most probably to allow the new bridge to be constructed 'in the dry' and the stream then diverted through it. This was a standard procedure where the topography permitted it. The original line, and the diversion, can be seen in Photographs 54 and 55.

Photograph 54 is a classic scene of the navvies at work. They are taking soil from part way up the embankment, which seems to be partly being used as a spoil heap at this stage and, by a barrow, down the plank run to the lower level where it was being used to infill the former stream bed. The new stream bed can be seen on the extreme right of the photograph and the two men on the right are standing in the old route.

The man walking along the plank is going back up with the empty barrow behind him. The same technique, but in reverse, was used when working in a deep cutting but in that case a horse would often be used to haul the barrow uphill with the navvy steering from behind. The empty barrow then would be taken back down the planking with the navvy again drawing it behind him. If he fell off he would jump one way and push the barrow the other to avoid it falling on top of him. The potential fall is not too far here but the planking was just as precarious wherever it was used.

This photograph also shows that the work to construct the embankment up to Bridge 9 on the right was taking place from the west, the material being brought from the cuttings on either side of Edmondthorpe and Wymondham station. Note that the embankment here is much lower at this stage and the end tipping wagons standing on the bridge are facing the camera. By contrast, the embankment on the left has reached a much higher level and is being tipped from the east (see also Photograph 53 above).

The portly gentleman and the dog also appear in the photographs of Bridge 3 under construction (Photographs 78 and 79). The dog appears again in Photograph 55.

Photograph 55 was taken at the same time as Photograph 54 and shows the same activity taking place, this time viewed from the embankment to the east of Bridge 10, the abutment of which can be seen on the left. The new cut for Wymondham Water can be seen running through the field above and to the right of the hut. The line of planks to the right of the hut follows the line of the former stream bed which is being infilled with soil taken from that tipped to form the embankment.

The timber hut is of some interest. It is a rather ramshackle and temporary affair with a sheet of corrugated

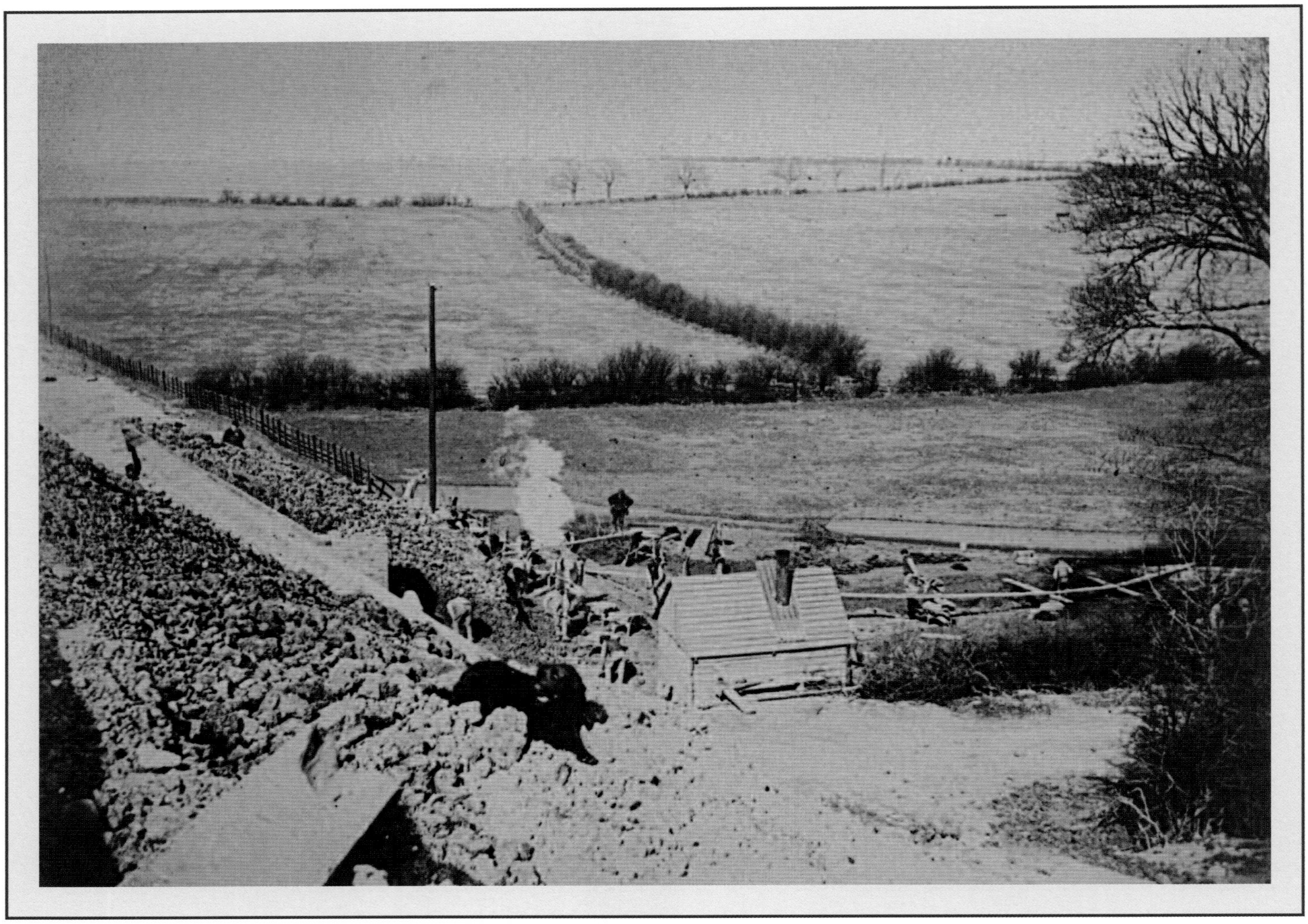

Photograph 55

iron to protect the roof from embers from the chimney. By the late nineteenth century, making shelters and huts had become as instinctive to the navvy as nest building to a bird. Their life in the open air was hard and such buildings provided shelter, rest and somewhere perhaps to heat some food.[58]

This photograph also illustrates the way that during the construction period a contractor would occupy ground on a temporary basis to facilitate the works. The fence line at the foot of the embankment marking the boundary of the railway can be seen in the centre right. The conversion of the stream required a temporary occupation. The Acts of Parliament and the Deposited Plans define the specific limits of deviation and working width.[59] Any land taken beyond these limits would have to be negotiated between the contractor and the landowner.

PHOTOGRAPH 56

Photograph 56, taken in 2008, shows a similar view to that in Photograph 54. This also shows how the ownership boundary would later be defined by the fence. What is not known is if the toe of the embankment extends into the field or if there was an existing knoll here before the railway came.

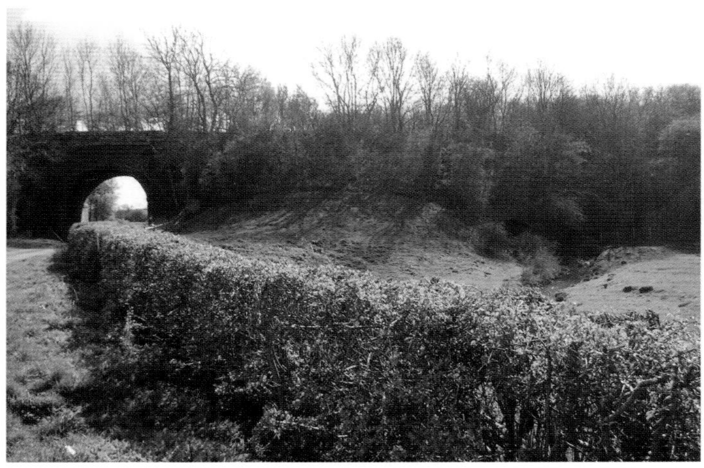

Photograph 56

[58] L. T. C. Rolt, *The Making of a Railway* (London, 1971), 77-86.

[59] Leicestershire Archives, Q5 73/273 (Midland Railway, Session 1889, Cottesmore and Bourne Deviations); Lincolnshire Archives, KP6/52 (Session 1888, Eastern and Midlands Railway extension to Midland and GNR).

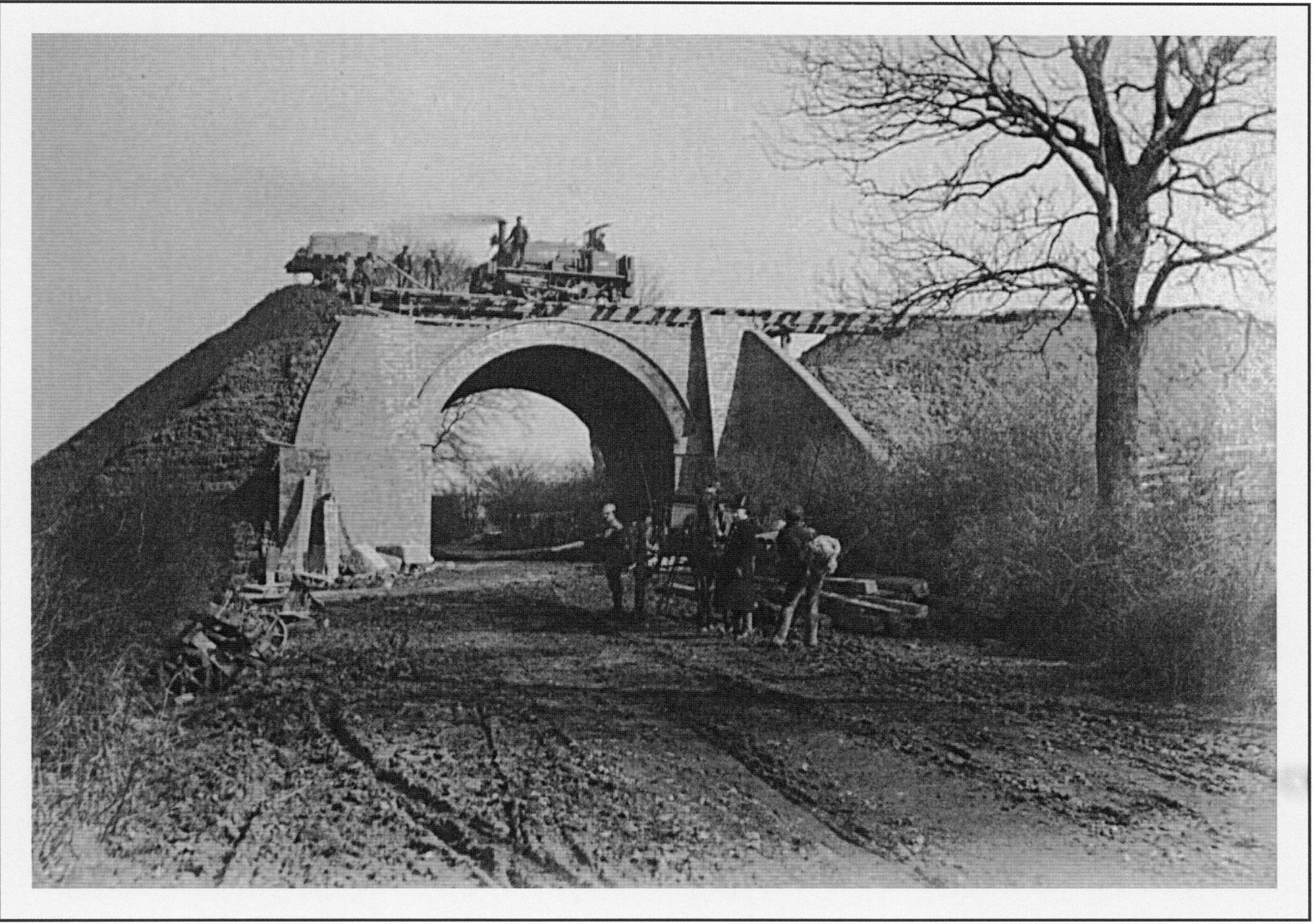

SEWSTERN ROAD BRIDGE, WYMONDHAM

PHOTOGRAPHS 57 AND 58

(Above and overleaf)

Photographs 57 and 58 both show Bridge 10, taking the line over Sewstern Road at Wymondham. The earlier is Photograph 57 which shows the construction phase of the embankment following the construction of the arch and abutments of the bridge. Spoil is being tipped on the left having been brought from the digging of the cutting to the east, about two kilometres away. Comparison with Photograph 58 shows that the embankment was to have about another 10 feet in height.

The 0-6-0 locomotive in Photograph 58 is probably the same one as seen in Photograph 64. That in Photograph 57 is a Manning Wardle 0-4-0, probably one of those referred to in the caption to Photograph 93 and also seen in Photograph 81. The condition of the locomotives is worthy of note (see caption to Photograph 36 above).

In Photograph 57, the locomotive has pushed an end tipping wagon to the end of the line from where its load was deposited. Although this was efficient mechanisation by the standards of the time, it was very poor compared to the standards of later generations. Here six men and one locomotive have been engaged in the transport and deposit of the load from one relatively small capacity wagon, and many thousands of such loads would be needed to raise such a high and long embankment as this one.

The operation of tipping was rather alarming by present day standards.[60] Usually, the wagons would be propelled by the locomotive to a point about 200 feet short of the end of the line. Here the wagons were detached individually and a horse attached to the first one. The driver would put him to a gallop, running alongside, and holding him by the head.

When about ten yards away from the tipping place, the driver would loosen the horse from the wagon and horse and driver would jump to one side. At the same time the tail board at the front of the wagon would be dropped by a second man jerking up a securing hook. A wooden sprag about three feet long and pointed at both ends would be thrust between the spokes of the rear wheels. The wagon would be brought to a sudden stop, the body would tip up from the wheels and the load discharged. Timing was the key but it was not uncommon for the wagon to drop down the embankment along with its contents. After each tip the ground would be levelled by navvies using spades.

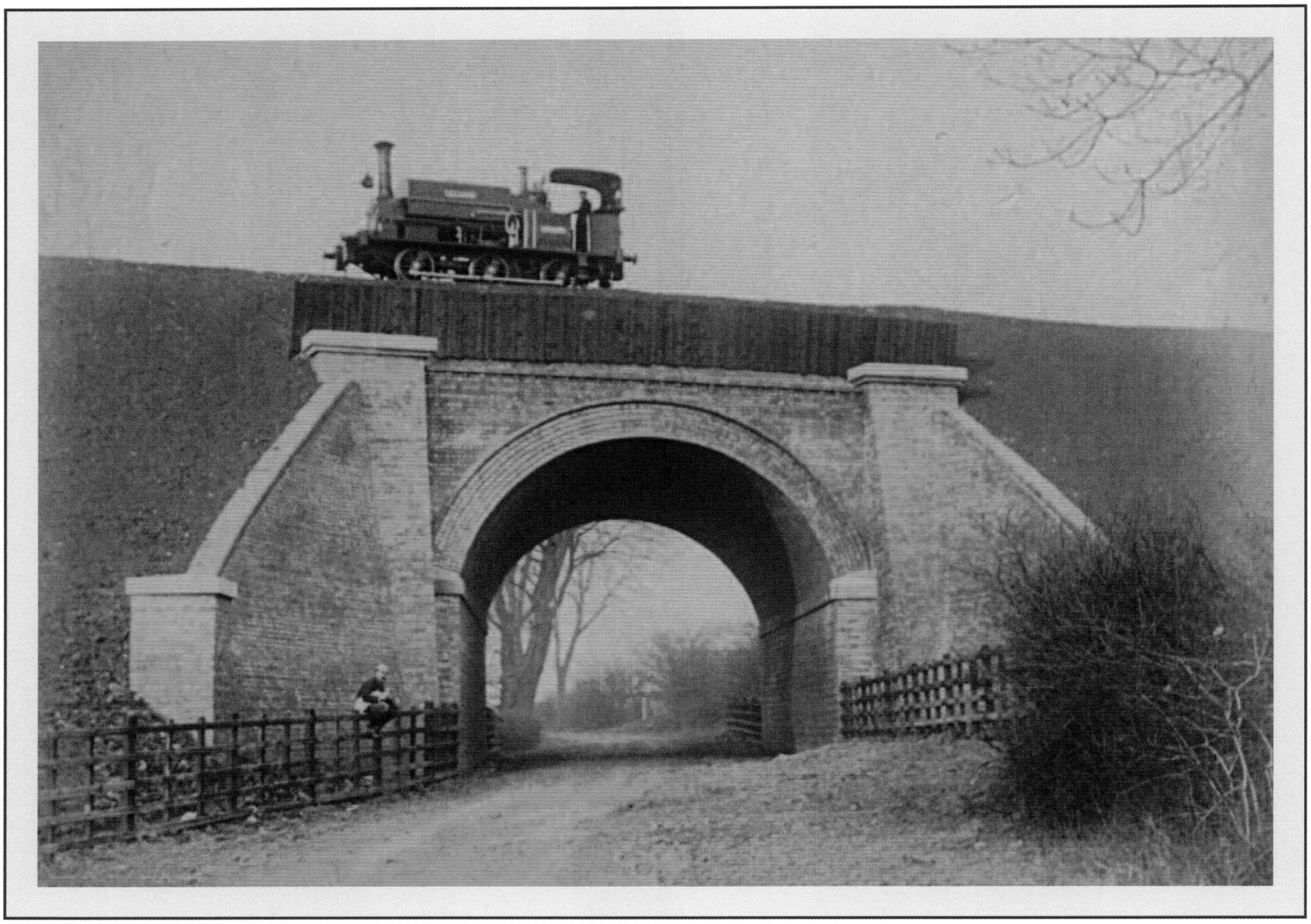

Photograph 58

In Photograph 57 it may be that the horse is not being used, but replaced by the locomotive propelling the wagon at the necessary speed and braking sharply at the appropriate point.

The line of the embankment was set out by using tall poles set into the ground along the centreline of the railway. To these were fixed horizontal boards set at the required finish level.

Note the baulks of timber in Photograph 57, carrying the rails from the embankment on the right to the top of the bridge. The smoke from the chimney indicates that there was a strong east wind blowing.

The uniformed coachman is patiently waiting for Charles Wilson with the pony and trap (see the caption to Photograph 24 for a further note on this).

PHOTOGRAPH 59

It looks as though the timber palisade seen in photograph 58 was originally meant to be a permanent feature as the piers have their stone cappings. The palisade was replaced with a conventional brick parapet, with the piers raised and the stones used to cap them at the higher level as seen in 2008 in Photograph 59.

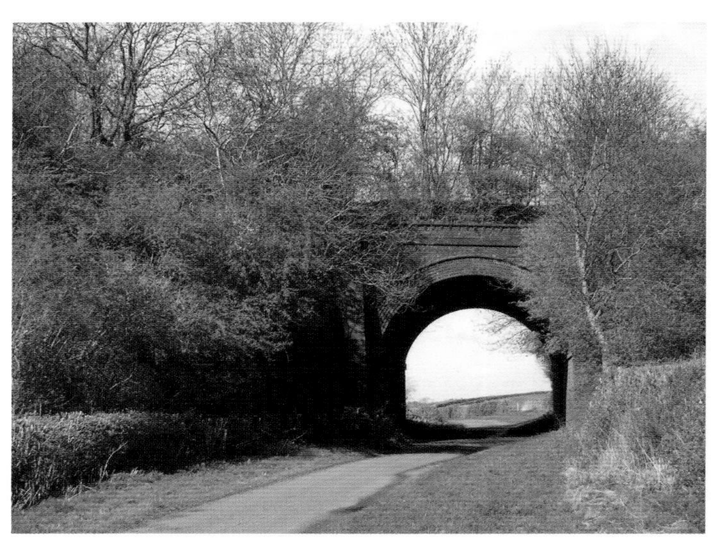

Photograph 59

[60] Notebook compiled by G. Anderson (Midland Railway Study Centre, Item RFBMCT 13316-1875).

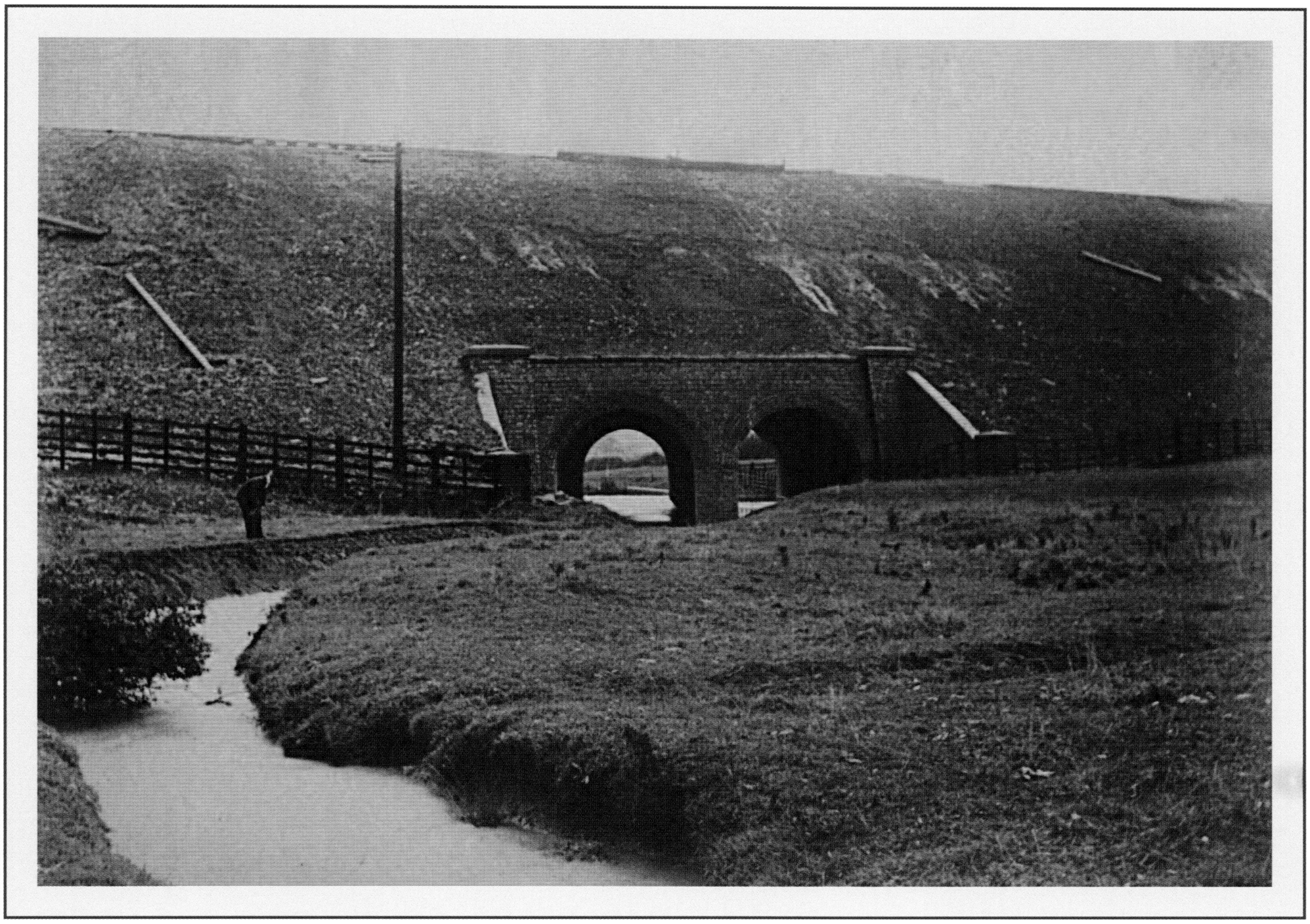

WYMONDHAM WATER BRIDGE, WYMONDHAM

PHOTOGRAPHS 60 AND 61

(Above and overleaf)

Photographs 60 and 61 are two views of the unusual double arched Bridge 9 through the tall embankment to the west of Sewstern Road at Wymondham. Photograph 60 is taken from the north side and shows the stream realignment referred to in the caption to Photograph 54 being inspected by the figure in the left centre. Photograph 61 is from the south.

PHOTOGRAPH 62

Interestingly, Photograph 60 has the stream, Wymondham Water, running through both arches while 61 has the water through the eastern arch only. The ground level through the other has been raised to provide for an occupation roadway, the situation that prevails today as shown in Photograph 62. This may have been done as an afterthought. Sewstern Road is very close and access could have been gained to the land across the stream, both north and south of the embankment, by farm access bridges.

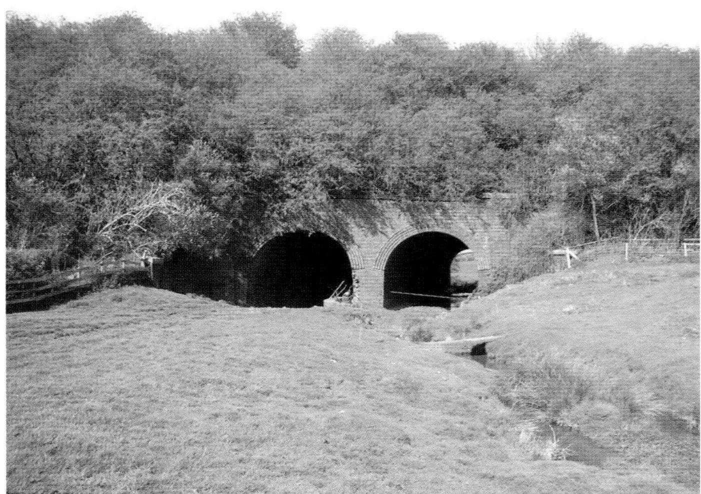

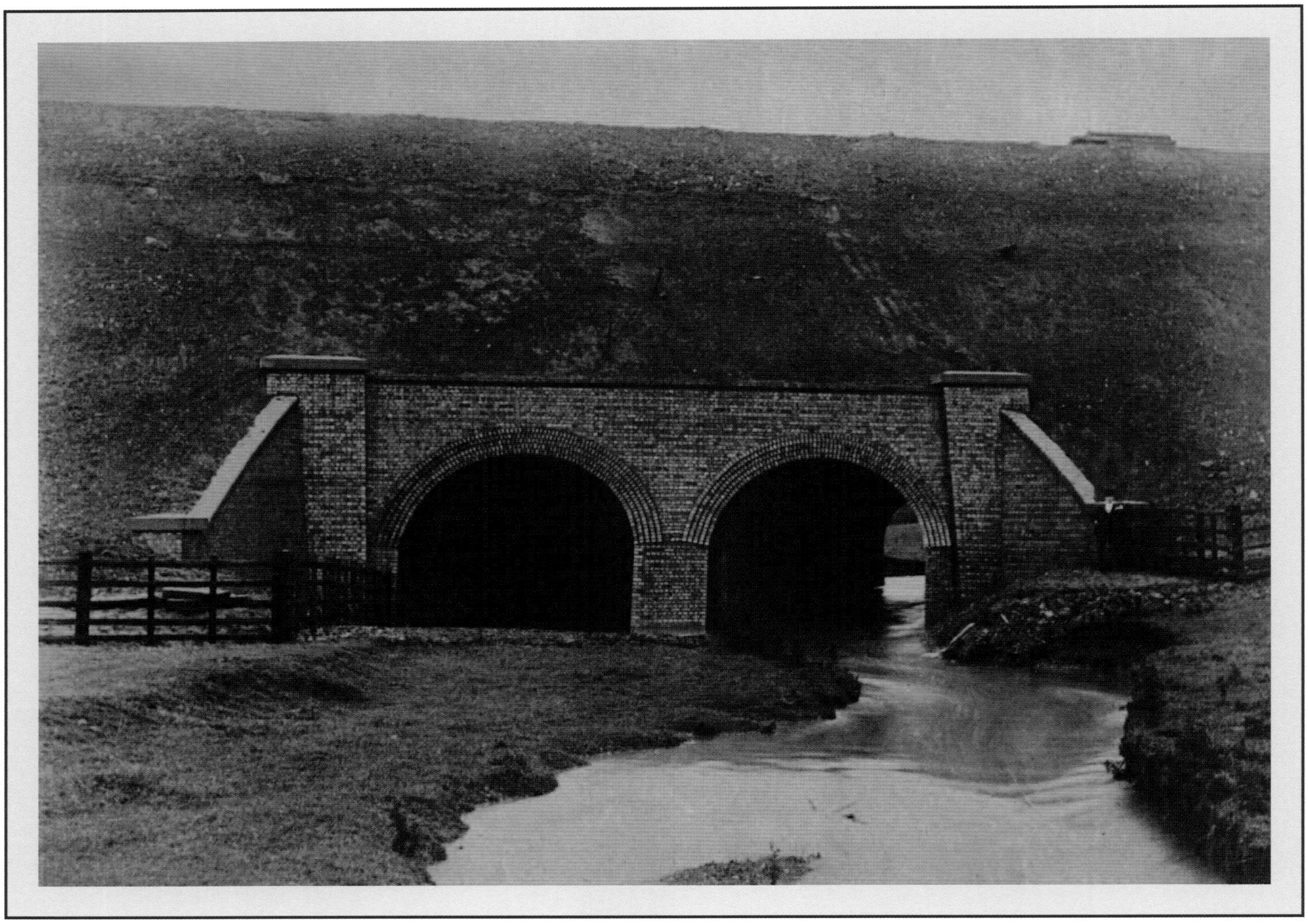

Photograph 61

MORTAR MILL

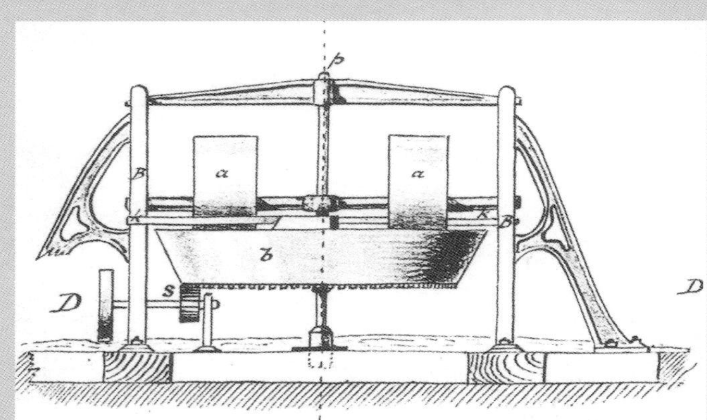

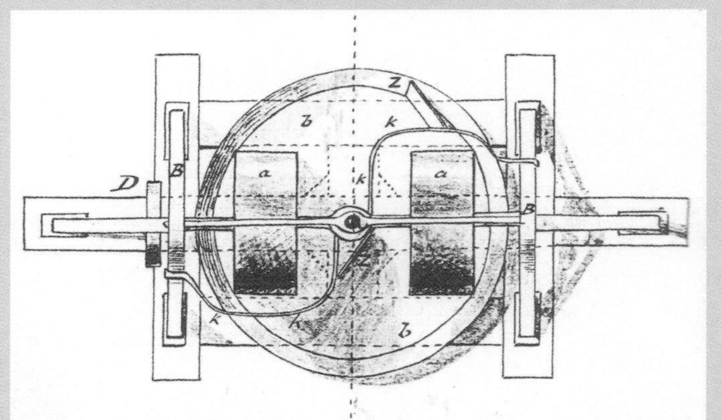

The Mortar Mill shown in Photograph 53 was just off to the right of Bridge 9 shown in Photograph 61. G Anderson, who worked under Charles Wilson in 1875 and compiled the notebook referred to on Page 14, described the function of the Mortar Mill and included the drawings reproduced here. The sketches show clearly the high standard of his work.

a a are a pair of heavy iron rollers supported by frame *B*. *b* is an iron basin, toothed on the underside to connect with the spur wheel *s*, itself connected to the drive wheel *D*. The drive wheel was connected to an engine by a strap. *k k* are iron bands connected to scrapers *z z*. The scrapers were to guide the mortar and ensure that it went under the rollers.

In the 1891 Census, in Wymondham, John Gould, lodging in a house in the Main Street, gave his occupation as Mortar Engine Driver. Presumably he was operating the portable steam engine which was driving the Mill at this site.

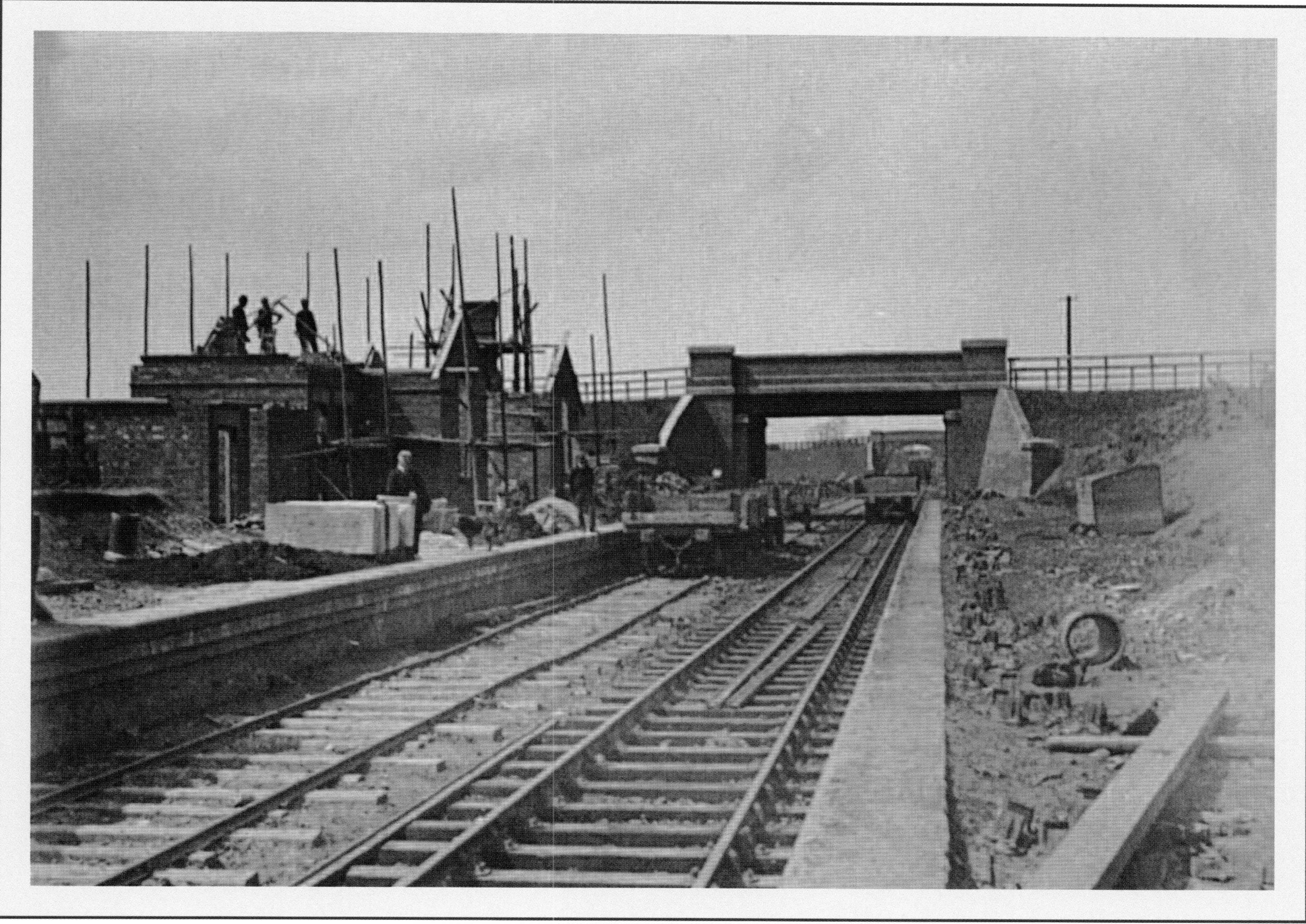

EDMONDTHORPE AND WYMONDHAM STATION

(see also Map 8)

PHOTOGRAPHS 63 AND 64

These show two views of Edmondthorpe and Wymondham station. Although the station is in Wymondham village it had to be given a name other than simply Wymondham as there was already a station of this name and spelling, but a different pronunciation (Windham), in Norfolk.

In Photograph 63, above, the station building is being built. This was to the same design as at Saxby and provided for a ticket office, waiting rooms and toilets. The builder was Mr C. Barnes of Melton Mowbray who also built the stations at Saxby and South Witham. The scaffolding is timber.

The right-hand platform has a number of rail chairs scattered along it. The track provides an interesting comparison of the permanent way, seen on the right, with the contractor's line to the left. The latter uses a very light rail by comparison, is not fully ballasted or particularly level, and is spiked to relatively rough timbers. The reason is that the contractor's track had to be portable as it was relaid several times, particularly on embankments and in cuttings. Also, speeds were very low.

End tipping wagons with dumb buffers are standing on both sets of rails. It is clear through the bridge arch that no work has started yet on the goods shed.

Bridge 7 is at the end of the platforms and has approach ramps but, even so, the height of the underside is restricted, hence the use of a girder to carry the road and maximise the headroom here. In 2009 the bridge is now suffering from a subsidence problem and is partly supported by large timber props. Through the arch, in the distance, is Bridge 6. This has been demolished since closure and replaced with an embankment.

Photograph 64, overleaf, shows the completed station, together with the new goods shed, seen through the arch of Bridge 7. Steps lead down to both platforms from the bridge and the contractor's line on the left has now been replaced by the permanent track. At the platform are two Midland Railway wagons, probably delivering materials from elsewhere on the MR system beyond the railway under construction. In front of the Midland Railway wagons is an 0-6-0 contractor's locomotive. This is probably the same locomotive as shown in Photograph 58 and may be Manning Wardle, Works Number 636 of 1876. This was

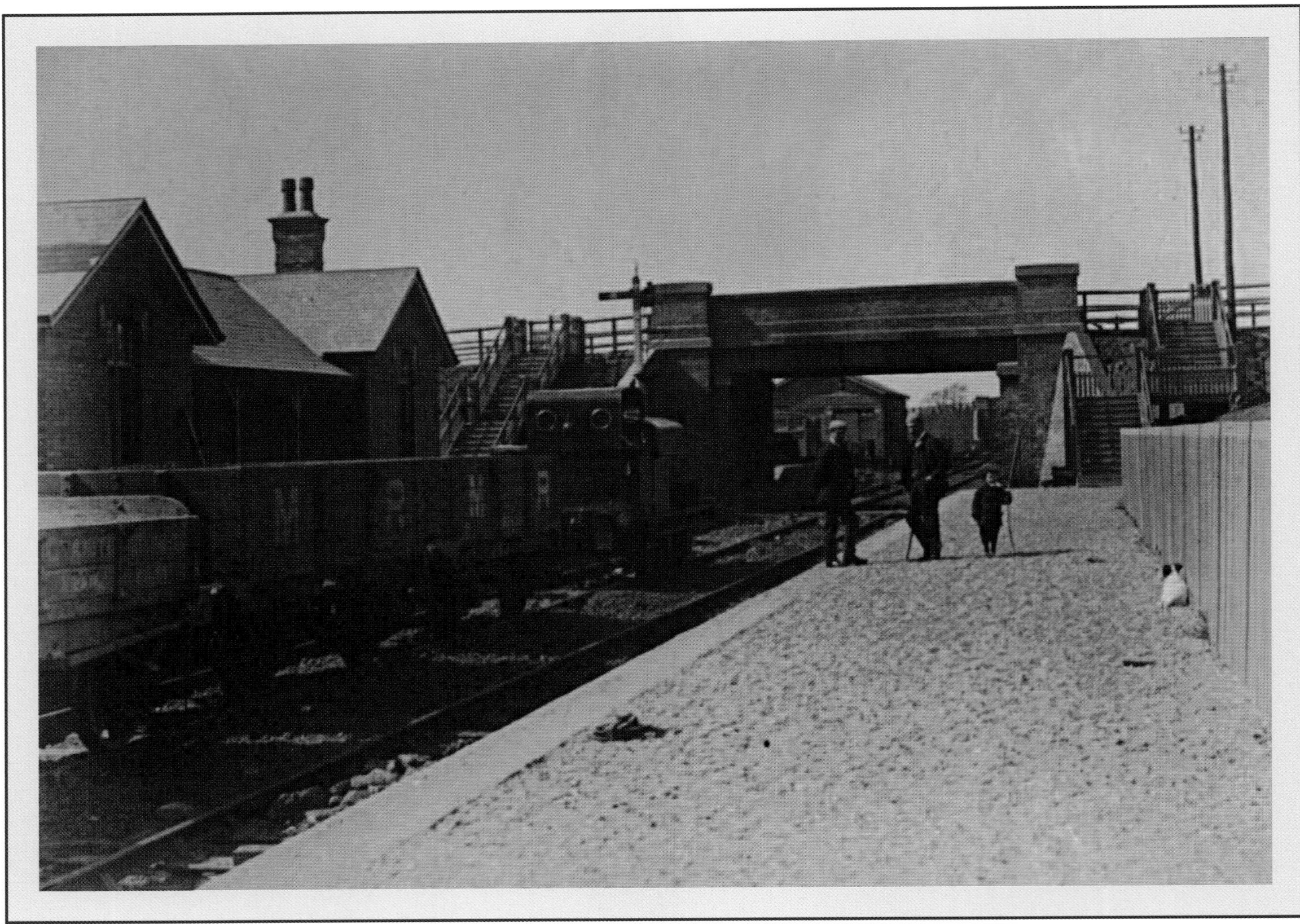

Photograph 64

delivered new to W. Moss but was later used by Holme and King, the contractor for this section of the line.[61]

The supply of Staffordshire Blue bricks for the contracted works is detailed in the caption to Photograph 20. Those used for the platform edgings at this station were supplied by Wood and Ivery from their Albion Brickworks in West Bromwich (see box on page 40).[62]

The small group of people is interesting. The men, and the dog, do appear on other photographs but here there is also a small boy. Charles Wilson had a son, Reginald, known as Rex, who would have been 4 in 1892 and this could be him.

[61] Correspondence from the Industrial Locomotive Society, April 2008.

[62] 'West Bromwich: Economic History' in M. W. Greenslade (ed.), *A History of the County of Stafford* 17 (Oxford, 1976), 27-43.

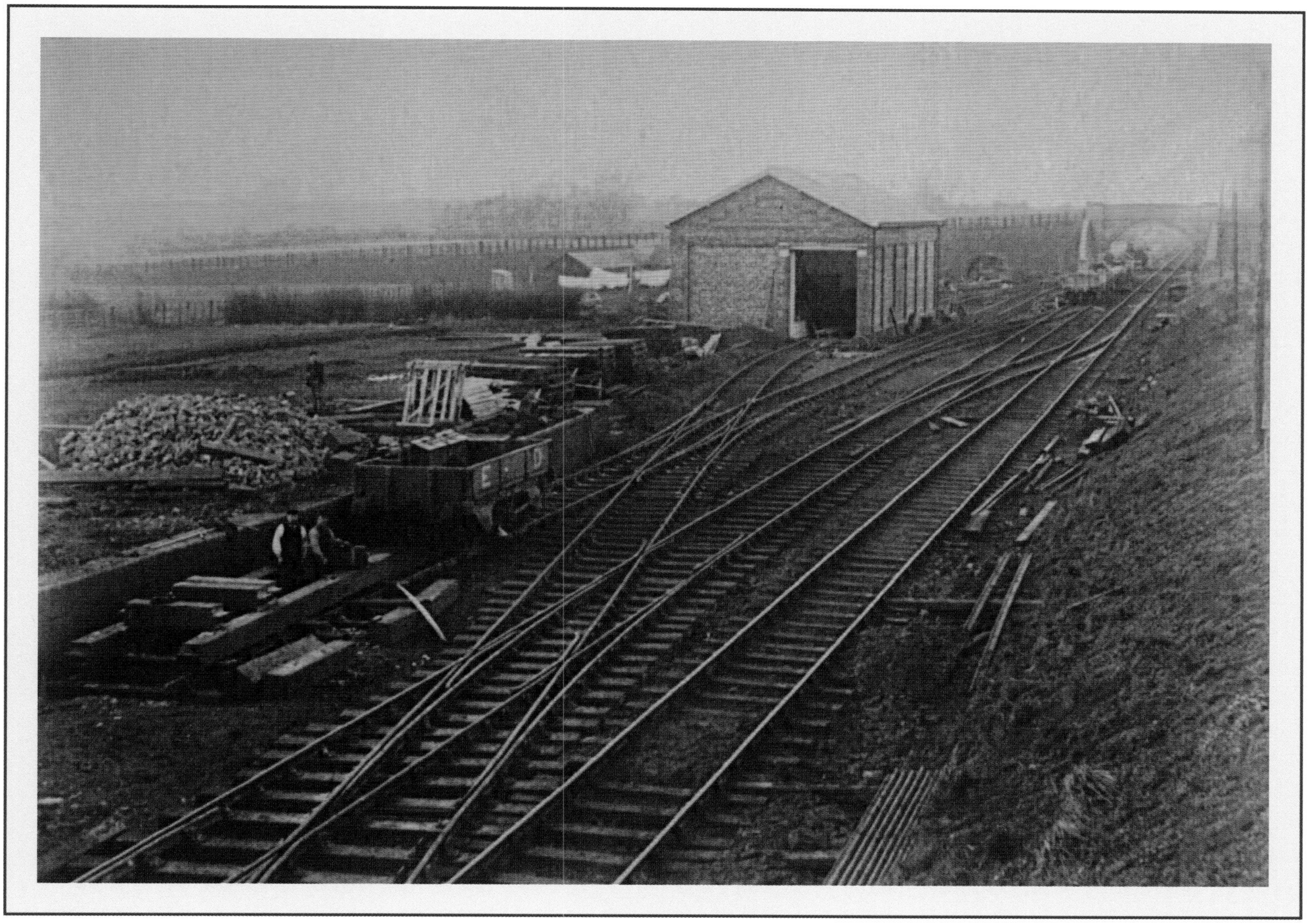

GOODS YARD, WYMONDHAM AND EDMONDTHORPE STATION

(see also Map 8)

PHOTOGRAPH 65

Photograph 65 is of the goods yard at Edmondthorpe and Wymondham, seen from Bridge No 7. The girl in Photograph 68 was standing approximately where the man at centre left is standing.

The goods yard here was to become a hive of activity. It handled coal, coke, cattle, cattle feed, farm seed and building materials.[63] Herbert Whait subsequently leased land here. He was a Coal Merchant and also dealt with corn and cattle cake.[64] The land taken for the goods yard was much greater in extent than would normally be expected. The mark in the field, just above the head of the man at centre left, defines the line of the only siding that crossed this land. This would have been used for unloading coal and loading or unloading other heavy items such as building materials or, if it were dry, grain or fertiliser.

In the foreground two men are working at what was to become the goods dock. This included a double cattle pen, constructed alongside where the wagon stands, the fencing and gates for which can be seen on the dock. Beyond the dock are what look to be piles of sleepers and the yard may have been used as a work site and depot for the distribution of materials such as these along the line. The dock itself is being used in the way it would after the line opened, that is, for the loading and unloading of railway wagons on the level.

Immediately beyond the wagon the dock turns at right angles. This is where horse-drawn carts, and later, lorries, could be drawn up alongside for them to be loaded or unloaded on the level.

Out of shot on the left is the east end of the dock. At the buffers was the cart loading dock, equipped with ramps to enable carts and machinery to be end loaded or unloaded from wagons. The goods shed appears to be almost complete. This would be used for the storage of items such as grain or fertiliser that had to be kept dry while it was waiting either for despatch or collection. As can be seen by the open door, a siding passed through it.

To the right of the line here was the brickyard of James Boam, established in about 1899, and to which a siding was subsequently laid. This was recorded as disused, and the siding shown as removed, in the Midland Railway survey of the line made in the period 1906-1912.[65]

PHOTOGRAPH 66

Photograph 66 shows the same view in 2009. The dock is partly hidden in the bushes to the left but the goods shed identifies the location.

On the far side of the site, to the left of the goods shed in Photograph 65, is a large shed with what look to be sheets hanging out to dry. This may indicate that it was a navvy house. Indeed, the existence of one hereabouts is known.[66] A surviving example can be found at the time of writing to the west of the stationmaster's house. These buildings were of timber, with a slate roof, and divided into three rooms. A large room in the centre was flanked by a similar room to one side with a smaller room to the other. The central and small room shared a chimney with back to back fireplaces. A married man and his family would live in the small room. The large unheated room would be a men's dormitory and the central room a communal sitting and dining room. The wife would keep the house, provide the meals and do the washing, and receive an income from the men for doing this.

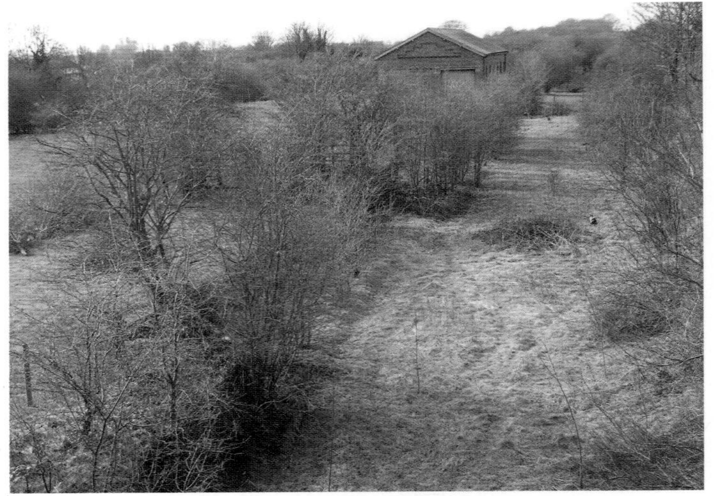

[63] R. Penniston Taylor, *A History of Wymondham, Leicestershire*, 2nd edn (Wymondham, 2004), 425.

[64] Personal correspondence, Trevor Hickman.

[65] Midland Railway Study Centre, Item No 00806.

[66] Penniston Taylor, *History of Wymondham*, 422.

NAVVY HOUSES OCCUPANTS

The 1891 Census recorded the names of those people living in the navvy houses. Three such houses are recorded on Butt Lane, that shown in Photograph 65 and the two adjacent to the Stationmaster's House, the survivor of which is shown in Photograph 67.

The Census Enumerator appears to have been working northwards from the Main Street and, if this is the case, the occupants of the hut shown in Photograph 65 were as follows. It is tempting to think that the men may have been at work when the Enumerator called and whoever provided the information, maybe Ann Smith, just did not know where her boarders were born. This is a not an uncommon feature of the recording of navvies in the Census. In some instances elsewhere, real names were not known and nicknames were given instead.

William Smith	Head	Aged 47	Public Works Ganger	born Whittlesea
Ann Smith	Wife	Aged 53		born Dudley
Job Smith	Son	Aged 25	General Labourer	born Burslem
Dan Smith	Son	Aged 17	General Labourer	born Burslem
Harriet Smith	Dau.	Aged 14		born Grimston
Alfred Thompson	Boarder	Aged 25	General Labourer	born London
William White	Boarder	Aged 24	General Labourer	born London
James Taylor	Boarder	Aged 42	General Labourer	born London
John White	Boarder	Aged 22	General Labourer	born London
Thomas Miller	Boarder	Aged 39	General Labourer	born London
Martin Hardy	Boarder	Aged 45	General Labourer	born London
William Jackson	Boarder	Aged 37	General Labourer	born London
Samuel Smith	Boarder	Aged 26	General Labourer	born London
Christopher Hughes	Boarder	Aged 50	General Labourer	born London

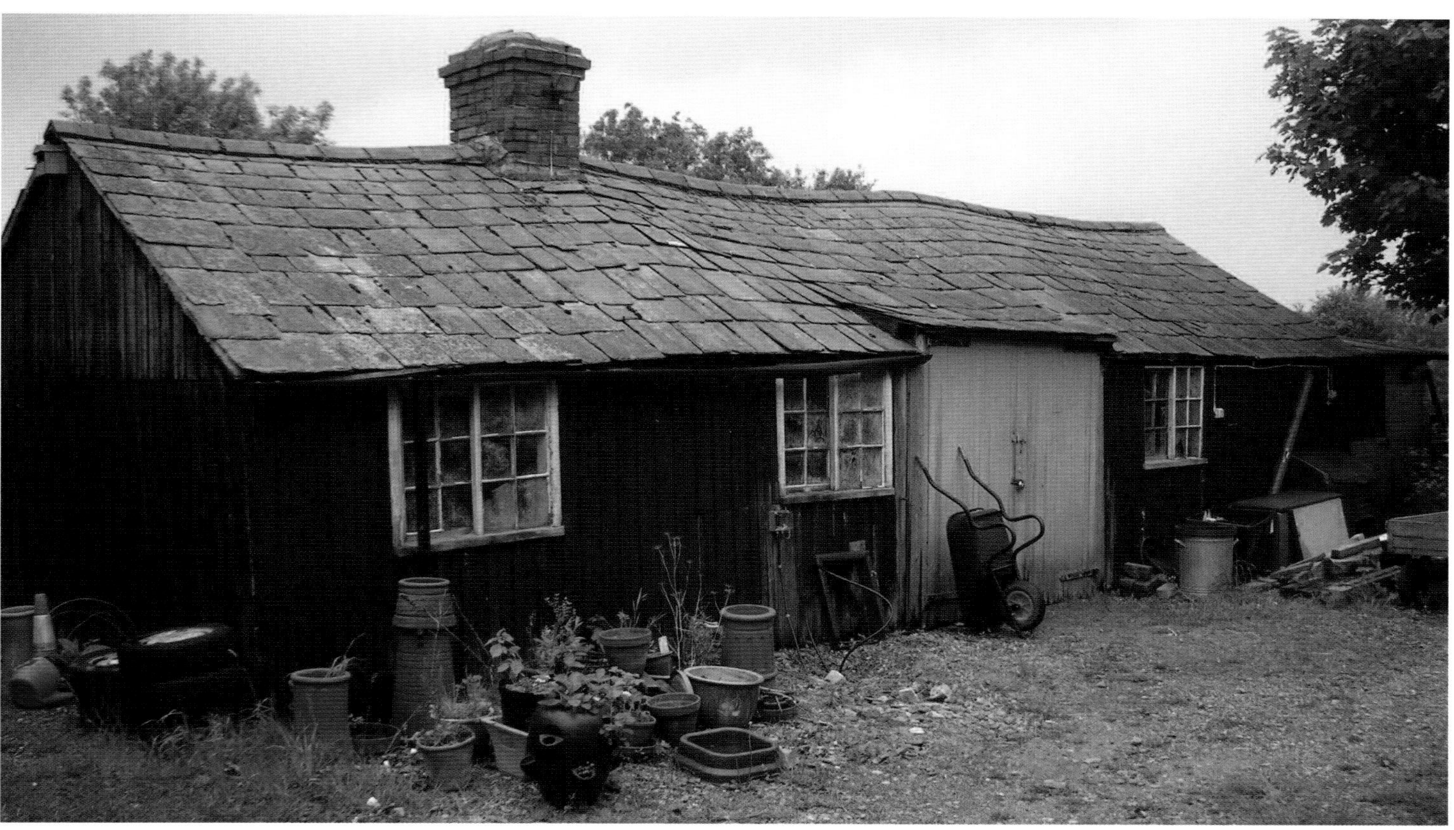

NAVVY HOUSING

PHOTOGRAPH 67

By the end of the nineteenth century, contractors provided relatively decent accommodation for their navvies and took some care for them, in contrast to the squalor of the housing they occupied in the middle years of the century.[67] Navvy housing was revolutionised by increasing concern about both the insanitary conditions the men lived in (together with their wives and children in the case of married men) and their moral and spiritual needs. The significant landmark was the construction of the Manchester Ship Canal from 1887 to 1894, followed by the construction of the Great Central Railway from 1894 to 1901. In both cases, purpose-built housing was provided, along with shops and tradesmen's deliveries. Spiritual needs were not overlooked and the Navvy Mission provided for this as well as recreational activities. In 1891 there was a Navvy Missioner, a Mr Eglington, stationed at Wymondham.[68]

The building of the Bourne to Saxby line was also undertaken during this period and the navvies here benefitted from this housing change. The housing may seem primitive by present day standards but in the late nineteenth century it would have been an improvement on the cottages of the rural poor.[69]

No building is shown to the west of the goods yard either on the Deposited Plan or on the 1904 OS map. Photograph 67 is of the surviving navvy house, adjacent to the station house. This is protected as a Grade II Listed Building and is believed by English Heritage to be the only surviving such house on its original site in England.[70]

The 1891 Census reveals the numbers of people accommodated at huts like these in the village: one hut housed nine; two others, ten each; another, eleven; another, twelve; two others, thirteen, and two more, fourteen.[71] In the hut shown in Photograph 65 there were fourteen. The Census also recorded at least 182 men living in the village who were working on the railway and, when their wives and children were taken into account the total increased the village population by some 270 souls. Seventy-five of the men gave their occupation as navvy, labourer, or excavator. Others were employed as gangers and foremen, brickmakers and bricklayers, blacksmiths, carpenters, navvy drivers and firemen, with a sprinkling of horse keepers, contractors assistants, surveyors, time keepers and cashiers.

This surviving house was one of a pair and both can be seen in the background of the photograph in Appendix C, page 129 below. The second house was demolished in about 1988.

[67] Michael Morris, 'Towards an archaeology of navvy huts and settlements of the industrial revolution', *Antiquity* 68 (1994), 573-584.

[68] *Grantham Journal* (5 December 1891). Elijah T. Eglington, Evangelist, is listed at Church Lane, Wymondham, in the Census Returns for 1891.

[69] Gary Boyd-Hope and Andrew Sargent, *Railways and Rural Life: S. W. A. Newton and The Great Central Railway* (Swindon, 2007), 198 - 211.

[70] English Heritage, Listed Buildings Register (Heritage Gateway, Listed Buildings Online).

[71] Penniston Taylor, *History of Wymondham*.

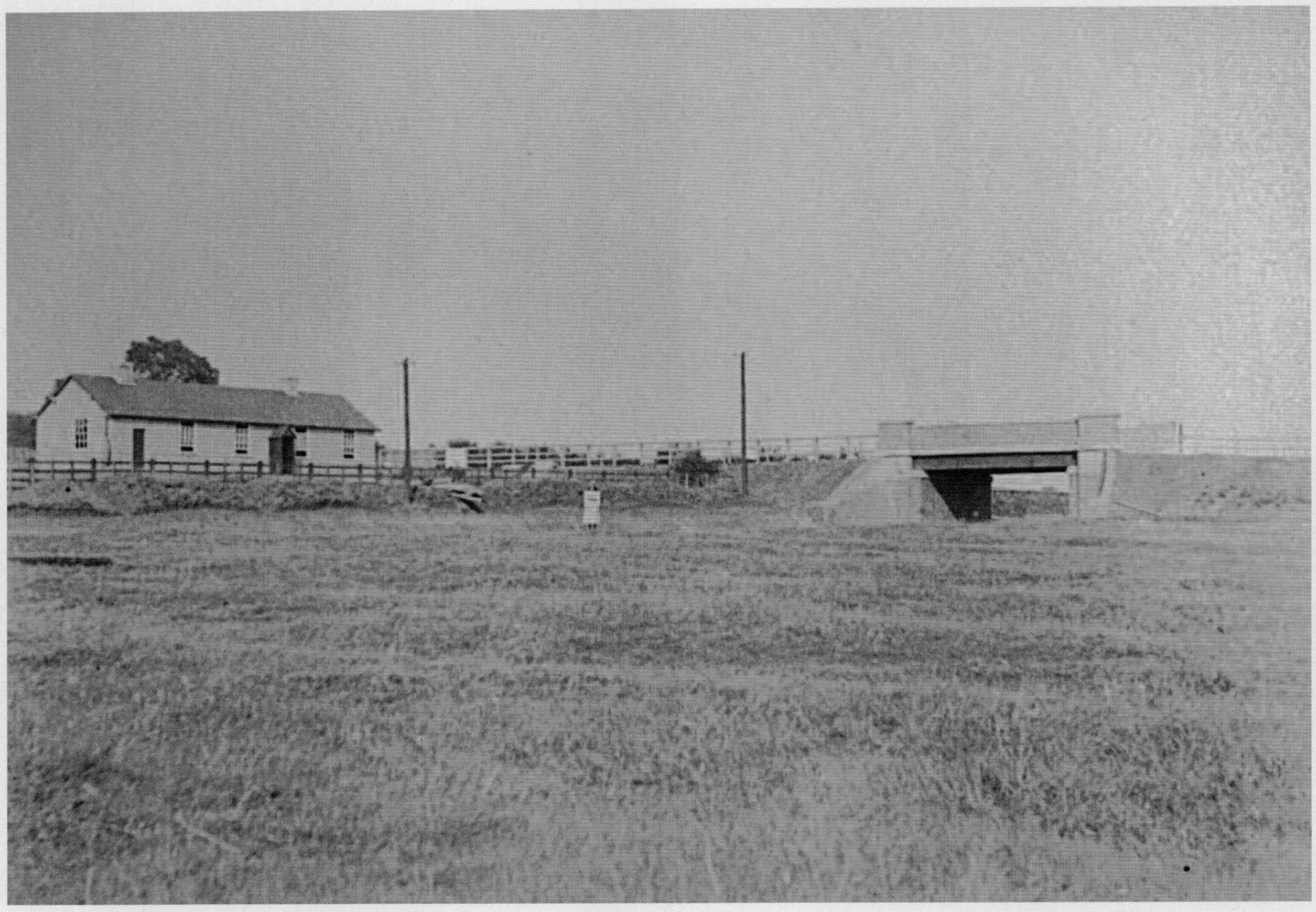

WYMONDHAM STATION MASTER'S HOUSE AND GOODS YARD

PHOTOGRAPH 68

Photograph 68 is a view across the field in which Edmondthorpe and Wymondham goods yard was built, with Bridge 7 on the right. The rails are out of sight as the line runs in a low cutting at this point.

The building was the station master's house. It is different to the house built for the station master at South Witham, which was a two storey brick building. Here at Wymondham is a timber clad bungalow. A comparison with Photograph 65 shows that this image was taken before the goods sidings were built. They were in the centre around where the girl is standing. Just out of shot, to the left of the house, were two timber navvy houses, one of which survives and is seen in Photograph 67.

PHOTOGRAPH 69

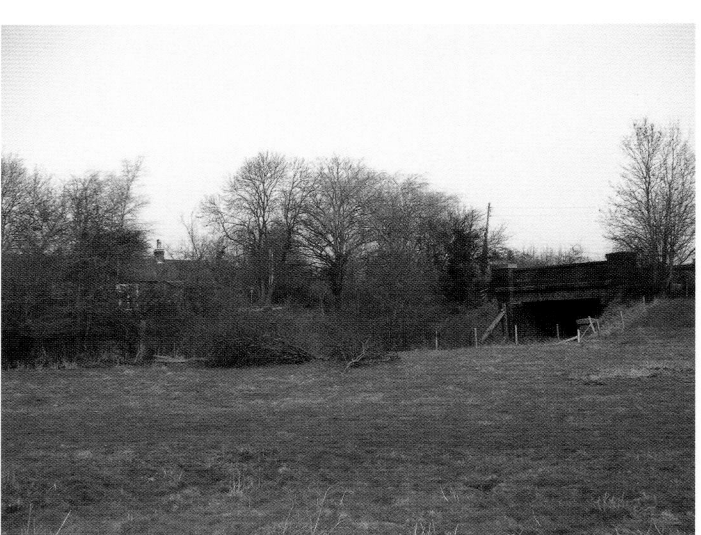

Photograph 69 is the same view as Photograph 68. Bridge 7 is to the right, with the Station House visible behind the trees. The trees in the centre have grown on the cattle dock and hide some of the fencing from view. The dock also retains a pump for providing water for waiting cattle as well as one of its end loading ramps.

PHOTOGRAPH 70

(above)

Photograph 70 is a closer view of the station master's house. It may well be that this house was built by the Midland Railway in advance of the construction work beginning, to house the station master eventually but in the meantime to provide accommodation, perhaps for their resident staff. The Great Central Railway provided differing grades of housing for managers during the construction of that line.[72] This theory is supported by the fact that these two photographs are examples of the very few in which women and children appear. Wilson may well have photographed his colleagues and their families as favours to them. Indeed, it is interesting to speculate that the girl in Photograph 68 may be one of his own daughters, either Edith (16 in 1892), Gertrude (14) or Mary (10). Wilson and his family were not living here, however, but at The Cottage, on the High Street in the village (see Chapter 2).

There is no entry for this house in the 1891 Census so it may not have been built or completed at that time.

PHOTOGRAPH 71

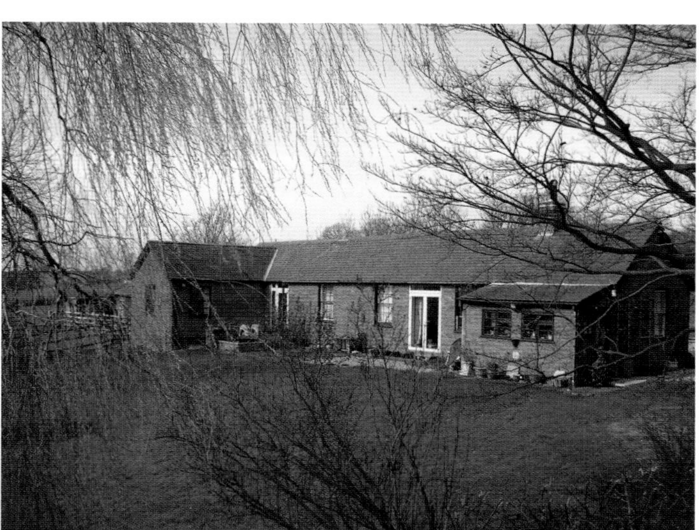

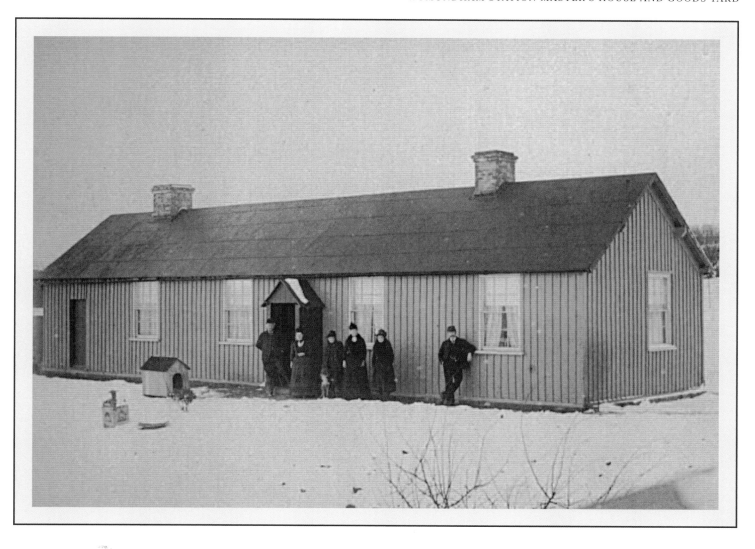

The view of the former Station House in 2009 (Photograph 71) shows a number of changes. The house now has a brick facade and extensions at both ends. Some of the original windows still survive and there is evidence on the ridge of the left-hand chimney.

[72] Boyd-Hope and Sargent, *Railways and Rural Life*, 198-211.

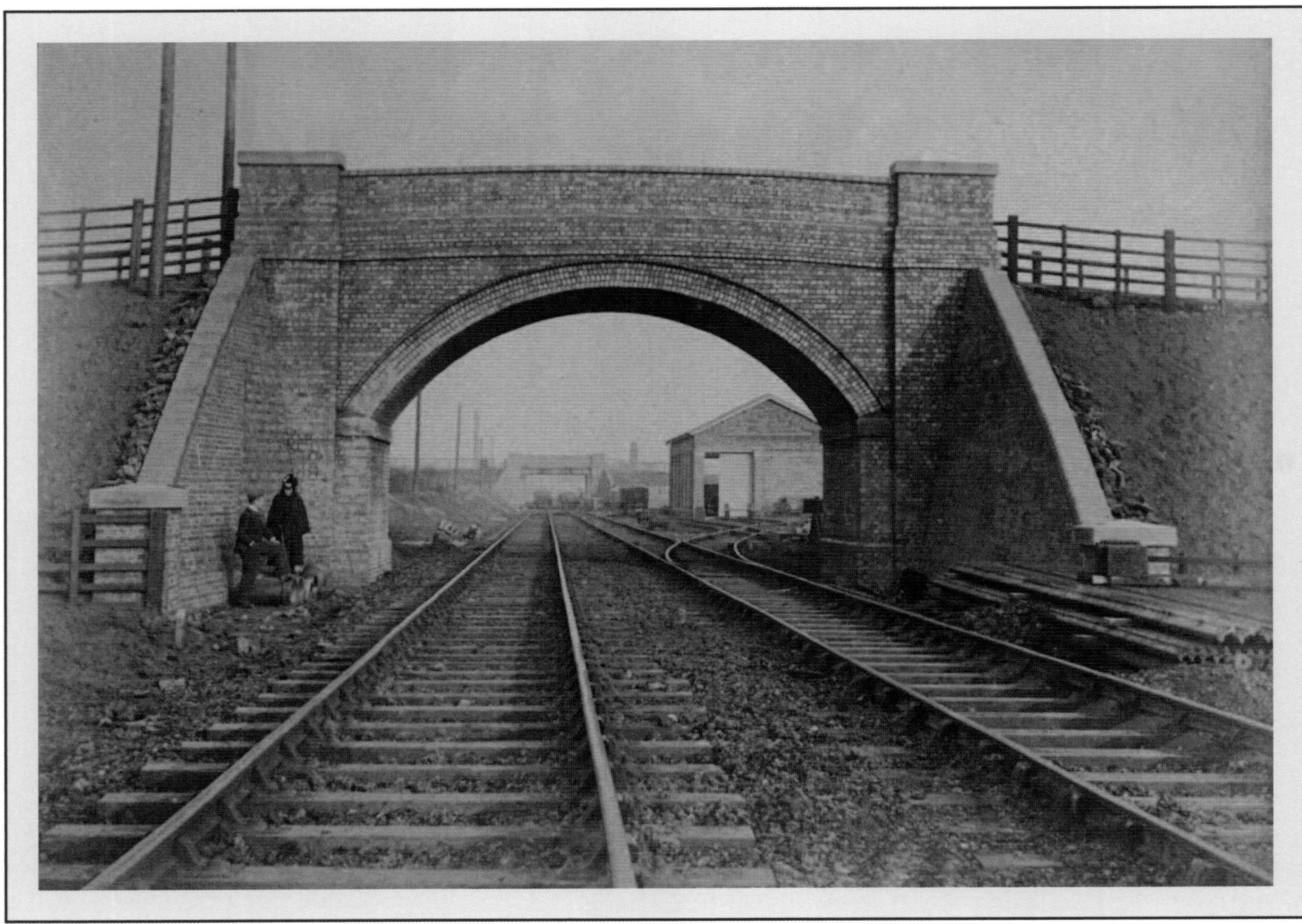

BRICKYARD LANE BRIDGE, WYMONDHAM

PHOTOGRAPH 72

Photograph 72 shows the goods shed and sidings at Edmondthorpe and Wymondham station, seen through the arch of Bridge 6. This bridge carried Brickyard Lane over the railway. Bridge 7 is in the distance. The platforms were on the other side of Bridge 7. The line was built as a double track through the station to allow for trains to pass.

Opportunities for trains to pass are always limited on a single line railway and it makes sense to do it at stations where trains will be calling at the platforms or carrying out shunting movements into and out of goods sidings. They were particularly important on this line because of the number of trains, including express trains, which passed through. In November 1904, for example, there were three local passenger trains in either direction scheduled to stop here, with two additional express trains in either direction between Leicester and Great Yarmouth.[73] In addition to these would be a number of local and long distance goods trains, added to in the summer months by additional excursion and holiday trains, many of them expresses, between the Midlands and the Norfolk coast. This passing loop was removed in the spring of 1962 and the rest of the rails removed after final closure in 1964.

Of the two men on the left, the one on the right hand is probably the coachman (see also Photographs 73 and 75 which were taken at the same time, as the same man appears in all the shots).

This bridge has been demolished and replaced with an embankment to carry the road which prohibits the taking of the comparison photograph.

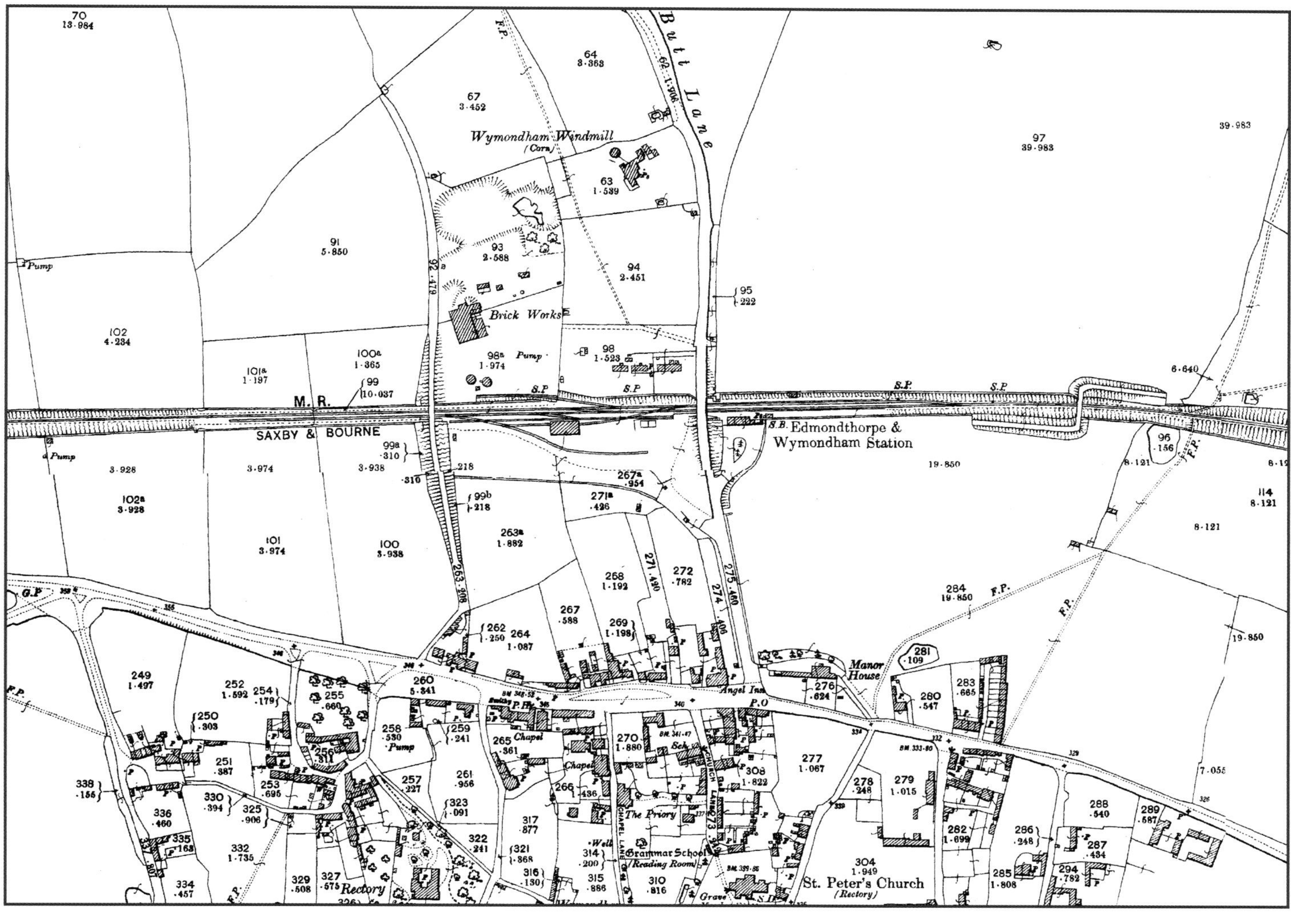

MAP 8

OS 1/2500 County Series Map, 1904. Edmondthorpe and Wymondham Station.

In the centre is Bridge 7 separating the station platforms to the right (see Photographs 63 and 64) from the goods sidings to the left. Through the station, the line is doubled to provide for a loop for trains travelling in opposite directions to pass. West of Bridge 7, the goods yard with its cattle pens and goods shed is to the south of the line (see Photographs 65 and 72).

To the north of the goods yard, three buildings lie parallel to the line. The larger one to the right is the Station Master's House (see Photographs 68 and 70). The other two are navvy houses. The one that survives (see Photograph 67) is that in the centre. Both of the navvy houses were retained as railway staff houses and were occupied up to the early 1950s. The plan form of the navvy houses is very similar to those shown on Map 3 and Map 6. In the field to the west of the houses is the brickyard of James Boam, with its own siding.

Bridge 6 carries the road to the brick works over the railway. The navvy house seen in Photograph 65 was situated in the field to the south east of this bridge. Bridge 8 is the occupation bridge on the right, with very distinctive S-shaped access ramps.

The house in which Charles Wilson lived during his time in the village is the large building on the north side the village green directly below the field number 269. The house itself is shown in Chapter 2 (see page 16).

[73] *Bradshaw's Railway Guide* (November 1904).

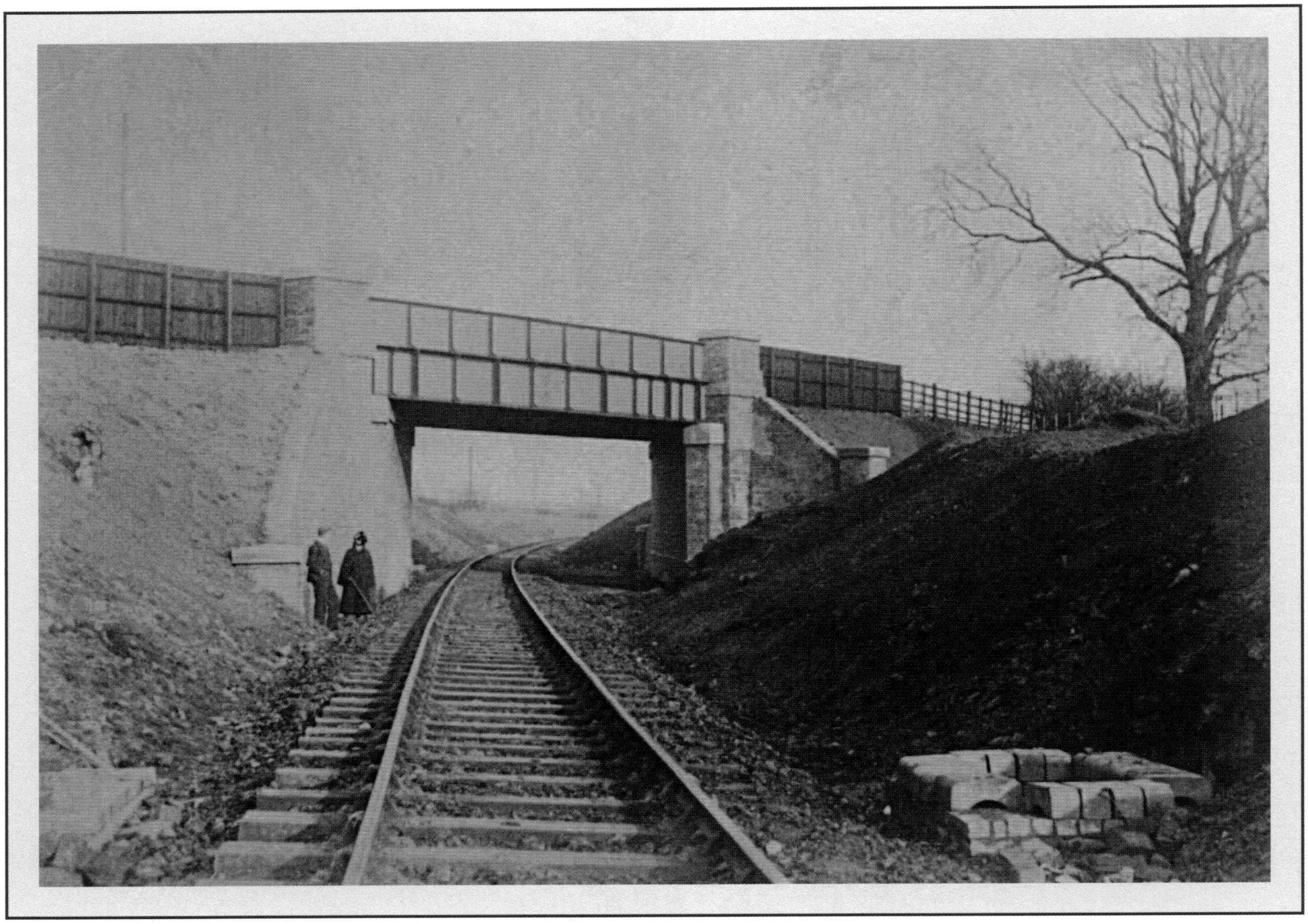

SAXBY ROAD BRIDGE, WYMONDHAM

PHOTOGRAPH 73

Photograph 73 shows the girder bridge, Bridge 5, carrying the road from Wymondham to Saxby over the railway. Here again space has been left for a double track. This bridge is unique on the line in having a girder to carry the road with a steel parapet on top. A girder bridge was required here because there would not be enough height between rail level and an arch to allow for a double line of rails without raising the road level excessively.

The person on the right is probably the coachman (see also Photographs 72 and 75, evidently taken at the same time, as the same man appears in each image).

The permanent way has been laid, but the ballasting has not been completed. The steel rails were 30 feet long and weighed 86lb to the yard. They were joined with plain fishplates, 40lb the pair, and carried in chairs weighing 50lbs. The chairs were bolted to creosoted sleepers with two trenails and two spikes.[74]

PHOTOGRAPH 74

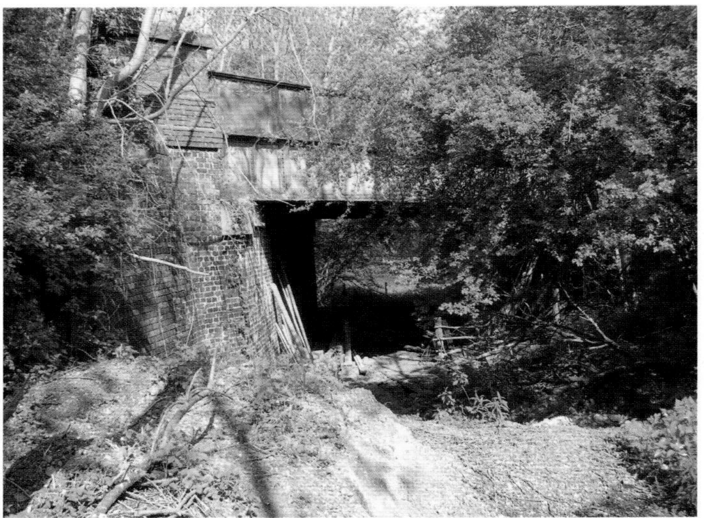

Photograph 74 shows this bridge in 2008. As a result of tree growth, as well as dumping on the trackbed, the view has had to be taken closer to the structure than Photograph 73. In 2009 the bridge itself was in a poor state of repair with the roadway narrowed to limit the weight imposed on the bridge.

[74] National Archives, RAIL 491/548.

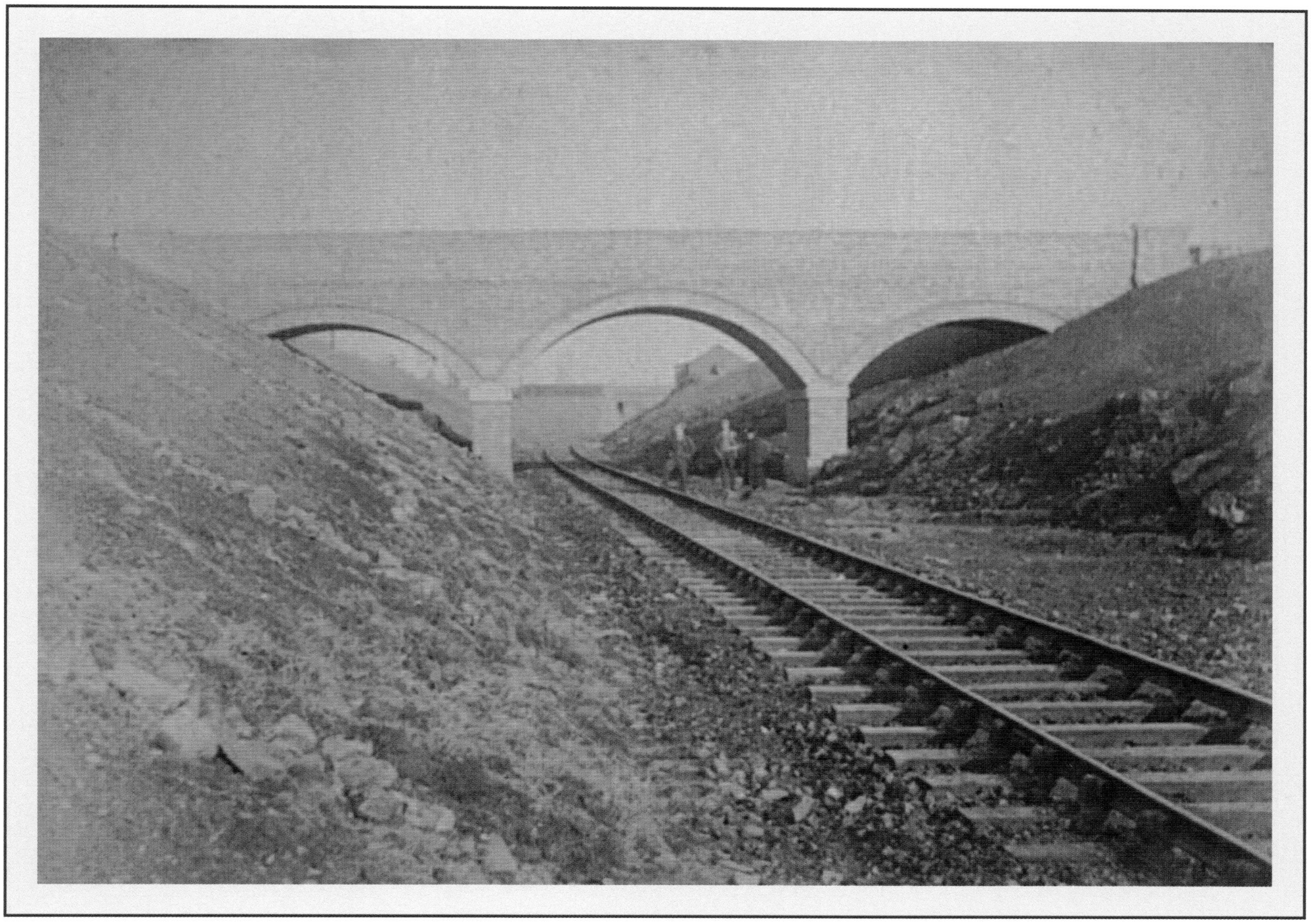

OCCUPATION BRIDGE WEST OF SAXBY ROAD, WYMONDHAM

PHOTOGRAPH 75

This shows the three segmental arches of Bridge 4, an occupation bridge, with the girder of Bridge 5 beyond. The men here are interesting. The two on the left, who appear elsewhere, may be Wilson's assistants. The third, who also appears in Photographs 72 and 73, may be a coachman. Charles Wilson had to have some form of transport to be able to carry out his duties and, as he was living in Wymondham at the time, the hire of a wagon or carriage from the village would be logical. (See also Photograph 25 for further information on this point.)

Between the two bridges, on the right, a hut can be seen. Neither the Deposited Plan for the line nor the OS map of 1904 shows a building here. There was a sizeable population of navvies in the village that had to be housed and temporary timber huts to live in were erected at convenient places along the line for them, several in Wymondham and some near to Bridge 5. This might be one of them. (See Photograph 67 for a description of these huts.)

PHOTOGRAPH 76

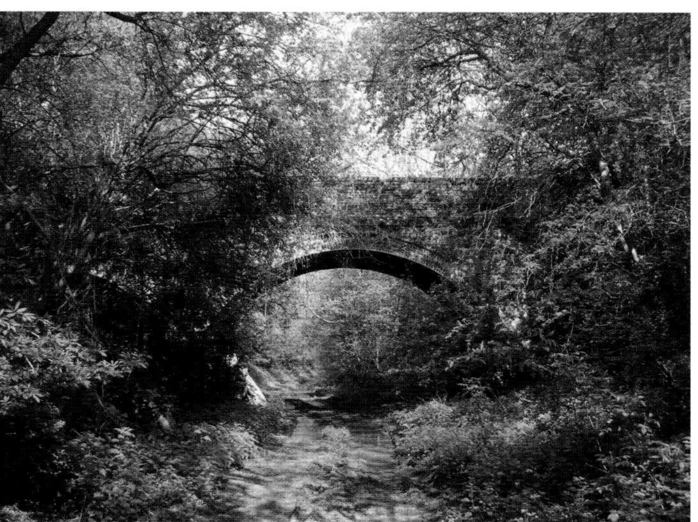

Photograph 76 shows the same, west, elevation of the bridge in May 2008, now in a more verdant setting.

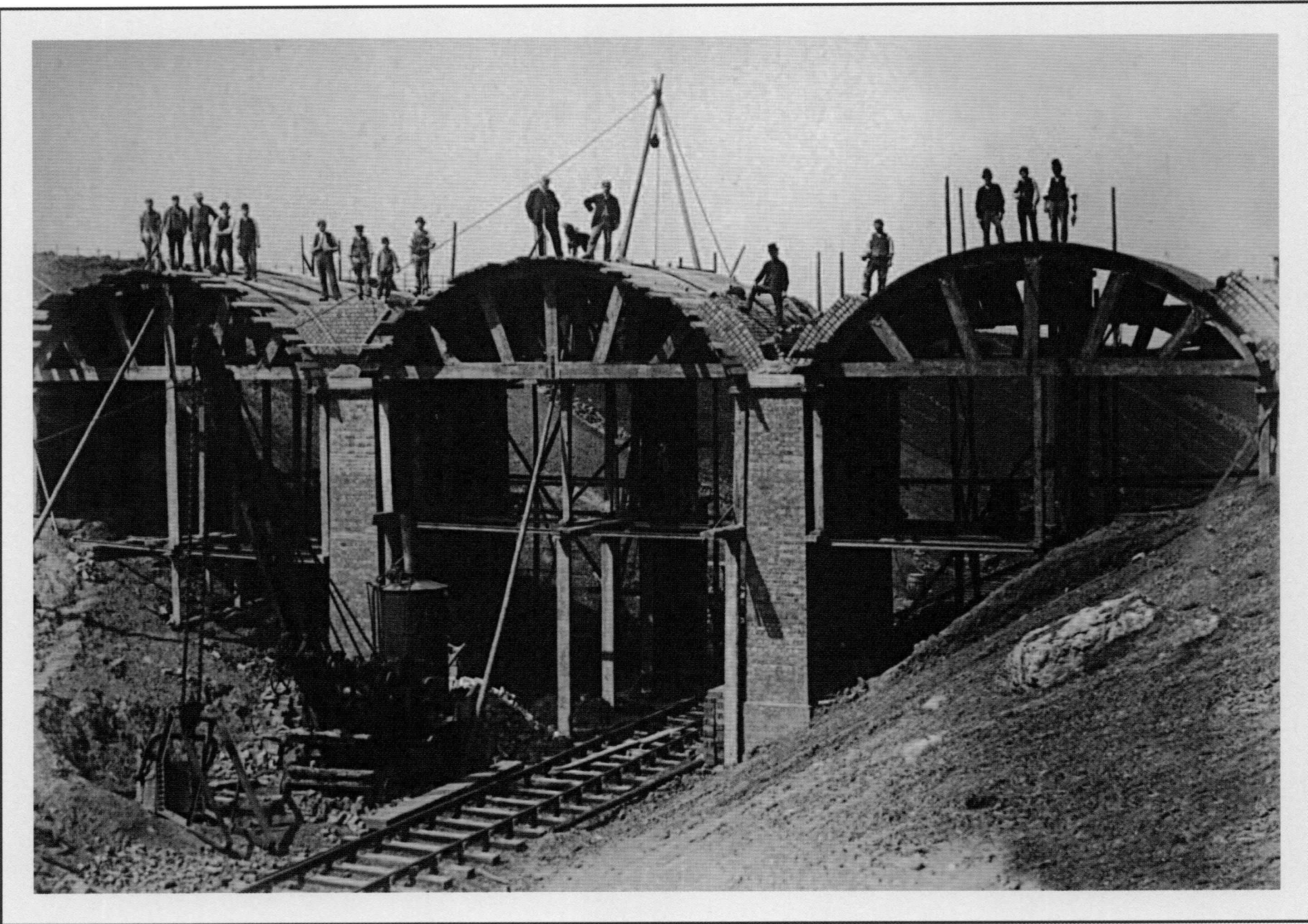

OCCUPATION BRIDGE, SAXBY PARISH

(see also Map 9)

PHOTOGRAPHS 77, 78 AND 79

Photographs 77 and 78 (opposite top) show Bridge 3 under construction, while Photograph 79 (opposite bottom) shows the completed bridge. The two former are of the east elevation, the latter of the west. Brick and stone arched bridges are only structurally sound when their arches are complete and the vertical and horizontal forces can be carried through the piers and abutments. The construction of timber centring, the framework to support the brick or stone arch rings during the construction period, enables the formation of the arch. Arches like this have always been built using this technique and still are today.

Photograph 77 clearly shows this process. The brickwork is being laid direct on to the timber arch. At the same time the arch ring is being raised on either side. A simple A-framed derrick on top provides a mechanism for the bricks and stonework to be hoisted up.

The excavator is a full circle crane excavator, made by Whitaker and Co. of Leeds. These were less efficient than the Dunbar-Ruston navvy seen in Photograph 30. However, the Whitaker could operate through a full 360 degrees whereas the Dunbar-Ruston was limited to 180 degrees. The first of the Whitaker machines was built in 1884 for work on the Manchester Ship Canal.

There are sixteen men in Photograph 77 and seventeen in Photograph 78. One of them is the portly gentleman referred to in Photograph 94, with a dog (perhaps that seen in Photographs 54 and 55). The other men might be considered to be navvies but this very general term included men with a variety of skills and trades. The men here will include some labourers but will be mainly bricklayers. The centreing also demonstrates why carpenters also formed part of the workforce.

Photograph 78 shows that the central arch was built with enough width to allow for a double track. The line was single here and the permanent track is being laid. The brick manhole in the bottom left corner has been built where any second track would have had to have been laid.

Photograph 79 shows the completed bridge from the other side. Because of the height of the piers they taper slightly towards the top. The depth of the cutting is clearly evident and it was the cut from here that was used to create the embankment further west on which the line dropped down to Saxby.

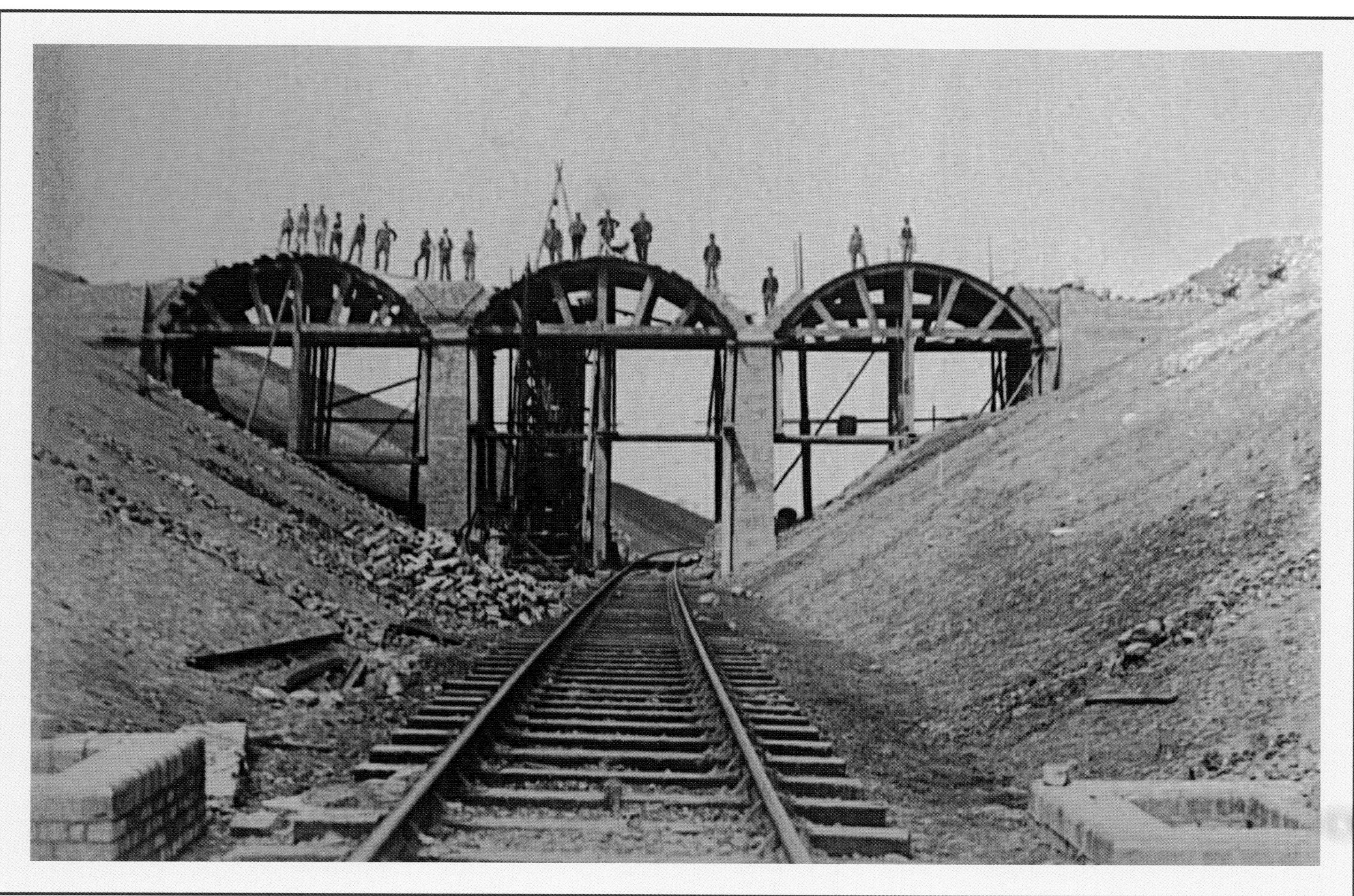

Photograph 78

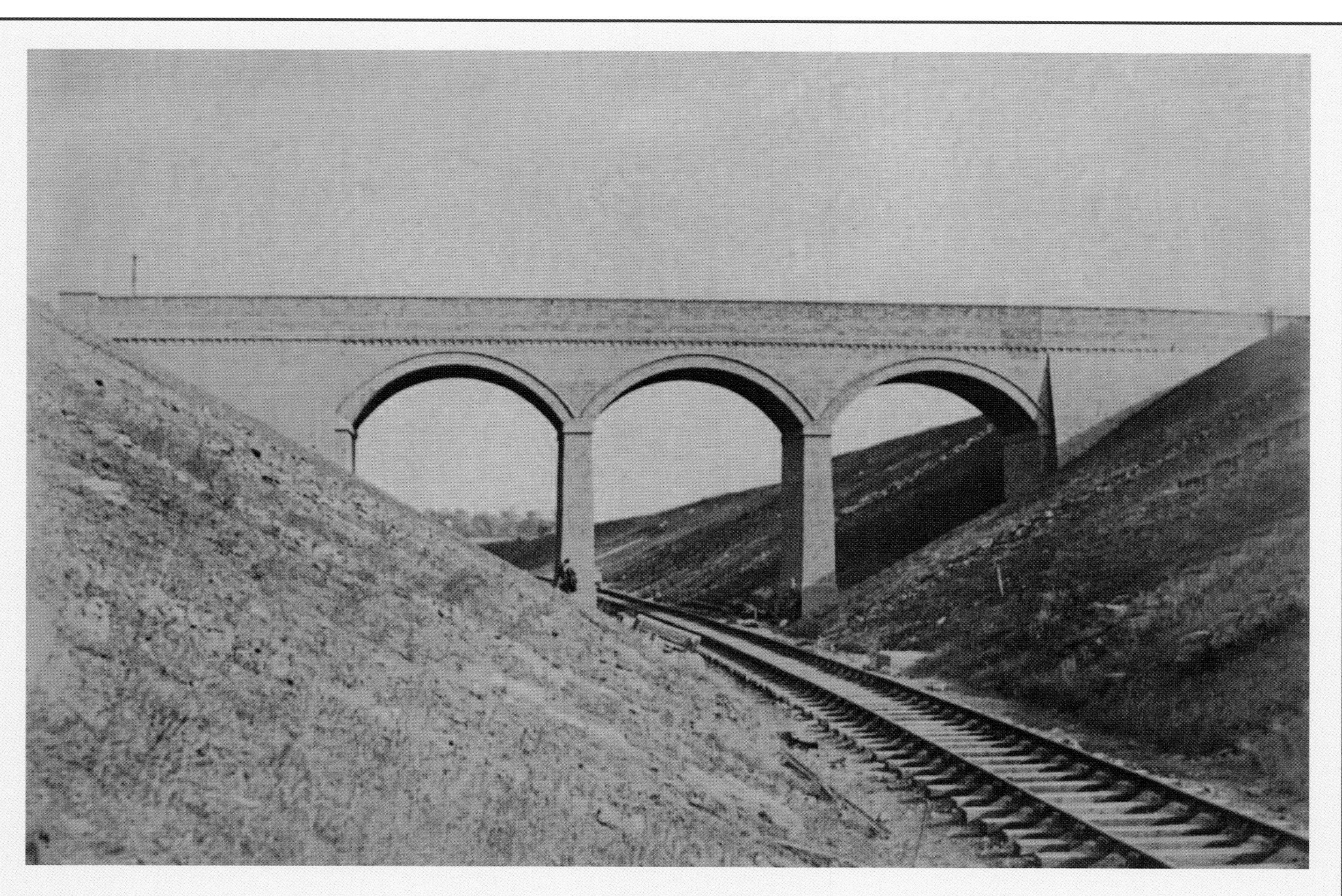

Photograph 79

PHOTOGRAPH 80

Photograph 80 shows the west elevation of Bridge 3, as it was in May 2008. The pier to the left is the northern pier against which the running line was laid. The line here closed for passenger trains in 1959; the last goods train ran in 1964, after which the track was removed.

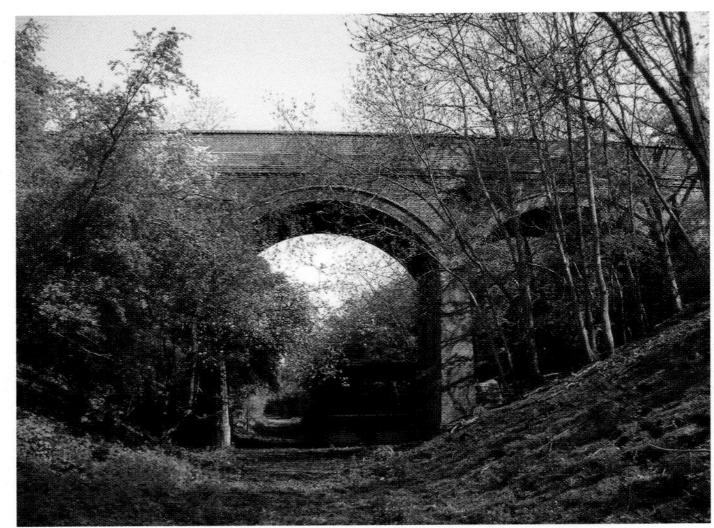

TEMPORARY BRIDGE OVER THE ORIGINAL SAXBY CURVE

(see also Map 9)

PHOTOGRAPHS 81 AND 82

(opposite)

To enable the railway construction works for the line to Bourne to go ahead, a temporary timber bridge was required over the original Saxby curve to maintain it in use until the new curve was opened. These two photographs show that bridge. When the new curve opened on 28 August 1892, the old curve was closed and this temporary bridge was replaced with an embankment.

Photograph 81 shows a contractor's locomotive, probably one of those referred to in the caption for Photograph 93 and also seen in Photograph 57. It has been used to bring an end tipping wagon down to the end of the line to tip its load to build the embankment. This tells us that the embankment here was built from the east to the west, the material for the embankment coming from the deep cutting to the east, over which Bridge 3 was built (shown in photographs 77, 78 and 79).

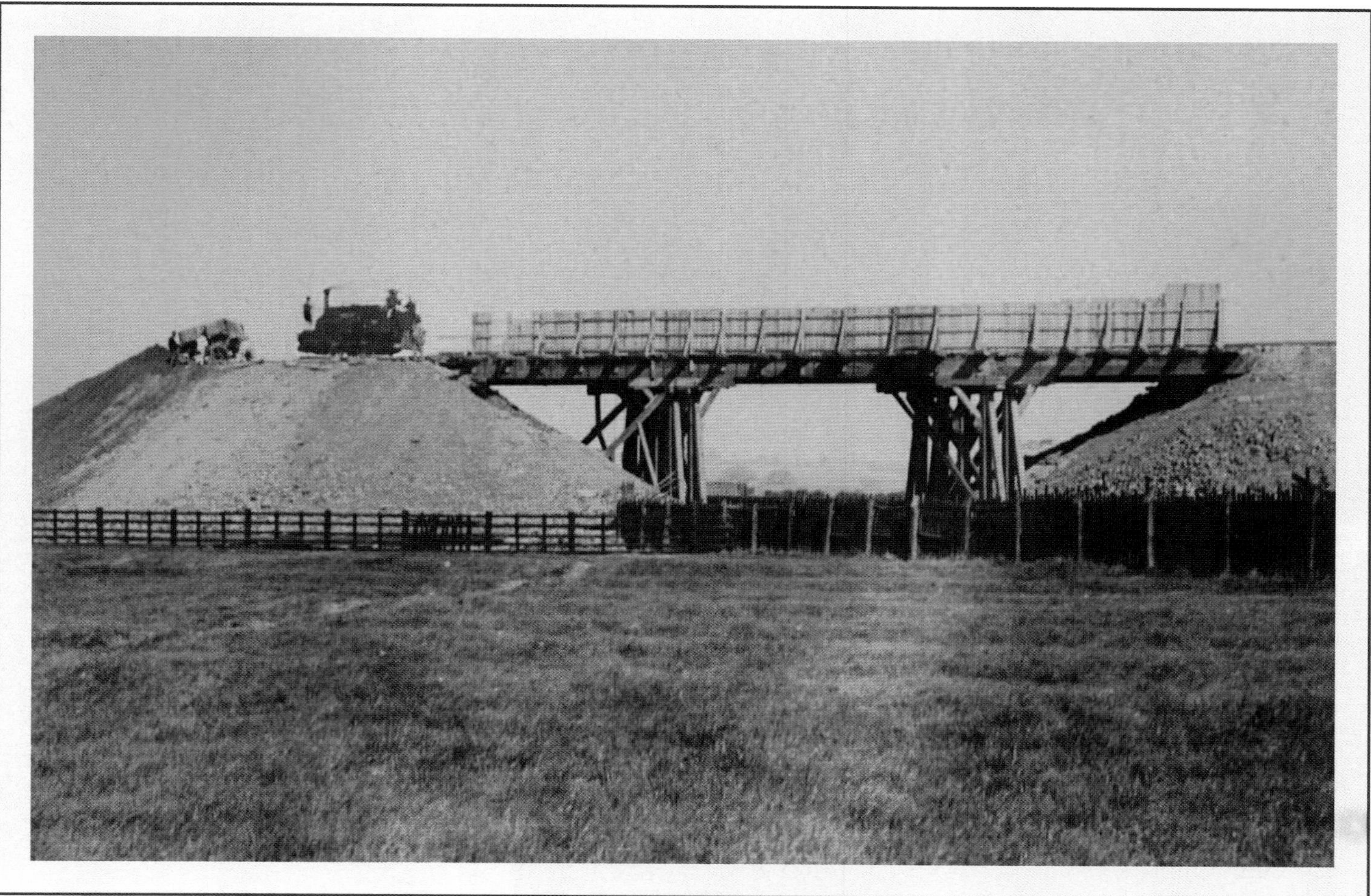

Photograph 81

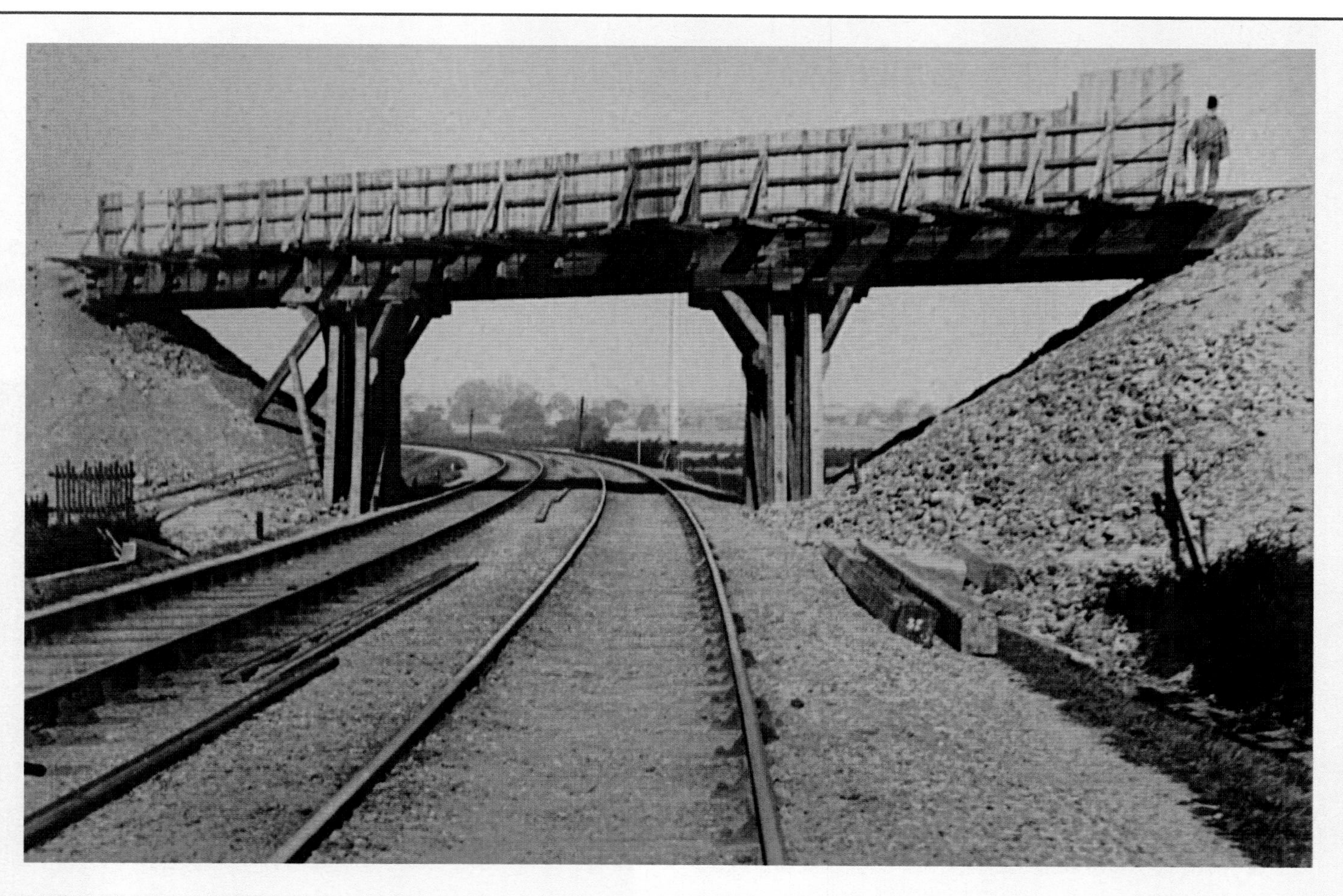

Photograph 82

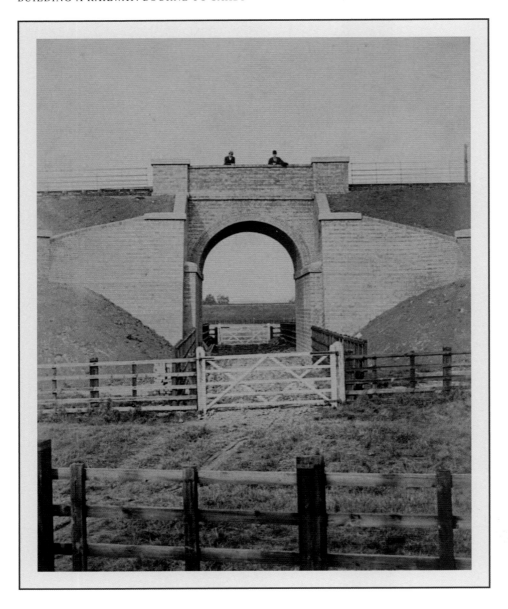

OCCUPATION BRIDGE, SAXBY

(see also Map 9)

PHOTOGRAPH 83

To reach Wymondham, the line had to cut through a spur of higher land, 30 metres above the level of the valley floor at Saxby. It crossed the valley on an embankment (seen here in Photograph 83), pierced by Bridge 2, an occupation bridge. This was built to carry a single line of rails. However, provision was made for the line to be widened if needed in the future. Forward of the parapet the abutment walls are continued down to additional piers from which the wing walls splay out on either side. If the line had been widened the abutments and piers would have been extended upwards and the embankment widened. The land within the railway ownership, up to the gate in front of the wing walls, would have allowed for this.

The fence in the foreground is that to the new Saxby curve, by what is now Bridge GSM2.36a in present day numbering.

PHOTOGRAPH 84

Photograph 84 shows that the bridge remained in a sound condition in May 2008, with some of the original fencing to the right.

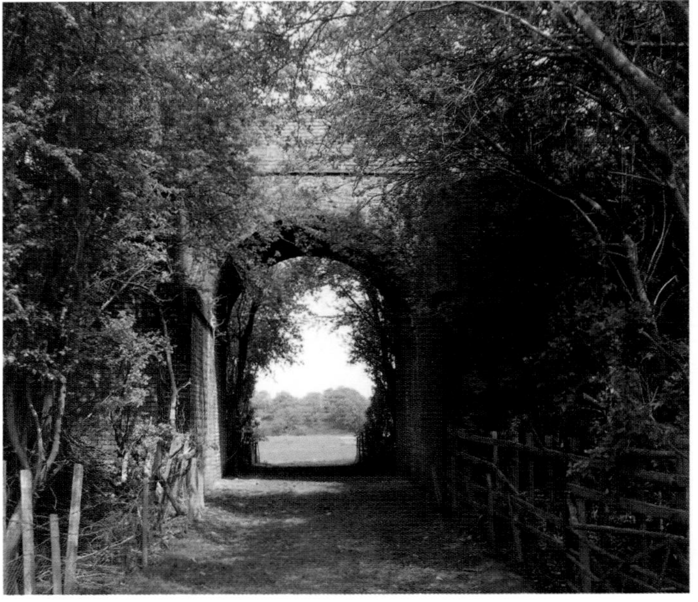

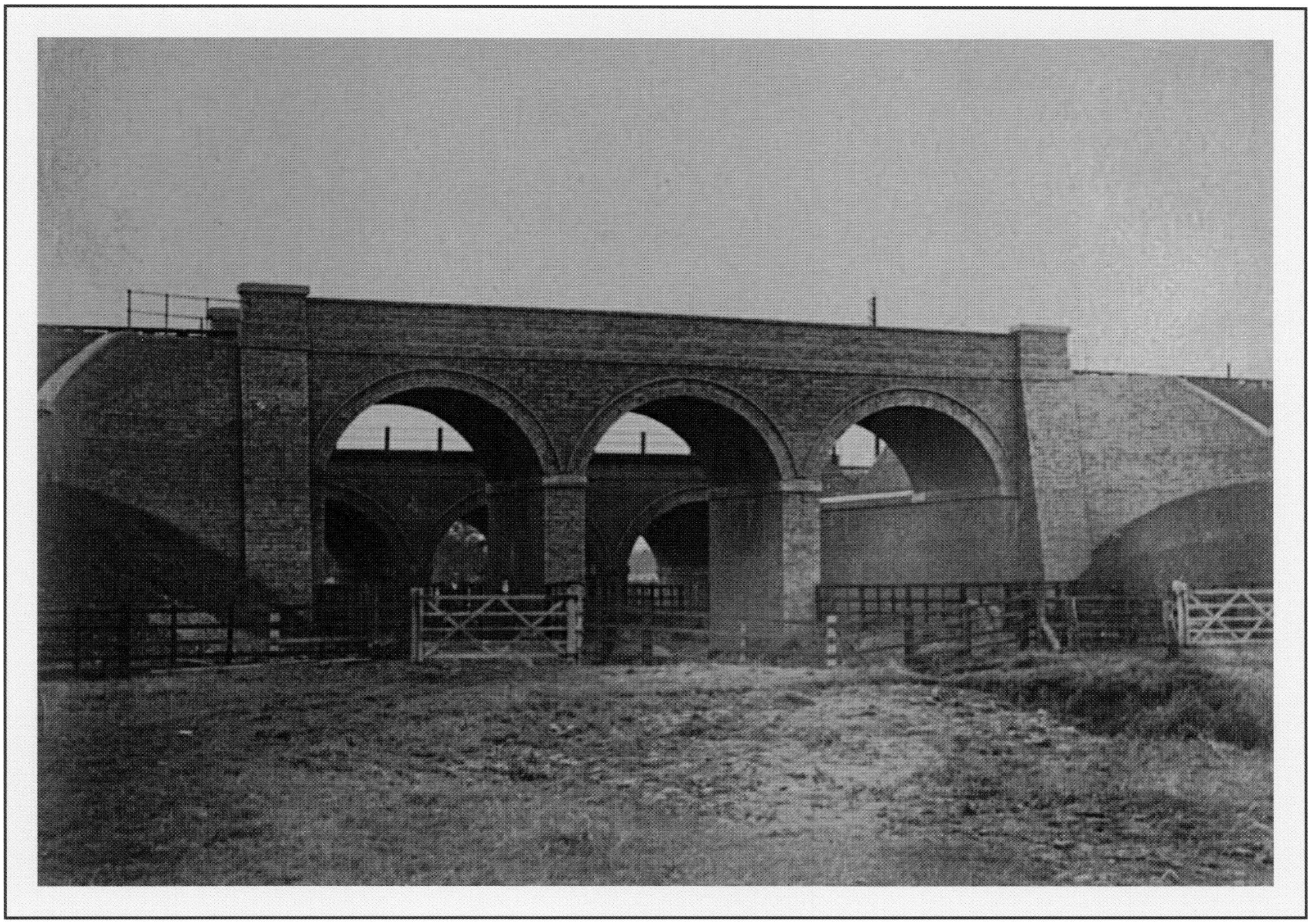

BRIDGE OVER RIVER EYE, SAXBY

(see also Map 9)

PHOTOGRAPH 85

This is Bridge 1 on the line to Bourne. The central arch carries the line over the River Eye and there are occupation arches to either side. On the far side, and at a lower level, a similar three arch bridge, but with railings rather than a brick parapet (now Bridge No GSM2.36) takes the new Saxby curve over the river and roadways.

Railway building works occasionally revealed archaeological remains. The construction of the Bourne line and the new Saxby curve resulted in only one such discovery, the site of an Anglo-Saxon cemetery. This was to the west of Bridge 1, about half way between here and Saxby station. In the late nineteenth century, notification of finds was dependent upon the goodwill of the workers. The find at Saxby was reported to Dr J. C. Cox, who recorded it. In his report he noted that he 'gained a good deal of information from Mr Wilson, the resident engineer, and from some of the gangers whom I interviewed'. [75]

PHOTOGRAPH 86

Photograph 86 shows the same view in May 2008. The far bridge is largely hidden by the subsequent tree growth. Some of the original fencing appears to have survived on the left.

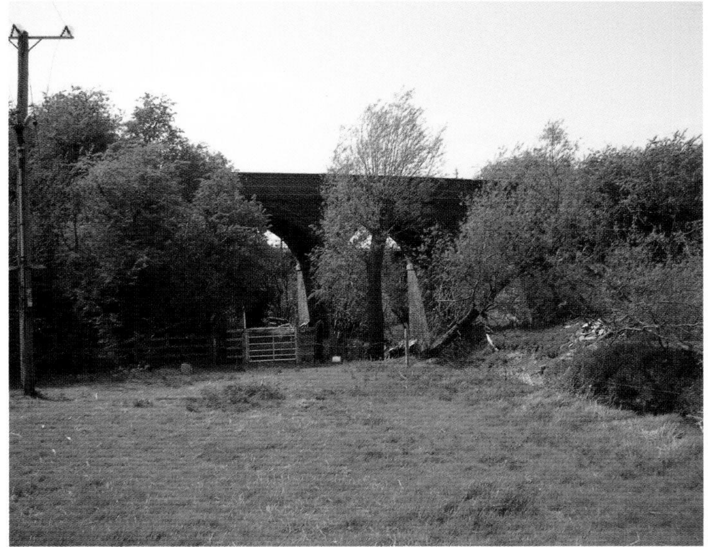

[75] J. C. Cox, 'On an Anglo-Saxon cemetery recently uncovered near Saxby', *Transactions of the Leicestershire Architectural and Archaeological Society* 8 (1899), 74-77.

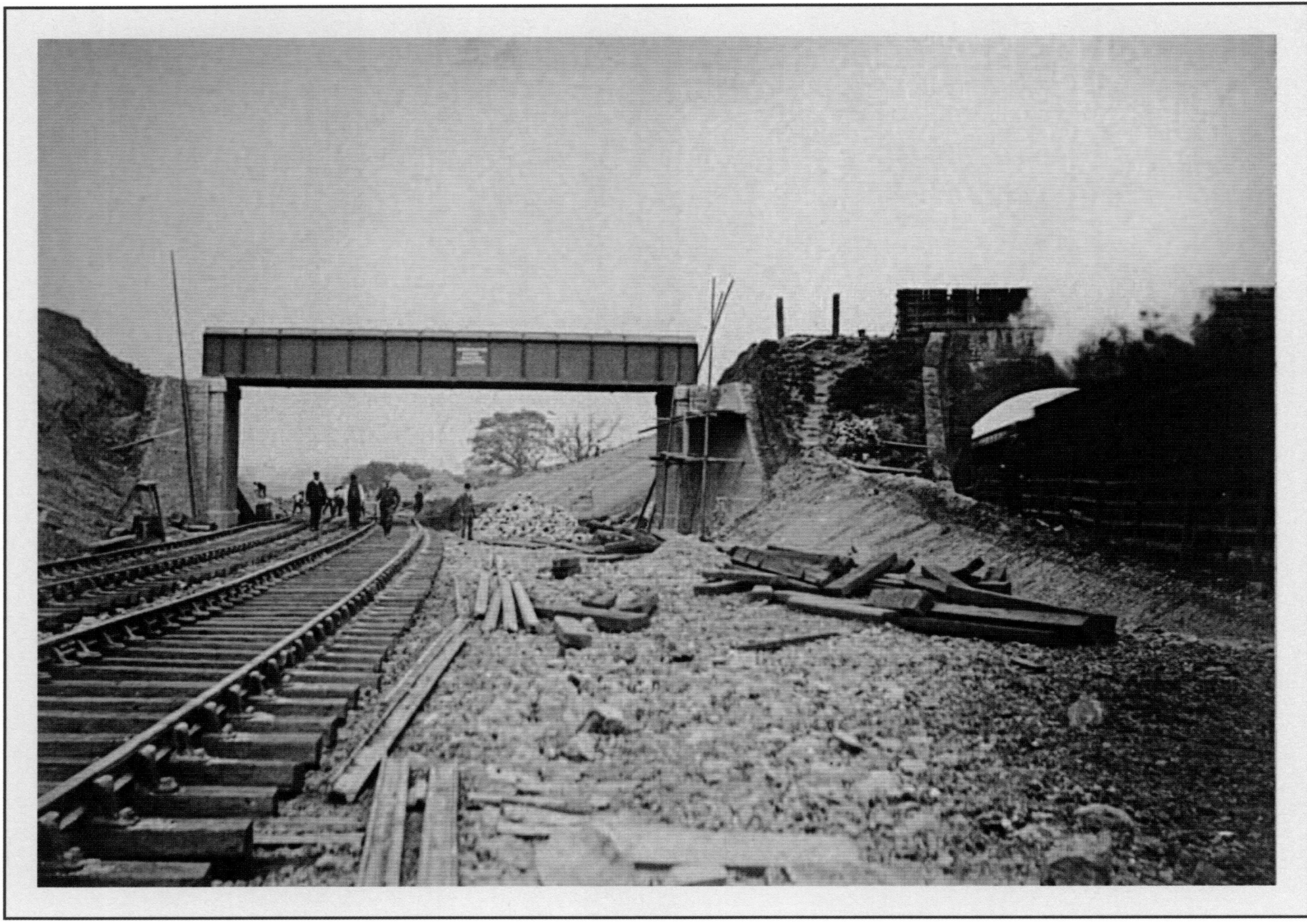

SOUTH END OF THE OLD AND NEW SAXBY CURVES

(see also Map 9)

PHOTOGRAPH 87

The new Saxby curve was just over one mile long. This view is of the southern end, looking north. On the extreme right is the original curve, with its brick occupation bridge over and a train bound for Leicester passing through the arch. To the left is the new bridge. As this had to span four tracks a girder was used here, supported on brick abutments. The abutments are still partly scaffolded with timber scaffolding and the permanent way for two of the tracks is being laid. Tantalisingly, the wording on the parapet is undecipherable.

PHOTOGRAPH 88

(opposite top)

Photograph 88 was taken at a later date. By now the dismantling of the track on the old curve is underway so the new curve must be open. The latter comprises the main running lines in the centre with loops for goods trains on either side. The entrance and exits for the loops at this end were controlled from the Wymondham Junction Signal Box which was behind the photographer.

Both of these bridges still survive but the working railway has precluded the taking of photographs. Now, the tracks along the new curve have been reduced to two with the removal of the goods loops.

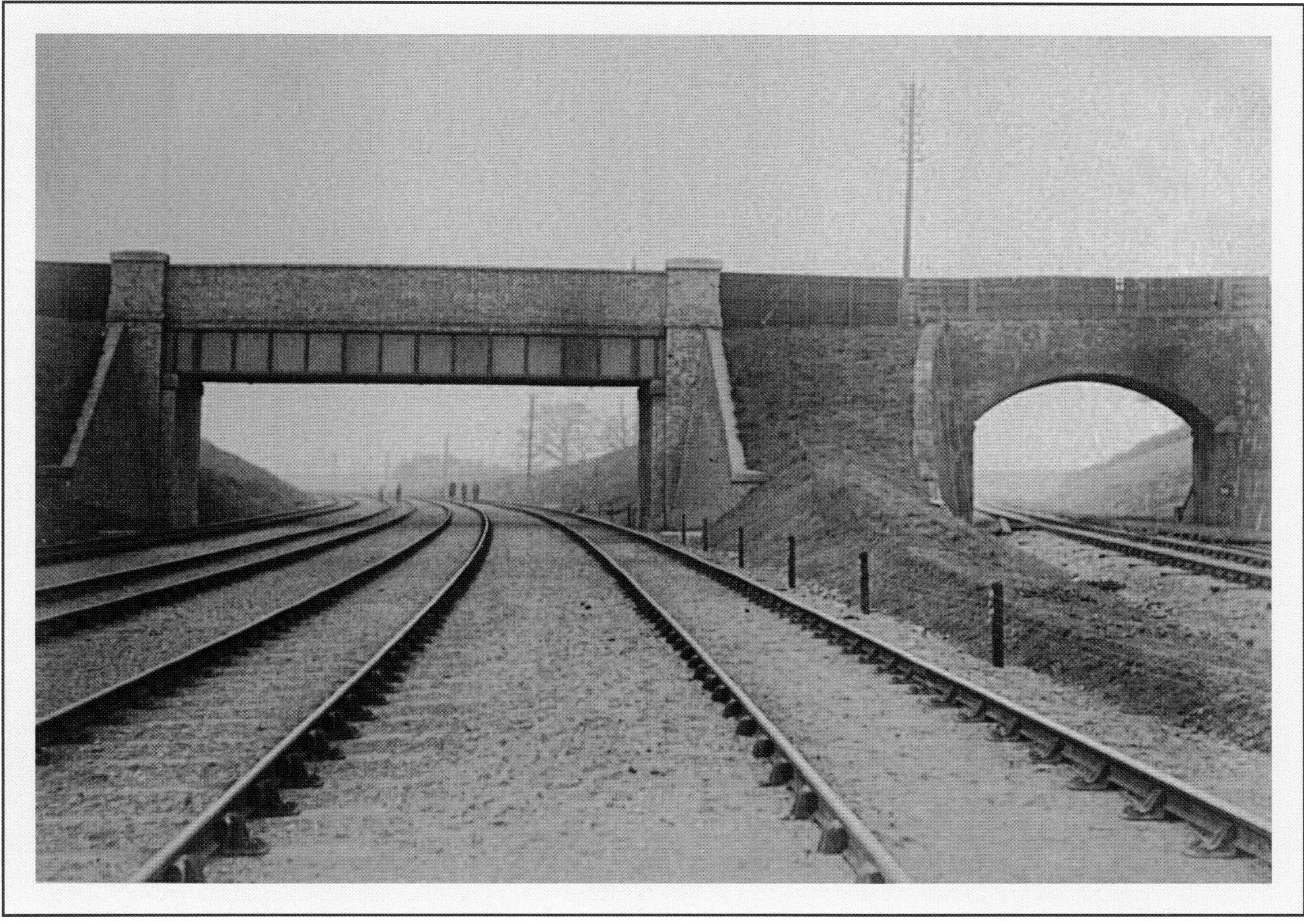

Photograph 88

OCCUPATION BRIDGES, NEW SAXBY CURVE

(see also Map 9)

PHOTOGRAPHS 89 AND 90

(overleaf)

Photograph 90 (overleaf, bottom) is of Bridge GSM2.36A and Photograph 89 (overleaf, top) shows the same bridge in the foreground with Bridge GSM2.36 in the background. The distinctive fencing and gates provided for Stapleford Park are very prominent.

The photographs were taken at the same time, as the four people on the bridge are the same in both; they include the portly gentleman seen in Photograph 94. On the track behind the men are Midland Railway wagons, one (partly hidden by the bridge parapet in Photograph 90) with '..ELL IRON COMPANY' and '..N MOWBRAY' underneath. This probably refers to the Holwell Iron Company Ltd. Their ironworks were at Asfordby Hill, near Melton Mowbray. Initially obtaining their stone close by the works, the opening of the Saxby-Bourne line gave rail access to large reserves of ironstone on the Buckminster Estate which they started quarrying in 1898.[76] However, as the line appears not yet to be open for traffic (as indicated by the isolated wagons standing between the two bridges), this wagon may have been used to deliver iron fixtures and fittings for the construction works.

The contract for the line required the 'best description of English iron' to be obtained from manufacturers approved by the Engineer and that the whole of the ironwork and other materials must be sent as far as possible by the Midland Railway.[77]

[76] Tonks, *Ironstone Quarries of the Midlands, VIII*, 13.

[77] National Archives, RAIL 491/548.

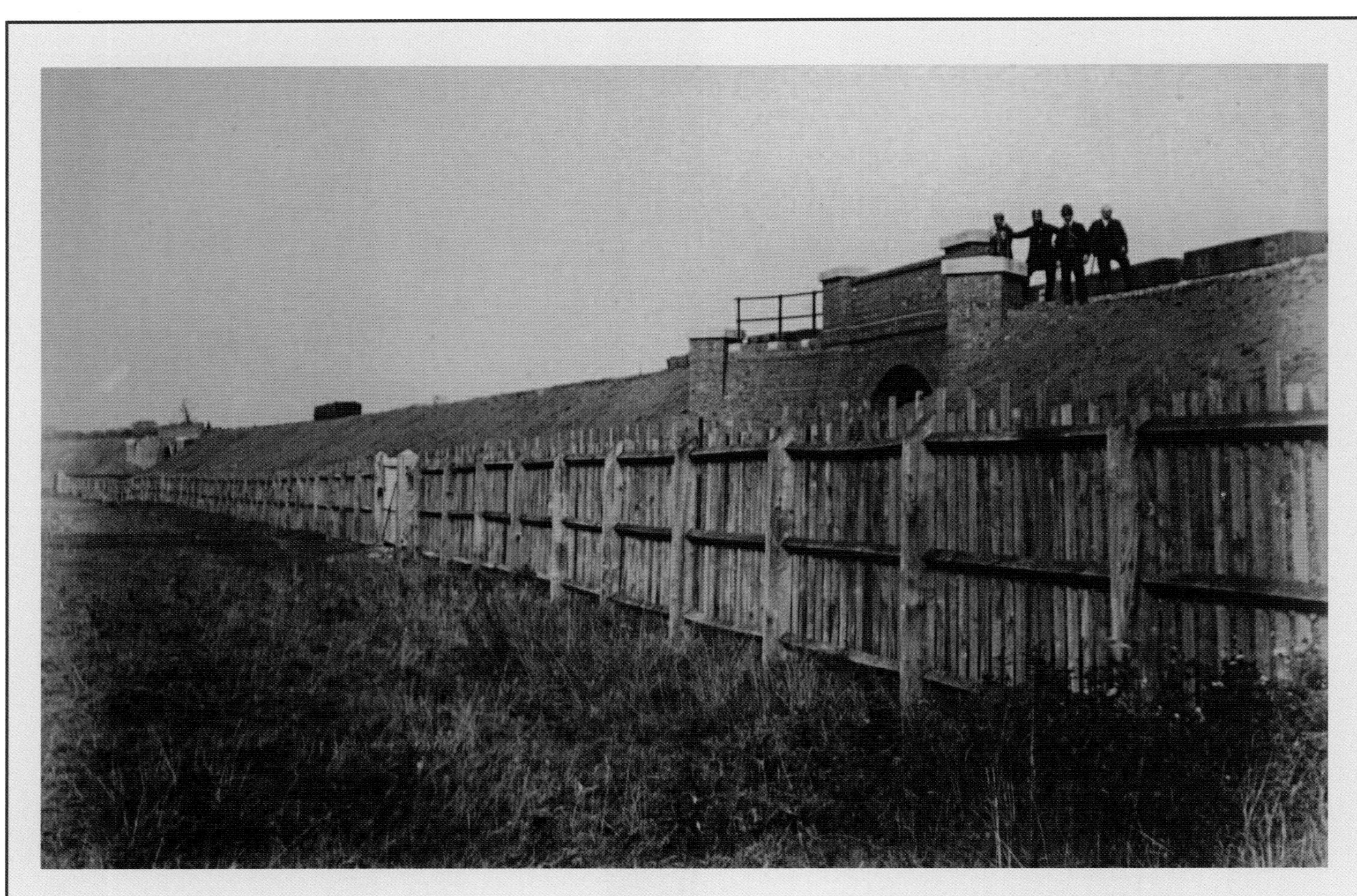

Photograph 89

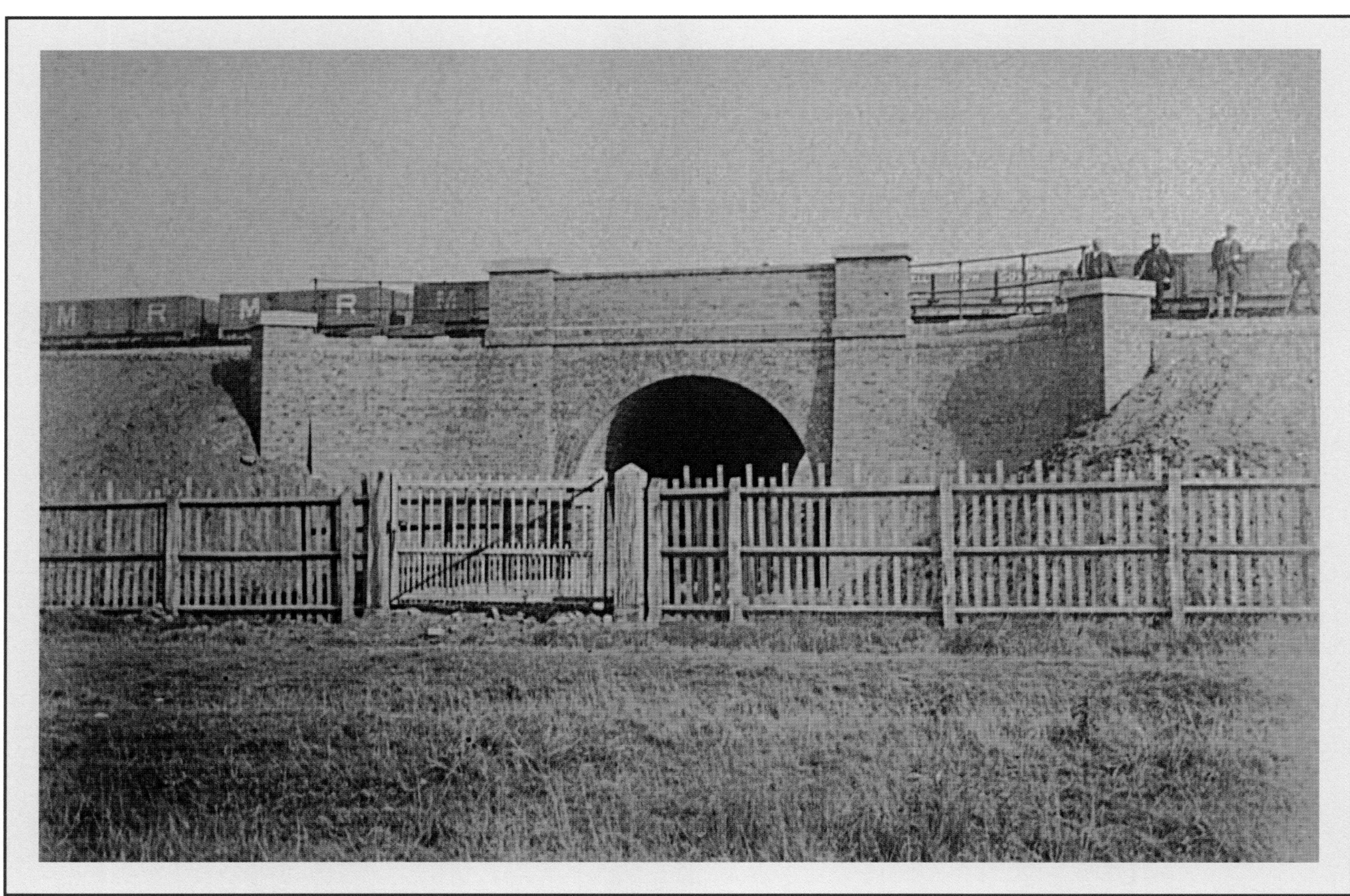

Photograph 90

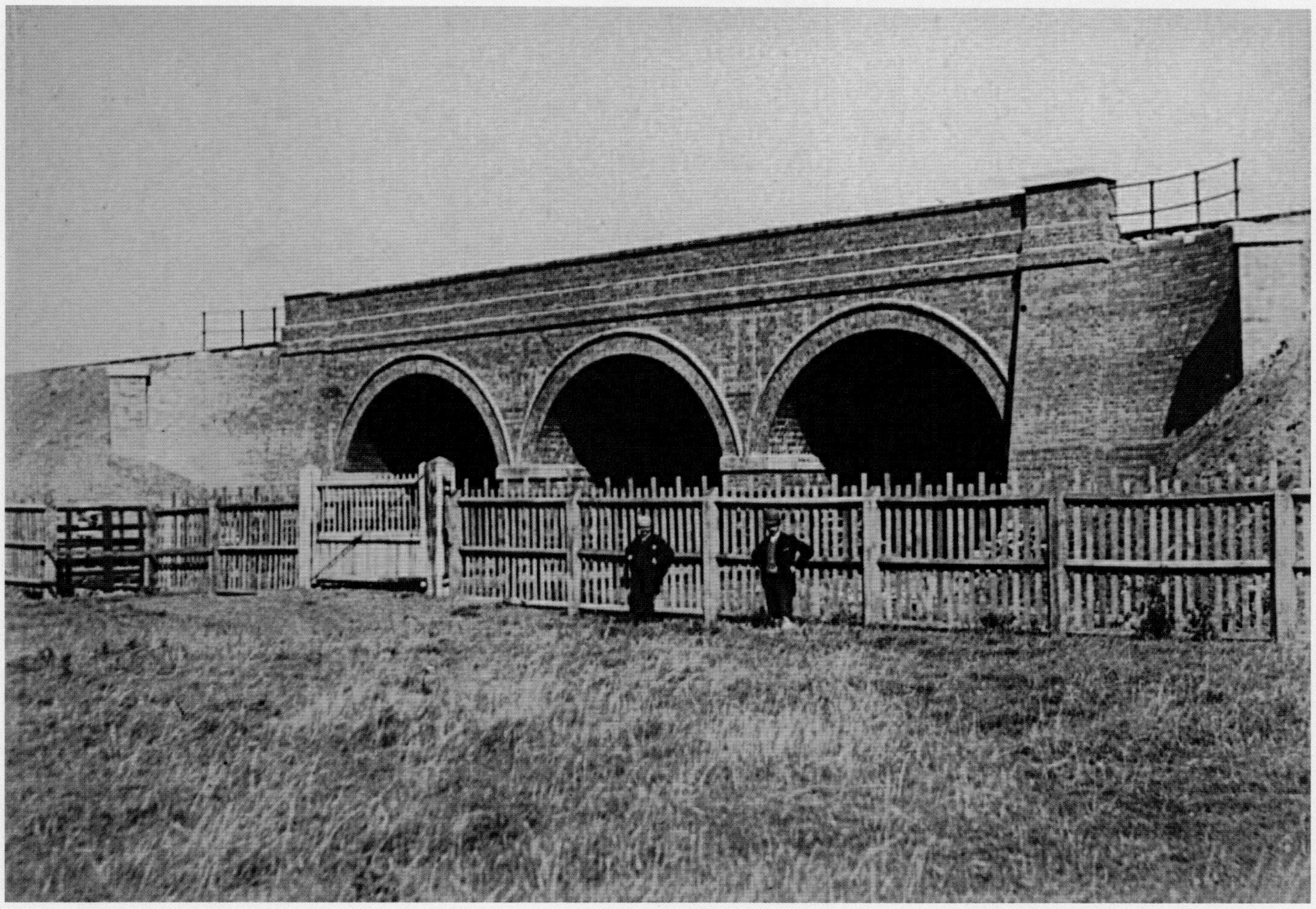

RIVER EYE BRIDGE, NEW SAXBY CURVE

(see also Map 9)

PHOTOGRAPH 91

Photograph 91 is of Bridge GSM2.36 on the new Saxby curve, from the south. To its north, but out of sight in this view, is a similar three-arched, but taller, bridge on the Bourne line (see Photograph 85). The infant River Eye runs through the central span with occupation arches to either side.

Very little survives of the fencing here. It was of a very distinctive style and ran the whole length of the new curve, facing Stapleford Park. Just one gateway can still be found, in a very dilapidated state, at the east end of Bridge GSM2.37 at the south end of the Saxby curve.

PHOTOGRAPH 92

Photograph 92 shows the surviving gate.

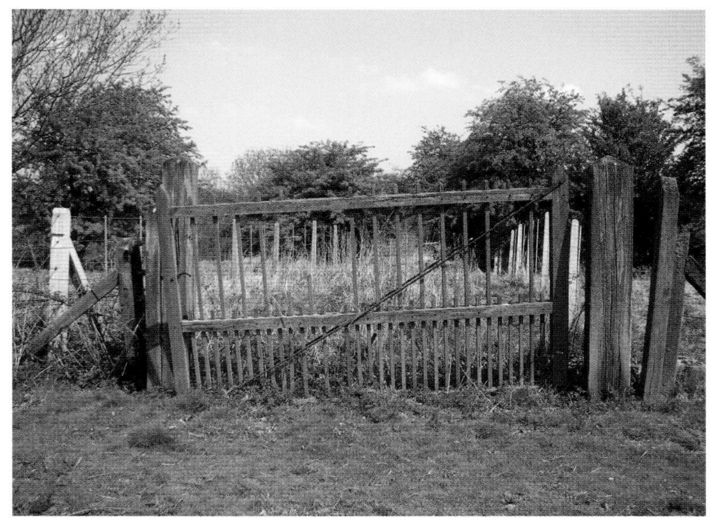

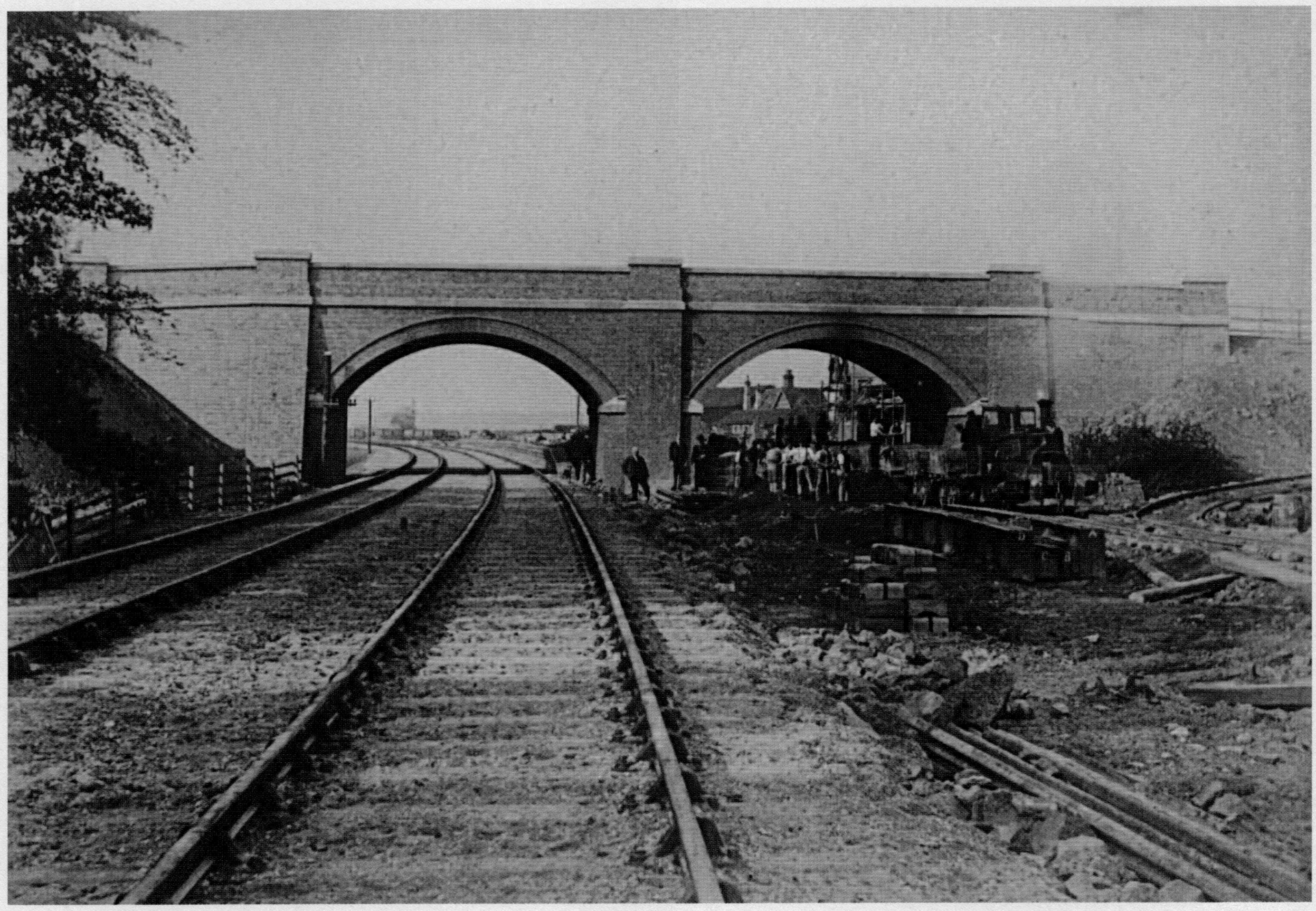

ROAD BRIDGE AT SAXBY STATION

PHOTOGRAPH 93

Photograph 93 shows the Saxby Station bridge from the east side. The permanent way has been laid on the new Saxby curve to the left. The covering of the sleepers with ballast was usual at that time. Although the track may be finished here the new station is still under construction. Through the right-hand arch the main platform building can be seen. The view through the left-hand arch shows that the island platform has been completed but no work has begun on the other platform here. Several goods wagons can also be seen in the station goods yard.

To the right a number of workmen have paused in their work to be photographed. They are standing near an outside cylindered, 0-4-0ST, contractor's locomotive with a train of tipper wagons. The contractor here was Holme and King of London and Liverpool, who was responsible for two contracts, the new Saxby curve and the section of line from Saxby to South Witham.[78] Three locomotives of this type, all built by the Hunslet Engine Co., are known to have been used on this contract: Works No 365/88, named PHYLLIS; 366/86, BEATRICE and 229/79, JOHN KNOWLES.[79]

The already disused Oakham Canal had to be infilled here and the locomotive is standing on the site where the earlier canal bridge carried the Stapleford-Saxby road. This was the start of the stretch of the canal towpath on which the Battle of Saxby was fought in 1844, between the railway surveyors and Lord Harborough and his employees. The result was the original Saxby curve, designed to keep the railway out of the parkland owned by Lord Harborough.[80]

Curving away from the front of the locomotive, off the picture to the right-hand side, is a contractor's line. This may have linked with the earlier Saxby curve, providing for the transfer of building materials to the contractor's works on the Saxby to Bourne line.

[78] Ronald H. Clark, *A Short History of the Midland and Great Northern Joint Railway* (Norwich, 1967), 51.

[79] Correspondence from the Industrial Locomotive Society, April 2008.

[80] C. E. Stretton, *The History of the Midland Railway* (London, 1901); Tim Warner, 'The battles of Saxby', *Backtrack* 2:4 (1988), 173-4; Geoffrey Body, *Great Railway Battles: Dramatic Conflicts of the Early Railway Years* (Peterborough, 1994), 14-23; Trevor Hickman, *Battlefields of Leicestershire* (Stroud, 2004), 146-158.

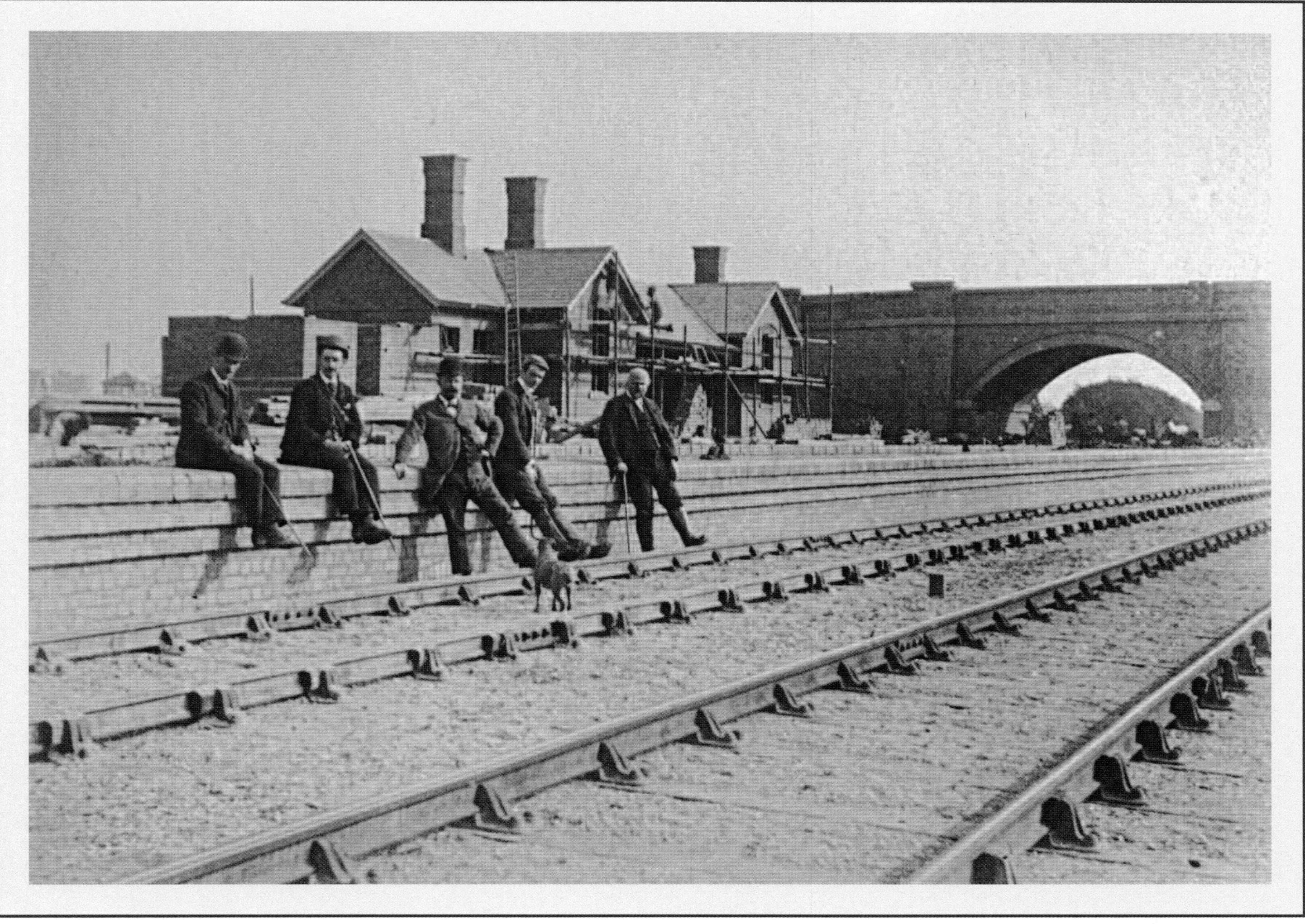

SAXBY STATION

(see also Map 10)

PHOTOGRAPH 94

Photograph 94 shows the station building at Saxby under construction. The builder for the three original stations, Saxby, Edmondthorpe and Wymondham, and South Witham, was Mr C. Barnes of Melton Mowbray.[81] Here the main platform building is almost complete, with scaffolding still in place and at least one workman on the scaffolding.

This building provided the booking office, waiting rooms and toilets. The Station Master continued to live in the original Station House, part of the earlier station buildings opened with the original Saxby curve on 1 February 1849. The former station became the new goods yard.

The bridge behind has been completed but the steps down to the platforms from the road have not been built. Indeed, there appears to be no provision for them in the bridge parapet (see Photograph 95).

Out of sight behind the platform is the double track in front of the building forming the new line to Bourne which headed away through the bridge arch in the background. The pair of lines in the foreground were those of the new Saxby curve, the route on the right being to and from Peterborough. Between the two routes was the island platform, the one on which the gentlemen are seated. The station layout was completed with a final platform built where the photographer was standing.

The five gentlemen, and the dog, were people who were clearly working closely with Charles Wilson. They appear in other photographs and the portly gentleman to the right is particularly recognisable.

The rails in the foreground are the permanent way, as opposed to the temporary contractor's lines which would have preceded them.

PHOTOGRAPH 95

(overleaf)

Photograph 95 shows the steps completed down to the north and the central island platforms. The bridge parapet had to be breached for them. The steps on the left led down to the Booking Office from where, if you had bought a ticket to Leicester or Peterborough, you had to climb back up to the road to get to your platform. The use of the road bridge in this way meant that a separate footbridge was unnecessary. It may have been that originally a separate footbridge was proposed to link the platforms. Such a late change to the plans would explain the need to breach the already-built parapets.

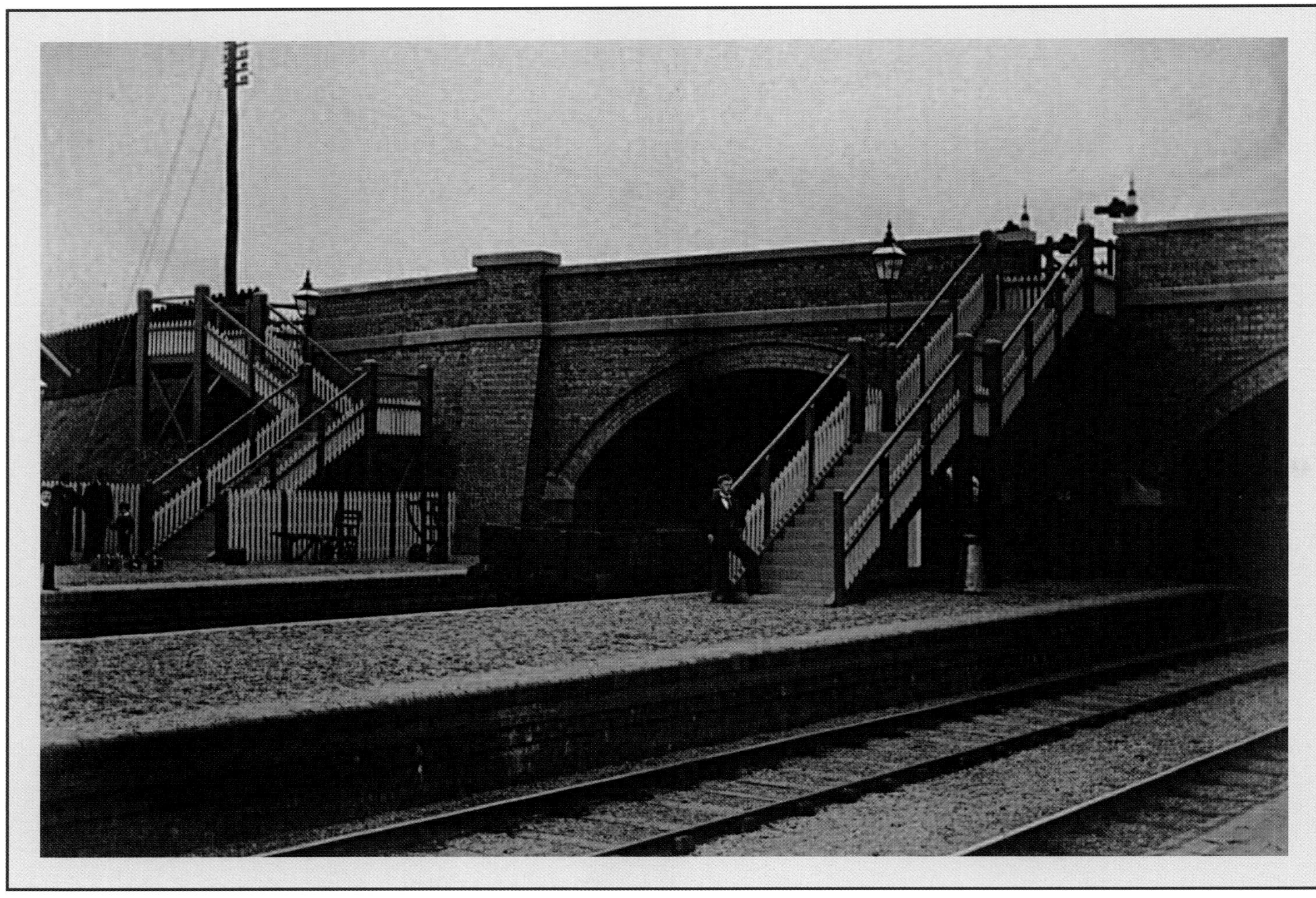

Photograph 95

The hand rails and balustrade are newly painted, lit by gas lamps. The presence of the milk churn at the foot of the steps to the right and the platform barrows on the far platform indicate that the station was probably open for traffic, certainly on the new curve, at this time. The Midland Railway wagon in the Bourne line platform is an indication that this part of the station was still not open for business.

The scene is completed with the telegraph pole and the signals peeping over the bridge. The former is carrying the telegraph network along the line, and is sited to carry the wires up and over the bridge, well clear of the public who would access the station. The signals are for the Bourne line and appear to be very badly sited, particularly for trains travelling to Bourne. From the station these would be hidden behind the bridge but there would have been duplicate or repeater signals, lower down the posts and visible to drivers through the arch. Those for the Peterborough platform can be seen through the right-hand bridge arch in Photograph 97.

PHOTOGRAPH 96

(opposite, top)

John Rhodes records that on 21 April 1893 a visit was arranged for the Directors of both the Midland and the Great Northern Railways to inspect the almost completed works.[82] Photograph 96 may be of that visit. They are standing in front of Saxby station building. This was identical to that built for Edmondthorpe and Wymondham station. Note how the end pavilions of the building are linked by a central recess, over which the roof is extended to form a veranda. Behind this the walls of the building are mostly glazed.

If this photograph was taken in April 1893 then it may have been after Charles Wilson had moved on to work in Yorkshire on the widening of the Midland Main Line at Millhouses, south of Sheffield, and after the new Saxby curve had opened, on 28 August 1892. As he had been a Resident Engineer, however, it is possible that he was asked to attend.

PHOTOGRAPH 97

(opposite, bottom)

The final image of Saxby station (Photograph 97) is rare among the Wilson photographs in that it shows the station in its completed form. This was one of the standard station building designs of the Midland Railway. Indeed, the stations on the line between Ilkley and Skipton, where Charles Wilson worked immediately before moving here, were exactly the same design. The only difference was that

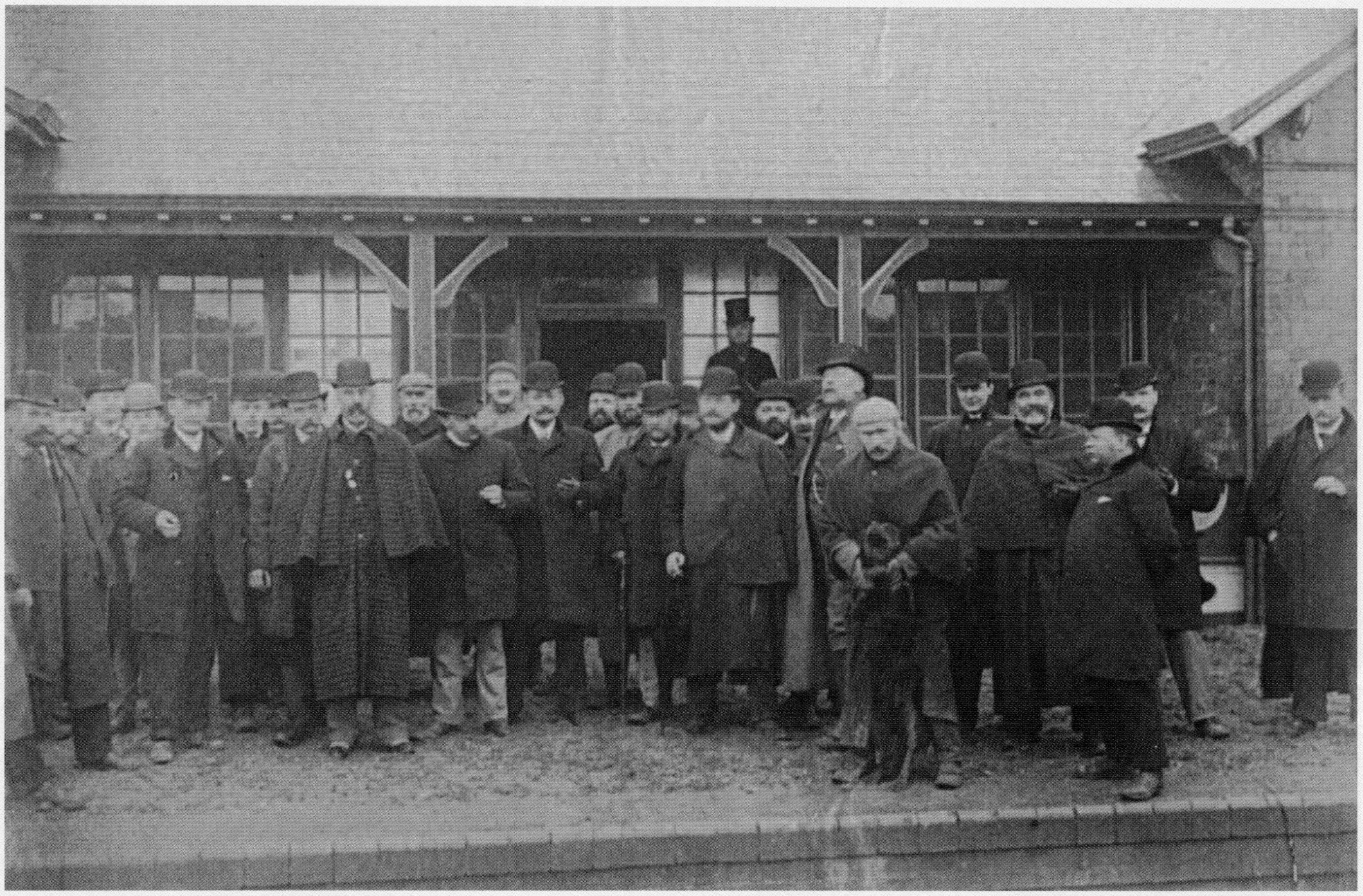

Photograph 96

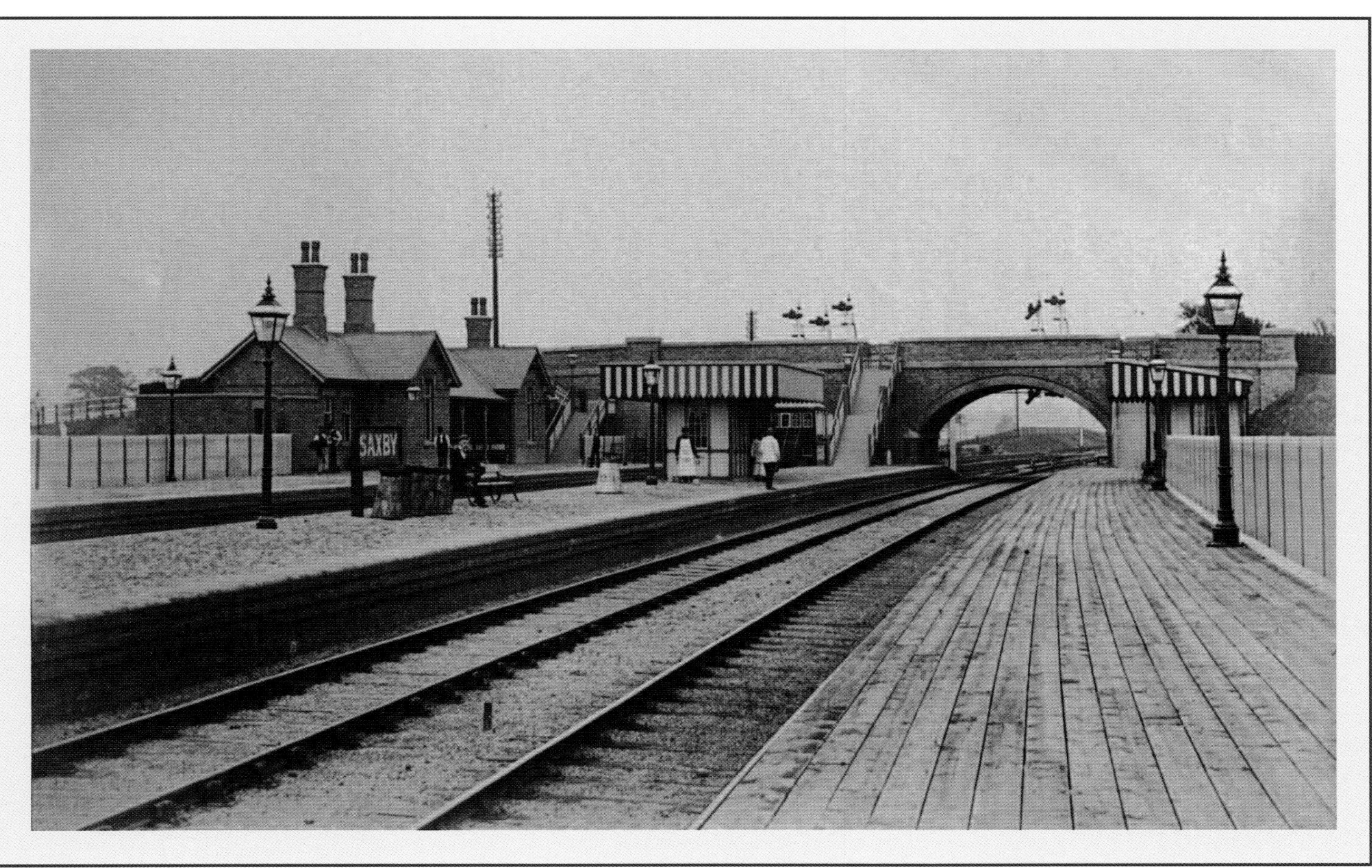

Photograph 97

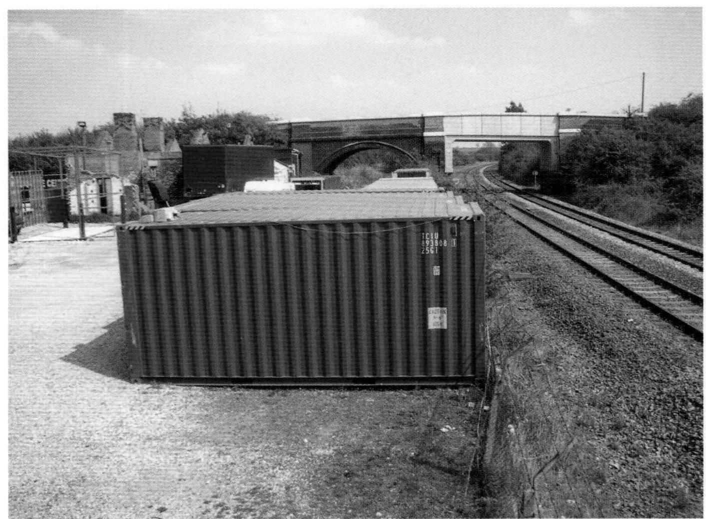

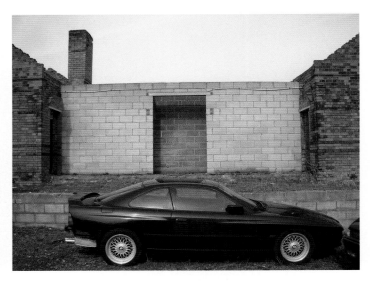

Photograph 98

Photograph 99

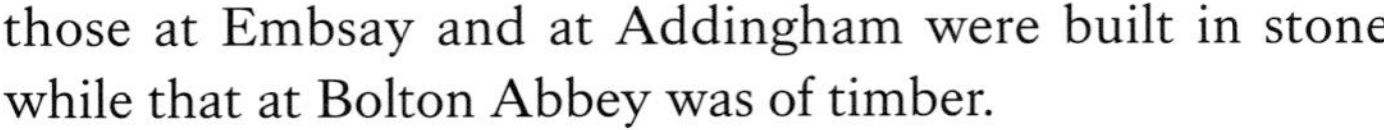

those at Embsay and at Addingham were built in stone while that at Bolton Abbey was of timber.

This photograph may well have been taken immediately prior to the visit of the Directors seen in Photograph 96. If required to attend, Wilson would have arrived before the important guests. On the island platform, by the small Waiting Room, there appear to be two painters working.

The painters are probably completing the striking pattern for the platform awnings. These colours were probably alternately Midland Railway maroon and cream. This colour scheme would have also been applied to the gas lamp columns which are of a standard Midland Railway pattern. It has been suggested that the waiting shelters here, with their extensive canopies, are reminiscent of Japanese teahouses.[83] The popular Japanese exhibition of 1885 in London and the first performance in the same year of the Gilbert and Sullivan opera, *The Mikado*, may have been the inspiration for this.

Through the left-hand bridge arch, to the right of the island platform Waiting Room, the Bourne line Signal Box can just be seen. Immediately in front of this box was a mile post recording 0 miles, as this was the starting point for the measurement of the line to Little Bytham. Underneath the right-hand arch the dark line across the track is the barrow crossing. The station staff would use these to move barrows of luggage and parcels between the platforms.

The platform on the extreme right has a timber plank decking. It may well be that a lighter form of construction was needed here as this platform was built over the bed of the former Oakham Canal.

PHOTOGRAPH 98

Photographs of this location in 2008 were not easy to obtain. The difficulties included the still working railway along the new Saxby Curve, and the use of the station site for commercial storage. Photograph 98 was taken from a point just above the surface of where the island platform was situated, a few yards west of where the men are sitting in Photograph 94. In May 2008 the station building was, by contrast, partly derelict, standing as a roofless shell. No sign remains of the former platform steps.

The original brick arch to the right has been replaced by a concrete structure. This may have been due to the fact that it had been constructed over the line of the Oakham Canal and suffered from subsidence as a result.

PHOTOGRAPH 99

Photograph 99 shows the location of the photograph of the Directors (Photograph 96). Work clearly started, at some time after 1985, to alter the building for a new use but this was never completed. The concrete block wall is approximately along the line of the glazed front screen seen behind the Directors in Photograph 96. New doorways have been cut through the side walls to the right and left, and stone corbels show where the beam rested that carried the front of the roof overhang.

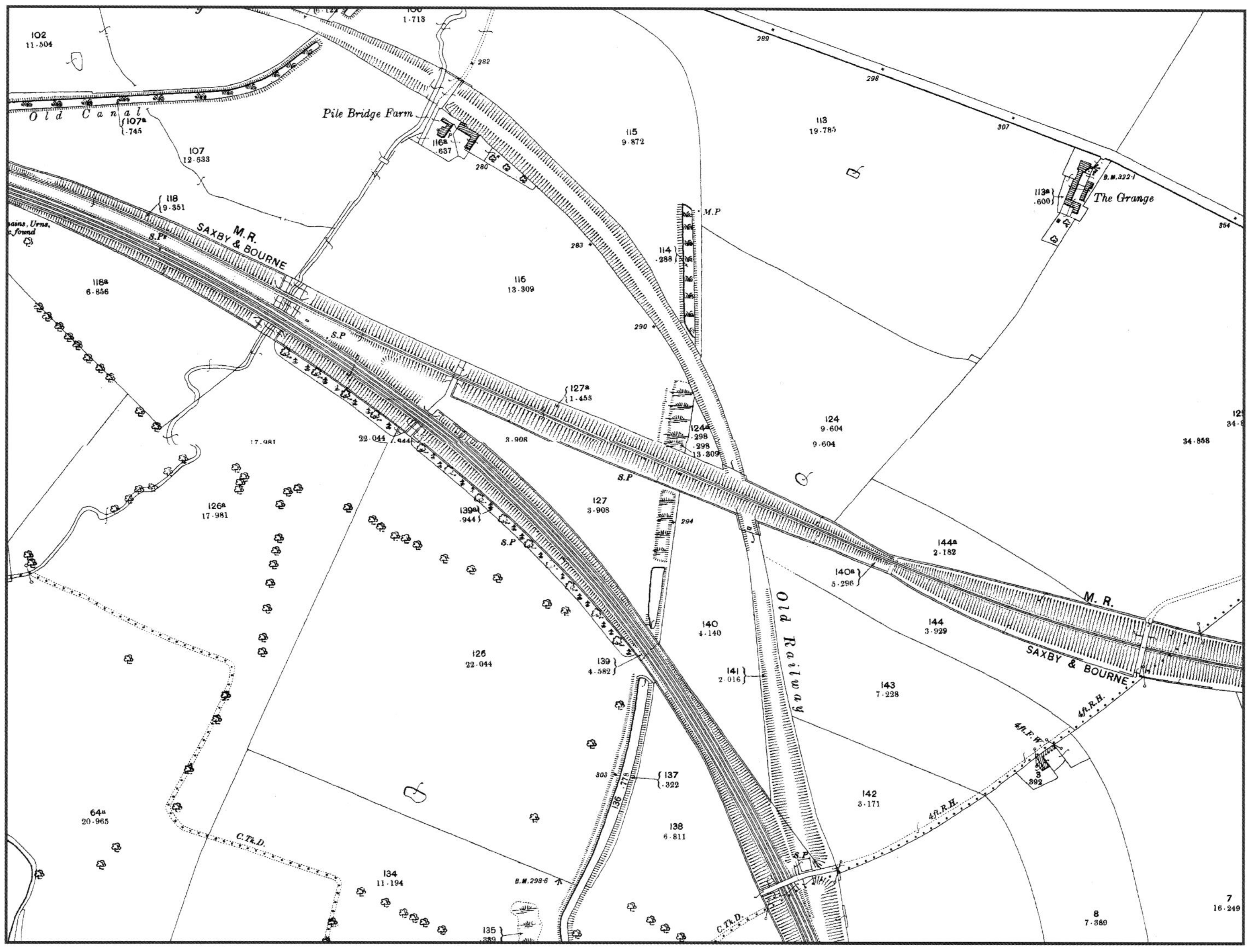

MAP 9

(opposite)
OS 1/2500 County Series Map, 1904. The Saxby Curves, Old and New.

The left edge of Map 9 overlaps the right edge of Map 10 to enable the whole of the routes of the old and new Saxby curves to be followed, as well as the junction with the line to Bourne. At the eastern edge of the map is Bridge 3, shown in Photographs 77, 78 and 79. Next west, the site of the temporary bridge over the Old Saxby Curve (shown in Photographs 81 and 82) is where the route of the 'Old Railway' crosses the route. The route of the Oakham Canal is next with the Bourne line embankment built across it. The Canal had been purchased by the Midland Railway in 1846 but it closed the following year.[84]

Now the new Saxby Curve and the Bourne line begin to converge, with Bridge GSM2.36A on the former (see Photographs 89 and 90) and Bridge 2 on the latter (see Photograph 83). On the left of this map the embankments of both lines are pierced by the River Eye with the bridges seen in Photographs 85 and 91. Finally, at the south end of the Saxby Curve is the pair of bridges seen in Photographs 87 and 88.

Pile Bridge Farm was named from the Pile Bridge which once carried the railway here over the farm access road.

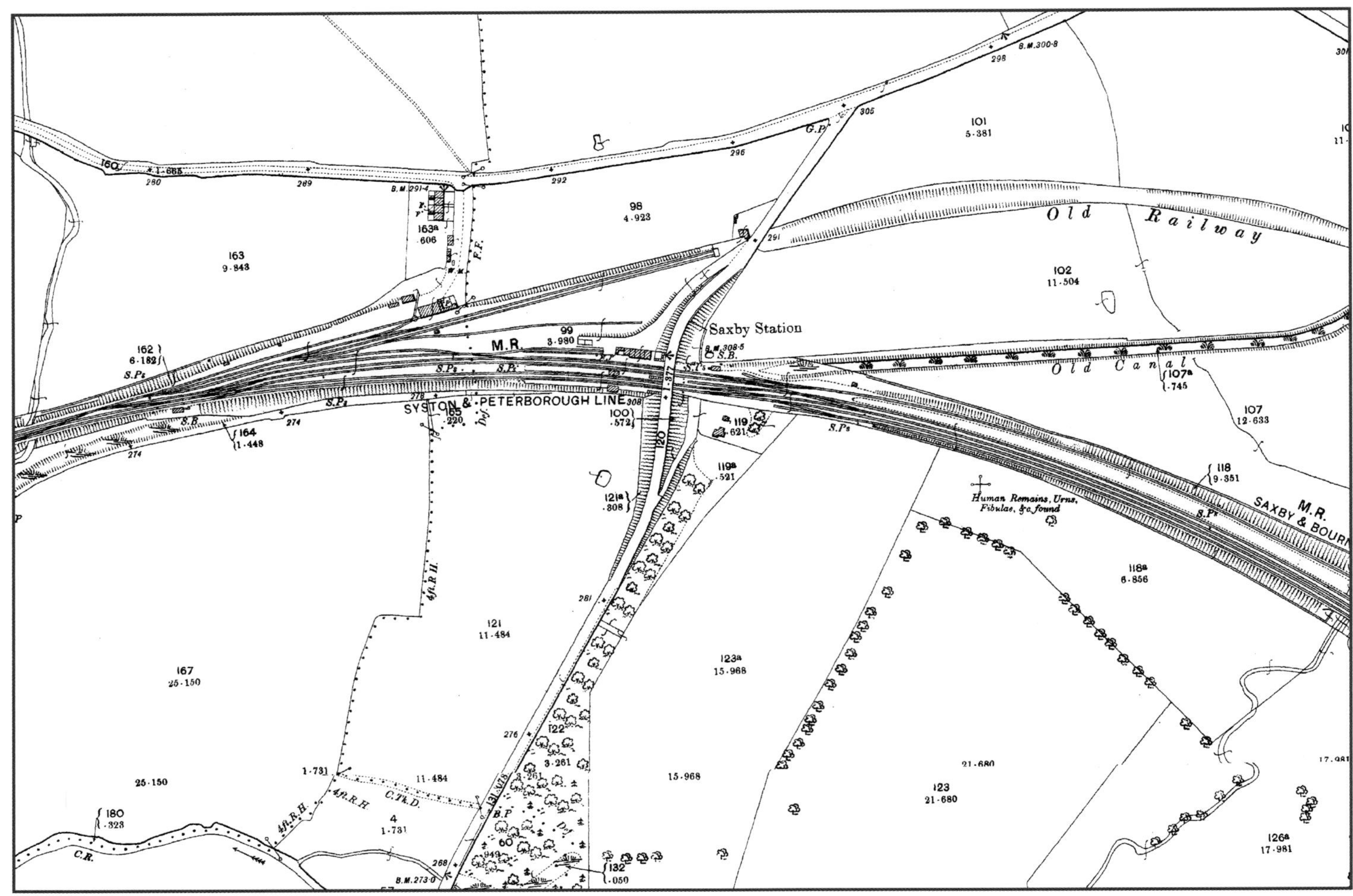

MAP 10

OS 1/2500 County Series Map, 1904. Saxby Station

The right edge of Map 10 overlaps the left edge of Map 9 to enable the whole of the routes of the old and new Saxby curves to be followed, as well as the junction with the line to Bourne. This shows Saxby Station and its road bridge, seen in Photographs 93, 94, 95, 96 and 97. The Old Curve can be seen as the 'Old Railway' with its remnants now included within the goods yard. The building along the north side of the old line here is the former station building which the Station Master continued to live in. At the north end of the access track to this is a row of railway workers' cottages.

The junction is immediately to the east of the bridge, itself built on the line of the canal. The centre of the site on which the archaeological remains were found during the construction works (referred to in the text to Photograph 85) is to the east of the station, on the south side of the line, marked with a cross and with the words 'Human Remains, Urns, Fibulae &c. found'.

81 *Grantham Journal* (10 September 1892), p.6, col.3.

82 John Rhodes, *Bourne to Saxby* (Boston, 1989), 17. See Appendix C.

83 Andrew Swift, 'Wish you were here? Railway postcards of Leicestershire', *Railway Archive* 4 (2003), 89.

84 Ronald Russell, *Lost Canals of England and Wales* (Newton Abbot, 1971).

APPENDIX A

National Archives RAIL 491/548
Extract from Contract No. 2

SUMMARY

	£	s.	d.
FENCING	5825	5	-
EARTHWORK	17688	4	8
OCCUPATION BRIDGE OVER LINE at 4 miles 9 chains [1]	463	5	-
OCCUPATION ROAD BRIDGE OVER LINE at 4 miles 51½ chains [2]	559	10	-
OCCUPATION BRIDGE UNDER LINE at 4 miles 74 chains [3]	473	-	-
PUBLIC ROAD BRIDGE UNDER LINE at 5 miles 24 chains [4]	1319	15	-
OCCUPATION BRIDGE UNDER LINE at 5 miles 44 chains [5]	486	-	6
OCCUPATION BRIDGE OVER LINE at 5 miles 74 chains [6]	510	10	3
OCCUPATION BRIDGE OVER LINE at 6 miles 6 chains [7]	489	-	3
OCCUPATION BRIDGE OVER LINE at 6 miles 12 chains [8]	497	-	3
OCCUPATION BRIDGE OVER LINE at 6 miles 20 chains [9]	497	-	3
PUBLIC ROAD BRIDGE UNDER LINE at 6 miles 63½ chains [10]	1332	5	-
OCCUPATION BRIDGE UNDER LINE at 6 miles 72 chains [11]	487	6	3
OCCUPATION BRIDGE UNDER LINE at 7 miles 8 chains [12]	528	13	9
OCCUPATION BRIDGE UNDER LINE at 7 miles 16 chains [13]	455	3	9
PUBLIC BRIDGE OVER LINE at 7 miles 34 chains [14]	1150	19	-
PUBLIC ROAD OVER LINE at 7 miles 52 ¼ chains [15]	928	9	-
OCCUPATION BRIDGE OVER LINE at 7 miles 65 chains [16]	600	7	6
OCCUPATION BRIDGE OVER LINE at 8 miles 6 chains [17]	494	10	-
OCCUPATION BRIDGE OVER LINE at 8 miles 20 chains [18]	573	19	-
OCCUPATION ROAD BRIDGE OVER LINE at 8 miles 40 chains [19]	419	10	-
OCCUPATION ROAD BRIDGE UNDER LINE (where directed) [20]	555	5	-
PUBLIC ROAD BRIDGE UNDER LINE at 8 miles 61 chains [21]	861	16	6
OCCUPATION BRIDGE UNDER LINE at 9 miles 11 chains [22]	432	8	-
OCCUPATION BRIDGE UNDER LINE at 9 miles 29¾ chains [23]	400	12	6
OCCUPATION BRIDGE UNDER LINE at 9 miles 4¼ chains [24]	415	12	6
OCCUPATION BRIDGE OVER LINE at 9 miles 79¾ chains [25]	593	10	-
CULVERTS AND DRAINS	3983	10	-
BALLASTING AND PERMANENT WAY	6588	-	-
ADDITIONAL WORKS	3279	5	-
DAY WORK	1367	10	-
MAINTENANCE FOR SIX MONTHS AFTER THE LINE IS OPEN FOR TRAFFIC	146	8	4
TOTAL AMOUNT OF CONTRACT	£ 54403	12	3

I AGREE TO EXECUTE ALL EXTRA AND ADDITIONAL Works or have deductions made from, or additions to my Estimate at the prices at which each item in the foregoing detailed Estimate is computed.

FOOTNOTES TO APPENDIX A

[1] Bridge 13, actually built at about 4 miles, 15 chains. See Photograph 50.
[2] Bridge 14, built as an under bridge. The description as an over bridge is an error.
[3] Bridge 15.
[4] Bridge 16, for The Drift. See Photograph 48.
[5] Bridge 17.
[6] Bridge 18. See Photograph 44.
[7] Not built.
[8] Bridge 19. See Photograph 45.
[9] Not built.
[10] Bridge 20, over Thistleton Lane. See Photographs 41 and 42.
[11] Not built. The consecutive number (21) was used for the culvert at about 6 miles 76 chains.
[12] Bridge 22. See Photograph 36.
[13] Bridge 23.
[14] Bridge 24, Broadgate Road. See Photographs 33 and 35.
[15] Bridge 25, Great North Road. See Photograph 31.
[16] Not built.
[17] Bridge 26, constructed at about 8 miles 12 chains. See Photographs 28 and 29.
[18] Not built.
[19] Bridge 27. See Photograph 27.
[20] Not built.
[21] Bridge 28, over Morkery Lane. See Photograph 25.
[22] Not built.
[23] Bridge 29.
[24] Bridge 30.
[25] Bridge 31. See Photograph 23.

APPENDIX B

ALBUM DETAILS

Album No.	*Book Photo No.*	*NGR*	*Description*
1	30		Dunbar Ruston steam navvy. Precise location not identified.
2	81	SK 8236 1892	Temporary bridge over the old Saxby curve from the south.
3	82	SK 8236 1892	Temporary bridge over the old Saxby curve from the south.
4	87	SK 8242 1856	New Saxby curve and old Saxby curve, south end.
5	41	SK 9250 1898	Bridge 20, South Witham.
6	93	SK 8138 1930	Saxby Station from the east side of the bridge.
7	94	SK 8138 1930	Saxby Station.
8	91	SK8192 1906	Bridge GSM2.36, new Saxby curve.
9	68	SK 8510 1908	Bridge 7, and the Wymondham Station Master's House.
10	89	SK 8210 1904	Bridge GSM2.36A with GSM2.36 beyond, new Saxby curve.
11	90	SK 8210 1904	Bridge GSM2.36A, new Saxby curve.
12	3	SK 0790 1906	Navvies at work, cutting east of Toft Tunnel.
13	33	SK 9350 1914	Bridge 24, South Witham, from the west.
14	70	SK 8510 1908	Wymondham Station Master's House.
15	57	SK 8585 1899	Bridge 10, Wymondham, from the south.
16	55	SK 8585 1899	Bridge 10, Wymondham, looking west.
17	54	SK 857 190	Bridges 9 and 10, Wymondham, from the north.
18	53	SK 857 190	Bridges 9 and 10, Wymondham, construction site from the south west.
19			Not on the Bourne to Saxby Line.

Album No.	*Book Photo No.*	*NGR*	*Description*
20	77	SK 8274 1876	Bridge 3 from the east.
21	78	SK 8274 1876	Bridge 3 from the east.
22	63	SK 8517 1900	Edmondthorpe and Wymondham Station, with Bridges 7 and 6 in background.
23	31	SK 9386 1921	Bridge 25, now the A1 road bridge, looking east.
24	75	SK 8406 1894	Bridge 4 with Bridge 5 in background.
25	4	TF 0795 1900	Toft Tunnel, east portal.
26	95	SK 8138 1930	Saxby Station.
27	28	SK 9468 1933	Believed to be Bridge 26 off Morkery Lane, looking east. See also Album No 33.
28	35	SK 9350 1918	Bridge 24 with Bridge 25 in background.
29	88	SK 8242 1856	Old and new Saxby curves, south end.
30	44	SK 9110 1876	Bridge 18, looking west.
31	45	SK 9146 1880	Bridge 19 with Bridge 18 in background.
32	8	TF 0278 1785	Bridge 245, looking east.
33	29	SK 9468 1933	Believed to be Bridge 26 off Morkery Lane, looking west. See also Album No 60.
34	14	TF 0164 1769	Bridge 43, East Coast main line crossing from the south.
35	85	SK 8194 1910	Bridge 1 with Bridge GSM2.36 beyond.
36	1	TF 0908 1930	Bridge 234 with Bridge 235 in distance.
37	27	SK 952 194	Believed to be Bridge 27 with Bridge 26 in background.
38	10	TF 0194 1776	Bridge 45, River West Glen tunnel from the south.
39	16	SK 9956 1794	Bridge 38 from the south.
40	42	SK 9250 1898	Bridge 20 from the south.

Album No.	*Book Photo No.*	*NGR*	*Description*
41	36	SK 9290 1906	Bridge 22, South Witham, looking north.
42	60	SK 8580 1900	Bridge 9, Wymondham, from the north.
43	65	SK 8508 1900	Edmondthorpe and Wymondham Goods Yard, with Bridge 6 in background.
44			Not on the Bourne to Saxby Line.
45			Bolton Abbey station, Yorkshire.
46	51	SK 8753 1889	Bridge 12 from the west.
47	39	SK 9246 1899	South Witham Station.
48	58	SK 8585 1899	Bridge 10, Wymondham, from the south.
49	64	SK 8517 1900	Edmondthorpe and Wymondham Station, Bridge 7.
50	96	SK 8138 1930	Saxby Station, probably the Directors' visit of 21 April 1893.
51			Bolton Abbey Station, Yorkshire.
52	79	SK 8274 1876	Bridge 3 from the west.
53	73	SK 8428 1900	Bridge 5 from the west.
54	12	TF 0172 1770	Bridge 44 from the south.
55	20	SK 9858 1834	Bridge 35 from the west.
56	50	SK 8835 1885	Bridge 13, looking west.
57	25	SK 9564 1945	Bridge 28 from the north.
58	38	SK 9246 1899	South Witham Station
59	97	SK 8138 1930	Saxby Station.
60	29	SK 947 194	Bridge 26. Additional copy of Album No 33.
61	72	SK 8517 1900	Edmondthorpe and Wymondham Station, Bridges 6 and 7.
62	23	SK 9754 1882	Bridge 31, looking west.

Album No.	*Book Photo No.*	*NGR*	*Description*
63	61	SK 8580 1900	Bridge 9, Wymondham, from the south.
64	48	SK 9010 1878	Bridge 16, The Drift, looking north.
65	6	TF 0622 1866	Bridge 239, Lound Viaduct, from the south.
66			Not on the Bourne to Saxby Line.
67	47	SK 9110 1876	Probably Bridge 18 or Bridge 19.
68			Not on the Bourne to Saxby Line.
69	18	SK 9900 1814	Bridge 37, Castle Bytham Station.
70			Not on the Bourne to Saxby Line.
71			Not on the Bourne to Saxby Line.
72	83	SK 8210 1900	Bridge 2 from the south.

APPENDIX C

BOURNE TO SAXBY

BY JOHN RHODES

Bourne
to
Saxby

By
John Rhodes

KMS BOOKS, BOSTON

This book by John Rhodes was published by KMS Books, Boston, in 1989 and has long been out of print. Any book about the construction phase of the line would have to include some subsequent history. The joint Editors were of the opinion that this earlier book was of a quality such that it merited a reprint and that by including that reprint in this book it would provide that subsequent history. The opportunity has been taken to include some very minor amendments from the original text.

CONTENTS

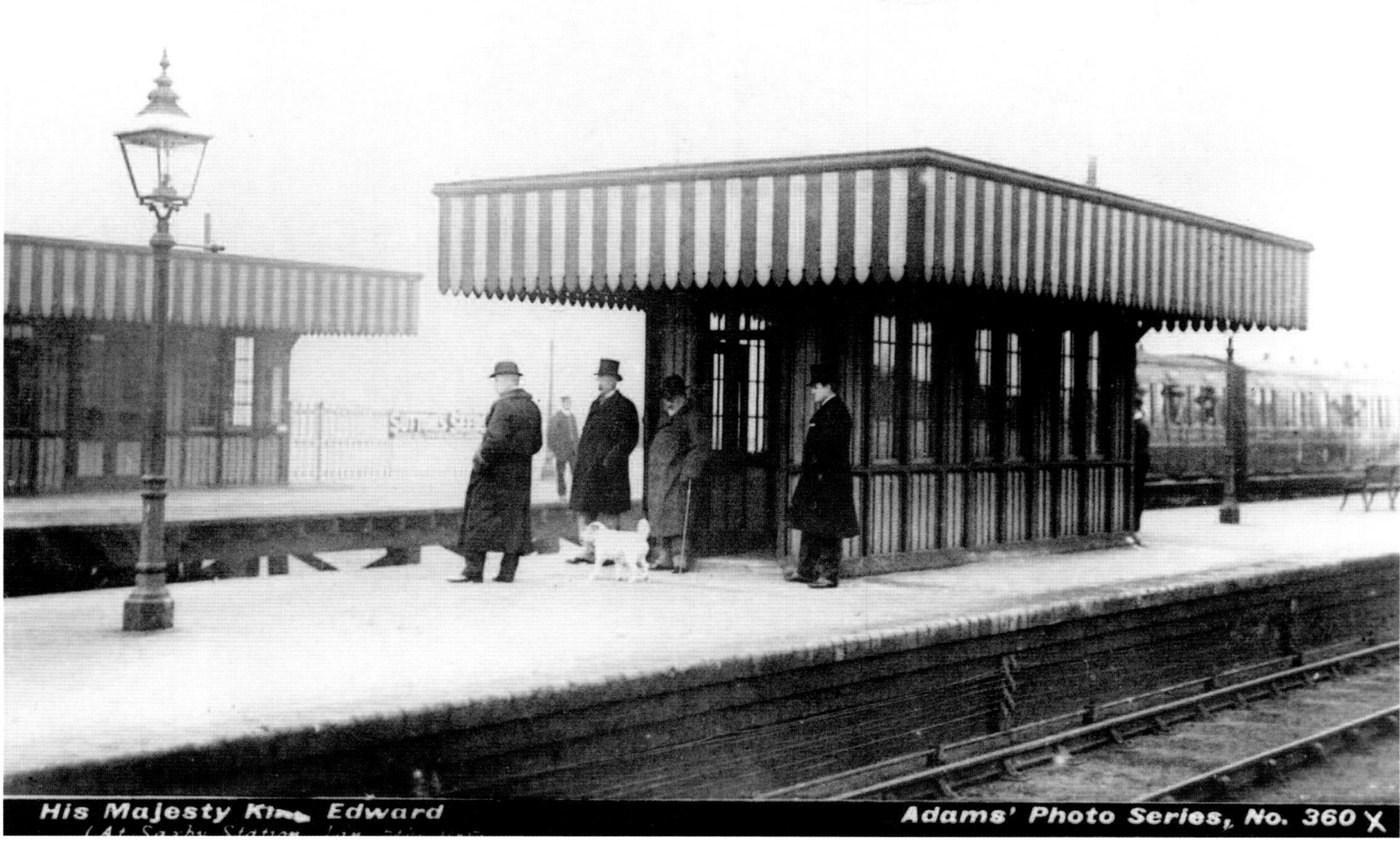

The ornate wooden shelters at Saxby station, photographed on the occasion of a visit by King Edward VII (and dog) in January 1907. The Bourne-Saxby line is in the foreground. (Lens of Sutton)

CHAPTER ONE

DEVELOPMENTS AT BOURNE AND SAXBY

Saxby

In the mid 1840s, the wily and unscrupulous George Hudson was at the height of his powers. As manager of the newly-formed Midland Railway he controlled over 1,000 miles of actual railway and was prodigiously inventive in his schemes for further proposed railways: in the space of two days in May 1846 he received approval for 40 different railway bills, with a total capital of ten million pounds. Nicknamed 'The Railway King' in tribute to his empire-building talents, he wielded immense influence locally and nationally, and he had amassed a personal fortune large enough to enable him to live an appropriately regal lifestyle. By a formidable blend of bluster, financial juggling and double dealing that amounted to genius, he had so far managed to out-manoeuvre most attempts from rival Companies to trespass on what he regarded as his Company's sphere of influence and area of operation. The proposal for a direct line between York and London by a Company which later emerged as the Great Northern, however, presented Hudson with a big problem. If the line were authorised, it would undoubtedly pose a serious threat to his own York-London route, which ran via the Midlands and was a rather circuitous way of reaching the capital. Faced with the prospect of major loss of traffic, Hudson turned his energies to countering, blocking and discrediting the rival scheme in an attempt to wreck it totally, and although he managed to delay the GN plans for a time, he ultimately failed, of course, to prevent their authorisation. The various ingenious, and sometimes underhand, ways in which he tried to stave off the opposition are irrelevant to this study, except for one scheme which brought a railway line to, among other places, the remote and insignificant village of Saxby, in Leicestershire.

In 1845 the Eastern Counties Railway, of which Hudson was later to become Chairman, had been authorised to build a line westwards from Ely to the cathedral city of Peterborough, and Hudson recognised that an alliance between his own Midland Railway and the ECR would be useful in pre-empting the London-York proposals by securing traffic from the Peterborough area before the London-York Company reached there. Accordingly, Hudson put forward proposals for a railway from Peterborough, via Stamford, Oakham and Melton Mowbray, to Syston, where it would join the Midland line

SAXBY JUNCTION
SOUTH WITHAM
CASTLE BYTHAM
EDENHAM BRANCH RLWY
EDENHAM
AUTHORISED 1888
EDMONDTHORPE & WYMONDHAM
1889 ROUTE
BOURNE
LITTLE BYTHAM
AUTHORISED 1889: ABANDONED
ASHWELL LT RLWY
GNR
ASHWELL
COTTESMORE
LOCATION MAP
1
2
3 MILES

SAXBY JCN SB
EDMONDTHORP& WYMONDHAM STN
PAIN'S SDG
BUCKMINSTER SDG
SOUTH WITHAM STN
CASTLE BYHAM STN
GN BRIDGE NO 43
LITTLE BYTHAM JCN
TOFT TUNNEL
BOURNE WEST JCN
100
L
264
100
L
132
L
200
132
L
100
L
200
L
110
L
100
440
100
0
1
2
3
4
5
6
7
8
9
10
11
12
13
14
15
16
17
18
MILES
GRADIENT PROFILE: SAXBY–BOURNE

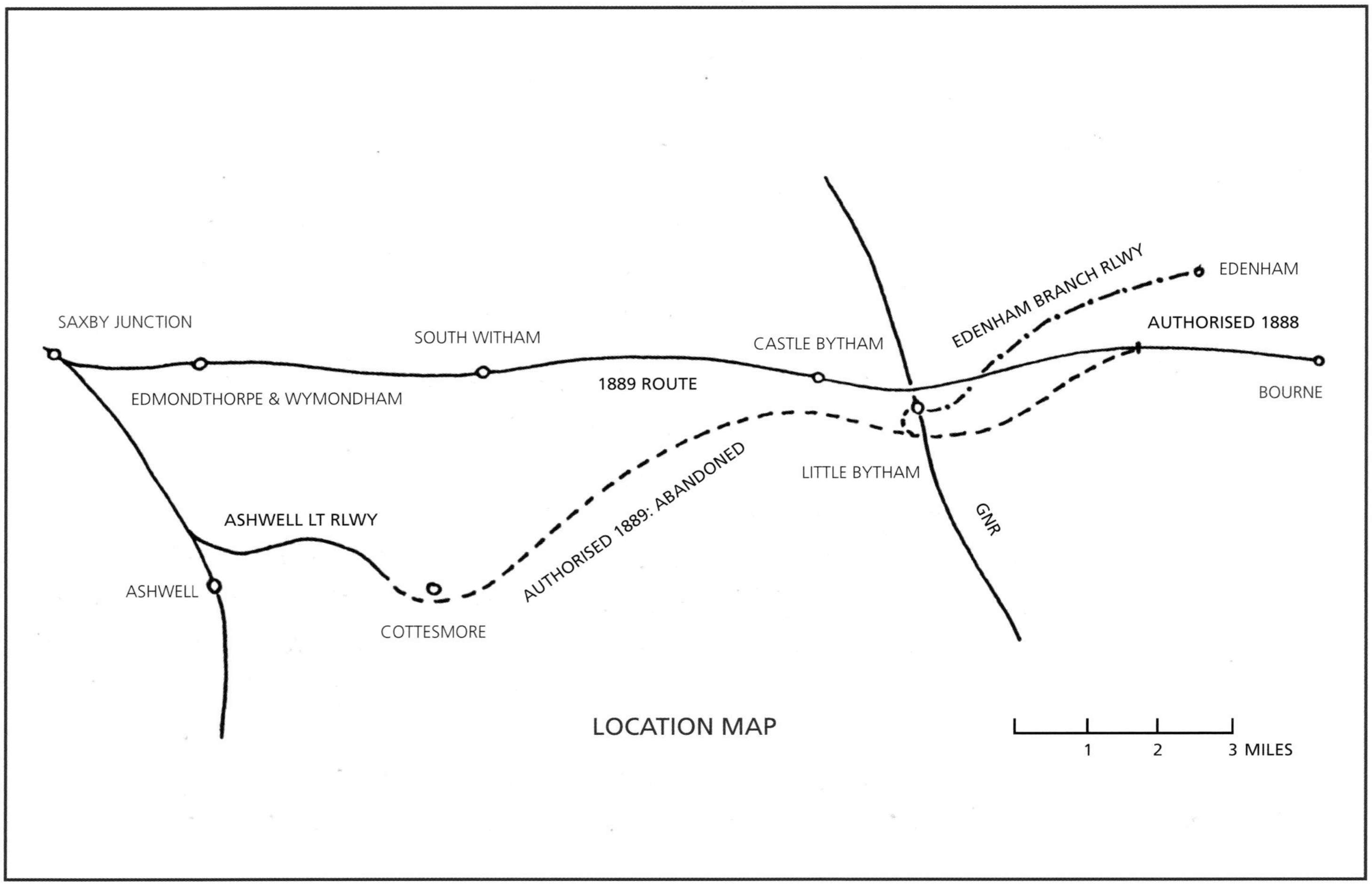

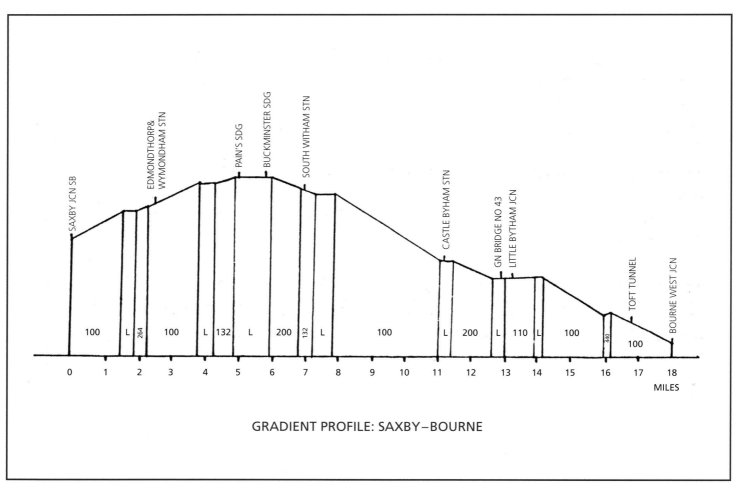

into Leicester. The route was sanctioned on June 30, 1845, but not before it had encountered some fierce and implacable opposition from a not entirely unexpected quarter.

Some miles north of Oakham, close to the village of Saxby, lay Stapleford Hall, the stately home of Lord Harborough. It was here that Hudson's route swung through ninety degrees to turn due west, skirting as it did so the extensive parkland, nearly a thousand acres, in which the Hall stood. Lord Harborough, a rather tetchy and irascible aristocrat, had for some time been a major shareholder in the Oakham Canal Company, which in 1802 had opened the 15-mile waterway from a junction with the Melton Mowbray Navigation to the town of Oakham. The canal's principal traffic was coal inwards and agricultural produce outwards, and even though it was always a shaky proposition financially, it did provide a useful service for the Earl's own estates, since there were wharves at both Saxby and Stapleford for the loading and unloading of goods. Lord Harborough's financial interest in the canal meant that he was inherently suspicious of railways, which were already beginning to kill off canal traffic up and down the country, and when he became aware that Hudson's proposed railway route not only ran in close proximity to his own stately home, but also intended to link the towns of Oakham and Melton Mowbray, which were already served by the canal, he was stung into active opposition.

The first moves in what was to become known as the Battle of Saxby came in November 1844, when seven of Hudson's surveyors arrived in the Stapleford area to reconnoitre the route and take the necessary measurements and levels of the land. Lord Harborough had already festooned the borders of his property with large notices threatening dire retribution on anybody attempting to enter his park for surveying purposes, and he backed up his threats by posting groups of estate workers at strategic points along his boundaries. As they approached the Park. the Midland surveyors were confronted by nine or ten of Lord Harborough's men, armed with pitchforks and sticks, and ordered away, even though they were still on public land. When they refused to turn back, they were set upon, herded into a farm cart, and driven off to the local magistrate. Since the Midland men had committed no crime, however, there was no legal action that could be taken against them, and the Earl's head keeper had to be content with venting his annoyance against them by tipping them out of the cart into the road. The surveyors were made of stern stuff, however, and, bruised but undaunted, returned the next day, prudently bringing with them a sizeable contingent of brawny navvies, borrowed from local railway workings, and some equally hefty prize-fighters imported from Nottingham. Lord Harborough's men, their numbers also reinforced, met them head-on, and a spectacular melée occurred as both groups shoved and pushed, crashed struggling into hedgerows, rolled furiously fighting in the mud of the roadway, or slid in a wild tangle of arms and legs into a dirty roadside ditch. The Midland contingent was eventually put to flight in a stirring chase along the canal towpath, to the cheers and excitement of a crowd of locals who had gathered. to see the fun. Violence escalated again a couple of days later in another unseemly brawl, during which a gigantic lock-keeper, hired by Lord Harborough, single-handedly knocked unconscious half a dozen opponents and smashed a valuable piece of surveying equipment said to be worth £32. The end product of all this mayhem was jail sentences for several navvies on a charge of riot, fines for some of Lord Harborough's men for damage they had caused, and a postponement of surveying activities in the Stapleford Park area until tempers had cooled.

Even after the MR had gained Parliamentary approval for its route in June 1845, Lord Harborough stubbornly refused to allow any construction work to be started anywhere near his estate. Tactfully, the MR agreed to re-route its line a little further away from Stapleford Hall, but when the surveyors arrived, with a bodyguard, to take new measurements and levels they were once again confronted by a group of Lord Harborough's men and the second Battle of Saxby was soon in full swing. Lord Harborough himself enlivened the proceedings on this occasion by driving his carriage, Boadicea-like, into the ranks of the hated railwaymen. The surveying did eventually get done, and the deviation was authorised on June 16, 1846, with the provision for a tunnel to be driven underneath a spinney of fine trees, Cuckoo Plantation, on Lord Harborough's estate so that the offending trains would be hidden from his Lordship's view. Unfortunately, during construction the tunnel collapsed, causing subsidence to the trees and apoplexy to their aristocratic owner. There followed a sharp legal battle, which ended in yet another deviation proposal authorised on July 22, 1847. By this time, the two sections of line on either side of the Saxby area had already been built and were in operation, that from Syston to Melton from September 1, 1846, and from Peterborough to Stamford from October 2 of the same year. Because of Lord Harborough's intransigence, it was not until May 1, 1848 that these two sections were linked, and the whole through route in operation.

At Saxby, a small station was built on the western end of the much contested curve, just off the main road and about half a mile from the village, almost on the bank of the Oakham Canal. The MR had agreed to buy the canal in April 1845 for the sum of £26,000 and 200 new Midland £40 shares, a decision the canal authorities (Lord Harborough excepted) were happy to accept since traffic was clearly on the wane: in the very dry summer of 1844 the waterway had been unnavigable for five months and goods had to be transported laboriously by road.

By the 1880s, when train speeds had increased considerably, the severe curve at Saxby was proving something of a restriction, particularly to express services, and the MR decided to re-route the line yet again in order to ease the situation. By this time there was a new incumbent at Stapleford Hall, who proved much more amenable than his peppery predecessor, and the MR was able to obtain approval for a new curve, of 56 furlongs 3 chains radius, on June 24, 1889, by the same Act that sanctioned most of the Bourne-Saxby extension, detailed later in this book.

Bourne

The first railway to reach the small market town of Bourne, on the edge of the Fens, was the short 6-miles terminal branch from the Great Northern main line at Essendine. The enterprise was a product of local initiative, organised by the vicar of Bourn and a retired Army general, who, together with a group of local worthies and landowners, formed the Bourn & Essendine Railway Company in 1857. The line opened, to the celebratory ringing of church bells, in May 1860, but was always under financial pressure, and was soon taken over by the GNR, which had operated the route from the beginning. Modest in scale the line might have been, but it did boast at its Bourne end a fine station building, the Red Hall, a former Elizabethan manor house thought at one time to have associations with the Gunpowder Plot (a claim recently shown to have been false), and which had passed through various ownerships, eventually becoming a private school for young ladies in the years immediately before the B & E took it over for use as station offices. A service of six passenger trains a day each way meant that Bourne was now in vital contact with the rest of the country, with easy access to London and the north, and with the benefit of cheaper coal and other goods being brought in, and agricultural produce going out to wider markets than was possible before.

Communications for the town improved even more a few years later, in 1866, when the Spalding & Bourn Railway reached there from the east, by a virtually dead straight, and single-track line which gave access to the junction station at Spalding, where routes from Peterborough, Boston, Lincoln and South Lynn converged. On January 2 1872, the GN opened passenger operations (5 trains a day each way) along a 17-mile branch from Bourne northwards to Sleaford, an event that was also celebrated by church bells ringing and large crowds of sightseers gathering at intermediate stations to cheer the first trains on their way. Thus, within a dozen years, Bourne had become an important railway junction, with something like 30 passenger trains a day, and a steady stream of freight to all parts of the country.

Station facilities had developed correspondingly to keep pace with the growth in traffic. The original B & E station had consisted of a single short platform in front of Red Hall; there was also a small engine and carriage-shed combined, a coal siding, and a 2-road goods yard. The arrival of the Spalding & Bourn had turned the station from a terminus into a through route, so an additional, island, platform was added (the Red Hall platform, being extended at the same time to double its length) and a third small platform, for the use of S & B trains only, added adjacent to South Street level crossing (although this probably only lasted for a few months). Siding space was increased. The S & B also had its own goods yard and shed to east of South Street. The opening of the Sleaford branch necessitated the installation of a signal box to control the junction, and a turntable was added to the engine-shed facilities.

By the 1870s, then, railway routes extended north, south and east from Bourne; as yet, however, there was no direct access available westwards, to give a link with the Midlands. It was possible to reach Nottingham via Essendine and Grantham, but this was something of a roundabout route and involved a change of trains at Essendine. A connection between Bourne and the MR Syston-Peterborough line would provide the best and most direct route, and it was, accordingly, in this direction that the next moves were made during the 1880s.

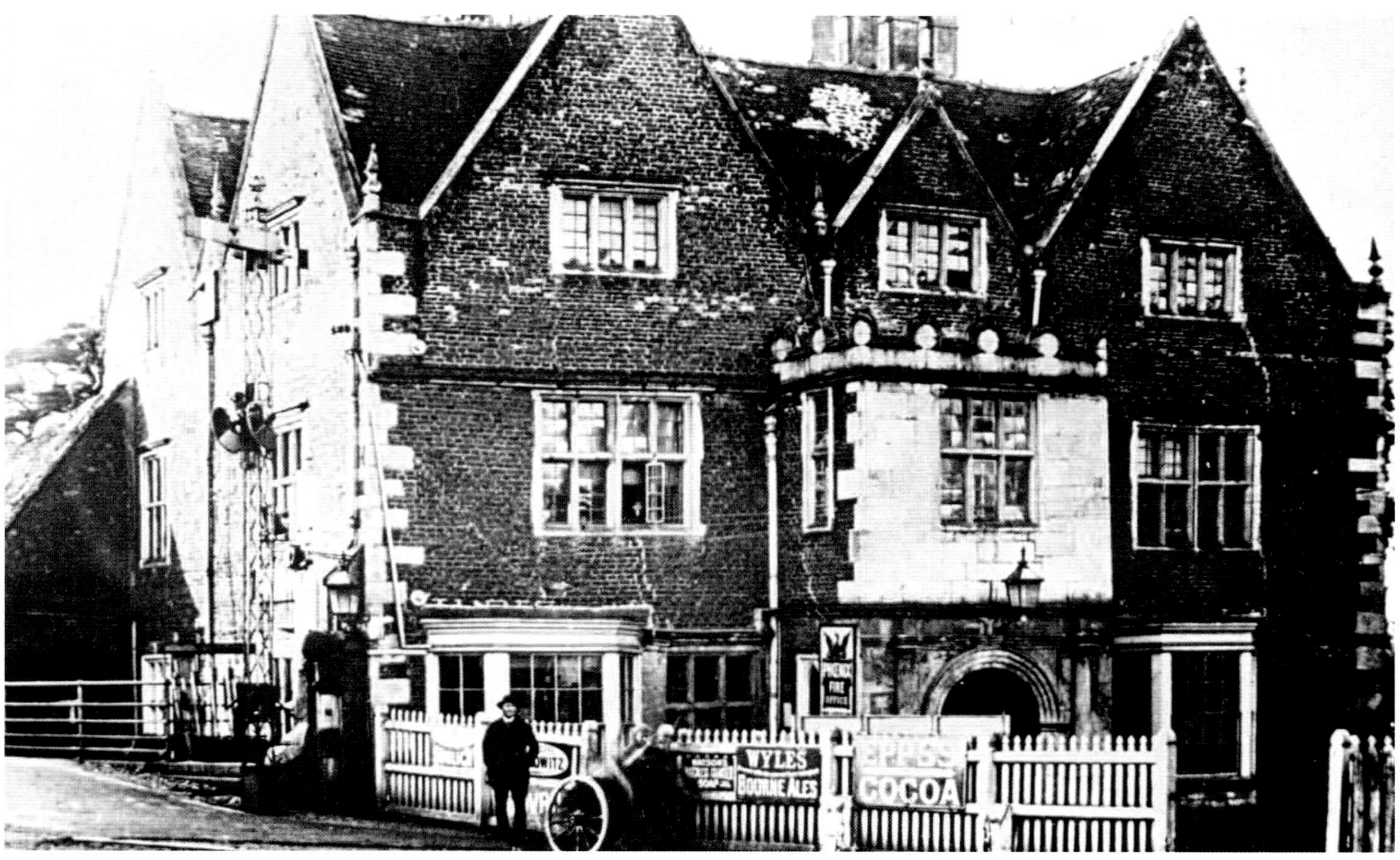

CHAPTER TWO

THE BOURNE- SAXBY LINK

Above: Red Hall, the original Bourne & Essendine station building, before the 1893 conversion. The platform ramp, later removed to make way for two sidings, can just be seen in the left foreground. (Welholme Galleries)

Although it was only in the last decade of the century that the Bourne-Saxby link was finally realised, it had been mooted as a viable proposition as far back as 1864, as part of the proposals for the line which eventually materialised as the Bourne-Spalding railway. The opening of that line in 1866 provided the link in a railway route that joined the GN main line at Essendine, via Bourne and Spalding, to Sutton Bridge and South Lynn in Norfolk. As yet, however, there was no possibility of through running since the component parts of the link were owned by four separate Companies: the GN (Essendine-Bourne); the Spalding & Bourn; the Norwich & Spalding (Spalding-Sutton Bridge); and the Lynn & Sutton Bridge. Two of these Companies, the Spalding & Bourn and the Lynn & Sutton Bridge, proposed an amalgamation into a new Company to be called the Midland & Eastern, which would then lease the Norwich & Spalding and build a new extension westwards from Bourne to join the MR at Saxby, thus linking the eastern counties and the Midlands by a more direct route than was then available. The MR, recognising an opportunity to extend its influence into GN territory, was quick to give its support to the scheme; the GN, seeing the Midland threat, was equally swift to oppose it. The conflict was resolved, when the Bill reached the Committee stage in the Commons, by a compromise between the two major Companies in which the Midland agreed to withdraw its support for the Saxby extension proposal in return for running powers over GN metals from Bourne to Essendine and from there, over a route then under construction, to Stamford, where a junction could be effected with the Midland's own Peterborough-Syston line. The formal agreement was ratified on July 1, 1866, and the first Bourne-Saxby link was thereby dropped, to lie in abeyance for more than 20 years.

The idea was resurrected in 1888 by the Eastern & Midland, a Company formed by takeover of all the smaller Companies formerly controlling the lines between Bourne and Lynn. Again in collaboration with the MR, the E & M proposed a line westwards from Bourne via Witham-on-the-Hill, crossing the GN main line south of Little Bytham station (where there would be a connecting junction) and then looping round to take in the villages of Clipsham, Stretton and Greetham before making an end-on junction with the existing MR mineral branch line at Cottesmore (see Location Map). Iron-ore had been quarried in this area since 1882, the ore at first being carried by horse and cart the couple of miles to Ashwell station, on the MR's Peterborough-Syston line, but the Midland soon found it more convenient to open a railway branch line to the edge of the ore field, where a network of tramways then led off into the quarries themselves. Since this branch was already laid to standard gauge, it would have been a simple operation to upgrade the track and adapt it for passenger working in order for it to become part of the through route to Bourne.

In return for Midland support of the scheme, the E & M agreed to route as much traffic as possible via the MR, rather than via the GNR from Bourne to Essendine, a proposal that was once again vigorously contested by the GN. Although the line received authorisation on June 28, 1888, the traffic agreement was thrown out by the Commons Committee and, again inevitably, the Companies concerned re-thought their positions and arrived at a compromise solution. The decision was made by the two large Companies, the MR and GNR, since the E & M was by this time sliding into deep financial trouble; the proposal was for a new route west from Bourne to cross the GN main line north of Little Bytham station (with, as before, a connecting junction) and then via South Witham to a junction at Saxby. The line would be under joint MR/GNR control from Bourne as far as Little Bytham (a double-track section), while the remaining, single-line, section would belong exclusively to the Midland. Plans for the new line (and also for the new, less severe, curve at Saxby, mentioned earlier) were drawn up by Alfred Langley, the Midland's engineer, and deposited on November 28, 1888, in order to meet the requirements for consideration in the 1889 Parliamentary session.

No problems were encountered in the Bill's progress and it passed smoothly through all stages, receiving sanction on June 24, 1889. By this time it was obvious that the E & M's financial problems were insuperable, and in 1891 the MR and GNR made an offer to take over the E & M route jointly, and, after some negotiation, this offer was accepted. The new Committee of the M & GN Joint took control of the E & M system from July 1, 1893, by which date the Bourne-Saxby line had been opened to goods traffic and trains were running between the Midlands and

Below: The signpost at Little Bytham Junction marking the point at which the Joint and Midland lines met end to end. (E. L. Back)

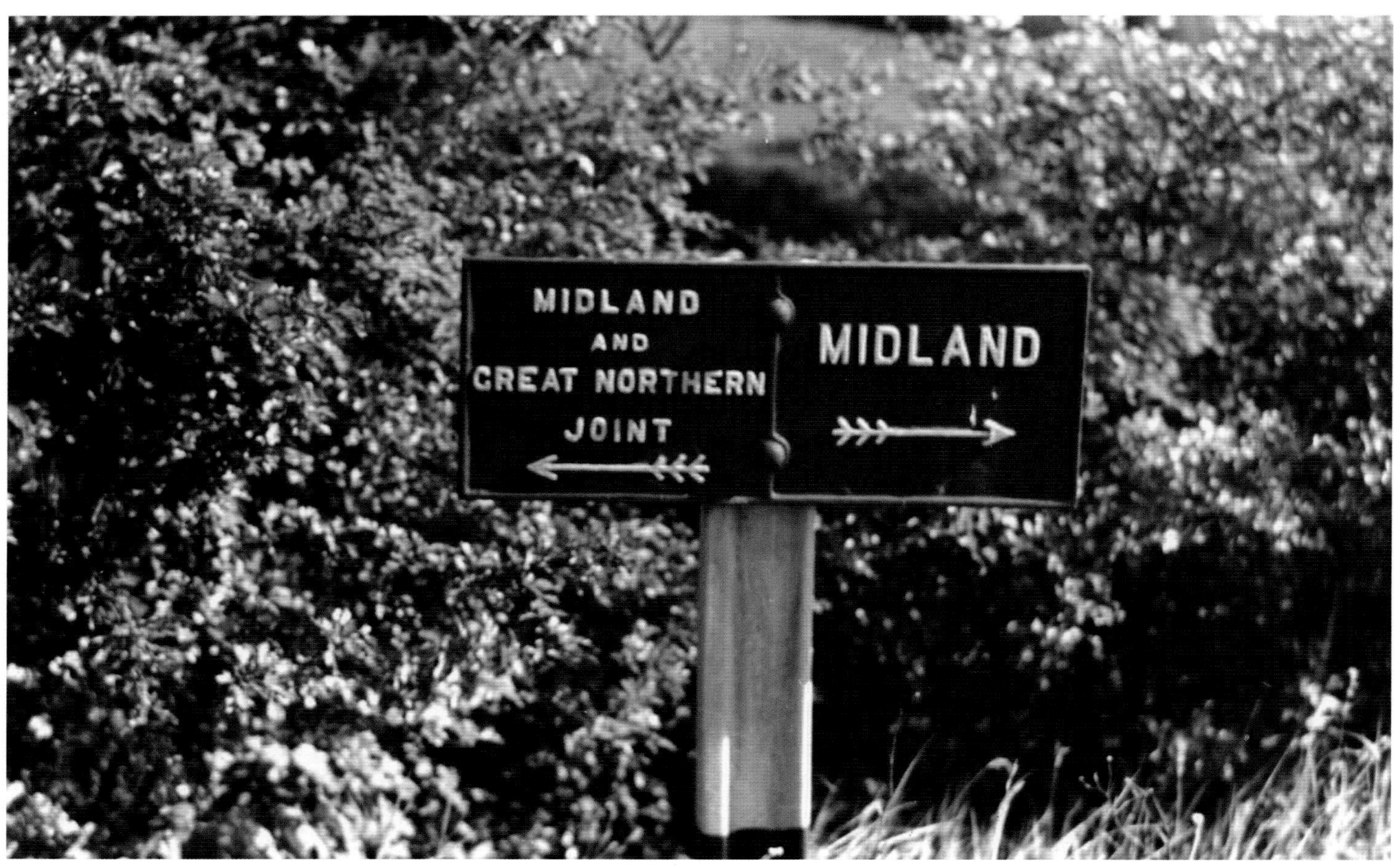

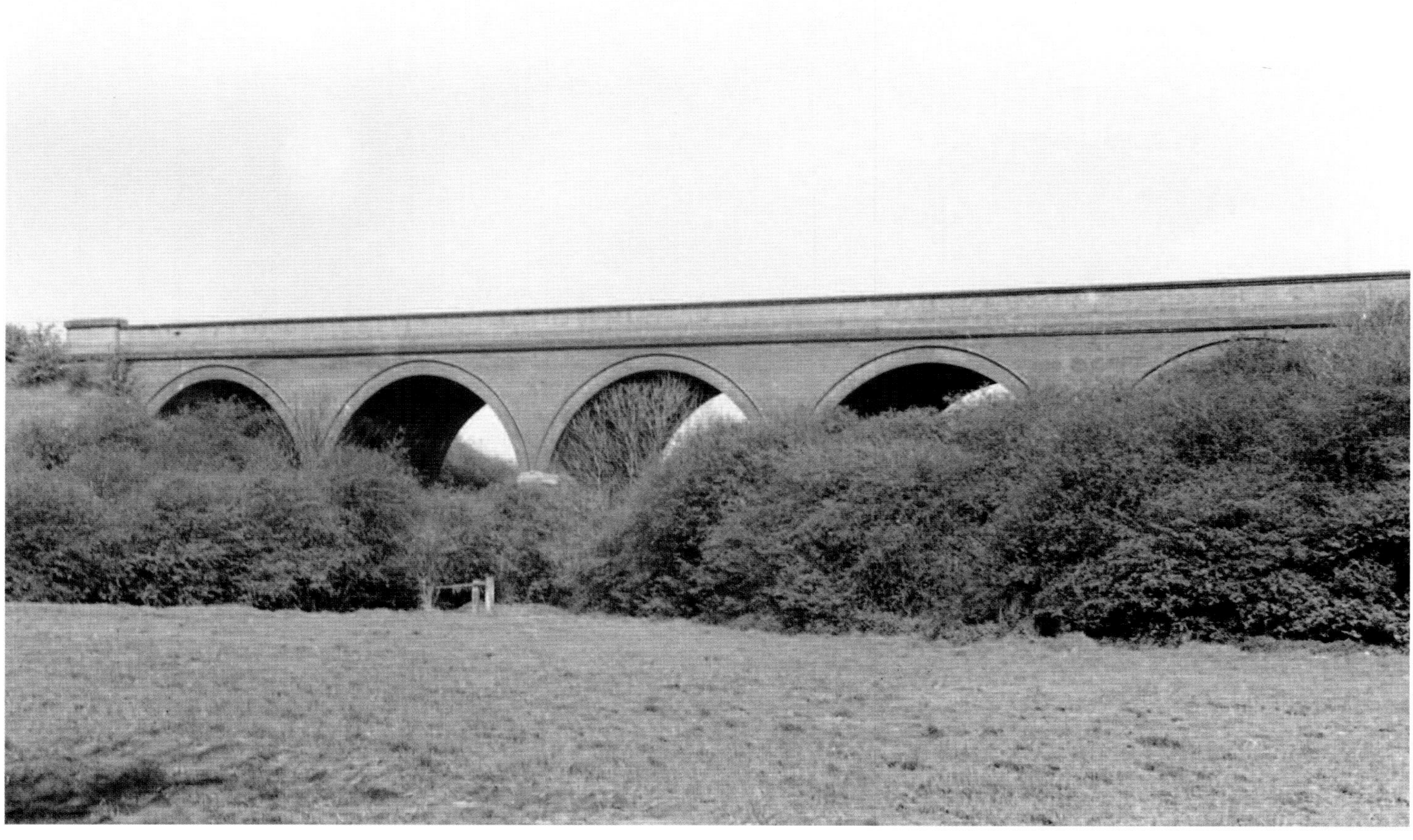

Above: The five arches of Lound viaduct, spanning the shallow valley of the Lound Beck about a mile west of Toft tunnel. (M & GN Circle)

Spalding, Lynn and the eastern counties. This, however, is to anticipate events a little; the next chapter backtracks a few years to detail the construction of the line itself.

CHAPTER THREE

CONSTRUCTION AND OPENING

The 18 miles of line, construction of which was under the overall charge of J. Allen McDonald, the Midland's Chief Engineer, were divided into three sections, and tenders invited accordingly. Eventually, the contract for the first section, Saxby to South Witham, including the new Saxby curve, was awarded to the firm of Holme & King, of London and Liverpool, with Mr. A. Wilson as their resident engineer; the middle section, from South Witham to Little Bytham, was given to Messrs. J.W. Nowell of Manchester, an old-established firm of railway contractors who had worked on the London & Birmingham line as far back as the late 1830s; and the final section, Little Bytham to Bourne, was taken by William Mousley of Eccleshall, Staffordshire, whose resident engineer was George McDonald. Mousley's firm was also awarded the contract for the new station at Bourne, and for the Spalding avoiding line, both being built at the same time. All contracts had been let by October 1890, when work was able to get under way along the route.

On the Saxby section, the first contract to be awarded, work had got off to a brisk start; by the beginning of November several miles of single line had already been laid. The track, in 30' lengths, was 85lbs to the yard, joined with plain fishplates wedged into 50lbs chairs, and ballasted mostly with broken stones and ashes. The land rose steadily between Saxby and a point mid-way between Wymondham and South Witham, where the summit of the line was reached, and a good deal of embanking and cutting was necessary to maintain workable gradients: the new Saxby curve and the junction with the Bourne line were carried on a 700-yard long embankment over a tributary of the River Eye, and there were two sizeable cuttings, one half a mile long, between Saxby and Wymondham.

On the middle section, six miles of route, work was under way by October 1890. South Witham became the headquarters of the navvy work-force, and a large settlement soon sprang up on the edge of the village, in a field belonging to a Mr Cooper, conveniently close to the Blue Bull public-house. Workshops for carpenters and blacksmiths were erected, equipped with a circular saw and a mortar-mill, both driven by steam power; a well was sunk to provide water for the engines. About a hundred men, divided into three groups, were employed on embanking work and shifting material, which was done initially by horse and cart. Stone for building work was dug from a local quarry in Mill Lane. Bad weather hampered progress at the beginning of December, when heavy snow made it necessary to suspend operations and lay off, albeit temporarily, a large number of navvies; by Christmas, however, conditions had eased and in order to make up for lost time the contractors, Messrs. Nowell (an aptly seasonal name) brought in digging machinery in the form of a Dunbar & Ruston "steam navvy". Steam-driven excavating machines were not new – the American railroad builders had been using them since the 1840s – but it was not until the end of the century that contractors in this country began to use them in any numbers. One machine, it was estimated, could do the work of between 30 and 80 men, and give a saving of up to 1/- a cubic yard of material removed. In such a quiet and remote rural area as South Witham, a steam navvy was a distinct novelty, and crowds of locals regularly turned out to gawp at the snorting monster biting its way through the countryside at a rate of 1,000 cubic yards a day.

The section between Little Bytham and Bourne was the most difficult on the route, and offered the most severe challenge to the contractor. The land to the east of Bourne is fenland, stretching out totally level for 25 miles until it reaches the waters of the Wash. West of the town, however, the terrain rises in a series of ridges, none of them spectacularly steep but between them combining to climb from a mere 35' above sea level to a high point of 439' between Wymondham and South Witham. The escarpment which overlooks Bourne was too steep to allow the line to be taken over it and so a tunnel had to be driven through it; even so, the line was still forced to climb at a steady 1 in 100 for four miles beyond the station with only a slight stretch falling at 1 in 440 at the halfway stage. Preliminary work on the tunnel started in November 1890 with the sinking of two shafts; for a depth of 50' the excavators worked through shale, but then struck hard rock, which slowed progress appreciably and necessitated the use of gunpowder to loosen it. At the other end of the section, however, round Little Bytham, work was carried on at a good rate, although the December snowstorms caused a similar laying-off of workmen here as at South Witham. Notwithstanding, the Chief Engineer was so satisfied with overall progress that by the end of the year it was being confidently forecast that the whole line would be ready for operation by August 1892.

1891 saw very solid progress made along the whole route. Tunnelling work got under way in earnest at the beginning of February, with the initial work-force of 100 men soon increased to about 400, most of them housed in a shanty settlement of temporary wooden huts. An order for one million of the two and a half million bricks needed for lining the tunnel was placed with the local brickmaker. Henry Kingston of Bourne, who made the bricks from clay dug from the foot of Stamford Hill, through which the tunnel was to be driven, where deposits lay 12' deep. A whole collection of workshops – a saw-mill, mortar-mill, smithies and carpenters shops – grew up around the workings. The tunnel shafts were served by two winding engines, while the air below was kept tolerably fresh by the use of a Roots patent blower to ventilate the excavations. Water was supplied at the site of operations by one and a quarter mile length of pipe fed by a bore-hole at Bourne. Spoil removed from the tunnel and from the cutting at its east end was taken to Spalding to form the embankment for the new loop line being built there; four trains of 20 wagons each made the journey every day, carrying between them 400 cubic yards of earth.

In order to facilitate the conveyance of material, such as bricks, from Bourne to the work-face, a two and a half mile tramway was laid to serve not only the tunnel but also the viaduct over the Glen valley at Lound, a little further down the line, work on which started in October 1891. The bridge was of five arches, each of 40' span and 44' from ground to rail level, and required one and a half million bricks in its construction. 200,000 cubic yards of soil from adjacent cuttings were tipped to form the approach embankments. In November, heavy rain caused the River Glen to burst its banks and flood a large area of the surrounding countryside. Part of an embankment was washed away, and work was suspended for a few days. throwing a number of men out of employment. Presumably they were easily able to find alternative jobs, since a local newspaper report had recently complained about the scarcity of labour in several parts of the district because of the demand for workers on the railway, where wages were much higher than could be obtained elsewhere; a railway labourer could earn £1 a week at this time, or even 25 or 30 shillings if on piecework.

When work resumed on the viaduct, a couple of men were injured in separate accidents; a stone-mason was hit by a falling block of stone when the shear-legs of some pulley tackle collapsed, and another man had his foot crushed by the contractor's engine while engaged in shunting operations.

Further westwards, towards Little Bytham, was another major cutting, 35' deep at its maximum, which

necessitated the removal of 200,000 cubic yards of spoil. Two steam navvies were employed on this at the height of operations, during the summer months, transferring the earth into wagons (about 450 loads daily), which were then hauled away by locomotives to be tipped to form embankments elsewhere along the route, mainly on the west side of Glen valley, on the approach to Lound viaduct. By the summer of 1891 work was advancing rapidly on the large cutting between Little Bytham and Castle Bytham, half a mile long and 30' deep. The underlying material here is rock, and it had to be removed by explosives; in June one navvy, Samuel Payne, was admitted to Stamford Infirmary with burns to the head and legs after injudicious use of gunpowder. A more serious accident occurred a few months later when a temporary bridge at South Witham collapsed and killed George Preston, known to all and sundry as Little Toby.

By mid-1891 the number of navvies at South Witham encampment had risen to 300, which had the startling effect for the 1891 Census of trebling the village's population. Such large concentrations of brawny workers, notorious for their drunkenness, strong language and immoral behaviour,were often looked upon with consternation by the inhabitants of the areas they invaded, but there does not seem to have been any unusual amount of trouble caused by the workers anywhere along the 18 miles of this line. There were the inevitable petty crimes: navvy John Smith charged with stealing a goose, value 7/6, from the Rev. Tollemache-Tollemache, rector of South Witham, and another navvy, William Goddard, charged with receiving said stolen goose; John Williams convicted of stealing a pair of scissors and other articles, valued at 5/-, and sent to prison for 14 days hard labour; Alfred Redgrave arrested for rather uncharitably absconding with the boots belonging to his fellow-lodger Frederick Kingston; a nameless ganger who even more uncharitably ran away with the navvies' sick-club money. Perhaps the low incidence of crime was partly due to the appointment by the MR of two special constables for six months in 1891, when the number of men employed was at its highest; these gentlemen, paid 30/- a week, patrolled the workings purposefully, keeping an eye open particularly for signs of drunkenness among the workers. Early in 1892 the MR terminated their appointment on the grounds of cost; ironically a few weeks later four navvies were before the courts charged with being roaring drunk at Little Bytham.

The most serious incident concerning navvies seems to have occurred when two labourers, James Hook and Thomas Smith, met in bare-fisted combat in a field near Wymondham. The two men had quarrelled some time before in a pub in Melton, and now Hook belligerently insisted on finishing the argument. Although Smith at first refused, Hook's taunts became too much for him and the pair of them slogged it out unmercifully until Hook was felled and collapsed in the shadow of a wall; he was later found to be dead. Smith gave himself up to the police and was sent for trial on a charge of manslaughter.

The morals and behaviour of the railway labourers were a keen concern of the Navvy Mission Society, a familiar presence on any large railway working in the latter years of the century. Local Mission Rooms were set up at Little Bytham in the Victoria Hall at Bourne, and at Castle Bytham (whose Mission was officially opened by Lady Frances Cecil), and regular meetings and "entertainments" were held; at Bourne, for example, Mr. A. Mousley, son of the contractor for that section, put together a programme of violin solos songs and recitations at which, we are told, "the humorous element met with hearty appreciation". In May 1892 the navvies at Castle Bytham were visited by Miss Spofford, fresh from her crusading among the wild workers of the Manchester Ship Canal, and who delivered a "very earnest and powerful address" on behalf of the Christian Excavators Society, apparently listened to with rapt attention by the Castle Bytham men.

That the majority of the navvies were well behaved and accepted by the villagers of the area was nicely shown on the occasion of the Village Feast Day at South Witham in 1891. Under a blazing blue sky, and to the accompaniment of the Castle Bytham Brass Band, the navvies entered fully into the festivities, organising a tug-of-war competition between the labourers and the gangers (the labourers won), and a cricket match between the representatives of the workers on the Castle Bytham and Little Bytham stretches of line. Mr Nowell, the contractor, and his wife were there, and Nowell donated many of the prizes presented to the victorious competitors.

By now it was apparent that the suggested opening date for the line of August 1892 had been too optimistic, since much work remained to be done. More severe weather at the beginning of the year, with hard frost and heavy snowfall, put 400 men out of work and brought progress to a halt on many parts of the route. The tunnelling at Toft continued, however, and by spring of 1892 the bore was almost complete. At Castle Bytham the deep cutting through the village was pushed forward slowly; a navvy was killed in June when he was struck by the contractor's engine during soil-tipping operations. In May an impressive party of 40 directors and officials of the GNR and the MR visited Bourne to inspect the site of the new station and to finalise plans for its construction.

Although autumn of that year did not see the completion of the whole line, it had by that time reached at least an approximate state of readiness throughout most of its length. On Nowell's section between South Witham and Little Bytham, work was almost finished except for the station buildings at South Witham, which was a separate contract let to Mr. C. Barnes of Melton, who was also responsible for the stations at Wymondham and Saxby. At the western end of the line the new curve at Saxby had been opened on August 28, and the station layout extensively modified and enlarged. The 1848 station building was retained in use for handling goods, and the trackwork of the original Saxby curve was terminated at the road connecting Saxby village with Stapleford Park to form a double siding. The new station boasted three platforms, the middle one being an island, all located directly beneath a road bridge from which access was gained to the platforms by flights of steps. The most northerly platform contained the main station building, a squat, single-storey brick structure, and perhaps not particularly eye-catching or impressive, but functional enough. The shelters on the other two platforms were of wood, and made to seem rather top-heavy by the canopy roof which projected over all four sides.

By the end of 1892 a total of £52,121 had been expended on the Bourne-Saxby workings, almost £20,000 of it in the latter six months of the year. By the end of February 1893 the Midland's Chief Engineer, Mr McDonald, was reporting that 18 miles of track had now been laid, and apart from large-scale operations still continuing on Toft tunnel and Castle Bytham cutting, most of the remaining work was minor; he expected the line to be open for traffic by the middle of the year. On April 21 the directors of the GNR and the MR were able to see the progress being made when they inspected the route by riding over it in a special saloon car. On Sunday, June 4, a large gang of men was put to work making the final connections between the MR and GNR systems at Bourne and Saxby, and on the following day, June 4, the line was finally opened for goods traffic. The first train from Leicester, came through early in the morning, reaching Bourne at about 7am on its way to South Lynn yard, and in the course of the day about 30 more goods trains rattled along the new line in both directions.

From the beginning, Midlands coal was an important commodity, and the first consignment, a modest two wagon-loads, was delivered on the first day of operations at South Witham, where two coal merchants, Messrs Ellis & Everard, and T.G. Bennet of Market Overton, had already made arrangements for business at the station. By October, the daily service of trains had been supplemented by a regular nightly service of Midland goods trains running from Spalding to London via Bourne and Saxby. The gradients which west-bound trains faced out of Bourne sometimes gave trouble, and there was a period in the autumn of 1893 when a stock of poor engine coal loaded into tenders meant that several trains ran out of steam on the approach to South Witham, with consequent delay to services. The approach of winter added the problem of severe weather; in late November a ferocious gale swept the whole country, with howling winds and heavy rain; buildings were damaged, trees uprooted, and off the coast ships were sunk - 20 vessels from Grimsby alone went down, with the loss of over 50 sailors. With the approach of night the temperature fell, and the rain turned to driving snow. On the exposed heights near South Witham and Wymondham the gale-force wind blew the snow into huge drifts, and a goods train heading west into the blizzard found itself brought to a halt, trapped in an eight-foot snowbank. The breakdown gang from Melton Mowbray had to be called out and struggled for several hours in the dark and cold before they could clear the line sufficiently for the train to resume its journey.

It had been expected that passenger services would begin soon after the inauguration of goods services - the last week of July had been mentioned – and in fact a special excursion train from the Midlands to Lynn did use the route on June 25; a general passenger service was, however, postponed, presumably because of the incomplete state of the line's stations, particularly at the Bourne end, where considerable re-modelling of the station site had only just begun, the existing station facilities being insufficient to cope with the expected increase in traffic consequent on the opening of the Saxby link. That a new station was to be built here had been decided back in 1890 and originally it had been announced that the old Red Hall would be demolished to make way for the improvements. Apart from being Bourne's very first station house, the Hall was, in itself, a very historic building, and there was considerable local agitation about its impending destruction. A local

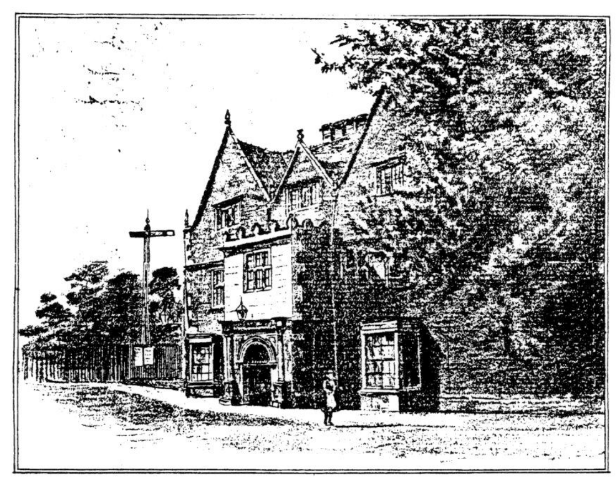

A Memorial from the Inhabitants of Bourne and Neighbourhood to the Directors of the Great Northern and Midland Railway Companies.

We the undersigned beg respectfully to approach you in the subject of the Old Hall at Bourne now used as the Railway Station, in danger of being pulled down to make way for the extension of the Railway from Saxby

The Old Hall is a red brick - Elizabethan Mansion with gabled roof and stone mullioned

architect, Mr John Traylen, of Stamford, enlisted the support of numerous tradesmen and influential members of the Bourne area in the presentation of a petition to the directors of the MR and GNR Companies which stated:

> We the undersigned beg respectfully to approach you on the subject of the Old Hall at Bourne now used as the railway Station, in danger of being pulled down to make way for the extension of the Railway from Saxby.
>
> The Old Hall is a red-brick Elizabethan Mansion with gabled roof and stone mullioned windows, once the residence of the Digby family, standing in Parklike grounds and forms one of the many interesting historical features of Bourne. The walls are thick and strong and the Roof watertight.
>
> It has formed the subject of Academy pictures and is still admired, measured and sketched by students, the fine oak stair-case inside and the venerable yew tree 300 years old being objects of peculiar interest.
>
> It has attracted the attention of the Society for the Protection of Ancient Buildings who unite with us in asking you to allow it to remain untouched that it may serve a useful purpose to your Company and still exercise its quiet influence as an antidote to the restless spirit of its surroundings.
>
> We can ill afford to lose such picturesque and historical relics of the past and your Memorialists therefore pray that it may still be preserved to them.

The appeal met with widespread support among the ordinary people of Bourne and attracted the attention of most of the London and provincial daily papers; periodicals such as the "Illustrated London News" featured drawings of the Hall in their pages. Recognising the strength of local feeling, the MR and GNR finally agreed to preserve the building and restore it, using it as the station master's residence. This was a decision welcomed by the "Grantham Journal", whose correspondent waxed nostalgic about the cosy informality of the Hall's main room, which did service as the waiting- room of the old station:

> There was always a delightful levelling of social distinctions in this dear old low-ceiled, thick-walled, rambling room. Duke and ditcher met on the same level; the invidious barriers of first, second and third class humanities were ignored. On a bitter winter day the roaring fire would be eclipsed by the opaque forms of as many honest Britons as could comfortably squeeze themselves into the charmed but limited circle.

Work on the new station, did not really get under way until June 1893, and entailed the building of a new goods shed and a larger, 2-road engine shed, as well as extensions to existing sidings and loading docks. The most noticeable improvement was to the platform and station buildings. With the abandonment of Red Hall as station offices, the 1860 platform in front of that building became redundant and was removed, being replaced by two sidings; the island platform was then considerably extended, to 700', and this contained all the necessary offices: waiting rooms, porters' rooms, parcels accommodation and booking office (although this was not actually opened for business until mid-July). It was originally intended to provide a subway from the approach road to the platform, but this idea was abandoned in favour of an iron footbridge, erected by Messrs. Arnold & Son of Doncaster at the end of 1894. The whole station works cost around £25,000.

Passenger trains eventually began to run between

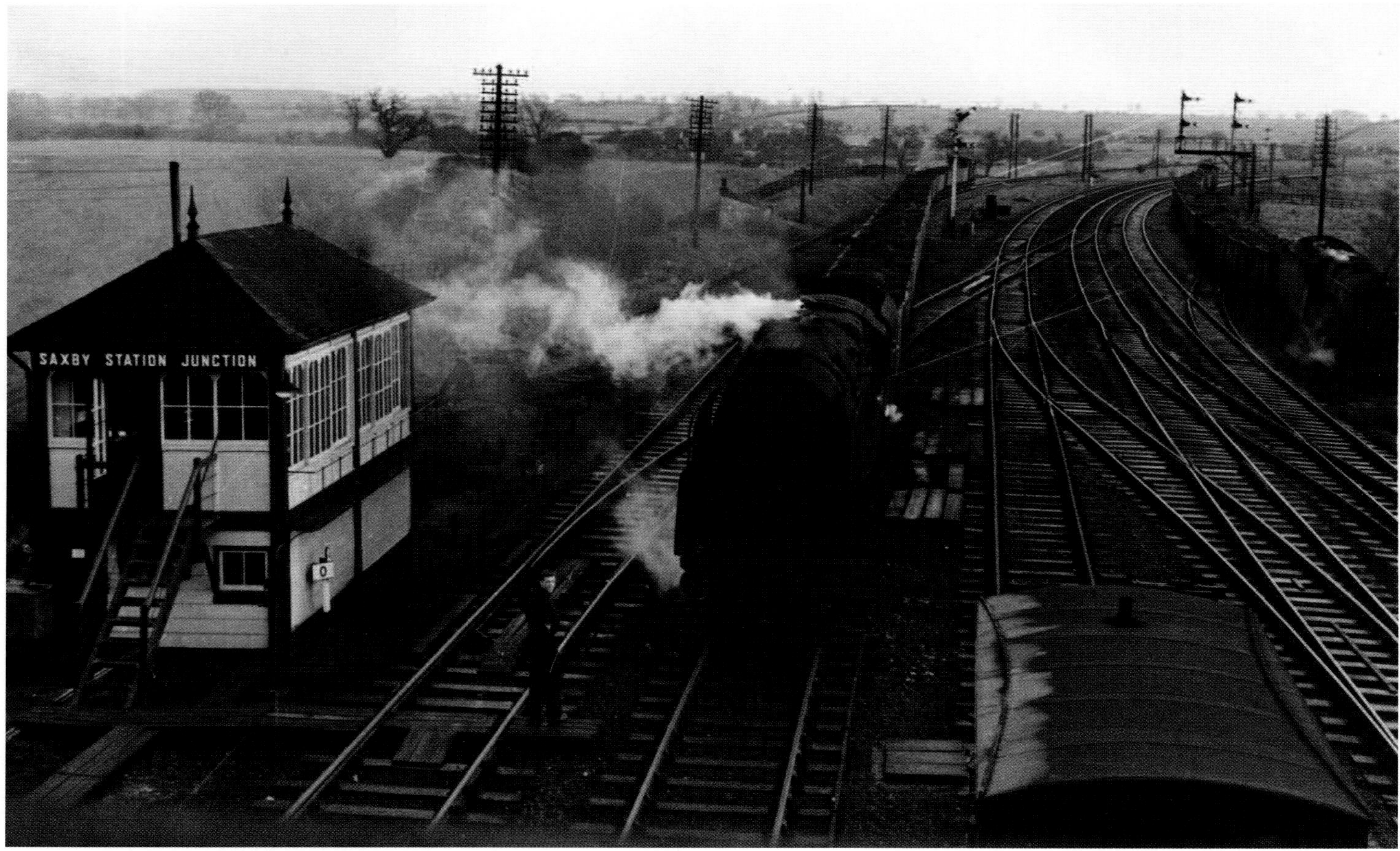

92121 approaches Saxby station in December 1960 with an ironstone train off the South Witham branch. On the right 8F 48361 simmers ignominiously after being derailed in the sand-drag, having passed signals at danger. Note the '0' milepost in front of the signal box, indicating the start of the Bourne line. (H. N. James)

Bourne and Saxby on May Day, Tuesday May 1, 1894. There was no official opening ceremony, but large crowds of people turned out to greet the first trains and at Wymondham the station was decorated with flags and banners. There were three trains a day each way: in the Up direction (Bourne-Saxby) arriving at Bourne from Spalding at 9.25am, 12.15pm and 5.20pm and on the Down line arriving at Bourne at 11.11am, 2.20pm and 8.25pm. Opening day was market day at Melton Mowbray, and so trains were well filled with farmers, with nearly a hundred people booked through to Melton on the first train. By July, special-rate market day tickets were made available for Leicester market, the cost from South Witham, for example, being 2/8 return.

From the beginning there was a thriving traffic to and from Spalding cattle market, held on Tuesdays; buyers of fat cattle regularly travelled from Leicester and Nottingham (an average of 250 passengers a week used the special Tuesday market trains in 1900), and the cattle themselves, herded through Spalding's main street to the station, would be loaded into cattle trains which then ran via Bourne and Saxby to the appropriate Midland stations. There was a similar weekly stock market at Bourne, on Thursdays, which also generated valuable traffic for the railway.

Other special excursions began almost immediately: early in June, Thomas Cook, the pioneering travel company, arranged an outing from Leicester to Holbeach, where a military tournament and sports events were being held. The return fare from South Witham was only 2/-, but the weather proved very unkind and only three people actually booked seats from that station. The first special train to be chartered by a private individual ran on May 24 and was used by Mr William Younger, the Unionist Parliamentary candidate for the Stamford Division, who required swift transport to take him to Melton Mowbray after a Conservative meeting in Bourne.

CHAPTER FOUR

THE ROUTE

The completed line, worked on the electric tablet system for the single-track section, and by block working for the double-track, was 18 miles 9 chains in length, measured between Saxby station and Bourne West Junction. The "0" milepost marking the beginning of the branch was actually located in front of Saxby Station signalbox, from where the Bourne line gradually diverged from the main Midland line, crossing the River Eye and climbing away at 1 in 100 for a mile and a half until a short level stretch was reached.

A further, less severe, climb brought the line to the first of two intermediate stations, at Wymondham, 2 miles

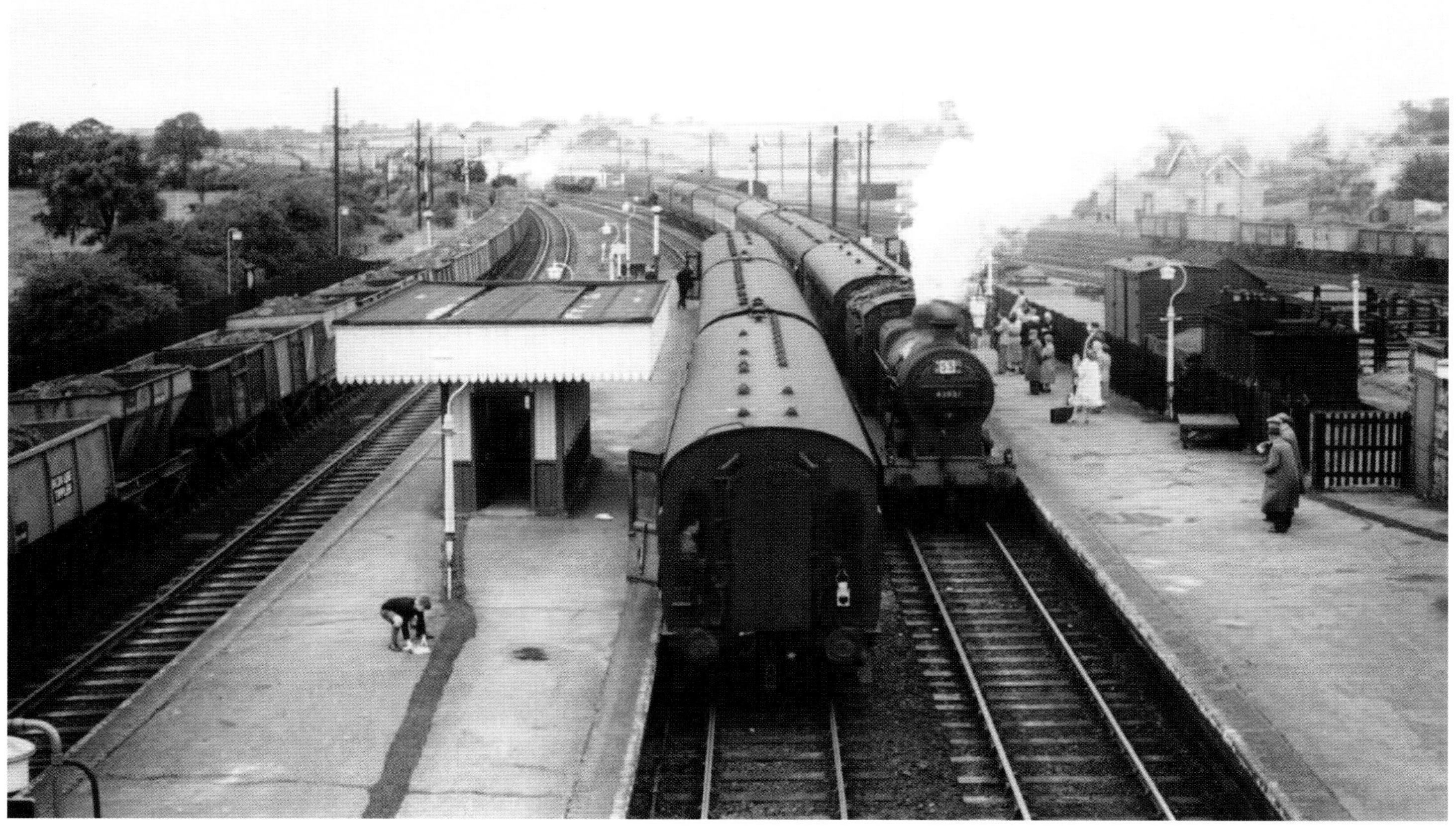

Above: Intense activity at Saxby Junction: 4F 43937 brings in a Leicester to Yarmouth excursion, an iron-stone train passes on the Peterborough-Syston line, and in the background two engines are in the process of changing trains. To the right half-hidden by smoke, is the 1848 Saxby station building, with a line of mineral wagons standing on the original Saxby curve, now a siding. (H. N. James)

34 chains from Saxby (the name was soon changed to Edmondthorpe & Wymondham to avoid confusion with Great Eastern's station at Wymondham, near Norwich). Station facilities here were of reasonable provision, with a separate goods yard (capacity 23 wagons) and shed to the south of the main line, separated from the 400'-long platforms and station buildings by an overbridge carrying Butt Lane, the main road north out of the village (later changed to Station Road). The main offices were housed in a single-storey brick building in the same style as that at Saxby, located on the Down side of the 676-yard long station loop; the Down side platform also contained the small signalbox, of standard MR design.

From Wymondham the line continued to climb steadily through a series of cuttings, emerging at about 5 miles from Saxby at the highest point of the route, 439' above sea level. From here it was almost all down-hill to Bourne, except for a few brief level stretches. At 6 miles 74 chains was located South Witham station, perched on a high, narrow embankment above the outskirts of the village, and this perhaps explains why the buildings and platforms were constructed of timber rather than brick, which would have needed substantial foundations difficult to provide on such a site. As at Wymondham, the platforms were 400' long; the passing loop was 279 yards, and the goods yard, also on an embankment behind the station, could hold 50 wagons.

From South Witham the line dropped through cuttings, passed underneath the Great North Road (which during construction of the overbridge, had been temporarily diverted at this point) and then through Castle Bytham village to level out again briefly at the bridge which carried the line over the Great Northern main line just north of Little Bytham station; the girder bridge was a single span of almost 100' between substantial brick abutments, and weighed 152 tons. Although the route here was still single-track, the bridge actually carried two lines, since a refuge siding, with space for 50 wagons, ran from Little Bytham signalbox for some distance west of the bridge.

The junction of the MR and M & GN Joint systems was located at 13 miles 7 chains from Saxby, near the isolated signalbox (Little Bytham Junction) of standard MR design and equipped with tablet-catching apparatus at the point where the single track diverged into double track for the rest of the distance between here and Bourne. A short distance east of Little Bytham box the line crossed the old trackbed of the former Edenham-Bytham Railway, built privately by Lord Willoughby d'Eresby to serve his estates at nearby Grimsthorpe. Opened in 1857, the line was actually authorised to carry passengers, but a combination of sharp curves, rough track and unreliable motive power meant that services were rather precarious; the railway

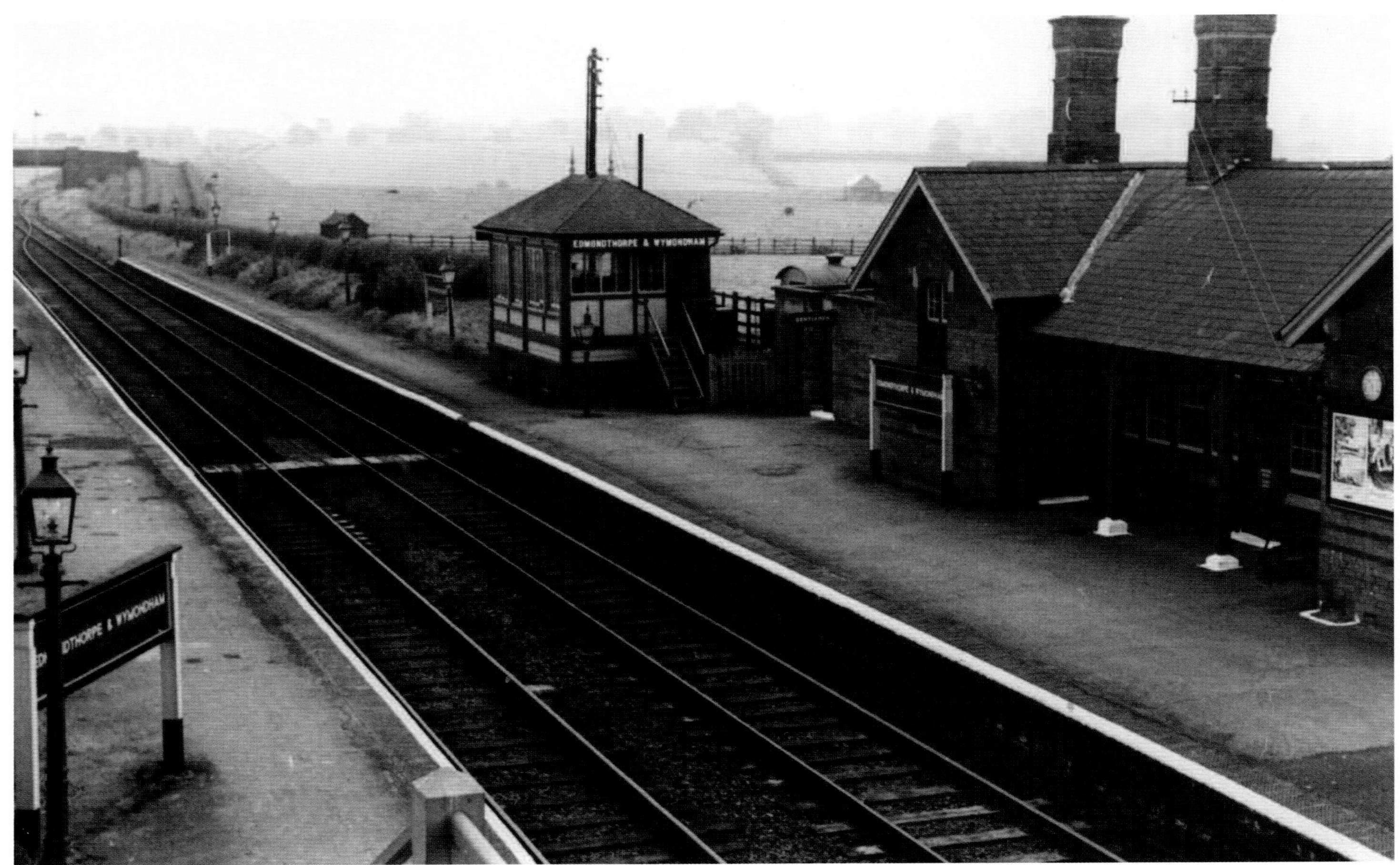

Above: Station layout at Edmondthorpe & Wymondham, showing main buildings in the same style as those at Saxby, with the signalbox half-way down the platform. In the left foreground, note the rails of the steps leading down from the road bridge. (F. Church)

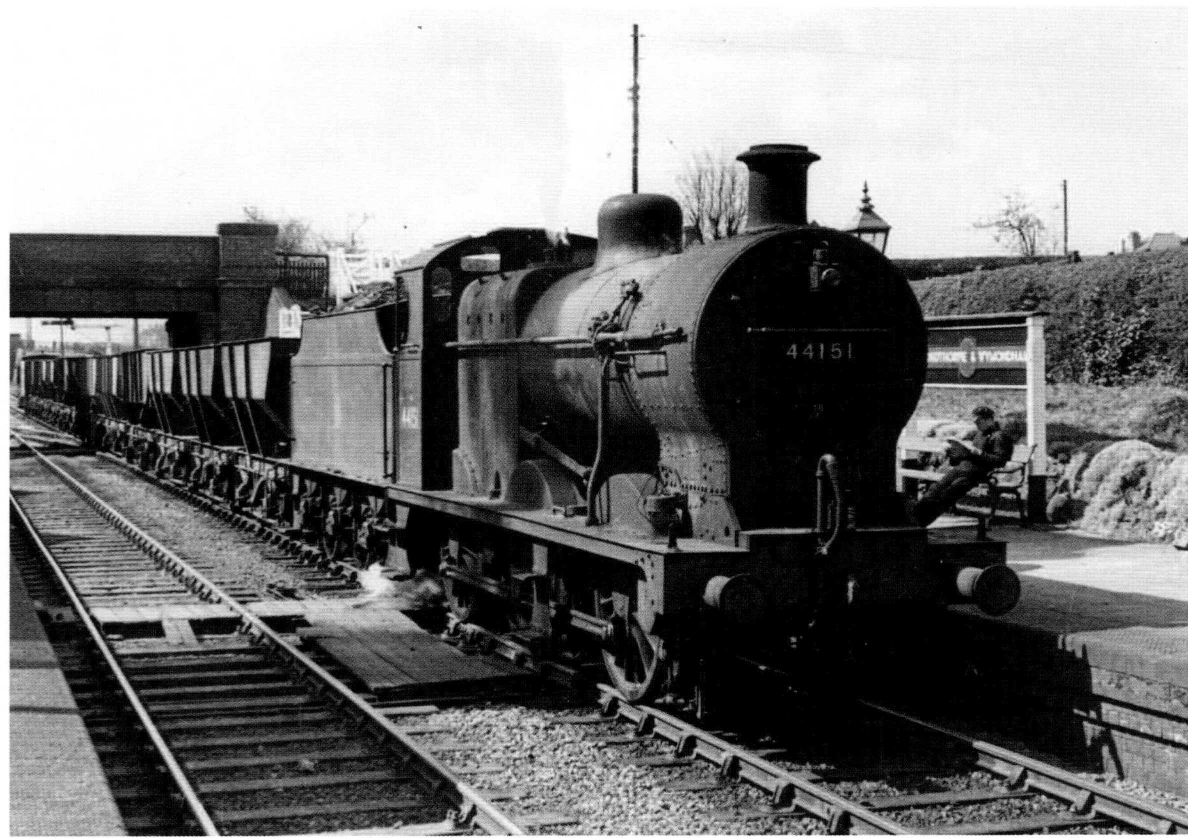

Above: The crew of 4F 44151, heading a string of empty iron-stone wagons, bask in the sunshine at Edmondthorpe & Wymondham, waiting in the station loop to be crossed by a west-bound train. (H. N. James)

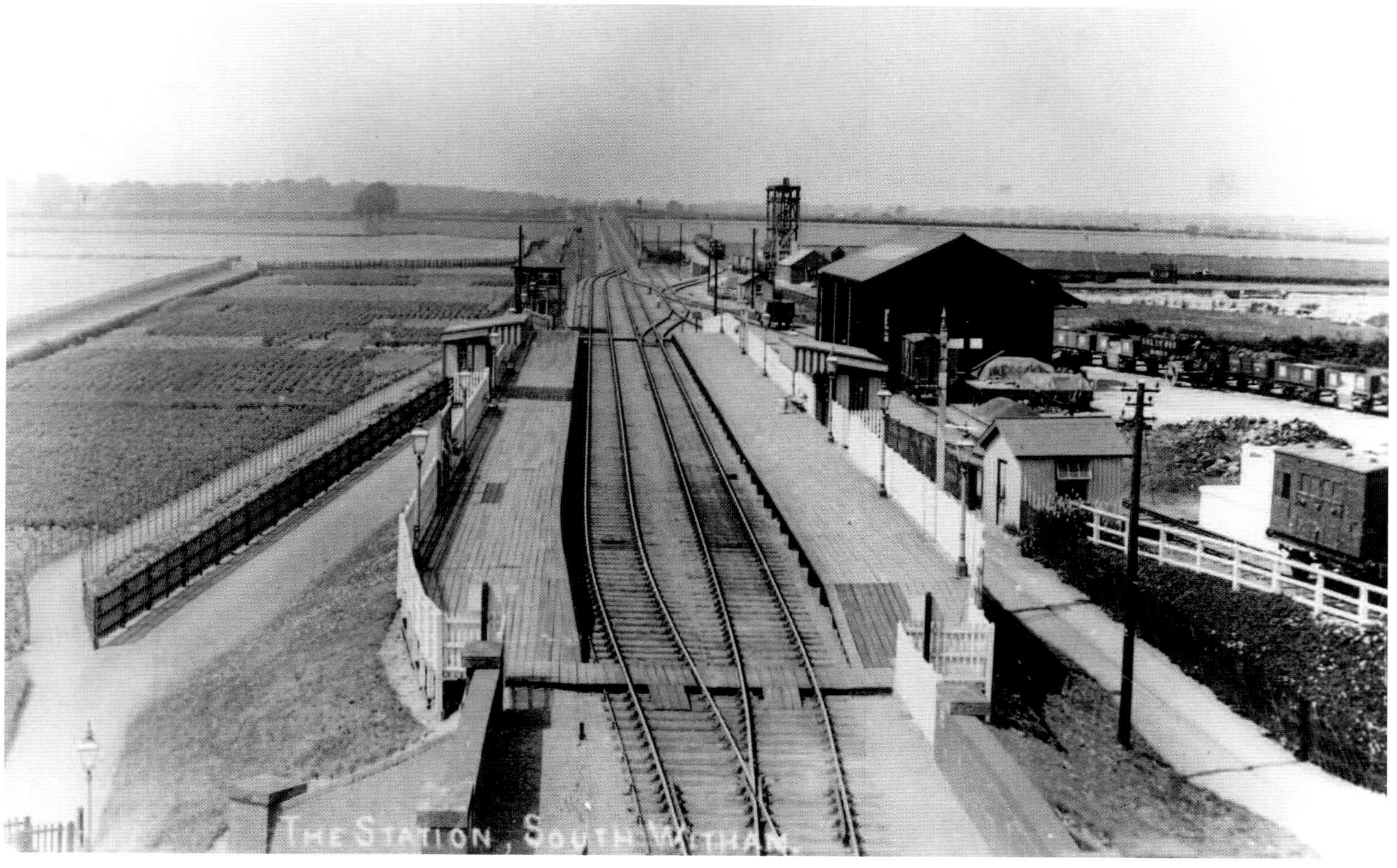

Above: Bird's-eye view of South Witham station, with its wooden platforms and station shelters. The signalbox can be seen just beyond the end of the Up platform, and to the right of the picture are the sidings and plant associated with the extensive iron-stone workings at South Witham. (Author's collection)

Below: A platform-level shot of South Witham station, looking west towards Saxby, in October 1958, a few months before the withdrawal of passenger services. South Witham, however, remained as a railhead for ironstone traffic until 1964. (F. Church)

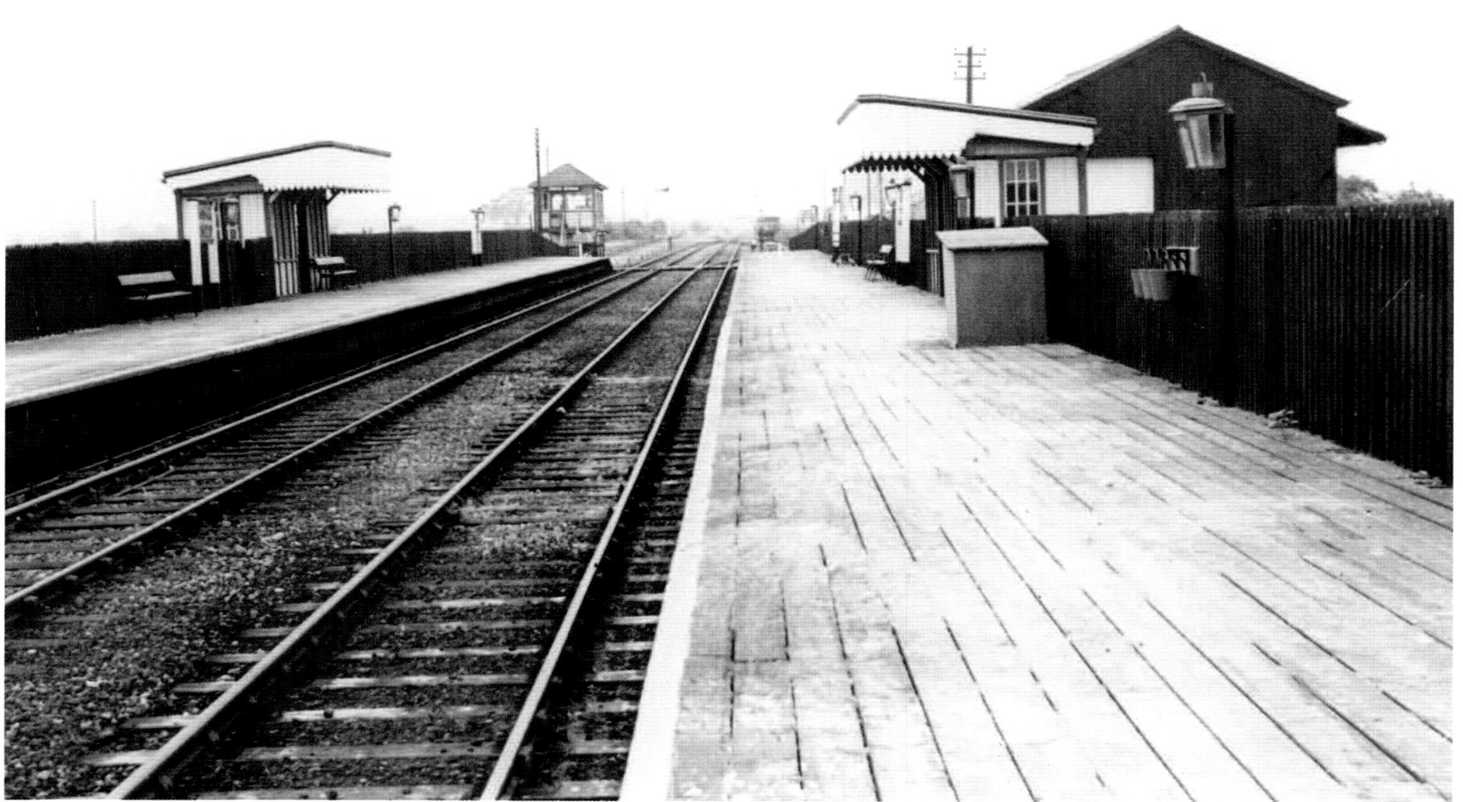

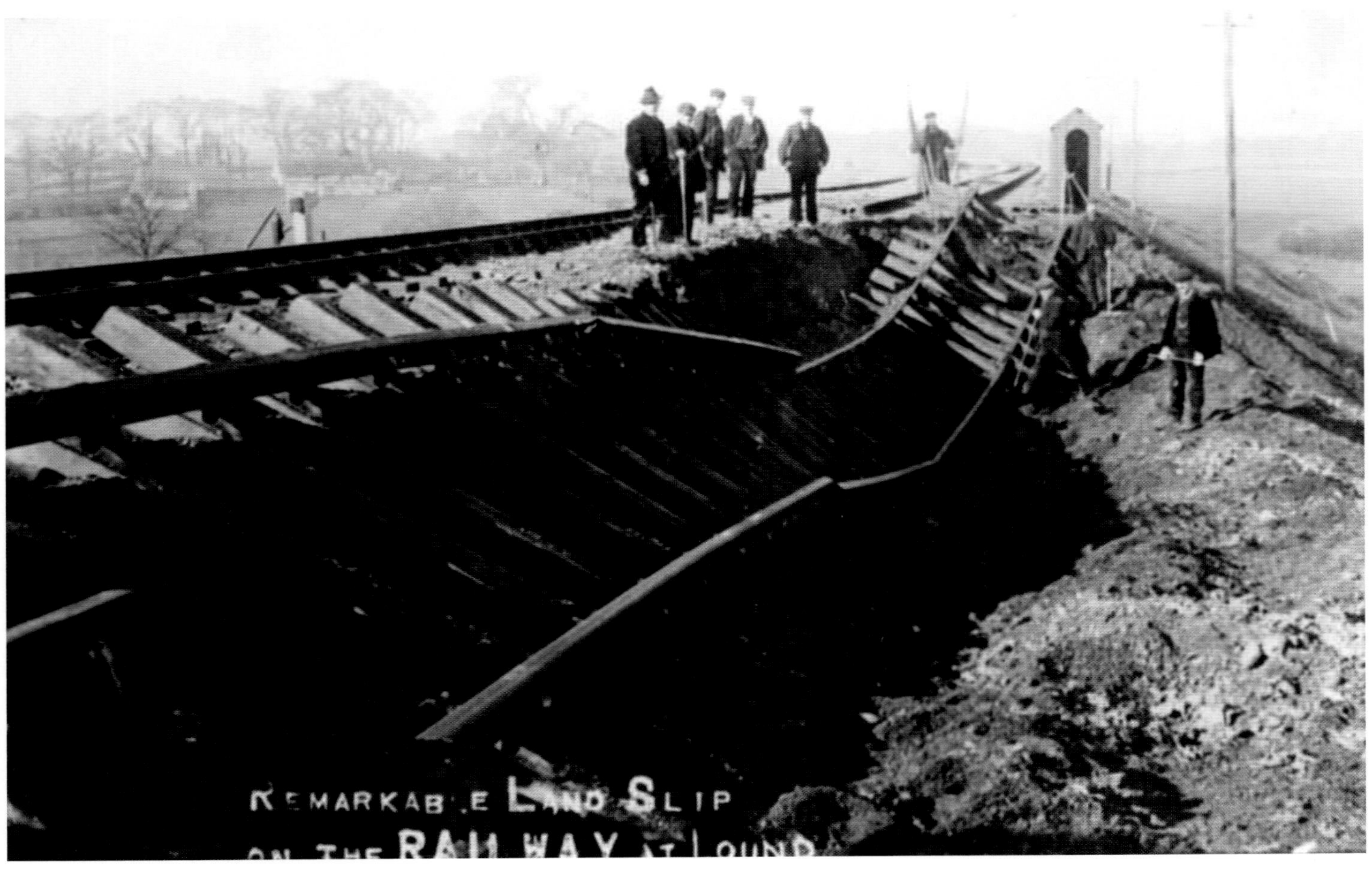

Above: A local postcard view, dated around 1910, showing a repair gang tackling a "remarkable land slip" on the embankment approaching Lound viaduct. (M & GN Circle)

Below: The east portal of the 330-yard long Toft tunnel, the only tunnel on the whole of the M & GN system. (E. L. Back)

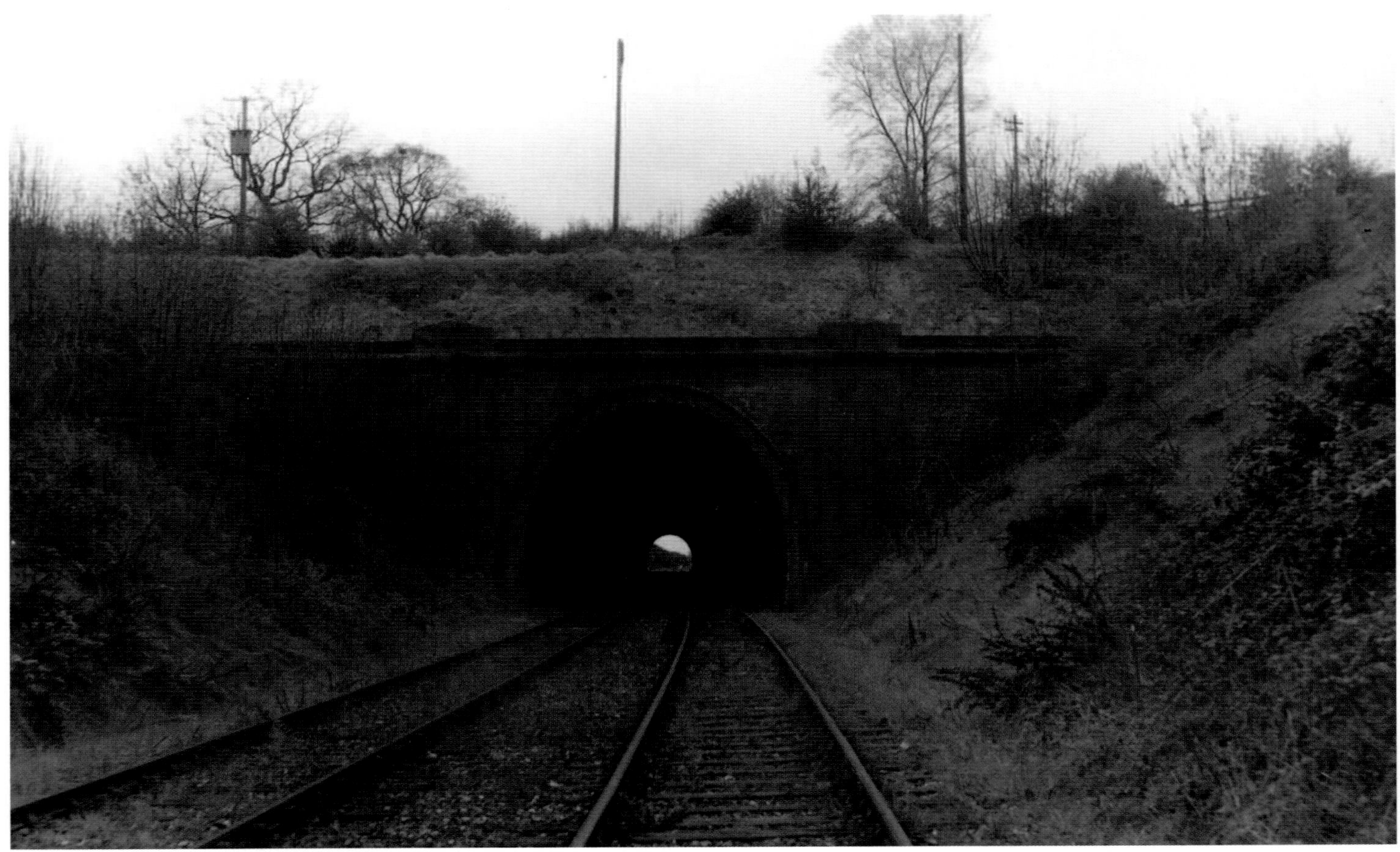

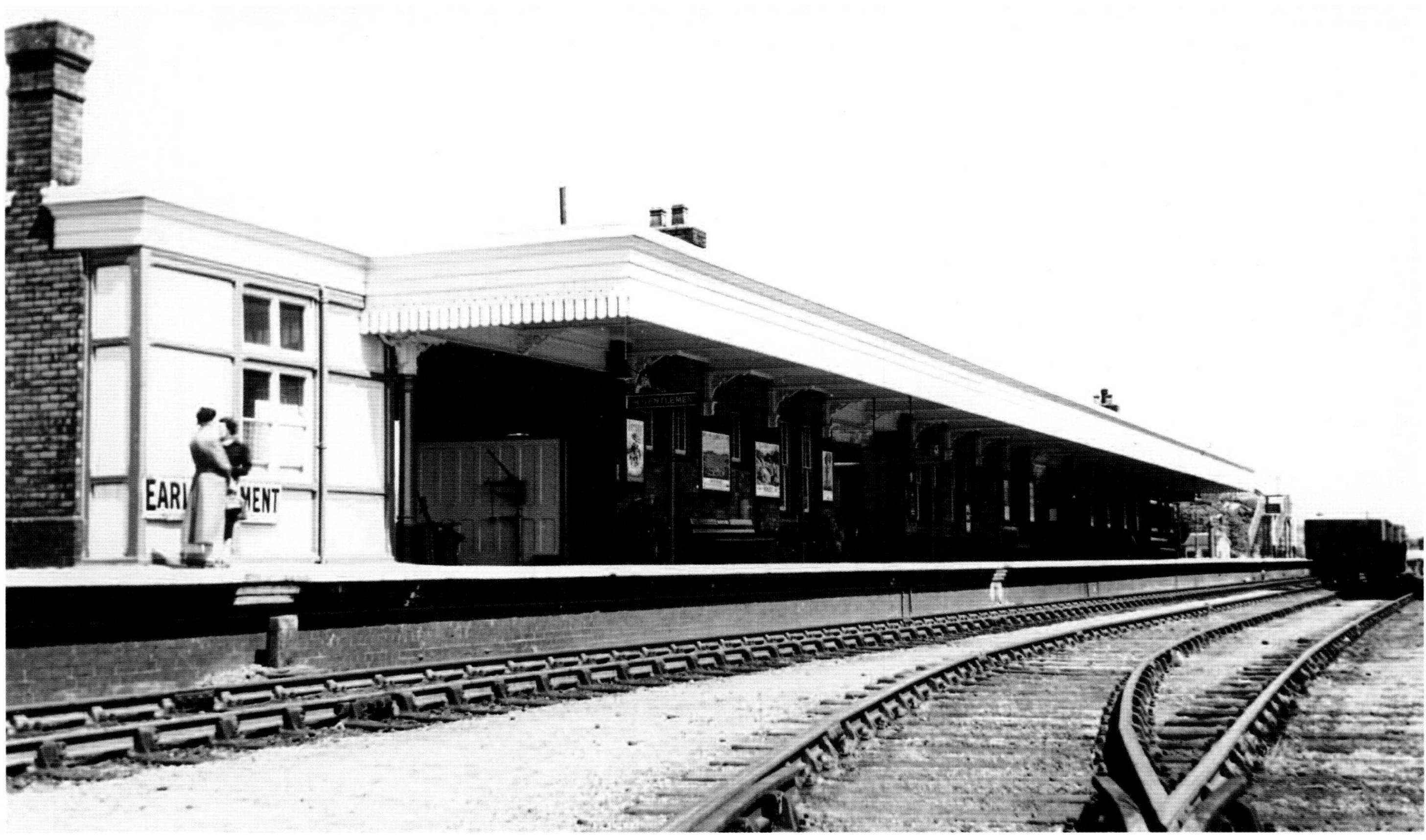

The Up side of the island platform at Bourne, used by most west-bound trains, photographed from the goods shed sidings. (Author's collection)

staggered on fitfully until the 1880s when it finally expired, having been reduced to using horse traction in its final years.

Skirting Dobbin's Wood, the Bourne-Saxby line curved gently into the Glen Valley, which it crossed by the Lound viaduct, longest and tallest bridge on the route, before passing under the Edenham-Toft road and reaching, at 16 miles 55 chains, the west portal of Toft tunnel. The tunnel itself was of modest dimensions, only 330 yards long, but had the distinction of being the only tunnel on the whole of the M & GN Joint system.

At the east end, trains emerged to run downgrade at 1 in 100, through a succession of overbridges carrying lanes and footpaths, to reach Bourne West signalbox, and the junction with the Bourne-Essendine line, before the final approach to Bourne station.

Castle Bytham

From the early days of the construction of the line there had been some surprise, and some concern, expressed that there was to be no station provided between Bourne and South Witham, a distance of 11 miles. At the beginning of 1892, a correspondent in the "Stamford Mercury" found the omission of the intermediate station "scarcely credible" and suggested strongly that "it would be in the interests of local trade" for the MR to modify its decision. It was true that the area between Bourne and Little Bytham was very sparsely populated, with only the very small village of Lound anywhere near the railway (Witham on the Hill, a more substantial settlement, was a good mile distant from the line) but Little Bytham and Castle Bytham had between them a population of well over a thousand and could claim to be worth the cost of a station in the amount of traffic, both goods and passenger, that they might generate. Little Bytham was, of course, already served by the GNR, and because of this the claims of the neighbouring Castle Bytham gradually gained preference. A local petition was presented to MR officials suggesting that coal traffic alone would provide sufficient business to cover costs; the point was also made that two thirds of the business currently done at Little Bytham's GNR station came from the villages of Castle Bytham, Clipsham, Holywell and Stocken Hall, a sure indication that there was a real need for station facilities at Castle Bytham itself. Hopes were high that this petition would produce results but it was with great disappointment that the villagers heard, in May 1893, that the MR directors had turned down the idea of a station there on the grounds that, contrary to what the locals might believe, in the Midland's view the district did not possess sufficient industry, outside of agriculture, to warrant the outlay on building and staffing.

Although this was a setback, pressure continued to be put on the MR even after the line was opened for passenger traffic, and there was some excitement in September 1894 when a party of MR officials arrived to inspect the site at Castle Bytham. Maybe their business was nothing to do with thoughts of a station, or maybe their deliberations

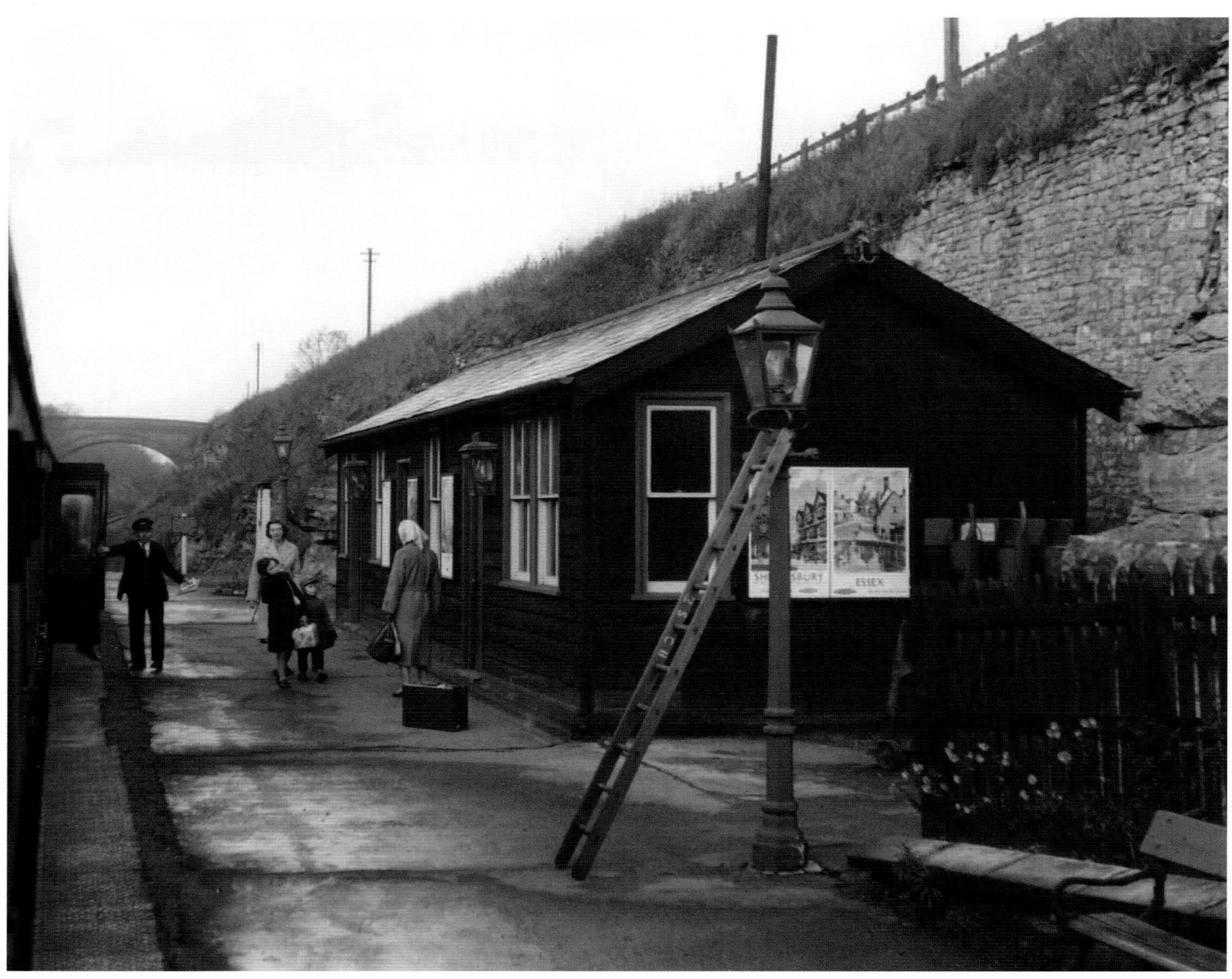

A shot of the wooden station building at Castle Bytham, taken from a carriage of the 10.22 am train for Bourne on December 29 1958. (M. C. Neale)

confirmed their original belief; either way, nothing came of the visit and the village had to be content to watch the trains steam through without stopping. Two years later, however, at the end of 1896, the persistence of the District Council, and of one influential member of the area, J. W. H. Davenport-Handley of Clipsham Hall, was rewarded when the MR finally agreed that there was sufficient traffic being generated along the line to warrant the addition of a station at Castle Bytham. Work began in the spring of 1897 at the chosen site, deep in the rock cutting that carried the line through the village. Because of the narrowness of the cutting at this point, the station was rather uncomfortably squeezed between track and sheer rock wall, with no room for a yard or proper approach road; a narrow path leading steeply down from the main road gave the only access to the 300'-long platform. A goods loop was also laid to the west of the station site, with a goods shed (later removed) and a loading dock. By the middle of 1897 it looked as if work was virtually complete, and opening for traffic was confidently expected at any time; unaccountably, the MR then announced that the station would not be ready until the end of the year. It was, in fact, January 3, 1898, before the first trains called, and these were only goods trains; there were further delays in completing the passenger accommodation (a strangely prolonged process, considering the rather primitive wooden structure that did service as waiting-room and booking-office) but eventually, on April 4, passenger services began. The first train to stop there was greeted by a crowd of locals, and as it left there was, one newspaper report said, "a shout of satisfaction from the grateful villagers".

The initial service was three trains a day each way, calling at Castle Bytham from Bourne at 9.42am, 12.28pm and 5.35pm and from Saxby at 10.55am, 1.58pm and 8.00pm. Goods traffic was stimulated by the opening by a Leicester coal merchant, Joseph Boam, of a coal depot next to the goods loop and a stone quarry on the high ground opposite the station itself, with a tramway running down to the loading dock. Soon after the opening to goods traffic, it was reported that coal sold in the area was already 3/- a ton cheaper than it had been previously.

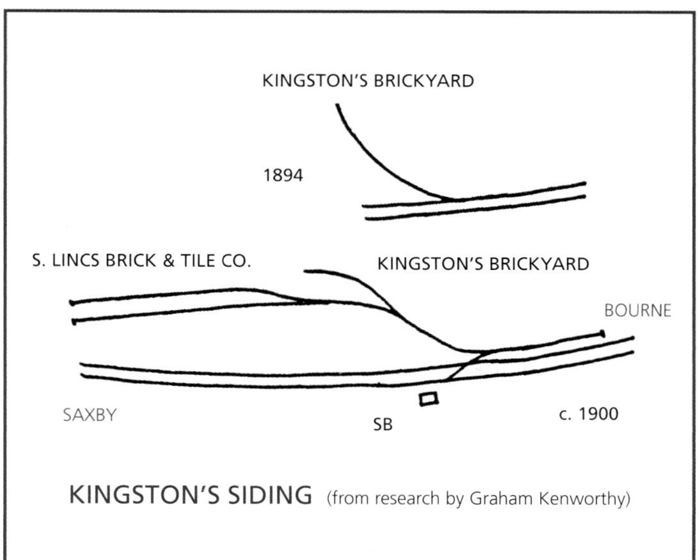

KINGSTON'S SIDING (from research by Graham Kenworthy)

CHAPTER FIVE

EARLY GOODS TRAFFIC AND PASSENGER WORKINGS

From the beginning it was agriculture, as expected, that provided the Bourne-Saxby route with its staple goods traffic outwards, and this was supplemented, for a short time after the line's opening, by regular consignments of bricks from small brickworks established at either end of the route. As has already been mentioned, many of the bricks required for the construction of Lound viaduct and Toft tunnel had been produced by Kingston's of Bourne, using clay from the foot of Stamford Hill. Bourne itself stands on the western edge of a huge belt of Oxford Clay which stretches from Dorset through Bedfordshire, Cambridgeshire, and Lincolnshire to the Humber estuary, and in the late 1880s Henry Kingston had exploited this natural resource and had opened brickworks on the edge of Bourne, a few hundred yards west of the station, near the wooden footbridge, erected later, which was known locally as the Red Steps. The opening of the Saxby line meant that the works was now conveniently sited next to the railway, which passed along the bottom of the yard, and it was a logical step for Kingston to request rail access to his premises for the easier conveyance of his bricks. By agreement of February 8, 1894, the new M & GN Joint Committee agreed to construct a single siding (known as Kingston's Siding, and worked by a 2-lever ground frame) as far as the boundary of Kingston's yard, while Kingston himself undertook to meet the cost of this construction and to provide on his own property "such other works as may be necessary to enable the works to be properly and profitably used." The siding was duly installed, and officially inspected on April 16, 1894.

By 1898 Kingston's yard had been taken over by the Bourne Brick & Tile Company (although Kingston himself was retained as manager); soon after, a rival concern, in the form of the South Lincs. Brick and Tile Company Ltd., opened on land directly adjacent to Kingston's site. Since the new Company also desired rail access, the existing single siding was modified to provide entry to both the Bourne and South Lincs, yards, while a crossover and headshunt were laid down on the main line and a small signalbox erected to control the junction (see diagram). In spite of the disappearance of his Company, Henry Kingston's name was perpetuated in that the new siding complex continued to be referred to as Kingston's Siding (as did the signalbox), even though the South Lincs. Company was served by what was officially known as Keeble's Siding. In view of the siding's proximity to Bourne station, wagons were allowed to be propelled to the site during daylight hours, provided that the front vehicle was a brake van with a guard riding in it.

The Bourne Brick & Tile Company went out of business some time just before the First World War, and on October 24, 1920, Kingston's Siding signalbox was closed, the lever frame being sent to Long Sutton station, whose signalbox was being renovated at the time. The sidings were then worked from Bourne West Box, and later, with the cessation of all brickmaking activity there, the layout was altered to a single refuge siding alongside the main line, with capacity for 50 wagons.

At the other end of the Saxby line, at Edmondthorpe & Wymondham, where a narrow belt of marlstone is present, the same Joseph Boam who had recently opened the coal yard and stone quarry at Castle Bytham's new station, developed, in 1899 or 1900, a small 2-kiln brickyard to the north of the main line and alongside a lane which became known as Brickyard Lane. A siding to serve the yard was accordingly laid in from the Up side of the station loop.

It was, however, the large-scale quarrying of limestone and iron ore that provided the line with outgoing traffic on a very significant scale, a traffic that lasted until closure of the whole route in the 1960s. The first workings in the area were those at Cottesmore, a few miles south of Market Overton which were opened up in 1882, and, from 1883, served by the MR's mineral branch from Ashwell which at one stage was intended to form part of the Bourne-Saxby through route (see Chapter 1). This particular area is rich in iron ore, and the ore-bearing seams proved capable of being worked well into the 1950s, by which time an extensive system of feeder lines and tramways had been constructed, snaking its way across the countryside. It was, of course, the MR's station at Ashwell that initially dealt with all mineral traffic from this ore-field, but the opening

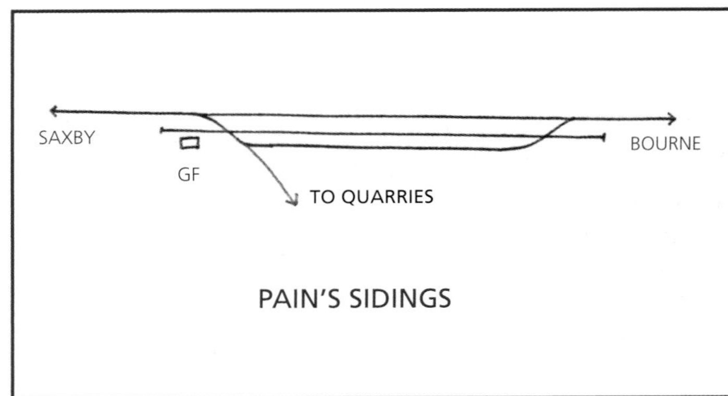

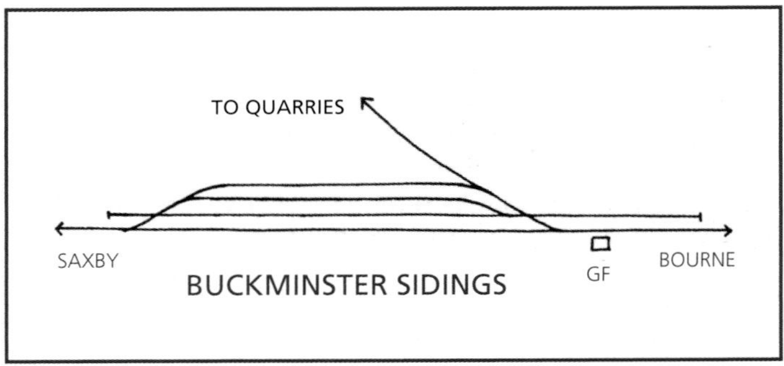

of the Bourne-Saxby line in 1893-4 prompted further exploration and quarrying to the north of the Cottesmore workings, which eventually produced their own system of tramways and interchange sidings at various points along that route.

The first development served by the Saxby line was at South Witham, where from 1895 the staple industry was the digging of limestone, at first on a site to the east of the station. By 1907 the area immediately behind the station had been opened up, and a standard-gauge tramway (utilising second-hand rails from the recently-abandoned Kettleby mines) was laid down to bring the quarried limestone to the station sidings. Because South Witham station was on an embankment, and therefore much higher than the quarry railway, a wooden-framed hoist, with a lift operated by a gas engine, was provided to take the limestone from quarry to station level, where it was loaded by conveyor belt into waiting wagons. The original hoist was burnt down in the 1930s and replaced by a more durable steel-framed construction powered by a diesel engine. In 1944 the quarries were extended westwards towards what became known as Thistleton Mines, whose principal industry was the extraction of iron ore rather than limestone.

In 1898 the Holwell Iron Co. Ltd., who owned the original workings at South Witham, built a standard-gauge line and interchange sidings on the windy heights between Wymondham and South Witham in order to serve an extensive system of ironstone quarries being opened up around the villages of Buckminster and Sewstern. Known logically enough as the Holwell Iron Company Sidings, the three lengthy sidings (including a loop and headshunt) were located on the northern side of the Bourne-Saxby line, at 5 miles 68 chains from Saxby Junction, and could hold nearly a hundred wagons. Access to the loop was controlled by a "stage", or ground frame, operated by the train crew and released by the section tablet. In 1899 the name of the sidings was officially changed to Buckminster Sidings, which it retained until closure.

Progressive extensions to the iron-stone workings eventually meant that by 1916 the whole quarry system had been pushed far enough north for its associated tramways to make an end-on junction with the GN's recently-opened High Dyke mineral branch, which left the East Coast main line about four miles south of Grantham. In 1918 the whole of the Buckminster Quarries, together with the South Witham mines, passed into the ownership of the Stanton Ironworks Co. Ltd.

The third, and final, development of ironstone loading facilities on the Saxby line came in 1906 when, at a remote and uninhabited spot a mile west of Buckminster Sidings, at the highest point of the route, a 2-road loop and headshunt was laid to allow the interchange of wagonloads from quarries at Market Overton. Known as Pain's Sidings, after the developer James Pain, they were, like the Buckminster system, controlled by ground-frame; as with the other two systems along the route, they were also taken over by the Stanton Ironworks Company, although not until 1928.

There were special instructions for working Pain's and Buckminster Sidings, as detailed in the Midland Appendix. At Pain's no vehicles were allowed to be shunted on to the main line at the west end of the loop, where the gradient fell away to Edmonthorpe & Wymondham station, unless there was a brake van with brakes fully applied, at the other end of the train. Trains which had proceeded to either Pain's or Buckminster Sidings for the collection or delivery of wagons were allowed to return in the direction from which they had come without going through the whole of the Edmondthorpe-South Witham tablet section.

The stone quarry at Castle Bytham, opened by James Boam, had, by the early years of this century, been taken over by Rippon's Lime and Stone Company, and was served by its own siding, with capacity for about 20 wagons.

Train services along the Bourne-Saxby route were mainly in the charge of MR engines; in the early years, for example, two Midland 0-4-4 tanks were stabled in the GN loco-shed at Spalding, together with an 0-6-0 for the through freight workings to London via Saxby. If MR locomotives worked east of Bourne they were retained overnight at South Lynn shed; for some time the local Saxby-Spalding daily passenger service (three trains each

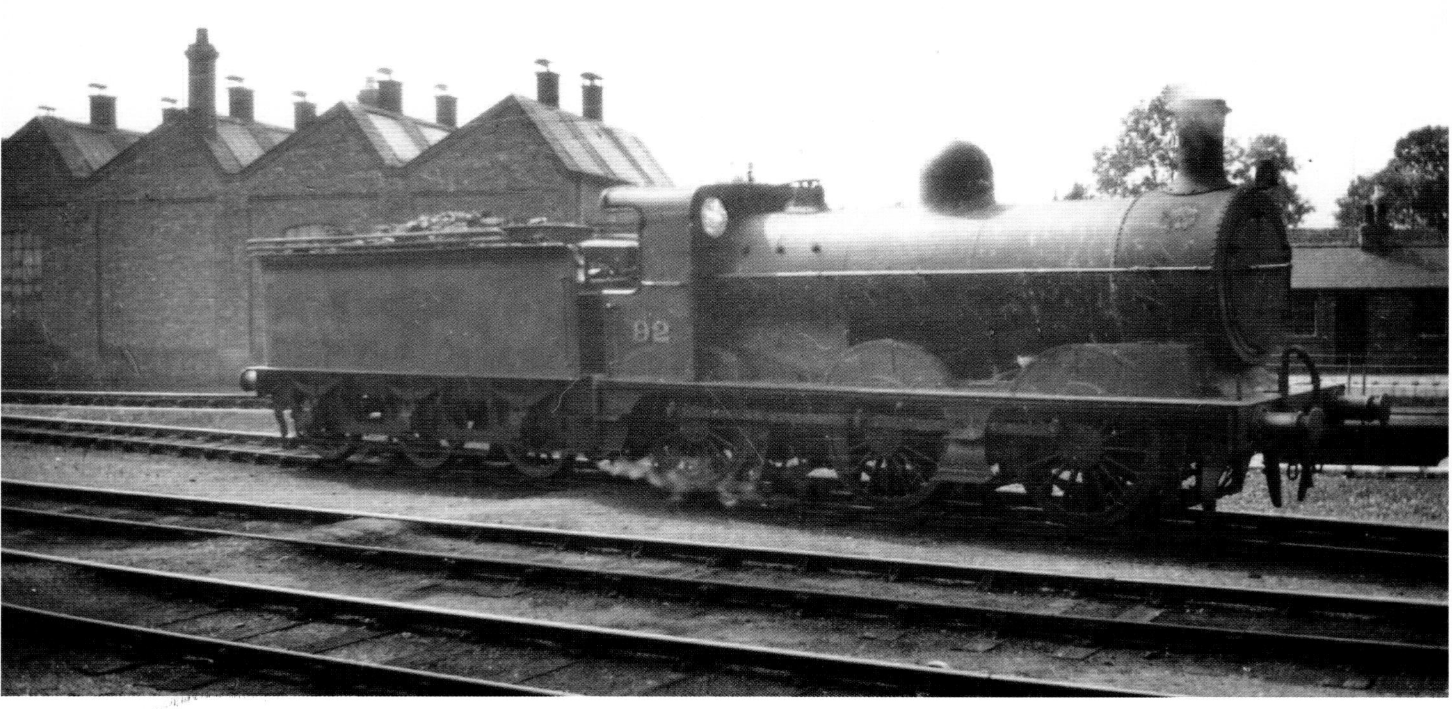

Above: 0-6-0 Locomotive No 92 simmers near Bourne locomotive depot. This shot was taken in 1933 and the loco was withdrawn in 1948. (Author's collection)

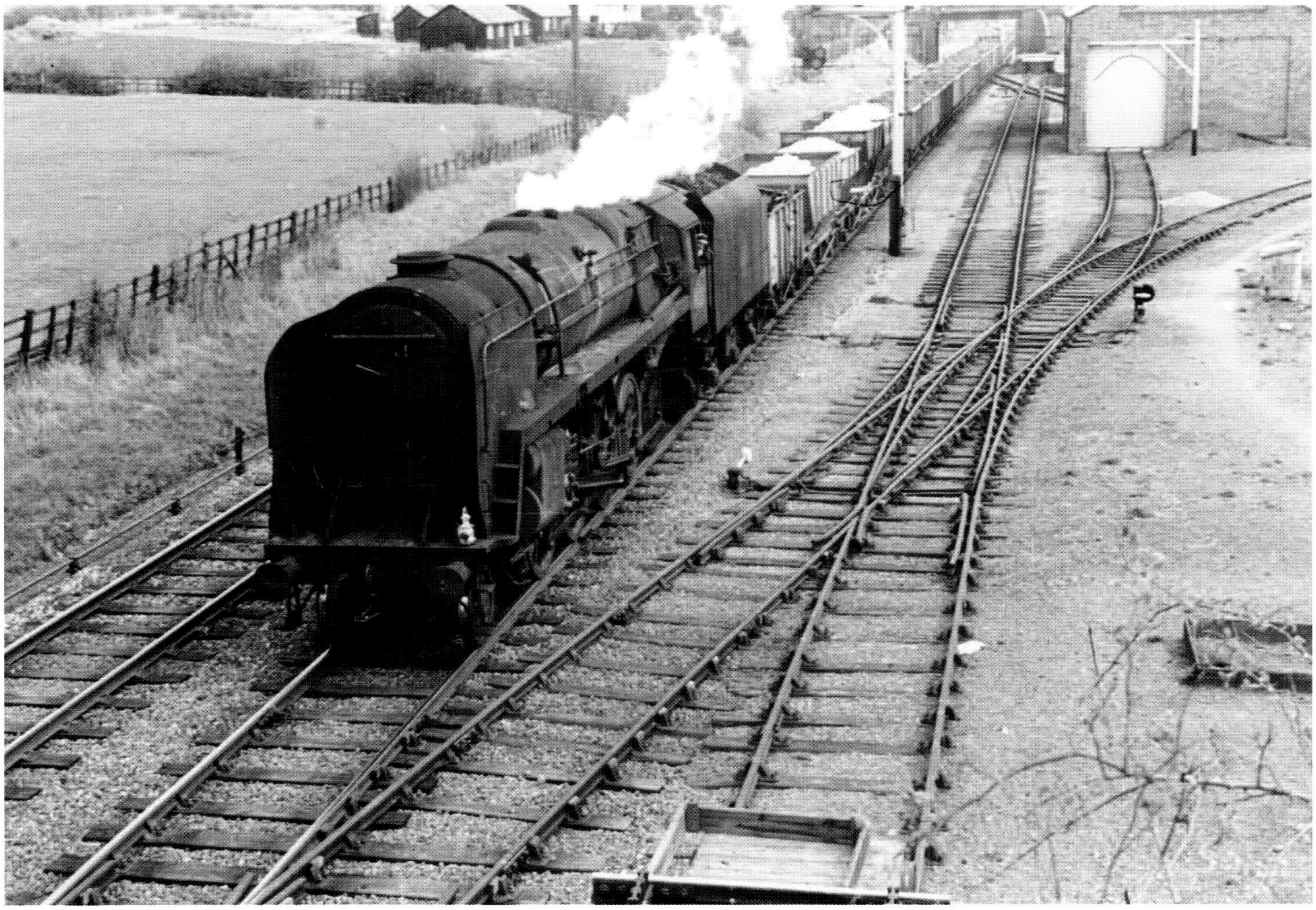

9F 92121, a regular engine on the South Witham spur in the early 1960s, coasts past the yard at Edmondthorpe & Wymondham. The train is using the extended station loop, lengthened in the post-1948 period. (H. N. James)

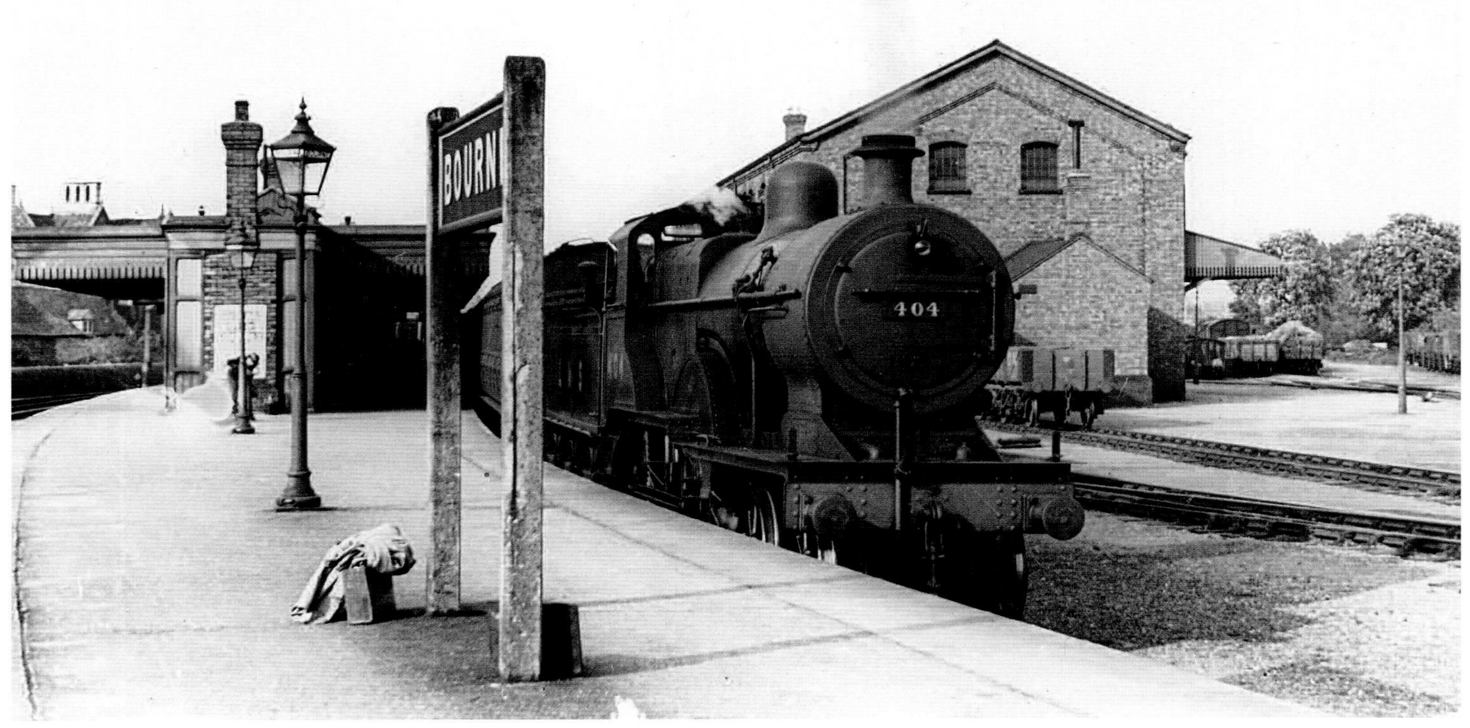

May 1937 and LMS 2P 404 prepares to depart from Bourne's Up platform with a King's Lynn to Nottingham train. The chimneys of Red Hall are visible above the station canopy on the left. (H. C. Casserley)

way) was worked alternately by both MR and M & GN engines on a yearly rota basis.

The passenger working that was to become known as the daily "Leicester", and which provided the line's most prestigious express service, began early in the route's history. In July 1894, only a couple of months after opening, a summer-only service of two trains east-bound and one west-bound was inaugurated to exploit the new link with the Midlands, running between Birmingham and Yarmouth, and usually conveying carriages for Norwich and Cromer, the train splitting into three sections at Melton Constable. In 1898 the service was extended to two trains in each direction, one daily, the other on Mondays, Fridays and Saturdays only, and by 1900 both trains were running daily. As they became more popular, the services were improved, with through Derby and Nottingham carriages added from the summer of 1902. which was also the year in which the service began to operate all the year round.

At first, MR engines handled the western half of the trip, changing at Bourne, but from the early years of this century M & GN locomotives (usually Johnson 4-4-Os) began to work through as far as Leicester (This explains an unofficial M & GN designation of the train as the "Leicester" even though its destination was Birmingham; early official timetables refer to it rather more accurately as the "Birmingham Express".)

For the summer months of 1903, a through MR/M & GN service from Manchester to Yarmouth via Nottingham and Saxby was introduced east-bound only; in the following year a balancing working appeared in the timetables.

CHAPTER SIX

DECLINE AND CLOSURE

Travelling through Kent on a Saturday afternoon in May 1939, the writer H.V. Morton was moved to comment with distaste on the change in the English countryside produced by the enormous increase in road transport:

> It was after the War that cheap motor-cars and motor omnibuses, and later coaches, began to transform the English road .... Inevitably the country has changed in appearance. Monotonous arterial roads take the shortest way from here to there; the petrol stations which punctuate them have developed a peculiar and horrible style of architecture which might have come from some alien planet ... I sometimes think it would be a good thing if every motor-car could be put out of action for six months to give us time to think where all this is leading us.

Whether you agreed with Morton's strictures or not, it was impossible to deny that road transport was posing a

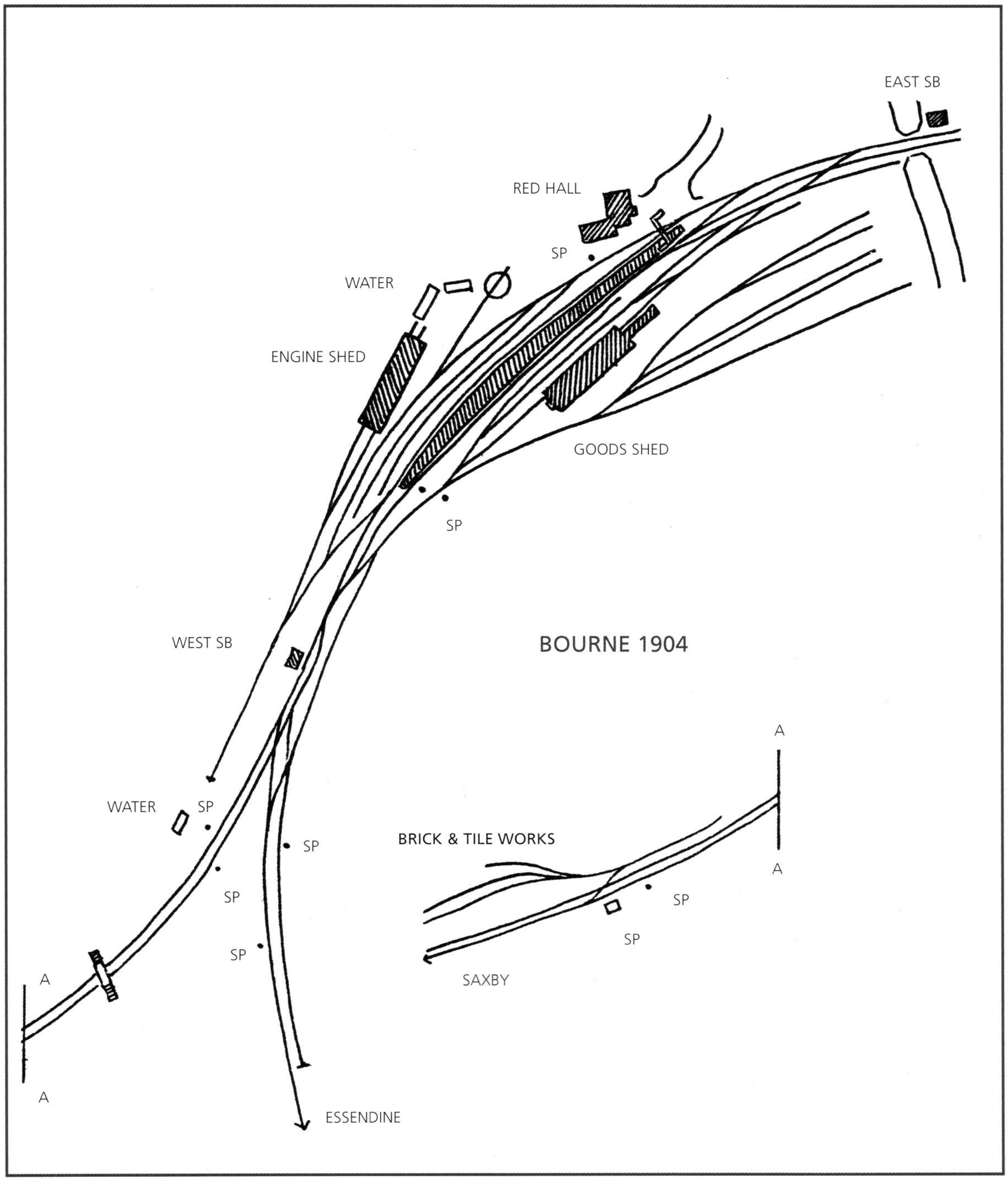

EAST SB
RED HALL
SP
WATER
ENGINE SHED
GOODS SHED
SP
WEST SB
BOURNE 1904
A
WATER
SP
SP
BRICK & TILE WORKS
A
SP
SP
SP
SP
A
SAXBY
A
ESSENDINE

QUARRY AREA
FURTHER SIDINGS ADDED POST-1907 AT WEST END OF STATION FOR QUARRY TRAFFIC
SP
GOODS
SAXBY
SP
SP
BOURNE
SB
SP
SOUTH WITHAM 1904

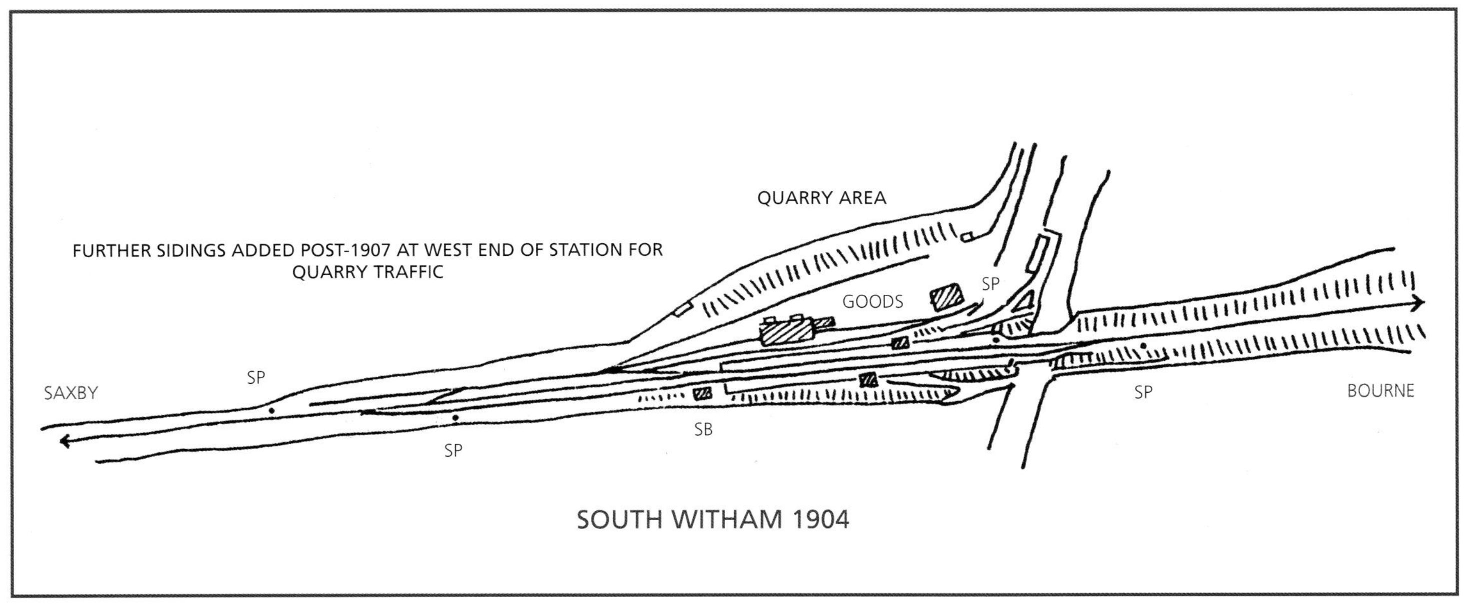

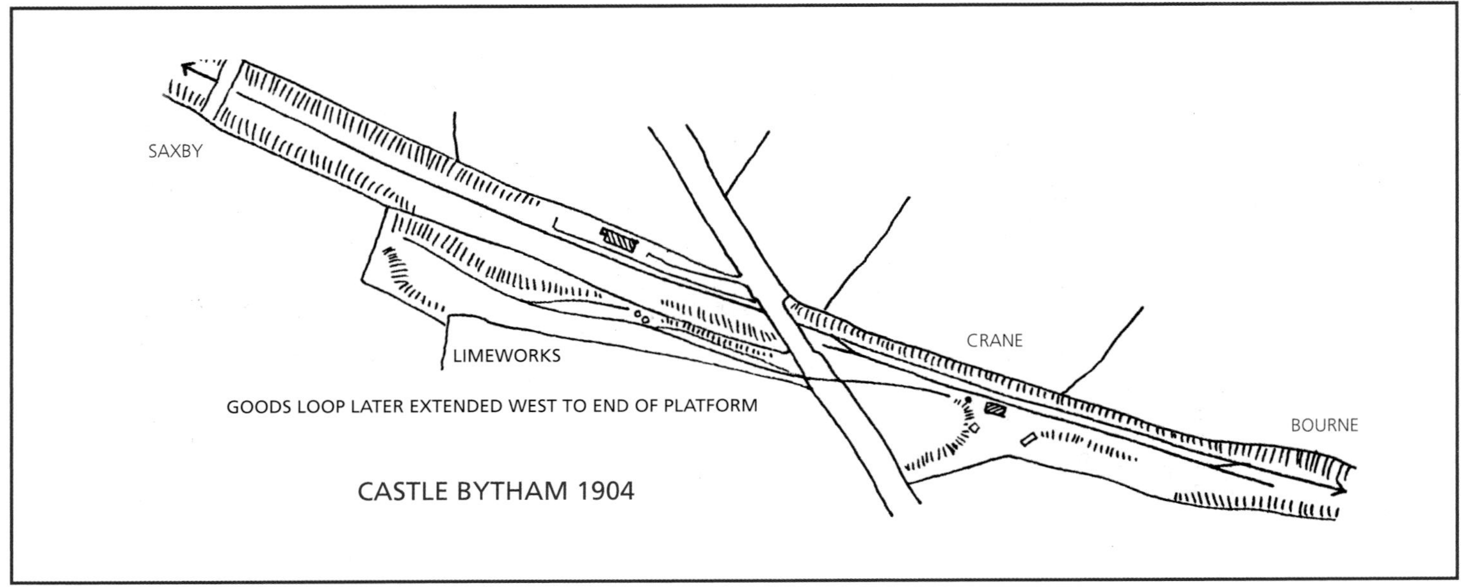

dangerous threat to the railways as the prime mover of goods and people. Although by today's standards private car ownership was on a modest scale, it was growing rapidly, and the motor-lorry, either in the hands of the small operator or as part of a large haulage concern, was making its impact felt on goods traffic. In rural areas, however, where wages were still low, the private car was much slower to make an appearance, and in the mid-1930s there were still large numbers of people for whom the railway continued to provide the most efficient and convenient form of transport for work or leisure. It was at holiday times, particularly August Bank Holidays, that lines such as the Bourne-Saxby link were impressively busy, with dozens of extra trains ingeniously slotted into a crowded timetable, most of them conveying Midlanders from their land-locked cities to the breezy and invigorating east coast where they could sample the bracing delights of Skegness, Cromer or Yarmouth.

During the August Bank Holiday of 1936, for example, sixteen extra excursion trains were routed along the Bourne-Saxby line between 1.00am and mid-day on Saturday, August 1, most of them heading for Yarmouth and Lowestoft, but a couple diverging to Skegness, one to Mablethorpe and one to Cromer. More than half were chartered by the Leicester Co-Operative Society to take their employees from Leicester, Coalville and Nuneaton to the coast, and there was a string of relief trains later in the morning to take up any surplus. Later in the day, in the other direction, empty coaching stock was returned to various Midland stations in time for further excursions scheduled for the following Monday.

Working with such a large number of trains in addition to the regular scheduled passenger services, and along a single-line route such as the 13 miles between Saxby and Little Bytham, could produce problems for operating staff if anything went wrong, and a hold-up to one train could easily have a "knock-on" effect to following trains, particularly those scheduled to cross at stations with trains from the opposite direction. On a July Saturday in 1937, for instance, a relief express from Leicester to Yarmouth was brought to a halt between South Witham and Castle Bytham by the expiry of its engine, blocking the line for some time before an assisting engine could be sent out. Further disruption of traffic consequent on the dropping of the single-line tablet at the distant Cuckoo Junction, near Spalding, caused repercussions as far back as Saxby, where an Up express was held at the Home signal for 20 minutes, which in turn delayed the 9.10am Leicester-Peterborough train. Late in the afternoon of the same eventful day, a 15-coach train, double-headed, was held in the loop at South Witham waiting to cross with a Down train; when the latter appeared it proved to be composed of two locomotives and 16 coaches, too long to be accommodated in the Down section of the station loop. The problem was solved by dividing the train and shunting part of it into the goods yard thus allowing the Up train to get on its way, but by this time the scheduled timetable was in some disarray.

Apart from holiday weekends, however, passenger traffic on the railways began to decline generally in the face of increasing competition from the private car, and although the 1939–45 war, and the consequent petrol rationing, forced many people to rely on rail travel once again, the post-war period saw the downward trend accelerated. This was reflected in the reduced traffic flow along the Bourne-Saxby route; the working timetable for September 1957 to June 1958 shows just four passenger trains between Bourne and the Midlands (6.45am King's Lynn to Nottingham, which stopped briefly at Little Bytham Junction to set down or take up permanent way patrolmen; 9.02am Yarmouth Beach to Birmingham; 4.00pm Spalding to Nottingham; 4.20pm King's Lynn to Nottingham), and four in the reverse direction (9.55am Saxby to King's Lynn. which picked up permanent-way men at Little Bytham Junction on Mondays, Wednesdays and Fridays; 1.45pm Birmingham to Yarmouth Beach; 4.20pm Nottingham to King's Lynn; 7.45pm Nottingham to Spalding). There was

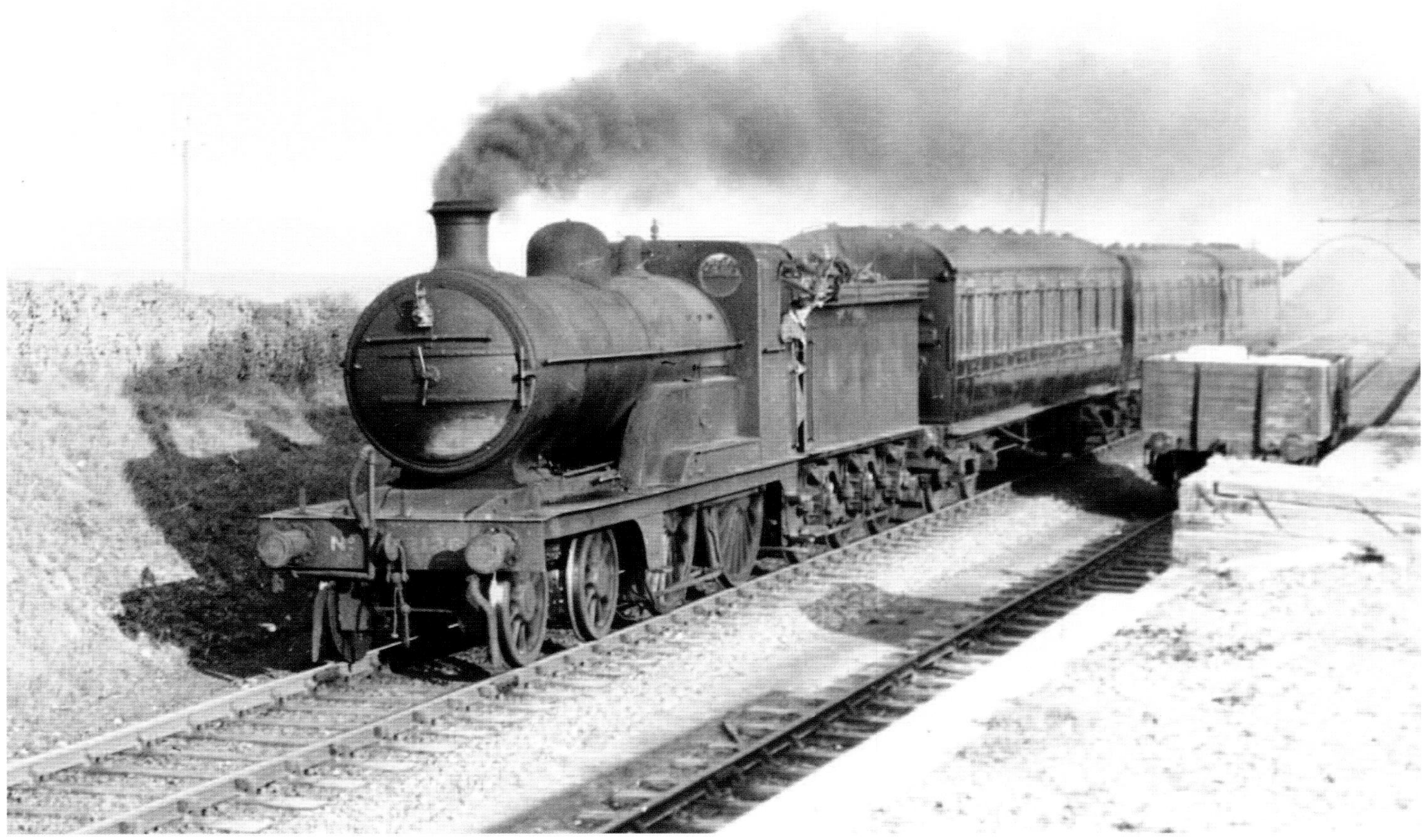

A 3-coach Spalding to Nottingham train with LNER D3 2128 in charge, passes the loading dock at Castle Bytham on September 27 1949. (P. H. Wells)

one Down freight Class J, which left Saxby at 6.15pm. stopping to shunt at South Witham for 38 minutes and at Castle Bytham for 10 minutes, and arriving at Bourne at 8.12pm. A single UP freight working, originating from Yarmouth Beach at 3.35pm (3.40pm on Saturdays), went through the Bourne-Saxby section without stopping, reaching Saxby at 10.21pm.

By the late 1950s the Eastern Region of British Railways was sufficiently concerned about the steady loss of traffic along the M & GN route to appoint a special committee to investigate the viability of the whole line. Its report, completed in May 1958, recommended closure of almost all the 180 route miles on the grounds of declining traffic, both goods and passenger, and the costly duplication of the route by the former Great Eastern lines which, in BR's words, "parallel it across the north of East Anglia."

Because of the scale of the proposed closure, and the numerous objections lodged against it, three TUCC inquiries were necessary, held at Norwich, Peterborough and Bourne. The arguments and counter-arguments concerning the M & GN line east of Bourne are not the province of this present study – I have dealt with them in detail in an earlier book (*The Midland & Great Northern Joint Railway*, Ian Allan, 1982) – and I shall accordingly concentrate here only on those points relating to the Bourne-Saxby stretch.

The TUCC inquiry at Bourne was held on October 27, 1958, when the case for retention of the rail link was put forward forcibly by Mr D. Reeson, the Clerk of the Bourne Urban Council. In essence, he made four main points.

First the closure of the M & GN would sever the main, and most direct, passenger rail link between the Midlands and the east coast, the connection between which areas was, it will be remembered, the main motive for the construction of the line in the first place. Secondly, the withdrawal of freight services would be detrimental to the agricultural and industrial economy of the Bourne area. Bourne was a growing town, and needed rail access; two of its other rail links had already been closed – that to Sleaford in 1930 and to Essendine in 1951 – and to remove its only remaining railway would cause considerable hardship to farmers and manufacturers who depended on the speedy and easy distribution of their products that the railway was able to offer. Thirdly, the argument that the M & GN route was duplicated by other lines was certainly not true of the Bourne-Saxby stretch, where there were no other railway lines within miles. Finally, Mr. Reeson was sceptical about the proposed substitution of bus services which, it had been suggested, would adequately bridge the gap left by the closure of the railway; these, he contended, were,

> to say the least, meagre in extent and frequency ... and even with the proposals put forward for new and improved bus services these services cannot take the place of the present rail services.

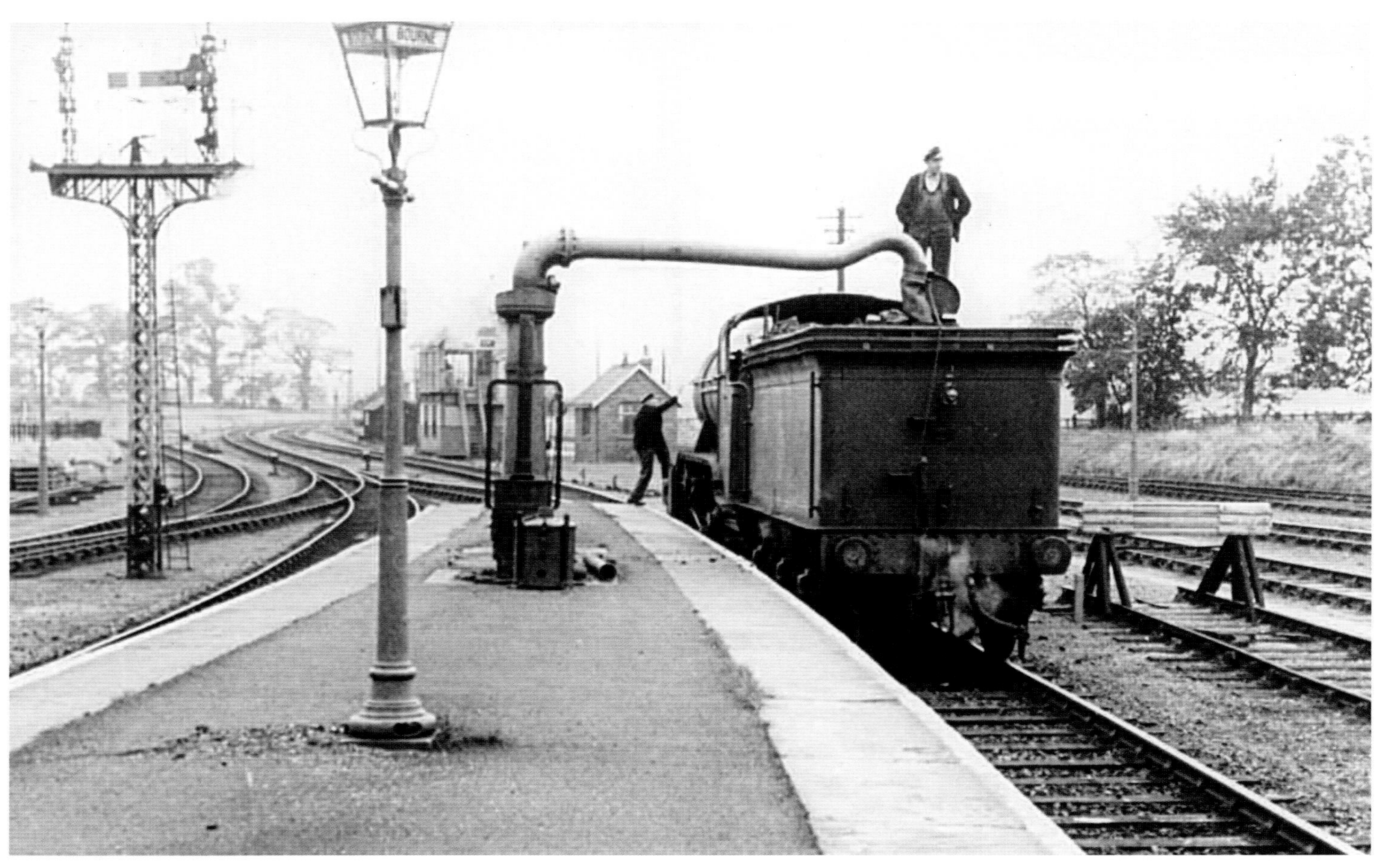

Above: Bourne station on October 18 1958, with K2 61771 taking water at the west end of the platform. (F. Church)

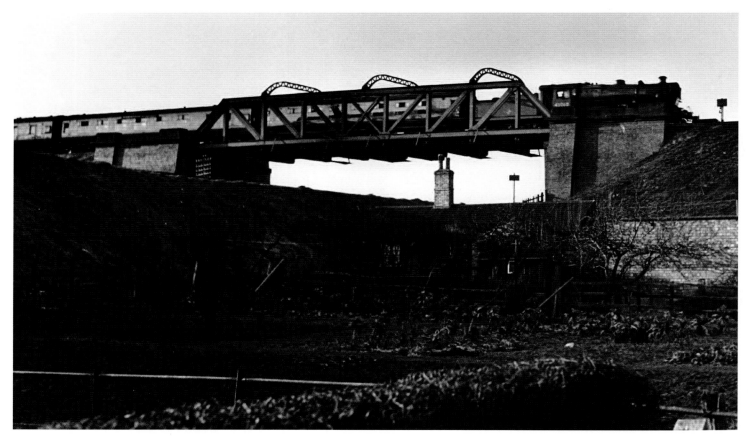

On the final day of passenger operations, February 28 1959, 4MT 43060 takes the last, east-bound, "Leicester" across the girder bridge which spanned the East Coast main line at Little Bytham. (P. H. Wells)

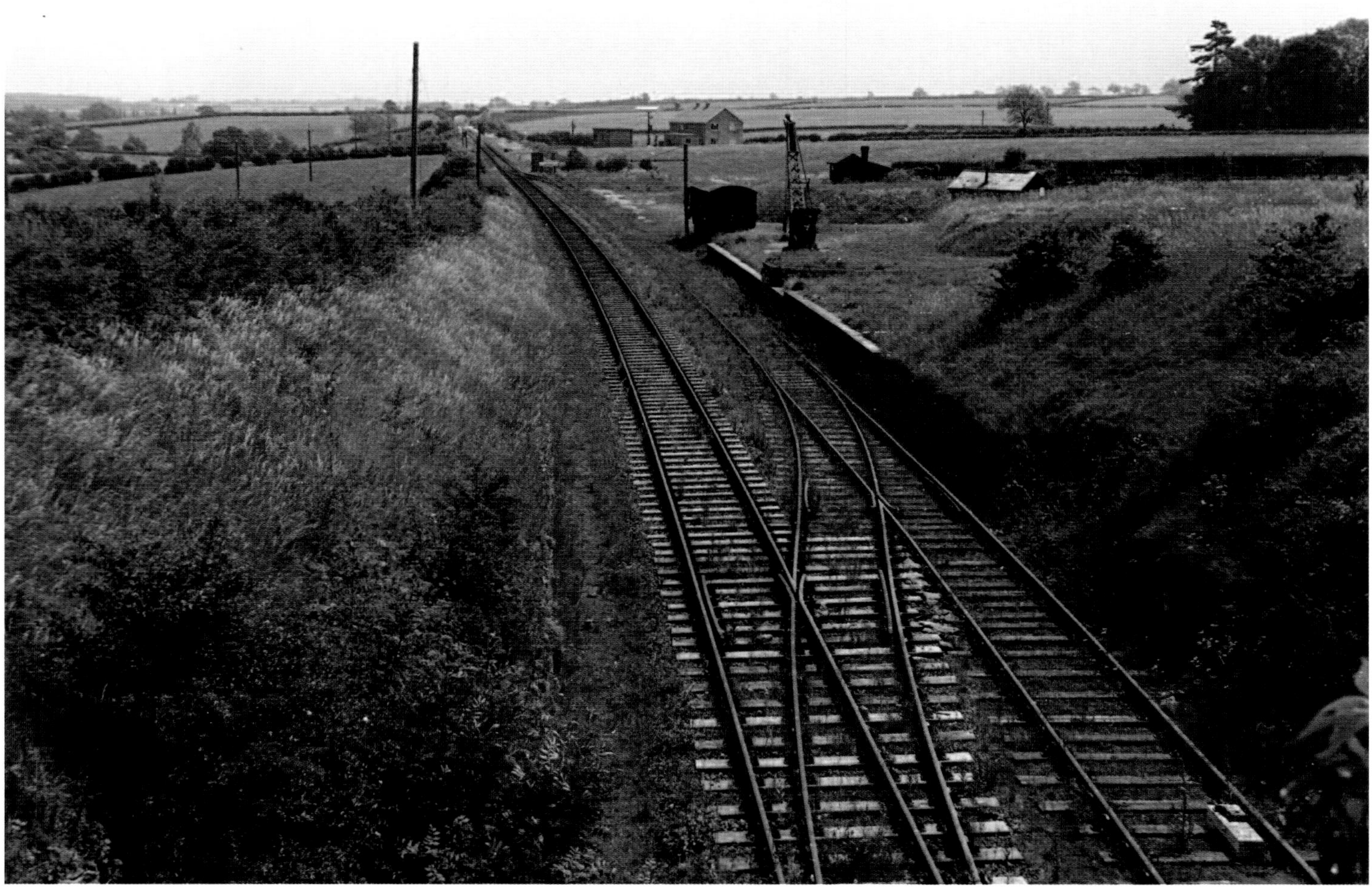

Above: A view eastwards from the road bridge at Castle Bytham, showing the weed-grown loop, crane and loading dock in June 1961. (H. N. James)

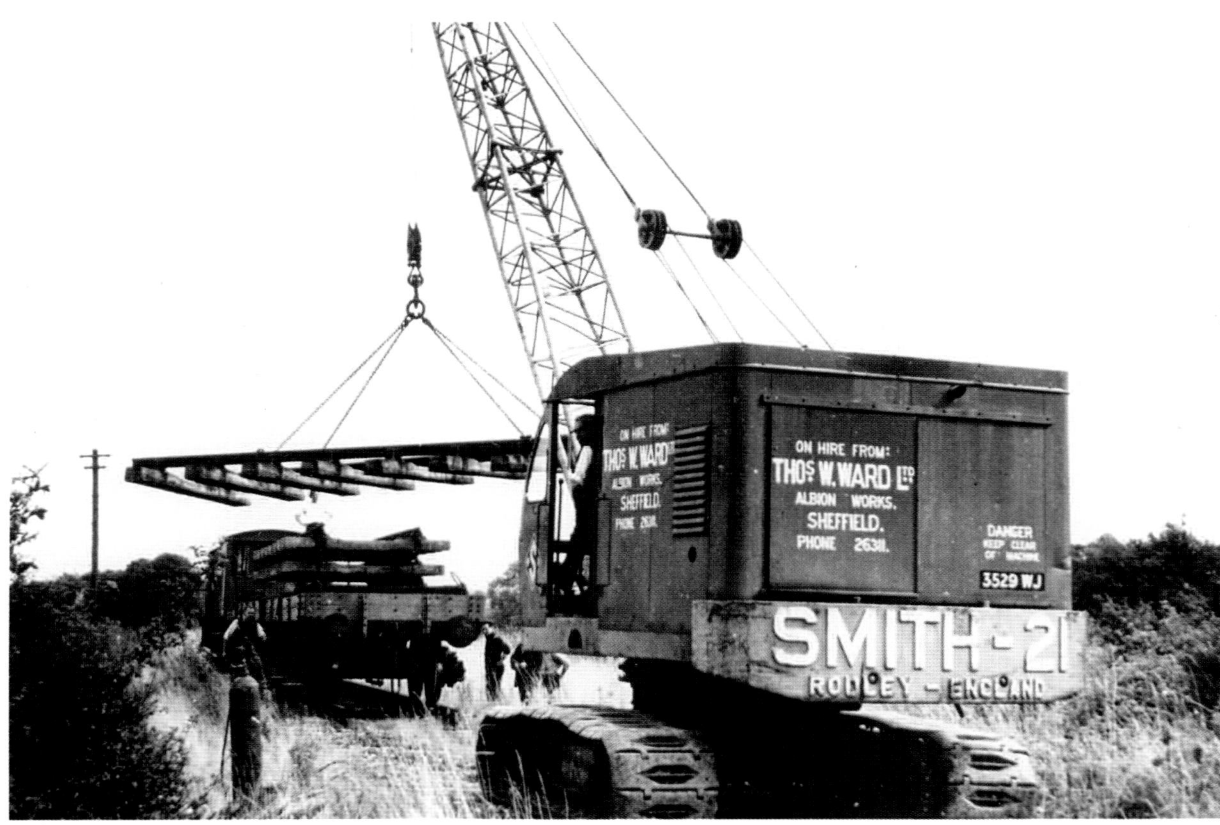

The end of the line; a contractor's crane lifts track panels at Castle Bytham in the spring of 1962. (E. L. Back)

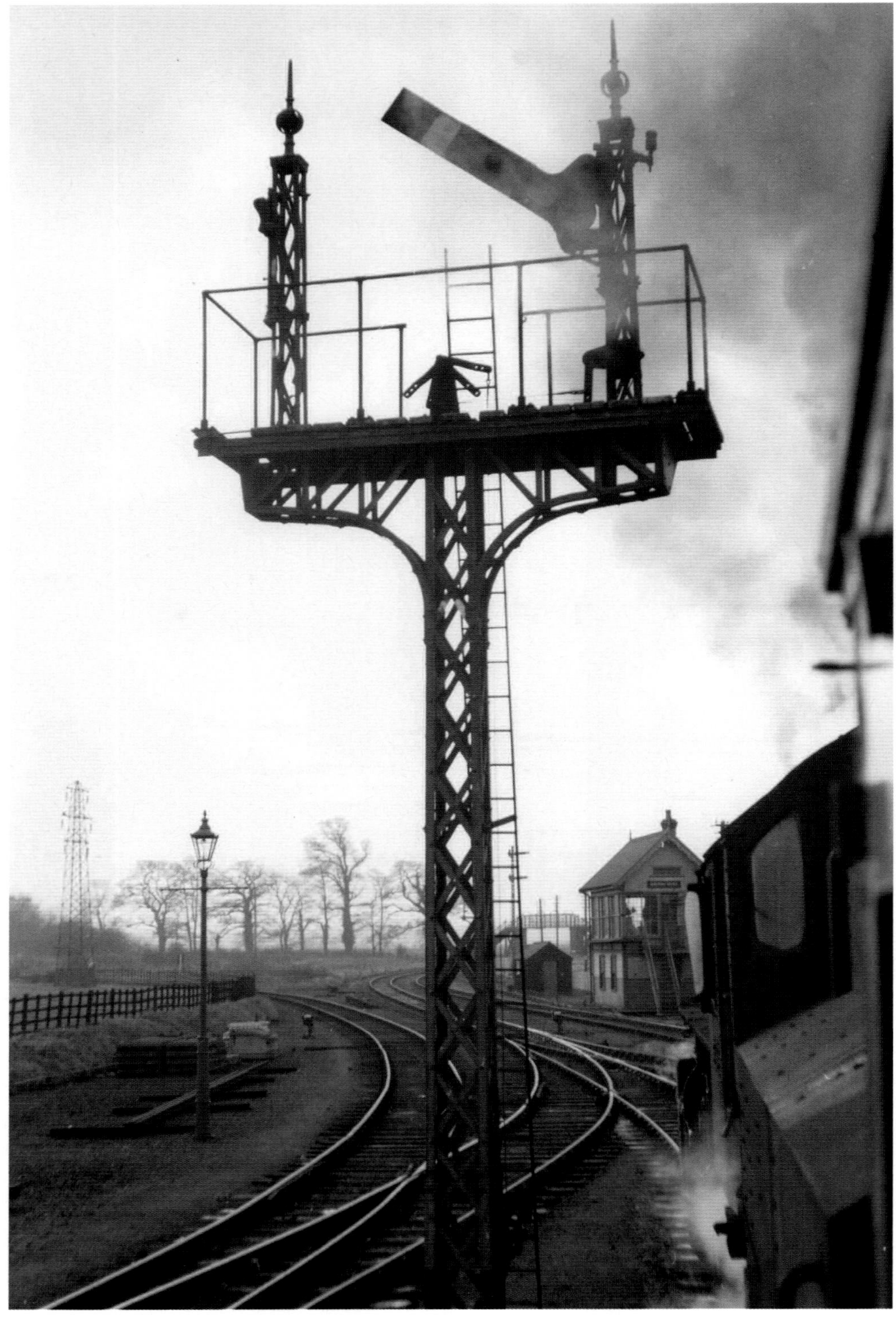

4MT 43066 takes the west-bound "Leicester" out of Bourne on December 29 1958. In the background are Bourne West signalbox and the Red Steps footbridge: curving away to the left is the headshunt for the goods sidings, along the outside of which ran the former Essendine Branch. (M. C. Neale)

Having heard the evidence from all three inquiries, the Central TUCC issued its decision at the end of November 1958. The Bourne-Saxby stretch, like most of the rest of the M & GN route, was to lose its passenger service, although the section between Saxby and South Witham was to remain open for freight only until the remaining ironstone deposits in the area had been worked out. Bourne itself retained a goods service eastwards to Spalding, and the station also served as the collection and delivery point for the Billingborough spur, the still-operational part of the former Bourne-Sleaford route. The final day for passenger services was set for Saturday, February 28, 1959.

An unusual surge of public interest in the line was evident in the final week of operations; at Saxby station, where weekly fare receipts were normally miserable £8, more than £20 was collected, and it was reported that Edmondthorpe & Wymondham station also saw more passenger activity than it had enjoyed for some time. On the day of closure itself, various small and unofficial ceremonies were held to mark the event: at South Witham the local vicar led a congregation of about 30 parishioners onto a Saxby train and completed a round trip by going back to South Witham immediately on the return service. For one Wymondham resident. Tommy Marriott, aged 73, whose father had been a signalman on the Bourne-Saxby line the occasion was a unique one: as a small child he had travelled to Melton on the very first train at the opening of the line in 1894, and he ceremonially repeated this journey

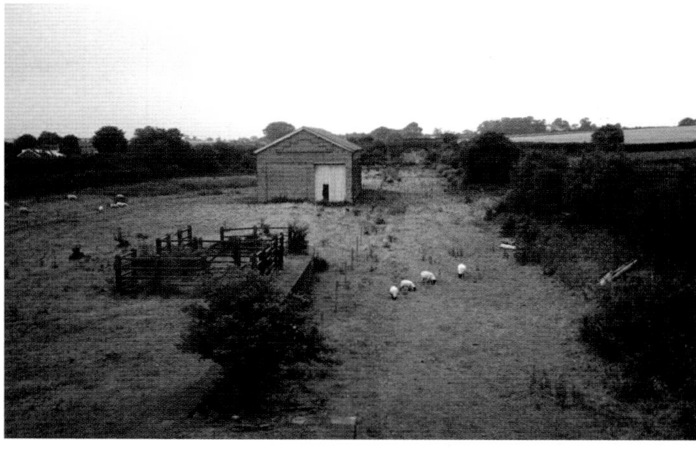

Sheep may safely graze... on the trackbed of the main line through Edmondthorpe & Wymondham. Goods shed, cattle pens and loading dock are still intact in the middle of what is now a field. (Author)

on the day of closure. At Castle Bytham, whose station was to close completely, the spectacle of trains blasting their way through the deep rock cutting for the last time attracted the particular attention of numerous photographers recording the day's activities for posterity.

The last Up "Leicester", hauled by 4MT 43060, and cheered on its way at the various stations en route, passed through Bourne at about 12.30 mid-day and had cleared Saxby by 1.10pm; the return working by the same locomotive, the last journey ever made by the route's crack express, reached Saxby at 3.48pm and Bourne by 4.20pm. The 7.45pm ex-Nottingham train, the very last through service on the route, carried about a hundred people (a considerable increase on normal loading), with another 20 joining the train at Saxby. Crowds of villagers at Edmondthorpe & Wymondham, South Witham and Castle Bytham, cheered and applauded as the train passed through their station and disappeared into the winter darkness. Bourne driver, Mr. S. Meeks, brought his train into his home station exactly on time at 9.04pm and completed his run a few miles further on at Spalding, reached at 9.24pm. The final train of all was a local service from Spalding, which ran into Bourne at 9.20pm.

No time was lost in putting into effect the closure of the line. On the following day, Sunday, March 1, a stop-block was erected across the line at South Witham, thus severing the route as a through link. Track was left in situ for some years, however, and it was not until the spring of 1962 that contractors moved in to lift the main line and sidings between Castle Bytham and Bourne. By October of the same year, Saxby Station signalbox had been taken out of service, and the passing loop and all sidings at Edmondthorpe & Wymondham had been removed.

The Saxby-South Witham section continued to provide regular ironstone workings, but this traffic was progressively wound down, and ceased in 1964, when Stewarts & Lloyds announced its decision to close the remaining Thistleton mines.

REMAINS

It is still possible today to follow the Bourne-Saxby route for a significant proportion of its length, and to find enough of its buildings remaining to make it of interest.

At Bourne, the station site has been cleared, apart from the brick-built goods shed, which stands close by the preserved Red Hall, the original station building. A short distance out of town is Toft tunnel, and the trackbed to

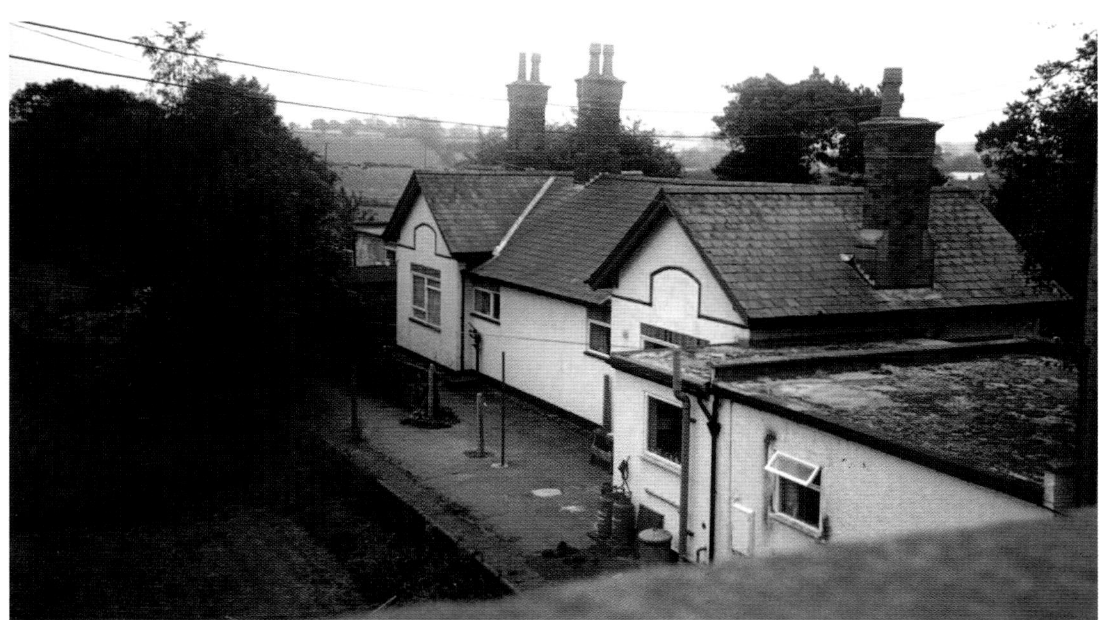

Edmondthorpe & Wymondham station buildings, converted to a private house with a lawn and flowerbeds where the train used to run. (Author)

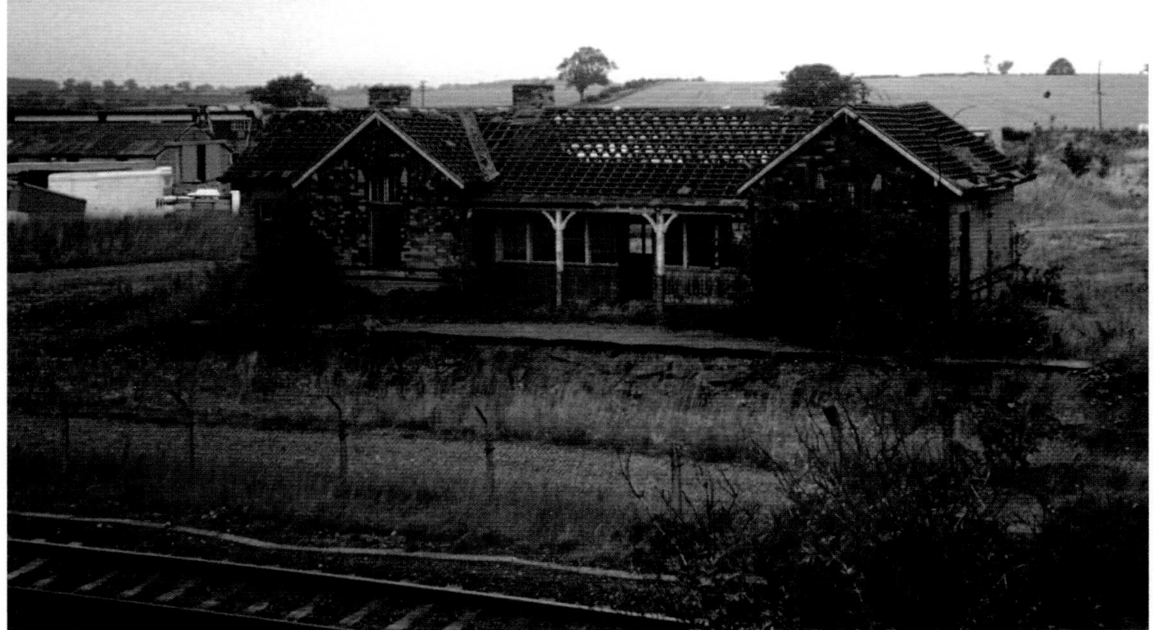

The shell of Saxby station buildings in August 1986. The Peterborough-Syston line, still in use, can be seen in the foreground. (Author)

Lound viaduct, which is still standing but accessible only by field walking.

At Little Bytham, the girder bridge over the East Coast main line was removed in March 1964, but the brick abutments remain. Castle Bytham's station has not survived intact (apart from the dilapidated platform) although the cutting can still be viewed from the road overbridge (No 37) in the village, and limestone working is still carried out on the site of Joseph Boam's original quarries. Amazingly, the 5-ton yard crane remains intact and rising incongruously from amongst the long grass and bushes that have overgrown the site.

At the point at which the line used to pass below the Al road, a short length of trackbed has been utilised as a new roadway, and the original railway bridge now carries the south-bound carriageway of the Great North Road. The station at South Witham has been cleared and built over (although the underbridge is still there); further westwards is the site of Buckminster exchange sidings and the trackbed and crossing gates for the Buckminster Quarries feeder line. Ironically, quarrying has been re-started around the site of South Witham station. Pain's Siding site is still visible, although the track of the tramway leading to the quarries is now part of a private field path.

At Edmonthorpe and Wymondham the station buildings have been preserved, and renovated as a private house, and in what was the station yard are the goods shed, weighbridge office and dilapidated cattle pens.

The Peterborough-Syston route is still in operation, of course, and trains continue to pass the site of Saxby Junction. Saxby's main station building has survived, although now in rather a derelict state, but all platforms have been removed. Most durable of all, perhaps, is the station house of the original Saxby station, and, at the point where the old Saxby curve crossed the road, the old gate-house; the route of the 1848 curve is also still clearly visible.

BOURNE–SAXBY: MAIN DATES

1848	May 1	Final section of Peterborough-Syston line opened
1860	May 16	Bourne-Essendine railway opened
1866	Aug 1	Spalding-Bourne railway opened
1872	Jan 2	Bourne-Sleaford railway opened
1889	June 24	Bourne-Saxby Act sanctioned
1892	Aug 28	New Saxby curve and station in use
1893	June 5	Bourne-Saxby line opened for goods traffic
1894	May 1	Bourne-Saxby line opened for passenger traffic
1898	Jan 3	Castle Bytham station opened for goods traffic
1898	Apr 4	Castle Bytham station opened for passenger traffic
	–	Holwell Iron Company Sidings (Buckminster) laid
1906	–	Pain's Sidings laid
1930	Sep 20	Last scheduled passenger service Bourne-Sleaford
1951	June 16	Last scheduled passenger service Bourne-Essendine
1958	Oct 27	TUCC Inquiry at Bourne to consider closure proposal
1959	Feb 28	Last scheduled passenger service Bourne-Saxby
1962	–	Bourne-Castle Bytham track lifted
1964	–	Saxby-South Witham section closed

TIMETABLES

BRADSHAW: AUGUST 1898

Down Trains			A		B	
BIRMINGHAM	dep	7.50	9.25	11.15	2.15	4.50
LEICESTER		9.35	10.45	12.50	3.20	6.25
SAXBY		10.30	11.15	1.35	3.53	7.35
EDMONDTHORPE		10.37	...	1.40	...	7.42
SOUTH WITHAM		10.45	...	1.48	...	7.50
CASTLE BYTHAM		10.55	...	1.58	...	8.00
BOURNE	arr	11.09	11.53	2.12	4.31	8.14

Up Trains				A		B
BOURNE	dep	9.29	12.07	2.30	5.22	6.20
CASTLE BYTHAM		9.42	12.28	...	5.35	...
SOUTH WITHAM		9.50	12.36	...	5.43	...
EDMONDTHORPE		10.00	12.46	...	5.53	...
SAXBY		10.06	12.52	3.06	5.59	6.51
LEICESTER		11.22	1.47	3.50	6.50	7.22
BIRMINGHAM		12.55	3.10	5.22	8.30	8.52

A: "Birmingham Express"
B: "Birmingham Express" Mon./Fri./Sat.

BRADSHAW: APRIL 1910

Down Trains						
BIRMINGHAM	dep	8.05	9.50	1.50		5.10
LEICESTER		9.30	12.05	3.06	6.43	
SAXBY		10.18	1.20	3.50	4.54	7.33
EDMONDTHORPE		10.23	1.26	...	5.01	7.39
SOUTH WITHAM		10.31	1.33	...	5.08	7.48
CASTLE BYTHAM		10.41	1.44	...	5.19	7.56
BOURNE	arr	10.55	1.57	4.20	5.32	8.10

Up Trains						
BOURNE	dep	9.14	12.15	12.25	5.15	6.07
CASTLE BYTHAM		9.28	...	12.41	5.29	a
SOUTH WITHAM		9.35	...	12.48	5.37	a
EDMONDTHORPE		9.46	...	12.59	5.47	a
SAXBY	arr	9.51	...	1.04	5.52	a
LEICESTER	arr	10.48	1.15	1.46	7.00	7.10
BIRMINGHAM	arr	12.58	3.12	3.12	8.45	8.45

a: Stops to set down from beyond Bourne

BRADSHAW: JULY 1922

Down Trains			SO	SX		SO	A		
BIRMINGHAM	dep	7.30	9.00	9.00	11.49		1.55	1.55	5.15
LEICESTER		9.06	10.45	10.45	1.00		3.22	3.22	7.25
SAXBY		10.01	11.15	11.25	1.50	3.50	4.03	5.11	8.25
EDMONDTHORPE		10.08	...	...	1.56	...	...	5.18	8.31
SOUTH WITHAM		10.20	...	...	2.05	...	...	5.27	8.40
CASTLE BYTHAM		10.31	...	...	2.14	...	...	5.36	8.50
BOURNE	arr	10.45	11.50	12.02	2.27	4.20	4.35	5.49	9.03

				A	A				
Up Trains				SX	SO				
BOURNE	dep		8.55	12.15	12.25	12.37	4.28	6.15	6.27
CASTLE BYTHAM			9.11	...	...	12.55	4.43	...	6.44
SOUTH WITHAM			9.21	...	...	1.05	...	6.38	6.56
EDMONDTHORPE		8.15	9.30	...	...	1.13	...	...	7.07
SAXBY	arr	8.21	9.35	12.50	12.58	1.19	5.06	6.54	7.14
LEICESTER		10.03	10.38	1.28	1.28	2.00	6.20	7.30	9.33
BIRMINGHAM		11.15	12.43	2.58	2.58	3.43	8.46	9.20	

A: Sheringham, Cromer, Norwich, Yarmouth and Lowestoft Express

OCTOBER 1943

Table 230 SAXBY, SOUTH WITHAM, and BOURNE

Miles	Week Days only	a.m		p.m
	Saxby .... dep	10 0	..	5 9
2½	Edmondthorpe C	10 7	..	5 16
7	South Witham	1019	..	5 26
13	Castle Bytham	1031	..	5 35
18	**Bourne** .... arr	1045	..	5 47

Miles	Week Days only	a.m		p.m
	Bourne .... dep	8 43	..	6 15
5	Castle Bytham	8 59	..	6 31
11	South Witham	9 9	..	6 42
15½	Edmondthorpe C	9 18	..	6 51
18	**Saxby** .... arr	9 23	..	6 56

C Edmondthorpe and Wymondham.

MARCH 1954

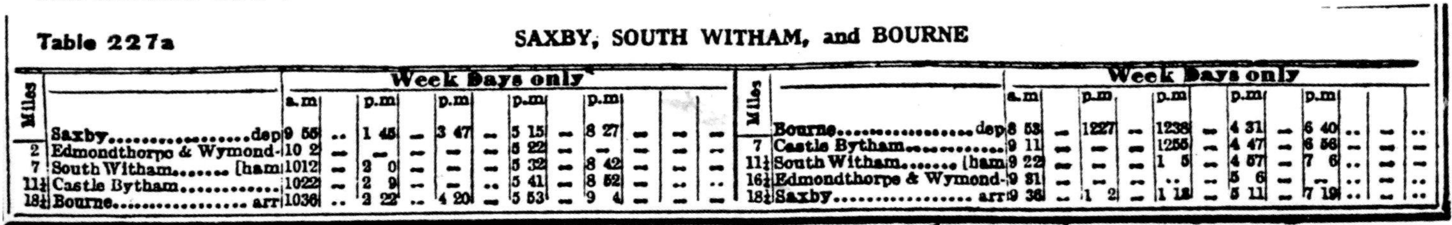

Table 227a SAXBY, SOUTH WITHAM, and BOURNE

Miles	Week Days only	a.m		p.m		p.m		p.m		p.m			
	Saxby .... dep	9 55	..	1 45	—	3 47	—	5 15	—	8 27	—	—	—
2	Edmondthorpe & Wymond-	10 2	—	—	—	—	—	5 22	—	—	—	—	—
7	South Witham .... [ham	1012	—	2 0	—	—	—	5 32	—	8 42	—	—	—
11½	Castle Bytham	1022	—	2 9	—	—	..	5 41	—	8 52	—	..	..
18½	**Bourne** .... arr	1036	..	2 22	..	4 20	—	5 53	—	9 4	—	—	—

Miles	Week Days only	a.m		p.m		p.m		p.m		p.m			
	Bourne .... dep	8 53	—	1227	—	1238	—	4 31	—	6 40	..	—	..
7	Castle Bytham	9 11	—	—	—	1255	—	4 47	—	6 56	—	—	—
11½	South Witham .... [ham	9 22	—	—	—	1 5	—	4 57	—	7 6	..	—	—
16½	Edmondthorpe & Wymond-	9 31	—	—	—	..	—	5 6	—	—	..	—	..
18½	**Saxby** .... arr	9 36	—	1 2	—	1 12	—	5 11	—	7 19	..	—	..

JULY 1957

Table 231 **SAXBY, SOUTH WITHAM and BOURNE**

Miles		Week Days only										
		a.m S	a.m S	a.m N	a.m L	p.m		p.m N		p.m P		
—	Saxby .... dep	7 44	9 39	9 55	1118	3 47	–	5 15	–	8 26	–	–
2	Edmondthorpe & Wymondham	..	..	10 1	..	–	..	5 21	–	..	..	–
7	South Witham............	–	–	1012	..	..	–	5 31	..	8 42	..	..
11¼	Castle Bytham.............	..	..	1021	..	..	..	5 40	..	8 51	..	–
18¼	Bourne .... arr	8 24	1017	1036	1154	4 20	..	5 53	..	9 4	..	..

Miles		Week Days only									
		a.m SN	a.m EN	a.m L	a.m S	p.m M	p.m E	p.m S	p.m S	p.m P	p.m N
—	Bourne .... dep	8 47	8 51	1132	1156	1222	1233	1245	2 55	4 25	6 42
7	Castle Bytham	9 6	9 9	..	..	..	..	–	–	4 41	6 57
11¼	South Witham ....ham	9 17	9 20	..	..	..	..	–	..	4 52	7 9
16¼	Edmondthorpe & Wymondham	9 26	9 29	..	..	..	..	..	..	5 3	..
18¼	Saxby .... arr	9 32	9 35	1213	1238	1 2	1 9	1 21	3 35	5 11	7Z22

E Except Saturdays
L Saturdays only. Runs until 7th September
M Saturdays only. Commences 29th June

N Through Carriages to or from Kings Lynn
P Through Carriages to or from Spalding

S Saturdays only
Z Arr 8 30 pm on Saturdays

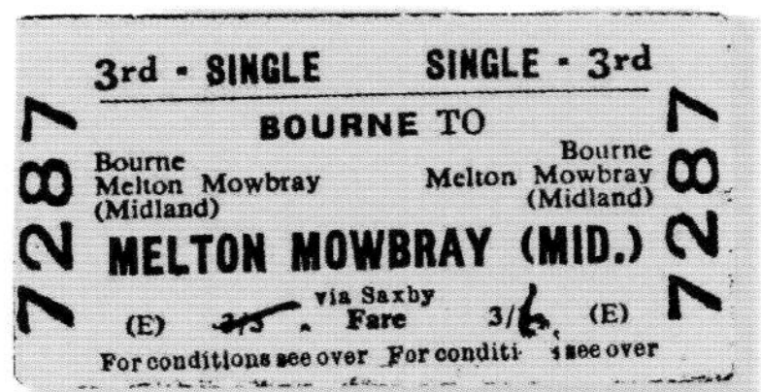

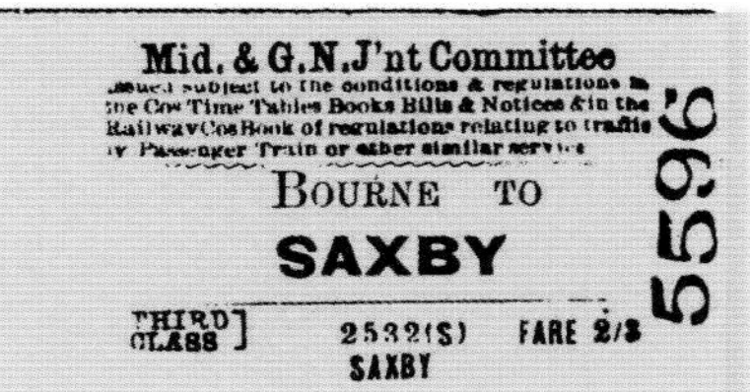

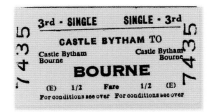

ACKNOWLEDGEMENTS

I would like to thank all the people who have helped me whilst writing this book, and in particular the following people for the use of their photographs:
M. C. Neale
F. Church
M & GN Circle
H. C. Casserley
E. L. Back
P. H. Wells
H. N. James
Lens of Sutton

Also thank you to:
The staff of the reference library at Peterborough and Stamford
The staff of the *Stamford Mercury*

SELECT BIBLIOGRAPHY

BACK, Michael.
Branch Lines Around Spalding: M&GN Saxby to Long Sutton.
(Midhurst: Middleton Press, 2009).

BODY, Geoffrey.
Great Railway Battles: Dramatic Conflicts of the Early Railway Years
(Peterborough: Silver Link Publishing, 1994).

BOWTELL, Harold D.
Reservoir Railways of the Yorkshire Pennines
(Blandford: Oakwood Press, 1979).

BOYD-HOPE, Gary and Andrew SARGENT.
Railways and Rural Life: S. W. A. Newton and the Great Central Railway
(Swindon: English Heritage, 2007).

BRUMHEAD, Derek and Jean and Ken RANGELEY.
The Kinder Reservoir and Railway
(New Mills: New Mills Heritage Centre, 2008).

BURTON, Anthony.
The Railway Builders
(London: John Murray, 1992).

CHORLTON, Martyn.
Danger Area: The Complete History of RAF South Witham 100 Maintenance Unit
(Spalding: Old Forge Publishing, 2003).

CLARKE, Ronald H.
A Short History of the Midland and Great Northern Joint Railway
(Norwich: Goose and Son, 1967).

CLINKER, C. R.
Clinker's Register of Closed Passenger Stations and Goods Depots in England, Scotland and Wales 1830–1980, new edn
(Weston Super Mare: Avon-Anglia, 1988).

COLEMAN, Terry.
The Railway Navvies, rev. edn
(Harmondsworth: Penguin, 1968).

COX, J. C.
'On an Anglo-Saxon cemetery recently uncovered near Saxby', *Transactions of the Leicestershire Architectural and Archaeological Society* 8 (1899), 74-77.

DIGBY, Nigel J. L.
A Guide to the Midland and Great Northern Joint Railway
(Shepperton: Ian Allan, 1993).

HADFIELD, Charles.
The Canals of the East Midlands
(Newton Abbot: David & Charles, 1970).

HARTLEY, Robert F.
The Medieval Earthworks of North-East Leicestershire
(Leicester: Leicestershire Museums, Art Galleries and Records Service, 1987).

HICKMAN, Trevor.
Battlefields of Leicestershire
(Stroud: Sutton Publishing, 2004).

HILL, Roger and Carey VESSEY.
British Railways Past and Present. No 27: Lincolnshire
(Kettering: Past & Present Publications, 1996).

LELEUX, Robin.
A Regional History of the Railways of Great Britain. Volume 9: The East Midlands, 2nd rev. edn
(Newton Abbot: David St John Thomas, 1984).

MANKTELOW, Peter.
Steam Shovels
(Princes Risborough: Shire Publications, 2001).

MAY, Trevor.
The Victorian Railway Worker
(Oxford: Shire Publications, 2008).

MITCHELL, William R.
Shanty Life on the Settle-Carlisle Railway
(Giggleswick: W. R. Mitchell, 1988).

MITCHELL, William R. (comp.)
How They Built the Settle-Carlisle Railway
(Giggleswick: W. R. Mitchell, 1989).

MOORE, Andrew.
Leicestershire's Stations: An Historical Perspective
(Narborough: Laurel House Publishing, 1998).

MORGAN, Bryan.
Railways: Civil Engineering
(London: Arrow Books, 1973).

MORRIS, Michael (Lord Killanin).
'Towards an archaeology of navvy huts and settlements of the industrial revolution', *Antiquity* 68 (1994), 573-584.

PEARSON, Rodney Edward and J. G. RUDDOCK.
Lord Willoughby's Railway: The Edenham Branch
(Grimsthorpe: Willoughby Memorial Trust, 1986).

POLS, Robert.
Dating Old Photographs, 2nd edn
(Birmingham: The Federation of Family History Societies, 1995).

RHODES, John.
The Midland & Great Northern Joint Railway
(London: Ian Allan, 1982).

RHODES, John.
Bourne to Saxby
(Boston: KMS Books, 1989).

ROBINSON, Peter.
Lincoln's Excavators: The Ruston Years, 1875–1930
(Wellington Somerset: Roundoak Publishing, 2003).

ROLT, L. T. C.
The Making of a Railway
(Bath: Hugh Evelyn, 1971).

RUSSELL, Ronald.
Lost Canals of England and Wales
(Newton Abbot: David and Charles, 1971).

SIMMONS, Jack.
The Express Train and Other Railway Studies
(Nairn: David St John Thomas, 1994).

SIMMONS, Jack.
The Victorian Railway, new edn
(London: Thames and Hudson, 1995).

SQUIRES, Stewart E.
The Lost Railways of Lincolnshire
(Ware: Castlemead, 1988).

STRETTON, Clement E.
The History of the Midland Railway
(London: Methuen, 1901).

SWAG.
South Witham in the Grantham Journal. Volume 1: 1854–1890
(South Witham: South Witham Archaeological Group, 2006).

SWAG.
South Witham Old and New
(South Witham: South Witham Archaeological Group, 2002).

SWAG.
South Witham: Stone Age to Space Age
(South Witham: South Witham Archaeological Group, 2004).

SWIFT, Andrew.
'Wish you were here? Railway postcards of Leicestershire',
Railway Archive 4 (2003), 89.

TAYLOR, Ralph Penniston.
A History of Wymondham, Leicestershire, 2nd edn
(Wymondham: Witmehà Press, 2004).

TEW, David.
The Melton to Oakham Canal, 2nd rev. edn
(Wymondham: Sycamore Press, 1984).

TONKS, Eric S.
The Ironstone Quarries of the Midlands: History, Operation and Railways. Part VII: Rutland
(Cheltenham: Runpast Publishing, 1989).

TONKS, Eric S.
The Ironstone Quarries of the Midlands: History, Operation and Railways. Part VIII: South Lincolnshire
(Cheltenham: Runpast Publishing, 1991).

VICTORIA COUNTY HISTORY.
'West Bromwich: Economic History' in M. W. Greenslade (ed.), *A History of the County of Stafford* 17
(Oxford, 1976), 27-43.

WALKER, Stephen (comp.)
Great Northern Branch Lines in Lincolnshire
(Boston: KMS Books, 1984).

WELLS, P. H.
Steam in the East Midlands
(London: Ian Allan, 1985).

WROTTESLEY, John.
The Great Northern Railway. Volume II: Expansion and Competition
(London: Batsford, 1979).

YORKE, Trevor.
Bridges Explained: Viaducts – Aqueducts
(Newbury: Countryside Books, 2008).

INDEX

Numbers in italic type refer to photograph numbers.
Numbers in roman type refer to page numbers.
In Appendix C the same convention applies.
Map numbers refer to maps within the text.